Child of Mine

Child of Mine

Feeding with Love and Good Sense

Ellyn Satter, R.D., M.S., M.S.S.W.

Bull Publishing Co.

Lovingly dedicated to my family. To my husband Larry, who shared the adventure of having and raising babies. To Kjerstin, whose winning ways showed us how—but tactfully. To Lucas, who was charming but firm about doing it *his* way. To Curtis, who was so enthusiastically persistent that there was never any question.

Cover design: Cindy LaBreacht
Interior design: Michelle Taverniti
Design assistant: Margaret Panofsky

Bull Publishing Co.
P.O. Box 208
Palo Alto, CA 94302-0208
(415) 322-2855

ISBN 0-915950-75-8 cloth
ISBN 0-915950-74-X paperback
Printed in the U.S.

Contents

Feeding—from Pregnancy Through the Toddler Period

Special Issues in Feeding

Of Current Interest

Acknowledgements

This book did not come from me alone. Many friends, associates and colleagues gave generously of their time, expertise and encouragement, and I thank them.

For professional technical evaluation of parts or all of the book:

Barbara Abrams, R.D., M.S.
Alfred Harper, PhD
Virginia Dykstal, R.N., C.P.N.P.
Patricia Joo, M.D.
Barbara Brew, M.D.
Ellyn Kroupa, M.A.
Terri Cohn, P.A.
Deborah Roussos, R.D., M.S.

Donna Oberg, R.D., M.S.
Gloria Green, R.D.
Laurie Fjeldstad, R.N., B.S.
Robert Jackson, M.D.
B. U. Li, M.D.
Marshall Cusic, Jr., M.D.
Albert Stunkard, M.D.
Donald Williams, A.C.S.W.

For help in reading the manuscript, editing, criticizing, reacting and supporting:

Laura Dennison
June Roffler
Elana Stern

Virginia Huber
Polly Colby

For expert and cheerful typing, always at the last minute:

Ruby Olson
Findley Cook
Clara Páez de Peña
Barbara Boyle

Pam Morgan
Kjerstin Satter
Lesley Rode
Joanne Prange

To the Reader

This is a book about feeding and the feeding relationship. It is a book that attempts to help you find the moderate middle ground between extremism and unconcern, between being domineering with your child's nutritional care and being neglectful. You need to know how to provide a nutritionally wholesome diet, but you also need to know how to feed in such a way that you nurture your child's sense of security, autonomy, and respect for himself and his body.

I intend this book to be a handbook and companion to you as you negotiate the four-year period from pregnancy through the toddler period (roughly age three). Because it should serve you as a reference book, I want you to be able to open it at any point and get the information you need. That means that some of the points must be made more than once. For instance, we will talk about calcium in the chapter on pregnancy and again, in greater detail, in the toddler chapter. Some subjects are covered in one place in considerable detail (not necessarily the first time the topic is raised), and at other times more briefly. Extensive cross referencing with page numbers or chapter names will help you to check back and forth as you go along.

I'm not going to tell you to change your child's diet to try to avoid cancer and heart disease. I don't think the evidence is good enough to give any clear direction. What I have done is give you advice about presenting a moderate and wholesome diet and guidelines to solving some of the nutritional problems of childhood: problems like selecting food that is appropriate for your child both developmentally and nutritionally; problems like feeding yourself well so you can produce a healthy baby and provide enough breast-milk; problems like doing all you can to prevent obesity; and problems like avoiding making the inevitable battles of the toddler period battles over food.

The three chapters of the book, Special Issues in Feeding, present information that will be helpful to you during the whole four years we discuss in the book. Chapter 9, Diarrhea, talks about managing diarrhea in children from infancy through toddlerhood. Chapter 10, Regulation of Food Intake, and Chapter 11, Obesity, discuss issues that are of major concern to most parents, are often misunderstood and mishandled, and can exert a major disrupting influence throughout your child's growing-up years. Read them early and often. You hear and read so much misinformation in this area that you will need to be reminded frequently about what is reasonable and real.

I have indicated scientific references so you can check out, if you want to, the evidence backing up what I say. While I have made some recommendations, the intent is to give you enough information so you can make your own decisions about your own child. As one young mother observed, "my baby sounds like all of those you talked about." Like the mothers I talk about, she had to make her observations and come up with solutions that were right for both of them.

Through it all, the important things to remember are 1) to enjoy your baby and 2) to trust yourself. If you do that, you can do a lot of things "wrong" and it won't make any difference.

Note on First Expanded Edition. In this First Expanded Edition of *Child of Mine*, the "Of Current Interest" section is new. This section includes two chapters, "The Feeding Relationship" and "Eating Disorders." The rest of the book remains the same.

In the three years since *Child of Mine* was published, I have learned more about feeding. Rather than waiting for a second edition, I want to share it now with you. There is a real need. Increasingly, parents and professionals tell stories about distorted feeding. Some of these situations are dreadful, and go on, with an enormous amount of pain and sacrifice, for years.

Parents are having trouble feeding themselves and feeding their children. They worry that their child eats too much or too little, grows too well or too poorly. Or they get caught up with their child in battles about eating that get bad enough to positively wreck meal time and other times. The struggle over feeding and growth can, at times, spoil an entire relationship.

Eating disorders in adults are on the increase, and they are having an impact on children's eating. Parents with severe difficulties with their own eating have a hard time parenting appropriately with food. Someone who doesn't know how to eat normally has great difficulty trusting a child to do so.

People not only need to know how to choose good food for their child, they need to know how to behave helpfully when they offer it. And they need to know when they are having serious difficulty in the area of feeding. I hope these two new chapters will help.

1
Introduction: History of Child Feeding

It is convenient, and sensible, to feed babies with food that is nutritionally appropriate and that they can ingest and digest most easily. The practical approach then, would be to nipple-feed breastmilk or another appropriate milk feeding as long as babies need to be held in a cuddling and supported position; and then, when they can sit up and can learn to swallow other foods, our practicality would lead us to progress them rapidly to table foods.

Unfortunately, this sensible approach has, as long as anyone can record or remember, been distorted by folk "wisdom," nutritional "knowledge" and social pressure. The attitudes of parents (which represent the attitudes of the times they live in) are evident from the way they feed their child. And, even in these enlightened times, our feeding attitudes and practices are often inconsistent with what we have (or should have) learned.

For me, one of the startling things about having a baby was coming slap up against what seemed to be the realization that I didn't know the simplest, most basic fact about taking care of one.

I knew I was *generally* ignorant. What I wasn't prepared for was the fine and exquisite detail of my ignorance. For example, I was very puzzled when the pediatrician told me that Kjerstin, my newborn daughter, would eat less frequently at night than during the day. How in the world did an infant know the difference between night and day? The pediatrician seemed to take it for granted that she would, so I didn't ask. I decided to wait and see. She slept longer at night (as do most, but not all babies). Fortunately Kjerstin seemed to know more about it than I did—a trend, I might add, that continued.

I thought I had her feeding regimen all figured out: I would breastfeed her and some day I would start feeding her solid foods. Just when, I didn't know, but I figured I would think about that when the time came. It had never occurred to me that I couldn't breastfeed, so I did. The obstetrical ward nurses helped us with some of the mechanics of it, and it went fine. Kjerstin seemed to know all about it. She cried when she was hungry, stopped eating when she was full, and even established herself on a nice feeding schedule. She knew the details, it seemed; all I had to do was provide backup and support.

It seemed to me that things were going well, particularly when we went to the pediatrician after the first month and found out that she had gained over two pounds. She was eating well and sleeping well and seemed to be satisfied and happy with her feeding regimen. She was waking up only once a night and eating at comfortably-spaced intervals throughout the day. Even though I knew little about feeding babies, that seemed right to me.

I must have led a very sheltered life. I was surprised when the pediatrician told me that it was time to start solid food. It hadn't occurred to me to even wonder about that yet. Breastfeeding seemed right for the way she was at that age. More ignorance, more details, I assumed, and went along with what the pediatrician said.

Solid foods, she said, would solve a lot of the problems that we were having. (We were having problems? I didn't know enough about the details to know we were having problems!) It was time, she said, that my daughter was sleeping through the night and she was just "putting something over on me" in insisting on getting up for that night feeding. (Actually, I was rather enjoying that night feeding, especially since my breasts got so full and uncomfortable I couldn't sleep.) Cereal would help that. Furthermore, Kjerstin was starting to get a little plump from "all that breastmilk," and was looking like a "fat little milk baby."

Cereal would take care of that, too, and I was to start her on it right away. It was to be given before the breastfeeding so she would be hungry enough to take it. Further, I was to get a demitasse spoon and put the solid feeding far enough back on her tongue so it would just slip right down and not be spit out on her chin. I was told to hold her on my lap with her head in the crook of my elbow, so she would be secure and at the right angle to let the mush slide right down her throat.

We worked very well at that, because by the second month Kjerstin was eating, two, two-ounce bowls of cereal a day and hardly spitting out a drop. She couldn't. I was practically putting it directly into her esophagus. The pediatrician praised us and rewarded us with another little tear-off sheet from the baby-food company, instructing me to now feed not only baby cereal, but also fruit and vegetable.

On the way home we made a quick stop at the grocery store, and the next day our family left for a three-week camping trip with Kjerstin, armed with an ice chest filled with milk, boxes of baby cereal, and dozens of little bottles with fruit and vegetables in them. What a trial it was to haul all that stuff along and keep it cool that whole time!

I can feel my blood pressure rising as I write this. Or maybe that flush spreading across my face is embarrassment, as I remember how guillible I was and how colossally ignorant, to accept that crazy, inaccurate advice in a field that was supposed to be my own. But at the same time I am struck by how much more sensibly I had been feeding her when I had been ignorant. I had been paying attention to her signals and feeding her in a way that seemed right for her developmentally. It was only after we got all those *details* that we really got off on the wrong track.

How my husband and I knocked ourselves out to push all that unnecessary food into that cooperative, vulnerable little baby. Well, my only reassurance is that I don't think it hurt her. She seemed to grow well and do well and had no major crises with diarrhea or dehydration, so I hope we did no harm. But we sure went to a great deal of unnecessary work, and we certainly gave her no positive benefit from the crazy, complicated feeding regimen we had her on.

By the time the boys, Lucas and Curtis, were born, I was able to defend myself against the details. I trusted my breastfeeding and delayed the addition of solids, even though they were both chubby, robust kids with great appetites.

I can remember going on a bike trip when Lucas was three months old. He rode on my back in a pack. When we stopped for lunch, he got off my back to breastfeed and that was that: not a spoon or a bottle in sight. How nice that was! All we needed was a few disposable diapers and we were ready for action. With Curtis, I was even more casual. Even though he ate often and irregularly and grew very fast, I knew breastmilk was all he needed at first. I had finally made my peace with the details.

The pediatrician has simplified things, too. In the time since my first-born in 1966, she has moderated her baby-feeding advice. The trend in baby-feeding has changed, and to a certain extent she has gone along with the trend.

Feeding babies is not complicated. Like me with my first baby, where most people get into trouble with feeding their children is in trying to make it more complicated than it really is. It seems that the most difficult task for a modern parent is to sort through the chaff of conflicting advice and information, to find the grain of common sense.

Most of us haven't experienced an infant until we have our own, so we must learn from relatives, from other parents, from professionals, from books. In raising kids, one of the easiest things to do is get advice. That's especially true about advice on feeding. Since everyone eats, everyone knows about feeding. A crowd gathers. What one person suggests, the other contradicts.

Feeding patterns for infants have changed so drastically in the last few years that you will probably get as many versions of appropriate feeding practices as people you consult. You can even find considerable variation in the recommendations of doctors, nurses, and dietitians.

You might say some people are more up-to-date than others. On the other hand, you might not want to say that, because sometimes being "modern" only means being fashionable. Some fashionable theories prove that babies have a remarkable capacity to adapt to the whims of their caretakers, and seem to do pretty well on a wide variety of feeding approaches.

Too often common infant feeding practice is based on only that—common practice. It need not be so. As with all other behaviors, as the infant grows and develops, abilities change and patterns of feeding change.

Nutritional needs vary as the child grows. The mouth muscle patterns vary at different ages—sucking patterns of early infancy give away to swallowing patterns, and finally chewing patterns appear. The digestive tract matures, from one adapted to milk digestion to one able to handle a wide range of food. The child continually develops her awareness and mastery of her environment. Along with this comes imitation of eating patterns of older people, and she will feel compelled at appropriate ages to adopt more-nearly-mature eating behaviors, just as she is driven to crawl, to stand and finally to walk.

To be able to know what you're doing and why you're doing it, as you feed your baby appropriately at different ages, you need to understand:

1. Your infant's nutritional needs at different ages.
2. How growth and development are related to eating.
3. Signals that indicate readiness for maturing eating styles.
4. Appropriate eating styles for a given level of growth, development and nutritional need.

Given this undertanding, you will be able to feed your infant with flexibility, based on a clear understanding of what he needs and is able to do at different stages of maturation. This is important, as different infants mature at different rates. You need to be able to adapt <u>your</u> feeding style to fit <u>your</u> infant.

When you match feeding practices to the child's developmental needs, the feeding regimen goes something like this:

- Give the baby breastmilk (supplemented with Vitamin D and flouride) or formula, only, for the first four to six months of life.
- When he can sit, supported, begin offering iron-fortified baby cereals mixed with formula or milk. Do this after the breast or bottle feeding.
- When your baby turns his head or otherwise indicates he's full, take his word for it.
- After he is taking about ⅓ to ½ cup of mixed-up cereal a day, gradually begin offering a variety of fork-mashed, unseasoned table foods, always after the milk feeding.
- At around 8–10 months when the baby is able to sit alone, shows an interest in the family table, and is adept at conveying things to his mouth, start putting him up to the table at mealtime, where he can

feed himself a variety of soft food that won't choke him. Offer an assortment that is likely to add up to a nutritious diet.

- At the same time (if he hasn't already) he is ready to start drinking with assistance from the cup.
- Now postpone the breast or bottle feeding until after the meal, and give formula or whole milk in a cup along with the meal.
- As he eats more at mealtime and drinks from the cup, he will gradually lose interest in the breast or bottle and can generally be weaned, one feeding at a time, with no hassle. At this point, he is getting more of his nutritional needs from a variety of foods, and formula or breastmilk becomes less important nutritionally.
- Once he is well-established on table food, it is all right to switch to whole milk, or to whole evaporated milk diluted one-to-one with water.

All of this development in eating takes place by age one year. About the only real change in eating you see after that is when the child gets his two-year molars, sometime in the second year, and can chew more efficiently. Then he can handle tougher, chewier foods.

And that's all there is to it: breast or formula alone for the first 4–6 months, beginning solids after that, and self feeding of table foods beginning around 8–10 months.

Working with Health Professionals

As my kids were growing up, I often got the feeling that pediatricians were putting themselves in charge of *my* children. It seemed that they weren't advising—they were dictating. I was expected to go along with their pronouncements without question. Those are the traditional roles of the patient and the physician: the physician is in charge of the patient's health care. The "good" patient has been the *compliant* one; that certainly has been an apt word, because being compliant means, "to accept or comply tacitly; to accept as inevitable or indisputable; to yield."

It's a good thing those times are passing. That kind of behavior by a parent may save time in the doctor's office, but it surely doesn't make a very good mental set for all the responsibility of raising kids.

It is kind of a chicken-and-egg question to try to decide which started to change first, patient or physician attitudes—but the relationship definitely is changing. People are expecting to retain responsibility for the health care of themselves and their children. They are looking to health care providers as consultants, as people to whom they can turn for information and recommendations. Along with that comes the patient's expectation that she will be able to understand the reasons for what she is doing, so she can take reasonably informed courses of action.

In their turn, health care providers are expecting to act more as consultants and resource people to parents. They are realizing that what the parent needs most of all is confidence in his or her own ability to make decisions. Therefore they are doing more informing, and educating, and giving advice, leaving the bulk of the decision making up to the parents. Nurses in pediatrics are doing what they call "anticipatory guidance"—telling parents ahead of time what to expect from their children, so parents will be prepared to interpret and handle changes.

Some parents don't like this approach any more than some health practitioners. They would much rather do it the old way. Here is hoping that those parents and practitioners find each other. Meanwhile, I am assuming that you want to be informed enough to make your own decisions.

In this book I will be your consultant as you struggle with this important business of caring for your child nutritionally. I will try to give you the nutrition information and tools you will need to make your own decisions. I want you to know the important nutritional issues and pros and cons about some of these issues. I will try to anticipate some of the problems you will be encountering and give suggestions about ways of handling those problems. I want to support you in developing your own confidence about caring for your child nutritionally.

All of this comes from my absolutely firm conviction that you are the person in charge, and that the rest of us are, at best, playing supportive roles.

Historical Perspective on Infant Feeding

It seems to me that a logical way to get started with the process is to take a look at what has gone before. Getting a perspective on infant feeding can help, I think, in a couple of ways. First, it can help you in fielding advice. Say, somebody is telling you that you should be doing something. If you can think, "Ah, yes, that is the way they did things back in the forties and the reason that they did that was this-and-this," you are going to be much more secure in accepting or rejecting that piece of advice. Second, a brief review of the recent history of infant feeding can provide us with an introduction to some of the important issues in infant feeding. It's kind of like telling a story to make a point: we can have some fun with this and conduct our business at the same time.

The recent history of infant feeding tells about the attitudes of parents toward babies, changing influences on families over the years, and the development of the science of nutrition and modern food technology. You will find remnants of some of the older ideas in a lot of the advice you get about infant feeding.

Until the early part of the 20th century, the infant who could not be breastfed usually could not survive. The technology was not available to provide the infant with a sanitary feeding that was digestible and nutritionally complete. It was not until the 1920's that a consistently safe and reliable substitute for breastmilk was available. By that time sanitation in milk production and handling had improved to the point where people had a better chance of getting fresh, wholesome milk.

Techniques of sterilization had been developed that prevented the bacterial contamination and dysentery that had been common in an artificially fed infant. Safer water supplies were developed. Easily cleaned and sterilized bottles and nipples were available. It was discovered that boiling cows' milk softened the milk curd formed in the infant's stomach, making it more digestible.

It was noted that since cows' milk is more concentrated than human milk, levels of calcium, phosphorus and protein were unnecessarily high, and that getting rid of the excess as waste products put an unnecessary load on the baby's kidneys. It was therefore helpful to dilute the formula with water. Then to make up for the calories lost through dilution, extra carbohydrate, generally sugar or syrup, was added. The diluted, carbohydrate-enriched mixture then more closely approximated human milk in composition.

In the 1920's and 1930's vitamin C was isolated and identified as the preventative of the scurvy possible in bottle-fed infants. Codliver oil came into use as a source of vitamin D to prevent rickets. The acceptance of canned, sterilized evaporated milk as the basis for infant formula (which, ironically, had been around ever since Gail Borden patented it in 1856) represented a great breakthrough in safety and convenience. Formula, based on canned milk, along with supplements of codliver oil and vitamin C, represented an artificial feed that was nutritious, convenient, safe and economical. (Later evaporated milk was fortified with vitamin D.)

It was the SCIENTIFIC AGE of feeding babies: formulas were adjusted to fit the age of the child, quantities to be fed were pre-selected in the doctor's office, and frequencies of feeding were rigidly controlled. Breastfeeding was considered old-fashioned and non-scientific, and the trend away from breastfeeding began. The percentage of newborns who were breastfed dropped to 65% in the 1940's and 25% in the late 50's.

The scientific age has continued, until now there are many commercial formulas on the market. They are based on pretty much the same principle: cows' milk modified by boiling, dilution, increase of calories with added carbohydrate, and supplementation with essential nutrients.

Trends in the introduction of solid foods have changed as rapidly as those related to the milk feeding. Early in the 1900's infants were kept on breastmilk alone until about age one year. However, as artificial feeding became more popular, some of the more adventurous parents and physicians began offering solids at an earlier age. The infants seemed to accommodate this, and continued to grow well, and therefore it was assumed to be appropriate. So experimentalists kept trying progressively earlier ages for solids introduction, until by 1960 it was common practice to offer cereals within two weeks to a month of birth, or even at birth, and other foods in rapid succession soon afterward.

The baby food market boomed, providing in convenient form the semi-liquid, super-smooth foods that the immature infant needed for swallowing without strangling. Instructions for introducing solids stressed thinning to a watery consistency, and putting the spoonful far back on the baby's tongue so she wouldn't just spit it back out. That was only logical, as the young infant's mouth is adapted to sucking, which forces the tongue up and against the roof of the mouth and propels anything not fed by nipple right back out. This mouth pattern is called the *extrusion* reflex. Once you get food far enough back on the tongue, it activates swallowing, so it goes down whether the infant wants it or not.

It appeared that infants naturally tolerated solid foods early in life, so it became common practice to give them, despite the fact that there was no evidence that early introduction was advantageous. Early feeding of solids was more costly and complicated, but people did it because they thought it was best for their babies.

Along with early progression to solid foods came early switching to pasteurized milk, most commonly 2% milk. This was presumably easier and cheaper than prolonged feeding of formula, which was said to be old-fashioned, and no longer necessary. Two percent milk was supposed to be helpful in preventing obesity, because it had fewer calories per ounce than formula. (This turned out to be an honest mistake resulting from ignorance, when it was shown in the late sixties[2] that babies over six weeks of age regulate food intake on the basis of calories consumed rather than on the basis of volume. Babies over six weeks had simply been drinking more of the 2% milk and gaining just as much weight.)

It was in this latter stage—of early addition of solid foods combined with switching to 2% milk—that the rational basis for infant feeding broke down. Feeding theory no longer matched infant needs. Babies still were more vulnerable than adults to contaminated food, and needed to be protected; they still had more immature stomachs and intestines that couldn't adequately digest a big, solid milk curd formed by pasteurized milk; their kidneys still didn't have the capacity to handle the overload of protein, calcium, phosphorus and sodium in 2% milk; and even after all those years of being dosed early on with solid foods, they still hadn't learned to get down a spoonful of runny cereal without pushing it out on their chins.

For twenty years health professionals were recommending feeding babies as if they knew nothing at all about nutrition and physiology.

It is only recently that nutritionists, physicians, nurses and other health professionals have been putting together what they know about babies, and coming up with recommendations for feeding babies that again make sense. I am perhaps too optimistic, but I don't think the trend will go back the other way. Developmental patterns of infants don't change, and nutritional requirements remain the same. Now that we are beginning to feed in a logical fashion in response to those considerations, I would hope that we have enough sense to continue to do so.

Right now, we have a particular problem, as we are at the transition between the old and the new. People I see in my practice have often been exposed to conflicting opinions and bits of information about feeding and are unsure of how to proceed. Some health workers still give strange and questionable feeding advice and parents are confused.

Social Perspective on Infant Feeding

Having taken this look back at some of those feeding practices from a nutritional and scientific perspective, I am struck with how many of the practices seem objectionable or even crazy. But when I stand back a little further and take a look at the feeding practices in the light of their social context, it begins to make sense why people did what they did. (It usually does, you know, if you can just get yourself adjusted to look at things in the proper perspective.) So let's establish a social perspective for that same period of time—the early part of the century.

The role of the family and the attitudes toward children have changed markedly since that time. In the early 1900's most women and children were involved in some concrete way with the family's means of making a living. The major occupations were the family farm or the small business or trade. Both parents were generally involved in those cooperative ventures, and child-raising had to be a part of other responsibilities. Children were expected to contribute economically from an early age, either by doing small essential tasks, or by taking care of younger children. The individual's well-being was assumed to be the result of the status of the whole family. Therefore, the welfare of the individual was less important than the maintenance of the physical, economic and social welfare of the family as a whole. At the same time, children were valued for the economic contribution that they could make to the family.

The attitude toward infants and children was that the will of the young child had to be tamed. "The right of the parent is to command, the duty of the child is to obey." Infant feeding times were regulated; parents were hesitant to respond to childrens' demands, lest their child become self-centered as an adult.

With the trend toward industrialization came a different pattern of family life. Now one or both parents, and often the older children as well, were working outside the home. Child care was delegated to a particular person in the family: the mother, older children, grandparents. Since most people working in industry had lower incomes, there simply wasn't enough money available to spare an employable family member for the express purpose of raising children. Families often lived in communities with relatives or close friends, so the community continued to act as a social network for the family, supervising and supporting the children. For the first time the family began to be somewhat isolated from the work place.

The attitudes toward children changed drastically with the industrial revolution. Industrial technology made intelligence the main skill for survival. So rather than continue to equip the child to live as part of a family, clan, ethnic group, religious group, or community, the family was called upon to equip the child to compete for a place as an *individual* in the larger society. Spontaneity and independence from the family became desirable traits. Parents were told by an emerging group of child care experts that emotional expressiveness and autonomy toward others were important for the individual who was to achieve independence as an adult. Independence was seen as the individual serving society. The person was being equipped to live as part of a technological, capitalist society.

By now pediatricians, too, were in the business of telling parents what to do about feeding their children. They had access to the unfolding body of information about nutrition. Since safe formula preparation was possible for families, the pediatrician had become able to control something he had never been able to control when babies were being breastfed: quantity and quality of their feeding. Parents were charging the pediatrician with the responsibility for taking care of children, so it seemed right that he should take charge of the important area of feeding as well.

The preoccupation with regularity in feeding had been around a long time; during those years it appeared to become a real obsession. It began to seem important to equip children from an early age with habits of regularity and punctuality, which would serve them in an increasingly technological age. Also, there was an increasing emphasis on the intellect; "experts" were coming into vogue, and the judgment of the pediatrician fit this new desire for expert opinion. The information coming from the child was less important. It was a matter of mind-over-body.

Therefore, although the emphasis was on the individual, the information that came from the child was less important than what was coming from the outside. The theme was to mold the individual from an early age, to fit into a certain pattern of society.

Along with the rigid formula routines came introduction of solid foods at earlier ages. The popular school of thought at that time, which went along with the increasing value placed on intelligence, was that the infant who could or would do something early, was displaying intellectual ability that would show up in all future activities. Thus, the willingness to swallow solid foods, or sit up, or walk at an early age predicted success later in adulthood.

Now we know that individual developmental differences in infancy are not preserved for very long. But parents were convinced of it then (probably by professionals), and acted out of genuine concern for the best interests of their children.

The separation between family life and community life which had started with the industrial revolution, became even greater after World War II. Families began moving to the suburbs, which isolated them not only from the work place, but also from their traditional social networks of kinship, and ethnic and religious groups. Since the people making this move were generally of the middle income or above, they had the means to support someone in the family for the business of child care. So raising children became, for the first time anywhere, the focus of women's full-time commitment and work—and the test of mothers' worth. In fact, it became a test of a woman's worth as a person, because the primary role of women was seen to be marrying and having children.

At the same time, the status and role of the children was dramatically changed. Having been removed geographically from day-to-day contact with the breadwinner, and having the mother in the full-time role of homemaker and child-care provider, essentially changed their economic status. For the first time children became a clear economic liability rather than an asset.

The child's task became to grow up in such a way that he could take his economic place in the outside world. Children were fed in a way that reflected the pressures being put on their mothers. Women were expected, or expected themselves, to do the best with their families—to provide for them and serve them. Children who "ate well" and "grew well" reflected well on their mothering. This put pressure on the feeding relationship that made it hard for mothers to be aware of children's innate needs and potential.

We are now at a point where once again, the family is changing. Increasingly mothers as well as fathers are going off to paid employment. Child care functions are being delegated to other people and organizations. Parenthood is seen as an option rather than an obligation, as more and more couples are choosing to remain childless. The people who do choose to have children are doing so deliberately and thoughtfully, accepting what they see as a considerable economic and social responsibility. An important part of making the decision is the struggle with the question of how to provide children with a nurturant, socializing environment, and still allow all family members what they see as appropriate opportunity and autonomy.

The attitude of society toward the individual is also changing. Rather than viewing the individual as responsible and subservient to society, it seems the other way around: society exists for service to the individual. Some alarmed critics have labeled the current mental set as narcissistic. Other more optimistic observers have called it an appropriate valuation of self. In any event, parents are responding by attempting to instill in their children a sense of personal competency and respect for their own and others' individuality. They seek to develop the capacity for flexible and responsible interactions with others and with the environment.

With respect to the feeding relationship, this has meant that parents are more willing than before to accept information coming from their children. They are attempting less to impose on their children external standards of schedule, quantity or food selection. They are beginning to feed their babies in a way that they see as being more functional, and responsive to the babies themselves. Breastfeeding is on the upswing, as mothers work out ways to continue the breastfeeding relationship even when going back to work.

Now, in addition to growing up to take her economic place in the world, the child must somehow do this in a way that allows her to maintain harmony with a *changing* world. Furthermore, given the optional nature of parenting, her "growing up well" becomes even more important to parents. Producing a good child validates their decision to have a child. How today's child manages to do all this represents a more complicated task than ever before. The purpose of this book is to be helpful to you as you find ways of supporting that growth.

Selected References

1. Cone, Thomas E. 200 Years of Feeding Infants in America. Ross Laboratories. 1976.
2. Fomon, Samuel J. Recent history and current trends. IN Infant Nutrition. W. B. Saunders, Philadelphia. 1974.

3. Greenleaf, B. K. Children Through the Ages: A History of Childhood. McGraw-Hill, New York. 1978.
4. Kagan, J. Overview: Perspectives on human infancy. IN The Handbook of Infant Development. J. D. Osofsky, (Ed). Wiley, New York. 1979.

2
Nutrition for Pregnancy

During pregnancy you are eating for two. Your need for all nutrients increases, both for maintaining the health and stamina of your own body and for providing for the growth of your baby. You need an additional 300 calories per day, your iron and folic acid requirements double, and your requirement for other vitamins and minerals increases by 25 to 50%. With the exception of iron and folic acid, you can get all the nutrients you need from a well-selected diet of ordinary foods.

Of all the nutritional considerations, however, the most critical is that of eating enough calories to maintain a slow and steady weight gain throughout pregnancy. This becomes difficult, but no less important, if you are nauseated and vomiting or have a poor appetite for any reason. At times it may become necessary to concentrate only on maintaining calorie intake—from whatever food source is tolerated.

People have always been fascinated by pregnancy and childbirth, and often have attempted to influence the outcome with dietary manipulations. In earlier times, when there was little information about nutrient composition of foods, dietary advice was influenced by the belief that obvious physical properties of different foods could produce specific effects on the mother and child. Pregnant women were sometimes forbidden to eat salty, acid, or sour foods for fear the infant would be born with a "sour" disposition. Eggs were sometimes restricted because of their association with the reproductive function.

On the other hand, certain foods were encouraged for their presumed beneficial effects. Pregnant women were often advised to eat broths, warm milk and ripe fruits, to soothe the fetus and ease the birth process.

Dietary recommendations for pregnancy were also influenced by current problems in obstetrical practice. In the early days of the Industrial Revolution, children in Europe had poor diets and worked long hours in dark factories. Rickets was a common nutritional disorder that impaired normal bone formation during the growing years; so when women became pregnant, contracted pelvis bones presented a major obstetrical risk. Physicians were unable to do cesarian sections or even use forceps delivery, and mortality of both mother and child during childbirth was very high.

Experience with his own patients in the 1880's led a German physician to advocate a fluid-restricted, low-carbohydrate, high-protein diet for women with contracted pelvis, to be followed for six weeks prior to birth. Women using such a diet produced smaller infants who were easier to deliver.[14] The diet may have had some justification in the 1880's, but it later gained in popularity and became a standard recommendation for women throughout pregnancy, even when the original rationale for it no longer applied.

This practice was consistent with the common view of the fetus as a parasite, bent on robbing from the mother the nutrients it needed for growth and development. "Responsible" nutritional practice was aimed at limiting maternal weight gain to that clearly needed by the fetus and its support systems, and did not allow for any accumulation in the mother's fat stores or tissue fluid. Eighteen pounds was the limit; anything over that was viewed as contributing to obesity in the mother.

In fact, an obstetrician who attended me during my first pregnancy and delivery adhered to this philosophy and practice. He insisted that a low-calorie, high-protein diet was necessary to prevent toxemia, or preeclampsia*. He also added sodium (salt) to the restricted list.

His reasoning was naive, similar to that of the early diets for pregnancy. A major symptom of preeclampsia, or toxemia, is fluid retention, which causes a sudden weight gain, usually about the 20th week of gestation. Since preeclampsia produced a weight gain, if you held down the weight gain and the salt intake, you would prevent the toxemia.

It didn't seem to affect his logic that the compositions of the two gains were not the same. Normal weight gain in pregnancy is made up of maternal and fetal tissue as well as some normal fluid retention. The weight gain of toxemia is water.

That obstetrician had the courage of his convictions—and was willing to get tough to enforce adherence to them. He put women on strict weight-control regimens, and set target weight gains, ranging from a high of 17 pounds to a low of no weight gain or even weight loss for the obese woman. And he used real strong-arm tactics, from an old-fashioned chewing-out, to threats not to deliver his patient. He wasn't alone in his goal of limiting weight gain. He was following

---

*Preeclampsia is a disorder found only in pregnancy, that can be dangerous to both mother and baby. To be identified as preeclampsia there must be three symptoms: Tissue fluid accumulation greater than that normal for pregnancy, elevated blood pressure, and protein in the urine.

common obstetrical practice, and the advice in standard obstetrical textbooks.

As a nutritionist, I questioned his logic, and certainly didn't like the looks of his rigid and boring diet. I knew women starved themselves for his appointments. But all he had to do to shut me up was to refer to his years of experience and superior knowledge about real-life practice.

It took another group of obstetricians, with further years of experience and better clinical information, to combat successfully his thinking and that of others like him. In 1970, a panel of respected obstetricians and nutritionists published a major reexamination of nutritional practices during pregnancy, *Maternal Nutrition and the Course of Pregnancy.*[3] Their consensus was that these routine weight, calorie and sodium restrictions during pregnancy were not only outmoded but potentially dangerous. They encouraged eating to appetite of a nutritious diet, aiming for an average weight gain of around 25 pounds, and no routine sodium limitations.

The Committee contradicted the parasite theory. They found that women with good diets tended to have superior infants and better obstetrical performance, and those with poor diets tended to have inferior infants and poorer obstetrical performance. "Superior" infants were healthy, robust babies with birthweights somewhere between six pounds ten ounces and eight pounds 14 ounces. (The generally accepted single figure of optimum birthweight is about seven and a half pounds.)

Our patients after 1970 were treated much differently than patients before that time. We began instructing them in normal nutrition, encouraging and supporting optimal weight gain (with the exception of one loyal nurse who persisted in sucking in her breath when patients gained well, and praising them when they gained poorly).

Three years later, we invited a graduate student in nutrition, Janet Valentine, to compare obstetrical performance before and after 1970.[5] She found that patients before 1970 gained, on the average, eight pounds less than those after 1970, 15.9 versus 24.2 pounds. She also found that the babies born to mothers who gained more were heavier by 159 grams—over five ounces. There were six mothers in the earlier study who gained less than ten pounds, and their babies were quite small—over 11 ounces less than the average babies. Women before 1970 reported for their 6 week postpartum check at about the same weight as before pregnancy. Those after 1970 were about five pounds heavier.

The five-ounce weight difference between the pre-1970 and post-1970 babies doesn't sound like much, and neither group had low birth weights. But it can be significant. For instance, babies from certain economically disadvantaged groups, on the average, weigh only ½ pound less at birth than babies from more prosperous groups; yet infant mortality in the poorer groups is two to three times that of the richer. You could blame this difference on factors other than nutrition, such as living conditions, until you realize that when poorer babies of adequate birth size are sorted out from the others, they do just as well as the more advantaged babies.[13]

To have a good diet during pregnancy you must have both good quantity and quality. You must have enough food, and it must meet your nutritional needs. The remainder of this chapter will deal with these issues.

However, as we do that, we must keep in mind that not every problem of pregnancy has a nutritional cause. It is likely that there are some circumstances in which nutrition plays a direct and critical role. But it is also probable that for some conditions, nutrition has little or no influence at all. In striving for good nutrition during pregnancy you are taking responsibility for those factors which you can control.

Weight Gain During Pregnancy

Everyone knows someone who has gained little weight during pregnancy, produced a seemingly healthy baby, and gone home from the hospital wearing her size-nine designer jeans. In our thinness-oriented society, that may seem like an admirable thing. But from the point of view of risk for the baby, it is anything but admirable. You have a slim chance of having good nutrition during pregnancy unless you eat enough calories and gain enough weight. Certainly, women have produced healthy, normal babies even though they have gained little weight, or perhaps even lost, but they have taken a risk.

During pregnancy you are in a state of growth. During growth, unless you are accumulating nutrients and putting on body weight, you are, essentially, starving. That starvation state carries two very real dangers for you and your baby. First, as long as you are not eating enough calories it will be very difficult for you to provide protein for your baby's needs. When calories in your diet are too low, dietary protein will simply be broken down and used for energy.

Second, if you are not eating enough calories, it will be easier for you to go into *ketosis*, a condition that is dangerous for your baby. Ketosis is an accumulation in the blood of the waste products of fat breakdown. It is caused by eating 1) a diet that is too high in fat, or 2) too low in carbohydrate, or 3) both, or 4) by not eating enough to maintain weight gain. When you are in a starvation state, your body starts to break down stored fat for energy. If there is too much fat breakdown, eventually the waste products start to accumulate, and you go into ketosis.*

Although there are some variations that we will discuss a little later, on the average women do best in pregnancy, and produce the best babies, when they gain about 22 to 28 pounds. You may shudder at this figure, especially if you are in that pre-maternity-clothes phase when your zippers won't zip, your blouses won't button, and you don't feel pregnant—just fat.

---

*Ketosis shows up in the urine. Your doctor is probably checking for ketosis by using a special dipstick in urine samples. If you are worried about undereating and developing ketosis, you can ask for your urine to be checked.

Dress yourself comfortably during this stage. Provide room for your hips, breasts and upper arms to expand as well as your abdomen. You'll be grateful for the clothes after you deliver, because you will have a good chance of being about the same size then that you were at three or four months gestation.

If you gain about 25 pounds during pregnancy, you will probably go back for your postpartum check at about six weeks within four or five pounds of your pre-pregnancy weight. Beyond that, it's hard to predict how quickly you'll lose after delivery. Some women lose promptly, others more slowly, still others seemingly hang on to much of their excess weight throughout breastfeeding. Continue with your moderate weight-control tactics of pregnancy (see pp. 34 and 50), dress attractively, and respect your own tempo. Eventually, it will come off.

Optimum Weight Gain. Whenever we start recommending optimum weight gains, there is a real danger that we will begin interfering with the normal process of food regulation during pregnancy. About the best we can do with weight gain recommendations is to give you an idea of what is "normal" and desirable.

You don't have to force weight gain. Starting in the second trimester you will be hungrier and, if you are willing to eat as much as your appetite indicates of generally nutritious food, you will gain weight appropriately, and the gain will be of healthy body tissue. Your body has its own wisdom about regulating your food intake and weight gain during pregnancy, and you should listen to it.

Weight Gain and Maternal Body Size. The best weight gain for you during pregnancy will depend on whether you are of normal weight or underweight or overweight. The best weight gain is that which produces the best fetus. Outcome of pregnancy is studied in two major ways: Birthweight and infant mortality. The two studies described below used the two different definitions of pregnancy outcome, but reached roughly the same conclusions about optimum weight gain.

At our clinic, we found what everyone else has found, that larger women tended to deliver bigger babies in all weight gain categories and that women who had a higher pre-pregnancy weight gain didn't have to gain as much weight for their fetus to be of adequate size. Conversely, women with low pre-pregnancy weights tended to have smaller babies, and had to gain more weight during pregnancy to allow their babies to achieve optimum size. In fact, if women achieved the "optimum" weight gains of the study below, their babies were of adequate size. (We defined women as overweight if they were 20% or more above normal, as defined in the Appendix (Table A-2), underweight if they were 10% or more below normal.)

A study of 53,518 pregnancies across the United States[8] based its outcome data on infant mortality, but also found that heavier women had to gain less weight to maintain a live birth average than did thinner women. This study defined overweight and underweight at 35%-above and 10%-below levels, respectively.

Figure 2-1. Optimum Weight Gain in Pregnancy.

Weight status at conception	Weight gain for lowest infant mortality
Normal weight	27 lb.
Underweight	30 lb.
Overweight	15 lb.

It is important to note, however, that in both studies, the overweight women's gain of less weight than optimum for her weight status appeared to have a marked effect on the fetus. Infant mortality in the national study doubled in overweight women who gained less than 15 pounds, and birthweights in our study of this same group fell off markedly. In other words, for the overweight woman it appears important to gain at least this minimum amount of weight.

Moreover, it is important for the overweight woman to avoid dieting during pregnancy as a way of regulating her weight. The many popular weight reduction diets that are high in protein and fat and low in carbohydrate increase the chances of developing ketosis. For all weight categories, but particularly for obese women, if weight gain is slow, the diet must be very carefully selected. It must be adequate in all essential nutrients, liberal in carbohydrate (preferably in the form of starch), and not excessive in fat.

Pattern of Weight Gain. Pregnancy brings little change in terms of calorie requirement and weight gain for the first 12 weeks. Then, beginning with the second trimester, calorie requirement increases by about 300 calories per day and weight begins to increase at the rate of almost a pound per week.

The graph on the next page shows distribution of "average" weight gain during pregnancy.

You are not very likely to gain in the nice, smooth pattern shown on this chart. Your weight gain from month to month will probably vary over and under the standard line. I found in my pregnancies that I lost two or three pounds immediately when I became pregnant, probably because of a shift in water balance, then gained seven pounds in each of the fourth and fifth months. I blamed that on a shift in body fluid as well, because I knew I wasn't overeating, at least to that extent. I kept my fingers crossed and tried not to do any mathematics in my head (you know, the type where you say "seven pounds times four more months is—"), and just kept on eating. Sure enough, by the sixth month the monthly gain had leveled off to a nicely respectable three pounds, and it actually dropped during the last trimester to only about two pounds per month. When it was graphed, my weight gain looked like the pattern in Figure 2-3—not really such an alarming picture, after all.

Women often will have a particular time in their pregnancies when they gain more than average or less than average. If your

Figure 2-2. Maternal Weight Gain in Pregnancy.

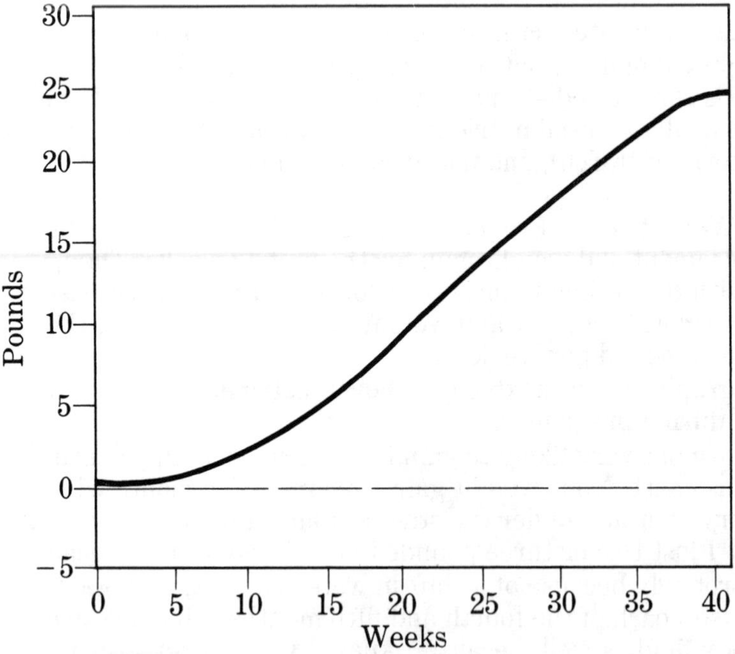

weight gain is generally varying over and under the standard line, don't worry about it. It is only when you go considerably above or considerably below the average that you may want to give some attention to your eating to see if you need to make some adjustments.

First Trimester. While growth of the developing fetus is small in actual size, its importance is very great. The beginning of all the baby's organ systems is being laid down at this stage, and the mother's body is preparing for pregnancy. Serum volume and blood

Figure 2-3. Weight gain in pregnancy: E.S.

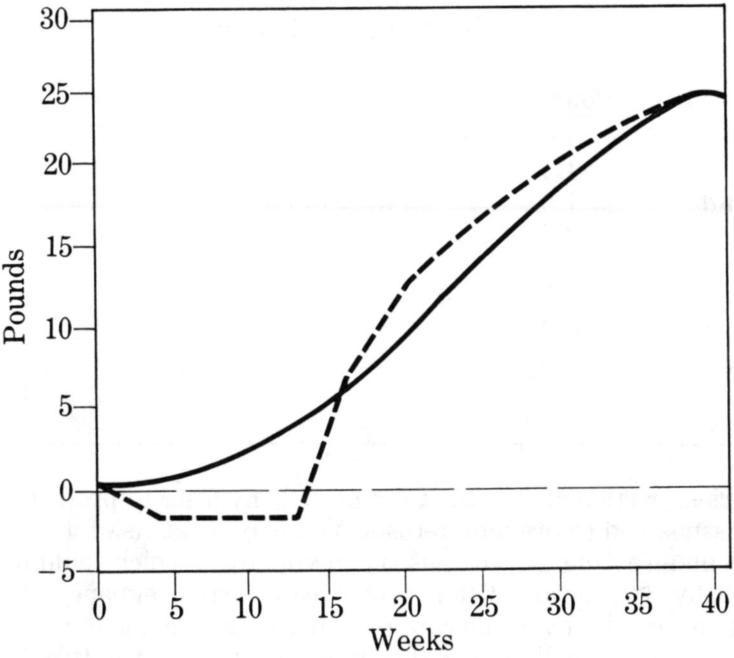

flow to the uterus both increase, there are changes in her breathing and digestive patterns, and adjustment in her pattern of carrying nutrients in the blood.

Because it is the time when the baby is basically being formed, any hazardous chemicals or severe infections are the most dangerous at this time. But because the absolute needs for nutrients is so small, any nutritional deficiencies won't have an impact unless they are particularly severe. It is primarily important during this stage to get

Figure 2-4. Components of Weight Gain.

This average weight gain is made up of the following:

	Pounds
Fetus	7.0
Placenta	1.4
Amnionic fluid	1.8
Uterus	2.0
Breasts	.9
Blood	2.7
Fat	8.0
Unaccounted	3.0
	26.8

enough calories, particularly in the form of carbohydrate to protect your body tissues and to prevent ketosis. You may be at risk for ketosis from undereating due to nausea and vomiting, which could be bad for the baby. If your appetite is poor during early pregnancy, it is important to eat whatever you can, even if you can't manage a well-balanced diet. We will discuss this in more detail later in this chapter.

Second Trimester. The second three months of pregnancy are the most important with respect to the changes in the mother's body that will support the pregnancy.

Blood volume increases by about four pints, to a total of around eight pints. Because the liquid fraction, or serum, increases in volume faster than the red blood cells are manufactured, you frequently see a drop in red blood cell count during this time. This isn't necessarily a sign of anemia. We will discuss this more in the section on iron.

Uterus and breasts grow and increase in size. It is important at this stage to have calories available to lay the groundwork for successful lactation. Placental growth during this stage is a vital part of a successful pregnancy; it is closely related to the size of the fetus.

Fat storage, to the regret of many women, is a normal and inevitable part of pregnancy. In fact a mother who is inadquately nourished will continue to deposit fat even though fetal growth is slowed.[14] This fat storage is insurance for the high energy costs of fetal growth in the last weeks of pregnancy, for labor and birth, and for lactation. In fact, it appears that depositing these energy stores during pregnancy is a very important part of assuring good lactation.

Third Trimester. The last three months of pregnancy is the time of maximum growth in the fetus and the placenta. If mothers undereat during the last 10 weeks of the pregnancy, they produce babies who are smaller in total body size. And the smallness does not just represent fat (although they do accumulate less). Babies who are underfed during the last 10 weeks of gestation have small organ systems; their heart, liver, kidneys, brains and other organs are smaller than in babies who have had access to more calories during that time.

In summary then, poor nutrition in the latter part of pregnancy affects fetal growth, whereas poor nutrition in the early months affects development of the embryo and its capacity to survive. Statistics on reproductive performance during the famine caused by the Nazi blockade of Rotterdam show this dramatically. Mothers going into the famine were generally well nourished, but once the blockade was imposed, average calorie intake dropped to less than 1000 calories per day, and protein was limited to 30 to 40 grams. Since the blockade lasted six months, babies were exposed to the famine for only part of their gestation; some pregnancies came to term during the blockade, some began.

Stillbirths and congenital malformations were highest for infants conceived during the famine. On the average, birth weights of infants exposed to the famine were reduced by 200 grams, or almost

½ pound. Weights were lowest for babies exposed to the famine during the entire last half of pregnancy.

Your Daily Food Guide

We'll begin by summarizing, in table form, the foods that are recommended for you to eat each day from the four major food categories.

There are separate outlines for adequate diets, (1) for pre-pregnancy and the first trimester (nutritional needs increase only slightly during the first trimester), (2) during the last two trimesters of pregnancy, and (3) during lactation.

The amounts are minimums—they are IN NO WAY INTENDED to dictate the total quantity of food that you eat.

In all of our discussion of nutrition, we will be talking about two major classes of nutrients: The macronutrients (nutrients needed in large amounts) and micronutrients (nutrients needed in small amounts). All foods contain both. The macronutrients, protein, fat, carbohydrate (and alcohol) make up most of the bulk of what we eat and are the calorie-contributers in our diet.* The micronutrients, the vitamins and minerals, are present in minute quantities and contribute no calories.

Unless you use alcohol, protein, fat and carbohydrate interact in providing all the calories in your diet. Generally, protein intake is fairly stable, with fat and carbohydrate varying in the proportion of calories they contribute to the diet.

Meal Planning; Food Distribution. Every meal should have a source of protein, some carbohydrate, preferably a starch (although sugar may also be included), and some fat. As we will discuss in more detail in the chapter on *Regulation of Food Intake*, these three sources of calories in combination will tend to be satisfying and

*The rest of the bulk comes from water and indigestible residue.

Figure 2-5. Your Daily Food Guide.

When Not Pregnant and During First Trimester	During Last Two Trimesters of Pregnancy	When Nursing
Milk or Milk Products		
2 cups Teenagers 4 cups*	4 cups Teenagers 6 cups*	4 cups Teenagers 6 cups*
Meat and Other Major Protein Sources		
2 servings, total of 4 ounces	3 servings, total of 6 ounces	2 servings, total of 4 ounces
Fruits & Vegetables		
4 servings vitamin C source daily	4 servings vitamin C source daily	4 servings vitamin C source daily
Vitamin A source every other day.	Vitamin A source every other day.	Vitamin A source every other day.
Breads & Cereals		
4 servings (enriched, fortified, or whole grain)	4 servings (enriched, fortified, or whole grain)	4 servings (enriched, fortified, or whole grain)

*See p. 37 for special requirements of very young teen-age mothers.

filling, and should stay with you long enough to keep you comfortable.

It is best to spread your calories and other nutrients fairly evenly throughout the day. Certainly breakfast for most people will be smaller, but don't let it be too small. In the morning you are likely to be coming off a 10 to 12-hour fast, and facing one of the high-energy-demanding periods of the day. Ideally, breakfast should account for a least 25% of your day's calorie intake, and provide at least one serving of a high-protein food, like milk or a meat group choice, along with two breads, some fat, and probably some fruit.

Protein is best utilized if it is distributed over several feedings. It is better, for example, to have an egg for breakfast, a meat and cheese sandwich for lunch and three-ounce steak for dinner, than it is to save up and have a six-ounce steak for dinner. Not only do you need those protein building materials throughout the day, but your body may have a limit as to how much protein it can use at one time.

Caloric Adequacy. If you follow the food guide on p. 33, the protein, vitamins and mineral levels in your diet should be adequate. It will not, however, be a truly adequate diet, because it will not contain enough calories.

The basic diet as outlined, even if you have four or five fat servings a day, will give you only about 1400 calories (1300 calories if you drink skim rather than 2% milk). While it is extremely difficult to estimate calorie requirement, we can guess that most women of childbearing age will require between 1600 and 3000 calories per day simply to maintain weight, and probably an additional 300 calories per day during the last two trimesters to achieve the appropriate growth and weight gain of pregnancy.

The best guide to how much you should be eating overall, is your feelings of hunger, appetite and satiety. Your body will regulate, if you let it, during pregnancy. Select a good well-balanced diet, provide yourself with regular meals and snacks, get a moderate amount of exercise, and trust yourself to eat the right amount of food.

Providing Adequate Calories. You can get the extra calories you need either by consuming more of the basic foods, or by consuming extra sugar and fat calories. Most people find it strange to be thinking about where the extra calories are going to come from to support a pregnancy. You may not in fact, have to think about it at all—you may simply find yourself eating a little more of everything from your basically adequate diet. That's a good way of doing it. Or you may want to be a little more deliberate about adding up your food choices. In case you do, let's discuss your options in more detail.

Eating more meat. The recommended amount of meat of four or six ounces, along with the protein in milk, will provide enough protein, but it is less than most of us generally eat. If you are accustomed to having more meat than that, by all means go ahead. Consuming more protein than you really need won't make your protein nutrition any better, but eating extra meat will help to insure that your diet will be adequate in minerals generally, and in some particularly important trace elements such as zinc.

Don't force-feed yourself with meat in hopes of helping to keep your weight down. A high-protein diet is no more slenderizing than any other type of diet. In fact, it almost inevitably will contain a lot of fat as well as protein, and its fat content makes it concentrated in calories. It is worth repeating that some of the popular high-protein, high-fat, low carbohydrate diets are absolutely inappropriate and even dangerous for pregnancy. They can send you into ketosis, and that is precisely what we don't want during pregnancy.

You should always have some substantial source of carbohydrate along with your meat—one or two servings of bread or fruit, to prevent ketosis and to keep the protein from being burned for energy. (Your body will fill its energy needs first, and if the only really good source of calories in a meal is the protein in meat, that will be used for energy rather than for building and repair of body tissue.)

Increasing Breads and Cereals. Once they get over their basic fear that eating starch will make them fat, many women find themselves eating two or more times the minimum number of servings from the bread group. They find starches filling and satisfying and, if anything, somewhat easier to regulate than some of the more concentrated foods such as meats.

Drinking More Milk or Higher-fat Milk. If you drink two extra glasses of whole milk per day, you will consume an extra 340 calories. It is up to you whether you want to drink more milk than that to get some of your extra calories. Unless you were calcium deficient to start with, the extra calcium probably won't do you any good.

Eating More Fruits and Vegetables. Like milk, fruit juices drunk for thirst can fool your natural sense of regulation. You will probably be safest if you avoid drinking any calorie-containing beverage, except as part of a nutritious meal or snack. That way, the calories will be consumed consciously as part of your food-regulation process, and you won't be so likely to take calories when you don't need them. Use good old-fashioned, cheap water for thirst.

Fruits and vegetables contribute moderate amounts of calories to your diet until you put extra sugar or fat on them. Apples baked in apple pie, or lettuce with roquefort dressing, are quite different in calories from their plainer counterparts. Whether you use extra sugar or extra fat will depend on how hungry you are and how your weight is responding.

Fats and sugars. Once you satisfy your requirements for *Your Daily Food Guide*, you can use sugars and fats for some of your extra calories. Sugar and fat, used to excess, can distort your diet; but used in moderation, they can enhance nutritious food and make it more appealing, and thus help you maintain the nutritional quality of your diet.

For example, you can probably afford butter on vegetables and on your bread. An oatmeal cookie has more fat and sugar than whole grain bread, but the basic vitamins and minerals of the bread group are still there. A cheese sauce may be just the thing to make the broccoli more interesting, and pumpkin pie, contributing a high-vitamin-A vegetable, milk and eggs, makes a great nutritional snack or part of a meal.

Making Up for Lost Time

You may be going into pregnancy poorly nourished. You might not have been too consistent in the past at feeding yourself well. You may have been a chronic dieter, willing to forgo nutritious food to keep your weight down. You may have had pregnancies close together and not have had time to recover nutritionally. You may have had twins.

Your nutrition before and between pregnancies has an impact on subsequent pregnancies. If you feel you have done less than well, you should make a special effort to eat nutritious foods during pregnancy. In fact, you should choose your extra calories more from the basic-foods groups, and less from the high-sugar, high-fat "extras" categories.

Teenaged Pregnancies

A girl continues to grow in height, skeletal, muscle and organ mass for about three years after she reaches menarche. If she becomes pregnant within two years of menarche, she is at particular nutritional risk, because she must provide calories and nutrients for her own growth at the same time that she must provide for her developing fetus.[1]

To get the large amounts of calcium, protein, vitamins and minerals she needs, the teenage mother should take six cups, rather than a quart of milk per day, and she should also pay particular attention to getting all of the foods in the daily food guide.

Given common teenage food preferences, this may seem unrealistic. However, being in the teenage group need not prevent a woman from enjoying nutritous foods. Assuming you are keeping within healthy limits on fats and over-all calories, you can include many common snack foods which are actually very nutritious (e.g., pizza, hamburgers, milkshakes and barbeques). More food suggestions that might appeal particularly to the teenage taste are included on p. 46.

Portion Sizes, Substitutes for the Daily Food Guide

Milk and Milk Products. Many women find their dislike or intolerance of milk changes during pregnancy, so give yourself a chance to like it, even it you haven't before. It is virtually impossible to get enough calcium and vitamin D from food unless you include milk and dairy products. If you can't drink milk, you will probably have to take a calcium supplement. Depending on what form of calcium you use, to get the 1200 mg calcium per day that you need, you will probably have to take six to twelve calcium pills.* You must also keep in mind that dairy products contribute 40% of the protein in your diet. If you omit them, you must increase your daily servings of meats or non-meat alternatives by two during the first trimester, and four during the second and third trimesters.

The following foods each gives as much calcium as you would get in a cup of milk.

Figure 2-6. Substitutes for Milk Calcium.

1 cup of milk	=	1 cup buttermilk or skim milk
		1 cup yogurt

*Avoid calcium diphosphate, as it can interfere with iron absorption. Also avoid dolomite and bone meal as calcium supplements; these contain excessive amounts of lead, as well as other toxicants.

1½ ounces cheddar-type cheese
1 cup custard or milk pudding
1½ cups ice cream
1½ cups cottage cheese
¼ cheese pizza (14 inch)

Check the *Toddler* chapter (p. 279) for a list of the calcium content of common foods. In the same section (p. 280) is a list of suggestions for including calcium in your diet.

Meat and Other Major Protein Sources. Meat and other major protein sources are good sources of protein, iron, B vitamins and trace elements. To help you estimate portion sizes, on the next page are some examples of one and three-ounce portions of cooked meat from the meat group, and also some non-meat alternatives, such as cooked dried beans and peanut butter. If you use cheese as a "meat" source, make sure you count it only once. That is, you can't count it as a milk serving and as a meat serving as well. Cheese is good for you, but it isn't that good!

Fruits and Vegetables. We depend on fruits and vegetables as the primary sources of vitamins A and C in the diet. They contain other nutrients as well, such as calcium, B vitamins, iron and trace elements, but in selecting fruits and vegetables we look particularly for the ones that are good vitamin A and C sources. If we provide those nutrients in natural foods, that is, vitamin C in orange juice rather than in a manufactured fruit drink, we can generally assume that other nutrients will be provided in adequate quantities. Here are charts to help you select fruits and vegetables. (They will be repeated in the *Toddler* chapter with different portion sizes.)

Vitamin A. During pregnancy your vitamin A requirement increases from 4000 to 5000 IU per day. A quart of milk will provide

Figure 2-7. Estimating Meat Portion

Meat Serving	Alternatives
1 oz. meat, poultry or fish	1 egg 1 slice (1 oz.) cheddar-type cheese ½ cup cooked dried beans, dried peas, lentils ¼ cup cottage cheese 2 Tbsp. peanut butter 2 slices (2 oz.) bologna 1 frankfurter (packed 8 per pound) ⅛ cheese pizza (14 inch) 4 slices bacon
3 oz. meat, poultry or fish—a piece of meat or fish about the size and thickness of the palm of your hand	One-fourth of a 2½ to 3-pound chicken (½ breast, or a leg and thigh) One medium loin pork chop, ¾-inch thick One lean ground beef pattie, made four to the pound*

*Meat shrinks about 25% with cooking, so a four-ounce raw patty cooks down to three ounces. Restaurants who sell "quarter pounders" are usually advertising raw weight.

you with 1000 IU, so you need to get 3000-4000 IU from fruits and vegetables. (We assume you'll be getting some vitamin A from miscellaneous sources like butter and margarine, and from fruits and vegetables not on this list.) Choose from the chart one excellent vita-

*Figure 2-8. Vitamin A in Fruits and Vegetables**

Excellent Sources More than 4500 IU per ½ cup	Good Sources 1500-4000 IU per ½ cup	Fair Sources Less than 1000 IU per ½ cup
Apricots, dried	Apricot nectar	Apricots
Cantaloupe	Asparagus	Brussel sprouts
Carrots	Broccoli	Peaches
Mixed vegetables	Nectarine	Peach nectar
Mango	Purple plums	Prunes
Pumpkin		Prune juice
Spinach, other greens		Tomatoes
Squash		Tomato juice
Sweet potatoes		Watermelon

*U.S.D.A. Home and Garden Bulletin Number 72

min A source every day, or a combination of two good sources, or at least one good plus one fair source.

Vitamin C is easier to get than vitamin A. You need about 80 mg of vitamin C daily during pregnancy, which is about 20 mg more than the non-pregnant level. From the chart on the next page, choose one excellent source of vitamin C or two good sources per day. Almost all fruits and vegetables have some vitamin C, so if you get your four servings of fruits and vegetables a day, you can assume that you will easily get the other 20 mg.

Breads and Cereals. I said it before, I'll say it again, and I am saying it right now: breads and cereals are important in your diet. Far from being the "filler," nutritionally-marginal food that many people think they are, they are good sources of B vitamins and iron, and

*Figure 2-9. Vitamin C in Fruits and Vegetables**

Excellent Sources— About 60 mg per ½ cup (One serving daily)	Good Sources— 25 to 40 mg per ½ cup (Two servings daily)
Broccoli	Asparagus
Brussel sprouts	Bean sprouts, raw
Cabbage	Chard
Cauliflower	Honeydew melon
Cantaloupe	Potato
Grapefruit; grapefruit juice	Tangerine
Kohlrabi	Tomatoes, tomato juice
Mango	Pureed baby fruits
Oranges, orange juice	
Papaya	
Peppers	
Spinach	
Strawberries	
Vitamin-C fortified infant juices	

*U.S.D.A. Home and Garden Bulletin number 72.

they provide valuable complex carbohydrate, or starch. If they are whole grain, they also provide fiber, and contribute trace elements, such as zinc and copper.

To get fiber and trace elements, it is desirable to use whole grain breads and cereals up to about half the time. (Beyond that, it may be that the fiber starts to interfere with mineral absorption—see the discussion in the *Toddler* chapter, p. 314.)

Read labels to be sure of what you're getting. The bread or cereal should be made with "enriched" or whole grain flour. "Enriched" means that iron and the B vitamins, thiamine, niacin and riboflavin have been added to restore that lost by refining. Many delicatessen and specialty breads are not made with enriched flour, so be careful. Some enriched products, rather than indicating "enriched" flour, list the nutrients separately, as in the following example:

Ingredients: flour, water, corn syrup, yeast, partially hydrogenated soybean oil, honey, molasses, wheat bran, crushed wheat, salt, wheat gluten, cornflour, oatmeal, soya meal, mono and diglycerides, barley malt, calcium sulfate, ethoxylated mono and diglycerides, vinegar, dry honey, dry molasses, inactive dry yeast, ammonium sulfate, niacin, ferrous sulfate, potassium bromate, thiamine mononitrate, riboflavin.

To get a whole grain product, read the label to be sure the first listed ingredient is whole wheat, or oatmeal, or whole grain of some other type. "Wheat flour" is not whole grain, nor is "unbleached flour." The following grain products are roughly equivalent with respect to calories, thiamine, riboflavin and iron content, but whole grains contribute additional vitamins, trace elements and fiber:

Figure 2-10. One-serving Equivalents of Breads and Cereals

Bread	
White, Whole wheat, Rye, Raisin	1 slice
Bagel	½
Biscuit, Dinner roll	1 (2″ diam.)
Buns	
Hamburger bun	½
Hot dog bun	1
Cereal, cooked	½ cup
Cereal, dry	
Flakes or puffed	¾ cup
Bran cereals	½ cup

Figure 2-10 (continued)

Natural cereals, Granola	¼ cup
Cornbread	1½″ cube
Crackers	
Graham	2 (2½″ squares)
Oyster	20 (¼ cup)
Saltines (2″ square)	5
Round thin (1½″ diam.)	7
English muffin	½
Grits	½ cup
Muffin	1 (2″ diam.)
Macaroni	½ cup cooked
Noodles	½ cup cooked
Pancake	1 (6″ diam.)
Rice	½ cup cooked
Spaghetti	½ cup cooked
Taco shell	1
Tortilla	1 (6-8″ diam.)
Waffle	1 (½″ × 4½″ × 2½″)

Fats. Fats contribute calories, flavor, and satiety value to the diet, as well as modest amounts of some fat-soluble vitamins like vitamin A. Because they are so concentrated in calories,* varying the fat content of your diet is a good way of adjusting calories to influence weight gain.

The following list of fat sources in the diet may be helpful to you. The portions are adjusted so that each choice contributes about 45 calories. From this list you can get an idea of the relative calorie

*1 gm. fat = 9 calories
1 gm. carbohydrate = 4 calories
1 gm. protein = 4 calories
1 gm. alcohol = 7 calories

concentrations of different kinds of fats, as well as some ideas for varying the fats you use in your diet. Keep in mind that with fats, as with other foods in your diet, it is probably safest, most nutritious and most enjoyable to use them in moderation and to select a variety, including vegetable oils as well as animal fats. If you have a particular concern about avoiding heart disease (see p. 311, *Toddler* chapter), have your doctor test your blood cholesterol, evaluate your risk factors, and help you decide whether you should go on a therapeutic diet.

Figure 2-11. One-Serving Equivalents of Fats.

Butter or margarine	1 tsp.	French dressing	1 Tbsp.
Bacon, crisp, drained	1 slice	Mayonnaise	1 tsp.
Cream, light (half & half)	2 Tbsp.	Nuts	6 small
Cream, heavy 40%	1 Tbsp.	Olives	5 small
Sour cream	1½ Tbsp.	Avocado	⅛ (4″ diam.)
Sour half and half	2 Tbsp.	Cooked salad dressing (Miracle Whip)	2 tsp.
Cream cheese	1 Tbsp.	Salad oil	1 tsp.
Bacon drippings	1 tsp.	Gravy	2 Tbsp.
Cream sauces	2 Tbsp.		

Combination Foods. People remain somewhat puritanical about good nutrition, assuming anything that tastes good must be bad for you, particularly if you can buy it at a "fast-food" outlet. They are always surprised when I show them the following list. They make comments like "but lasagna is so starchy—I didn't know it was *good* for you" or, "it never occurred to me that tacos could be nutritious, but I guess they are." For the part of you that remains a puritan about food selection, here is a list of combination "fun foods" that can perk up your food selection. You may not have considered how many nutrient food groups are represented. Bon Appetit!

Figure 2-12. "Fun Foods" that Make Nutritional Sense

	Meat/ Protein	Milk	Fruit & Veg.	Bread	Sugar Fat
Barbeque on bun	√		√	√	√
Hot dog on bun	√			√	√
Corn dog	√			√	√
Coney (chili dog) on bun	√		√	√	√
Hamburger delux (with lettuce and tomato)	√		√	√	√
Cheeseburger	√	√		√	√
Hero, torpedo, submarine	√	√	√	√	√
Fish sandwich (with cheese)	√	(√)		√	√
Steak sandwich	√			√	√
*Bratwurst on bun	√			√	√
Gyros sandwich (a Greek specialty)	√	√	√	√	√
Other sandwiches					
Peanut butter and jelly	√			√	√
Grilled cheese or plain	√ or	√		√	√
Salami, bologna, etc.	√			√	√
Tuna salad, egg salad with lettuce	√		√	√	√
Fried egg	√			√	√

	Meat/ Protein	Milk	Fruit & Veg.	Bread	Sugar Fat
Ham with lettuce	✓		✓	✓	✓
Bacon, lettuce, tomato	some		✓	✓	✓
Chili	✓		✓	✓	✓
Tacos	✓	✓	✓	✓	✓
Burritos, etc.	✓		✓	✓	✓
Pizza	✓	✓	✓	✓	✓
Spaghetti—Meat balls or meat sauce	✓		✓	✓	✓
Lasagna	✓	✓	✓	✓	✓
Beans: Bean soup	✓		✓		✓
Bean salads (cheese)	✓		✓		✓
Refried beans	✓		✓		✓
Pork and beans	✓		✓		✓
Eggs: Hard, deviled, pickled	✓				✓
Pickled herring	✓				✓
Sardines and crackers	✓			✓	

*You may have to come to Wisconsin for this one!

Miscellaneous Foods. What about "junk foods?" Nutritionists are fond of saying, "there are really no junk foods, only junk diets." Translated, that means that there are really no good or bad foods, it all depends on the context.

Say you still need more calories, you have satisfied all of your other nutritional requirements for the day and you get a yen for potato chips. Those chips will provide you with calories you need and not replace any needed sources of nutrients. Thus, potato chips in that instance are not "junk foods." In fact, if your diet is lacking only in calories, the chips would be better for you than something like carrots because the chips would give more calories. If, on the other hand, you have had nothing to eat all day but coke and candy bars, those potato chips would definitely fall into the junk (or, more junk) category.

Keep in mind that incidence of tooth decay increases with your frequency of eating sugar. Also keep in mind that a very high fat diet is a distorted and potentially unhealthy diet. Because you want your diet to be as good as possible during pregnancy, for the most part, it is better if you choose fairly nutritious food for your meals and snacks.

Enriched snack crackers or chex snack mix are more nutritious than potato chips and give you the same salty crunch. An oatmeal cookie or some raisin spice cake (perhaps made in part with whole-grain flour) provide more nutrients than a sweet like a snack cake (like Twinkies®, for instance). A whole grain coffee cake with nuts is more nutritious than a doughnut. But, if it's potato chips or snack cakes you love, you had better allow yourself a treat now and then, if only to keep from being obsessed with them (and ending up on truly stressful eating binges). Only you know how often that is!

Selected Nutrients in Detail

The need for all nutrients is increased during pregnancy. As a new cell is formed in your baby's body, all the nutrients must be there to build the cell and allow it to function biochemically. You have to have the structural nutrients like protein (and calcium for bone cells) to build the framework of the cell. Then you have to have the functional nutrients, like vitamins and minerals, to provide for the chemical reactions that take place within the cell and give it life.

In all there are over forty nutrients that we know to be essential for good health. Of those forty nutrients, there are a few that we single out for particular attention during pregnancy and that we will be discussing in this section. Some nutrients, like iron and folic acid, are selected for "special attention" because they are difficult to get in adequate quantities in the American food supply. Others, like fluoride and B_6 are controversial, and you may have questions about them. Still other nutrients like protein, and also calories, are not that difficult to get, but bear discussion because they occupy such a centrally important role in the healthy pregnancy.

Some nutrients, like calcium and iron, are more immediately important for mother than baby. Zinc and other trace elements are included because of the problem of nutrient interaction. Fiber is discussed along with the nutrients, because of the common problem of constipation during pregnancy.

Calories. As we said earlier, it is difficult to predict the calorie requirement for a healthy pregnancy. Not only do women (like people generally) vary a great deal in their ordinary energy requirements, but in addition their bodies change during pregnancy in ways that influence energy needs. During the last half of pregnancy, the basal metabolic rate increases, using energy at a faster rate. At the same time, the intestine slows down, increasing the efficiency with which it extracts energy and other nutrients. In normal digestion, a certain percentage of available calories, and of nutrients in the diet "slip through." That percentage drops during pregnancy.

Women's activity levels vary. Some women react to pregnancy with increased energy and activity. Others, particularly during the last trimester, are tired, feel heavy and don't move around as much.

Some people try to calculate calorie requirement during pregnancy and prescribe a calorie requirement. In view of what I have just said, it is pretty obvious that this is not only difficult but perhaps foolhardy. About the only safe way to regulate food intake during pregnancy is with a healthy and well-functioning appetite. The only reasonable way to assess adequacy of calorie intake is by measuring weight gain.

As I've said repeatedly, you mustn't diet during pregnancy. Instead you should help yourself to regulate well. You can do this by:

1. Providing yourself with regular and satisfying meals, and devoting time and attention to eating them.
2. Providing snacks, if you are hungry for them, making them significant by choosing good food, and taking your time with it.
3. Getting moderate and regular exercise. Your body regulates better if you aren't too sedentary.
4. Paying careful attention to your body's signals of self regulation; that is, hunger, appetite and satiety. (Satiety is the feeling of fullness and well-being you get after a filling and tasty meal or snack.)
5. Varying the caloric density of your foods. If you must attempt to slow weight gain, you can increase your proportion of bulky and relatively low-calorie foods, like fruits and vegetables, breads and cereals and broth soups. To increase weight gain, do the opposite: hold down the low caloric density foods and eat more high caloric density (like fatty and sugary) foods. (Nutritious foods that are high in calories include ice cream, peanut better, sweetened yogurt, cheese, fruit and custard pies, etc.)

Protein. Protein provides the basic structure for all cells in the body. You need extra protein for the changes taking place in your own body (increase in blood volume, breasts, uterus, nutrient storage), plus protein to build your baby's body.

Protein requirement. In the *Toddler* chapter (p. 276) there is a table summarizing the protein content of different foods. Seventy-four to seventy-six grams of protein per day is recommended during pregnancy at any age.[2] Most people in this country eat about 100 grams per day, which probably shouldn't be discouraged. While the excess protein won't do any good, high-protein foods are important for other reasons: they are good sources of B vitamins and trace elements. As we said earlier, however, don't go overboard on the protein.

Protein and calories. Protein nutrition depends on calorie intake. If calorie levels in the diet are insufficient to support the growth of pregnancy, the protein will be sacrificed to provide energy.

In a study in Guatamala with a group of women whose diets appeared to be poor in all nutrients,[9] supplemental calories from non-protein sources produced as much of an improvement in the outcome of pregnancy as did calories plus protein. It appeared that the mothers could get by on relatively low amounts of protein in their diets as long as they were getting enough calories.

It may be, although this is not proven as yet, that those Guatamalan mothers who didn't get the extra protein were depleting their own muscle and organ tissue to provide for their babies' protein needs. That certainly isn't desirable for the mothers, particularly when they are facing the stress of lactation. However, it appeared that as long as the calorie levels were adequate, their babies came through the pregnancy in good shape.

Non-meat Protein. The non-meat sources of protein we referred to earlier, cooked dried beans, peas, lentils and peanut butter, all give fairly concentrated amounts of protein. However, these proteins are "incomplete." They must be properly planned into meals to make them good protein sources for you, because with incomplete protein you must match foods, compensating with one food for the protein deficiencies of another.

If you plan to eat a vegetarian diet, you should study the subject in detail. (The *Toddler* chapter, p. 312 discusses the subject a little more thoroughly.) It might be a good idea to consult with a good dietitian about the quality of your diet. However, to briefly summarize, there are two ways you can utilize plant protein so it will supply your protein needs:

1. Consume plant with animal protein, at the same meal or within about two hours of each other (e.g., chili with ground beef or navy bean soup with bits of ham).
2. Eat grains and legumes or grains and nuts at the same meal (e.g., lentils and rice or peanut butter on bread).

Iron. Iron is essential for the formation of hemoglobin, the red substance in blood which carries oxygen from the lungs to the body tissues. During pregnancy, your iron requirement increases markedly, as you make up to four pints of additional blood, provide iron for your baby's iron reserve, and fortify yourself against blood losses during delivery.

Iron is one of the few nutrients in which the fetus acts as a parasite—it assures its own availability of iron by drawing from the mother. If you don't have enough iron during pregnancy, you could become anemic, but it is unlikely that your baby will be anemic. The most common cause of iron deficiency anemia in the infant is prematurity. The infant who has a short gestation misses out on at least part of the time when most nutrient storage takes place.

Providing iron for pregnancy. You can use a combination of strategies to provide for the considerable iron demand of pregnancy:

- Make sure you have good iron stores going into pregnancy. Eat a nutritious diet (following the suggestions below). Give yourself two years between pregnancies to get your iron storage up to normal.
- Keep your diet adequate in all essential nutrients. You can't build red cells with iron alone; you have to have enough food energy (calories), protein, vitamins, and minerals.
- Eat meat, poultry and fish. Iron from these sources is absorbed by your body several times as well as plant iron. These foods also contain something known as "meat factor," which improves iron absorption from other foods eaten at the same time.

- Eat a good vitamin-C source along with the meal. This improves iron absorption from the whole meal. Keep in mind the many vegetables and fruits that are rich in vitamin C, such as broccoli, spinach, and cantaloupe. (See the list on p. 42)
- Eat meat, poultry or fish and a vitamin C source at the same meal. Each helps iron absorption of the other. Spaghetti and meat sauce made with tomatoes is an example of an iron-containing meal with meat factor and vitamin C.
- Choose snack foods that provide some iron, such as fruits and vegetables, enriched or whole grain breads and cereals, nuts and seeds. Many times meals give adequate iron but snacks are poorly chosen.
- Take an iron supplement of 30 to 60 mg. per day.*
- Cook with cast-iron pans, to enrich your food with iron.
- When you eat, avoid consuming substances that are known to impair iron absorption, such as tea, antacids and calcium phosphate. (Calcium diphosphate is sometimes used as a calcium supplement.)

The chart in the *Toddler* chapter (p. 282) shows amounts of iron in common foods. The most iron you can reasonably expect to get from your diet is about 12 to 15 mg. per day. Liver is a rich source, but you should limit your liver consumption to twice monthly; eating too much liver will give you too much vitamin A. (Three ounces of beef liver can have about 45,000 IU of vitamin A.)

Supplementation with Iron. There is a long-standing nutritionists' and physicians' hassle about iron supplementation during pregnancy. Most accept the 30 to 60 mg. supplementation level[3] as reasonable, although a few argue that we are supplementing unnecessarily. They point out that blood levels of all nutrients tend to decrease during pregnancy. Generally, small women, those who have

---

*Most iron in supplements is combined with other elements. Common forms of supplemental iron, ferrous sulfate and ferrous fumarate, are about ⅓ iron; ferrous gluconate contains 11% iron. Ask your pharmacist to calculate the elemental iron in your supplement.

had several pregnancies, and those with multiple births show the greatest drop.[3] Most blood levels, including those of iron, can be increased if oral supplements are given, but whether these increases are normal or even desirable is the question—one that will require additional research.

Generally, it appears that this modest supplement of 30–60 mg. per day does no harm and may do some good, particularly for women who have low iron stores or iron-poor diets. But the controversy focuses on *levels* of iron—many physicians respond to dropping blood values of iron (the hematocrit and hemoglobin) by prescribing supplementation with an additional 100–200 mg. iron per day.

This practice, in my view, is unwise and not helpful. In the first place, these high levels of iron cause constipation and sometimes stomach upset. In the second place, too much iron interferes with absorption of trace elements such as zinc.[12] Thirdly, it is generally unnecessary.

Low blood values are generally caused by an increase in blood volume rather than a drop in number of red blood cells.[3] During the second trimester, blood serum production gets ahead of red cell formation and hematocrit drops. During the third trimester, with or without supplements, red cell formation catches up, and blood values approach the levels of the first trimester. And finally, the clincher is that those big doses of iron don't help anyway. They just pass through the intestine without being absorbed. Pregnant women absorb as much iron as they can and make red cells as fast as they can.[3] Additional iron can't speed up the process.

Folic Acid. The demand for folic acid doubles during pregnancy—in contrast to the requirement for other nutrients, which increases by 25 to 50%.[2] That, in combination with the low folate content of the typical American diet, leads to the standard and desirable practice of supplementing the diet with 200–400 micrograms of folic acid per day.

Folates play a central role in all cell synthesis. They provide the raw materials for DNA and RNA, the genetic messengers of the cell. Because of this central role of folic acid, a deficiency can have far-reaching consequences. The most common symptom is megaloblastic anemia, a type of anemia characterized by accumulation of large, immature red blood cells. Excellent food sources of folic acid include liver, kidney, brewer's yeast, and dark green leafy vegetables. Good sources are lean beef, veal, eggs, orange juice and whole grain cereals.

Vitamin B_6. Some people take vitamin B_6 in high doses to help control the nausea of early pregnancy. While some women who take it say it helps, there are no controlled studies to support its effectiveness.

Calcium. If you are over 18 years old, your base requirement for calcium is 800 milligrams per day. Younger women need 1200 mg. daily. For pregnancy and lactation you need to add 400 mg. per day. You need calcium during pregnancy to keep your bones strong and to build your baby's bones and teeth. You also need calcium circulating in your blood to allow normal blood clotting and muscle contraction.

The Baby's Need for Calcium. The fetus needs most of its calcium during the last trimester, when skeletal growth is maximum and the teeth are being formed. During that time the infant requires about 250 to 300 mg. calcium per day from the maternal blood supply. As with iron, the fetus appears to act like a parasite with respect to calcium. If you do not provide calcium from your diet, your bones will be robbed to provide calcium for your baby. (The saying, "a tooth for every child" accurately describes the process, though not the source.) The fairly common increase in dental caries during pregnancy probably has more to do with a slight increase in mouth acidity[11] (which gives a good reason for cautioning against too-frequent sugar consumption and for encouraging regular toothbrushing and flossing).

The Mother's Need for Calcium. Although the fetus is protected, this process of "robbing mother's bones" could have severe consequences for your own bone health. Maintaining strong bones is particularly hard for women. Women over age thirty gradually begin losing calcium, and in older life, many women have thin, weak, demineralized bones—a condition called osteoporosis. It appears that consuming adequate calcium and vitamin D throughout early life establishes good calcium stores prior to age thirty, and protects them after that time (though it isn't clear right now whether the process of bone demineralization can be stopped completely by good calcium nutrition).

Calcium and Leg Cramps. Many people think milk consumption has something to do with the muscle spasms and leg cramps that often appear during the last trimester. The problem seems to be that pregnant women have trouble maintaining serum calcium, which can make muscles more irritable. This problem can be worsened by exceptionally high intakes of phosphorus in the diet, because too much phosphorus can interfere with calcium absorption. Because milk is a source of phosphorus as well as calcium, some clinicians reason that the way to prevent cramps is to omit milk and substitute calcium pills. However, it does not appear that milk intake is the culprit, nor can leg cramps be prevented if milk drinking is curtailed. It is better to limit high phosphorus foods such as processed meats, snack foods and cola drinks.[14]

Sodium. Along with the strict limitations on calories, for many years sodium restriction was a part of the routine dietary management of pregnancy. That practice has pretty well been eliminated. More and more clinicians are realizing that sodium, like any other nutrient, is necessary during pregnancy.

A mild degree of fluid retention is a normal part of pregnancy. At times, however, the fluid retention becomes more marked, blood pressure goes up and there may even be protein in the urine. These are all the symptoms of preeclampsia, which we mentioned earlier. The treatment of choice for such marked edema and other symptoms, is bed rest—not diuretics, or sodium restriction.[10]

However, on the general principle that any nutrient used to excess can be harmful, sodium can be abused. In particular, high sodium intake is associated in some people with elevated blood pressure.

Fluoride. The estimated safe and adequate intake of fluoride for adults is 1.5–4.0 mg. per day. Fluoride in drinking water may be helpful in maintaining strong teeth and bones in adults. It is certainly beneficial in children for developing strong, caries-resistant tooth enamel. Municipal water supplies are generally fluoridated to the level of one part per million or 1 mg. per liter. Check with your health department to ascertain your local levels.

There are a very few studies of fluoride supplementation in pregnancy above that found in drinking water. One study showed prenatal exposure to 2.5 mg. supplemental fluoride per day to be helpful in reducing decay in the child's permanent teeth. Children of fluoride-supplemented pregnancies had thicker, more caries-resistant tooth enamel, with less pitting and ridges.[4] Because of the limited studies it's hard to tell if prenatal fluoride supplementation helps children's tooth enamel without doing any harm.

Fluorine, like other trace elements, is toxic if you take too much of it. The first symptom of excess intake is mottling (white, opaque spotting) of the tooth enamel in children. True toxicity in adults doesn't show up until you take 10 to 40 times the usual supplementation amounts for several years. In the few current studies of standard supplementation, there have been no signs of toxicity in either mother or infant.[4]

You certainly should drink plenty of fluoridated water during pregnancy and, if your local water is *not* supplemented, it could conceivably help your baby's teeth if you take a supplement, probably no larger than 1 mg. per day (2.2 mg. sodium fluoride).

Fiber. Making sure you get enough fiber will be helpful for preventing the constipation that often accompanies pregnancy. As we said earlier, the speed with which food moves through the gastrointestinal tract decreases during pregnancy. At the same time, the fetus grows and causes crowding in the abdomen. Both these factors appear to contribute to constipation.

Good sources of fiber in the diet are plant foods—whole grain breads and cereals, bran, dry beans and peas, nuts, fruits and vegetables. Of these, the whole grains appear to help the most. If you decide to increase the fiber in your diet, however, you should do so gradually, because you can cause diarrhea if you overdo it. Add on one serving of whole grain at a time until you find your bowel function is improved.

Generally, we call it good bowel function when you have a formed stool that you can pass without excessive straining or discomfort. You don't have to go daily—every two, three or even four days is OK. Stop your whole grain intake at 3 or 4 servings, or about half of your total bread and cereal intake. After that, if your bowel function is still not what you want, you can add a couple tablespoons of bran to your diet. The miller's bran that you get in the health food store is a good choice, as are bran cereals.

Zinc and Other Trace Elements. We have mentioned zinc in connection with several other nutrients, notably protein, iron and fiber. In every case, zinc absorption and utilization is affected by intakes of the other nutrients. These nutrient interactions are typical of nutrition in general and of trace element nutrition, in particular—an excess of one nutrient can interfere or even prevent the absorption of another. Zinc is also typical of other trace elements such as copper, fluoride and selenium, in that a certain small amount is necessary for good nutrition, but an excess amount can be toxic. And the difference between a safe dose and a toxic dose is, for the most part, very small.

Because overdosing is so easy and so dangerous, your best bet, with zinc as with other trace elements, is to count on a wide variety of foods to provide them in your diet.

The people in danger of developing trace element deficiencies are those at the dietary extremes—on extremely high fiber diets, or on limited and extremely refined diets. People who exist on low meat diets and eat primarily white bread, snack cakes, toaster pops, breakfast drinks, space food sticks and the like are in the greatest danger of developing trace element deficiencies. Most fabricated foods like these are enriched, or supplemented with only a few nutrients, leaving trace element nutrition untouched.

Supplements. There are something over 40 nutrients known to be essential for humans. Of those, a maximum of about 15 are provided in an "all-purpose" vitamin-mineral supplement, even in the wide-range supplements that are sometimes prescribed during pregnancy. To repeat, with the exception of iron and folic acid, which are probably desirable as supplements during pregnancy, your best bet for getting a nutritionally adequate diet is in consuming a wide variety of food—ordinary food from the ordinary grocery store.

The so-called "natural" vitamin and mineral supplements are very expensive and no more effective than the synthetic preparations. In fact, "natural" supplements frequently are mixtures of synthetic and natural substances, a step necessary to guarantee potency, since natural food substances vary widely in their nutrient density.

If you must take nutritional supplements during pregnancy, keep the total level of supplementation down to that of the Recommended Daily Allowances in the appendix. You should consult with a dietitian if you need help with your figuring. (While you're there, have her evaluate your diet.) REMEMBER: A LITTLE BIT IS

GOOD, BUT A WHOLE LOT MORE CAN BE HARMFUL, ESPECIALLY IN PREGNANCY.

To repeat, taking excessive quantities of some nutrients can be harmful. This is particularly true for the fat-soluble vitamins A and D. Both are toxic in high amounts, and both can produce fetal deformities, including urinary tract anomolies, abnormal skull development, and calcium deposits in the arteries.

High doses of water-soluble vitamins are not toxic, since the fetus can excrete unneeded amounts, but high doses given to the mother may have other undesirable consequences. Too much of any nutrient can take up more than its share of the carrier system that transports nutrients across the placenta, and thus cause a deficiency of another nutrient. Excessive vitamin intake can also promote a higher-than-normal requirement for the vitamin in both mother and baby. An infant born of a mother on high vitamin C doses can temporarily show deficiency symptoms on otherwise adequate amounts, until he adjusts to the more normal intake. The bodies of people on vitamin C supplements become so accustomed to wasting the excess vitamin C that they continue to do so for a time after the supplement is discontinued.

Food-related Problems in Pregnancy

Nausea and Vomiting. "Morning sickness is a myth . . ." The face of one knowing husband lighted up during a counseling session when I pointed this out to his suffering wife. But his face fell when I went on to add, ". . . Actually, it lasts all day." His wife, however, was delighted.

As far as she was concerned, I had tweaked him, however unwittingly, in exactly the right place. She had been getting little sympathy for her struggle with the very common discomfort of early pregnancy: the moderate, but (if you have it) always-present nausea and stomach uneasiness.

It seems that this nausea is relieved by eating, but often only while you are eating and immediately afterward. About the only things that really seem to help are sleeping and getting your mind off it. Some women are sick in the morning and get it over with; others don't get sick at all.

Some women have a marked nausea almost all the time, and may vomit seemingly every time they eat. One woman reported that it made her so mad that she went right back to the table and ate again. That was probably not such a bad tactic, unless it aggravated the vomiting. The digestive process appears to be pretty quick and resourceful about capturing nutrients even under such adverse conditions. To use a macabre example, women who vomit intentionally as a way of losing weight usually don't, even though to all outward appearances they are getting rid of all the calories they consume. Their digestive systems manage to extract the calories even though much of the food bulk is forcefully ejected.

If your problem is severe nausea, remember that your major nutritional concern during that first trimester is to prevent ketosis. Small, regular, high-carbohydrate meals will keep you from falling back on your fat stores as a source of calories. Breads and cereals and fruits are good sources of carbohydrate, as are soda pop and candy. Some few women can't eat at all, and have to depend on constantly sucking on hard candy and popsickles and sipping Seven-Up to get their calories. If that is all you can manage, you had better go with it. The alternative may be hospitalization and intravenous feeding.

Many women worry because they lose their interest in meats and vegetables during the early months. This is really less of a concern than maintaining carbohydrate intake; most people have plenty of nutrients stored in their bodies to provide for the small early demands of the fetus.

But there are some tactics that seem to help maintain nutritional balance. It seems that meats and vegetables are more acceptable if they are laced liberally with starchy foods. Many times a casserole or sandwich will taste good, and can give the same nutrients as plain meat and vegetable. Surprisingly, even people who are nauseated can sometimes enjoy spicy foods such as pizza or chili. Beyond keeping the carbohydrate intake up, there are really no rules about what you should eat. You simply have to respect your appetite.

Many women say the smell of cooking bothers them, and that they can eat better if they don't have to do the cooking. And many men, in contrast to our earlier example, are very understanding and supportive about taking over the cooking for a time. You may feel better if you eat very small, regular meals. It might also help to eat meals dry, that is, without any beverage, and drink your fluids in between meals.

Gas, Bloating and Indigestion. Gas, bloating and indigestion increase in frequency during the last months of pregnancy when the baby begins to compete for space in the abdomen.

Heartburn. Many women complain of heartburn, which is an irritation caused by the stomach contents rising into the lower esophagus. During pregnancy the regulatory valves, or sphincters, relax in your digestive tract, including the one at the junction between your esophagus and stomach. This allows the acidic stomach contents to back up into the esophagus and cause irritation.

You may be able to control this problem chemically and mechanically. In the first place, avoid stimulating excess acid formation by avoiding caffeine and excluding stomach irritants like aspirin, pepper and nutmeg. Drinking milk and eating other protein and fat sources may help control stomach acid. Relax at meals and chew your food thoroughly. Avoid filling your stomach too full; eat small frequent meals and limit fluids at meals. Don't bend over or lie down after you eat, or do anything that will allow the stomach contents to flow up your esophagus.

It may be, however sadly, that nothing will help your heartburn (except for delivery). Even the antacids that are often prescribed to control the problem may not help (and some kinds of antacids may combine with calcium to make it less available to the body). An occasional use to allow you to sleep or to reduce a marked discomfort may be all right, but don't get in the habit of taking them regularly.

Gas. Stomach and intestinal gas are generally more of a social than a physical problem. For you, it might not even be a problem. If you would like to control belching and flatus with diet, it might help you to avoid certain foods that are generally thought to be gas-forming.

Figure 2-13. Foods That May Be Gas-forming

Raw apples
Melons
Onions, garlic
Cabbage
Cucumbers
Dried beans, split peas, baked beans, etc.
Spiced luncheon meat items
Chili, Mexican food
Italian food, pizza
"Hot" spices

Also keep in mind that much gas in the gastrointestinal tract comes from swallowed air. Make sure you relax when you eat and don't gulp your food.

Loss of Appetite. There are a few times in pregnancy when your appetite is not an appropriate guide to food intake. This will show up in a weight gain that is too low. Typically, women have problems with poor appetite when they are: 1) just getting over nausea from the first trimester; 2) have been ill and not eating well; 3) are in the third trimester and finding that the physical size of the fetus is affecting their appetite.

Start out by cutting down on bulky low-calorie foods. Filling up on broth soups or salads will interfere with your ability to consume more-concentrated foods. Another approach would be to eat somewhat more often. This is especially helpful during the last trimester when your stomach capacity is lower. Sometimes it is necessary to deliberately eat more than you really want to for a while to stimulate your appetite. Women report that after a week or two of "overeating" their appetite improves and they can again regulate their eating automatically.

Constipation. See the discussion on fiber (p. 314).

Excessive Weight Gain. It is very difficult to make general statements about what constitutes excessive weight gain in pregnancy as far as the *mother* is concerned. (The earlier discussion was from the infant's perspective—how much weight gain does it take to produce a healthy *infant.*) Some women have told me they gained forty pounds in a pregnancy and had absolutely no difficulty getting it off. These tend to be women who are good regulators when they aren't pregnant—who seemingly can eat to appetite and maintain a stable body weight. Others report gaining modest amounts of weight and having terrific problems getting it off afterwards. These are often women who generally struggle with their weight, supervise every bite and every ounce they gain, and gain at or below the bare minimum. I have often suspected, but can't prove it, that the pregnant metabolism simply becomes very efficient under these circumstances and squeezes all the juice it can out of every single calorie.

Still other women clearly overgain. They put on weight very rapidly during pregnancy and have a great deal of difficulty getting it off afterwards. These tend to be women who are chronic dieters, who are used to depriving themselves and supervising their weight very carefully—when they get advice to stop dieting and gain weight during pregnancy, they really don't know how to go about it, and overdo it.

If you're in the easy gain-easy loss group, you probably don't need to worry. Your body seems to have a great deal of reliable wisdom and I prefer not to disrupt that. If you're in the modest gain-difficult loss group, you may benefit from relaxing your standards a bit, allowing more food and more weight gain. In the long run I would hope that your body would come through pregnancy not quite so conserving and somewhat better at being able to let go of the extra weight.

The group I think that should give careful attention to food regulation during pregnancy is the third group, the chronic dieters. If you are in this group, you may be malnourished going into pregnancy, because of the frequent dieting and chronic struggles with weight. If you are, the excessive weight gain may not be all bad, because it at least helps to restore depleted nutritional stores. However, coping with major weight gain after pregnancy can be a real burden, especially to the women who depend too much on skininess to feel good about themselves.

Generally, if you are a chronic dieter and are constantly working against your body's natural tendencies of appetite and weight, it is probably wise to gain on the high side of average—more in the area of the high than the low twenties. (This is particularly true if you are underweight going into pregnancy.) However, you should also be wary of finding yourself on the way to super gains of forty and fifty pounds. And in control lies the rub.

From the "bad old days" of strict weight control during pregnancy we found out what women do when they are trying to hold down on weight. They starve themselves for three days before they go to the doctor, and then after their appointment they go out for french fries. Or they cut themselves down so low at meals they are starving, and then knuckle under at break time and raid the candy machine. That is precisely the kind of behavior we don't want to touch off by prescribing weight control.

During pregnancy is a good time for you to learn to eat normally, and to find out what happens with your weight when you do that. You need to know that your body will regulate if you let it—and give it *reasonable* help. You need to learn what it is like to sit down to the table hungry and eat slowly until you are satisfied. And you need to learn to manage, appropriately, foods that you have long denied yourself permission to eat, such as bread, potatoes, or even sweets.

You can get some clues about how to go about helping yourself to learn this process by reading the sections in this book on food regulation and obesity. In some ways you may have to treat yourself like a child as you learn, or relearn the whole process of tuning in on, and trusting, your body's cues of self regulation.

And don't forget to get enough exercise (if there is no physical problem which rules out exercise). Regular exercise will make your appetite a more trustworthy guide to how much you should be eating, will burn off excess calories, and will enhance your feelings of well being so you may be less dependent on food for emotional reasons.

A Few Cautions

Saccharine. If you give mice enough saccharine, they will develop cancer in their bladders. We don't know whether malignancies will develop in humans (and don't experiment by force feeding them the substance). However, it is important to keep in mind that a potentially carcinoginic substance is most dangerous during cell division, when its presence can distort and disrupt the division process—in other words, its danger is greatest during the growth of the fetus and in young children. While there are no studies available relating saccharine-related injury to this group, it still seems wise to avoid saccharine during pregnancy and during the rapid growth of childhood. Diet soft drinks are the primary source of saccharine in the American diet.

Caffeine. Any substance consumed by a pregnant woman will appear in some form in her fetus. Caffeine appears to be transported particularly well, and achieves the same concentration in the baby's bloodstream as in the mother's. That gives reason for pause. It is unclear what harm, if any, caffeine does to the fetus. A recent study in mice, that found birth defects in fetuses of mothers receiving 600 mg. caffeine per day, has been reinterpreted to indicate no damage to the fetus. Human studies show no association between caffeine intake in pregnancy and fetal abnormalities.[6, 11]

We do know, however, that caffeine can cause a variety of problems, from agitation and sleeplessness to excess stomach acidity. It is probably wise to avoid overdosing yourself, and your baby, with what is really quite a powerful drug. The following list shows major caffeine-containing foods and their approximate caffeine content.

Figure 2-14. Caffeine Content of Foods and Beverages

Food Source	Amount	Caffeine Content
Regular Coffee	8 oz.	100-500 mg.
Instant Coffee	8 oz.	80-100 mg.
Decaf. Coffee	8 oz.	3-5 mg.
Tea	8 oz.	60-65 mg.
Regular Cola	6 oz.	36 mg.
Diet Cola	6 oz.	18 mg.
Chocolate Bar	1 oz.	20 mg.

Read the fine print on the labels for the caffeine content of other soft drinks, such as Mountain Dew, Dr. Pepper, etc.

Nicotine. A discussion of smoking may seem out of place to you in this book. Perhaps it is. Nicotine consumption, however, can negate the effects of a careful and nutritious diet. Infants are smaller if their mother smokes during pregnancy. Smoking is also associated with increased frequency of stillbirth, and mortality during the newborn period.[14] DON'T SMOKE during pregnancy, and while you're about it, stay off it after your baby is born. The evidence is accumulating that non-smokers subjected to tobacco smoke suffer many of the same ill effects as smokers.

Alcohol. If a pregnant woman drinks alcohol in large and regular amounts, it is likely to cause birth defects in her baby. Fetal Alcohol Syndrome (FAS) is a well-known pattern of physical, mental and behavorial problems found in infants of drinking mothers. In addition, there is accumulating evidence that even moderate alcohol intake during pregnancy can be harmful: it can lower birth weight and increase the number of birth defects.

It is hard to say what constitutes "moderate" intake. It appears that regular daily use of as little as one or two ounces of absolute alcohol (equivalent to two to four ounces of hard liquor, two to four bottles of beer or the same number of three-ounce glasses of wine) can be harmful.[14] It also appears that saving up the alcohol for an occasional binge is worse than regular moderate intake.

Clearly, the safest course during pregnancy is to avoid alcohol altogether. A daily or occasional glass of wine or other alcohol-containing beverage will probably do no harm. However, there is a disturbingly small difference between a safe and a toxic dose.

Medications, Drugs. Don't take any medications or drugs without the approval of your doctor. This includes over-the-counter preparations such as antacids, headache remedies, and laxatives as well as prescription or non-prescription diet pills and diuretics.

PCB's. The toxic industrial chemical, polychlorinated biphenyl (PCB), accumulates in the fat of fish living in waters which have received discharges of waste containing PCB. Pregnant women, nursing mothers, and children under six should not eat fish from areas known to be contaminated with PCB. Since these are inland waters and streams, these fish would not generally be found in commercial trade. You would only be exposed to them if you are eating the catch of a hobby fisherman. The Wisconsin fishing license booklet has a listing of rivers and streams known to be contaminated with PCBs. Your local fishing booklet may have the same, or you might check with your department of natural resources or state health department.

If you have been heavily exposed to PCB, your breast milk may be sufficiently contaminated to discourage your breastfeeding. If you suspect you have been heavily exposed, it is wise to have your milk tested.

There is a great deal of basic nutrition information tucked away in this chapter, so I hope you won't put it away when you get through your pregnancy. I also hope you don't put away your emphasis on feeding yourself well, once you get through pregnancy.

If you are planning to breastfeed, you will need a good diet to support that. But more than that you, personally, need a good diet to remain strong and well. Don't turn all of your attention to nourishing your child. Remember to nourish yourself.

Selected References

1. Beal, V. A. Assessment of nutritional status in pregnancy—II. The American Journal of Clinical Nutrition. 34:691–696. 1981.
2. Committee on Dietary Allowances, Food and Nutrition Board, National Research Council, National Academy of Sciences, Rec-

ommended dietary allowances. U.S. Government Printing Office. 1980.

3. Committee on Maternal Nutrition, Food and Nutrition Board, National Research Council, National Academy of Sciences: Maternal nutrition and the course of pregnancy. Washington, D.C. 1970. U.S. Government Printing Office. 1970.
4. Glenn. Immunity conveyed by sodium fluoride supplements during pregnancy—II. Journal of Dentistry for Children. January–February 1979. p. 17.
5. Gormician, A., J. Valentine and E. Satter. Relationships of maternal weight gain, prepregnancy weight, and infant birthweight. Journal of the American Dietetic Association. 77: 662–667. 1980.
6. Linn, S., S. C. Shoenbaum, R. R. Monson, B. Rosner, P. G. Stubblefield and K. J. Ryan. No association between coffee consumption and adverse outcomes of pregnancy. The New England Journal of Medicine. 306:141–145. 1982.
7. Monson, E. R., et al. Estimation of available dietary iron. The American Journal of Clinical Nutrition. 31:134–141. 1978.
8. Naeye, R. L. Weight gain and the outcome of pregnancy. American Journal of Obstetrics and Gynecology. 135:3. 1979.
9. Naismith, D. J. Maternal nutrition and the outcome of pregnancy—a critical appraisal. Proceedings of the Nutrition Society. 39:1–15. 1980.
10. Pike, R. L. and D. S. Gursky. Further evidence of deleterious effects produced by sodium restriction during pregnancy. The American Journal of Clinical Nutrition. 23:833. 1970.
11. Rosenberg, L., A. A. Mitchell, S. Shapiro, D. Slone. Selected birth defects in relation to caffeine-containing beverages. Journal of the American Medical Association. 247:1429–1431. 1982.
12. Solomons, N. W. and R. A. Jacob. Studies on the bioavailability of zinc in humans: effects of heme and nonheme iron on the ab-

sorption of zinc. The American Journal of Clinical Nutrition. 34:249–258. 1981.

13. Winick, Myron. Growing Up Healthy. William Morrow. New York. 1982.
14. Worthington-Roberts, B. S., J. Vermeersch and S. R. Williams. Nutrition in Pregnancy and Lactation. C. V. Mosby. St. Louis. 1981.

3
Breastfeeding Versus Bottle Feeding.

Breastfeeding is better than infant formula for most babies. But formula feeding, appropriately conducted, is a highly acceptable substitute. Babies fed both ways can be appropriately fed—or overfed—or underfed. Breastmilk is undeniably more sophisticated nutritionally, and will continue to be because it is a living substance. Babies appear to have less stomach and intestinal upsets on breastmilk than they do on other kinds of feeding. Other arguments can support either breastmilk or formula—these include considerations of convenience, immunity to disease, working, economy, appearance and sexuality.

Your first task in feeding your infant is to decide which kind of a milk feeding you will use. I will be discussing the nutrition of the milk feeding in a later chapter. For now it is enough to say that the only food that an infant needs for the first five to six months of life is a properly-constituted milk-based feed, either breast milk or a formula.

I want you to know my bias right from the beginning, and that is that if at all possible I would like to have you breastfeed your infant. Breastmilk has some characteristics that cannot be duplicated by even the most sophisticated formula. But formula feeding, appropriately conducted, is a highly acceptable substitute.

In this country, as in other technologically advantaged countries, we have access to refrigeration and are generally able to maintain adequate standards of sanitation. Most people can read and follow directions and are able to afford enough formula for their babies.* All these factors have allowed successful artificial feeding. Breastfeeding is not the life-or-death matter it is in some developing countries.

Right now it is in vogue to strongly encourage breastfeeding. To listen in on some circles of nutritionists and pediatricians you would think breastfeeding was right there next to godliness. While this is all very nice for people who want to and can breastfeed their baby, it can represent nothing but a big guilt trip for people who can't. Forget about that. You will have plenty of opportunities to feel guilty as a parent without feeling guilty about *that*, too.

However you decide to feed your baby, give yourself the credit of having reached a carefully-considered decision that is best for you and your family. You can feed your infant well (or poorly) either way. You can have a warm, close feeding relationship either way.

My task, then, becomes one of helping you make a decision, based on your knowledge of the needs of your family.

---

*For families who are economically limited and at nutritional risk, the Women, Infants and Children program (WIC) provides food for breastfeeding women or formula for infants.

Producing an Adequate Amount of Breastmilk

One of the very common reasons women give for deciding to bottle feed is that they think breastfeeding is hard. They think it is difficult to provide enough milk for the baby, and they don't know if they can do it or not. Often they have heard stories of someone whose milk supply was inadequate, or who simply "dried up" and was forced to wean her infant from breast to bottle. And that can be a realistic picture. In some cases breastfeeding isn't successful—but usually not for physical or physiological reasons.

There seem to be a couple of major factors involved in breastfeeding failure. The most important one is lack of knowledge. Breastfeeding is not difficult, but there are a few basic principles that you do have to know. Let's look at them in general terms. (I'll discuss these principles in more detail in Chapter 6.)

Breastfeeding is not entirely instinctive. Primates as well as people learn how to breastfeed by observing the process in others. We have had little such opportunity in our society. Most of our mothers and even grandmothers did not know how to breastfeed. When they were having their babies, bottle feeding was popular and breastfeeding was considered slightly disgusting and/or too difficult. If they did try to breastfeed, failure rate was high, partly because it was just too easy to supplement with a bottle. They had seen their siblings and cousins being bottle fed, so they knew how to do that.

They also had little confidence in their physical ability to provide enough milk for the baby—which brings us to the other major factor in breastfeeding failure, and that is self doubt. If parents are overly hesitant about the mother's ability to breastfeed, it can impair her breastmilk supply and bring about a failure.

That's because breastmilk is produced according to a law of supply and demand. Emptying of the breasts stimulates them to produce more breastmilk. If a mother is <u>too</u> anxious (most beginners are <u>somewhat</u> anxious), it can impair letdown of breastmilk, the mechanism that gets the milk from the production to the delivery area in the breasts. The milk is there, at least initially, but anxiety, suspicion and self doubt make the mother tense, and impair its delivery to the infant. The milk stays in the breasts, the biological message is relayed to the mammary tissue to make less, not more milk, and milk supply does, indeed, decrease.

It is also important to have reassurance that the ability to produce breastmilk has nothing to do with the apparent size of the breasts. It appears that there is no correlation between breast size and amount of glandular (milk-producing) tissue in the breasts. Larger breasts contain more fat and fibrous tissue than smaller breasts, but not necessarily any more glandular tissue.

The breastfeeding mother needs two important things: information and support. Most women *can* breastfeed their infants. Some of our best statistics on this come from the developing countries, where twenty years ago even under conditions of poverty, over 90% of mothers were successfully breastfeeding their infants.[4] I say *were*, because with the advent of western ideas and customs, and planting of the seed of doubt, breastfeeding "failure" is on the increase, as is bottle feeding. There are other factors involved, such as movement away from family support, and imitation of western patterns of infant feeding, but the basic fact remains that before these intrusions, a very high percentage of women were breastfeeding successfully.

Now that women are receiving support and information from each other, from well-informed health professionals and from well-written books, the success rate in this country is again rising. If you want to breastfeed, chances are very good that you will be able to do it.

Nutritional Desirability

We are sophisticated enough to admit that we don't know all there is to know about nutrition. Attempts of nutritionists and formula manufacturers to duplicate nature, i.e., breastmilk with formula, are constantly improving, but all must still acknowledge that there is more to be known. Research on breastmilk components continues to turn up remarkably sophisticated and intricate interactions between infant need and nutritional provision. For example, colostrum (the yellowish fluid produced before breastmilk) and early breastmilk are relatively high in zinc.[3] This high level is provided at a time when the "still-unfinished" newborn has special needs for zinc—while rapidly synthesizing zinc-containing enzymes. (Nutritionists are still debating optimum levels of zinc in formulas.) In addition, colostrum and early breastmilk contain proteins which give the baby immunity from organisms that enter through the intestine.*

Breastmilk also contains lipase, an enzyme that helps the infant's immature intestine digest other fats. Breastmilk is living, and those immunoglobulins and the lipase can be destroyed by heating. So taking it unpasteurized, directly from the breast, is a benefit formula can't duplicate.

Breastmilk is constantly changing: Breastmilk for the newborn is different in some ways than that for the child a few months old; a specific example would be the variation in zinc levels. Also, within each breastfeeding, the first milk is quite low in fat and looks thin and bluish. Then as the feeding progresses it contains more and more fat, until most of the fat is produced in the last minute of nursing. The infant then stops nursing and will only resume with the lower-fat milk from the other breast. This may have something to do with signaling the infant to stop nursing, and could have an impact on food and weight regulation.[2]

---

*As a matter of fact, factors in breastmilk that appear to confer immunity from viruses and bacteria are amazingly diverse. One that appears particularly interesting is the form of fat in the breastmilk (monoglycerides and free fatty acids of a particular chain length[6]). This appears to destroy certain viruses and bacteria by dissolving the fatty sheath around them.

Breastmilk is nutritionally very nearly complete: it needs only to be supplemented with vitamin D and fluoride to make it nutritionally complete for the full-term newborn infant.

Commercial proprietary formulas are good imitations of breastmilk. They are digestible, we can generally keep them sanitary, and we are able to give them to our infants in adequate amounts to allow appropriate growth. Their nutritional adequacy is demonstrated by the healthy and robust babies they produce. Commercial formulas are complete to the limits of present knowledge—no supplements are necessary. Formula manufacturers respond to research on breastmilk by duplicating insofar as possible breastmilk components.

The "old fashioned" evaporated milk formula is still a good substitute for breastmilk and is a good feeding choice for many families who need to control costs. If it is made with vitamin D-fortified evaporated milk, it needs only to be supplemented with vitamin C to be nutritionally complete.

We could debate endlessly on the convenience-breast-versus-bottle topic. It's handy to take the breastfed baby and disposable diaper and be all set for an outing. For long trips it's even better. However, if you leave the baby at home with a sitter, the bottle-fed baby may give you more flexibility for coming and going.

Convenience

There is also the consideration of *where* you can breastfeed your baby. Social custom allows you to bottle feed a baby in a restaurant, a waiting room, or any public place. It is ironic that social custom is not as free in defining acceptable locations for breastfeeding. You may be adroit enough or uninhibited enough to feel comfortable about feeding your infant almost anywhere, and I say, "Good for you!" But the fact remains that at some times and in some places, some people will frown at your breastfeeding your infant. And that also has something to do with convenience.

Is it more difficult to prepare bottles or to learn how to breast feed? You'll need to pamper yourself a bit to help establish and maintain a breastfeeding relationship. A matter of individual judgment and preference, don't you think?

Working

Since about 50% of women with children under six years of age are now working, this has a major impact on the decision as to whether to breast or bottle feed. Many women are able to breastfeed even if they are working full time. It takes a cooperative baby, however, and sometimes babies wean themselves abruptly to the bottle. It appears to be most successful if Mom can have a pregnancy leave of at least a month to six weeks when she breastfeeds totally, to get her breastmilk supply well established. Then when she goes back to work her supply has a better chance of maintaining itself with the nursing during the times she's at home. (I will discuss working and breastfeeding in more detail in the *Breastfeeding* chapter, p. 204)

Working women who bottle feed feel bottles are more desirable because their baby won't have to make a transition in feeding. They think they would end up bottle feeding anyway, and don't think it's worth the trouble to get their breast milk established. Both groups include parents who are concerned about their babies and come to thoughtful and considered decisions about the feeding style that is best for their family.

Weight Gain in Infants

A common argument is that breastfed babies are leaner than bottle-fed babies, which supposedly confers an advantage in terms of potential obesity in adult life. Some large and well-conducted studies done in the early 1970's have supported that, others have not.[1] A possible explanation for the discrepancy is the wide variation in the way breastfeeding is conducted. A child who is fed casually on demand is going to have quite a different breastfeeding experience than the one whose parents are very insistent on adhering to something that resembles a schedule.

Early in the '70's, many parents and professionals didn't know much about breastfeeding, and the tendency was to be more rigid. As parents have become more knowledgeable on how-to-breastfeed, they have become more casual about scheduling. More have been having a successful breastfeeding experience because breastfeeding depends on frequent stimulation.

Growth rates have improved as people have become more knowledgeable and successful. From my observation of my own children and those of friends, this has certainly been the case. We have all produced chubby little breastfed babies who later slimmed down into just-right toddlers and preschoolers. Pediatricians and nurse practitioners, too, have commented on the chubby-appearing (though weight-appropriate) breast babies thay have been seeing, and have observed informally that those babies pretty consistently slim down by the time they are three or four.

You will note that I am speaking of my observations. That has a value, particularly when one has had considerable experience and there is a scarcity of evidence from solid scientific research. I have not done a controlled study of a large group of breastfed babies who were being well and generously fed in response to demand, and followed them through their growing-up years to see what happens to them, weight-wise. Until I do, or unless I cite the scientific findings of others, you should be aware that I am giving you my opinion only. You should also keep this in mind the next time you get advice from someone based on their "long experience." In most cases what we're all talking about is a preconceived idea, supported by years of selected observations!

Economy

Evaporated milk formulas are least expensive, followed by breastfeeding, then commercial formulas. It costs more for you to eat when you are breastfeeding. It costs ⅓ to ½ more than breastfeeding to buy commercial formula—the lesser amount if you are purchasing it in powdered form, the greater if you are buying the liquid ready-to-feed. Cost of liquid concentrate formulas, which you mix with equal parts of water before feeding, is in between. (I will go into all of this in more detail in Chapter 5.)

Sexuality

One thing that you and your mate definitely need to discuss is your thoughts and feelings about how breastfeeding is going to affect your personal and sexual relationship. There is no denying that the infant-mother breastfeeding relationship represents a unity that can be seen in some ways as excluding the father. The mother may be giving the infant time, attention and emotional involvement that would have been previously reserved for her mate. It's important for the father to be able to talk about how he reacts to this. There may be little that can be done about changing the situation, but talking and sharing feelings can help a great deal to relieve anxiety and help keep you close.

Both men and women fear that breastfeeding will be an intrusion on the sexual relationship. Men think that a woman who is breastfeeding won't be as interested in sex. Also at times it is disturbing to them to see their mate's breasts, which they consider to be a sexual organ reserved for their erotic pleasure, used in a fashion which seems to be divorced from sexuality.

The truth of the matter is that breastfeeding is <u>not</u> divorced from sexuality, either emotionally or physiologically. Masters and Johnson[8] found that post partum women who breast fed had more rapid return to nonpregnant levels of sexual interest. Some also reported significantly higher levels of sexual tension than in the non-pregnant state.

This breastfeeding-sexual association can be a cause for concern. Some women experience sexual arousal from nursing, some don't. Those who do may worry that they are somehow abnormal. They aren't. All women, with the initiation of suckling, release certain hormones from the pituitary gland. These hormones cause uterine contractions that go on during the feeding and for about 20 minutes after the feeding. (This is one of the advantages of breastfeeding, as it enhances the return of the uterus to a more nearly pre-pregnant size.) Some women experience sensations from the contractions as sexual, some do not, others are not even aware that there are contractions. All are normal perceptions.[9]

The breastfeeding-sexual association can go the other way as well. Sexual arousal and orgasm frequently are accompanied by milk dripping from the breasts. That is because breastfeeding and sexual arousal use the same nerve pathways and hormones. The hormones prolactin and oxytocin are secreted in response to suckling, and allow milk secretion and milk let-down by the breast. The same hormones are released in response to sexual arousal.

The possibility of having nursing stimulate you erotically may be perfectly logical and acceptable to you. On the other hand, it may be alarming and even disgusting. Having milk drip from your breasts while you are making love may be a real turn-on for you—or a real turn-off. It's hard to know how you *will* react. It may be better just to take a wait-and-see attitude: try out breastfeeding, let yourselves feel what you feel, and then discuss it.

Personal Preference

Some people get a real emotional and physical high from breastfeeding. Others see it as all in a day's work. Some people think it's disgusting and can't imagine doing it.

It's important to consider and respect your own feelings in making your choice of infant feeding. A good feeding relationship with your infant is all-important, and if you hate it, you won't be able to hide it from yourself, your baby, or anyone else. Even the sophisticated components of breast milk can't make up for that.

As I said earlier, the father's feelings come into play here, too. Some fathers feel breastfeeding is just great, and encourage it strongly. Others have reservations. They might see breastfeeding as being too much of a burden for the mother. Perhaps they would like to feed the infant themselves, and feel left out. Or, as I have discussed, they may feel that breastfeeding is an intrusion on the sexual relationship. Possibly they would like to have a little more social freedom, and dislike the thought of being tied down to a feeding schedule. These feelings all need to be considered in making the choice of feeding.

Particularly if this is your first child, you can't really anticipate how you and your mate will react to feeding your infant. You might become so involved that you won't even want to leave her. On the other hand, you may feel hemmed in, and really feel you need some time to get out.

Your baby will have a lot to do with your feelings about needing to get away, as well as your feelings about the feeding relationship. Your baby may be so placid and well-mannered that you can take her anywhere; being around her may be so easy that you won't feel tied down. On the other hand she might be a dissatisfied little barracuda who makes her presence known at all the worst times. Having an opportunity for a breather from a difficult child can be wonderful. (A hasty word of encouragement: children change.)

If you remain undecided, you might consider trying out breastfeeding right after you deliver. If you decide you don't like it or it's not working out, it's much easier to switch to the bottle than vice versa. In some maternity wards well over 50% of infants are now being breastfed. Health professionals are now more supportive of breastfeeding, and better at helping you get started.

Appearance

Most women are concerned about their figures. They are eager to return as quickly as possible to their prepregnant weight and shape, and wonder how breastfeeding will affect that. Some have heard that they have to gain weight to breastfeed.

Breastfeeding allows you a normal physiological process of using calories in breastmilk production to help you lose the weight. It also forces you to be patient in your attempts to regain your figure. One of the ways that your body apparently prepared for lactation is by fat deposition during pregnancy. About eight pounds of the average 25-pound weight gain during pregnancy is fat, which represents a calorie store of roughly 28,000 calories. Breastfeeding allows you to utilize this calorie store in providing some of the calorie demands of lactation, which for the newborn can range from 400 to 700 calories per day. As you draw on this calorie store you will lose weight gradually.

Breastfeeding, however, makes it important not to lose weight too fast, as that can impair your breast milk supply. Generally, we recommend a weight loss of no more than one pound per week. That should enable you to eat enough to maintain both your energy level and your breastmilk supply.

From a physiological standpoint, you don't have to be as patient in waiting to diet when you are bottle feeding. But I still have my reservations about your dieting right after delivery. Physically and emotionally I doubt that it is generally wise to be cutting down on food intake at a time when you have so many new demands on you. But in any event, dieting while bottle feeding won't impair the baby's milk supply.

Mother-infant Bonding

It appears that formation of intense attachment between mother and infant, and father and infant, occurs readily during a sensitive period in the first 24 hours of life,[7] and in the early days after birth. The beginning of this bonding may have a long-term impact on the relationship between parent and child.

Certainly bottle feeding as well as breastfeeding parents can insist on extensive contact with their infant during this important time. Whether breastfeeding increases the intensity of the attachment is not really known. Because breastfeeding forces a close contact and interdependence of mother and child, however, the mechanics do promote proximity. In cases where there is a high risk of "disorders of mothering," health professionals in pediatrics are particularly likely to encourage breastfeeding to promote this contact and interdependency.

Safety

A certain very small and variable percentage of every drug taken by the mother will show up in the breastmilk. For that reason caution in drug selection and consumption during breastfeeding is extremely important. Certain of the antacids, anticoagulants, hormones, anticonvulsants, laxatives and other drugs are absolutely contraindicated for use while breastfeeding. Indeed, any drug, over-the-counter or otherwise, should be carefully checked before use by the breastfeeding mother. There are also a few foods, such as rhubarb and chocolate, that are inadvisable during breastfeeding because they contain an active ingredient that is laxative.[1]

Environmental contaminants are another major consideration for the breastfeeding mother. Certain chemical pollutants in the food chain are excreted in the fat of breast milk. The insecticide DDT was banned from general use years ago but is still present in breast milk. It appears, however, that the maximum likely to be ingested is several hundred times less than that known to cause acute intoxication in humans.

Additionally, it is somewhat cold comfort to know that the newborn already has more insecticide stored in body fat from intrauterine exposure than he is likely to acquire if suckled. In other words, the exposure is unavoidable, and it is unlikely that you will exacerbate the problem by breastfeeding.

More recent has been the concern about polychlorinated biphenyls (PCB's) and polybrominated biphenyls (PBB's). The first is a heat-transfer agent, the latter a fire retardant. They are present in the food supply purely by accident, sometimes as a waste discharged into water from factories. These, too, are carried in body fat and transferred to the fetus and to breast milk. Currently most health authorities, on the basis of absence of evidence of harm to infants from present levels of PCB's and PBB's in breastmilk, are recommending no change in current nursing practice. However, they are recommending that young women, especially if they are pregnant or lactating, limit their consumption of game fish from PCB-containing waters. Further, they are recommending that if a woman has been exposed to known contaminated areas that she get her breastmilk analyzed and decide on an individual basis whether or not to continue breastfeeding.[10]

Cows' milk contaminated with PCB is simply not allowed on the market. Further, these substances are stored in fat, and milk fat is replaced with vegetable fat in formulas, eliminating a substantial source of these contaminants.

Commercial formulas, however, are not without their dangers. Unless handled properly, they can be contaminated bacterially. Also, unless mixed properly they can be diluted too much and cause retarded growth or, at the other extreme, diluted too little and cause dehydration of the infant.

There have been mistakes over the years in proprietary formula production. Nutrients have been present in inappropriate amounts. When this has happened, babies have not done well, and the error tracked down and corrected.

In summary, then, there are three major factors to be considered in making the decision about breast or bottle feeding for your infant:

1. Your home and work demands.
2. Nutritional and physiological considerations for you and the baby.
3. Your feelings.

All three are important. But because it is sometimes harder for people to pay attention to their feelings, I would like to close by emphasizing those.

All your logic may tell you that breastfeeding is the most desirable alternative. But your feelings may say you don't want to. Don't let anyone (not even yourself) tell you you shouldn't be feeling that way. They are your feelings and they are valid.

If you would like to change your feelings, that's another matter. Think about how you feel, and talk about it with your mate. Really explore your feelings and see if you can find out where they come from. Step back and try to get a broader perspective on the matter. Your feelings may have something to do with the way you see yourself in relation to each other or in relation to the world in general.

Find out how your partner is feeling. Keep in mind as you listen to him that there is room for you each to have *different* feelings. You can only acknowledge and accept. You can't persuade or argue someone out of their feelings. Nor need you somehow change things to make the feelings go away. (Sometimes that's possible, but often it's not.) If you feel that you are really struggling or reacting in a way that puzzles or distresses you, you might want to get professional help.

Spending some time exploring in this fashion *before* the baby comes, as you both decide on a milk feeding, is good preparation for *after* the baby comes. Then you may have ambivalence about many things, and you certainly will have feelings and reactions to your changed status. To keep you together at that time it is important to keep you talking to one another. A major key in caring for your child is caring for your relationship.

Selected References

1. Fomon, Samuel J. Infant Nutrition. 2nd ed. W. B. Saunders. 1974.
2. Hall, B. Changing composition of human milk and early development of an appetite control. Lancet. April 5, 1975, 779–81.
3. Hambridge, K. Michael. The Role of Zinc and Other Trace Metals in pediatric nutrition and health. IN Pediatric Clinics of North America: Nutrition in Pediatrics. February 1977, 95.
4. Jelliffe, D. B. Infant Nutrition in the Subtropics and Tropics. 2nd ed. World Health Organ. Monograph Ser. No. 29. Geneva, 1968.
5. Jelliffe, Derrick B. and E. F. Patrice Jellifee. Breast is Best: modern meanings. New England Journal of Medicine. 297(17):912–915. 1977.
6. Kabara, Jon J. Lipids as host-resistance factors of human milk. Nutrition reviews 38(2):65–73. February 1980.
7. Lozoff, Betsy, Gary M. Brittenham, Mary Anne Trause, John H. Kennell, and Marshall H. Klaus. The mother-newborn relationship: limits of adaptability. The Journal of Pediatrics 91(2):1–12. 1977.
8. Masters, W. and V. Johnson. Human Sexual Response. Little, Brown and Company. Boston. 1966.
9. Weichert, Carol. Breast-feeding: first thoughts. Pediatrics 56(6):987–990.
10. Wisconsin Dept. of Health and Social Services. Statement on Chemical Contaminants in Breastmilk. Madison, WI 53701. October, 1977.

4
Calories and Normal Growth

Your child is born with a certain growth potential, and with the ability to appropriately regulate his food intake to support that growth potential. You can trust him to let you know how much he needs to eat, and you can trust him to make up for his errors in eating. He may overeat at a feeding and spit up, then go longer before he gets hungry again. He may undereat for a whole day, or several days, then make up for it by being extra-hungry for a time.

Your baby will grow by getting taller, heavier and fatter. It is generally safe to let that process take care of itself—to feed him and see how he grows. However, growth charts are generally used in the doctor's office as a way of evaluating normal progress in height and weight. Understanding how to read and interpret them can be helpful and interesting for you. However, to be useful, and not harmful, they must be based on accurate height and weight measurements. It is also helpful to maintain a somewhat detached attitude in following your child's growth, and not to overreact to normal variations in growth patterns.

Nourishing a young infant presents very specialized nutritional considerations. A newborn has an extremely high nutrient requirement per unit of body mass. Due to his rapid growth rate, the newborn has relatively higher requirements for calories and for all nutrients, including water, than at any other time in his life. At the same time, excesses in total food, or in any one of the nutrients, can be harmful and even dangerous. Not only do there have to be enough nutrients in the baby's diet, but they have to be there in the right quantities and in the right balance to each other. Managing all that can be complicated, given the day-to-day fluctuation in food intake of a normal infant AND the gradual increase in nutrient needs as the child grows.

Given the complexity of the nutritional puzzle, the solution is remarkably simple. Your infant regulates his total calorie intake, using his hunger and satiety. And if his food is appropriate, as with breastmilk or a carefully-balanced infant formula, he will be getting the right relative amounts of each of the necessary nutrients with each calorie of food. At the same time that he takes enough calories to satisfy his hunger he will automatically be taking enough of all the nutrients necessary for growth. As he gradually gets bigger and needs increasing amounts of nutrients for growth and development, his hunger will increase and he will get those nutrients. Again, the nutrients will be in proper quantities and in proper balance to one another.

As we pointed out in previous chapters, for the first few months, either breastmilk (with supplemental fluoride and vitamin D) or a properly-constituted commercial formula will provide all required nutrients in the proper balance for the growth and health of your infant. So, having made that important decision early on, you will need to know two things:

1. How to provide the proper amount of food to allow your baby to grow properly.
2. How to interpret his growth.

The calorie* is an important base unit of the science of nutrition. Calories are a measure of the energy that is essential for life to exist. The average calorie requirement for a newborn is about 45 to 50 calories per pound of body weight. (The adult calorie requirement is about 10 to 15 calories per pound of body weight.) Of these calories, during the first four months, about one-third go for growth; about two-thirds go for maintaining the moderate physical activity of the newborn and his physiological processes: breathing, digestion of food, circulation of blood, and the various metabolic processes necessary for life.

The Growth Process

The infant usually doubles his birthweight within four months. Most infants this age spend much of their time sleeping. Between four and twelve months the calorie requirement remains about the same: between 45 and 50 calories per pound of body weight. After four months of age the infant usually spends only about 10% of calories for growth, but uses a higher proportion of calories for physical activity.

Along with body size in general, the brain and nervous system in particular do a great deal of growing during the first 24 months of life. The most active phase of brain growth in the human infant begins during the last trimester of pregnancy, and continues until about two years of age. It would seem logical to assume that this would make the malnourished infant very vulnerable to retarded intellectual capacity.

Studies have failed to support that point of view; some apparently malnourished infants who are in socially rich and stimulating environments seem not to show the intellectual effect of malnutri-

*I will use the word "calorie" in the way it is popularly understood. It actually refers to the "kilocalorie," which is a unit of scientific measurement.

tion. That was the situation during the World War II blockade of Rotterdam in 1944–45. Despite the fact that food was severely limited, to the point of famine, males born during that famine had scores on intelligence tests at age 18 similar to babies born in non-famine areas.

But usually the malnourished infant is also in a limited social environment. The malnourished infant is usually also intellectually under-stimulated and socially deprived, and develops an impaired intellectual capacity because of the combination of these factors. The undernourished infant is often in the care of an undernourished mother. Because of low energy levels caused by their lack of food, each of them fails to provide much stimulation for the other, and the environment of the infant, as well as the nutritional status, becomes limiting. So, in such cases you could say that the nutritional status does have an effect on the infant, but that it seems also to involve social and environmental factors.

Now, I am not telling you that good nutrition is unimportant for intellectual growth. It can be one of the factors, but to have a negative impact, other factors must be present as well. What I am saying is: RELAX. Children have ups and downs in food intake. It is not necessary to entertain yourself with visions of an intellectually defective child each time your infant eats poorly.

Obesity. Simple survival, and laying the basis for healthy mind and body is the vital nutritional goal in the early months. In practice sometimes I wonder if this consideration is overlooked or forgotten among all the publicity about obesity prevention.

The beginnings of adult obesity are said to be laid in infancy. Since concerned parents and professionals are eager to avoid the social, psychological and emotional consequences of obesity, I see them worrying more about overfeeding than about underfeeding their infant. They wonder how much they should be feeding their baby and worry that they might be feeding too much. Sometimes I see a baby who seems to be positively underfed, and usually find I am talking to a parent who is extremely concerned about overweight.

I think, however, that many of us have begun to pull back some in our alarmist tactics about preventing obesity. There is a very low correlation between excessive fatness in infancy and overweight in older children, and possibly in adults. Not every fat baby is a fat adult, but there is some risk so some prevention seems appropriate.[10] It seems to me that in most cases this prevention can take the form of setting things up so the baby can achieve normal growth and food regulation. And, in the few cases where this normal process must be modified, the prevention must not be so vigorous that the infant simply isn't allowed to grow normally. (See the more detailed discussion of these questions in Chapter 11.)

Slow or Inadequate Growth

It is easy to get caught in a feeding struggle with a slow-growing child or with one who appears to eat poorly because of illness. My neighbor, David, had some problems with asthma when he was about a year old and his chest congestion, occasional pneumonia, and frequent ear aches would repeatedly put him "off his feed," usually just about the time his parents were feeling good about his eating and hoping he could catch up a bit on his weight.

I warned them that a major risk for them was getting too anxious about his eating and trying too hard to feed him. His mother acknowledged that already at 14 months he was getting a wicked little gleam in his eye when she would try various food tactics to get him to eat. (David, like most children, is no dummy and knows when he has the upper hand.)

Hard as it is, you have to feed a child like David the way you would any other child—present appropriate food in a supportive fashion and allow him to make the choice about eating. As we will discuss in the chapter on *Regulation* (p. 345), the more you pressure, the more poorly they will eat.

Getting the Right Amount of Calories

So it becomes a balancing act: enough calories to allow optimum growth, but not so many that the baby gets too fat. That sounds difficult enough—but we must also consider other factors: some infants eat more and grow faster than others; every infant eats more some days than others. Also, infants vary widely in their caloric requirements. If you have a big, wide awake, demanding baby who grows very rapidly, he will probably have a higher calorie need than a small, sleepy, placid baby who is growing very slowly.

In addition to variation in rate of growth and differences in personality, there seems to be a definite relationship to physical activity. A number of years ago, Rose and Mayer[3] did a research project where they strapped tiny pedometers to the arms and legs of young infants. They found consistently that the more active babies tended to be thinner and to eat more than the less active babies, who had a higher proportion of body fat and ate less. It appeared that these activity levels were the result of innate characteristics of the infants and could not be attributed to external circumstances.

There is even beginning to be some evidence that there is variation in calorie requirement between infants who appear to be the same in size, growth and activity. One infant will be comfortable, healthy and normal on food intake that is significantly less than that of another.

Variation in Calorie Requirement. The following chart gives you some idea of the variation in calorie requirement at different ages.[4] The energy requirement figures were calculated by taking standard weights at different ages and figuring 50 calories per pound of body weight. The calorie figures were converted to formula intake by figuring 20 calories per ounce of formula.

Figure 4-1. Spread of Daily Calorie Requirements During First Year (Courtesy the Gerber Company).

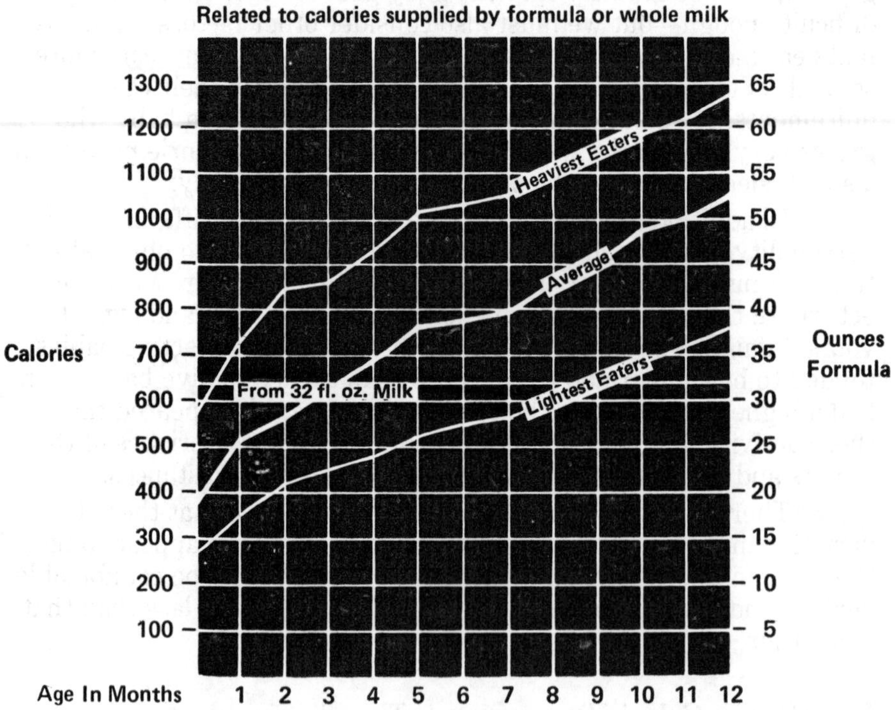

As you can see, there is a wide variation in calorie intakes among normal infants at a given age. At age three months, for example, the smallest, least-hungry baby will be consuming about 500 calories, or about 25 ounces of formula per day. If that baby is eating as few as six times per day, the average amount of formula per feeding will be a little over four ounces. By contrast, the largest, possibly most active baby will be taking almost twice as many calories, about 860 calories, and about 43 ounces of formula per day. If that hungry baby can get by on six feedings a day, he will be getting an average of over seven ounces of formula or breastmilk per feeding. If you are breastfeeding one of the big, active, hungry babies, you may need more frequent feedings to keep up with his needs.

The charts can give you an idea of the range of food intakes for different infants. How much a given infant actually eats depends on his size, activity, growth rate and metabolic rate. It can also depend on the digestibility of the food, a subject I will discuss in the *Milk Feeding* chapter. It's difficult to predict exact calorie requirements at any age, but with the infant it is particularly so.

Variation in Day-to-day Intake. Not only do infants vary from one another in food intake, but the individual infant also varies on a daily basis. Back in 1937, Arnold Geselle and Francis Ilg demonstrated that point very nicely.[5] They fed babies on demand, allowing sleeping and waking times, as well as eating times and quantities of formula to shift at the will of the infant. It became apparent from these observations that babies, like big people, are not consistently hungry from one day to the next. This chart plots the milk intake in ounces per day of baby "J," who was followed through his sixth, seventh and eighth weeks.

In day one of week six, little "J" consumed 23 ounces of formula (460 calories). On the next day he took 24 ounces (480 calories). The third day his milk intake went up to 29 ounces (580 calories), then 25, 30, 23, 28. The fluctuation in the eighth week was even greater. On the fourth, fifth, sixth and seventh days of week eight, the milk intake was 26, 21, 28 and 32 ounces, respectively. The pattern seemed to be that a hungry day was often followed by a less-hungry day, which in turn preceded another hungry day. Despite all that fluctuation, though, baby "J" grew at a consistent rate, as you can see by the following chart, which shows the body weight in pounds for those same three weeks.

Figure 4-2. Formula Intake of Baby "J" (Courtesy J. B. Lippincott)

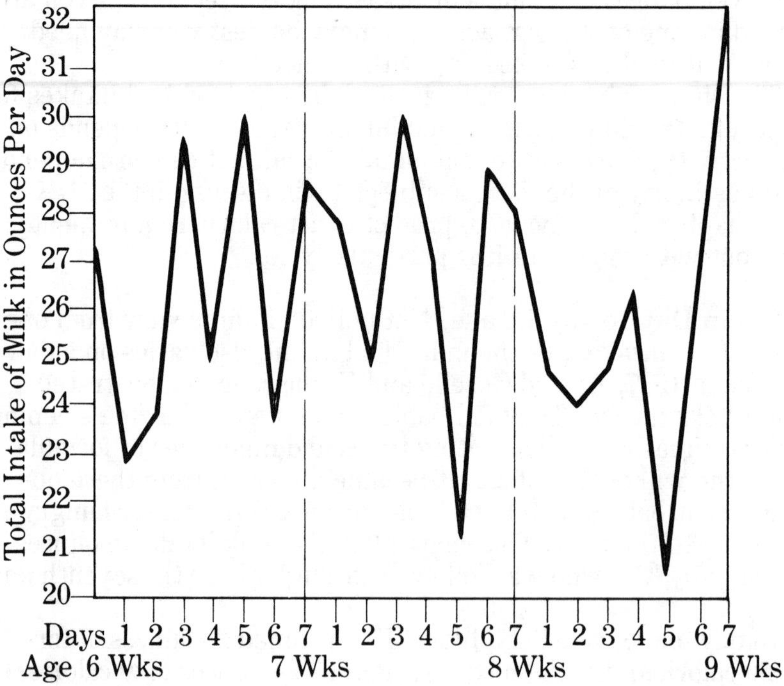

During that three-week period "J" increased his weight from 9 pounds 12 ounces to 11 pounds. He was weighed daily, and his weight fluctuated by no more than two ounces on a daily basis. Even in week eight, when his food intake fluctuated wildly, his weight increased at a steady rate.

Figure 4-3. Growth of Baby "J" (Courtesy J. B. Lippincott)

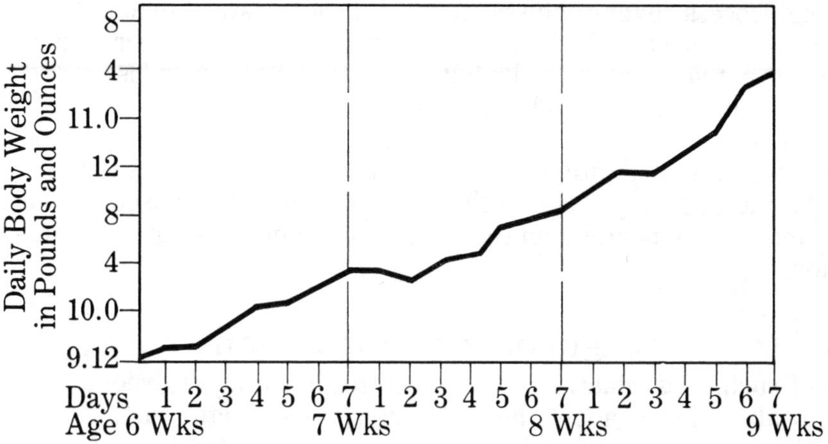

It appears not only that the child was regulating food intake on a daily basis, but also that his process of food regulation was somehow able to accommodate for daily fluctuations in food intake. His caretakers made no attempt at all to regulate the quantity of food that he took. They simply responded to his cues of hunger and satiety with a nutritious milk feeding, being sure that they gave him enough time to eat until he was satisfied, but at the same time taking care not to urge him to eat.

Feeding intervals were irregular, with some naps going longer than others. At times little "J" probably drained his bottles and wanted more, and at other times refused part of the bottle.

These studies were done in 1937, when the then "modern" physicians, using the then-perfected evaporated milk formulas, calculated "appropriate" ounces of formula on the basis of babies' weight. Babies were expected to eat that amount, no more, no less, and to take it at regular intervals and in regular amounts. Parents were expected to see to it that they did. Geselle and Ilg called that feeding process "over-sophisticated . . . if the constitutional indicators are ignored in the interests of inflexible schedule there ensues a contest between infant and adult . . . with unnecessary losses and emotional disturbances on both sides."

There had to be a better way—there was, and there is, to help babies regulate food intake. Ironically, the way was, and is to be <u>un</u>sophisticated, to go back to the method parents have used forever: seek-and-find, depending on the infant for the major source of information.

Origin of Food Regulation

Hilde Bruch, a psychiatrist who specializes in eating disorders, has an appealing theory about the beginnings of food regulation.[1] She says that a newborn infant is presented with a variety of sensations from his body, some pleasant and some unpleasant. He has no way of sorting out one sensation from the other or identifying a source of appropriate comfort for the feelings of uneasiness or distress. It is up to the discerning parent or caretaker to take the time with the infant to figure out what is bothering him.

If the parent is able to do this with reasonable accuracy and consistency, eventually the child, too, will come to the point where he can accurately identify what is bothering him and fulfill his needs appropriately. That is, as an older person, if he is hungry he will eat, if he is bored he will find something to do, etc. If, on the other hand, the parent consistently misidentifies the source of the infant's discomfort, the child too will learn to confuse one sensation and source of gratification with the other. If the parent offers bottle or breast in response to any signal of discomfort or distress, she will probably teach the infant that the way to fix any problem is to eat.

So the idea, then, is to correctly identify and respond to your infant's discomfort signals. With some babies it is easy; they only cry if they are hungry or wet, and sometimes not even when they are wet. Other babies are not so easy. They cry a lot and seem to complain about every little thing—boredom, gassiness, loneliness, temperature, heaven only knows what all, maybe even politics and the weather.

Soothing the Fussy Baby

The fussier infant may also want to eat fairly frequently, as his wide-awake lifestyle makes him more active and he may need more calories. For a child like that you will need more flexibility in care, comfort and entertaining tactics. Talk to friends and professionals, read books, and experiment. (My favorite tactic was to put the baby in a soft backpack with good head support and just "wear" him while I went about my work.) Don't feel you are doing something wrong if you feed a child like that quite often. Once you have burped, changed, cuddled and entertained, if your baby is still pressing, you had better go ahead and feed him, even if it seems like an unlikely time. These same babies seem to take a long time settling down to any kind of routine.

Feeding Schedules

One of the things that could sabotage your response to your baby's needs is trying too hard to follow a schedule. I have not talked to any professionals or read a book in years that recommends a feeding schedule. But, generation after generation of young parents (including me, when I was at that stage) have somehow preserved the myth of the every-four-hour feeding schedule as some kind of a standard for which they should strive. It is remarkable to me that that should be so, since it has been over 30 years since rigid schedules were professionally in vogue.

But persist it has, and it causes parents lots of unnecessary discomfort. There is nothing magic about an every-four-hour feeding schedule. Certainly it is much more convenient for parents to be able to anticipate when their child will be able to eat next, and some children adapt themselves to this very nicely. Others just don't make it. Some won't settle for *any* sort of regularity with their feeding schedule. They may, for example, manage to make it for five hours from one feeding to the next, and then demand two feedings an hour apart.

That is really all right as far as the infant is concerned. He just has some residual hunger that he needs to have satisfied. Whether or not it is all right with you is another matter. You may find this irregular feeding pattern absolutely maddening, and feel you must persist in your efforts to regulate your infant's schedule.

Most times I find the source of a lot of the parents' discomfort with eating patterns like this coming from the outside: other people are pressing subtly (or not-so-subtly) for the parent to get the child on a "regular schedule."

I see many parents who seem to be in this predicament, but I am thinking particularly about Mrs. Washburn as I write this. She and little Daniel stopped into my office one day after their pediatrician's appointment. She wanted to know what she could do to get her baby on a different feeding schedule.

Dan was a big, active, wide-awake two-month-old baby. He had gained five pounds since birth and had done it all on breastmilk. He was eating at frequent and irregular intervals and was still getting up twice a night to nurse. It was apparent that Mrs. Washburn was a conscientious and concerned young mother who enjoyed her infant, but it was also apparent that she was feeling very upset about their feeding relationship.

Before I responded to her request, I asked her, "What is there about the way he is eating that bothers you?" She looked a little startled and then became thoughtful. "I really don't mind feeding him that often," she said. "He nurses well and I am enjoying having him around. But everyone keeps talking about getting him on some sort of schedule. And the doctor asked me if he wasn't sleeping through the night yet. I just think that I must be doing something wrong."

I asked her what she did when he woke up, fussing. "At times he seems very hungry, almost frantic, so I feed him right away. Other times I cuddle him and play with him. I change him and put him in his swing for a while. Or he sits up in his infant seat and watches me while I do my work. But nothing works for very long. He just starts fussing again and doesn't seem like he is happy until I feed him. Maybe I should put him on a bottle or something to see if I can get him to be on some sort of schedule."

"Is a schedule important for you?"

"Well, it would be nice at times. But no, I can really manage without it. I just want to do the right thing for Dan."

What an easy case to solve! I was able to reassure Mrs. Washburn that she was doing exactly the right things for her baby. He was clearly an exceptionally hungry, fast-growing little guy, very bright and curious. It *was* possible to overfeed him, as he could get in the habit of using eating for entertainment, but she was forestalling that by going through the list of other possibilities before she fed him. In short, she was following a rhythm that was right on target for her particular baby.

What a shame that she was being made to feel uneasy by the subtle demands for an external schedule! How ironic that she would consider weaning him to formula in an attempt to satisfy something as unnecessary as a regular schedule!

With Mrs. Washburn it was easy, as she really didn't want a regular schedule. She needed support for doing it the way she was doing it. For others it is not so easy, as they really *are* disturbed by the irregularity and frequency of the feedings. That is, in fact, the way I was with Lucas, my second child.

Given my experience with Kjerstin, our oldest, who was a placid, compliant, regular little baby, I figured I could shape Lucas' habits into some sort of schedule right away. (Always be wary of advice from parents who have had easy babies.) So I tackled Lucas with a fair amount of vigor and self confidence.

He was an entirely different kid from his sister. In fact, he was a lot like little Daniel: hungry, curious, active. What a character he was! And could he eat! He would nurse about every two hours, on the average, then take a little catnap and be up again, wanting us to entertain him. He would wait five hours to eat and then want two feedings, one right after the other. Some days seemed like they were a hundred years long; I was either caring for him or trying to predict when I would care for him next.

I was absolutely insistent that I would get him on a schedule. Not only did I think we were doing something wrong in allowing this non-schedule, it was driving me bananas. So struggle, we did. I staved him off when he was hungry, and woke him up when I thought he should be having a feeding. Some days he would behave in a way that approximated regularity and my hopes would rise, only to be dashed by his subsequent return to his random patterns. I think, short of allowing him to scream from hunger, I was about as close to a rigid, insistent parent as you would find. And all to no avail. It was clear that my most persistent efforts were not working.

So I gave up. He wasn't about to change, so I changed. I fed him when he wanted to be fed and forgot about scheduling. And it helped! Once I stopped fuming and fussing about needing the schedule, I began to learn to be more casual.

When Curtis was born he was even bigger, hungrier and more irregular than Lucas. So I gave up from the very start. It seemed to me with three children the only answer was to HANG LOOSE—a philosophy that has yet to fail me.

I was committed enough to breastfeeding that I wasn't about to give it up on the gamble that bottle feeding would make them more "manageable." I figured that they would probably keep their same habits, and meanwhile I would be struggling with bottles as well.

Some parents choose to switch to the bottle with kids like this. Then, at least Mom can get some help with some of the feedings. Again, I think that is pretty much an individual decision, that only you can make in your own situation.

I wasn't alone in my concern about feeding intervals. A common reason that parents over-encourage their children to eat at any given feeding is they are hoping to prolong the interval between feedings—if they can get in a few more swallows, it should hold them longer. Parents do this for a variety of reasons: to make child care less time-consuming, because they think it is somehow better for the infant; or the way it "should" be done; or because they are afraid of making their infant too spoiled and demanding if they respond to his needs too often.

There is nothing to suggest that widely-spaced feeding intervals are any better for the infant physiologically, nutritionally or socially. In fact, the infant's small digestive system, her high calorie needs, and the rapid digestibility of breastmilk and formula would all seem to encourage relatively frequent feedings.

Carrying *vs* Caching. People evolved, in fact, as mammals that eat often. Babies have probably been carried and nursed frequently for over 99% of the human species' existence.[7] As the story goes, there are two different infant-rearing patterns in mammals: carrying and caching. The carrying kind, like the human, keeps the infant near at hand at all times, responding to and feeding the infant as his needs occur. The caching kind parks the infant somewhere and goes off to forage for food, coming back periodically to feed.

There are differences in milk composition that correspond to these differences in nurturing patterns. The milk of the carrying mother is lower in fat, so it is utilized more rapidly, causing the infant to demand to be fed more frequently. Milk of the caching mother must stay with the infant longer, so milk is relatively concentrated, especially in fat.

Since the human approach to child rearing fits the carrying pattern, you would expect to see more frequent feeding and interacting. And that is what you do see, in some infants more than others. Daniel and Lucas and Curtis, for example, insisted on being involved and cared for frequently. Others are more cooperative about allowing themselves to be cached, in bed or elsewhere, and cared for more intermittently. The former are defined as being difficult, troublesome children and the latter as better, easier babies. It seems that despite the fact that people are generally fascinated with their children, they also feel uncomfortable about giving them too-frequent attention and stimulation.

I have wondered if the myth of spoiling has something to do with that discomfort. People fear that too-close attention to infants' needs, or too-great readiness to respond to them will cause them to be "spoiled." You really can't spoil a little baby. The fear of spoiling is based on the philosophy that if you give in to a child's demands too readily and too consistently, that will cause her to be even more demanding, that somehow she will generate even more reasons to keep you coming back.

That presumes that the child is involved in some sort of struggle for dominance with his caring adults. And of course that's not true. The infant is aware only of his feelings and responses and can only communicate those. If he is calling for attention, it is because he has a real, genuine need, not a manufactured one.

The newborn infant and young child have a great need for closeness, warmth and nurturing. While the older child and adult have the same needs, they can be satisfied with more intermittent contact. In order for a child to make that transition, he must have his needs responded to consistently so he can feel satisfied and secure. Then he can move on to his next developmental stage, secure in having accomplished his previous tasks.

Signs of Satiety

Babies have many different ways of showing they have had enough to eat: they spit out the nipple, they doze off with milk drooling out of their mouth, they start to play with or bite on the nipple rather than suck. Many babies have an appealing little face-squeezing maneuver they make when they have had enough to eat. For some babies satiety comes abruptly and absolutely, and they quit nursing suddenly. Others taper off, eating more and more slowly as they kind of drift into satiety.

In summary, then, we can say your best tactic in feeding your infant is to tune in on and trust his signals of self regulation.

Your child's response to that feeding approach will be growth that is optimum for him. How large a person he will become depends on his genetic potential. Whether or not he grows to the limits of his genetic potential depends primarily on how he eats throughout his growing years. Your goal then, in feeding your child is to enable him to eat in such a way that he can get the body that's right for him.

Growth Curves

I am so convinced of the infant's ability to regulate his own food intake and growth that I would feel comfortable in stopping right here with our growth discussion. As long as you are giving a good milk feeding in a friendly and supportive way, you generally don't have to worry about normal growth: it will happen. But, there are a few exceptions, and there is the curiosity and fun of evaluating that process as it takes place. So, in the rest of the chapter I'll be interpreting for you the method that your health professional uses in monitoring your child's growth: the use of growth curves.

Some health workers feel very strongly that parents who are not trained in interpreting normal growth should not be given growth curve charts. They fear that the parent will weigh and measure and plot their child's growth compulsively, overreacting to every little variation. So, don't do that. Realize that there will be trends and variations over time, and that generally there isn't too much to get excited about.

Also realize that properly interpreting these growth curves is a complex process that requires schooling in growth and development, and experience with many infants. The health professional is definitely the person with whom to consult in evaluating the growth curves, AND THAT'S IMPORTANT. But they will be giving you information from the growth curves, and you will have to know some basics in order to interpret them properly to yourself. It's the basics that I propose to give you in the following discussion.

Standard growth curves are graphs of the variation in normal growth of normal children. They have been constructed by weighing and measuring large numbers of children and noting the variations in height and weight that occur in different age groups. Once the growth patterns of all these children are plotted, you come up with a series of normal curves that look like the ones on the next pages. These charts were published in 1976 by the National Center for Health Statistics.[6] They are the growth standards recommended at this time for general use.

Types of Growth Curves. There are separate graphs for heights and weights of boys and girls of different ages, as well as graphs that plot the two together. There are graphs for head circumference, as well as graphs that correlate weight and height, and special graphs for prepubertal boys and girls. For our purpose we will use about four (see Figures 4-4 through 4-7).

1. Girls: Birth to 36 months—Physical Growth
   a. Length-for-age/weight-for-age. (Figure 4-4)
   b. Head circumference/weight-for-length. (Figure 4-5)
2. Boys: Birth to 36 months—Physical Growth
   a. Length-for-age/weight-for-age. (Figure 4-6)
   b. Head circumference/weight-for-length. (Figure 4-7)

All four figures show two graphs in one, which is somewhat confusing, and I apologize. However, this is probably how you will see them in the doctor's office, so I will present them that way to you here. On Figures 4-4 and 4-6, the upper left-hand graph is the length graph (we measure children lying down until they are about three years old, when we start standing them up to be measured), and the lower right-hand graph is the weight graph.

On Figures 4-5 and 4-7, the upper left hand graph is head circumference (your doctor will take this from time to time, but we are going to overlook it) and the lower right is weight-by-length. This latter graph ignores age and plots only according to weight and length.

The small numbers within the lines at the right-hand side of the graphs refer to percentile: "5" means fifth percentile, "10" means tenth percentile, and so on.

If you want the charts for older kids, they are constructed as weight and stature charts for boys and girls from 2 to 18 years, and are available in pediatricians' offices.

Typically you will encounter these charts when you take your child in for regular checkups. He will be weighed and measured and the figures plotted on growth charts that will be inserted in his medical record. Each time you will be told his position in the percentile ratings for growth. (For example, your child might be 50th percentile for height and 60th percentile for weight.)

Reading the Growth Curve. Let's discuss this in more detail, using the chart in Figure 4-4: *Growth chart for infant girls—Length-for-age and weight-for-age.* As you look at the chart, you will notice that

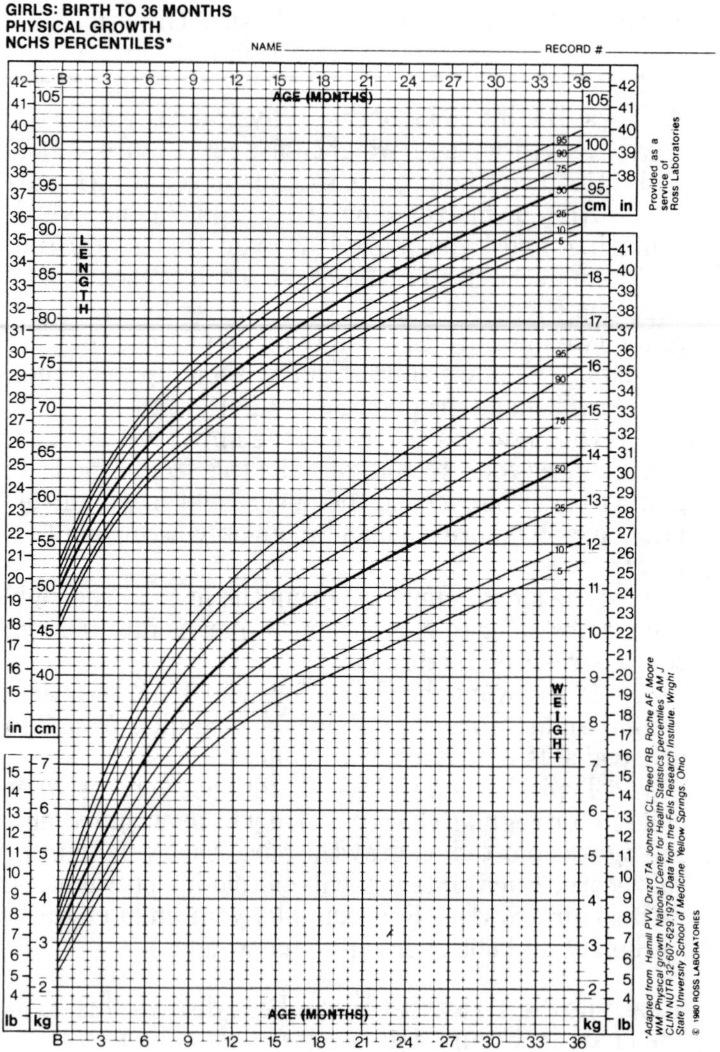

Figure 4-4. Growth Chart for Infant Girls. Length-for-age and Weight-for-age (Courtesy Ross Laboratories).

GIRLS: BIRTH TO 36 MONTHS
PHYSICAL GROWTH
NCHS PERCENTILES*

NAME ________________ RECORD # ________

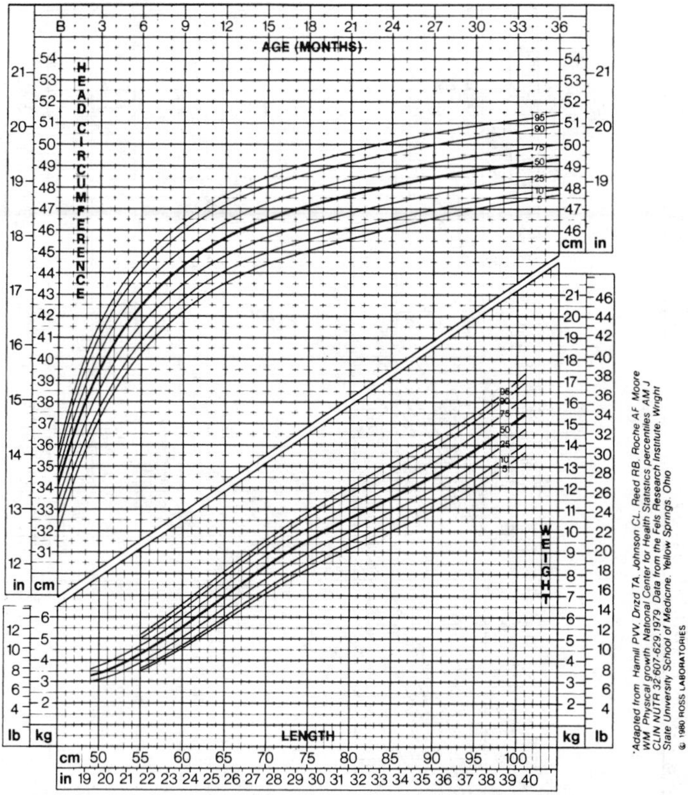

DATE	AGE	LENGTH	WEIGHT	HEAD C	DATE	AGE	LENGTH	WEIGHT	HEAD C.
	BIRTH								

Figure 4-5. Growth Chart for Infant Girls. Head Circumference and Weight-for-length (Courtesy Ross Laboratories).

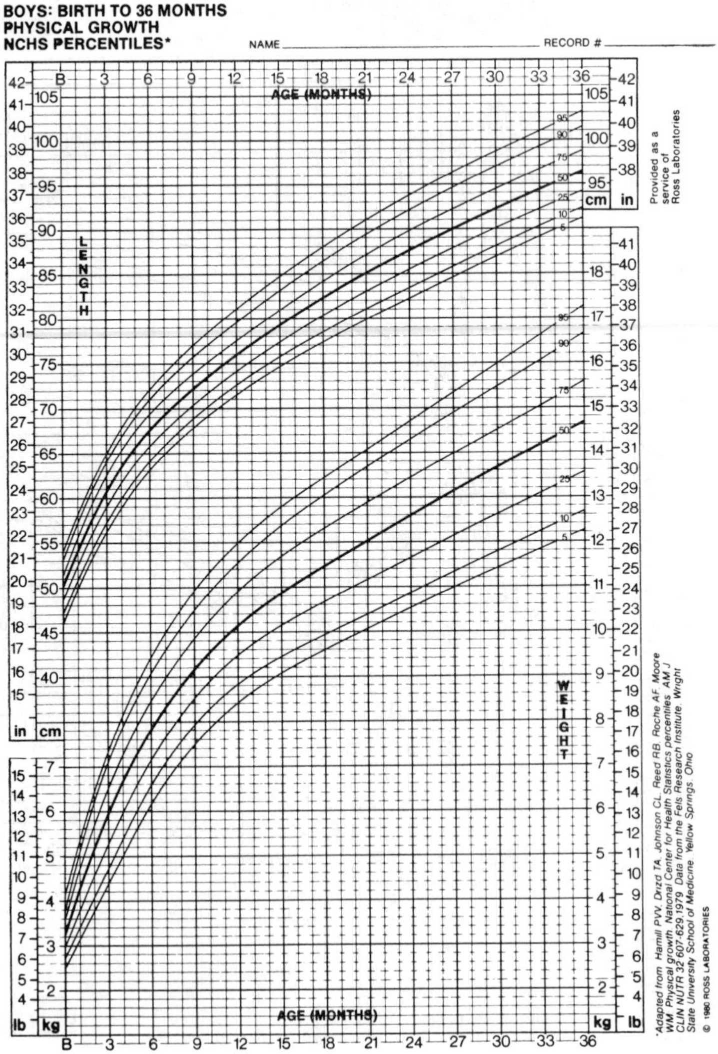

Figure 4-6. Growth Chart for Infant Boys. Length-for-age and Weight-for-age (Courtesy Ross Laboratories).

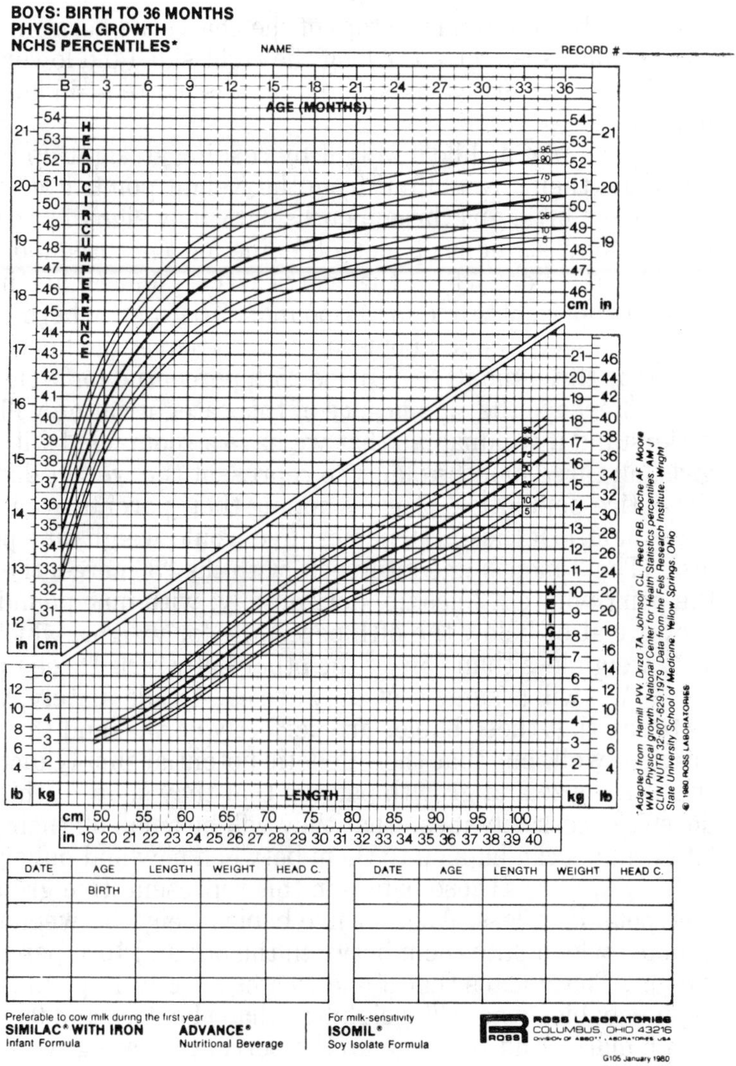

Figure 4-7. Growth Chart for Infant Boys. Head Circumference and Weight-for-length. (Courtesy Ross Laboratories).

along the bottom (and the top) of the chart, the horizontal axis, the *age* in months is plotted. Along the right side (and lower left side) of the chart, the vertical axis, the *weight* is plotted—in kilograms, and in pounds.

You plot a child's weight by reading straight up from the age point and then straight out from the weight point. For instance, if you have a little girl three months old who weighs 11 pounds, you would follow straight up along the line for age three months. You would make a dot where that vertical three-month line intersects with the horizontal line for 11 pounds. That dot, where those two lines intersect, is just about on the 25th percentile line. That means that that three-month-old girl is 25th percentile for weight.

Perhaps the significance of this categorization will be easier to understand if we imagine that we have a room filled with 100 baby girls, all three months old, who represent the weight distribution of the entire population. (Here's hoping their parents are in that room with them!) Of those 100 babies, five would weigh nine pounds or less. (The 3-month line intersects with the "5" percentile curve line at the point where it lines up, horizontally, with nine pounds.) We say they are at or below the fifth percentile for weight, which means that they weigh less than 95% of the other baby girls three months old.

We will assume that they are eating adequately, which allows us to say that these babies are perfectly normal and that they are growing well, but that their genetic potential simply dictates that this is the size and growth pattern that they show at this time. It doesn't necessarily mean that they will be small all their lives, as a lot of things can happen to them between now and puberty.

So, five of those babies in this representative group weigh nine pounds or less. Another five babies weigh between nine and ten pounds, which puts them between the 5th and 10th percentiles for weight. That means that if one weighs exactly 10 pounds, there will be nine babies who will weigh less than she does and 90 who will weigh more. And so we go up the percentile ratings.

When you get up to the one baby on the 50th percentile rating line, she will be smaller than half the babies and bigger than the rest. Fifty percent of the babies will weigh between 11 and 12.5 pounds; they will be between the 25th and 75th percentiles on the weight curve. Those babies "tend toward the average." That doesn't necessarily mean their growth is any more or less desirable than that of infants weighing more or less than those in this mid-range. It simply means that they are closer to the midpoint of weight, so they have more company in their weight range than do the infants at the outside extremes—in the 75th-and-above or in the 25th-and-below percentile ranges.

When you use the growth charts in this way—to compare an individual child's growth with that of other children—you are primarily satisfying your curiosity. Don't get caught up in treating growth curves like grades in school. A child growing at the 95th percentile isn't doing any better than the one growing at the 5th percentile. The most important aspect of the growth curve is to be able to compare each individual child to herself—to evaluate her growth as it progresses from one month to the next.

Evaluating Your Child's Growth. In most cases, once a child is established in a percentile rating of growth, she will remain in that percentile track. For instance, Jane started out in the 25th percentile range. She weighed 9½ pounds at two months of age and around 11 pounds at three months, and we predicted that she would stay in the same 25th percentile track from month to month (see Figure 4-8). However, at four months her growth rate started to slow. She weighed 11½, 12 and 12½ pounds respectively, at her fourth, fifth and sixth month checks, and her percentiles fell from the 25th to the 5th. We started looking around for causes.

Had she suddenly become more active? Was breastmilk production falling off? The change in percentile rating gave us a clue that something was going on that could be affecting her health

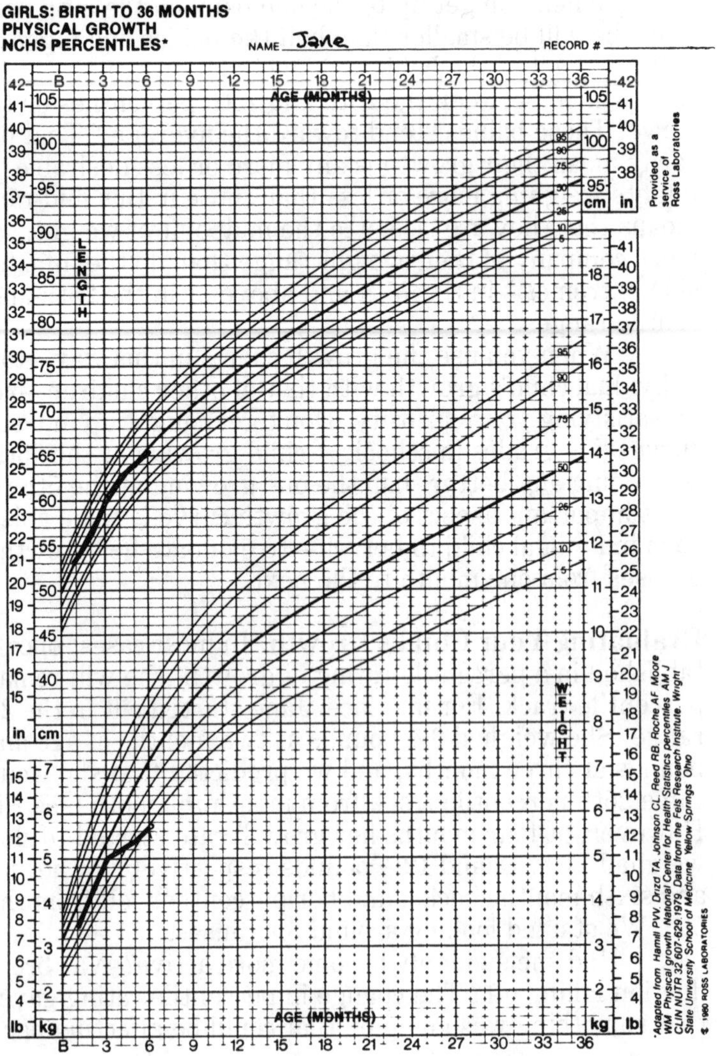

Figure 4-8. Inadequate Weight Gain of Jane.

status. In her case, it turned out to be the beginnings of asthma, which was causing chronic lung infections.

Jane continued to grow smoothly in height, even though her weight was falling off. Generally height increase will continue smoothly; the weight is the most immediate and reliable signal of a change in nutritional status.

Using the growth curves for height as well as for weight gives some further information. Each time your child is weighed and measured, he will be plotted on both curves, and you will be given a report that could say, for instance, 60th percentile for height and 60th percentile for weight. That would mean that your child is somewhat larger than the average child and that she also has an average body build: her height and weight percentiles are balanced.

Jane was a tall slender baby from the start. She was 50th percentile for height and 25th for weight. And, of course, as her weight dropped off, she got even more slender.

Weight-for-length graphs. The weight-for-length graphs use a single figure to give you information on your baby's relative weight and length. Figure 4-9 shows this relationship for Jane using the data plotted on Figure 4-8. If we plot Jane's length at 3 months, which was 23½ inches, against her weight, which was 10¾ pounds (both shown on Figure 4-8), she comes out (on Figure 4-9) a little below the 25th percentile, weight for height.* You can use this figure to compare Jane with other children and find out what we already know, that she is on the slender side. More importantly, you can use it to assess her growth progression and will be able to see that her weight for height dropped from a little below the 25th percentile to below the 5th percentile by the time she was six months old.

In interpreting these percentile ratings, take a look at yourself. Do you have an average body build or do you have more of a

---

*Children below the 50th percentile are relatively taller and thinner, those above are relatively blockier.

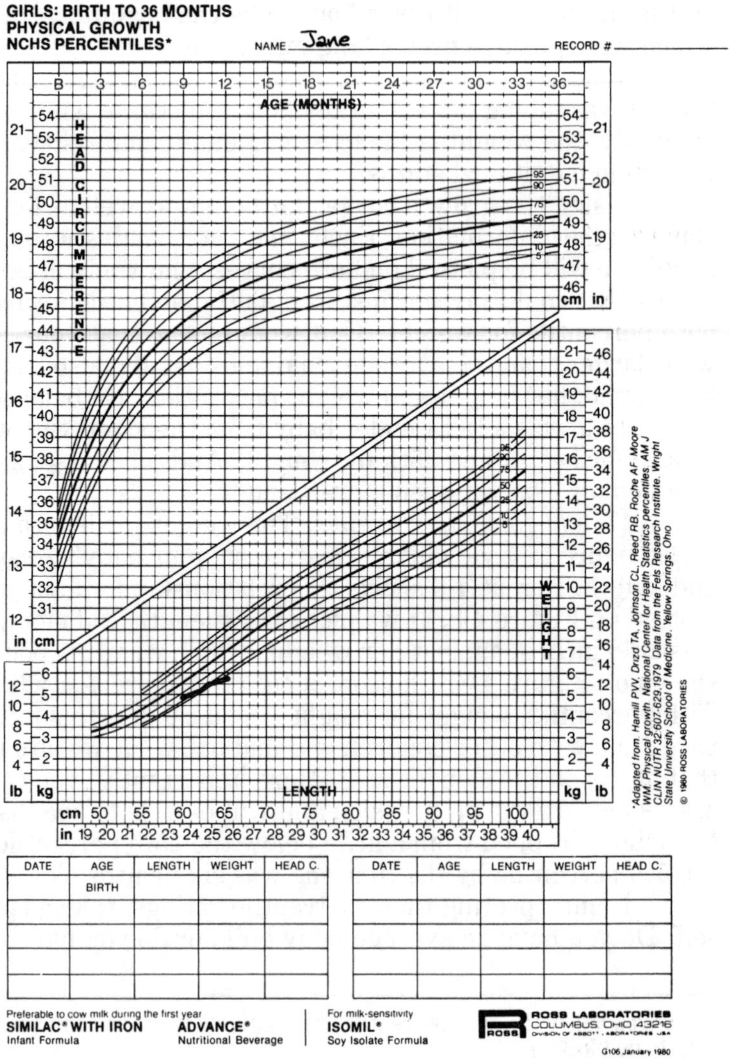

Figure 4-9. Inadequate Weight Gain of Jane, Plotted on Weight-for-length Graph.

blocky, chunky build? Or perhaps you are tall and slender, with longer, thinner bones and longer, more slender muscles. Your child's body build may reflect your body build.

Physical vs Aesthetic Standards. One of the things that you must watch out for as you evaluate your child's growth is that you don't confuse standards of normal growth with standards of fashion. The "ideal" body, according to the dictates of fashion, is a fairly slender body. That is very nice, if you or your child happen to have a naturally slender body. But it is not so nice if you are dealing with a more blocky body build. All too often what is happening then is that someone is trying to get his child to conform to the fashionable slender standard—to get thinner. In reality, what that does is try to force that person to be thinner than is really right or natural for him.

To achieve and maintain this abnormally low weight, it will be necessary for the person to give quite a lot of attention to an otherwise automatic process: that of food regulation. The person tries to be thinner than his body is really set up to be. To accomplish this, he will have to eat less than his body tells him to eat. In other words, he will have to stop trusting his appetite and his internal cues of hunger and satiety, and will have to start regulating his food intake with his head. He (or someone making his decisions for him) will have to use some system of deciding how much food he should be having, and he will have to limit himself to that. And, he will have to adhere to that system of regulation for as long as he wants his weight to remain at what for him is a lower-than-normal level.

If you are the parent, and trying to force this slimming regimen on a child who is constitutionally more heavy, you really have your work cut out for you. You essentially will be trying to get the child to eat less than he really wants, and you will have to keep it up for a very long time.

The same kind of struggle can occur when people are trying to manipulate their weights the other way. Anyone who has tried to gain weight can tell you that it can be as involving and discouraging as trying to lose. And it is just as difficult to try to adjust a natural weight upward as it is to try to adjust it downward.

It seems to me to be the more reasonable and logical approach to allow the child to achieve the growth pattern and body that is right for her. Then, the next step is to allow or encourage her to feel good about her body. You need to let her know that it is a good body, and allow her to develop an aesthetic appreciation of her body that is broader and more flexible than this crazy, rigid norm that we now glorify. You need to help her to realize that her health and physical capability are as important as the way she looks.

I am using "her" intentionally in this section, because I think that it is harder to provide this for girls than for boys. There seems to be a narrower and more rigid standard of appearance for girls. This is changing, but girls are encouraged less to participate in sports, so they get less of a sense of themselves physically and functionally than boys do.

I was reminded the other day of how difficult this is for kids when I went to an office picnic. As I played volleyball with the kids, I watched them. I was intrigued by two of the girls in particular, because their bodies (and, it seemed, their personalities) were in such a contrast to each other. The older girl, who was 13, was a tall, very slender girl. Aesthetically, she was just right. She moved somewhat slowly after the ball if it came near her and had about average coordination for a kid her age.

The other girl, age 11, was about average height and was one of the most muscular little girls I have ever seen. She had wonderful strong little legs, heavy legs, with hardly any fat on them. She had a square compact little body and arms that were well-shaped and solid-looking. She was dodging and diving for the ball and doing very well—her coordination was remarkable. It was so much fun watching her. She simply had a great body and she could handle it very well.

I was surprised after the game ended to find out that the two girls were sisters. Their mother confirmed my suspicions that the older one had primary interests other than sports, and that the little one really went for physical activities of any sort. She apparently was doing very well in gymnastics and goes out for any sport that she can. But, her mother said, the little girl gets lots of teasing from the other kids because they say she is too fat. And the gymnastics teacher keeps telling her that she should cut down on her eating because to be really good at gymnastics she should be more slender. Her mother thinks that all that emphasis on being thinner is stupid, so she's not about to pressure her daughter to slim down. Here's hoping that despite all that social pressure, the little girl can hang on to a sense of her own body as being good.

We have wandered into a considerably older age group in our discussion of growth curves. I hope you agree that the digression was valid. Parents' standards and preconceptions of appropriate growth are going to have an impact on how they feed their infant, right from the start. We will discuss this topic in more detail in chapters 10 and 11.

Improper Use of Growth Curves. But let's go back to infancy. I want to spend some time alerting you to how the growth curves can cause problems if they are used improperly. One big hazard comes from inaccurate measurements. Weights are generally measured accurately. Usually doctors' offices will use the beam-type baby scales for weighing, and that's good, though even those scales should be checked periodically for accuracy. In a very few cases you will see the spring-type scales and that is not good. Readings from those scales frequently vary considerably, depending on the vagaries of the machine.

Heights, however, are generally done poorly. Accurate length measures of babies are difficult to take, and typically are not taken in the doctors' offices. To do it right you need to have the baby resting on a rigid surface, and you need two experienced people to do the measuring. One person uses both hands to hold the baby's head straight and against a vertical headboard. The other person holds the feet, knees and hips completely extended. Applying gentle traction, this latter person brings a movable footboard to rest firmly against the baby's heels. (It sounds awful, doesn't it? But it is really quite humane.) Then you get an accurate measurement that can be charted with some reliability on the percentile curves.

I have never seen it done that way. What I have seen is done by one person, who lays the baby on the paper-covered pad on the examining table. He takes a pencil and makes a mark at the top of the baby's head. Then he pulls down one of the feet and makes another mark on the paper. Finally, he moves the baby and measures between the marks. A well known authority on infant nutrition says, "measurement of length is difficult and should not be attempted unless satisfactory equipment and two trained examiners are available. In many instances, it will not be practical to measure length routinely."[3]

It is unfortunate that this is the source of the height data you will probably have available for your child, because height is the measurement that indicates long-term nutritional status. Further, these inaccuracies in height measurements make it very difficult or even futile to attempt to interpret weight-for-height measurements. For example, if we go back to our three-month-old baby girl, we will figure that at age three months she is right on the 25th percentile line for weight and height: she weighs 10.8 lb and she is almost 23 inches long.

Say when we check her three months later her weight is still on the 25th percentile line: she now weighs a little over 14½ lb. But this time, using the paper and pencil system of measuring height, she now appears to be 24½ inches tall, or right on the 10th percentile line. To be on the 25th percentile line, she would have to be 25¼ inches long, an error of only ¾ inch. That error is quite possible, given a standard squirmy baby with typically elastic legs. So now it looks like our baby, who was so well-balanced before, is doing one of two things: falling off the growth curve for height, or getting fatter. Either can be alarming for parents. Both are entirely unnecessary conclusions, based on the available evidence.

What I have seen happen, on the basis of results like this, is the parent will become alarmed about excessive weight gain and attempt to cut back on the child's food. As is absolutely predictable when the parent tries to intrude on the child's business of food regulation, a struggle ensues. Everyone becomes too preoccupied with eating, and what was an easy, natural process gets invested with all sorts of anxieties.

The maddening thing about all this is that it is so absolutely unnecessary. Measurements of height that casual, simply should not be used as a basis for any kind of recommendations. But they are used in exactly that way, and more. I was horrified to hear of a health professional advising parents that they should shoot to keep their child's weight at about 10 percentile ratings lower than the height, because it was really better to have a child who was a little leaner than a little fatter. In other words, normal growth is invalid, and one should try to modify it to fit these arbitrary standards. It is exactly that kind of advice that makes parents rigid and preoccupied with feeding, and involved in a struggle in which they are essentially encouraged to deprive their child of food.

I see harried parents who come in complaining that they are concerned about their child's weight, and reporting that they are trying to get her to eat a little less. But, they explain, their child will *not* be satisfied on smaller amounts of food. She fusses and complains until she gets as much as usual and continues to gain at her regular rate. The parents typically feel ambivalent but always guilty: guilty at not being able to restrict their child's food intake more effectively, guilty at trying to be stingy with food for a little baby.

At that point I would say that it is better to burn the charts than to cause that kind of crazy and unnecessary anxiety and conflict.

What I have given you is a very mixed review of growth charts. I have introduced them to you and explained how they can be used productively, and I have spent a fair amount of time pointing out the harm that can be done if they are used poorly. So what, you may ask, is the point?

The point is that they will be used. In most cases your child's growth will be plotted on these charts, and you generally will be given the percentile information. It's what you do with the information that will make all the difference.

Information on the growth curves is only one of the pieces of information you will have on your baby, and not the most important one, at that. You can do one of two things with it. You can put yourself in the position of monitoring and manipulating your child's growth, responding to apparent changes with changes in feeding. Or you can keep your fingers crossed and trust that growth will proceed appropriately, meanwhile feeding in response to your baby's demand. I would encourage the latter.

If your child seems to be demanding and getting enough to eat, and seems to grow and be reasonably happy and content, that is an important piece of information. If the weight is being accurately checked and is increasing at a fairly smooth rate, that is an important piece of information. But as long as heights are being taken improperly, you have no choice but to be very cautious in drawing any conclusions using height data.

Your Child's Appearance

In addition, of course, you will be evaluating your baby's growth the same way parents have always evaluated their infant's growth: by looking at him. He'll usually be getting longer and heavier; his body and arms and legs will be filling out. He'll develop a round stomach that sticks out, and the shape of his face will change and probably get rounder and fatter looking. In fact, compared with what he looked like as a newborn, your infant may just look fat to you. That's fine. Babies normally put on a lot of fat in the first year of life.

At birth the infant has only about 11% body fat. By age one year, the percentage of body fat has increased to 24%. (Subsequently this decreases to about 21% by age two and 18% by age three.)[2] This accumulation of body fat is normal and desirable. Fat functions importantly in the little body as a source of calories in case of illness. With the high metabolic demands and calorie requirement of a person that small, even a short-term illness could be dangerous if it weren't for that calorie store. Fat also functions to protect the baby's organs and as an insulator to help maintain normal body temperature. Fat stores in the human body are functional. It is only when the fat stores become excessive that they should be a cause for concern.

This chapter is intended to help you understand, not manage, the process of growth. Your baby is the one with the information about *his* normal growth and *his* process of food regulation. In the very great percentage of cases, your best and safest approach is to support that regulatory process with appropriate food, offered in response to the infant's signals of hunger and satiety.

Enabling your child to get the body that is right for him is your important task. The way you accomplish that task is through paying attention to information coming from him.

Selected References

1. Bruch, Hilde. Eating Disorders. Obesity, Anorexia Nervosa and the Person Within. Basic Books. New York. 1973.
2. Fomon, Samuel J. Infant Nutrition. W. B. Saunders, Philadelphia. 1974.

3. Fomon, Samuel J. Nutritional Disorders of Children. Prevention, Screening, and Followup. DHEW Publication No. (HSA) 76-5612. DHEW Rockville, Maryland. 1976.
4. Gerber. Current Practices in Infant Feeding. 1980.
5. Gesell, Arnold and Frances L. Ilg. Feeding Behavior of Infants J. B. Lippincot, Philadelphia. 1937.
6. Hamill, P. V. V. *et al.* NCHS Growth Charts. 1976. Vital and Health Statistics-Series II. Health Resources Administration, DHEW, Rockville, Maryland. 1976(a).
7. Lozoff, Betsy, *et al.* The mother-newborn relationship: limits of adaptability. The Journal of Pediatrics 91:(L) 1-12. July. 1977.
8. Rose, H. E. and J. Mayer, Activity, calorie intake, fat storage and the energy balance of infants. Pediatrics 41:18. 1968.
9. Stein, Z. A. *et al.* Famine and Human Development: The Dutch Hunger Winter of 1944–45. New York: Oxford University Press. 1975.
10. Weil, William B. Current controversies in childhood obesity. The Journal of Pediatrics. 91(2):175–187. 1977.

5
The Milk Feeding

The newborn infant imposes some stringent demands on his milk feeding. It must be very easily digestible, it must not disrupt the relatively fragile balance of his body chemistry, and, because it is the major, or only food for the first six months, it must be absolutely appropriate for his nutritional needs. Breastmilk, commercial formulas (both cow's milk and soy based), and evaporated milk formula all adequately fill these specifications. Other formulas, such as the hypoallergenic formulas and the premature infant formulas, are more highly specialized, to provide for infants with the special needs they are designed for.

Although modern formula feeding is convenient and safe, it is important not to become casual about the mechanics of preparation. The water supply must be clean and safe, the nursing equipment sanitary and comfortable (for both feeder and fed), and the formula prepared precisely according to directions.

A newborn baby has special nutritional and feeding needs. To grow and thrive, he requires more gentle and specialized handling than an older child. But at the same time, feeding behaviors are like other behaviors: as your baby grows and develops, his abilities change and his patterns of feeding change. To feed your baby appropriately at different ages you need to observe his ability to eat and you need to choose food and feeding methods that he can handle. You also need to understand nutritional requirements and to know and respect his limitations, so you can select foods that are both developmentally and nutritionally appropriate.

During his first year, your baby will pass through three fairly distinctive feeding patterns:

Feeding Periods

0–6 Months—Milk feeding	4–12 Months—Transition (beginning solids)	8 Months on—Adult-like

The ages in the chart overlap, as babies spend varying amounts of time in each of the feeding periods.

In this chapter and in the chapter on breastfeeding we will be discussing only the milk feeding. In chapter 7 we will get into the transition period, where your baby works his way into and through the beginning solid-foods stage and up to the beginning adult stage.

Feeding recommendations for the milk feeding stage are short and to the point.

The vitamins mentioned in the feeding recommendations come in liquid form. You give them to the baby with the calibrated eyedropper that comes with the bottle. We will talk further about this in "nutritional supplementation" later in the chapter.

Figure 5-1. Feeding Recommendations for the First Six Months.

The Milk Feeding	Nutritional Supplements
Breastmilk	Vitamin D—400 IU Fluoride—0.25 mg
Commercial formula	Fluoride if none in water—0.25 mg Iron—5–10 mg—at four months*
Evaporated milk formula	Fluoride if none in water Vitamin C—35 mg or 3 ounces orange juice Iron—5–10 mg—at four months

Avoid pasteurized milk. This is inappropriate for infant feeding.

*The preterm baby on all feedings needs iron at two months.

Milk feeding recommendations and feeding practices for babies have changed considerably in the last few years, as you can see by the table on the next page.[10]

Breastfeeding is definitely on the increase, both in incidence and duration. Most physicians have discontinued the undesirable practice of switching young babies from formula to 2% milk, and babies are being kept on formula longer. Pasteurized milk use for the young infant is considerably below earlier figures.

Figure 5-3 summarizes infant behaviors and abilities that have an impact on feeding.

As you can see from the table, in those early months, the young infant's only feeding skill is his instinctive suckling ability. He can't sit up, or, early on, even hold his head up, and he can't control

Figure 5-2. Infant Formula and Milk Use.

	Percentage of infants receiving*			
	In Hospital		At Age 5–6 Mo.	
	1971	1979	1971	1979
Breast	24.7	51.0	5.5	23.0
Whole cows milk and evaporated milk	0.9	0.1	68.1	25.2
Total prepared formulas	77.4	54.1	28.0	57.6
Without iron	56.5	26.8	14.6	17.3
With iron	20.9	27.3	13.4	40.3

*The figures do not add up to 100% because some babies were taking more than one type of milk feeding.

the motion of his hands. He has the digestive ability only to handle a milk feeding that is properly catered to his needs. His homeostatic ability (his ability to protect his body from dehydration and disruptions in chemical imbalance) is low, and his milk feeding has to be modified to help him.

It is clear that only a milk feeding fed by nipple is developmentally and nutritionally appropriate during this early stage. It is further clear that the newborn baby, with his special needs, imposes some very rigorous demands on the milk feeding.

Digestion

The milk feeding must set up a soft and easily-digestible curd when it is mixed with the acid in the baby's stomach. Breastmilk, formula, or milk that has been heat treated in some way (heated to boiling) sets

Figure 5-3. Developmental Patterns and Feeding Style in the First Six Months

	Birth	1 mo.	2 mo.	3 mo.	4 mo.	5 mo.	6 mo.
Mouth Pattern:	Sucking, "extrusion" pattern.				Beginning swallow pattern. Can transfer food from front of tongue to back	Beginning of drooling	
Hand Coordination:	Random motion of hands.				Hands beginning to go to mouth.		Palmar grasp.
Body Control:	Prone on back. Can raise head when on stomach.				Sits supported. Loses balance when reaches.		Sits unsupported. Can balance while manipulating with hands.
Digestive Ability:	Can digest appropriate milk.				Intestinal amylase begins to increase to allow starch digestion.		
Homeostatic Ability:	Low. Needs carefully-adapted formula.						
Nutritional Requirements:	Relatively high nutrient requirement for rapid growth.		Iron stores depleted in premature infants.			Iron stores begin to be depleted in term babies.	
Feeding Style:	Nipple-feeding by breast or bottle					Beginning spoon feeding.	
Food Selection:	Breastmilk or formula.					Beginning solids: Iron source.	

up a soft, custard-like curd that is easy to digest. In contrast, pasteurized milk, or, worse yet, raw cow's milk, sets up a tough cheesy curd that is very difficult to digest. Protein and fat absorption from non-heat-treated milk is lower. It is so low, in fact, that some babies have to consume 25 to 50% more milk than usual to satisfy their nutritional requirements. This problem persists as long as milk is the sole or primary food.

Homeostasis

The milk feeding must compensate for the young infant's limited ability to maintain homeostasis (balanced body chemistry).

A diet that gives a baby way too much protein or salt or potassium for the amount of water it contains can draw too much water out of her body and make her dehydrated.* Breastmilk and formulas (if they are properly measured and mixed) have a good balance of water to other nutrients and you won't have to worry about maintaining homeostasis.

Straying from the standard milk feeding could cause trouble, particularly if your baby is losing more water than usual in other ways (if she is sweating a lot or is vomiting or has diarrhea). Pasteurized 2% or skim cow's milk, for example, could disrupt homeostasis because it is too concentrated in both protein and sodium for the amount of calories it contains. Commercial formulas that are inadequately diluted can offer the child too much of all nutrients in relation to her fluid intake. Meats offered too early can overload her ability to get rid of nitrogen. All of these feeding practices are common, poor, and unnecessary.

---

*Excessive sodium, potassium and nitrogen are waste products that have to be carried from the cells and excreted in the urine. The young infant has a limited ability to concentrate his urine, meaning he has to put out a high fluid volume for a given amount of waste products. The older child or adult can be much stingier with the water, so doesn't run the same risk of dehydration.

Nutritional Requirements

The milk feeding must carry virtually the whole nutritional load for the infant up until age six months. Because of that, it must be absolutely appropriate for his needs and provide optimal nourishment. Breast milk and standard formulas are both balanced, so that a given volume of milk will provide the proper proportion of calories, water, protein, fat, carbohydrate, vitamins and minerals. (Tables of nutrients in breastmilk and formula are in the Appendix.) When calorie needs are high, other nutrient needs are also high, so the infant can regulate them all appropriately with his signals of hunger and satiety.

If any nutrient is too high or too low relative to all the rest, the whole balance can be disrupted.

Calories. Breastmilk and formulas each give 20 calories per ounce; the comparison with other milks is shown in the table below.

Figure 5-4. Calories per Ounce in Common Infant Feedings

Milk feeding	Caloric density (Calories per ounce)
Breast milk	20
Standard milk-based formulas	20
Soy formulas	20
Whole milk	19
2% milk	15
Advance (formula from Ross "for older children")	16
Skim milk	10

Source: Formula manufacturers; U.S.D.A. Home and Garden Bulletin #72.

The milk feedings that are lower in calories, such as overdiluted formula or 2% or skim milk, give the baby too much volume for the calories he needs, and make it harder for him to grow and gain properly.

Protein, fat and carbohydrate. Each of these three calorie sources in your baby's diet has a nutritional role to play. Since each contributes a percentage of total calories, varying one will vary another. For example, a diet that is too high in protein is likely to be too low in fat or carbohydrate, or both.

Figure 5-5. Protein, Fat and Carbohydrate in the diet.

Nutrient	Function	Too Much	Too Little
Protein	Builds body tissue	Dehydration	Nutritional inadequacy
Fat	Provides long-lasting energy Carries essential nutrients	Ketosis* Poor appetite	Unsatisfying: baby hungry soon
Carbohydrate	Provides quick energy Spares protein for building and repair Helps burn dietary fat	Diet not satisfying	Allows ketosis Energy low Protection for protein low

*We talked about ketosis in the chapter on pregnancy. It is the accumulation of waste products from the incomplete burning of fat. It is like soot from a poorly-burning fire. Carbohydrate helps the fire burn well.

All standard infant formulas have a good proportion of protein, carbohydrate and fat. However, pasteurized milk, whether it is whole, 2%, or skim, is too high in protein for this age, with the protein excess going up as the fat goes down. Whole milk contains enough fat but, as we said earlier, the baby has a hard time digesting and absorbing the fat.

To this point we have demonstrated that breastmilk or formula, and those foods alone, are appropriate in the early months for your baby's developmental and nutritional needs.

The issues remaining to discuss in the rest of the chapter are:

- Types of milk feedings
- Cost of feeding an infant
- Nutritional supplementation
- The nursing equipment
- Position, timing, temperature of feeding
- Safety, sanitation and dilution
- Promoting good feedings
- Quantity of formula
- Feeding frequency

Types of Milk Feedings

Several types of infant milk feedings and the types of protein, fat and carbohydrate they contain are listed in the table on the next page. When we discuss special nutritional needs you'll be able to see how this protein, fat and carbohydrate information is helpful.

Cow Milk Based Formulas

Commercial. Enfamil®, Similac® and SMA® are the most commonly used formulas. They are highly satisfactory for most babies. Enfamil and Similac come with or without iron.

SMA® and Similac with whey® are based on protein that has been modified, ostensibly to make it more like the protein in human

Figure 5-6. Protein, Fat and Carbohydrate in Common Infant Milk Feedings.

Milk Feeding	Protein	Fat	Carbohydrate
Breastmilk	40% casein* 60% whey	Reflects mother's diet	Lactose
Cow Milk Formulas			
Standard commercial Enfamil® and Similac®	82% casein 18% whey	Vegetable oil	Lactose
Whey-based commercial SMA® and Similac® with whey	40% casein 60% whey	Vegetable oil	Lactose
"Homemade" evaporated milk formula	82% casein 18% whey	Butterfat	Lactose/sucrose
Soy-based formulas	Soy isolate	Vegetable oil	Sucrose or corn syrup solids, or both
Predigested Formulas			
Nutramigen®	Predigested casein	Vegetable oil	Modified tapioca starch and sucrose
Pregestimil®	Predigested casein and amino acids	Corn oil and medium chain triglycerides	Corn syrup solids and modified tapioca starch

*Casein and whey are Miss Muffett's "curds and whey." Cow milk's high casein content is responsible for the tough curd it forms unless it is heat treated.

milk, by decreasing the casein and increasing the whey. It appears the premature infants do better on high-whey formulas.[5] While manufacturers imply that these formulas, which some call "humanized," are better than the "standard" formulas for all infants, in reality term babies grow and thrive well on both types. For these babies, "humanized" seems to be really little more than a buzz word to give the impression that the unique characteristics of breastmilk can somehow be duplicated. They cannot.

Manufacturers frequently change their formulas. The information here may be out of date by the time you read it. The trend appears to be to whey-based formulas and you will likely see the standard (casein-based) formulas being changed to whey-based. You may see adjustments in the amount of iron or other nutrients.

Recipe: Evaporated Milk Formula

One 13-ounce can whole evaporated milk, fortified with vitamins A and D
Nineteen ounces tap water
One ounce (two tablespoons) sugar (either table sugar or corn syrup). Do NOT use honey.

Mix well, portion into sterilized individual bottles, cover and refrigerate. May also be refrigerated in a covered, clean bulk container,

Evaporated milk formula. Infant formula made from evaporated milk is an "old-fashioned" homemade formula that is still a good, low-cost choice for the term infant. Evaporated milk* is a canned cow's milk product that has been concentrated by removing

*An improved can design for evaporated milk has brought the lead content down to the acceptable level of about 0.08 parts per million. This compares with the lead content of concentrated commercial formulas of about 0.02 parts per million.

half of the water. (It is *not* the same as condensed milk, which has sugar added and is used for baking.) It is better for babies than pasteurized milk because the canning process boils it long enough to make it digestible.
Be sure that you use WHOLE evaporated milk and that it is fortified with vitamins A and D.

Since most nutrients are provided by the milk, this formula needs only to be supplemented with 35 mg. vitamin C per day. You can give this in three ounces of orange juice per day or in the form of drops.

Simple as it is, the evaporated milk formula has been calculated very carefully to give an appropriate calorie and nutrient density and to provide the proper proportions of protein, fat and carbohydrate. So if you choose to use it, you must follow the formula absolutely slavishly. Do not substitute other milks or change the proportions of milk, sugar and water. Again, do not use honey as a sugar source (much honey is contaminated with botulinum spores).

The standard proportions of milk, sugar and water are appropriate throughout the time the infant is kept on formula. In the fifties pediatricians would shift the proportions of milk, sugar and water depending on the age of the child, with the water and sugar decreasing as the child got older. That practice was probably based on the inability of health workers, and possibly parents, to tolerate simplicity in infant feeding.

Soy based formulas. Isomil®, Prosobee®, and other soy-based formulas are used for the infant who is sensitive or allergic (or potentially so) to cow milk protein, or who is having trouble digesting lactose (milk sugar). Babies may be chronically sensitive to cow's milk protein and have to stay away from it for the first several months. Or they may be sensitive only for a few days, after they have had diarrhea, and need to use soy formula just for a few days.

Babies are often put on soy formula on the assumption that they cannot digest lactose, but other sugars, such as sucrose, can be a problem as well. Usually, intolerance for these sugars is temporary and appears after an infant has diarrhea from a viral or bacterial infection.

To avoid sucrose as well as lactose you need to read the ingredients list on the label, and select a soy formula that contains corn syrup solids, and/or another carbohydrate source like modified tapioca starch, rather than sucrose.

While soy formulas are used for the infant who is allergic, or potentially allergic to cow's milk protein, it is important to know that soy protein can cause as many allergies as cow's milk. In fact, quite a few babies are allergic to both. For the infant who has allergic reactions to both cow's milk and soy milk or extreme reactions to either one, or who has a strong family history of allergies, it is probably wise to use one of the hypoallergenic, "predigested" formulas described below.

Soy formulas are safe. Many people are afraid of them because they have read about the infants taking Neo-Mull-Soy® who got sick from chloride deficiency. The manufacturer, Syntex Laboratories, had not maintained proper quality control in preparing their infant formulas, and some containing inadequate chloride were put on the market.* The Food and Drug Administration is now required by law to test formulas for proper nutrient levels.

Soy milk is not a substitute for soy formula. Nutrient density, as well as proportions of protein, fat and carbohydrate are inappropriate where used as the sole food of a young infant.

Predigested formulas. The protein, fat or carbohydrate, or all three, in predigested formulas are modified to make them more manageable to the infant with allergies or with digestive problems. The two major specialized formulas, Pregestimil® and Nutramigen®, are based on a protein that is non-allergenic and highly digestible. Pregestimil, however, goes two steps further than Nutramigen in cater-

---

*Syntex Laboratories no longer makes infant formulas.

ing to special needs, in that it modifies the fat and carbohydrate as well as the protein.

The carbohydrate in Pregestimil comes from corn syrup solids and modified tapioca starch, both of which can be handled by most babies who have trouble with other sugars. Much of the fat in Pregestimil (medium-chain triglycerides) needs no digestion and is well-absorbed by the infant who can't manage other kinds of fat, such as infants who have had part of their intestine removed, or who have cystic fibrosis, or for some unknown reason get diarrhea from other dietary fat.

To summarize, Nutramigen and Pregestimil have important, if limited, uses:

- For babies who are allergic to cow's milk and soy protein. (See p. 306 in the *Toddler* chapter for a more-detailed discussion on allergies.)
- As a supplemental feeding for breastfed babies who have a good chance of being allergic.
- For babies who have had a severe reaction to cow's milk formula—severe diarrhea, lots of mucous in the stools. These babies are also likely to react to soy protein.

Premature infant formulas. The pre-term infant must grow and gain at the same rate as if he were still in the uterus. Such babies have missed acquiring the great deal of lean and bony tissue and mineral stores which are put on during the last portion of a term pregnancy. To provide for these special needs, premature infant formulas contain more protein and minerals per calorie than standard formulas.

These formulas are only available to hospitals and are given only under careful medical supervision. They are not suitable for a term infant, and, at a certain point, the premature infant must be switched from his "special" formula to a standard formula. To give him a somewhat greater nutritional margin of error, the pre-term infant should be kept on a commercial formula for the whole first year and should not be switched to evaporated milk or pasteurized milk. In fact, if a baby has been struggling nutritionally all along, I don't think it would hurt to keep on with commerical formula, even up to 18 months.

I hope you never need most of this technical information about formulas. Ideally, you will be able to select a good formula and stick to it throughout your baby's early months. You only need to worry about the more detailed information if he develops special needs, if he has a good chance of becoming allergic, if he has a viral or bacterial infection, or if he can't tolerate the standard protein, fat or carbohydrate.

But don't be too ready to switch formulas. Not all upsets are of the sort that require special feeding. It appears that, regardless of feeding, about 40% of babies have colic, or inconsolable crying after feeding, and about 40% vomit from time to time, or even frequently, after they are fed. By age one year, studies show that 14% of babies have had at least one episode of marked vomiting and diarrhea and 16% are still waking up at night.[1] Probably in most cases these problems would have persisted despite a change in feeding.

Cost of Feeding an Infant

The cost of the milk feeding varies by as much as four-fold, depending on the type and form of feeding you choose. Formulas come in ready-to-feed liquid form, liquid concentrated form (which has to be diluted one-to-one with water), and in powdered form. They come packed in single-serving containers, including single-serving containers that are all ready for you to simply screw on the nipple and feed.

I made a survey in September of 1982 of the local grocery stores and drug stores and came up with estimates (Figure 5-7) for one quart of infant formula or milk.

These prices are going to be out-of-date by the time you read this. However, we can make some generalizations that will probably remain valid for some time.

Figure 5-7. Costs of Infant Milk Feedings—1 quart

Specialized Formulas		
Powdered Pregestimil, Nutramigen		$2.76–$3.47
Standard Commercial Milk- or Soy-Based Formula		
Ready-to-feed		$1.63
Concentrated		1.22
Powdered		1.32
Breastfeeding (Mother's extra food)		
2 cups milk	.22	
1 fruit or vegetable	.20	
250 extra calories	.20	
	.62	
Nutritional supplement for infant	.10	
Total		.72
Evaporated Milk Formula		
1 can evaporated milk	.59	
2 Tablespoons sugar	.03	
3 ounces orange juice or nutritional supplement	.10	
Total		.72

The specialized formulas are extremely expensive and something that you would probably use only if your infant was highly likely to benefit from them. Secondly, the prices vary, so it is worth shopping around. Some pharamacies are willing to sell these at a little above wholesale price, realizing what a special need they fill.

Comparing ready-to-feed formulas with concentrated formulas, you pay about 20% more for the convenience of not having to mix with water. It may be worth it to you, particularly if your water supply is unreliable. Suprisingly, the powdered formulas cost about the same as the concentrate. The price is kept high by the low demand. Our local grocery stores carried only the liquid formulas; I had to search through several drug stores before I found one that carried the powder. You might get a good price on the powdered formula if you are willing to have the druggist order and buy it by the case. But unless there is a definite price advantage, I would encourage using the liquid formula. Powdered formulas are hard to mix accurately.

Breastfeeding is not free. To produce a quart, or 600 calories of breastmilk, the mother will have to consume about 750 more calories. She will need to provide herself with more protein, calcium and all other nutrients. She will need to supplement her infant with flouride and vitamin D. The cost of these foods and supplements will vary, depending on her food choices. If the mother is taking some sort of vitamin and mineral supplement to support the breastfeeding, that will further increase the cost.

Evaporated milk formula is remarkably inexpensive—this formula, plus the nutritional supplement (which is included to provide the vitamin C lacking in evaporated milk), costs about half as much as the least expensive commercial formula. Evaporated milk formula is almost as cheap as pasteurized milk, and offers a real option to parents who have felt forced by cost to switch from commercial formula to pasteurized milk.

Nutritional Supplementation

Figure 5-1 gave recommendations about supplementing vitamins C and D, flouride and iron. You will need additional information about the needs for some of the vitamins and minerals, and may have been confused by what you have heard in the past. Among other possible sources of confusion, you may have received inconsistent advice from "experts." Health workers don't agree on the timing and level of iron and fluoride supplements; they argue about vitamin D supplementation of the breastfed infant, and are confused about the need for vitamin C supplements.

I am recommending what I consider to be ideal supplementation. Others will disagree. Your doctor might disagree, and you may end up not knowing what to do. I don't want you to worry unnecessarily, if you have your baby on a pattern of supplementation other than the one I am outlining here. The disagreements show that the answers are not clear-cut. The practices you should avoid, however, are: 1) Giving too much vitamin A, vitamin D and fluoride, and 2) Failing to provide iron—much beyond age six months.

Iron. As with other nutrients, you want your baby to have the right amount of iron, neither more nor less than he needs. Giving too much iron can decrease zinc absorption. Giving iron too soon to a breastfed baby can interfere with his unique intestinal immunity. Giving too little can limit red blood cell production.

Again, the schedule for beginning iron supplementation is:[3]

Premature baby, breast or formula	2 months
Formula-fed term baby	4 months
Breast-fed term baby	6 months

Regardless of maternal iron status, term infants are born with a good supply of iron. The newborn has need for, and utilizes very little dietary iron before age four months.[4] Up until that time he gets his iron from breaking down the extra red blood cells he was born with. Breastmilk iron, although in low concentrations, is about 50% absorbed (a relatively high absorption rate), and provides some protection against iron deficiency anemia. Furthermore, breastmilk iron is carried in a form, lactoferrin, which prevents its use as a nutrient by undesirable intestinal bacteria and protects against infestation by those bacteria. Supplemental iron, on the other hand, nourishes intestinal bacteria as well as the child, and also changes the type of bacteria.

Addition of any type of solid food also changes the intestinal bacteria. Since you have to change the intestinal bacteria anyway at age six months, when you start giving solid foods, you might as well accomplish two goals at one time and make the first solid food one that is high in iron. The best choice is iron-fortified infant cereal.

In contrast to breastmilk iron, the iron in cow's milk is only about 10% absorbed.* Furthermore, the bottle-fed infant already harbors a variety of bacteria in his colon. Since he has been able to absorb little dietary iron, and since there is little to be lost (in terms of increased bacterial activity) from the addition of iron, the bottle-fed infant should be started on iron at about age four months. This can be in the form of iron-fortified formula, or as iron drops.

The amount of supplementary iron depends on the size and maturity of the child.

10-15 pounds	5 mg.
15-20 pounds	10 mg.
Premature infant	10 mg.

Iron-fortified formula has 12.8 mg. iron per liter. Generally the child will consume about the right amount of formula to give him the recommended levels of iron.** Many health workers and parents hesitate to use iron-fortified formulas because they think the iron

---

*Cow's milk feeding may actually undermine iron nutrition. Some young infants (up to 140-days-old) who consume large amounts of pasteurized milk bleed a little from the intestine. Although the amount is small (about 3 ml per day in some cases—less than a teaspoon—which means the loss of 0.9 milligram iron per day), it could cause anemia.

**There is some talk of reducing the level of supplemental iron in fortified formula to 6 or 7 mg per liter. This is probably desirable, as the lower level of iron reduces the potential interference with trace element nutrition. The amount of iron absorbed at this lower level of fortification is almost as high as that from the more-heavily fortified formula.

causes stomach aches and intestinal problems. Apparently this is not the case: all infants experience these problems, those on iron-fortified formula to no greater extent than those on regular formula.[11]

Give the amount of iron your baby needs, but no more than that. Again, if you give too much supplemental iron, it may interfere with absorption of zinc[15] and possibly of other trace elements. Although you should always read the label on your particular package, generally iron drops have 10 mg. iron per milliliter, the amount that you administer from the little dropper that comes in the package. If your child needs only 5 mg. iron, you will have to eyeball the dose by filling the dropper only halfway.

Iron-fortified baby cereal provides 7 mg. iron per four-tablespoon serving (three level tablespoons of dry cereal mixed with milk or formula).

Once a child is well established on iron-fortified cereal he will be getting adequate iron for his needs and should be taken off the iron-fortified formula or the iron drops.

A good source of iron should be continued until the child is about 18 months old or gets through the high-risk period for iron-deficiency anemia.

Vitamin D. Vitamin D is necessary for the proper absorption of calcium and phosphorus, in the formation of teeth and bones. We get vitamin D in commercial formulas, evaporated milk and vitamin-D-fortified pasteurized milk, and in egg yolks. Our grandmothers dosed their children with cod-liver oil as a source of vitamin D, and our skin can make vitamin D if exposed to sunlight. A deficiency of vitamin D causes rickets, a softening and malformation of the bones. Bones that aren't properly mineralized with calcium and phosphorus can become deformed, causing the bow legs and beaded ribs of the child with rickets.

Health workers are too casual about vitamin D supplementation, particularly for the breastfed infant. Breastfed babies can, and do, get rickets, particularly if their skin is dark and if they are exposed to very little sunlight. For a while we thought there was significant vitamin D activity in breastmilk, but it turns out there is really very little—too little for a baby's needs. For the first month or two it does appear that babies can get along without vitamin D, but certainly by age three months they should be supplemented.[13] The breastfed infant needs 400 units of vitamin D per day.[6]

Rickets has also been reported in children with milk allergy, who (in lieu of the nutrients they would ordinarily have received in milk) received a calcium supplement but not additional vitamin D, and in children who receive anti-convulsant medication. Children who drink very little milk or who consume milk not fortified with vitamin D should have a supplement of 400 IU of vitamin D daily. (Farm children often get their milk out of the dairy milk cooler, and that is not fortified with vitamin D.)

You also must be careful not to give too much vitamin D. Because it is a fat-soluble vitamin, excessive amounts can be stored in the body and cause toxicity. However, do not panic. Your child will not get vitamin D toxicity the minute he exceeds 400 IU per day. (In fact, if he is taking more than a quart of formula per day he will be getting more than 400 IU.) Generally, you are safe with fat-soluble vitamins if you do not exceed twice the recommended level. I would, however, be very careful to avoid giving vitamin in concentrated drop form to an infant who is also getting it in his formula.

Vitamin C. Vitamin C is probably our most overused vitamin. Not only do we adults dose ourselves to ridiculous extremes with vitamin C, we do the same thing with our infant children. The young infant needs, roughly, 35 milligrams of vitamin C per day. The breastfeeding mother who is drinking four to six ounces of orange juice per day can easily provide that amount in her breast milk. Commercial formulas provide about 35 mg of vitamin C per quart. The only infant who really needs to be supplemented with vitamin C is the one taking an evaporated milk formula, or, heaven forbid, trying to get by on pasteurized milk. Those infants need a supplemental source of vitamin C.

There is a drop that provides vitamin C, alone, but you have to look for it and insist on it. Generally vitamin C comes in combination with vitamins A and D. Those drops are not appropriate for the infant who is already getting ample amounts of vitamins A and D in his formula or milk.

A good way of providing vitamin C for the evaporated-milk-fed baby is in three ounces of orange juice a day. Some babies, however, can get a rash or a stomach ache from orange juice. If you notice signs of sensitivity, switch your child to three ounces of the infant-pack apple juice, which is fortified with adequate vitamin C. Apple juice isn't as nutritious as orange juice, but the infant pack is well fortified with vitamin C, and most babies don't have any problems with it. Notice I specified *infant pack* apple juice. Apple juice does not naturally contain vitamin C, and most "adult" apple juices and cider are not supplemented.

Fluoride. Children who get the recommended amounts of fluoride from birth have an average of 60% to 65% fewer cavities than children who do not get the recommended amounts. Fluoride in your baby's diet must come either from fluoridated drinking water or from fluoride supplements. Breastmilk contains little fluoride, even if the mother is drinking fluoridated water. Commercial formulas and evaporated milk do not naturally contain fluoride, nor are they supplemented.

The infant who is getting no fluoride in his diet and consuming only small amounts of water (the breastfed infant or the one on ready-to-feed formula) should be supplemented with 0.25 mg. of fluoride per day.[2] Take special note of the dosage, as some drops contain double that amount—0.50 mg. That is too high, as it can cause mottling, or white opaque spotting of the tooth enamel.

If your child is taking a concentrated, powdered, or evaporated-milk formula, he may be getting enough fluoride, provided the water you use for mixing contains at least 0.3 parts per million fluoride. However, if the level is less than 0.3 ppm, you should supplement with 0.25 mg. fluoride per day.

Fluoride drops are available by prescription, either alone or in combination with vitamins A, C, and D. The latter is an appropriate choice for the breastfed infant. (Although the breastfed baby doesn't need vitamins A and C, there are no formulations with only vitamin D and fluoride.) Fluoride alone is a better choice for the child on a ready-to-feed formula. If your problem is insufficient fluoridation of your local drinking water, you can get fluoride tablets to treat your water. Call your local department of health for more information.

Water should be fluoridated to a level of somewhere between 0.3 and one part per million. Levels above this can cause mottling or staining of the teeth; levels below may not give optimum protection against decay.

The Water Supply

The ideal water for the young infant is clean, low in nitrate and sodium, and fluoridated. Most of our city water supplies and local wells are sanitary and safe. If you have any doubt at all about the bacterial content or nitrate or sodium levels in your water, you should contact your local department of health and have it tested for cleanliness and levels of nitrate, sodium and fluoride.

Excessive nitrate intake is dangerous for the young infant because his body can change it to nitrite, and nitrite can displace oxygen in the red blood cells and interfere with oxygen-carrying capacity. Boiling the water doesn't help; it only concentrates the nitrates. If the nitrate level is 10 mg. per liter or more, you will need some other source of water until your baby is on a mixed diet.[5]

The concern with sodium in drinking water relates to possible long-term effects of excessive sodium intake, such as increased blood pressure. Sodium in water may occur naturally or it may be added by the water softening process. Have your water tested if you suspect it is salty. Use only the unsoftened water to dilute formula or juice.

The Nursing Equipment

There are some gadgets that are helpful for breastfeeding that we will discuss in the next chapter. For now we will be discussing bottle feeding.

You need equipment that works well, and that you and your baby can manage well. A nipple that is comfortable in your baby's mouth, and that feeds the formula at a manageable rate, has everything to do with establishing smooth and comfortable feeding. If your baby either is working too hard to get the formula, or is getting strangled by a too-fast flow, he will repeatedly pull off the nipple and fuss. That will frustrate both of you.

There are three main types of nipples: the traditional Evenflo® type, the Playtex® nurser type, and the Nuk® type. The latter is the one that is "orthodontically" shaped, and it looks like it has been left too close to the stove. Usually, babies are pretty flexible about taking up with the nipple you offer, but occasionally you'll find an infant who has a very marked preference. Many breast-feeding parents say their baby can only manage the Nuk, which supposedly most closely duplicates the breast nipple shape in the infant's mouth.

Nipple openings are either holes or cross-cut. It doesn't matter which you use as long as the nipple flows well. When you hold the bottle upside down, the formula should come out in steady drops that follow each other closely, but not in a constant flow. If it comes out too slowly, you can enlarge the opening with a hot needle, checking it to get the proper flow. Discard the nipple if the flow is too fast. Also discard cross-cut nipples when the opening becomes flabby.

Bottles can be the traditional rigid glass or plastic types, or the sort that have a throw-away plastic liner. The liners are sterile, so with those only the nipple and nipple cover have to be boiled.

In choosing between the rigid-sided bottles, I prefer the glass because I think it is easier to clean and dries faster after it is rinsed. Glass also keeps its shape better than plastic, so it makes a more-reliable measuring tool. Although it is true that the plastic bottles won't shatter, it really takes quite a bit to break a glass bottle. Since glass holds the temperature better, a feeding stays warm longer, and a cold bottle in a diaper bag stays cold longer. Do stay away from those cutsey animal-shaped nursing bottles; all those little curves and corners are just too hard to keep clean.

During the feeding you must provide for air flow into the bottle. If the ring of a traditional rigid-sided bottle is screwed on too tightly, no air will be able to get in around the ring. The baby will be causing a vacuum as he sucks, the nipple will collapse, and he will be forced to pull away before he wants to. On the other hand, if the ring is too loose, the flow will be too fast, and he may choke or overfeed himself and spit up. Loosen the ring just enough to get a good air flow (but not so much that you get formula all down the baby's shirt-front). As the baby sucks you should be able to hear the air feeding into the bottle and see the air bubbles. Air flow isn't a problem with plastic liners, as the liners simply collapse as they empty. You don't even have to hold them upright.

The rigid-sided bottle has to be properly tilted so the nipple is well-filled with formula throughout the feeding. Otherwise the infant will suck in air, certainly become frustrated, and possibly get a stomach ache.

Position, Timing, Temperature of Feeding

Hold your baby while you feed him so his head is a little higher than the rest of his body. If he is lying too flat, the milk can come back up in his throat, get into his eustacian tube, and cause earache.

Don't ever prop your baby's bottle and let him feed himself in bed. Cuddling while feeding is a vital part of nurturing; also, in addition to depriving you of important contact with each other, bottle propping can cause earache, bottle mouth, and choking. Bottle mouth is rampant tooth decay, predominantly of the upper teeth, that comes from letting a child go to sleep with milk, juice, or any caloric liquid pooling in his mouth. If your baby has teeth and is dozing off with the nipple in his mouth, you should remove the nipple, then straighten him up and stimulate him a bit so he swallows before you put him down for his nap.

Babies don't seem to mind too much whether their milk feeding is warmed or cold, as long as it is consistent. If you warm his bottle you should do it immediately prior to feeding. Don't let bottles stand out of the refrigerator to come to room temperature between feedings.

Safety, Sanitation and Dilution

One of the advantages of breastmilk is its safety. It comes straight from the source, so it doesn't have a chance to get contaminated. It is always properly mixed; it is not overconcentrated or underconcentrated. On the other hand, carelessly-prepared formula can get contaminated, or it can be improperly diluted. You must take particular care to see that your baby's formula, like breastmilk, is sanitary and properly mixed.

Modern formula preparation is deceptively simple—so simple, in fact, that it is easy to become lax and inattentive, and to begin to make some serious errors. There is no way of knowing how often babies get sick from contaminated or overconcentrated formula. Most babies who are hospitalized for vomiting and diarrhea are bottle fed.[9] Part of the difference may come from the handling rather than the formula.

While we don't know how many times formulas are contaminated, we do know that in many cases formulas are improperly diluted. A check on waiting room bottles in a pediatric clinic in England[16] showed over half of the feedings to be overconcentrated, with some of them triple the proper concentration.

Overconcentrated formula can overload the infant's ability to excrete waste products, and produce varying degrees of dehydration. Underconcentrated formula can impair growth rate and, in certain susceptible children, lead to water intoxication. Water intoxication, or overloading with water, puts a burden on the circulatory system and causes a too-great dilution of the bloodstream minerals that the body needs for normal function.

When you prepare your baby's formula, you have to pay scrupulous attention to detail in measuring, mixing, sanitation and refrigeration.

Sanitation. It is worth taking some extra care to see that your baby's food is safe and clean. Babies have less immunity to bacteria in the digestive tract, and are more sensitive to irritating substances than the older person. The baby who has diarrhea or is vomiting from a food infection risks dehydration. In our clean environments there is no excuse for food infections. In this section we will be talking about the principles of preparing and handling food in a way that will make and keep it safe.

Health workers' recommendations vary as to the degree of sterilization needed in the preparation of infant formula. Some instruct parents to boil water, bottles, nipples and all equipment used in preparation of formula. Others say good dish washing and clean water supply is enough, given our generally clean home conditions.

That might be all right if parents were as scrupulous as the health workers expect them to be. I have observed, however, that people can be woefully casual about food-handling (for adults as well as children). Unless they are taught, people don't think to wash their hands before they start working with food, they don't know about proper dishwashing techniques, and they leave food standing out at room temperature.

I think you should sterilize for the first three months. That should get your infant through the time of highest incidence of gastrointestinal upsets, and allow him to develop some tolerance for bacteria before he is exposed to them in the potentially large doses common in contaminated formula. I will describe three approaches to sterilizing, and also go into some detail about good hygenic technique in food handling. If you know all this already, bear with me. In this area I would rather tell too much than too little.

The formula manufacturers provide some very nice, free booklets with instructions and pictures detailing proper formula preparation. You can get one of these booklets from your physician, or by writing to Ross Laboratories or Mead Johnson. I will summarize and highlight some of the instructions.

Bacteria need three things to grow: food, water and the proper temperature. It is our job to see to it that they are deprived of one, two, or all three. To keep food safe we must reduce bacterial numbers as low as possible, and then make the environment for those remaining as unpleasant as possible.

Infant formulas and evaporated milk are sterile as they come from the can. That is, the bacteria have been destroyed by the heating process during manufacturing. The water supply and carefully washed utensils, bottles and nipples are clean but not sterile. Boiling equipment in water sterilizes it: it reduces the number of bacteria to a very low level, and thus decreases the amount of contamination that milk gets from these sources.

You can sterilize either by using the *aseptic* method, through *terminal heating*, or by the *single bottle* method. If you use the *aseptic method*, boil everything before you assemble it: the water used in formula preparation, the bottles, the nipples and nipple covers, and the measuring and mixing equipment. Don't forget to boil the can opener. Boil the water used in the formula for five minutes, the equipment for twenty. Then, being careful not to touch or contaminate, fill the bottles either one at a time or in a batch sufficient to last a day. Cover and refrigerate any prefilled bottles and the unused liquid formula. Use within 48 hours.

If you use *terminal sterilization*, clean but do not boil the equipment and ingredients. Prepare formula to the proper dilution, fill the bottles, invert the nipples, cover with the nipple discs (or leave nipples upright and cover with dome covers), and loosely screw on the rings. Then place the whole bottle-and-formula assembly in a pot with water about three inches deep. Cover and boil 25 minutes. (You can buy a sterilizer, but any big pot with a rack and a tight lid will work.) Remove the pot from the heat and let it stand, covered, one hour. Then take out the bottles, tighten the nipple rings and refrigerate. These filled bottles should also be used within 48 hours.

Once you get the hang of it, the terminal sterilization method is easy and quite foolproof. You don't have to be so careful about handling your bottles as you fill them, plus you don't have to preboil all the components.

For the *single-bottle* method, wash the bottles, fill each bottle with enough water to properly dilute the formula for one feeding, cap loosely and terminally sterilize. When the bottles cool, tighten the rings and store for no more than three days at room temperature. When you are ready to make the feeding, put in the right amount of concentrate or powder, shake it well and feed. (You can prepare a single eight-ounce bottle of evaporated milk formula by mixing three ounces evaporated milk, four and one-half ounces of water, and two teaspoons corn syrup or sugar.)

Of the three methods, the single bottle method is the best and easiest. You decrease the risk of bacterial contamination because you don't handle the equipment after you sterilize it, plus the germs simply don't have a chance to grow in the milk medium before the bottle is fed to the infant.

Sterilizing does not make up for sloppy habits. Your technique and handling of equipment and formula must be consistently excellent in any event, but particularly if you choose not to sterilize. First of all, your hands must be clean. To get rid of as many bacteria as possible you must wash your hands with soap. Simply rinsing them off with water doesn't do much but rearrange the bacteria. If you must dry your hands after washing, dry them on a clean towel.

Then, your sink must be clean. Take the time to scrub your sink with fresh, hot water and detergent and rinse it well with clear, hot water. Sinks can become contaminated with all sorts of undesirable bacteria. For instance, almost all raw chickens have salmonella on them, and fresh vegetables have botulinum spores on them. Any grease or food particles left in a sink will probably be kept moist by frequent tap usage, providing a perfect medium for bacterial growth.

Once you get your sink clean and rinsed, you can get started cleaning the top of the formula can, the bottles, nipples, measuring cups and spoons and stirring spoons, the can opener, and other equipment you use in formula preparation. Use a clean dishcloth. Use a bottle brush only for the baby bottles; wash and rinse it carefully after each use and put it where it can quickly dry and stay dry. Remember, any time you leave things wet you are providing a good medium for bacterial growth.

As you carefully wash the bottles and nipples, scrub the insides of the bottles and be sure to get all the milk drips from around the rims. (It's a good idea to rinse bottles and nipples with cool water right after use—this prevents formation of a milk film.) Give special attention to the nipples, wiping off the milk spots and forcing wash and rinse water through the holes in the nipples. Rinse carefully in water as hot as your hands can stand. Be sure that you get all the suds off, as dried scum from soap contains food particles and, again, provides a good medium for bacterial growth. Invert the bottles in a drying rack, put the nipples in a clean strainer, and let them air dry.

Automatic dishwashers generally do a good job of cleaning bottles and equipment. You need to be sure, however, that the water is getting up to about 140 degrees, and that the rinse cycle is doing a good job of getting off all of that caustic detergent. Check the instruction booklet on the dishwasher to be sure that you are using the correct amount of detergent, and carefully measure that amount into the machine. Use the full cycle, including the pre-rinse, when you wash the bottles. If the milk is really dried onto the bottles, soak them first and manually remove the residue.

Even if you are not planning to sterilize the other equipment, I would encourage you to boil up the nipples, let them dry, and store them in a clean, dry fruit jar.

Once the bottles are clean and dry, store them, inverted or covered, in a clean place. Again, if the bottles are not sterilized, it is probably better to fill them one at a time just before each feeding. Carefully cover any unused milk or formula and refrigerate, or, if it is powder, store in a cool, dry, place.

Keeping Formula Cool. Check your refrigerator temperature to see that it is somewhere between 35 and 40 degrees fahrenheit. Food keeps best when it is kept as cool as possible without freezing.

If you decide to warm your baby's bottle, do so only immediately prior to feeding. Generally we say that if a food is held between 40 and 140 degrees (optimum temperatures for bacterial growth) for two hours or more, it is contaminated and should be discarded.

Keep time and temperature in mind when you carry bottles in a diaper bag. Have the formula very cold when you pack it, and wrap it with a thick cloth to help keep it cold. If you are going to be away from refrigeration for a particularly long time, you might consider carrying along an ice chest or buying the single-feeding bottles or cans of formula.

I am not encouraging you to become a fanatic about cleanliness. You would be going too far if you imitate a fabled professor of mine and wash your door knobs with alcohol.

It certainly would be going too far to yell at big brother or sister about touching the baby's hands with their grubby little paws or sharing their toys with him. Your baby will naturally get exposed to germs in his environment, and he will gradually develop resistance to them. As he becomes exposed, his intestine will become less sensitive and react less. With your careful handling of formula, you are keeping the bacterial level down and giving him a chance to gradually develop his ability to live with the germs in his environment.

Proper Dilution of Formula. Unless your child is under very close medical supervision, it is extremely important to accurately follow standard directions in making up infant formulas. People not only make mistakes, they even vary concentrations intentionally. Some parents want their child to grow faster so they concentrate the formula. Or they want to have longer intervals between feedings, or less wet diapers. Occasionally someone will feed concentrated infant formula full strength (the liquid that you are supposed to dilute one-to-one with water), by accident or otherwise. The results can be tragic.

DON'T EXPERIMENT. FOLLOW DIRECTIONS. Use standard measuring cups and spoons, or the equipment provided with the formula. For measuring liquids, use the clear measuring cups with the volume marked off on the sides. Get your eye down even with the mark on the side of the cup to make sure you are measuring liquid accurately. Use aluminum or plastic nesting cups for dry measures. If they give you a little scoop for measuring formula for a single bottle, use it. The diameter and depth of the scoop are carefully selected to allow you to measure as accurately as possible. If you change to another brand of formula, use the scoop that comes with the new brand, and again read the package directions. Don't assume the procedure is the same for all brands.

For making up several bottles at a time, you may have to use a measuring cup. Again, follow the instructions. Some say to pack the formula into the cup, others simply say to spoon it. If it says to spoon it, do so—don't dig the cup into the powder. After you fill the cup according to directions, level off the top with a spatula or straight-edged knife. Do not level by shaking or tapping the cup. That changes the way the formula packs and makes for inaccurate measurement.

If you are making up one bottle at a time, you may use the measurements on the baby bottle, *provided it has rigid sides*, and you follow the package directions. DO NOT measure in the baby bottles that have disposable plastic inner liners; you simply cannot get an accurate measurement.

At the same time that you are being careful not to make the formula overconcentrated, be sure that you are not underconcentrating it. While too much water in the formula is not as dangerous as too little water, it can affect your baby's growth, especially if he is under six weeks of age. The baby over six weeks simply demands a larger volume of the dilute formula to satisfy his energy needs. The disadvantage is getting the child accustomed to taking great quantities of food. (Some have speculated that this is a habit that could carry over into adult life.)

The point then: when making up baby formula, don't get it close, GET IT RIGHT.

Quantity of Formula

As we discussed in the chapter on calories and normal growth, the amount of formula that your baby takes will be an individual matter, depending on his age, growth rate, activity level, and efficiency of metabolism. He can be trusted to regulate his food intake with his own cues of hunger and satiety. Your role is to learn to detect these cues and respond to them appropriately.

For your own interest and reassurance I am going to give you some figures on typical formula intakes, ranging from the 10th to the 90th percentile.[12]

Figure 5-8. Range of Daily Formula Intake

Age*	Percentile 10th	50th	90th
One month	14 oz.	20 oz.	28 oz.
Two months	23 oz.	28 oz.	34 oz.
Three months	25 oz.	31 oz.	40 oz.
Four months	27 oz.	31 oz.	39 oz.
Five months	27 oz.	34 oz.	45 oz.
Six months	30 oz.	37 oz.	50 oz.

*Formula intakes are reported for only the first six months because that is generally the time that a child is kept on formula alone.

At the 10th percentile the baby is taking as much or more formula than 10% of all infants. At the 50th percentile he is about in the middle, and at the 90th percentile he is taking as much or more than 90% of infants. Don't become immediately alarmed if your infant's food intake is outside these ranges. Keep in mind that 10% of infants are consuming more even than those in the 90th percentile and 10% are consuming less than those in the 10th percentile. Also keep in mind that these intakes are weekly averages. Your baby's day-to-day intake will vary.

It is remarkable that the highest-consuming newborn eats twice as much as the lowest-consuming one. At all ages, the child at the 90th percentile takes at least half again more formula than the one at the 10th percentile.

Feeding Frequency

As with quantity, you must give your child a say in determining the frequency with which he is fed. Physicians will often ask about the number of times a child is fed in a day (some even have the audacity to dictate the number of feedings). Parents often appear startled by the inquiry and will respond with something like, "well, let me see, he wakes up in the morning and wants to be fed, that's one time, and then sometimes he wants to be fed again about 9:00, but sometimes he doesn't, and then. . ." Unless they are put to the test, they simply don't know. If you regularly prepare a batch of bottles for a day, you will have to have some general idea of the number; but, beyond that, I don't really think it is important.

Your baby will feed as often as he needs to. As he gets bigger and his stomach holds more, and his digestive process accomodates more, he will eat less frequently. By the time he is a toddler he will probably be eating about six times a day: three meals and three snacks.

I will acknowledge that once in a while baby and parents get on a too-frequent pattern. By that I mean an almost-hourly feeding pattern. I would guess that parents or baby are over-interpreting hunger, and would suggest trying some other methods of comforting or entertaining. But if the infant is truly hungry he should be fed, even if the frequency is higher than some standard, somewhere, says he should be fed.

Promoting Good Feeding

The best feeding approach is one that is controlled by the baby rather than controlled by you. You let the baby control things when you pay attention to information coming from him and try to interpret and respond in a way that will allow him to eat well. Here are some examples of infant-controlled and parent-controlled feeding behavior.

The "infant-controlled" column describes how you behave when you are paying attention, and responding appropriately, to information coming from your baby. The "parent-controlled" column describes the behavior of a parent who is running the show with feeding, and ignoring or overruling information coming from the baby.

Infant controlled	Parent controlled
Attentive to infant behavior—allows quantity to vary	Ignores infant behavior Enforces externally-determined quantity
Holds bottle still at an appropriate angle	Rotates, tilts, jiggles bottle
Feeds according to baby's times or evolves a routine	Imposes feeding routine
Poises nipple over lips and allows baby to open up	Pushes nipple in
Problem solving, using trial and error	Assigns traits for problems—"He doesn't like his bottle"
Allows pauses—gives time to decide to finish feed	Terminates feeding abruptly at pauses
Soothes fussiness—finds reason for discomfort	Interprets infant fussiness as a sign of satiety

Weaning

We have to jump ahead now, to talk about weaning from the bottle or breast, as that generally becomes a concern somewhere between age eight months and a year.

Weaning at the appropriate time is important for a couple of reasons. First, the infant approaching 12 months is usually physically ready for a changed feeding style. He can feed himself chopped or mashed food and he can drink from a cup. He may even be ready to begin awkward experimentation with holding the cup and drinking from it himself. Second, excessive and overly prolonged bottle use and breastfeeding can promote some undesirable nutritional habits. He can overdemand milk, replacing other needed nutrients in his diet. Older babies often carry their bottles around and sip along, thus keeping their teeth exposed to calorie-containing liquids that can cause tooth decay.

I would like to avoid giving any hard-and-fast rules about weaning. In some cases there is a real, pitched battle between parent and child as the parent insists on eliminating the bottle or breast and the child begs and cries to have it. It does not have to be that way. Weaning is a process of gradually replacing nipple feeding of milk with other modes of eating and sources of nourishment. It does not have to become a process of depriving a child of something she holds near and dear.

You actually begin the weaning when you introduce your child to solid foods and get her started drinking from the cup. As she eats more solids and consumes more liquid from the cup, you can often drop out the mealtime nursing and she won't even miss it. When you start juices, you should do it with a cup, not by bottle, and that will reinforce her cup-drinking skill and keep her from building any more dependency on the bottle.

Babies sometimes get ready before their parents do to give up breast or bottle. The baby takes less formula and parents become alarmed. Or the baby has a bout of teething and loses her appetite for a time. Or parents are frustrated over lack of interest because they have gotten in the habit of offering a bottle as a way of calming her down. Or, most poignant of all, parents simply don't want to give up this sign of infancy. For whatever reason, missing the naturally presented opportunity to wean increases the chances that parent and child will later get into a struggle over it.

Many times children will continue to take an early morning or late night bottle or breastfeeding past the time when they are essentially weaned the rest of the day. I don't have any problem with that (as long as they are not dozing off with the liquid still pooling in their mouths). Generally, morning and evening nursings offer the equivalent of snacks and aren't replacing any meals, so they are really no problem.

Often during an illness or a bout with teething a child who is virtually weaned will want to return to nursing for a while. I think there is room for flexibility in that case; generally when the upset passes they will again lose interest in the breast or bottle.

We have worked very hard in this chapter. It worried me a bit as I finished it off, wondering if I had overloaded you with too much technical information. I reassured myself that you really needed the detail to help you deal with your advisors and make wise decisions.

However, I wasn't totally convinced until I read an article in the *American Journal of Disorders in Children*[14] about five babies in California who were suffering from kwashiorkor. Kwashiorkor is a severe malnutrition in children characterized by thin, reddening hair that falls out easily, failure to grow, irritability, sensitivity, lethargy and major swelling of the whole body. Why were these children so malnourished? They had been suspected of having a cow's milk allergy and had been taken off their formula and put instead, on *non-dairy creamer* as a substitute. The article did not identify the advisor.

In developing countries, people who know nothing about nutrition will feed babies anything that looks like milk and expect them to survive on it. In the United States, that that kind of thing should happen is absolutely astounding. With that kind of ignorance around SOMEBODY has to know what they are doing. Now you know. Defend yourself accordingly.

Don't get so buried by the technical information that you forget to establish a good feeding relationship with your baby. Start out with a good feeding, and then trust yourself to feed it—in a way that works for you and your own child.

Selected References

1. Boulton, T. J. C. and M. P. Rowley. Nutritional studies during early childhood. III. Incidental observations of temperament, habits and experiences of ill-health. Australian Paediatrics Journal 15:87–90. 1979.
2. Committee On Nutrition. Fluoride supplementation: revised dosage schedule. Pediatrics. 63:150. 1979.
3. Committee on Nutrition. Iron supplementation for infants. Pediatrics. 58:765–768. 1976.
4. Dallman, P. R., M. A. Siimes and A. Stekel. Iron deficiency in infancy and childhood. The American Journal of Clinical Nutrition. 33:86–118. 1980.
5. Fomon, S. J. Infant Nutrition. W. B. Saunders. Philadelphia. 1974.
6. Fomon, S. J., L. J. Filer, T. A. Anderson and E. E. Ziegler. Recommendations for feeding normal infants. Pediatrics. 63:52–59. 1979.
7. Fomon, S. J., E. E. Ziegler, S. E. Nelson and B. B. Edwards. Cow milk feeding in infancy: gastrointestinal blood loss and iron nutritional status. The Journal of Pediatrics. 98:540–545. 1981.
8. Johnson, G. H., G. A. Purvis, R. D. Wallace. What nutrients do our infants really get? Nutrition Today. 16(4):4–10. 1981.
9. Larsen, S. A., and D. R. Homer. Relation of breast versus bottle feeding to hospitalization for gastroenteritis in a middle-class U. S. population. The Journal of Pediatrics. :417–418. 1978.
10. Martinez, G. A. and J. P. Nalezienski. 1980 update: the recent trend in breast-feeding. Pediatrics. 67:260–263. 1981.
11. Osaki, F. A. Iron-fortified formulas and gastrointestinal symptoms in infants: a controlled study. Pediatrics. 66:168–170. 1980.
12. Owen, A. L. Feeding guide. A nutritional guide for the maturing infant. Health Learning Systems, Bloomfield, New Jersey. 1979.

13. Reeve, L. E., R. W. Chesney and H. F. DeLuca. Vitamin D of human milk: identification of biologically active forms. The American Journal of Clinical Nutrition 36:122–126. 1982.
14. Sinatra, R. R. and R. J. Merritt. Iatrogenic kwashiorkor in infants. American Journal of Diseases of Children. 135:21–23. 1981.
15. Solomons, N. W. and R. A. Jacob. Studies on the bioavailability of zinc in humans: effects of heme and nonheme iron on the absorption of zinc. The American Journal of Clinical Nutrition 34:475–482. 1981.
16. Taitz, L. S. and H. D. Byers. High calorie/osmolar feeding and hypertonic dehydration. Archives of Disease in Childhood. 47:257–260. 1972.

6
Breastfeeding How-to

Breastfeeding works on a law of supply and demand. Emptying the breasts stimulates them to make more milk. A hungry infant eats more often, empties the breasts more completely and promotes more milk production. The reverse is true for the less hungry infant, who leaves milk in the breast and signals it to make less milk.

Thriving while breastfeeding depends on both maternal and infant factors. The mother must eat enough, rest enough, and condition her letdown reflex. The baby must be alert and active enough to demand to be fed. She must also have a good suck and enough strength to get the milk out of the breasts.

Problems in breastfeeding are really more "bugs in the system" than signs of impending failure. Breast problems (like engorgement and soreness) as well as infant problems (like fussiness or a poor suck) can generally be solved without resorting to weaning.

Breastfeeding doesn't just happen; it has to be learned. It is striking to me how many parents get intimately involved with the whole birthing process through classes and reading, but assume that the part of the reproductive cycle that takes place after birth—lactation—will somehow or other happen naturally or instinctively. Quite the reverse is true.

There is a whole range of understanding and behavior that makes up successful breastfeeding. In our society, we have to go to some trouble to provide ourselves with that understanding and behavior. The situation is improving, but most people haven't had a chance to see a baby being breastfed. Or, if we are lucky enough to have seen the process, most of us have not been privileged enough to really look closely at a breastfeeding couple. We are too shy or constrained to be able to know how the baby's mouth fits the mother's breast, and how the two of them behave in that very intimate feeding relationship.

There are many good breastfeeding books around, books that offer you emotional support as well as information. One of my favorites is Eiger, M. S. and Olds, S., *The Complete Book of Breastfeeding*. New York, Wodman. 1972. I like that one for its emphasis on considering your own needs in the breastfeeding relationship as well as those of the baby. Another favorite is Karen Pryor's book, *Nursing Your Baby*, New York, Simon and Schuster, 1973. Ms. Pryor talks to you like a calm, supportive, and experienced friend, giving a wealth of detailed information and problem-solving tips, both for breastfeeding and for parenting in general. Her book is, however, somewhat dated by her assumption that physicians won't be supportive of, or knowledgable about, breastfeeding. That has definitely changed in the last 10 years. Physicians now are highly committed to breastfeeding, and many are good at supporting the process. Also, the La Leche League International's newly revised *The Womanly Art of Breastfeeding* (1981) is a big (350 pages) and detailed book. You might like it for its enthusiastic parent-to-parent exchange and dedication to breastfeeding, as well as its discussion of parenting topics in general.* All three are available in paperback.

With all of this good information around, our goals in this chapter are going to be:

1. To select out and emphasize what's most important for you to know.
2. To emphasize the maternal-nutritional aspects of breastfeeding.

The main and most important thing you have to know about breastfeeding is that it works on a law of supply and demand. IF YOUR BABY NEEDS AND DEMANDS MORE MILK, HE WILL WANT TO NURSE MORE AND YOU WILL MAKE MORE.

To be able to respond to the demand, however, you have to be eating enough food so you can make milk. YOU HAVE TO FEED YOURSELF IN ORDER TO BE ABLE TO FEED YOUR BABY.

Hang on to those principles as the two to take away from this chapter. Hang on to them now as we turn to our next order of business, again diving into the detail.

A Tale of Two Babies

The stories of Janet and Martha will serve as a useful introduction to our topic. Both women were first-time mothers. Both had good pregnancies, carried their babies to term and had good normal deliveries. Both delivered in a hospital with a supportive nursing staff who helped them with the details of getting started nursing. The nurses were understanding and didn't seem to be at all surprised that Martha didn't even know how to hold her baby and that Janet had a rather difficult time knowing how to position herself comfortably.

Each woman needed the nurse's encouragement to go through the process of getting well-settled in a comfortable chair, putting a

---

*I don't agree, however, with what any of these books have to say about solid foods selection. If you compare their recommendations with my solid food discussion in chapter seven, I think you'll see why.

pillow on her lap, and settling the baby in the crook of her arm to nurse. Janet appreciated being helped to nurse while she was lying down. Both had read about these positions and preparations in books, but were surprised at how awkward and self-conscious they felt as they actually went through the motions.

They were also surprised to see their babies behaving in such predictable ways. The nurse showed them how to stroke the baby's cheek nearest the nipple to get her to turn toward the nipple, and right on cue, each did, mouth open, searching for the nipple. Martha was particularly startled when her baby latched on to the breast. It was remarkable to her to see so much of her nipple and areola disappear into that tiny mouth. And she was surprised at the strength of the pressure. In fact, the baby seemed to know all about getting properly attached to the nipple and suckling.

Janet's baby was not quite as quick getting going. She seemed to be satisfied to take just the very end of the nipple in her mouth, and Janet had to pull her back off again, and flatten out her nipple and areola to fit better into her baby's mouth. It also seemed to help if she extended the baby's neck and tipped her head back a bit.

They were both surprised at their baby's willingness to nurse just to get the small amount of yellowish colostrum they had available early on. Then, when their breast milk came in, they were further interested to see that it was, indeed, thin and bluish-looking, and that the milk toward the end of the feed was creamier and more-opaque looking. The nurses confirmed what they had read about the variation in fat content between the "fore" or early milk in the feed, and the "hind" or later milk.

By the time they went home from the hospital, both babies and both mothers were doing fine with nursing. There, however, our stories diverge. Martha's baby became increasingly active, demanding, and dissatisfied. She seemed to want to nurse at least every two hours all day, and was getting her mother up at least twice nightly to feed her. She was an eager nurser and had a powerful suck. She had no patience with an empty breast, and would quit nursing abruptly and start chewing energetically on the nipple until her mother switched her to the other breast; then she would also rapidly empty it, and seemingly look around for more. She would take short cat naps and be up again, demanding to be held and comforted and entertained, and, soon nursed again.

Martha was really getting worn out. Her husband and mother were complaining because her baby ate so often, and one well-meaning advisor even suggested that her milk disagreed with the baby, and that she should try giving her a bottle. But Martha persisted, even though at times she, hereself, felt like she was just being stubborn and a little crazy to do so.

Janet, on the other hand, had an easier time of it. Her baby remained quiet and placid. She would wake up to lie quietly in her crib, and seldom made much of a fuss about eating. When she nursed, she did so politely, often drifting off to sleep before she even got to the second breast. She woke up only once nightly from the early days on and adjusted during the day to three or four-hour feeding intervals, occasionally even going five hours at a stretch before she asked, politely, to be fed again. Janet and her husband felt comfortable and easy with their new baby, and congratulated themselves on doing so well with her.

It was an exhausted, harrassed and insecure Martha who presented her baby for the one-month checkup. To her astonishment, she found that her baby had gained two pounds in that short time. She protested that there must be a mistake, pointing out how unsatisfied she seemed to be, and how frequently she wanted to nurse.

Janet received other news. She was sadly jarred from her confidence and sense of well-being to discover that her baby, although she had grown nicely in height, had barely regained her birth-weight. Her baby had been so placid that she had not even been demanding enough to get her calorie needs met.

Fortunately both mothers had supportive and knowledgeable health practitioners, who were able to help them get on the right track with their breastfeeding. Martha needed mostly to be reassured that things were going well. Her schedule, although it seemed hectic and demanding, was just right for her baby and was apparently helping her to thrive. Knowing that, she was able to relax and quit feeling like she was doing something wrong. As a result, the schedule, even though it didn't get any better, wasn't as wearing on her.

Janet needed some help stimulating her baby—and herself—to encourage a more frequent feeding schedule. She had been losing weight fairly rapidly, and her doctor encouraged her to eat more, rest more, and to begin waking her daughter up at frequent intervals to feed her. She had to learn some tricks to stimulate her baby, like unwrapping her feet, moving her around, jack-knifing her,* and taking advantage of any wakefulness to feed before cleaning or dressing her.

Her baby did start to eat more and to be more demanding. Her weight was better two weeks later, and by the time another month had passed, the baby had taken over demanding to be fed, although Janet still had to be careful not to let her sleep beyond four hours at a stretch during the day.

From these stories emerge the three themes about breastfeeding that we will be following in this chapter:

1. It takes two to breastfeed. To produce an adequate quantity of breastmilk depends on infant as well as maternal factors.
2. There is an important role to be filled in breastfeeding relationships, that of support and teaching.

---

*This is also called the "China doll" maneuver—you repeatedly bring your baby from a lying to a sitting position or from a sitting position to a "flopped over" position, where the baby bends over her lap.

3. In most breastfeeding relationships, as with other relationships, there will be problems while the partners work things out.

Maternal and Infant Factors in Breastfeeding

Breastfeeding takes two. Thriving while breastfeeding depends on the child's ability to stimulate the breasts and ingest, digest and assimilate the breastmilk, as well as the mother's ability to produce breastmilk and make it available to her baby. The many factors in the breastfeeding relationship are outlined on the next page, in the *Thriving Chart.*

Thriving While Breastfeeding

Before we can take a look at the specific factors in successful breastfeeding, we have to know what we mean by a thriving baby. Your baby's growth and weight gain is your most concrete way of assessing your breastfeeding regimen. (This is not, however, to say that your breastfeeding is unsuccessful if you have not provided fully for your baby's nutritional needs . . . more about this in our discussion of relactation and induced lactation.)

Like Janet's baby, breastfed infants may have inadequate weight gain or even weight loss, without showing the signs of hunger or fussiness you would expect in an underfed infant. In fact, now that breastfeeding is on the increase, while the systems for supporting it are not yet very well established, increasing numbers of babies are arriving for their first checkup with "failure to thrive."*

Part of the problem is the delay in checking. Breastfeeding babies should be weighed after two weeks, instead of waiting for the

---

*Failure to thrive is clearly inadequate growth, as distinguished from the normally slow-growing baby we will discuss later.

Figure 6-1. Thriving Chart (Modified from Laurence, R. Breastfeeding: a guide for the medical profession. St. Louis. C. V. Mosby Co. p. 178. 1980.)

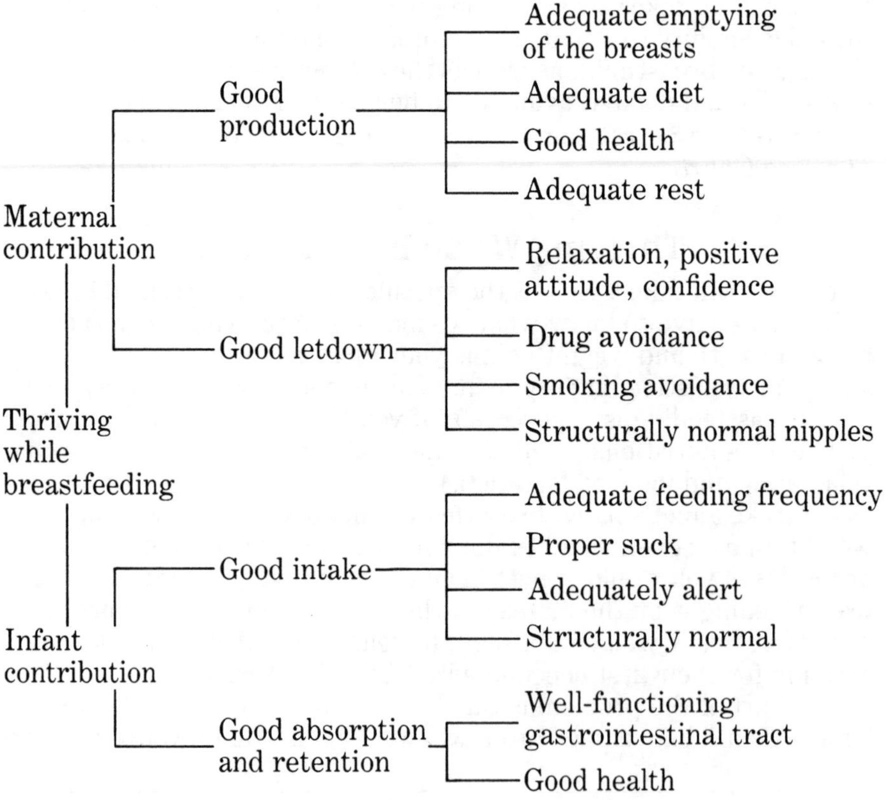

usual new-baby visit at one month. Part of the problem is that parents are not aware of risk. Babies who grow poorly are often placid babies of first-time mothers, like Janet's baby. Babies like Martha's do not grow poorly. They keep after their parents until they get enough to eat.

It is difficult to define adequate infant weight gain, especially for breastfed infants. In a study done in Iowa in 1970, at least 10% of 149 normal breastfed infants had not regained their birth weight by age 14 days. Generally, full-term babies are expected to regain their birth weight by 10 days of age and then gain about 5 to 7 ounces per week during their first month or two.[5] It can be reassuring to know that gain velocities fluctuate; the slowest growing infant one month may be the fastest growing another.

The Slow-growing Baby. However, when you assess a slow weight gain in an infant, you always have to wonder if the gain is "normal" for this particular baby. Some babies simply grow slowly but very consistently and achieve a growth that is, for them, very satisfactory.

Janet's baby was probably growing too slowly. Her infrequent feeding and low demand indicated that she was not stimulating her mother's breastmilk production enough. With other babies who are growing slowly, however, there is nothing so clearly wrong with the breastfeeding routine. They are adequately alert and show a good breastfeeding pattern. At times, these babies have been weaned to the bottle in an attempt to increase their growth rate, only to continue the very slow rate of gain.

A baby who is truly failing to thrive at the breast will show a decreased frequency of feeding, sleepiness, a weak suck, and lack of interest in feeding. If the condition is severe, he will have a lack of urination and bowel movements, his skin will be cool, and he may show some of the symptoms of dehydration.

If your baby is gaining slowly, it helps to keep a daily record of wet diapers—6 to 8 per day is a good sign. It also helps to ask an experienced person to observe a breast feeding, looking for things like infant alertness, sucking pattern and signs of milk flow. Your observer should also note your awareness of milk letdown, and involvement and relaxation with the baby. Check to make sure you are optimizing the factors important for good breastmilk production and letdown that we will be discussing soon, emphasizing frequent nursing and eating enough food.

Just as Janet's baby was running behind, so Martha's was running ahead. Fortunately, it did not occur to Martha to be concerned about overgain, but many parents do worry about that. At that early age, it is wise to concentrate on establishing the breastfeeding relationship, and let the growth take care of itself.

Martha's baby appeared to be pressing because she was hungry. The fact that she was nursing for nourishment, not entertainment, was evident from her hungry response to the breast, and lack of patience with an empty breast. Martha was wise to feed her and trust that her growth would be appropriate for her.

Let's go into more detail about the factors in adequate milk production.

Adequate Breast Stimulation. Adequate breast stimulation is essential and depends on maternal as well as infant factors. Looking at our *Thriving Chart* (p. 172), the first factor in good production is adequate emptying of the breasts. (This, in turn, depends on letdown, which we'll discuss in the next section.) As our stories have demonstrated, production also depends on infant factors, namely an infant who is alert enough to stimulate lactation by demanding a high feeding frequency.

Any rules that limit your baby's sucking and your contact with your baby will get in the way of breastfeeding. We have plenty of rules. We have prescriptions about intervals (every four hours), about duration (three minutes or five or seven), about number (six in twenty-four hours), and about amount of mother-baby contact (you will spoil him).

Frequency of Breastfeeding. Parents are often concerned about the frequency with which they nurse babies, and rightly so, because the breastfeeding baby will probably need to nurse 8 to 12 times per day in the early weeks. That is tiring, especially when you combine it with all the other care required by a new baby. I once figured out that, on the better days, the feeding, changing, washing, cleaning, caring and adoring of a new baby takes about six hours.

A study in 1950[14] of 100 newborn breastfed infants on a self-demand schedule showed the average number of feedings per day throughout the first week:

Day	1	2	3	4	5	6	7
Feedings	6.2	6.9	8.1	8.6	8.5	8.3	7.0

Remember that these figures are averages, and that averaging numbers smooths out the variation. In other words, although there is an apparent variation in feeding frequency in that first week, the *actual* variation for any given baby was even greater.

It is just coincidence if the intervals between feedings show any consistency. Your baby may want to eat every two or three hours,* and then have one or two sleeping periods each day when he goes four or even five hours. Then he will want to eat right away, and then again an hour later want to make up for lost time.

Emptying the breasts stimulates them to make more milk. As your baby grows and requires more milk, he will signal his need by more thoroughly emptying your breasts and by wanting to eat more

---

*Feedings intervals are timed from the beginning of one feeding to the beginning of the next.

often. Increased emptying and sucking stimulation will increase the amount of breastmilk you make. If, on the other hand, your baby needs less milk than you are making, which is typical of that time in early lactation when breastmilk first comes in, the leftover milk in the breast will shut down manufacture, and you will make less, to match your baby's needs.

Sometimes this shutdown happens inappropriately, as it did with Janet's baby or when a baby is sick for a time. Then it is necessary to increase nursing frequency for a while to again stimulate increased production.

Hungry Days. During the weeks and months of nursing, the times when you are in balance with your baby's needs will alternate with times when his needs increase and you fall behind in breastmilk production. His growth spurts, and hungry days, may take place at fairly predictable times, such as at seven to ten days of age, five to six weeks, and at three months. Other growth spurts, however, are not so predictable. Some appear to have one hungry day a week, while others seem to be pressing all the time. It may be that Martha's baby was like that.

"A continually fretful baby" who is calmed by nursing is most likely hungry, which is good, because his hunger is a stimulus for milk production. Contrast him with Janet's too-slow-growing infant who became lethargic. That baby was not even getting enough to be demanding.

Generally you can get your milk supply up if you increase your nursing frequency for about 48 hours. Those are tough, tiring days, when your baby seems dissatisfied and unhappy and you seemingly do nothing but nurse. You may even ask yourself what you are doing to your child by persisting in the process. It appears, however, that those hungry days have a developmental as well as a nutritional function. Often you will find that after hungry days, your baby has increased the time of his quiet alert state. Being hungry and dissatisfied for a time may help stimulate his interest and awareness of the world around him.

Carrying him around in a back- or front-pack, while you do your chores, seems to help comfort him and get him through those days. Outside help with chores can be a life-saver during those times; barring that, you may need to develop the ability to let everything else go and make nursing the highest priority in your life for a couple of days.

Once you get past the newborn period,* lest you should end up spending almost all your time nursing, you should know that a hungry, vigorously-sucking baby can get most of the milk from a breast in four to five minutes. He can totally empty a breast in seven to ten, so there is really no need for you to make the feeding more than 20 minutes in length. Knowing that is a great help. Some mothers think they should nurse 45 minutes or more, and if their baby wants to be fed every two hours or so, they really spend almost all of their time nursing.

Don't overdo the ritual that goes along with feeding. Elaborate hand and nipple washing may just be wearing you out. You also might consider double diapering, especially at night, to cut down on the amount of fussing that goes along with feeding time.

The most common explanation for prematurely stopping breastfeeding is the belief that the baby is not getting enough to eat. Uninformed parents get into trouble with breastfeeding because they do not know the law of supply and demand. Then, when their baby has his first hungry days, they assume that the breastmilk is drying up and hasten to offer a bottle. The satisfied infant then fails to give stimulation to the breasts, and milk supply does, indeed, fall behind the infant's need. With each hungry day, more bottles are offered, the breasts get less stimulation, and eventually many babies begin to

---

*A newborn feeding can take an hour by the time you feed, burp, change and play.

show a preference for the bottle. The bottle delivers more milk with less effort than breastfeeding.

Meanwhile, the mother becomes increasingly frustrated and insecure with her nursing, feels a lot of conflict about the bottle, and eventually gives up altogether, feeling disappointed and like a failure. It is easy to see how lack of information about breastfeeding can make success difficult.

As your baby gets older, his nursing intervals may lengthen and his nursing times may shorten. This depends at least in part on how much food he needs. The chart, *Spread of Caloric Requirements During the First Year*, in the chapter *Calories And Normal Growth* (p. 88), shows the wide variation in infant calorie requirement. A big-eating fast-growing baby will have to provide more breast stimulation than a baby who needs less food. There is undoubtedly also a variation in the frequency of breast emptying a woman must have in order to maintain her breastmilk supply as her baby gets older. Thus, feeding frequency is a highly individual matter that can only be determined by mother and baby.

The Middle-Aged Baby. Middle-aged babies (4–6 months) nurse very fast, and get on with what they were doing. They will often come off the nipple to crane their necks and look around at any distraction, or, worse yet, try to look around without letting go. Because babies at this age can often empty a breast in five minutes or less, their mothers worry that they are not getting enough to eat. (They also miss the long, quiet intimate feedings.) But babies that age seem to be able to maintain and even increase milk supply on fewer feedings and still benefit from the intimacy, even if it is brief.

It is important to continue to keep an eye on growth rate in these middle-aged babies. At times we see an inappropriate falling-off in growth at about three months. If this happens with your baby, you may have to take the lead in resting more, nursing more frequently, and perhaps in cutting down on distractions while you nurse.

Good Letdown. In the last section, we alluded to good letdown as being important to adequate emptying of the breasts. To clearly understand that point, you have to know a bit about breast anatomy and physiology. Here is a picture of the structure of the lactating breast.[14]

Figure 6-2. Structure of the Lactating Breast (Courtesy of Worthington-Roberts[12]).

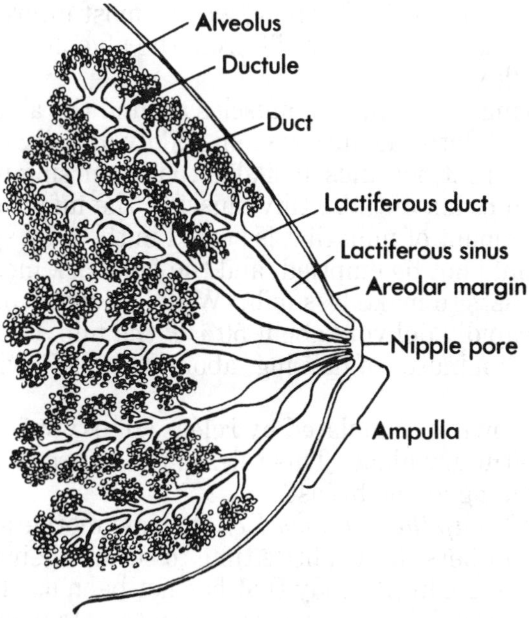

From Worthington-Roberts, Bonnie S.: Lactation and human milk: nutritional considerations. In Worthington-Roberts, Bonnie S., Vermeersch, Joyce, and Williams, Sue Rodwell: Nutrition in Pregnancy and Lactation, ed. 2, St. Louis, 1981, The C. V. Mosby Co.

The milk-producing parts of breasts resemble a series of bunches of grapes. The "grape" is the alveolus, which is the milk factory of the breast. The stems leading from the grapes are the ducts that carry the milk to increasingly larger "stems" or channels until each "bunch" of alveoli feeds the milk into the large lactiferous duct. Each of these channels carries its milk to a pore, or opening in the nipple. About an inch or inch and a half back from the nipple pore is an enlarged part of the lactiferous duct, called a lactiferous sinus. This bulging area in the duct is important to note for our later discussion of the infant suck. For now, we are most interested in the process that releases the breastmilk from the alveolus to the nipple: the letdown reflex.

During letdown, tiny muscles around the alveoli contract and force the milk into the duct system and eventually to the lactiferous sinuses, where it becomes available to the nursing infant. Without the letdown reflex of those tiny muscles, the infant could only get at the small amount of milk that is stored in the duct system, the breasts would not be emptied, and the feedback message would signal the breasts to make less milk. With letdown, you get a flow of milk that rapidly delivers about 50% of the milk to the baby within the first two minutes of nursing, about 80 to 90% within the first four minutes.[14]

Letdown is stimulated by release of oxytocin from the mother's pituitary gland. This release is, in turn, stimulated by the infant's sucking at the breast.

Setting up the Letdown Reflex. New mothers, particularly first-time mothers, take a little time to set up their letdown reflex.[5] Like any system in the body that has not been used before, it takes a while to get it going. And you can learn to help yourself to let down your milk.

Establishing Letdown. To begin with, you may need to take pressure off yourself by identifying, and perhaps, adjusting, your goals. Is your goal to produce a lot of breastmilk, or is it to have a warm and close breastfeeding experience? Women who have partially nursed adoptive babies, or have provided for part of the needs of an ill or uncooperative baby, seem to feel their nursing was successful, irrespective of the amounts they produced. This is not to say that you won't produce enough or that it's not a reasonable goal to produce enough. What it is saying is that you can get some pressure off yourself about achieving letdown, and can relax and enjoy the experience, by concentrating on the nursing, not on the quantity of milk.

Keeping your mind on the process itself, and not so much on the outcome, is a well-proven tactic that behaviorists have used for enhancing people's success with all kinds of pursuits, from weight loss to becoming a better golfer; and along with keeping your mind on the process goes congratulating and supporting yourself for good performance. Olympic divers, rather than berating themselves for errors, pay attention to the positive aspects of position and movement that they would like to repeat. You aren't trying to be an Olympic nurser, but the technique can be helpful.

A couple of the key behaviors we're going to emphasize in establishing letdown are a) knowing your baby, and b) relaxing yourself. When you accomplish that, give yourself some recognition. And let the letdown take care of itself.

Here are ways of setting up a routine for yourself that will condition the milk letdown, as well as make the experience more meaningful for both of you. They are listed in the order you will probably do them, not in order of importance.

1. Maintain a relaxed life style. Don't let yourself get rushed or overtired. This is particularly important early on when you are establishing the reflex. Later on the reflex can function despite some disruption, but at first you really have to protect yourself.
2. Pick up your baby; watch and hold him at times when you don't feel pressure to nurse.
3. Set up the environment. Provide yourself with a comfortable nursing spot, get something to drink, maybe something to eat.

4. Relax yourself. Take a couple of deep breaths, or use your regulated breathing exercise that you used during labor and delivery.
5. Take time to center yourself. Bring your attention to yourself, your baby and your shared activity. Be aware of the very real pleasure and satisfaction of sharing that time with your child.
6. If you're not letting down, massage your breasts as the baby nurses. Once the baby has exhausted the readily available milk supply, massage that breast gently in a circular pattern with the fingertips of your free hand, emptying first one quadrant and then another. This does externally what the letdown reflex does internally—moves the milk from the alveoli to the ducts and sinuses, where it can be readily removed. (To know when massage is necessary, you have to be able to distinguish between your baby's long, rhythmic suck and swallow when he is getting milk, and the short, choppy jaw movements when he is not. We'll talk more about this later.)
7. Take advantage of letdown that takes place at odd times. If you have leaking, you are probably having a letdown. Pick up your baby and feed her if you think she is likely to be hungry enough to cooperate.
8. Read a book or watch TV, if that helps you relax. This is contradictory to the earlier advice about focusing attention on the baby. However, it may work for you to turn your attention away in a relaxed fashion and trust your body to take care of the process by itself.

How Can You Tell if You're Having Letdown? Awareness of letdown varies. Some women have very strong physical sensations, while others have little or none. Some women are aware of a feeling of pins and needles, a kind of pain or tingling sensation, beginning shortly after nursing starts, and disappearing gradually thereafter. Sometimes women can feel uterine contractions, ranging from mild to painful. Other women get a sensation of intense thirst. With letdown you will probably get dripping or even spurting of milk from the alternate breast. And the character of the baby's sucking, as we said earlier, will change.

In the early feedings after birth, the letdown reflex may not occur for three minutes or longer after nursing begins. Later, after the learning period, the reflex usually begins within 30 seconds of starting nursing, or after hearing your baby (or someone else's baby) cry. You may find yourself letting down at odd times and not even be aware of what has stimulated it—maybe a subtle smell or sound.

We have said that frequent emptying of the breasts is essential to stimulating them to produce breastmilk, and we have discussed the importance of the letdown in releasing that milk from the breasts. Our next order of business is discussing the other major factor in breastmilk production: your consuming enough food.

Eating Well While Breastfeeding. You have to feed yourself if you are going to feed your child.[9] Feeding yourself means, most importantly in lactation, eating enough food so you can make milk and lose weight no more rapidly than one-half pound per week, *provided you have it to lose.* If you have gained insufficient amounts of weight during pregnancy, you probably should eat enough so you don't lose weight at all. Calories to support lactation come from your fat stores of pregnancy as well as from your diet. If you have stored little or no fat, you will have to make it up from your diet.

Lactation failure with low energy intake. A number of studies of lactation failure and failure to thrive in infants[3,4,8,10] have pointed to some characteristics of mothers and babies that are related to the mother's energy intake:

1. Babies of low birth weight. (Is this secondary to poor maternal weight gain in pregnancy?)
2. Mothers who were dieting to lose weight, both during pregnancy and lactation.
3. Women with poor eating habits in general.
4. Women who were very tired and seemingly experiencing some

loss of appetite associated with their fatigue.
5. Women who were "too busy to eat."
6. Women who were very concerned over what foods to avoid.

It appears that women who eat too little during lactation produce breastmilk that is lower in quantity, although quality remains the same,[8] except perhaps for fat content. If the mother's diet is low in calories, she may have a reduced total milk fat in her "hind" milk.* With poor fat content, the amount of the resulting high-water, high-protein milk that the baby must consume to satisfy his calorie requirement is tripled or even quadrupled. In such cases, regardless of whether the problem is reduction in total quantity of milk or reduction in fat content, the solution is the same: increasing the mother's calorie intake, including fat as well as protein and carbohydrate sources.

Calorie intake. Your best guides to how how much you should be eating are your own hunger and appetite, and your own and your baby's weight response. You may not even be aware of eating more than usual—most women are not. However, for the part of you that wants to run things with your head as well as with the rest of your body, the figures on estimated calorie requirements for producing breastmilk are in Figure 6-3.[13]

If you have gained adequately during pregnancy, you can probably lactate well by providing yourself with 50 to 75 percent of the extra calories necessary for producing milk, and depend on the stored fat in your body for the rest. Women seem to continue to lactate well if they lose about one-half pound per week (again, provided they have a healthy amount of fat to lose), and in some cases can even lose as much as a pound a week without problems.

However, it is important to be very cautious about accelerating weight loss when you are breastfeeding. Even women who are very well established in lactation find that if they cut down their food

---

*This is the high-fat milk secreted in the last few minutes of nursing.

intake and try to lose more weight, their babies become irritable and fussy and fail to gain weight. When they again increase the calorie, including fat content of their diets, the babies become satisfied and resume their normal weight gain patterns.

Figure 6-3. Energy cost of Producing Breastmilk

Age of baby (months)	Volume of milk taken (ml/day)	Oz/day	Energy value of milk (calories/day)	Total energy cost of producing milk assuming 90% efficiency (calories/day)
0–1	600	20	402	446
1–2	840	28	563	626
2–3	930	31	623	692
3–4	960	32	643	714
4–5	1010	34	677	752
5–6	1100	37	737	819

Fluid Intake. Be sure to consume enough liquids to quench your thirst. You do not, however, have to force yourself to drink more than that. One of the myths about breastfeeding that has been passed on in the best circles for years and years is the idea that if the mother markedly increases her fluid intake, it will increase the amount of milk she makes. Twenty years ago, two British physicians tested this theory and found that drinking water or other fluids in amounts larger than those the mother wishes to drink to quench her thirst actually impairs lactation.[6]

On the other hand, if the mother is clearly dehydrated, her milk supply will go down. Or if she is depending on fluids for calories to support her lactation, fluid intake can have an effect on lactation.

But simply forcing fluids in an attempt to increase lactation is apparently a tactic that backfires.

Quality of the Mother's Diet During Lactation. Choosing a good quality diet during lactation is more for your benefit than the baby's. Unless you are extremely poorly nourished and depleted in some nutrients, lactation will draw on your nutrient stores to make your breastmilk adequate in protein, vitamin and mineral content.

Accordingly, your diet during breastfeeding should protect you against depleting your own nutrient stores. You shouldn't rob your own bones of calcium to get the calcium for milk. And you shouldn't have to break down your own muscle and organ tissue to get enough protein for manufacturing breastmilk.

An optimum diet for lactation is very much like an optimum diet for pregnancy except it is higher in calories and lower in protein.

Figure 6-4. Food for lactation

Milk and milk products	4 cups (six cups for teens)
Meat and other major protein sources	2 servings (total of four ounces)
Fruits and vegetables	4 servings Vitamin C source daily Vitamin A source every other day
Breads and cereals	4 servings

This basic diet will not give you enough calories—perhaps only half of what you need for lactation. Check back to the discussion in the *Pregnancy* chapter. (p. 35) to get some suggestions for increasing your total food intake to an adequate level.

Vitamins and Minerals in Breastmilk. The mother's intake of some vitamins and minerals is reflected in breastmilk content; others appear not to be. Figure 6-5 summarizes what we know about this topic:[2]

Figure 6-5. Effect of Maternal Intake on Milk Content of Vitamins and Minerals.
(Copyright, American Academy of Pediatrics. 1981.)

Minerals	Effect of intake on milk content
Sodium	None
Calcium	None
Iron	None
Zinc	None
Copper	None
Manganese	Yes
Selenium	Unknown
Iodine	Yes
Fluoride	None

Fat-soluble Vitamins	Effect of intake on milk content
D	Unknown
K	None
A	Yes
E	Unknown

Water-soluble Vitamins	Effect of intake on milk content
Ascorbic acid	Yes
Thiamine	Yes
Riboflavin	Yes
Niacin	Yes
Panthothenic acid	Yes
Pyridoxine	Unknown
Biotin	Unknown
Folate	None
Cyanocobalamin	Yes

As you can see, the nutrients that can be affected by maternal intake are manganese and iodine, fat soluble-vitamin A and the water-soluble vitamins with the exception of folate and possibly pyridoxine and biotin. Manganese is found in whole grains and nuts. Iodine should be no problem if you use iodized salt; it is also present as a byproduct of the production of milk and commercially-baked bread.

Breastmilk is not a good source of vitamin D, so I will not recommend supplementing your diet to provide it.[11] Also, there should be no need for concern about vitamin K because it is routinely supplemented as an injection for all newborns.

Ample supplies of vitamin A and the water-soluble vitamins can be maintained with wise selection of a good quality diet as outlined in the table on p. 186. Generally vitamin and mineral supplements are not necessary for women eating a nourishing well-balanced diet.

The nutrients listed as "unknown"—selenium, vitamins D and E, pyridoxine and biotin—have not been researched enough to know whether or not the mother's intake influences breastmilk composition. All can be provided in adequate amounts from a well-selected diet.

Foods to avoid while breastfeeding. Traces of anything you eat can show up in breastmilk. If you eat a lot of onion or garlic, chances are your breastmilk will taste like onion or garlic. Most babies do not seem to mind.

Some babies, however, appear to get fussy or have some congestion when their mothers eat certain foods. Some clinicians associate the mother's consumption of cow's milk (or occasionally, of eggs) with infant colic. They have observed that the colic in babies they have tested has disappeared when cow's milk was removed from the mother's diet and reappeared when the mothers again drank milk.[7]

It is probably the unusual child who reacts to his mother's diet. Further, it is hard to sort out whether infant behavior is a true reaction to food or simply a coincidence, since all babies are fussy, get congested, or appear colicky at times. But if you have a fussy or colicky baby, it is probably worth a try to see if your food could be causing it. Try by removing the food from your diet, but check to make sure you are not unnecessarily limiting your food selection before you cut it out completely.* (Stop eating it a couple of times, see if symptoms disappear, then reintroduce it and see if they reappear.) Often babies will develop a tolerance for most foods by the time they are four or five months old.

Other Factors in Production and Letdown.

Being good to yourself. We have touched on adequate rest and a positive mental attitude as being factors in good breastmilk production. Babies respond to their mothers' tension and fatigue with fretting and crying. If you are getting too strung out, your baby's fussing may be telling you that you are too tense, or that you are over-working. In a sense, your baby is telling you to take better care of yourself.

Smoking and drug and alcohol abuse may also impair milk production and letdown. Some drugs in the mother's milk, such as painkillers and tranquilizers, may sedate the baby and make him less insistent on nursing.[5]

From the physiology of the mother's milk production and letdown, we can now move to the mechanics of getting the milk into the baby. The whole process of suckling is again a topic in which infant and maternal factors are interrelated. The milk delivery system depends on an infant who can suck properly—who has a mouth that is

---

*As with all cases of allergy, if the original reaction to the food has been extreme or violent, do not challenge unless there is a physician supervising. It is highly unlikely, but I suppose not impossible to get a reaction of this magnitude to breastmilk.

adequate structurally, and who can learn the patterns necessary for appropriate suckling. It also depends on the mother's having a nipple that protrudes enough so the baby can grasp it and hold it in his mouth.

The Mechanics of Suckling. Breastfeeding is a three-fold action of suction, chewing and compression by the tongue and lips.[12] It is a process of suckling, which differs basically from the sucking that a baby does at a rubber nipple. The picture below demonstrates why breastfeeding is sometimes called a "pump suck."

The properly-grasped nipple is drawn into the mouth, and up against the roof of the mouth with the aid of the tongue. Suction is important, not to remove milk from the breast but to hold the nipple in place in the baby's mouth. The tongue is in the front of the mouth and strokes the bottom of the nipple.

The baby in Figure 6-6 is properly positioned on the nipple, with his lips almost completely encompassing the areola. His jaw is in a position to apply pressure on the lactiferous sinuses. As he nurses, his lower jaw squeezes the lactiferous sinuses against the roof of the mouth and forces the milk out through the pores in the nipple. The tongue, in turn, moves backward and forward in a swallowing action that is well-coordinated with the suckling.

In Figure 6-7 the baby is poorly attached to the nipple. Because his mouth is not placed far enough back on the areola, his jaws cannot compress the lactiferous sinuses, and the whole position and movement of his tongue are disrupted.

Evaluating your baby's suck. Some mothers report that the baby's ears wiggle when he is nursing appropriately. This is probably a good sign, as it lets you know he is using his jaw in an appropriate up and down motion. The temples near his upper jaw will also move in and out. Here are some additional signs that your baby is suckling properly:[12]

1. Is his lower lip out and not tucked in?
2. Are his cheeks rounded and firm? If they are drawn in too much, he may be maintaining inadequate suction.
3. Is his tongue visible when you draw his lips aside? If not, it may be curled backwards instead of being placed properly beneath the nipple.
4. Can he be easily removed from the breast? If he is properly attached, you will have to put a finger in the corner of his mouth to break the suction in order to remove him comfortably from the breast.
5. Is there a noisy "drawing" sound of milk being removed from the breast during suckling? If he is improperly positioned, you will hear a soft, clicking sound.

To correct faulty positioning, depress the baby's tongue immediately before inserting the nipple. You might squirt a little milk into his mouth to get him to open up further. Another help may be tipping his head back just a bit, to position the nipple well up against the roof of his mouth.

Another approach to teaching your baby to suck is to encourage him to use an orthodontic rubber nipple, such as the Nuk®, between breastfeedings.

Proper Nipple Shape. The most important question for you in nipple preparation is to find out whether you have properly protractile nipples. There are tiny muscles around the nipple that contract with stimulation and allow the nipple to stick out for the baby to grasp it. You probably know if your nipples become erect when they are stimulated or cold. If the nipple remains flat, or shrinks in when it is stimulated, you may have inverted nipples. The test is to pinch your nipple (where it meets your breast) with thumb and forefinger. If the nipple contracts or shrinks back, it is considered inverted. One nipple may be inverted, the other not.

Figure 6-6. Proper infant suck.

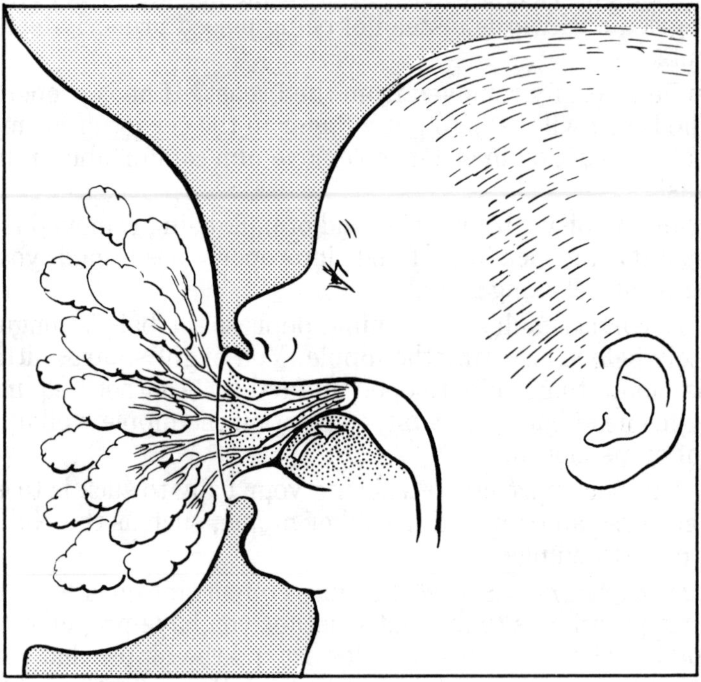

From Worthington-Roberts, Bonnie S.: Lactation and human milk: nutritional considerations. In Worthington-Roberts, Bonnie S., Vermeersch, Joyce, and Williams, Sue Rodwell: Nutrition in pregnancy and lactation, ed. 2, St. Louis, 1981, The C. V. Mosby Co.

Figure 6-7. Improper infant attachment to nipple.

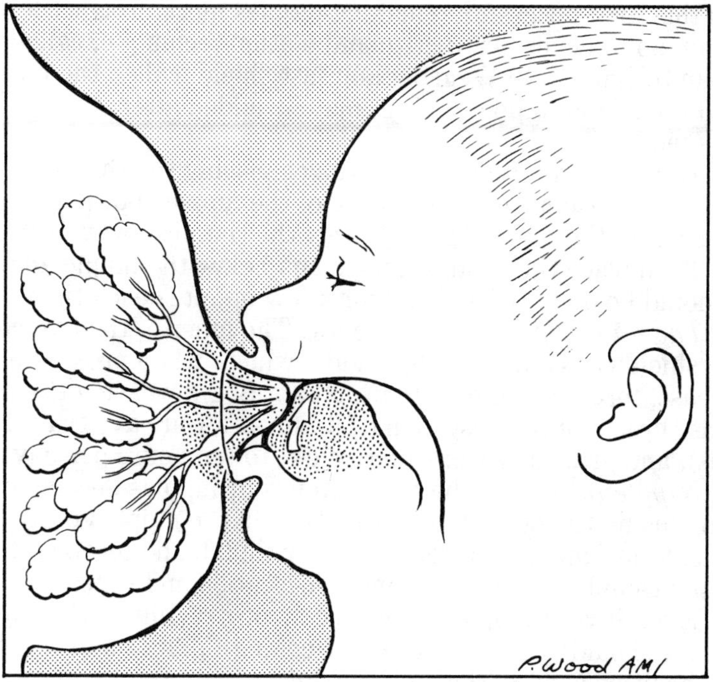

From Worthington-Roberts, Bonnie S.: Lactation and human milk: nutritional considerations. In Worthington-Roberts, Bonnie S., Vermeersch, Joyce, and Williams, Sue Rodwell: Nutrition in pregnancy and lactation, ed. 2, St. Louis, 1981, The C. V. Mosby Co.

Many times inverted nipples become protractile during pregnancy. However, if nipples are still flat or inverted during the third trimester, it will certainly be helpful and may be essential to work with them to make them more protractile. There are several techniques that are successful in making nipples more protractile. The two main approaches are, 1) A manipulation technique, called the Hoffman technique. 2) Wearing a breast shield, called the milk cup. A third technique, nipple rolling, may be added after the nipple can be grasped.[5]

The Hoffman Technique involves placing the thumbs opposite each other on either side of the base of the nipple and, pressing firmly against the breast, gently draw the thumbs away from each other. Then place the thumbs above and below the nipple and repeat. This should be done twice a day for a few minutes each time.

The milk cup is pictured below. The inner of the two concave plastic shields has a hole in the middle which, when pressed against the breast, forces the nipple to protrude. Begin wearing the cup as early as three months gestation (if it appears you have truly inverted nipples), and gradually work up to eight to ten hours per day.

Nipple rolling can be done after your nipples become protractile from using the other two methods. Pull the nipple gently but firmly outward and roll it between your thumb and forefinger. Then move the thumb and finger to another location and repeat.

Even if your nipples aren't nicely protractile by the time you deliver, it should not rule out breastfeeding. Many times a baby with a good healthy suck can bring them out.

Other Factors in Breastfeeding. Sometimes you can do everything right and breastfeeding simply will not work, for reasons that are outside of your control. If you are very sick, or your baby is very sick, it may make it impossible to breastfeed. Babies with heart defects sometimes don't have enough energy to take on the extra work of breastfeeding. Babies born with structural abnormalities, like cleft

Figure 6-8. The milk cup (Courtesy of Goldfarb and Tibbetts[3]).

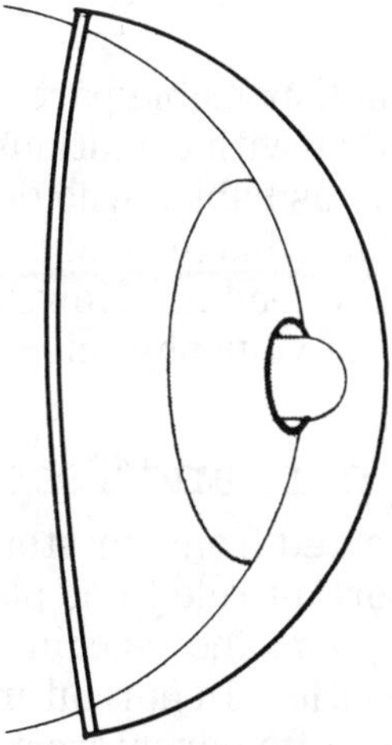

palate, have a harder time breastfeeding. If the cleft is severe and extensive, breastfeeding may even be impossible.* Tragically, some babies are born with insufficient neurological or muscular control to be able to breastfeed. And some babies have inborn errors of metabolism that demand highly specialized diets.

Sometimes babies who do poorly on breastfeeding will also do poorly on bottle feeding. Looking back at our *Thriving* table (p. 172), you will note that part of the infant contribution to breastfeeding is good absorption and retention, which, in turn, depend on a well-functioning stomach and intestine. Babies who have pyloric stenosis (nar-

*It may be possible for you to hand-express breastmilk and give it to your baby with a nipple especially designed for a cleft palate.

rowing of the passageway between the stomach and intestine), or who spit up excessively, may grow less rapidly than other babies, at least for a time. Often you will see catch-up growth once the problem is resolved.

Good health is an indispensible part of thriving. Babies with infections, lung problems, or with conditions requiring surgery, will not thrive in the same way as babies who do not have to struggle against such problems. These babies will likely do as well with breastfeeding as with bottle feeding. However, you must carefully evaluate this with the aid of your physician.

Support and Teaching

A second theme we extracted from our stories early on in the chapter was that there is an important role to be played in breastfeeding relationships—that of support and teaching. Breastfeeding goes better in more primitive societies. In our culture we say a baby is "born"—the child's birth shifts our interest away from mother to baby. In many cultures, it is said that at delivery a woman "becomes a mother," which keeps the emphasis on the mother.

In those cultures where breastfeeding is common and successful, there is a special system of support to help the young woman learn to mother. However, in those same cultures, with urbanization and mobility and moving away from traditional support systems, breastfeeding failure is increasing.

Dana Raphael, an anthropologist who has made a detailed study of lactation in primitive societies, calls this supportive function the *doula* role.[5] The doula is the supplier of information, the giver of physical and emotional support and the engenderer of confidence.

Unfortunately, we are too sophisticated in our society to have maintained this doula role. You may find, however, that it is worthwhile creating for yourself. You may be fortunate enough to have a mother or a special friend or a nurse, who can move in with you and provide for you for the first weeks after your baby is born. Most new parents, however, will have to draw on several resources to put together a well-functioning doula system for themselves.

Where would you find such resources?

1. Obstetrical care that informs, encourages and supports breastfeeding, both before and after delivery.
2. A hospital setting that will teach and support your early experiences with your baby and with breastfeeding.
3. A pediatric staff that is enthusiastically pro-breastfeeding, but also realistic enough about nutrition and lactation to provide careful follow-up of your breastfeeding experience.
4. A person experienced in lactation who is willing to talk with you before delivery about breastfeeding, and to stop by at frequent intervals afterwards, just to find out how things are going, and to offer information, encouragement and support.
5. Someone who is willing to point out to you over and over again how well you are doing.

Supportive Obstetrical Care. Because the whole birthing experience is such an intense one, the obstetrician, midwife, nurses, and nutritionists with whom you work before delivery become very important people in your life. If those people feel breastfeeding is important, their attitudes will provide good support for you. They are the ones who should begin to inform you about what to expect, and who should be able to help you if your nipples are flat or inverted.

Find out in detail about the routine at delivery. Breastfeeding goes better if you hold down on sedation and anesthesia, and if you have access to your baby early and often. Ask about sedation and make sure your baby can be with you in the delivery and recovery room.

Keep in mind that during labor and delivery you are likely to be very sensitive. Even a casual comment may seem to you to be serious criticism; conversely, a simple gesture of praise may be reassuring out of proportion. You are justified in looking for an obstetrician who seems supportive to you, and who is sensitive to your emotional as well as physical needs.

The Hospital Setting. Don't take anything for granted. Talk to the head nurse, the obstetrician, and the pediatrician to find out about hospital routines. Specifically, you need to find out if they encourage parents and babies to be together in the delivery room and right afterwards, whether they allow rooming in, whether they know how to instruct you in breastfeeding, and whether they refrain from giving formula to breastfed babies.

The most helpful hospital routines are the ones that encourage you to nurse according to the baby's needs, both while you are in the hospital and at home. Until about ten years ago, however, hospitals whisked the baby away immediately after birth, bathed him, and then popped him into a little warming oven to make sure his temperature was stabilized before he was returned to his parents. But routines are changing and you can likely find a hospital that encourages you to have access to your baby during that important, exciting, and extremely receptive time, right after birth.

Rooming in, as you probably already know, is having the baby in your room with you at the hospital. This is very important to you for getting comfortable with your baby and finding out you can soothe and comfort her and take care of her needs. If it is your first baby, you probably won't know the simplest tasks like diapering, holding, and burping. It may be terrifying to you to be left alone with your baby, and you may feel helpless at first about knowing what to do with a tiny baby.

You need a caring and supportive person to be there to coach you while you learn about breastfeeding and child care. This is the role that is best played by an obstetrical nurse.* About the only way

*Don't depend so much on the nurse that you don't really learn to do it yourself. Ask all the questions you can.

you can find out whether the attitude of the nurses is respectful and supportive is to talk with other mothers who have delivered and breastfed in the hospital. If you don't know anyone personally, ask for the names of some women who have delivered there recently, and talk with them about how they felt about their care and instruction.

Some hospitals give their nursing babies sugar (glucose) water during the time they are waiting for the breastmilk to come in, and sometimes even afterwards. The biggest problem this presents is that the rubber nipple on the glucose water bottle demands a different sucking pattern from that of the human nipple. It can be confusing to the baby. Water given from a spoon or through an eyedropper is much better.

While it may be better for the hospital to use plain water rather than glucose water, it may not be worth getting too excited about it. The five percent glucose water that is generally used has only about 20 calories in three ounces. Most babies won't take much more than half an ounce. (They seem to hold out for breastmilk, even if they get hungry before it comes in.) Using the water might help if it is reassuring to you to know that your baby is hydrated during that time, especially if your milk is somewhat slow to come in. And it certainly helps pediatricians relax.

The Pediatric Staff. The physician you choose to care for your baby is the person who will be most directly involved with your breastfeeding experience. About the only time your obstetrician will get involved, after birth, is if you have some problem with your breasts, like an infection. (If this fragmentation of professional relationships bothers you, you may find that you prefer to go to a general practitioner or a family practitioner.) The local breastfeeding grapevine will be able to tell you which physicians are knowledgeable and supportive with breastfeeding, and which ones merely tolerate it and tell you to give a bottle for every little thing that goes wrong.

Get acquainted with that person before your baby is born, discuss your plans to breastfeed, and get some of his ideas and attitudes about breastfeeding. Find out whether he is willing to do a two-week check, how he follows up on breastfeeding couples (does he call you or wait until you call him), and what he thinks about supplementing breastmilk and starting solids early.

Find out precisely who will be giving you the care at your doctor's office. You may spend more time in the office and on the phone with nurses or pediatric nurse practitioners or a physician's assistant than you will with the doctor. You may or may not like that. In any event you need to check out that person to make sure that you like her and find her knowledgeable and supportive. And don't hesitate to ask to speak and work with the person you want.

The Weight Check. Doctor's offices vary in their recommended frequency of well-baby exams. Around this area, it is fairly standard practice to give a baby a complete exam at age two weeks to a month, exams every two months after that until age six to seven months, then wait for the next examination until age one year. The nurse practitioners and office nurses also offer brief weight checks. These cost about one third to one half as much as the complete exam, depending on how much time the health worker spends counseling with the parent.*

While breastfed babies don't need any more well-baby exams, they may need more frequent weight checks than bottlefed babies. (Growth is, after all, your major measure of quantity of food intake.) Waiting to schedule the first well-baby exam at age one month is postponing it too long for a breastfeeding baby. You need to get in by two weeks to have your baby weighed and to get some feedback on your breastfeeding relationship.

Martha could have been helped greatly in getting through those difficult early weeks if she had come in two weeks earlier. And

---

*If you have an accurate beam (not spring) scale, you could do these in-between checks yourself at home and plot them on your own growth chart. If you feel, however, that you need support or information, it is worth the trip and the cost.

Janet could have found out her baby wasn't doing well, and adjusted her baby's breastfeeding routine, before she got so far behind. If your doctor doesn't regularly schedule a two-week weight check or well-baby exam, ask for it. It is probably also wise to get another weight check at age one month, and monthly after that until six months. As I said earlier, the three-month-old baby occasionally will fall off on weight gain. Further, the four- to six-month-old baby often changes his feeding patterns so dramatically that you will appreciate the reassurance of knowing things are actually going well.

Try to look at this weight check as an important help to you, and not as the product of a suspicious mind that thinks your breastfeeding is not going to work out. More and more physicians are becoming pro-breastfeeding. Making sure your baby is growing properly is a vital part of their role in caring for your little one. It is also an important way of assessing how well the breastfeeding is going and picking up on any problems.

Even if your pediatrician suggests a bottle at times, don't automatically assume that he is out to make your breastfeeding fail. Sometimes you just get so tired and worn out and tense and nervous that a relief bottle can help you rest and let your nerves unwind.

An Experienced Teacher and Support Person. You can do all of your studying and homework about breastfeeding, but once you get into the situation, you will still benefit from having someone to tell you what you already know. You need someone you know and trust to keep in touch with, by telephone or in person.

She should start when your baby is about a week old, when you are likely to be feeling isolated after leaving the hospital. Then she can remind you that it is normal for new babies to eat frequently, and reassure you that the decrease in the size of your breasts is not loss of milk, but only loss of the engorgement that goes along with early lactation. Or, better yet, she can listen to your concerns and allow you to figure all of that out for yourself.

It would be great if she would show up again at two to three weeks to find out about the weight check and help you deal with, or celebrate, your appointment with the doctor. Your baby is likely to be getting more alert and demanding about that time, and also you may be starting to put more demands on yourself, assuming that you are through the postpartum period. Both of these can combine to make a fussy baby, and may make you question whether breastfeeding is really worthwhile. Then it's important to have a gentle reminder to take care of yourself, and to remember that it really takes at least a good six weeks to get through that intensive new-baby learning experience.

It is also helpful to be reminded that the new-baby adjustment period is, even under the best of conditions, rather a challenging time. One woman observed that, for her, getting through that newborn time was no easier with her fifth baby than with the first. At six weeks postpartum, you can be usefully reminded that you are likely to encounter some hungry days, and be counseled about how to respond to them. You may see your breast size continue to dwindle, and appreciate the affirmation that mammary tissue is still there and functioning.

Your support person may be a good friend, a relative, a nurse or dietitian in the doctor's office, a community health nurse or nutritionist, or a member of a breastfeeding support group such as La Leche League. You may, in fact, find that going to breastfeeding support group meetings is a good way of getting the contact and reassurance that you need.

If you choose the support-group approach, it is best to get started going to the meetings before your baby is born. Generally, however, it works better during that early postpartum period if you have someone who will seek *you* out. (The support group might help provide you with this person.) You are likely to be shy and not too assertive during that early postpartum time, and perhaps a bit embarrassed about asking questions that you fear may be naive. Watch out, however, for advice and "support" from women who did not breastfeed their own babies, or who had an unsuccessful breastfeeding experience. They could be unintentionally but ever-so-subtly undermining. And feel no pressure to accept any advice you don't agree with—whether the advisor is experienced with breastfeeding or not.

If you are fortunate enough to have a helper come to the house, remember that you need someone to focus attention on *you* so you can learn to be a mother. Your helper should encourage you to relax, to nap when the baby does, and to let her take care of the house, laundry and cooking while you devote yourself to your baby's and your own well-being.

Someone to Prop You Up (Advice to Fathers). A new mother is in an emotionally and physically dependent position and needs to be mothered. This role is often played by the father, and if you are a new father, you know it is not an easy role to play. You are doing your own adjusting about that time. Your responsibilities have increased tremendously, your life and schedule have been disrupted, and in most cases you are naive about what to expect or how to cope with a new baby. At the same time, you may find your partner to be experiencing considerable psychological and physical changes, and in many cases, having difficulty adjusting to the tremendous responsibility of the new baby—and being depressed or emotionally labile.

If the baby is being breastfed, your role is even more important and difficult, because you will have to be reassuring and supportive about a process about which you probably know little.

To negotiate all of this successfully, you need to be informed about breastfeeding. You can read and talk to health professionals, to make yourself knowledgeable about the process and about what to expect. Other experienced fathers can be a good help to you if you know how to ask. Men often are not as good at this as women; they tend to joke about their difficulties, rather than seek other men's help in finding their way out of them. But if you let other men know that you value their experience and sincerely want some advice in problem solving, I think they will come through for you.

You will be a big help to the breastfeeding if you offer reassurance and comfort at the tough spots. Both of you may know you are ignorant and inexperienced, but still your opinion that things appear to be going along just fine carries a lot of weight. You can help your partner gain confidence as a parent and breastfeeder. And you can also expect some help with that process for yourself.

It helps a great deal if you can just be there. Having you in the house to fall back on when things get tough is tremendously comforting and reassuring, even if you don't do anything. And of course, you can help out in a very concrete way by regulating the phone calls and the visitors, and protecting your partner from advisors who are critical of breastfeeding. You can also pay lots of attention to any older children, and see that meals are on the table, the laundry done and the house is reasonably picked up.

Breastfeeding While Working. You may be able to breastfeed your baby when you go back to work or you may not. I think it is worth making the effort. At the very least, you will be able to postpone the time when you will have to wean your baby totally from the breast. At the very most, you will be able to work full time, and provide your baby with enough breastmilk to fill all (or almost all) of his milk-feeding needs. Most likely your experience will turn out being somewhere between the extremes—you may be able to breastfeed totally, if you work less than full time, or be able to provide less than all of your baby's nutritional needs if you work full time.

You will need to think about a couple of things if you are planning to work and continue breastfeeding. First, is it your goal to provide your baby with breastmilk, only, and not use formula at all? Or is it acceptable to you to allow your baby to have formula at times when you can't be there, and maintain your breastmilk supply for the regular times when you will be with him?

Insisting on breastmilk only will mean that you must learn to hand-express your milk and to store and handle it properly for bottle or cup-feeding. Stimulating your breasts with hand expression on work days, when you are separated from your baby, will help maintain your breastmilk supply so you will be able to breastfeed totally (perhaps with some catch-up increase in frequency), on weekends and days off.* If you decide on a combination of formula and breastmilk, you will probably have to continue with the same schedule of formula substitutes and bottle feedings on days off that you follow on work days.

Keep in mind that it isn't totally going to be your decision about how you manage your working and breastfeeding. Babies respond in a variety of ways when their mothers go back to work. One will go on a virtual hunger strike during the day, seemingly refusing to eat until mom shows up, then nurse and make up for it at night. Another will begin to prefer the bottle and wean himself from the breast (this occasionally happens during the distractible four to six-month age range). But most babies will take a bottle willingly—as long as it is offered by someone other than mother—and nurse happily when they get the chance.

Managing the feeding schedule. Assuming that your breastfeedings while you are working will be more limited, it is most important that they be as calm and unhurried as possible. It is ideal if your baby is ready to eat as soon as you get home, and if you are able to sit down and relax and feed for as long as you both want to. Morning feedings should be equally unhurried. Particularly if you have older children, accomplishing that demands a cooperative partner who is willing to take on child care and food preparation at those times.

Some working mothers increase the number of evening, night and morning feedings to compensate for absences during the day.

---

*You have a better chance of eliminating bottles on days off if you are working less than full time.

They might take the baby to bed with them to allow more-frequent feedings during the night. While that can be effective, you might not be comfortable about having your baby in bed with you. But at least one middle-of-the-night feeding is important to help you to keep up your breastmilk supply after you return to work.

An ideal situation, of course, is to have your child-care setting close enough to your work place so you can go and nurse when your baby needs it. But even if your baby is not that handy, you still might be able to reach him over the lunch hour. Babies can be quite adaptable and patient at waiting to be breastfed at certain times, if it becomes clear to them that their only other alternative is the bottle.

In any event, you will need a cooperative and supportive child-care person to work with you; to persuade your baby to wait a little longer until you get home to breastfeed; to encourage a reluctant baby to take a bottle when he would rather be breastfed (and to reassure you through those first difficult days that "things will get better"); and perhaps to provide a quiet place for you to breastfeed.

If you are relying on frozen breastmilk, have your sitter plan to start out by thawing about four ounces of breastmilk. Most babies take somewhere around this amount, and you don't want to waste the precious stuff. If that amount is too little for your baby, he will let you know—by asking for more right away, or, by demanding to be fed again after a relatively short time.

Making the transition to work. If your goal is to manually express and provide for all of your baby's nutritional needs, study the information in the next sections. If you are planning to use formula during your working hours, select one of the formulas we discussed in the *Milk* chapter (chapter 5).

Be sure your baby knows how to take a bottle by the time you return to work—your partner will likely have to undertake that teaching project, as most babies won't take a bottle from their breastfeeding mothers. It is a good idea to start to feed your baby a bottle once or twice a week by the time he is three to four weeks old. By that time your milk supply should be established, and your baby will still be flexible about switching from breast to bottle. Some breastfed babies do better with a Nuk® nipple. Have the sitter feed breastmilk or formula on demand through most of the day, but hold off toward the end of the day so your baby will be ready to nurse soon after you get back.

When you get back to work, your breasts will feel overfull and may leak during the day, but quite soon your daytime supply will adjust to the demand, and you will be comfortable again.

Storing breastmilk. Breastmilk is extremely perishable—it must be properly handled and stored to keep it safe and nutritious for your baby. Probably the best and easiest approach is to store it in new plastic bags (these are sterile). Some people have found the disposal liners from baby bottles to be cheap and handy; others use Ziploc® or other food storage bags.

Breastmilk stored in plastic bags freezes quickly and can be thawed quickly under cold running water. New plastic bags have the advantage of being sterile, cheap and available. Some of milk's anti-infective properties will adhere to glass, but not to plastic, but that's really only a consideration for the baby who gets most of his breastmilk by bottle (e.g., an ill or premature baby).

Breastmilk may be kept unfrozen for no more than 24 hours. If you are planning to freeze it, you should do so immediately after you collect it. Freeze and store breastmilk at 0 degrees fahrenheit or lower, and keep it for no longer than a month.* If breastmilk is stored too long, the fat separates out, the protein clumps, and it gets bad-tasting. Rotate your supply of breastmilk in the freezer, using the oldest first.

---

*This storage time is recommended by Robert Bradley, Ph.D., a food scientist, on the basis of his research on freezing milk.

You may pour it into a regular bottle to feed it, or use one of the bottles intended for the disposable liner, if you have used that for storage. Discard any unused breastmilk after the feeding.

Some women can get eight ounces of breastmilk at a time when they hand express. Most express only a couple of ounces at a time and accumulate breastmilk stores gradually. You can freeze small amounts as you go along and combine them in the same container, as long as the quantity you are adding (the just-collected, liquid milk) does not exceed the amount you have frozen. Putting too much liquid milk in with the frozen milk will thaw it, impair the quality, and may even allow a small amount of bacterial growth.

You can manually remove milk from your breasts by hand expression, or you can use a breast pump. Either method starts with breast massage. For either method, express for three to five minutes on each breast at first and work up to ten to fifteen.

Milk will initially be ejected in small spurts and then will flow freely. But don't worry if nothing comes out the first few times you try—you'll soon get the knack of it.

As you express, you may find that repeating the massage briefly helps to work the milk down. You may also find it helpful to switch from one breast to another, as one breast lets down milk in response to stimulus from the other.

Breast massage. Wash your hands and expose your breasts. Stroke from the outside edge of the breast toward the nipple, applying gentle but firm pressure with the palms of your hands. Alternate your hands as you work around your breast, stroking from the shoulder down, the side in, the waist up, and the breastbone in. Massage around each breast several times before you make any attempt to manually express milk.

Hand expression. Some people feel that hand expression is faster and easier than using a breast pump, while others argue the opposite. It appears to be a matter of individual preference and capability, and is really up to you which you prefer.

Leaning over a sterile container for catching the milk, place your thumb and index finger on your areola behind the nipple, about an inch back from the nipple (this will be right over the lactiferous sinuses). *As you press gently inward toward the chest wall*, squeeze the thumb and finger together gently: push back and squeeze.

Keep that thumb and finger in the same position until no more milk comes out, then rotate to another position and repeat.

Repeat the massage on the other breast before beginning to express from that breast.

Breast pumps. All breast pumps have a funnel-shaped flange that comes in contact with your nipple. The flange is placed against the breast and the milk removed by suction. The source of power used to provide the suction may be electricity, water, or manual (using a squeeze ball, a squeeze gun, or a piston action).

Electric pumps are efficient, but expensive, so you are better off renting rather than buying. Hospitals, clinics, breastfeeding support groups and hospital supply stores often have electric breast pumps for rent. A popular new hand pump is sold both as the Happy Family® breast pump and as the Marshall® breast pump. This uses a cyclinder and piston action, and costs between $20 and $30.

To use a breast pump, first massage your breast before you start expressing milk. Moisten the flange of the pump with water or the first few drops of milk to lubricate and to allow the flange to make a better seal with your breast. Let your nipple slide along the inside of the top part of the flange of the pump. This sliding is important for contact to stimulate the letdown reflex.

Hold the flange just tightly enough against your breast to make a good seal, but not so tightly that you dig the flange into your breast and pinch off the flow of milk. Stop pumping one minute after the milk has slowed, and break the seal by pressing your finger against your breast where it contacts the flange.

After each use, make sure that you thoroughly wash all parts of the collecting apparatus that comes in contact with the milk. Rinse thoroughly, and allow to air dry.

As with breastfeeding in general, you cannot predict or force an ideal experience with breastfeeding while working. Some babies won't cooperate. Manual expression doesn't provide enough stimulation to maintain breastmilk supply in some cases, and some mothers find they don't like manual expression. But even if you have to provide less breastmilk or stop nursing earlier than you want to, remember that your baby benefits from any breastfeeding, whether it is partial or full, or continued for a day, a week or several months. Any time you have spent nursing is important and worthwhile: don't let the fact of a limited experience spoil that for you.

In all cases, the important thing is providing your baby and yourself with a positive and productive experience.

Problems With Breastfeeding

Breastfeeding is an association between two people which, like any other intimate relationship, may take some negotiating and managing if it is to work out well for both parties. The fact that problems crop up is no sign that breastfeeding is going poorly, but rather a common part of the process that you can hope to more-or-less take in stride as you work out your system.

Many women are finding they have to work out a method for breastfeeding while working. This is a "problem" that has a number of satisfactory solutions. Working or not, you may have problems with your breasts. You may have to work with your baby to encourage an optimum response to breastfeeding. You may have to use medications, or you may have to deal with relactation or inducing lactation.

Breast Problems. You may have problems with your breasts and nipples like leaking, engorgement, soreness, caking, plugging, and infections. Keep in mind that it is common to have these problems simultaneously, and that most or all of them can be related to failure to empty the breasts adequately. Inhibited letdown leads to engorgement, which, in turn, causes nipple soreness as the infant chews at the nipple to get at the milk. Many times caking and plugging, which refer to blocking of a duct with hardened milk, is caused by failure to adequately and completely empty an area of the breast.

Milk staying too long in a particular area of the breast can lead to breast infections. If, in turn, the infection is not controlled, it can get worse and cause an abscess or breakdown in breast tissue. This last condition is very serious indeed, and can be one of the few conditions that demands weaning.

To prevent most problems, nurse more frequently and for moderate lengths of time, especially early on, and use both breasts at most feedings. Most breastfeeding problems can be prevented or cured with frequent and adequate emptying of the breasts.

Leaking. Some women leak more than others, and some are more annoyed and embarrassed by it than others. To manage leaking, you can learn the tactic of putting firm pressure against your nipples to stop the leaking.* Fold your arms across your breasts and press them firmly toward the chest wall. You may also press with your thumbs and forefingers directly on the nipple. Some women use a breast cup to catch the leaks. (Don't use the cup to collect milk for feeding—it's too easy to let it become contaminated.) It is better to use absorbent pads than plastic liners to protect your clothing, but either can hold moisture on your skin and cause irritation.

Engorgement. This is the accumulation of milk in early lactation. Engorged breasts are hot, heavy and hard, with milk, but also

---

*Although this may not be such a good tactic if you are prone to plugged ducts.

probably more with the swelling that accompanies the beginning of lactation. This usually occurs on the first full day of milk production and lasts about 24 hours. Again, your best approach is to nurse early and often. To help your baby attach to the nipple, which may be stretched flat by the swelling, you may have to hand express some milk. You certainly will have to compress the areola just under your nipple between thumb and forefinger to help it raise up and allow the baby to grasp it well.

Sore Nipples. The parts of the nipple that get the greatest stress during nursing are: a) the points at the corners of the baby's mouth that are compressed by nursing and b) the part of the nipple and areola that is stroked by the baby's tongue. Varying the nursing position (sitting, lying, football hold*) is important to vary the points of stress. You can also lie down and put your baby upside down to nurse, that is, with his feet up toward your head. This is awkward and somewhat unsatisfying, but helps put the stress in a completely different place. You also get a closeup view of your baby's toes wiggling with the pleasure of nursing.

Also check to make sure that your baby is getting the nipple and areola well into his mouth and that he is not hanging on to the nipple.

Plugged Duct. This will show up as a red and tender area on the breast, behind the areola. To help unplug that area of the breast, take a hot shower and massage the breast from well behind the plugged area toward the nipple while the hot water flows over the breast. Nurse immediately afterward, again massaging the affected area, and the nursing will probably dislodge the plug.

Breast Infections. The first symptom of a breast infection may be like the flu: generalized aching and fatigue and elevated temperature. In fact, if you have flu-like symptoms, you should assume you

---

*Hold your baby on his back under your arm, head forward, as if he were a football.

have a breast infection until you have seen your doctor. After several hours an area of redness and soreness may develop, although this generally appears before the other symptoms.

Don't wean. The infection is best handled, and a more-serious condition more-likely prevented (such as breast abscess) if you keep the milk moving and keep on emptying your breast. In fact, some people even avoid antibiotics, and recommend the same treatment for breast infection as for a plugged duct. If you choose this approach, however, you should keep in touch with your doctor and look for improvement within 24 hours. If the infection doesn't get any better by then, you would be wise to begin taking antibiotics while continuing with the other suggestions. Again, you don't have to wean. The quantity of antibiotic that the baby will get is unlikely to cause a problem, but ask your doctor and your baby's doctor to OK the medication.

Breast Abscess. This is a pronounced infection in a local area of the breast, accompanied by flu-like symptoms and a clearly-defined, red, hot, painful area in the breast. Breast abscess is an infrequent problem that almost always follows abrupt weaning in the face of mastitis. It is a condition that is very serious indeed, and requires surgical drainage (like opening a boil) for treatment. You probably won't be able to nurse from an abscessed breast until it is completely healed.

A breast abscess is best avoided by continued frequent nursing and prompt treatment of mastitis.

Relactation. This is resumption of breastfeeding following cessation or significant decrease in milk production. To accomplish this requires time, patience and a cooperative baby. Babies under three months are generally more willing to cooperate with the required sucking than older babies.

While you wait for your mammary tissue to get started functioning again, you will have to use some system of feeding your baby formula. You may want to breastfeed, then offer a bottle afterwards. The exceptional baby may be able to take a good amount of formula from a cup. Or you may want to use the Lact-Aid® nursing trainer (see picture below). These devices are a bother to clean and fill, but they do have the advantage of nourishing the baby at the breast, eliminating prolonged feeding times, and stimulating the proper suckling reflex.

Success of Relactation. A study in Nebraska of 366 women who attempted relactation[1] showed varying degrees of success. However, most women who went through the process felt positive about it, and their good feelings really had very little to do with either the length of time they nursed their baby or with their baby's need for supplementary formula.

Most mothers stressed as important the impact that nursing had on their relationship with their baby. When the mother stressed milk production itself as a goal, she was less likely to have been satisfied with her relactation experience. In fact, striving to produce a certain amount of milk was more likely to present a barrier to her in increasing her milk supply.

Induced lactation. Most adoptive parents choose to bottlefeed their baby, and that's fine. Breastfeeding an adoptive child, without benefit of the priming of pregnancy, is a more difficult process. But given a healthy newborn with a strong sucking need, and a truly committed mother with patience and understanding, apparently it is possible to provide at least part of the baby's milk requirements through induced lactation.[5]

A Lact-Aid® nursing trainer (figure 6-9)* appears to be a very helpful part of the process, with quantities of formula adjusted to mandate a frequent nursing schedule. You can tell by the character

---

*Lact-Aid is available through the mail from Lact-Aid, Box 6861, Denver, CO 80206, or through authorized Lact-Aid representatives.

of the baby's stool when breastmilk is being produced (it gets less formed and less smelly on breastmilk), and can gradually decrease on the amount of formula, until you are providing your maximum amount of breastmilk—which may or may not satisfy all of your baby's need.

Figure 6-9. Lact-Aid® nursing trainer (Courtesy of Goldfarb and Tibbetts[5]).

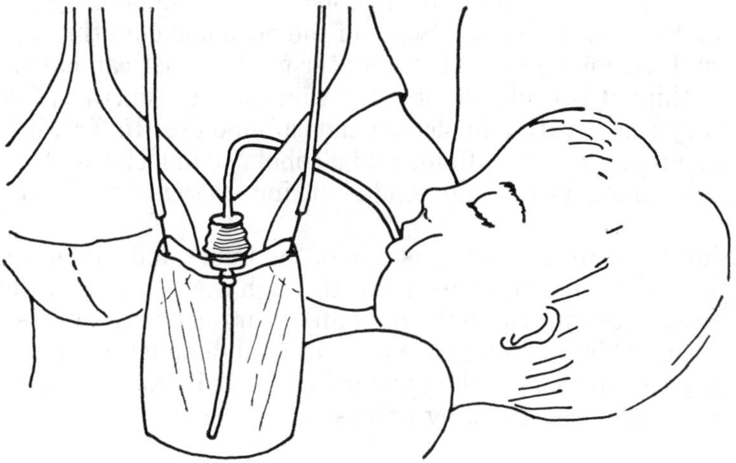

Again, don't judge your experience as a success or failure solely by the amount of breastmilk you produce. Your baby may need to get all or nearly all of his nourishment from supplementary sources, and yet still be benefitting psychologically from nursing at the breast.

Drugs. It is best to use *all* drugs as little as possible during nursing. You'll need to avoid a few drugs that present a significant risk to a breastfed baby. These are listed below in Figure 6-10. All other drugs are best consumed right after nursing, so your body has some time to clear them away before the next feeding. Still other common drugs in low doses, such as caffeine, alcohol, and oral contraceptives, deserve special consideration.

Caffeine may interfere with relaxation, both for you and the baby. Alcohol does get through to the baby, and how much is a reasonable dose? We don't know. Birth control pills, especially the higher-dosage ones, have been accused of (and defended against) decreasing breastmilk supply. Some of the hormone gets through to the baby, and we don't know what long-term effect that can have.

I think it is probably best to avoid the oral contraceptives and to be very conservative in alcohol and caffeine use. In fact, it is probably wise to limit your caffeine and alcohol use in lactation to no more than those amounts I recommended during pregnancy (pp. 67-8).

Cesarian Section. It is the passage of the infant and the placenta from the uterus, not the movement through the birth canal, that stimulates lactation. Breastfeeding after surgical birth differs from that of vaginal birth only in the amount of abdominal tenderness you are likely to experience when you hold your baby for breastfeeding. Otherwise, the breastfeeding process is the same.

Baby Problems. With breastfeeding, you have breast problems and you have baby problems. Some babies may need a little different strategy in management. For their benefit, here are a few tips you may find helpful.

The Fat Baby. As you read the chapters on *Calories and Normal Growth*, *Food Regulation*, and *Obesity*, you will find a consistent emphasis on not getting all excited about the baby who appears to be fat. However, some babies do seem to want a lot of sucking, and

Figure 6-10. Abbreviated Guide to Drug Therapy in Nursing Mothers.

Drugs viewed as safe if used in moderation	
Aspirin	Most antihistamines
Antidiarrheal agents	Insulin
Most antibiotics	Epinephrine

Drugs viewed as potentially harmful if used recklessly	
Sulfonamides*	Steroids
Oral contraceptives**	Diazepam (Valium)
Chloramphenicol**	Diuretics
Lithium carbonate	Nalidixic acid
Reserpine	Barbiturates
Theophylline	Phenytoin
Narcotics (including codeine)	

Drugs contraindicated for nursing mothers	
Iodides	Atropine
Radioactive agents	Metronidazole (Flagyl)
Anticoagulants	Bromides
Tetracycline	Propylthiouracil
Antimetabolites	Dihydrotachysterol
Ergot preparations	Most cathartics***

From Worthington-Roberts, Bonnie S., and Taylor, Lynda E.: Guidance for lactating mothers. In Worthington-Roberts, Bonnie S., Vermeersch, Joyce, and Williams, Sue Rodwell: Nutrition in pregnancy and lactation, ed. 2, St. Louis, 1981, The C. V. Mosby Co.

*Probably contraindicated during the first month of the infant's life.

**If utilized at all, the "Minipill" is suggested, with observation of the baby for possible hormone effects.

***Milk of magnesia and nondigestible fibers are safe; mineral oil in moderation is also safe.

some do seem to fill up a lot of their spare time by demanding to be fed. With such a child, you will want to be sure that you are not overfeeding. These tactics may be helpful:

- Nurse on one breast instead of two at a feeding—if your baby will stand for it.
- Learn and use a variety of soothing and entertaining techniques for your baby between feeds.
- Before you feed, routinely sort out the other possible reasons for fussing, such as wetness or loneliness.
- Offer water between feedings.

If, however, you do all these things, and you find your baby is still hungry and pressing to be fed, go ahead and feed. You are not trying to deprive him of food with these tactics; you are simply making sure that it *is* food that he wants and not simply more sucking, more soothing or more entertaining.

The Colicky Baby. Some babies cry and appear to be in pain for part or almost all of the time they are awake. They apparently have nothing wrong with them, but they are not to be comforted, seemingly no matter what you do. Other babies are fussy, more or less all of the time. They tend to do well physically, because they often are fed in response to their fussiness.

With fussy and irritable babies, it is important to know a lot of soothing and comforting techniques, such as swaddling, rocking, short-term crying, music, noise, carrying in a baby carrier, or using a pacifier or baby swing. Search baby books, talk to health workers and other parents, and see if you can come up with some helpful techniques. Sometimes, however, the only helpful technique is giving your baby time to grow out of being a newborn and into being an older, more organized and more placid baby.

The Placid Baby. This baby, like Janet's baby, is often "so good" that she makes poor weight gain. With this child, rather than soothing, you need stimulating techniques.

Increase your contact with your baby, and try not to leave her in her crib when she is awake. Nurse frequently, even if it has to be your idea. If your baby drifts off before nursing well, stroke her under the chin, from throat to mouth, while she nurses. Interrupt the nursing with diaper changing to get her more wide awake, or give her a bath before nursing to stimulate her a little bit.

The Main Points

Once again, we are back where we started. Remember, to do well with breastfeeding,

- Nurse early and often
- Take care of yourself by eating well and resting well
- Enjoy your baby

Selected References

1. Auerback, K. G. and J. L. Avery. Relactation: a study of 366 cases. Pediatrics 65:236–242. 1980.
2. Committee on Nutrition. Nutrition and lactation. Pediatrics. 58:435–443. 1981.
3. Cunningham, A. S. Morbidity in breast fed and artificially fed infants. Journal of Pediatrics 95:685–689. 1979.
4. Gilmore, H. E. and T. W. Rowland. Critical malnutrition in breast-fed infants. American Journal of Diseases of Children 134:885–887. 1978.
5. Goldfarb, J. and E. Tibbetts. Breastfeeding Handbook. Enslow. New Jersey. 1980.
6. Illingworth, R. S. and B. Kilpatrick. Lancet. 265:1175. 1953.
7. Jakobsson, I.and T. Lindberg. Cow's milk as a cause of infantile colic in breast-fed infants. Lancet 26 August 1978.

8. Naismith, D. J. Maternal nutrition and the outcome of pregnancy—a critical appraisal. From Symposium on Nutrition of the Mother and Child. Proceedings of the Nutrition Society. 39: 1980.
9. Nichols, B. L. and V. M. Nichols. Human milk: nutritional resource. In Nutrition and Child Health: Perspectives for the 1980s. 190–246. 1981.
10. O'Connor, P.A. Failure to thrive with breast feeding. Clinical Pediatrics 17:833–835. 1978.
11. Reeve, Lorraine E. R. W. Chesney and H. F. DeLuca. Vitamin D of human milk: identification of biologically active forms. The American Journal of Clinical Nutrition. 36:122–126. 1982.
12. Riordan, J. and B. A. Countryman. Basics of breast-feeding Parts III–VI. Journal of Obstetrical and Gynecological Nursing 9:273–282, 357–366. 1980.
13. Widdowson, Elsie M. Nutrition and lactation. In Winick, W. Nutritional Disorders of American Women. Wiley. New York. 1977.
14. Worthington-Roberts, B. S. and L. E. Taylor. Guidance for lactating mothers. In Worthington-Roberts, B. S. et al. Nutrition in Pregnancy and Lactation. C. V. Mosby. St. Louis. 1981.

7

Introduction of Solid Foods to the Infant Diet

The infant makes a transition in feeding, between ages 4 to 12 months, from all breastmilk or formula to table foods. Foods added during that transition period must be appropriate both nutritionally and developmentally; they must provide the needed nutrients as well as textures and consistencies that will stimulate the child to learn more mature eating styles.

Iron-fortified infant rice cereal, added at 4-7 months, is a good first solid food; it gives iron, and provides a smooth, semi-liquid texture that is helpful as a first food. Later it can be thickened up, as the child's mouth skills progress. The next addition, at 6–8 months, of cooked or soft fruits and vegetables that are mashed or chopped, offer vitamins A and C and a lumpier texture that encourages more tongue control and chewing. "Finger" breads and cereals added about the same time encourage finger dexterity and hand-mouth coordination, as well as supplementing the B vitamins and iron in the diet. The change to "table foods" at 7–10 months is a change in degree only, since the child should be increasingly encouraged to eat family fare and helped to adhere to the family eating schedule.

The final transition, from breastmilk or formula to whole pasteurized milk, can be made once a child is eating three meals a day (plus snacks as needed), and getting a good assortment of foods from the basic-four food plan.

People behave as if there were rules, carved in stone, about feeding solid foods to infants. Each culture and age has had a protocol for guiding the nursing infant through the transition from suckling and milk-feeding to an eating style that resembles that of the adult. And each age has had its prejudices about what is good and bad for infants.

In the early part of this century infants were kept on breast milk until they were about a year old.[6] People were afraid to feed their babies solid foods: they thought the babies would get sick, or at least not do as well on anything but breast milk. Maybe they were right. At that time many were dependent upon an erratic food supply, and unreliable sanitation and refrigeration: depending on solid foods was dangerous for some.

Gradually, people began to get a little more adventurous about earlier introduction to solid food—as they looked for a substitute and a supplement for breast feeding. Nutrition was a developing science, bringing with it an awareness of the importance of a diversified diet. In 1923, a German doctor published a paper describing his rearing of 12 infants on a completely milk-free diet. The infants ate well and developed normally. There was scientific support for the new concept.[6]

During the mid-1930's people began to overcome their earlier fear of feeding solid foods before age one year. During that period one vitamin after another was being discovered, and the role of nutrition in deficiency illnesses began to be understood. Finally, in 1936 the American Medical Association recommended the introduction of solid foods by age four to six months to provide vitamins, iron and "possible other factors," and because of "psychological benefits on food habits."[6]

In 1943, a physician searching for ways of supplementing breastfeeding created a sensation when he successfully fed babies four to eight weeks old sardines in oil, creamed tuna fish, salmon, shrimp, and mashed peas and carrots.[6]

People didn't stop at just pushing children in their food selection; they also pushed their feeding in other ways. A 1956 article in a professional journal recommended beginning feeding of solid food on the second or third day of life, and encouraged omitting the night feeding by age 15 days. After that, the infants were to continue on three meals per day.[6]

The trend to early solids was so energetic that the *Committee on Nutrition** issued a position paper in 1958[6] cautioning against early supplementation with solid foods. They argued that feeding solids before four to six months really didn't accomplish much, and they gave three months as the earliest starting date. But even that recommendation was viewed as calling for an incredible delay. It was ignored until the 1970's, when the trend shifted in the opposite direction. Now the 1958 paper seems conservative. Pity the poor Committee that got caught in the transition.

Now the nursing and milk-feeding period is again being prolonged. Solid foods introduction is being postponed until four to six months of age, or even later. Once again, people are fearful of changing, and worried that perhaps this "new" feeding style will be wrong or bad for their babies.

---

*The Committee on Nutrition of the American Academy of Pediatrics is made up of physicians. They regularly review topics of nutritional concern and publish position papers in the journal *Pediatrics*.

Perhaps parents are looking for what they simply can't have in that age between four months and a year: predictability. In truth, the whole time from the end of the nursing period, which is signaled by the introduction of solid foods, to the establishment of the child on table foods, is one of constant transition, as you can see by the table below.

Developmental Patterns and Feeding Recommendations

During the period from six to twelve months, the baby adds mouth skills. He must first learn to transfer "prechewed" food from the front of his mouth to the back. He progresses until eventually he can take in, or even bite off, pieces of soft food and use his tongue to position the food so he can crush and pulp it with his jaw. He adds hand coordination, as he first learns to capture things by folding his fingers over his palm in a palmar grasp, and then uses his finger and thumb independently and in opposition to each other in the pincer grasp. He learns to control his body so he can sit to be fed and eventually feed himself. His digestive ability and homeostatic ability become more flexible and less prone to disruption. And as the result of all these developmental changes, he adds eating styles, as he struggles with accommodating to spoon feeding by someone else, and, eventually, to being able to feed himself.

The infant in transition changes his feeding schedule from one that caters to his hunger rhythm to one that interacts with and is affected by the family eating schedule. And his eating progression reflects his growth in other ways. Eating becomes more of a social event, and the baby's attention broadens out from his primary caretaker to other members of the family and other aspects of his environment. He becomes aware of the texture of the food, the splash it makes when it drops on the floor, the way the dog darts after it, and the way his parents jump up and run for a cloth.

Figure 7-1. Developmental Patterns and Feeding Recommendations

	6 mo.	7 mo.	8 mo.	9 mo.	10 mo.	11 mo.	12 mo.	13 mo.	14 mo.	15 mo.	16 mo.
Mouth Pattern:	Beginning swallow pattern. Can transfer food from front of tongue to back.		Beginning chewing pattern: side-to-side motion of tongue and mashing food with jaws.				Continuing maturation of biting, chewing, swallowing.				
Hand Coordination:	Palmar grasp.	Pincer grasp beginning.	Grabs spoon		Can get spoon in mouth but generally turns it over.		Beginning mastery of spoon—still spilling most times.			Spoon to mouth—with load intact!	
	Urge to put anything in mouth continues until about age three. Increases risk for poisoning throughout this time.										
Body Control:	Sits unsupported. Can balance while manipulating with hands.		Continuing improvement in balance while sitting.								
		Begins to stand. Can pull self to feet and move around.					Beginning and increasing mastery of walking				
Digestive:		Gastric acid volume begins to increase.			Can handle balanced amounts of all reasonably soft, moderately-seasoned family food.						
Homeostatic Ability:		Increasing ability to maintain hydration and chemical balance.									
Nutritional Requirements:	Iron stores begin to be depleted in term babies.		Gradually increasing proportion of adequate diet offered by foods other than milk feeding.							All daily nutritional requirements provided by a mixed table food diet: Primary source of nutrients and calories is table food and cup.	
Feeding Style:	Spoon feeding.	Introduce cup at meals.		Begin self-feeding with cup. Beginning proficiency with spoon.						Reasonably adept with spoon and cup. Can feed self with spoon, drink from cup. Weaned from bottle. Continuance of breast-feeding up to baby and parents.	
Food Selection:	Semi-solid foods	Increase texture, stiffness of solids			Pieces of soft, cooked foods						

The remarkable thing about all of this changing is that he does it in such a short time. The four-to-six month old is still being cuddled for nursing. He may be wolfing down his feeding, or periodically jerking his mouth off the nipple and craning his neck so he won't miss out on what is going on, but he is still, essentially, being suckled. However, by the time he is 10 months old, or even eight months old, he is probably sitting up at the table with the rest of the family, eating what they eat, and quite possibly even feeding himself.

When we encounter feeding problems during this stage, it is often because parents aren't aware of the transitory nature of it all. They allow themselves to get into a feeding routine, and fail to progress when their child is ready. You simply must not allow yourself to settle down to any feeding routine during this stage. The only thing you can plan on is change.

Let's get to work. We are going to discuss when, what and how: *When* to start and progress with solid foods and feeding styles; *what* are appropriate food choices to satisfy nutritional and developmental needs; and *how* you go about starting and progressing with solid foods. Again, to give you a road map so you don't get lost in the detail, here is a feeding chart that summarizes the basic recommendations.

Solid Foods Addition in Brief

You can get through the transition period with a minimum of hassle if you start solid foods late and progress quickly to table food. It is only when you start early—say before five months of age—that you have to struggle with feeding spoons and baby-food warmers, little jars of baby food, and pureeing your own.

It's a lot easier on you, and better for your baby, if you wait to start solid foods until she is ready for them. Somewhere between four and seven months of age your baby will be sitting up, drooling, and opening her mouth when she sees something approaching. Those

Figure 7-2. Feeding Schedule: Six to Twelve Months

	4–7 months*	6–8 months	7–10 months	10–12 months
Milk Feeding	Breastmilk or Formula	Breastmilk or Formula	Breastmilk or Formula	Breastmilk or formula Evaporated milk diluted 1:1 with water Whole pasteurized milk OR COMBINATION
Cereal and bread	Begin iron—fortified baby cereal mixed with milk feeding	Continue baby cereal. Begin other breads and cereals	Continue baby cereal. Other breads and cereals from table	Continue baby cereal until 18 months. Total of four servings bread and cereal from table
Fruit and vegetables (including juice)	None	Begin juice from cup: 3 ounces vitamin C source Begin fork-mashed, soft fruits & vegetables	3 ounces juice Pieces of soft & cooked fruits & vegetables from table	Table-food diet to allow 4 servings/day, including juice
Meat and other protein sources	None	None	Gradually begin milled or finely-cut meat. Casseroles, ground beef, eggs, fish, peanut butter, legumes, cheese	Two servings daily; one ounce total, meat or equivalent

*ages overlap and are given as ranges because of variations in rate of infant development.

are all signals for a change in eating style: a progression to solid foods.

Start out with one of those little long-handled demitasse baby-feeding spoons so you can both handle it well. You might have to hold her while you introduce solid foods, to reassure her that it is really all right. Later on you can go to a comfortable high chair that supports her feet.

Introduce one new food at a time, trying it out for perhaps two or three days, and checking for reactions like stomach aches and diarrhea, skin rashes, or wheezing. Then go on the next food. If she dislikes or rejects something, take no for an answer for a while, and try it a bit later. If she still says no, take her word for it; everyone is entitled to some food dislikes. You can still check out occasionally to see if she feels the same way about it.

The best first food is iron-fortified infant rice cereal mixed with milk or formula. This provides a good source of iron, as well as a good distribution of calories among protein, fat and carbohydrate. Rice cereal is the least likely of the grains to cause an allergic reaction. Start out with one cereal feeding daily and work up until she is taking two meals daily and getting a daily total of ⅓ to ½ cup. By that time she may be somewhere between six and eight months old and capable of eating even stiffer and lumpier cereal.

The next step is to begin to offer fruits, fruit juices and vegetables, as sources of vitamins C and A in preparation for the day when formula consumption will drop too low to provide these nutrients. There is no rush about this, nor is any particular order better than any other.

Given the stimulation of the thicker cereal, your baby will start to show some up-and-down chewing motions of her jaw, and will start manipulating her tongue to guide the food. If that's the case, it is probably a good idea to give her a little more to work on: fork-mashed cooked, or even diced fruits and vegetables. Baby foods are all right nutritionally, but they don't teach chewing skills.

During the fruits-and-vegetables stage it is also a good idea to start offering dry cereals, bread and crackers. Your baby will enjoy manipulating them and to the extent she gets it down, she will take in a few nutrients.

Cereal made with milk and fruits and vegetables, along with breastmilk or formula, really provide an adequate diet. You can start shaping these foods into meals, offering cereal and fruit for one meal, cereal and vegetable for another.

Since your child has no nutritional need for more protein, you really don't have to worry about introducing meat until she is ready to go on to table food. It is generally at that point that babies start eating considerably more solid foods, their milk consumption drops, and they need that meat protein to keep their diet adequate.

By the time you have worked your way through a series of fruits, fruit juices and vegetables, your child may begin to show an interest in what is going on at the table. He may be grabbing the spoon from you and clamming up when you try to feed him. He is giving you a clear message that it is really time to let him do it himself.

You'd better let him. Mash up his food, thicken it so it will hang together, put it on the high chair tray, get out of the way and let him go after it. He may not even need his food mashed if he is able to handle pieces of cooked vegetables and fruits, breads, or noodles and macaroni. Meat, however, is one food that cannot be gummed well. It doesn't soften up in the mouth. Meat needs to be chopped or cut up very fine, and may still need to be moistened a bit with meat or vegetable juice to make it palatable for your baby.

You can begin offering a milk beverage from the cup any time during the transitional period. In fact, many breast-fed babies learn to take a cup early on, rather than an artificial nipple, as a way of getting relief feedings.

By the time he is between ten and twelve months, and perhaps even earlier, he should be sitting in a high chair eating family-food meals and drinking a milk beverage from a cup. Satisfying his hunger and thirst at the table will allow him to omit the nursing at that feeding. From then on he will increasingly resemble an older child in his eating style, as he takes his meals and snacks "just like the rest of the family."

Babies progress at different rates and in different styles through these feeding stages. One young friend of mine took to cereal so enthusiastically at his very first solid feeding (at five months) that he set up a terrific howl between bites, complaining because his mother wasn't getting the food there fast enough. Another, at age six months, did not approve at all, pursed his lips and would on no account open up. It took his mother two weeks of gentle persistence before she could persuade and teach him to eat solids. She *was* persistent, because his growth on breastfeeding seemed to be falling off. Otherwise she could have dropped the subject and tried again later.

That is what another mother ended up doing with her son—he never would try out solid foods until one day she let him do it himself. She set him up to the table and he ate everything he could get his hands on. He was so insistent on eating that she had to throw caution to winds and simply feed him all his new foods at one time.

Each of them had a different experience on their way to achieving their feeding goal: Making the transition from nursing to table food.

It all sounds very simple, doesn't it? Well, it is and it isn't. Starting solids later simplifies things. But children vary widely, and feeding information varies from one doctor's office to another and from one social group to another. Your child care worker may have a different idea about feeding solids than you do. There are many ideas, myths and persuasions about solid foods introduction. That makes it confusing and hard, and the synopsis I've just given you won't seem to cover some of your day-by-day questions. To help you cope with it all, we again have to go into more detail.

Before we can get into our sequence of when to do what and how to go about it, however, we have to lay to rest the issue of when to get started. That is a very hotly-debated topic.

When To Start Solid Foods

The most reasonable and logical time to begin introducing solid foods into your baby's diet is when he needs them and is ready for them. (That reasoning and logic, unfortunately, is not always applied.) Babies generally get ready for solids somewhere between four and six months of age.

Breastmilk or formula, with appropriate vitamin supplementation, is nutritionally complete for your baby until four to six months. If he eats anything else, he will consume less of his milk feeding: he will replace it with food that is for him, at that time, nutritionally inferior.

As I described earlier, somewhere between four and six months your baby will probably begin to show developmental patterns that indicate he is ready for solids. If you are unsure about what you are seeing, or think your baby is developing skills faster than average, you can try some test feedings. Other than possibly compromising the intestinal immunity of totally breastfed infants (by changing the type of bacteria in their intestines), there is probably nothing wrong with experimenting with small amounts of cereal by age four months. If you give the milk feeding first, and offer the cereal feeding afterwards, your baby can indicate his own readiness for cereal introduction. He might not eat much at most of those earlier sessions, but they are still good practice.

But even as his calorie needs and hunger levels increase at about this time, you should still continue to depend primarily on greater quantities of breastmilk or formula. Up until your baby is well-established on table foods it is too early to allow calories from solids to replace too many milk feeding calories.

Once in a while we start a baby somewhat early on solids because he has to depend on them to give him enough to eat. His growth rate on breastfeeding may be falling off, or he may be bottle-fed and simply not take his bottle very well. After an initial learning period, that baby will probably take to solids pretty well. Then it is particularly important to choose solids that provide well for his nutritional needs.*

The 32 Ounce Rule. Some physicians automatically use the rule-of-thumb of putting a baby on solid foods when he is taking more than a quart of formula per day. (More recently, it has become the "one liter" recommendation, which is 1.06 quarts.) I don't know where that idea originally came from. I suspect, in my darker moments, that it was based on the evaporated milk formula, which made up to 33 ounces: If your baby took more than that amount, you had to make another batch. Now that old recommendation is being kept alive by, among other people, the Gerber baby food company, in advertisements to parents and in informational material for health workers.[8] (If you review Figure 5-8 in the *Formula* chapter, you will see that infants reach the 32-ounce level of formula consumption at widely differing ages. The infant in the 90th percentile for formula consumption could manage 32 ounces some time before he was two months old, whereas the one in the 10th percentile could not even at six months.)

The Committee on Nutrition has recommended that milk or formula consumption be limited to one quart per day FOR THE INFANT OVER AGE SIX MONTHS.** That's logical. The high-consuming baby probably won't drop back to a quart right at six months,

---

*I would be sure to offer cereal two, or even three times a day, and hold off on fruits and vegetables.

**The Gerber company cites this recommendation but neglects to mention the reference to age.

but by the end of the first year he should have replaced most of his formula calories with solid foods. Using one quart as the milestone for solid foods won't have anything to do with a baby's developmental or nutritional needs—except coincidentally. But it surely sells baby food.

Sleeping Through The Night. Parents think about starting solid foods because they have heard that solids will make their baby feel "more satisfied" (perhaps meaning sleep longer, or maybe be less fussy and demanding). I won't argue with your desire to make a demanding infant a little less demanding, or to get a good night's sleep. But studies don't give much cause for hope.[9, 12] Your baby will sleep or be content for longer periods only when his stomach can hold more and his nutritional needs aren't so pressing.

Despite those wretched stories by proud parents who boast that their baby slept through the first night she came home from the hospital, most babies don't get to the point where they can sleep six or seven hours at a stretch until 12 to 16 weeks.[12] That coincides with a drop-off in their very-rapid growth rate, and the decrease in the total calories they need for growth. Most new parents will need to get up to feed babies twice a night in the early weeks. If you find that hard, it's because it is hard.

There will come a time, however, when feeding solids does have something to do with contentment, particularly for the breastfed baby. Increases in appetite in the younger breastfed baby can generally be met by stepping up the nursing frequency to stimulate increased breastmilk supply. However, as the child approaches six months, it is likely that he will continue to be hungry despite increased nursing frequency, and he should be started on solid foods. (If those persistent hungry days appear considerably before six months, and particularly before four months, it is better nutritionally to give supplemental formula.)

Feeding Frequency. Some guidelines say solid foods should be introduced when the baby regularly eats more often than every three hours. I don't think that's right. Some babies, especially breastfed ones, regularly eat every two hours. I think, however, that if a baby is eating more than every two hours, *or* if his growth starts to fall off on ANY feeding frequency, that you had better do some problem-solving.* He may not be getting enough to eat or be properly utilizing his food.

"Opinionated" Babies. Back when I was young and naive, one of the ways a doctor persuaded me to start solid foods early was by warning me that if I waited too long, my daughter would get opinionated and hooked on breastfeeding, and wouldn't eat anything else. My doctor said she "knew" what she was talking about because she had seen it happen in her practice.

However, when the question was subjected to careful scientific inquiry, it appeared that my doctor's perception and what actually happened were two different things. A public health nurse[1] observed many infants over a ten-year period from 1940 to 1950 and found that babies under three or four months old really didn't seem to want much to do with solid foods. In fact, they and their mothers were getting into some real hassles over solid food introduction and, despite earlier struggles, the babies first really cheerfully accepted solid foods at around four months.

Solid Foods In The Bottle. Some people get around the acceptance problem by putting solid foods in the bottle. They mix a thin gruel of cereal, widen the hole in the nipple, and get the "solids" in that way.

The tactic is nothing more or less than forcefeeding and should be avoided. The cereal will increase the caloric density of the for-

---

*Even this suggestion is too rigid for some cultures, where babies are given breastfeeding "snacks" at very frequent intervals.

mula, and could force the baby to take too many calories in his attempt to get his water needs satisfied.

Then there is the syringe-action nipple feeder for young infants; I haven't seen these around lately, so I hope they've gone away. These gadgets have no value for the child with normal mouth patterns. The child who is not developmentally ready to eat from a spoon is unlikely to need solid foods.

Safety. We can also cite food safety as an argument for postponing solid foods. Some people are starting to question the safety of common food components such as salt, sugar, nitrate and various stabilisers and emulsifiers. Without taking sides on the issue, I can point out that the younger the child, the greater the vulnerability to questionable dietary components. An older infant will be better able to metabolize and get rid of toxicants in foods.

A good example is salt, which can be toxic, especially for infants, if you get the levels high enough. Some solid foods that I occasionally see parents choosing for their children, like hot dogs, canned spaghetti dinners and canned soups, put an additional load on the baby's kidneys, because of their high salt content.[17] The older child can handle additional salt better than the younger one, because his kidneys are more mature and capable of concentrating his urine more. An older child is also better at letting you know when he is actually thirsty, and can refuse milk when he really wants water.

Some parents simply like the idea of feeding their baby solid foods, and get a lot of satisfaction out of spoon-feeding. Others feel proud if their children are advanced in any way, and are prone to push up all schedules. In any event, try to control your impulse until your baby is at least four months old. Then, as I said earlier, be particularly careful to start out on infant rice cereal, mixed with formula or milk, and offer it only <u>after</u> you give the milk feeding.

Allergy. Estimates of the percentage of infants subject to allergic reactions to foods range from 0.3 to 55%, depending on who is being studied and how you define an allergic reaction.[13] Incidence of food allergies is greatest during infancy. Children whose parents have allergic reactions to food are at a greater risk of having food allergies than are others.

If you are particularly concerned about avoiding allergic reactions, it is probably better to wait a little longer to introduce solid foods. Any new food is a potential allergen. The younger baby is more likely to react allergically, before his immune system is fully operational.* If you keep him away from highly-allergenic foods, such as wheat, egg white, citrus and cow's milk, until 7–9 months, you may be avoiding some problems. This won't prevent you from introducing solid foods, starting with rice cereal diluted with whatever milk or formula you are using, or with one of the hypoallergenic formulas we discussed in the *Milk Feeding* chapter.

Some people argue that six months is too *early* for starting solid foods. They point to potential allergic reactions, not realizing that they can get around that by careful food selection. Or they are convinced that solids introduction will make the baby gain faster and increase the chances that he will get too fat. I don't think that's really a valid concern. Unless babies are really being force-fed with solids, it is likely that they will simply compensate for solids by taking less milk and gain at about the same rate.

As with most everything, however, there can be too much of a good thing. Now that the trend to later introduction of solid foods is becoming pretty well established, we are finding some parents and babies so comfortable with nursing that they are postponing solids introduction too long. Once your child is six months old, I would start practicing regularly with solid foods, even if he doesn't seem too taken with it. Don't get panicky or desperate, just be gently persis-

---

*The intestine develops resistance to large protein molecules as your baby gets older. Resistance significantly improves by seven to nine months, and continues to improve until up to 12 to 24 months of age.

tent. Somewhere between four to seven or eight months he is going to become developmentally ready for solid foods, and you don't want to miss it. If you do, you are going to have a child who is really hooked on nursing and doesn't want any part of any other form of getting nourishment.

When and What To Feed and How To Go About It

If you haven't figured this out already, as you begin giving your baby solid food, I think you will become aware that if you're going to get into conflict with relatives or child care workers, it will be about food. Keep in mind that you are the parent, and while you will benefit from feedback and constructive criticism from other people, the final decisions, and the responsibility for making them, rest with you. You are the one who should first introduce your child to new foods and changes in feeding routines. You are the one to decide and determine how your child will be fed.

You are introducing solid foods for two reasons: 1) To provide for your infant nutritionally; and 2) To encourage and support developmental changes. The following sequence generally satisfies both requirements.

Figure 7-3. Food Additions During the Transition Period

4–7 months	6–8 months	7–10 months	9–12 months
Infant cereal	Fruits and vegetables. Juices "Finger" breads and cereals.	Table foods Meats	Weanling milk

Once again, the times vary and overlap as infants move through these stages at different rates.

This little table is a rearrangement and condensation of the one we looked at before (Figure 7-2). You can refer to it as an outline for the rest of this chapter. The whole transition period is such an eventful time that it helps to have a clear overview of where we are and what we're doing.

Iron-fortified Baby Cereal. Iron fortified rice or barley baby cereal, mixed with formula or milk, is the best first solid food, both developmentally and nutritionally. Its texture can be varied to fit the mouth skills of the baby. (Some babies do better with it very thin, others manage it better if it's thicker.) The infant cereals contain a good amount of iron that is well absorbed by the baby. In addition the high-carbohydrate cereal, mixed with milk, gives a good proportion of protein, fat, and carbohydrate that won't disrupt the balance of the diet. Finally, rice and barley are the grains which are least likely to cause allergic reactions.

Other first solid foods have shortcomings. Some that are fine developmentally, like yogurt, cottage cheese, pureed meat, egg yolks and pureed fruits and vegetables, are all wrong nutritionally. Yogurt and cottage cheese are low in iron and simply give more of the same milk nutrients that the baby has been getting all along. Pureed meat is a pretty good source of iron, but it is so high in protein that it can imbalance the diet. Egg yolk gives way too much fat and the iron isn't absorbed well. Vegetables and fruits offer most of their calories as carbohydrate and can push dietary carbohydrate up too high, and, while they give a little iron, it really isn't enough.

We'll be making reference as we go along to keeping an eye on the protein, fat and carbohydrate in the solid foods so you don't imbalance the diet. As we said in the *Milk Feeding* chapter, excesses or deficiencies in any of these calorie-contributing nutrients can have a variety of undesirable consequences (see Figure 5-5).

To help you know what we're talking about, here is a chart that shows concentrations of protein, fat and carbohydrate in the various food groups.

Figure 7-4. Protein, Fat and Carbohydrate in Foods

	Protein	Fat	Carbohydrate	
			Starch	Sugar
Milk	✓	✓*		✓
Vegetables			✓	
Fruit and fruit juice				✓
Breads and cereals			✓	
Meat, fish, poultry, eggs, cheese, peanut butter	✓	✓		
Cooked dried beans	✓		✓	
Butter, margarine, salad dressing, cooking oils		✓		
Sweets, pop, fruit drinks				✓

*Unless it's skim milk

Once your baby is regularly on baby cereal, gradually work up from one feeding to two, until she is taking a total of about ½ cup per day—that will give her the 7 mg. of iron that she needs daily. At that point make sure you take her off any other iron supplementation because that will push her iron intake up too high. Continue to give a good iron source until your baby is about 18 months old, to get her through the high-risk period of iron deficiency anemia.

Iron in the Diet. People argue about food sources of iron in the baby's diet, and use a variety of foods that they think will give iron. Iron-fortified baby cereal is the only adequate food source of iron for the young infant. However, so you don't just have to take my word

Figure 7-5. Iron Content of Selected Infant Foods

Food	mg. Iron/3 ounces Food
Milk and Formula	
Human milk-cow milk formula unfortified with iron	.05
Iron—fortified formula	1.3
Cereals	
Iron fortified (dry) mixed with milk	7
Bottled pre-prepared cereal—fruit	5
Malto-meal, Cream of Wheat, cooked	2–3
Strained and Junior Foods	
Meats, poultry	1–2
Liver	4–6
Egg yolks	3
High meat dinner	less than 1
Vegetables, fruits	
Vegetables	less than 0.5
Fruits	less than 0.5
Standard Meat Cuts	
Beef, pork, lamb	2–3
Poultry	1.5
Beef liver, chicken liver	8.5
Calf liver	14.2
Pork liver	24.7

Source: U.S.D.A. Home and Garden Bulletin #72

for it, the amounts of iron in common infant foods are shown in Figure 7-5.

Iron in dry-packed infant cereals is in the form of very fine iron particles, and the iron in the bottled, pre-prepared cereals is in the form of ferrous sulfate. They have five and seven milligrams of iron per three-ounce serving, respectively. About 10% of each of these forms of iron is absorbed, which is a satisfactory amount.[4] In contrast, "adult" cereals that recommend themselves as good sources of iron for babies, Maltomeal and Cream of Wheat, have only two or three milligrams of iron per three-ounce serving. Furthermore, it is in the form of iron phosphate, which is only about 1% absorbed. In reality, that iron is there more for the label than for nutrition.

Meat and liver are good sources of iron. Even though the concentration of meat iron is relatively low, it is about 20% absorbed.[4] What is more, meat mixed with a meal helps absorption of all iron from that meal. However, there is the factor of calorie distribution: that amount of meat would contribute too much protein and make the overall diet too high in protein. Liver is very high in iron, but a daily serving of liver would provide too much vitamin A.*

Egg yolks traditionally have been added to babies' diets as a source of iron. However, we now discover that the iron in egg yolk is very poorly absorbed unless you take a good source of vitamin C at the same time. Without the vitamin C, egg yolk mixed with a meal that has other sources of iron will actually decrease the absorption of other food iron. In addition, egg yolks are too high in calories and too high in fat.**

---

*Not too long ago, there was a report in the *Journal of Pediatrics* about twin seven-month-olds who got vitamin A intoxication from eating chicken liver every day for three months.[10]

**Unless his diet is very low in fat. If a parent is determined to feed skim milk I may try to get her to feed egg yolks as a fat source. However, in general it is better to wait with egg yolk until the child is ready to eat the whole egg. Because egg white is a common allergen, we delay that until age nine months.

The Milk for Mixing Cereal. I have said, repeatedly, that the cereal should be mixed with milk or formula. Cereal mixed with water will provide carbohydrate only. The same is true, in spades, if you follow the recommendation of the Gerber company and mix your baby food with (Gerber) apple juice. The juice gives even more carbohydrate and no protein or fat.

Finding a milk for mixing the cereal is no problem for the formula-fed baby: just use whatever you are putting in his bottle. However, it is a little more complicated for the breastfed baby. For him, you can mix the cereal with hand-expressed breast milk, with pasteurized whole milk, with formula (either regular or hypoallergenic), or with diluted evaporated milk.

For some women, who are good enough at hand-expressing and have enough breastmilk, the first alternative works well. From the standpoint of preventing food reactions, that is certainly a good choice, particularly for the child with a strong family history of allergies. If allergies are less of a concern, one of the cow-milk-based approaches might work as well.

If you use formula, you will have to keep in mind that you will be using only a few ounces a day for diluting cereal so you will need to open, or prepare only a small amount at a time. (You could buy the powdered formula or the small individual-serving size of the liquid formula.) Use any liquid formula within one or two days. Pasteurized whole milk is probably not such a bad choice if you keep the quantities to below eight ounces a day (poor digestibility of pasteurized milk is not as much of a problem if it is well-diluted with other foods), and as long as you are not starting too early with cereal feeding. (Some infants under age six months lose small amounts of blood in their intestine when they take pasteurized milk.)

In general, I think the best choice is evaporated milk, diluted one-to-one with water. It is heat-treated, so it is very digestible and won't cause intestinal bleeding. You can buy it in five-ounce cans, so once you dilute it you only have ten ounces.

Alternatives to Infant Cereals. For a while, people were hesitating to use infant cereals because they contained salt, modified food starch, and a whole list of stabilisers and emulsifiers that combined to produce a rather ominous-looking label. Now, however, as with many commercial baby foods, the formulation has been changed. Baby cereals contain primarily the cereal flour, an emulsifier (soy lecithin), and a source of calcium. The salt has been taken out, as have the other emulsifiers and stabilisers.

If, however, "baby foods" are objectionable to you on general principles, there is an alternative. Use Malt-O-Meal or Cream of Wheat or, better yet, Cream of Rice that you have made with formula or whole milk (the cooking will boil it). Then provide the iron either with iron drops or iron-fortified formula.

Fruits and Vegetables. Somewhere in the range of six to eight months, once you get your baby well-established on iron-fortified baby cereal, you should start to work on adding fruits and vegetables to her diet. Your nutritional goal in adding fruits and vegetables is to get your baby accustomed to taking good sources of vitamins A and C in preparation for the time when her formula or breastmilk consumption drops too low to provide them in adequate amounts. Fruits and vegetables also give other vitamins and minerals, which may or may not be needed by this time. Diversifying the diet increases our chances of giving the baby everything she needs.

Your developmental goal is to introduce her to lumpier foods and foods of a different texture and flavor and to work her up, when she is ready, to finger-feeding herself chunks of soft and cooked fruits and vegetables.

Fruits and vegetables are primarily sources of carbohydrates, and are relatively low in caloric density (calories per ounce). They make good next additions to the diet after infant cereal, which is relatively high in caloric density, high in protein and low in carbohydrate.

Don't overdo it with fruits and vegetables, however, or you could dilute out the caloric density of the diet or distort the relative protein, fat and carbohydrate distribution. Three ounces of juice a day, or one or two two-tablespoon servings of fruit or vegetable is enough. Overfeeding with juice is an extremely common error. I often see mothers in the waiting room giving their babies eight-ounce bottles of juice. They shouldn't do it! Babies don't need the juice—it spoils their appetite, and sipping along on juice from a bottle can also spoil their teeth. Children who eat poorly often are filling up by drinking juice between meals. DON'T OVERDO THE JUICE. Three ounces per day is enough.

Caloric Density. Since we'll be making further references to caloric density as we go along, the chart below will be helpful to you in getting an idea of how the calories in fruits and vegetables compare with those in other common infant foods.

Figure 7-6. Caloric Density of Standard Infant Foods

Category	Calories per Three Ounces
Formulas and breast milk	60
Infant cereal made with whole milk or formula (1:6)	110
Baby cereals in jars	55–70
Infant cereal made with water (1:6)	50
Infant cereal made with juice (1:6)	85
Fruits and juices	40–80
Vegetables; plain, buttered, creamed	25–70
Meats	90–135
High-meat dinners	75–105
Egg yolks	195
Infant desserts	60–95

Source: Gerber Products Company, U.S.D.A. Home and Garden Bulletin #72.

Egg yolks have roughly eight times the calories of plain vegetables. Theoretically, a baby should be able to accommodate by simply eating less egg yolks and/or more vegetables. However, life is not theoretical, and you will want to know what you are doing with calorie concentrations in case your baby has special needs.

If your baby is a slow gainer, you want to go easy on the vegetables. If his rate of gain seems a little rapid, you would want to avoid egg yolks. (Actually, you should avoid them anyway, for reasons I will get to later.) Fruits and vegetables are quite interchangeable nutritionally and developmentally, so if you have a baby who refuses to take one or the other, you can be flexible. Furthermore, the order in which you introduce them really doesn't matter. People make up elaborate arguments for starting with one or the other, but don't worry about it.

Give Fruits and Juices in Moderation. To get a nutritionally-adequate serving, ⅓ cup of vitamin C-rich fruit or juice will do the trick very nicely. One or two tablespoons of other fruits is a nutritionally adequate serving, although children are generally willing to eat more than that because they like them so much. However, I would put an upper limit on fruit and fruit juice of about ¼ cup per serving (except for the C-rich fruit or juice) for the child under age one, because overdoing it can cause stomach ache or diarrhea. If he wants more juice than that, dilute it with water to make the small amount go farther.

Sources of Vitamin A. Infants and children ages six months to three years need about 2000 International Units (400 Retinol Equivalents) of vitamin A per day. A quart of formula or breastmilk contributes about 2000 to 2600 IU vitamin A, a quart of cow's milk about 1000 IU. The greatest need for non-milk sources of vitamin A will come after we make the transition to cow's milk, and milk consumption drops to two to three cups per day. Then your child will be getting only about 500 to 750 IU of vitamin A in milk, and we'll have to depend on vegetables and fruits to provide the other 1250 to 1500 IU.

Vitamin A is found in varying concentrations in a variety of fruits and vegetables.

Figure 7-7. Vitamin A in Fruits and Vegetables

Excellent Sources (More than 3500 IU per 3 ounces)	Good Sources (1000–3000 IU per 3 ounces)	Fair Sources (Less than 1000 IU per 3 ounces)
Apricots, dried	Apricot nectar	Apricots
Cantaloupe	Asparagus	Brussel sprouts
Carrots	Broccoli	Peaches
Mixed vegetables	Nectarine	Peach nectar
Mango	Purple plums	Prunes
Pumpkin		Prune juice
Spinach, other greens		Tomatoes
Squash		Tomato juice
Sweet potatoes		Watermelon

Source: U.S.D.A. Home and Garden Bulletin #72

The excellent sources would need to be given only every other day. (That works because vitamin A is a fat-soluble vitamin and is stored in the body.) To get enough vitamin A from the "good" sources you will have to use them every day. The "fair" sources have enough vitamin A to contribute significantly to the diet, but shouldn't be depended on as the sole sources.

If you give too many dark green and deep yellow vegetables, like broccoli, sweet potatoes, carrots and squash, your baby might turn yellow. This is a condition called carotenemia, caused by accumulation of the yellow coloring that the body converts to vitamin A. Carotenemia doesn't hurt him and it goes away if you take him off so much carotene. But there is really no reason why you should let your beautiful baby turn all yellow, so try not to give high-carotene vegetables and fruits more than every other day.

Limit potentially high-nitrate vegetables, like beets, carrots and spinach, to one or two tablespoons per feeding. Because of low stomach acidity, the young infant may convert nitrate to nitrite, which can displace oxygen in hemoglobin. The rapid breathing, lethargy and shortage of oxygen that results is called methemoglobinemia (and can actually be fatal if the dose of nitrate is very large). A while back there was a report of twin boys who were fed bottles of homemade carrot juice made from a batch of carrots that happened to be very high in nitrate. One of the babies refused the bottle, but the other took a large serving of high-nitrate carrots and became very ill from methemoglobinemia.

By age six months stomach acidity increases and nitrate overload is less of a problem, but I still wouldn't take chances with carrot juice.

Sources of Vitamin C. In contrast to vitamin A, vitamin C is a water-soluble vitamin that is not stored well in the body. You need to provide either one "excellent" or two "good" vitamin C sources every day. The infant up to one year needs about 35 mg of vitamin C per day, and from one to three years about 45 mg.

Many, if not most fruits and vegetables supply small amounts of vitamin C—on the order of five or ten milligrams per serving. We will call these the "fair" sources and it is reassuring to know they are there as a back stop if you miss with your primary sources; but do not depend on their vitamin C contribution to the diet.

Some very tasty fruits and vegetables did not appear on our vitamin A and C lists, for example, peas, beets, bananas and apples. As I said, these and other fruits and vegetables generally have vitamins A and C but in quantities too low to be considered "good" or "fair" sources. In addition, like the foods listed, they contribute other nutrients to the diet. For example, bananas have folic acid, and fruits

Figure 7-8. Vitamin C in Fruits and Vegetables

Excellent Sources (More than 35 mg per three ounces, one serving daily)	Good Sources (20 to 30 mg per three ounces, two servings daily)
Broccoli	Asparagus
Brussels sprouts	Bean sprouts, raw
Cabbage	Chard
Cauliflower	Honeydew melon
Cantaloupe	Potato
Grapefruit; grapefruit juice	Tangerine
Kohlrabi	Tomatoes, tomato juice
Mango	Pureed baby fruits
Oranges, orange juice	
Papaya	
Peppers	
Spinach	
Strawberries	
Vitamin-C fortified infant juices	

Source: U.S.D.A. Home and Garden Bulletin #72

and vegetables in general are good sources of potassium. Most will give some trace elements like zinc and copper. All have some plant fiber. They contribute to the diet, and, once the requirements for vitamins A and C are satisfied, make worthwhile choices to fill out the two or three servings a day your child will be working up to.

Don't get panicky if your child doesn't consume optimum amounts of vitamin C and A-rich foods. The recommended nutrient intake allows him to provide for his daily need as well as to store some nutrient in his body. If he doesn't drink his orange juice today, he can fall back on the vitamin C he stored yesterday.

Digesting and Ingesting Fruits and Vegetables. Don't get excited when pieces of fruits and vegetables and the stains from beets and other foods start to come through in your baby's diaper. Unless someone chews very thoroughly, those are the waste products of normal digestion. Stools of older children and adults look the same way; we just don't pay so much attention to them.

Once you get to the point of introducing fruits and vegetables, your baby is probably going to be able to digest any reasonably-bland food that he can gum well. In fact, chewing and swallowing probably represent the major limitation in his digestive system. Again, your developmental goal in introducing fruits and vegetables is to introduce him to different textures and flavors, and to get him used to the idea of handling the pieces of food you get when you mash or dice cooked fruits and vegetables or offer a chunk of banana or apple. You can use the bottled baby foods if you want, but they are really too thin and smooth to provide much developmental stimulus.

Selection of Fruits and Vegetables. Depending on your baby's oral ability and hand coordination, you may need to fork-mash fruits and vegetables such as carrots or bananas, and feed them to her. Or you may simply give her a chunk of banana to bite off and gum. If she has developed a pincer grasp, she may delight in picking up whole peas and gumming them. Any tender, cooked vegetable is appropriate at this age. Fruits canned in juice, water, or light syrup and then drained and mashed, chopped or chunked are fine. Many fresh fruits, such as peaches, pears, and plums (all with skins removed) are also good choices. You can mash, dice or chunk, depending on your child's ability. Many babies are good at sucking on an orange or grapefruit section and, surprisingly, really seem to love the sour taste. Some can gum a peeled apple wedge or a carrot, while others haven't gotten the hang of it and bite off too-big pieces.

If your baby can't handle apples, make scrapings: using a carrot peeler, remove and discard the peeling; then keep right on peeling until you have a little pile of scrapings. Cut them up, as some of the strips may be long, and let your child eat them with her fingers. Or feed them by spoon.

Try to give your baby the vegetable you are having at the family dinner table. Prepare frozen or fresh vegetables without added salt and give part to the baby. She can handle diced or mashed peas, cooked cauliflower, broccoli flowerettes, corn, mixed vegetables, etc. It's better to stay away from canned vegetables, as they really are quite high in salt.

If your baby is having trouble with pieces of food, you might consider buying a little hand baby-food grinder. You can take this right to the table and quickly reduce the family fare to a thick pulp that your baby will find delectable.

Baby Foods. Once we get into the fruits and vegetables stage we have to resolve the question of whether or not to use baby food. Actually it is probably already resolved: by starting solids late and progressing rapidly to table food, you really side-step the whole issue of baby food, and whether to make it or buy it, because the baby doesn't need it.

Making Your Own Baby Food. Generally, when people inquire about making their own baby food, they are thinking about pureeing and freezing. Whole books deal with recipes for baby, the art of blending, and freezing the puree in ice cube trays to provide "convenient" blocks of foods that can be simply thawed and fed.

Frankly, I view that as a lot of unnecessary work, a potential source of contamination, and as accomplishing very little. The infant who still needs the pureeing doesn't need the fruits and vegetables. And the infant who is ready for the fruits and vegetables doesn't need the pureeing.

The sooner you get your baby to the point where you perceive him as a participant in the family eating style, the better it is for all of you. He needs and wants to be able to imitate your eating habits;

you won't be able for long to get away with feeding your baby one way and yourself another.

Bottled Baby Foods. As I said, if your baby is old enough to take fruits and vegetables, he won't get much developmental benefit from bottled baby foods. Using the somewhat-lumpier "junior foods" helps a little, but they are still pretty thin and smooth compared to table food.

Nevertheless, there are a few times I see a need for bottled baby food. For parents who insist on starting early, the child under six months taking fruits and vegetables may need a silky-smooth texture to avoid choking. He also may need protection against botulinum spores.* Occasionally we see a developmentally delayed child who, due to a problem with muscle control, needs to be worked up through pureed food and introduced very gradually to thicker, lumpier food. Also, baby foods come in handy when you are traveling and having a hard time getting access to other appropriate foods. And then there is the occasional meal, like salad, that just doesn't work for the baby.

And of course there is the problem of the meals in the child-care setting when you are working. At times, especially in the early solid foods stage, you may find it easier to send a jar of baby food. Then, as you introduce appropriate foods at home, like hard-cooked eggs, crackers, and sandwiches, you can pack a lunch more like one you would use for an older child. (I think you should be the one to introduce new foods, not the sitter. You are the parent and you are entitled to share your child's new experiences—first.)

Bottled baby foods are safe and nutritious. They are sanitary, carefully handled to preserve nutritional quality, and they are low in

---

*Any fresh or frozen fruit or vegetable—indeed, anything that has come in contact with the ground—is potentially contaminated with botulinum spores. These can only be destroyed by pressure canning. Since "adult" canned vegetables are too high in salt, baby foods are the other alternative.

salt and sugar. The manufacturers claim that they are equal to or lower in cost than the ones you prepare yourself by pureeing. Plus, you get all those nice little jars. If you use bottled baby foods, make sure the jars are sealed. The dome on the cover should be pulled down by the vacuum inside the jar and you should hear a pop when you open it. (Incredible as it seems, shoppers will open jars, smell or taste, and then close them and put them back on the shelves.)

The Meal Pattern. As you work with adding fruits and vegetables to your baby's diet, you will be working toward a two-meal-a-day pattern. It's a good idea to continue giving cereal morning and night, or any two times when it seems like a meal-type feeding fits in well. Then, as you introduce fruit and vegetables you can, perhaps, give fruit or fruit juice with one cereal feeding and a vegetable with another.

Finger Breads and Cereals. Sometime during the fruit and vegetable stage and as you go into the table food stage you are going to find yourself giving your baby crackers, pieces of bread, and dry cereals to pick up and eat. In doing that you will be responding to his developmental needs, as he'll be right at the stage of practicing his pincer grasp, putting everything in his mouth and trying out his chewing skills. Those foods are also appropriate nutritionally. They provide B vitamins and iron and, if you are using whole grains, they also give some trace elements and fiber.

You have to keep in mind, however, that along with bread or crackers you may also be introducing wheat, which is one of the more common allergens. (Incidence of allergic reactions to all foods ranges from 0.3 to 10%.) If your baby is at least seven months old, wheat introduction is probably OK. However, if you, yourself, are particularly sensitive to wheat, your baby has an increased chance of having a wheat sensitivity and you may want to wait longer. To avoid wheat you can choose things like rice crackers, corn and rice chex, corn flakes and the like. Read the label and avoid anything that has wheat flour, wheat starch or wheat gluten in it. Generally, if a label just says "flour," it means *wheat* flour.

Probably by nine months it is as safe as it is going to be to begin experimenting with wheat in small quantities. Do keep a sharp eye, however, for such reactions as a skin rash, wheezing, stomach aches or diarrhea. If your child seems to react, take her off the wheat for a couple of weeks and then try again. It is easy to think she has an allergy when she really doesn't, because such symptoms are so common. You certainly don't want to burden yourself with avoiding wheat if you don't have to.

Making the Transition to Table Food. Somewhere between seven and ten months of age you will probably find your baby sitting in the high chair, showing good hand-mouth coordination, developing a pretty dextrous palmar grasp or perhaps even a pincer grasp, and beginning to show "adult" chewing patterns: side to side movements with her tongue and mashing her food with her jaws. You may have her entertaining herself with dry cereal and crackers while you eat your meal.

It is time that she joins you for dinner. She can by that time progress very nicely from semi-solid mashed or pureed food to pieces of soft food that she can feed and chew herself.

It's nice when the ability and the impulse to self-feed come along at the same time. Sometimes, however, the mind is willing, yea eager to self-feed, but the body won't cooperate yet. That is when your baby starts to refuse spoon feeding but can't quite manage to pick up or chew finger food. He gets frustrated at his failed attempts, his mother or father gets frustrated at having the spoon refused, and mealtime deteriorates. Take heart, this is only temporary. The skills will come and the situation will resolve itself. The most important thing is to avoid forceful spoon-feeding and to minimize the frustration for all of you.

If the grasp is still palmar, try giving your baby one spoon and feeding with a second spoon. Or use sticky foods (see below) and load the spoon for him to self-feed. Consider giving strips of toast, peeled apple wedges, long crackers, etc. for a short time until the pincer grasp appears. This may produce a limited diet, but it's only for a short time. Nutritionally, you must still be depending heavily on breastmilk or formula while you make this transition.

If the grasp is there but he is still gagging on pieces of food, go to thick mashed or milled foods. (Don't resort to baby foods unless there is a real chewing-swallowing problem; they will only slow his development.) Mix baby cereal thick, and break the mass apart so he can pick it up. Mash or mill fruits and vegetables and thicken with some baby cereal. Or put some potato and another vegetable through the baby food grinder and moisten it just enough to make a thick, gluey mass that can be picked up. This is wonderfully messy and dries to the high chair very much like cement.

What about messing and playing with the food? At first you will probably see quite a lot of this. The Arabs have a saying, "you taste with your fingers." I wonder if our sterile eating arrangements are depriving us of some eating satisfaction! In any event, the infant has a real need to feel, see and smell the food before deciding to eat it. In fact, the concept of eating that strange-looking stuff is one that is learned gradually. It's wonderful to watch the expression of amazed delight on a child's face when something tasty finally does make it into his mouth.

So at first you will see more messing and exploration than eating, but usually this stage passes quickly. The transition to table food is often abrupt and enthusiastic, particularly if the child is at the table with other family members and allowed to eat the same foods.

Meat. When your baby goes on table food (somewhere between seven and ten months), you should start adding meat to her diet. It hasn't really been necessary before then, because she has been experimenting texturally with cereal, fruit and vegetable, getting iron from cereal, and getting plenty of protein from formula or breastmilk. However, once she starts eating from the table, and works up to three meals a day, her quantity of solid foods will increase and her breastmilk or formula consumption will begin to drop. In fact it is a good idea to encourage the drop by skipping the milk feeding before the meal—or if your baby won't stand for that, giving only part of it. In other words, it is time to encourage her to replace breastmilk or formula with solid foods. At this point she will need other, non-milk sources of protein, such as meat, poultry or fish, or concentrated vegetable sources such as cooked dried beans and peanut butter.*

Introducing meat is a bit of a problem as, in some ways, your baby isn't really ready to handle it developmentally. She doesn't have the right teeth. But you can't wait until she is 18 to 24 months old to get her molars, so you will have to modify the texture of the meat to fit her capacities. Of course hamburger, in a patty or meatloaf or casserole is no problem. Neither are fish and tender poultry. The steaks and chops and roasts, however, call for some special handling.

If you have a baby food grinder, here is one place it may come in handy. You will have to cut the meat up rather finely, and moisten it a bit to get it through the grinder, but with some persistence, it will go. It also helps to mix the chunks of meat in with the mashed potatoes, and to keep stirring the mixture as you work it through the grinder. Or you can simply cut up the meat, if you cut it very fine. Using a sharp knife, cut the meat, across the grain, into about ⅛-inch fibers. Moisten it and let your baby pick it up with her fingers, or mix it in with other foods.

Your baby might take her meat and other foods better if you make her a little mixed dinner.

Treasure the recipe—it is the only baby-food recipe you will get from me. It is intended to be something you can mix up from

---

*See the discussion in the *Toddler* chapter on non-meat protein.

whatever you happen to be making for dinner. It is not intended to be multiplied and made in great vats and frozen. If you want to do that, you will have to find instructions in another book.

Recipe for Mixed Dinner

2 tablespoons chopped or ground meat, poultry, fish or grated cheese—or ½ egg
¼ cup cooked rice, noodles, macaroni, or potatoes
2 tablespoons vegetable: pieces, chopped or mashed
Liquid to moisten: broth, milk, low-fat gravy.

This works as a finger food—if you use our broader definition of a finger food as anything that sticks together long enough to get it from plate to mouth. (Or high chair tray, for that matter; most plates end up on the floor.)

If your baby has developed a palmar grasp, self-feeding will involve pushing the heel of his hand against the food and closing his fingers over it, scraping it into his palm. To eat it, he will scrape the palm of his hand against his lip. (That is, he will eat it after he enjoys squishing it a few times in his hand, letting the wonderful goo ooze out between his fingers.) It isn't pretty, but it works, and he will think he is just the smartest person ever.

Once he gets that pincer grasp going and gets interested enough in eating so he no longer experiments as much with his food, his eating will be prettier. Eventually he will even want to use a spoon, but you will probably have to wait a few months for that.

You may be surprised at the small amount of meat I recommend in the mixed dinner. It is equivalent to a ½-ounce serving, and it is really enough for a baby. If she has two ½-ounce servings of meat per day, and continues to take at least 16 ounces of formula or milk per day, that will give her enough protein. The older infant and toddler require roughly 21 grams of protein per day. An ounce of meat and a cup of formula or milk each provides seven or eight grams protein.

The following list gives protein values of common foods:

Figure 7-9. Quantity of food that gives seven to eight grams of protein

Food	Amount
Milk or formula: cow, soy	8 ounces
Egg	1
Soybeans, cooked	⅓ cup
Cooked dried beans	½ cup
Cottage cheese	¼ cup
Peanut butter	2 Tablespoons
Other nut butters	3 Tablespoons
Cheese: cheddar, American, etc.	1 ounce

Source: U.S.D.A. Home and Garden Bulletin #72.

The Three-meal-a-day Pattern. If it seems to you that we just talked about the meal pattern, you're right, we did. But once your baby starts eating from the table, it's time to change it again. She will begin to take a main meal, eating the same foods at the same time as the rest of the family. She should continue to get her ½ cup of baby cereal a day (measured after it is mixed), taking it in one or two meals or snacks. So, breakfast isn't hard to plan, and dinner isn't hard to plan, but what about lunch? That's the meal that many families find difficult.

My favorite and easiest lunch suggestion, is leftovers. Cook a bit extra the night before, put aside enough for the next day, refrigerate it promptly, and reheat it for your baby's (and your) lunch.

Also, by this time eggs are another possibility. Once your baby gets to seven to nine months old, he will be past the high-risk period for egg allergy and ready to eat a scrambled or soft-cooked egg. Don't forget to give him some bread or other starch with it: combine that with a fruit or vegetable and you have a nice meal. People worry about the cholesterol in eggs. Unless you have a family history of major heart disease, 3 or 4 eggs weekly should be all right for him.

Also, though it may surprise you, your baby is now ready for a peanut butter sandwich or some peanut butter on toast. You should wait a while to use lunch meats or hot dogs, and then use them only sparingly. The baby-food meat sticks are a low-salt, low-nitrate, convenient (if expensive) meat source for lunches. They give about 10 grams of protein per jar.

I will go into meal planning in more detail, and offer more food suggestions, in the *Toddler* chapter.

Keep in mind at this stage that you are helping your child make the transition from the demand feeding pattern of infancy to the meals-plus-snacks routine of the toddler. In order to allow him to fit into the family meal pattern, you may have to make some adjustments. You may find yourself eating a light breakfast and then having lunch at 11:00, so the two of you can eat together. Or you may rely on snacks as a way of tiding him over between meals. If you have a very long afternoon and late dinner, you may want to give two snacks.

At first, the snacks will be breastfeedings or bottle feedings. As your baby approaches a year, however, it is probably better to make those snacks the same that you would feed to an older child: crackers and cheese, fruit or peanut butter, apples, etc. See Figure 8-7 in the *Toddler* chapter for a list of some nutritious snacks.

Overall, you are going to have the best luck selecting food for your child at this age if you stop thinking of him as a baby and start thinking of him as a toddler. (How's that for a heart-rending statement?) You might not be ready for him to be that grown-up: but he is ready, and you had better let him go. You can baby him in some other way.

The Weanling Milk. For the child who is well established on table food, including meat, there is only one transition left to make: the shift from the milk feeding of infancy to some other kind of milk. He no longer needs the extra vitamins and minerals provided by an infant milk feeding, nor does he need so much help with digestion and maintaining homeostasis.

A child is well-established on table food when he is sitting up, three times a day with the rest of the family, primarily self-feeding with his hands, and drinking, with assistance, from the cup. He should be taking at least three ounces of solid foods at each meal, with a good selection from the basic-four food plan, and his formula or breastmilk consumption should have dropped off, most noticeably through elimination of some of the nursing sessions.

Once his formula consumption drops below 32 ounces, or he has eliminated two or three of his daily breastfeedings, you may quite safely go to whole evaporated milk that has been diluted one-to-one with water. If you are switching to whole pasteurized milk, wait until the formula amount drops to between 16 and 24 ounces. Then use whole milk.

After you reach the table-food stage, you have several alternatives open to you in choosing the milk feeding for the rest of the first years.

Breastfed Infant. I think even a breastfed baby who is 10 to 12 months old should be drinking his mealtime milk from a cup. If the breast is too-freely offered at mealtime the baby won't be as hungry or as interested in table foods. That is not to say, however, that the breastfed baby that age should be completely weaned from the breast. Breastfeeding is still good for snacks and for late-night and early morning feedings.

The milk used for cup drinking can be one of the following:

Commercial Formula. The baby formula manufacturers very-energetically encourage keeping infants on formula for the whole first year. Since the product representatives from the companies are consistent and energetic teachers of physicians, this recommendation has been pretty widely accepted by health professionals and passed on to parents. However, unless there is a specific reason for staying on formula for that long I really don't think there is any need for it. By the time they are set on table foods, most babies no longer need the nutritional help that is provided by commercial formulas. Formula can cover for a variety of nutritional errors, but its use can also cut down on your motivation to teach your child to eat a variety of nutritious foods.

However, a baby who is very small or grows unusually slowly, or who has a lot of digestive upsets, should be left on his formula.

Pasteurized Whole Milk. Pasteurized milk is an acceptable choice at this point. Digestion of pasteurized milk is less of a problem for an older child, not because his stomach is older, but because he is getting a mixed diet. Dilution of milk in his stomach with other foods makes it set up a softer, more-digestible curd.

We are counting on milk to provide fat, so babies should be kept on *whole* milk until they are about two years old. Young children don't get that much other fat: they eat very little meat, they love low-fat foods like breads, cereals, and fruits, and even if their vegetables are buttered, they don't eat that many of them.

Remember that to form our well-balanced diet, we are counting on milk to provide vitamins A and D, as well as calcium and protein. Most milk that is currently on the market, even powdered milk, will give you those nutrients. Do read the label, however, because there are a few milks that are not fortified with vitamins A and D, and there are some imitation milks and milk substitutes that are simply not equivalent to milk, nutritionally.

If you use fresh milk, it must be pasteurized. There is a small risk of unpasteurized milk carrying brucellosis or tuberculosis, although dairy herds are now carefully checked for these diseases. A more-likely risk is that the milk will contain germs from undetected mastitis, or that the milk is contaminated from the barn or from the handling. There are no nutritional advantages to using raw milk.

Evaporated Milk. Particularly if your baby is still taking over 24 ounces of milk a day, you should consider using whole evaporated milk, diluted one-to-one with water, as a weanling milk. It is heat-treated, contains vitamins A and D, and is priced about the same as whole pasteurized milk. Since many families buy only 2% or skim milk for adults and older children, they will have to get a special milk for the baby anyway, and it could just as well have evaporated milk's advantage of heat treatment.

Fluoride. You can discontinue the fluoride supplement after your child is eating foods from the table and drinking water and juice, provided your water supply is fluoridated at least to the level of 0.3 p.p.m. If the water contains less than 0.3 p.p.m. fluoride, continue with the 0.25 mg supplement. Foods cooked with fluoridated water provide significant amounts of fluoride, as do juices that are mixed using fluoridated water. You should also remember to teach and encourage your child to think of water for thirst.

You should probably avoid fluoridated toothpaste for the child under age three years. Since small children generally swallow, rather than spit out toothpaste, they could ingest enough to cause fluorosis of the tooth enamel.

Fat, Sugars and Salt. I will have more to say about all of these in other chapters. For now, we'll talk about them only as they relate to the infant under a year of age.

Fat. Fat in the diet of the young infant comes mostly from milk and formula. Concern about heart disease, however, introduces a controversy about the kind of fat and amount of cholesterol in children's diets.

Breastmilk and cow's milk contain saturated fat and cholesterol. Consuming both tends to increase blood cholesterol, which may, in turn, have something to do with increasing risk of heart disease. (This is one of the points the experts debate when they argue about whether or not diet can contribute to heart disease.) Commercial formulas contain no cholesterol, have polyunsaturated fats, and tend to lower blood cholesterol.

Studies have shown that infants who are breastfed, or who get butterfat in their formulas, have higher blood cholesterols than those who are fed commercial formulas. However, infants weaned from formula or breast milk to diets that are pretty much the same have similar cholesterol concentrations at ages three and four.[13] The Committee on Nutrition, based on this evidence, has said that in view of the good growth and performance of children on current feeding regimens, there is little basis for recommending changes in fat selection before age one year, even in children who are at risk of developing heart disease.[2]

Some argue that formulas should contain cholesterol. They speculate (without clear research evidence) that babies need dietary cholesterol to properly form the fatty sheath around their nerves. Others maintain that a person's later ability to get rid of excessive cholesterol in his body can be dependent on the exposure he received to cholesterol in his early diet. The evidence of similar cholesterol levels in the 3–4 year-old preschoolers would dispute this theory.

The heart disease question aside, as your infant makes his transition to table food you will probably wonder whether you should be buttering his bread or adding fat to his vegetables. I would go by his preference. If he seems to prefer a little extra fat, then add it. He doesn't really need the fat, as long as he continues to take whole milk. If he drinks 2% or skim milk, you should see to it that he gets one teaspoon of fat (for 2%), or two teaspoons (for skim), for each eight ounces of milk that he consumes.

If your baby isn't growing or gaining as well as he should and you do add extra fat, use polyunsaturated margarine or vegetable oil rather than butter. Babies digest and absorb vegetable oils better than animal fat.

Sugar. Sugar is easy enough to avoid while your child is small, and adds nothing except calories to the diet. As long as your baby doesn't know what he is missing, you might as well keep him away from added sugar. Sooner or later someone will come along to introduce him to sweets and he will probably develop a taste for them, just like the rest of us. Until then, hold off.

There is no reason for you to sweeten his food. He may start eating his cereal sooner if it is sweetened, but it is better that he gets a chance to experience and enjoy the good taste of grain, even if it takes him longer to get going on it. (I think adding sugar to food is different from adding fat. Fat enhances food flavor; sugar disguises it.) He may like desserts and seem to go for those unnecessary little baby desserts; but he doesn't need the variety, and he will be forfeiting the pleasure of learning about other foods.

Honey. Particularly avoid honey in any form for the first year. This includes honey that has been baked into a cookie or bread, or honey for dipping a pacifier. Honey at times is contaminated with the spores of clostridium botulinum. If allowed to grow in an airtight place, these spores produce clostridium toxin, which can cause severe illness and even death. Generally this is a problem only in improperly-canned, non-acid foods, like green beans. But it can happen in the young infant's intestine, which is also an air-tight place. The spores grow, produce the toxin, and poison the infant.

The bacteria and chemicals in the intestines of older people change in some way to prevent the spores from growing. Clostridium poisoning from spores is generally found only in babies under age six months, but to be on the safe side we say that honey should first be given only after age one year.

It is no great loss. The practical fact is that honey is not more nutritious than sugar. The same goes for raw sugar, and other forms of sugars that are touted as nutritious alternatives to table sugar. The amount of worthwhile nutrients in these foods is so small that if you were to consume enough to give you any significant amount of a nutrient it would give you too much sugar.

Salt. Salt should be held to a low level in the baby's diet. He won't miss it. Salt added to baby foods is there more for the feeder than for the fed: babies accept unsalted baby food just as well as salted. Breastmilk, formula and unsalted foods in their natural state have enough sodium in them to satisfy essential nutrient requirements.

It is generally agreed that there is an advantage for many people in keeping the dietary sodium low, particularly those specifically at risk for heart disease. (Life-long low sodium intakes are correlated with lower blood pressures.) However, at the same time you have to remember that sodium is an essential nutrient, and should not be eliminated completely from the diet. In fact, in some cases your doctor may even feel it is necessary to supplement with salt if, for example, your baby is feverish and perspiring a great deal or is losing sodium for some other reason. But let your doctor decide—don't do it yourself.

Baby foods no longer have added sodium. Home-prepared foods of course have varying amounts of salt, depending on the preference of the cook. Canned foods (except for fruits), pre-prepared, "convenience" soups and dinners, snack chips and crackers, lunch meats and cured meats are all generally high in sodium. To keep down on levels of sodium for your baby, avoid high-salt foods, take out the baby's portion before you salt for the family, or cook salt-free and let everyone salt to taste.

The Overview

Having worked our way through each of the additions, it is time to take an overall look at the balance of your baby's diet. Maintaining a proper diet is considerably more complicated now than when she was on just breastmilk or formula, because you have the challenge of keeping a reasonable proportion between the several food groups. I will be discussing this whole topic in more detail in the *Toddler* chapter, and I would encourage you to read that right now, even if you aren't ready to start thinking of your baby as a toddler. For the time being, I will confine my discussion to a few general observations about dietary balance.

At the end of the transition period, all of your baby's daily nutritional requirements will be provided by a mixed table food diet. The MINIMUM amount of food from each of the food groups she will need in order to have a nutritious diet are:

Milk	16–24 ounces
Fruits and vegetables	Four servings, each 1–2 Tbsp. vitamin C source: 3 ounces daily vitamin A source: 3 times weekly
Bread and cereals	Four servings daily, each about ¼ the adult serving size
Meats, poultry, fish, eggs	Two servings daily, each about ½ ounce

Your baby will vary on a day-to-day basis in the quantities she eats from each of these food groups. Generally that is no problem as long as, on a weekly average, she satisfies her minimum requirement from each of the groups. Babies will often eat disproportionately large amounts of breads and cereals, and that is fine, provided everything else is there in minimum amounts. However, if she is using a particular food group to the exclusion of the others, it can get to be a problem.

Babies will occasionally prefer to drink their meals, insisting on more and more milk and showing little interest in solid foods. If that is the case, you should impose an upper limit on the milk of three or even two cups a day, and try to get her to save some of her hunger for solid foods. The same goes for juices. If allowed to, many babies will drink so much juice that they spoil their appetite for other foods. Be sure you are regularly offering water—it may be that you just have an extra-thirsty baby.

Now you can heave a big sigh of relief. You have come through the constant changes of the transitional feeding period. From now on, your little one will be polishing his skills—getting better at drinking from the cup, chewing, finally even learning to use a spoon and fork. He'll be interested in his food and pretty accepting of a variety of foods. You can look forward to more of a regular routine as you include him in your family eating pattern. You even get a little breather before your beginning toddler starts to develop the more-limited appetite and contrariness of that age group. ENJOY!

Selected References

1. Beal, Virginia A. On the acceptance of solid foods and other food patterns of infants and children. Pediatrics 28:448–456. 1957.
2. Committee on Nutrition. Commentary on breast-feeding and infant formulas, including proposed standards for formulas. Pediatrics 57(2):278–285. 1976.
3. Committee on Nutrition. Fluoride supplementation: revised dosage schedule. Pediatrics 63:150. 1979.

4. Committee on Nutrition. Iron supplementation for infants. Pediatrics. 58:765–768. 1976.
5. Committee on Nutrition. On the feeding of supplemental foods to infants. Pediatrics 65(6):1178–1181. 1980.
6. Committee on Nutrition. On the feeding of solid foods to infants. Pediatrics 29:685–692. 1958.
7. Fomon, S. J., L. J. Filer, T. A. Anderson and E. E. Ziegler. Recommendations for feeding normal infants. Pediatrics 63:52–59. 1979.
8. Gerber Products Company. Current Practices in Infant Feeding. Freemont, Michigan. 1980.
9. Grunwaldt. Edgar, F. Bates and D. Guthrie. The onset of sleeping through the night. Pediatrics. 31:667–668. 1960.
10. Mahoney, C. P., M. T. Margolis, T. A. Knauss & R. F. Labbe. Chronic vitamin A intoxication in infants fed chicken liver. Pediatrics. 65:893–896. 1980.
11. Osaki, F. A., and S. A. Landaw. Inhibition of iron absorption from human milk by baby food. American Journal of Diseases of Children. 134:459–460. 1980.
12. Parmelee, A. H., W. H. Wenner and H. R. Schulz. Infant sleep patterns from birth to 16 weeks of age. Journal of Pediatrics. 65:839–848. 1964.
13. Pipes, Peggy L. Infant feeding and nutrition. IN Nutrition in Infancy and Childhood. C.V. Mosby Co., St. Louis. 1981.
14. Taitz, L. S. and H. D. Byers. High calorie/osmolar feeding and hypertonic dehydration. Archives of Disease of Childhood. 47: 257–260. 1972.

8
Feeding the Toddler

It is your job as parent to avoid, whenever possible, making the inevitable battles of the toddler period battles over food. During the time from 18 months to three years, your child's rapid infant growth rate slows down, she becomes a "demon explorer," and she shows, at times, a fierce contrariness in her attempts to establish that she is a person separate from you. Her food intake decreases, and you will naturally become concerned. However, if you emphasize or enforce eating too much, you will arouse her need to exert her individuality and the battle will be on. Toddlers would rather exert their independence than eat. Successfully negotiating this tricky time demands a division of responsibility: you are responsible for what your child is presented to eat, she is responsible for what and how much she eats.

I could almost write the script for a toddler consult. When parents come to see me with a child 12 to 30 months old, they come with an all-too-familiar list of concerns and frustrations about feeding. They tell me that their child is not eating enough, especially of meat and vegetables and fruits. They complain that their child will only eat a few foods, and that he wants those foods again and again. They object to his dawdling with his food and they are concerned about milk consumption. Some worry that their child drinks too little milk; about an equal number worry that he drinks too much.

Developmental Changes

These typical food problems have everything to do with what is happening to and with the toddler socially, physically and behaviorally. To get a better feeling for that, let's first broaden our perspective and look at toddler developmental changes.

Psychological and Social Changes. The theme of this chapter is "managing toddler eating behavior." Actually, that is rather a silly theme, because NOBODY manages a toddler. There is a story about a powerful Norse god who was boasting that he could get anyone to do his bidding. A woman responded that she knew of someone whose will and strength were greater than his. She was referring to her two-year-old son. Foolish god, he didn't believe her and it was left to the son to prove the truth of her words. And, of course, he did.

That mother knew what you and I know: You can prevent a toddler from doing what you don't want him to do, but you can't force him to do what you want him to do. And you had better not try, or you'll simply have a profitless fight on your hands.

The toddler's task is to find out and prove to himself and to you that he is a separate person from you. He finds out that he is a separate person by saying "no" a lot, because whenever he resists what you want he proves to himself that he is separate from you. He has a tremendous need to be independent, to be successful, to explore, and to have limits. And he feels absolutely ambivalent about it all.

He needs to know that he is an individual, but he also needs to know that he can't dominate you. Unless you let him know clearly that the limits exist, he will become more and more provocative, until you finally move in and stop him. He also has an exuberant and unrestrained curiosity, and seems to need to make the same sort of impact on his environment that he does on you.

Dr. Spock called the child at this age a "demon explorer." He and Arnold Gesell described toddlers as demanding, assertive, mercurial, precooperative, contrary, obstinate, exasperating, imperious, balky, negativistic, bossy and over fussy. Hardly encouraging. But notice they said *precooperative*. That should give you hope.

Your role as a parent during this period is very tricky. You need to provide for exploration and independence. You need to set things up for him so he can be successful; but at the same time you have to avoid giving in to unreasonable demands. You have to keep trying to distinguish appropriate limits, and to separate them from mere reactions (although sometimes your emotional reaction is the best signal that your child is going too far).

You are also experiencing a loss. You are losing your baby and all the intense intimacy of that early period. Your child stops being a cuddly, loving, responsive person and turns into the embodiment of all those negative adjectives we strung out earlier.

With food, your child will be testing and waging a campaign for control, just like with everything else in his life. He will look to you for limits, and you must provide them without being too controlling. Your job is to strike the same balance you are struggling for elsewhere: to find the middle ground somewhere between rigidity and overpermissiveness.

Finding this middle ground is important, not only in establishing good attitudes about eating, but also in insuring a nutritionally adequate diet. Children's diets suffer when parents go to the extremes of over-rigidity or overpermissiveness.[8] Parents who criticize or manage or intrude on eating too much have children who don't eat well. Children eat poorly when parents disagree too much about how they should be managed. On the other hand, if parents ignore food selection, or leave too many decisions to children, they also eat poorly.

Physical changes. The child this age is growing more slowly than at an earlier age. In fact, as you can see from the chart on the next page, the rate of growth of the child one and two years old is only half to a third that of the infant up to age 12 months.[6]

The child this age grows in height more quickly than she gains weight, and she loses body fat, using her stored fat for part of her energy needs.

The toddler won't be as hungry, so she will eat less overall. Her appetite will be erratic and sporadic; she apparently can overwhelm any desire to eat with struggles with her parents, with excitement, and with fatigue. She is still hungry and wants to eat during this time, but she wants more to be independent.

If she is well nourished, she is likely to be troublesome, demanding and energetic. Poorly nourished children sit in the corner and don't cause anyone any problems.

Behavioral Changes. The toddler period is a thrilling, frustrating time of skill building. Your toddler will be learning to crawl, walk and run, to climb and to manipulate objects around her. She will be gaining even more control over the fine muscles in her hands and arms, so she can manipulate her food better and can learn to use eating utensils and drink from a cup. She will spill and drop a lot, won't be able to cut up her food, will have a hard time chasing and balancing peas, and won't be able to chew very tough things. She will still choke somewhat more easily than an older child, although she

Figure 8-1. Comparative weight gain of an infant during the first, second and third years of life (Courtesy Gerber Products Co.).

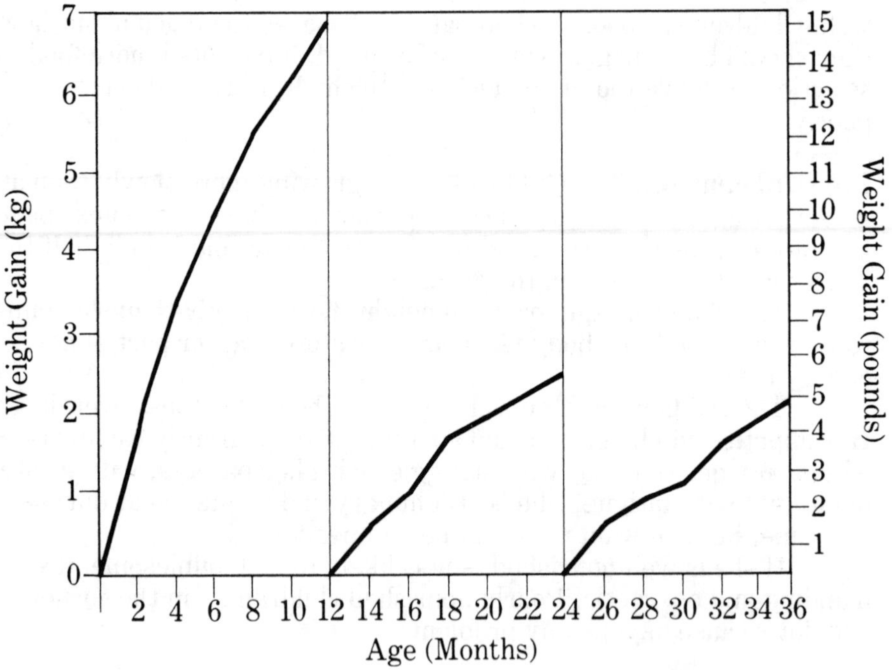

will likely take the difficult food out of her mouth, rather than allowing it to strangle her.

She needs to feel successful, and her tendency to feel embarrassed when she is not successful will show in her habit of slipping the difficult food under the edge of the plate, or sticking it in her pocket. Sympathetic food selection can help the toddler feel more competent and proud of herself. Providing her with eating utensils that she can manage easily will also help toward that goal—as will ignoring her sloppiness and contrariness.

Her skills and interest in self feeding will vary. At times she will absolutely insist on doing everything herself, and do rather an expert job of it; at other times she will drop things, or will want to be fed.

So how are you going to care nutritionally for this contrary, demanding, mercurial creature? In the following sections, I will attempt to define your job for you. I will try to give you some ideas about what you can be doing to promote good eating—and also to alert you to when you may go too far.

We will talk about nutritional adequacy, food selection, mealtime psychology, and other topics. But as we discuss these areas, there is one vital and central point that will come up again and again—in "managing" toddler eating, you must be aware of the division of responsibility:

You are responsible for <u>what</u> your child is offered to eat, <u>where</u> and <u>when</u> it is presented.

She is responsible for <u>how much</u> of it she eats.

If you cross these lines, you are going to get into trouble. You are setting limits for your toddler when you let her know that she can't bully you into offering different food than what you had planned. You are promoting her independence by allowing her to pick and choose from what is available.

Getting Enough of the Right Kind of Food

My major goal in this section is to reassure you that your child is actually doing OK. It is not to pressure you more to see to it that your child eats right. If you feel the pressure, let it be with respect to your family meal-planning. You can only expect yourself to get the right foods on the table. You can't expect yourself to get your child to eat them.

Often parents can relax once they know how little food children really need to eat. At the end of our solid feeding chapter, we talked about the basic four-food plan for the older infant. These same guidelines are appropriate for the toddler.

It is most important to be aware of child-sized portions. Too often we judge what a child "should" be eating by the quantities we, ourselves eat. It's easy to put too much on the plate and make the child feel overwhelmed by the amounts, sometimes to the point where he won't even try to eat.

Figure 8–2. Basic Four-Food Plan

1. *Milk—2–3 cups per day.* Two cups is adequate; more than three is inadvisable because it is then replacing other foods in the diet.
2. *Fruits and vegetables—4 servings per day.* An average adult serving is generally ½ cup or 1 piece (as commonly served). For a child we can say that a nutritionally-adequate portion size is one tablespoon per year of age or one fourth of the adult serving. Thus a child two years old will be taking two tablespoons of fruit or vegetables per serving, or a quarter of an apple or banana.

   An exception would be orange juice, which should be ⅓ cup daily, or the equivalent of another vitamin C source.
3. *Breads and cereals, enriched or whole grained—4 servings per day.* A child's serving is ¼ to ⅓ the adult portion size. The adult serving would be one slice of bread, five crackers, or ½ cup rice, cereal or pasta. Many children will eat disproportionately large amounts from this group, but that's no problem as long as minimum requirements from other groups are being met. Whole grains are appropriate and nutritionally desirable at this age; use them about half the time.
4. *Meats, fish, poultry, eggs, peanut butter, cooked dried beans—2 servings per day.* An adult's serving of meat is 2 to 3 ounces at a

meal. A child's serving is about ½ ounce, for a total of one ounce per day. If the child under age 3 is taking 2 cups of milk per day, 1 ounce of meat or equivalent is adequate to provide the protein requirement. A good source of protein should be offered at each meal.

Meat is often a problem for the infant and toddler, possibly due to difficulty of chewing and swallowing. Casseroles, hearty soups, eggs, fish, hamburger patties, barbecues, peanut butter and legumes* are often accepted better than plain meats.

Hot dogs and lunch meats are fine if limited to once or twice a week. High levels of salt, fat and nitrate make too-frequent consumption a concern.

*Cooked dried beans and peas such as navy beans, pinto beans, lima beans and split peas.

Let me emphasize some things about portion size. I said a good rule of thumb to use is one-fourth to one-third the adult portion size, or one tablespoon per year of age, whichever works better for the particular food. If you are judging bread or a piece of fruit, use the fraction. If you are portioning vegetables or say, rice, the tablespoon might be the easier guide. Give less than you think your child will eat and let him ask for more.

Most people are surprised at the small amount of milk and meat and other protein sources that are required to give enough protein. If there is any nutrient that is likely NOT to be deficient in the American diet it is protein. To repeat, 16 ounces of milk, plus one ounce of meat or meat substitute, provides an ample amount of protein for children up to three years of age. (After that the meat should go up to two ounces per day.)

Restated in more detail, the child one to three years of age needs about 23 grams of protein per day.* The amount of protein, in grams, in typical food sources is listed in the following table:

Figure 8-3. Levels of Protein in Commonly-used Foods

Milk	Grams Protein
Milk, 8 oz.	8
Cheese, cheddar, swiss, etc., 1 oz.	7
Cottage cheese, ¼ cup	7
Meat Group	
Meat, fish, poultry, 1 oz.	7
Egg, 1	7
Cooked dry beans & peas, ½ cup	7
Cooked soybeans, ½ cup	11
Peanut butter, 2 Tbsp.	7
Peanuts, 3 Tbsp.	7
Cashews, 5 Tbsp.	7
Almonds, 5 Tbsp.	7
Breads and Cereals	
Bread, 1 slice	2
Buns, biscuits, muffins, 1	2
Cooked cereals & grain, ½ cup	2
Breakfast cereal, 1 oz.	2
Vegetables and Fruits	
Vegetables, ½ cup	.5-1
Fruits & juices, ½ cup	.5

*All recommendations for levels of nutrients are taken from the Recommended Daily Allowances of the National Research Council, 1980. A table with the complete recommendations is in the Appendix.

Your child will probably eat more than this, and that is fine. Those portion sizes are intended to let you know the minimum he needs to eat to achieve a nutritionally-adequate diet. They are in no way intended for you to use in holding down the amounts he eats.

Evaluating the Diet. To evaluate your child's diet, give some casual attention to the distribution of choices among food groups to be sure that he is not consistently eating one group of foods so enthusiastically that he is completely excluding another group. This might happen on an isolated day or two, which is no problem, but if it happens too often, it could unbalance the diet.

Expect Variation. Many of us eat a nutritionally adequate diet on a weekly average, but few will meet all the minimum requirements every day. Even adults will eat significantly more calories one day than another. We might miss some vegetables or milk one day but consume extra the next. These same variations show up in children. When we discuss the daily food plan, interpret that as being an average of intake for several days, up to a week. Ideally, though, all the food groups should be offered every day; that way your family can regulate themselves in eating appropriate amounts.

Calorie Intakes. They will vary from day to day, and your child will eat as many calories as he needs. The child between one and three years of age will consume about 40 calories per inch of height. This will come out to be somewhere between 1,000 and 1300 calories per day. If you have ever dieted, you know how those seemingly small quantities of food add up. If your child is offered food at reasonably regular intervals, he will eat. No healthy child has ever voluntarily starved.

Milk Intake. Some children drink more milk than they should and will need to be limited so as not to spoil their appetite for other foods. Put a glass of water along with a glass of milk at your child's place, and then put the milk carton back in the refrigerator. That will encourage him to drink water for thirst, and begin to treat the milk as what it is: a food, not a beverage.

Some children do not drink enough milk. Most children, in fact, go through a time when they don't drink much milk. Generally, if you don't make a big issue of it, they go back to it eventually. If you worry or force or tell other people that Suzie won't drink milk, however, she will be reminded and taught that she doesn't like milk, and she might even feel she has to avoid milk on general principles.

Left alone, she will probably go back. While you are waiting for her to do so, you can utilize some information about calcium nutrition. Children from ages one through ten need about 800 mg. of calcium a day. They can get calcium from a variety of foods, although dairy products provide the best food sources, as you can see from the chart on the opposite page.

I will list (Figure 8-5) some tactics you can use for getting calcium into your child's diet, but don't go to great lengths to prepare special food. The chances that a child will refuse a food increase in direct proportion to your effort to provide it.

The footnote on p. 280 suggests using lactase to break down milk sugar for the lactose-intolerant child. Before and during the toddler period you will most likely only see lactose intolerance as a temporary problem following a major intestinal upset like viral enteritis. Even in groups of people who are extremely likely to become lactose intolerant as adults, lactase insufficiency doesn't appear before ages four or five.

Even relatively lactose intolerant children (who are not sick or recovering from acute diarrhea—see *Diarrhea* chapter) can drink some milk. They might get a little gas from it, especially at first, but the gas doesn't hurt them. (It's normal to have a variation in intestinal gas, even if there are no particular intestinal problems.)

If your child cannot tolerate something about the milk other than the lactose,* you should either try to substitute soy formula, or

---

*See the section on allergies at the end of the chapter.

Figure 8-4. Calcium in Foods.

Food	Amount	Calcium (mg.)
Dairy products		
Milk, fluid	1 cup	300
Milk, powdered	1 Tbsp.	60
Cheese, natural or processed	1 ounce	200
Cottage cheese	¼ cup	60
Yogurt	1 cup	300
Ice cream	½ cup	110
Cream cheese	1 Tbsp.	10
Meat and other protein sources		
Meat, poultry, fish	3 ounces	10–20
Canned fish with bones	3 ounces	250
Egg	1	30
Cooked dried beans	½ cup	70
Nuts and seeds	2 Tbsp.	20–40
Peanut butter	2 Tbsp.	20
Bread, cereal, pasta		
Bread	1 slice	25
Biscuits, rolls	1	25
Corn tortillas	1	60
Cooked and dry cereals	1 serving	15
Noodles, macaroni	½ cup	15
Vegetables and fruits		
Vegetables, average	½ cup	20–40
Green leafy vegetables, average	½ cup	100
Fruits, average	½ cup	20–40

Table 8-5. Suggestions for Increasing Calcium in the Diet

Use Dairy Products*

Make fortified milk: Combine 2 cups fluid milk, ⅓ cup powdered milk. Refrigerate before using. Substitute wherever you use milk. One cup fortified milk = 1½ cup regular milk.

Add flavorings to milk: strawberry, chocolate, soft-drink powders. Make eggnog, cocoa, milkshakes.

Make a "smoothie": Blend milk with fruit to make a milkshake-like beverage.

Use milk in some cooking instead of water: cooked cereal, soups, gravies.

Put powdered milk in baking: Add 2 Tbsp. powdered milk to each cup of flour. Store and use for all baking.

Put powdered milk in other cooking.
Ground beef: ½ cup per pound. Add water.
Casseroles: 2 Tbsp. per cup.
Vegetables: Make cream sauce.

Make desserts (use fortified milk): custard, pudding, rice pudding, pumpkin custard, cheese cake.

Use cheese in cooking: Macaroni and cheese, lasagna, tacos, grilled cheese sandwich, cheeseburgers, pizza.

Use High-Calcium Vegetables

Use legumes: bean or split pea soup, chili, three-bean salad, pea-pickle-cheese salad, kidney bean with cheese.

Use greens: In salads, soups, as a vegetable in casseroles.

*If your child gets intestinal gas or diarrhea from drinking milk, she may have a deficiency of lactase, the intestinal enzyme that digests milk sugar. You can buy lactase to pretreat milk. Use the brand name Lact-Aid®. Ask your pharmacist.

one of the hypoallergenic formulas. Both of these will give the calcium and vitamin D that you are counting on milk to provide. Don't use soy milk; it doesn't have the vitamin D of milk and is unpredictable about providing other nutrients.

Pasteurized goat's milk is a substitute for cow's milk that some people can tolerate. This may or may not be fortified with vitamin D; read the label. It is also low in folic acid, but this should not be a problem if a child is eating a variety of foods.

Calcium supplements don't work very well for the infant and toddler. Most supplements come in the form of tablets and the daily dose is four to six or more. It is an exceptional child who can, and will, swallow several pills a day. The only chewable I can find contains calcium phosphate, which interferes with iron absorption. Calcium in tablets is usually in the form of calcium lactate, and you will generally pay about the same amount for a day's calcium in tablet form as you do for milk. Calcium pills come with or without vitamin D. Which you should choose depends on whether your child is getting another good vitamin D source. Avoid bone meal and dolomite; they are contaminated with excessive amounts of lead and other trace elements.

Iron. Another nutrient that concerns us with the toddler is iron. Iron deficiency anemia continues to be a problem up until about age two years, particularly for children living in poverty.

There are two common nutritional errors that contribute to iron deficiency anemia in older infants and toddlers: 1) Overconsumption of milk (more than 16 to 24 ounces per day), with resultant low intake of iron-containing food; and 2) Poor snack selection; whereas meals commonly provide appropriate amounts of iron, snacks may provide calories with few nutrients of any sort.

The child who is one to three years old needs 15 mg. iron per day. With the exception of milk, the foods listed on the next page, eaten in child-size portions, provide significant iron.

Figure 8-6. Iron Content of Selected Foods

Food	Amount	Iron (mg.)
Meat and other protein		
Beef, pork, lamb	3 ounces	2–3
Poultry	3 ounces	1.5
Beef or chicken liver	3 ounces	8.5
Calves liver	3 ounces	14
Pork liver	3 ounces	25
Clams	3 ounces	5
Oysters	3 ounces	13
Other fish, shellfish	3 ounces	1–1.5
Egg	1	1
Nuts, average	2 Tbsp.	1
Seeds (sunflower, squash, pumpkin, average)	2 Tbsp.	2
Breads and Cereals		
Enriched or whole-grain bread	1 slice	0.7
Noodles, spaghetti, etc.	½ cup	0.7
Cooked or dry cereals	½–¾ cup	0.7
Multi-vitamin and iron supplement cereals	Iron content varies; read package.	
Fruits and Vegetables		
Green leafy vegetables	½ cup	2
Peas, mixed vegetables	½ cup	2
Other vegetables, average	½ cup	0.8
Prunes and dates	½ cup	2
Other fruits and juices	½ cup	0.6
Milk		
Whole, skim, 2% milk	1 cup	0.1 mg.

Miscellaneous		
Blackstrap molasses	1 Tbsp.	3
Sorghum	1 Tbsp.	2.5
Molasses, medium	1 Tbsp.	1

Iron in meat, poultry and fish is absorbed several times as well as iron from vegetable sources.[9] It seems that these animal protein foods contain something we call a "meat factor," which also improves absorption of vegetable iron eaten at the same time as meat. Similarly, vitamin C sources consumed at the same time as other iron-containing foods will improve iron absorption.[9] "Meat factor" and Vitamin C also help each other out in iron absorption: if you take both at a meal, the iron absorption will be even further improved.[9] Examples of meals that would have both meat and vitamin C include hamburgers and coleslaw, spaghetti with tomato sauce, hot dogs and orange wedges.

Iron in egg yolk is poorly absorbed. In fact, unless you take vitamin C at the same time, egg yolk will actually impair iron absorption from other foods. Milk apparently neither enhances or blocks iron absorption from other foods.[9]

Limit liver consumption to twice a month. Eating too much liver will give too much vitamin A.

Vitamins A and C: As you run a rough check on your child's food intake, you will want to make sure that his food sources add up to a good amount of vitamin C almost every day (see p. 248 for a list of foods containing vitamin C), and a good amount of vitamin A every other day (see p. 246). Don't worry unnecessarily about temporary short-falls, however; as long as he is not suffering from any major illness, his food intake can drop 25 to 50% below the recommended allowances, and he will still be doing pretty well. Our nutrient requirements build in a "fudge factor," which means that we can eat somewhat less than prescribed quantities of nutrients and still be all right nutritionally.

If it seems like he just isn't eating any, say, high vitamin-A vegetables, you might want to see to it that he is offered some cantaloupe or apricot or peach nectar for a snack. But be subtle about it; you must not let him know that you are willing to substitute other foods for those he refuses.

Vitamin and Mineral Supplements. If your water is inadequately fluoridated, your child may need to take a fluoride supplement.* Beyond that, if you are preparing a nutritionally adequate diet, eating it yourself and presenting it in a neutral and matter-of-fact fashion, your child will not need to take vitamin-mineral supplements. Sooner or later he will eat well and will provide himself with an adequate diet.

Don't get too caught up in evaluating your child's diet. *Pay attention to whether he seems energetic and is growing well.* If observing his food intake and assessing it for nutritional adequacy is making you nervous, stop. He is probably doing OK. When I actually sit down to calculate nutrient intake in detail, I am always surprised at what odd diets add up to nutritional adequacy.

Pay at least as much attention to what you are offering (and the way you are offering it) as you do to what he is eating. Over-all, that will reflect his nutritional status much more clearly than any analysis of what he happens to accept on a few isolated days.

Food Selection

Before we get started on this section, let me issue a word of warning: Don't get so involved with planning and preparing nutritious food for your child that you forget that your ultimate job is *to parent.* Providing food will take some time and attention. Don't let it take too much.

---

*See the Supplemental Fluoride Schedule, table A-6 in the Appendix.

If you are running yourself ragged providing superior, homemade, delectable everything for your family, you may be sacrificing something else that is more important.

If you love to cook and it gives you more energy for other things, that is one thing. But if you see it as just another job, you will be perfectly justified in finding shortcuts, using good-quality mixes and convenience foods, and even taking in an occasional "fast-food" franchise.

Frozen vegetables are just as nutritious as fresh, and they take a lot less preparation time. It's great if you love to bake bread. You can, however, find good breads on the grocery-store shelf that are just as nutritious as the ones you bake yourself. It's fun to make yogurt and grow your own sprouts, but if you are getting up in the middle of the night to attend to them, the juice might not be worth the squeeze. And speaking of that, frozen orange juice is just as nutritious as juice you make yourself from fresh oranges.

Meal Planning. A meal should provide—

Protein: Meat, fish, poultry, egg, cooked dried beans, seeds or nuts.

A bread or cereal: Bread, bun, noodles, spaghetti, etc.

A fruit or vegetable or both.

Milk.

A nutritionally complete meal might contain only two food items, such as a tuna noodle casserole with peas and a glass of milk. Or everything could be separate, as with meat loaf, mashed potatoes, broccoli, bread and milk. Vegetables might be part of a combination dish, as in spaghetti and meat sauce. Fruit can be served as part of dessert, as in oatmeal raisin cookies, or given as a juice along with a meal.

You can evaluate some convenience foods, such as canned or frozen dinners or hearty soups—good menu choices for you and your toddler. You can just look at the product to see if it has vegetable and starch in it. To find out if it has enough protein, however, you will need to check the nutritional labeling. A toddler should be able to get about five grams of protein from a half-cup serving of main-dish food.

If everything doesn't fit into the meal, you can count on the snack to provide part of it. A fruit juice at a snack can help make up for a fruit or vegetable that wasn't eaten at the meal.

The hamburger, fried chicken, pizza and taco places offer nutritious choices for an occasional meal. If your child has milk or a milkshake (instead of pop) and some french fries or coleslaw, he can really come out quite well in getting a nutritionally-complete meal. These fast-food meals have two main drawbacks—their high sodium content and their lack of fruits and vegetables. (With the exception of batter-fried food, the fat content of fast foods is not too bad.) But such drawbacks do not become major problems if you don't go there too often.

Catering to Likes and Dislikes. In planning meals for your family, you will probably want to treat your child just like you do everyone else—by catering to a reasonable degree to her food preferences as you plan menus. But don't limit your menus to just the foods that you know your child will like. One good strategy is to include one food he likes with each meal; if the vegetable is a less-favorite one, have a bread or salad that your child usually likes.

I say *usually* likes, because another feature of this age group is that they will eat a food enthusiastically one time, and completely shun it the next, which is frustrating to say the least. You'll run out at one meal and have way too much at the next.

Short-order Cooking. You have the meal on the table, the toddler whines he doesn't like it, you insist he eat it, he refuses, and you say,

"All right, what will you eat?" That is short-order cooking. Don't do it. In fact, don't even get close to it. When your toddler complains he doesn't like something, ignore it. Don't give him the idea that you are concerned or upset about it or willing to substitute. Have his milk on the table when he arrives, put some bread on the table so he won't starve, give him some support in getting himself served, and leave him to his own devices.

Making Food Easy to Eat. Your toddler needs some help with certain foods. He can't chew tough and fibrous food too well, like meat, and too-dry food seems to get stuck in his mouth. Here are some suggestions to help the eating process along:

- Cut foods into bite-sized pieces, preferably before he gets there. He won't be able for some time to handle a knife, and is likely to have a tantrum about not being allowed to try—and another one about trying and failing.
- Make some foods soft and moist. If you have dry meat, have creamed peas. Make the mashed potatoes a little softer than you would for adults.
- Allow him to eat his foods at room temperature. Perhaps you can dish his up in a separate serving bowl so it can cool off or warm up a bit before he tries to eat it.
- Keep ground beef patties in the freezer to substitute when you have roasts or steaks that your child can't handle easily. Cook patties only long enough for the color to change to brown so it is still juicy. Meat is hard to eat, even for older children.
- Give salads without dressing and serve them as finger food.
- Make soups thin enough to drink from a cup or thick enough to spoon easily.
- Cook strong-flavored vegetables, such as brussels sprouts, in about an equal volume of cooking water and then throw away the water. You will be throwing away nutrients, but there's a better chance that they will be eaten.
- Prepare food well. Children accept foods better when they are

properly cooked with natural colors and textures preserved.
- Put a little extra color in foods. Children are interested in a little parsley in the hot dish or some carrot grated into the coleslaw.
- Put up with their idiosyncrasies about shapes. Children will often insist on having their sandwiches quartered, and if they are halfed, they will throw tantrums. Or they will think carrot sticks are inedible but will eat carrot dollars very happily. Orange wedges with the skins attached are often eaten better than sections.

You may delight in making little orange section boats and little gingerbread man sandwiches. I think that's fine for a party or special occasion, but not as a regular thing. I suspect parents who are willing regularly to go that far of having too much anxiety about their child's eating. I also know from experience that if I have gone to some trouble to make food cute and my child won't eat it, I feel disgusted and it is hard to ignore his refusal. Regularly providing cute food tends to confuse food with playthings. Food should look like FOOD, not like toys.

Mealtime Environment

To promote good attitudes about food and good nutrition, it is important for your meals to be significant, and pleasant.

By significant I mean that there needs to be a meal on the table. Someone in the household has to take responsibility for planning, purchasing and preparing the food. Significant also means expecting the family to show up to eat the meal, to pay attention to it, and to spend some time over it. Of course there are those unavoidable times when meals will have to be rushed, but if that is happening too often, you need to do some problem-solving.

Make mealtime pleasant. Don't argue, fight or scold at mealtimes, and don't let anyone else do it either. It is tempting to ventilate gripes at mealtime, because that may be the one reliable time when the family is together. Don't do it!

Consider Timing. Have your meals at whatever time works in your household. Don't be too concerned if your family eats at an unusual time—say has the evening meal quite late. The child this age is beginning to fit into the family's routine (instead of vice-versa). You can control the child's hunger with judicious use of snacks, so he will be able to wait and eat along with the rest of the family. This is important; one of the most powerful influences on your child's food acceptance is eating with you and seeing you enjoy a wide variety of nutritious food.

Seating Arrangements. Make any adjustments that may enhance everyone's comfort. Use whatever seating arrangement allows your child to sit at a convenient height in relation to the table. Her feet should be supported, as it is uncomfortable for anyone to have his feet dangling for any length of time.

Use a child-sized plate and utensils. A plate with low edges will give her a bang-board for pushing the food onto her fork or spoon. A smaller plate will help you regulate your portioning. Junior-sized silverware is a good size for this age, or a broad salad fork and a spoon work well. She should have a glass with a broad base that sits firmly on the table, and it should be small enough so that she can encircle it with her hands. If you are concerned about your floor, protect it some way, as there will be inevitable spills and dropping.

Occasionally children will ask to be allowed to sit at their own small eating table and chairs. That is fine and also comfortable for them, as long as they don't abuse the privilege by getting up and running around during the meal.

Eating Mechanics. Give her silverware, but don't insist that she use it. If she is allowed to look, feel, mash and smell while exploring new food, she is more likely to accept it. You'll be able to tell if she is truly exploring a new food, or just playing or messing around to get you to react. Once she stops eating, it is time to let her get down from the table.

Don't worry too much about the mechanics of eating. Parents who make frequent demands on their children to eat, sit properly and use the napkin, interrupt their child's eating. Children either become rebellious or so preoccupied with the mechanics that they lose their interest in food. As your child matures, her dexterity will develop, and the spills, dropped food and utensils, and general mess will decrease. Developing wholesome attitudes about eating is more important, at this stage, than the niceties of table manners.

Enforcing Food Consumption. Don't do it! Your job is to get food on the table and to make it clear to everyone that they are expected to come to the table. Your job is not to enforce, cajole, trick or persuade them to eat. I often see fathers getting into the act as eating enforcer, particularly at dinner time. They take a hard line, insisting that the child will eat. In defense of fathers, I most often see them doing this when the mother is being overly-solicitous, worrying over food refusal, cajoling the child to eat, or even falling prey to short order cooking; because mother is so mushy, father has to be extra tough.

The role of disciplinarian is an important one; there are good and bad ways of filling it. You must not force, cajole, trick or otherwise interfere with your child's prerogative of deciding how much she will eat. What you CAN do is insist that she come to the table, be firm about limiting food availability to what is on the table, and refuse to allow her to complain about and criticize the food. And if mother shows signs of weakening and running for the peanut butter and jelly, you can remind her (diplomatically) that there will be another meal, and that your child is likely to survive very nicely until then.

Then you can go ahead and enjoy your own food, and refuse to allow your child to behave in a way that interferes with your own mealtime enjoyment. And don't forget to eat your vegetables.

Acknowledging Eating

You can acknowledge your child's willingness to try a new food, but don't praise him for eating a lot of it. That is interfering with his self-regulation. Giving him enthusiastic approval for his eating may teach him to eat just to please you. You want him to eat to please *himself*. Don't laugh at his mistakes, either. That is also paying too much attention to his eating, and will encourage him either to show off or to be embarrassed.

Reinforcing Desirable Behavior. Ignore undesirable behavior respecting food or eating, even if it means you have to remove your child from the table. Whenever you pay attention, or praise, coax or beg, or give in to his demands for food, you are paying attention to and rewarding bad behavior. Observe what you are doing that may inadvertently give attention to bad behavior. When you respond to his grocery-store crying and whining by buying him a candy bar, you are supporting his misbehavior. (You are also supporting your own weakness, because *you* get rewarded by *his* stopping crying.)

You can reinforce by paying attention, recognizing, and acknowledging appropriate behavior. Take time to eat and chat with your child at mealtime. Don't reserve your mealtime attention for the times when he is being naughty. If he misbehaves, put him down. When he behaves well, welcome him at the table and include him in the conversation.

Getting Ready to Eat. Children at times will get so tired or stimulated from play that they don't feel like eating. If you can manage it, a few minutes spent with him before offering the meal, perhaps reading a book to get settled down, can pay off in an improved appetite.

Other times they get so involved in their play that they don't want to come to the table. A five minute warning may help. Sometimes nothing helps, and your child will tell you he's not hungry anyway and will, on no account, eat. Tell him that that is his choice, but that you expect him to come to the table whether he eats or not and that you expect him to stay a while.

How long depends on your child. It needs to be long enough for him to get settled down and bored enough to realize that if he is going to have to sit there anyway, he might as well go ahead and eat, but not so long for it to seem vicious and punitive. (This situation is different from letting a fed child down from the table when he starts to misbehave. Here we have a hungry child who needs to be deprived of his other activity so he can know he's hungry.)

Food Acceptance

Depending on how much your child has to test you, you will probably have some showdowns over food. Don't, however, have them over what he will eat. Have them about what you will provide. You can't force him to eat his peas, but you can refuse to get up and make string beans as a substitute.

Your child may, or probably will, invite you to fight over his eating by refusing certain foods or whole meals. If you let him know you are concerned, he will get the upper hand, and manipulate you into doing all sorts of objectionable things to get him to eat. Don't overreact. Your only recourse is to ignore his food refusal and then decline to feed him when he comes around later panhandling for food. Don't order, beg, punish, force, reason or coax. You will always lose. And your child will lose, too, because he will be so busy struggling with you that he won't be able to eat well.

You won't avoid struggles by giving in to his demands. You will only postpone them. He needs to know he can rely on you to set limits on his behavior. If you give in, he will simply become more and more provocative until you are *forced* to have a confrontation with him. You might as well do it sooner rather than later.

Eat a Variety of Foods. If you are a finicky eater, you are likely to teach or allow your child to be the same way. Try new foods and attempt to teach yourself to eat a variety of foods. But go slowly; don't push it. Start out with a goal of taking one bite of a food you don't like. Once that becomes really quite tolerable, go to two bites. Don't expect yourself to eat a whole serving until you really like it. If you force too much on yourself too soon, you will feel revolted.

Change Undesirable Eating Behavior Slowly and Expect Setbacks. This goes for your own eating as well as that of your child. If you whittle away at undesirable behavior a little at a time, you will probably make major advances over time. If you try to do too much, too fast, you will relapse and may never make it.

Use Good Tactics for Introducing New Foods. Introduce new foods early. Acceptance of new foods is age-related. The older children get, the more likely they are to refuse new food. Observe the time of day when your child takes a new food most easily and give it to him then. This may be when he is most hungry. He may also accept new foods better if he is not too tired or excited. He will certainly accept them better if he doesn't feel pressure about it. The first time he is introduced to a new food, he may only look at it and not get around to eating it until the second or third time he sees it.

Do serve very small portions of a new or unpopular food. One pea or green bean has a better chance of being eaten than a whole big serving. Be judicious about demanding that he taste everything. This often works with minimum fuss, but be careful about establishing requirements. You'll lose. On the other hand, you might have a child who is suspicious of anything new, and then likes and eats it very well once he tastes it. Experiment and see what works for you.

Separate Rejection of You from Rejection of Your Food. Don't confuse the reason for your child's food rejection. That is easier said than done, particularly if you like to pay a lot of attention to what your family likes, and struggle to find things that you think they will eat. You have to find a balance here, and one of the best ways I know of achieving it is to pay attention to your *own* preferences. Treat your own food likes and dislikes with as much respect as you do those of the rest of the family. Expect them to eat a less-favored food at times, simply because you *love* it. And if you make something you don't like, say so politely—to yourself.

Set realistic standards for yourself. You have to keep a lot of things in mind as you prepare your menus: cost, food availability, nutritional balance, the time you have available for preparation. With your busy life, you are simply going to have to resign yourself to the fact that some meals are not going to be all that hot.

Keep in mind that their not eating is not *your* failure. If you prepare acceptable food, it is not your fault if they won't eat. It's not their fault either. They just happen not to like it or not to feel like eating it. Children need to learn at home to cope with food they don't particularly enjoy. (From working in cafeterias, I know too many adults who throw tantrums when presented with food that doesn't happen to match their expectations.)

Don't Promote Food Jags. Don't ask your child what he wants for lunch. Make it and put it on the table. If he wants to eat a particular food every single day, let him ask for it ahead of time, and give it to him at snack time. Don't let him come to the table and refuse what you have prepared and demand the other food. Many times if you don't give children the idea that they have a choice about food selection, it won't occur to them. But at the same time, they need to learn to do some selecting. Snack time is a good time for that.

Snacking

People often think that snacking is bad for their children, and try to prevent eating between meals. That really isn't necessary or even helpful. *Children's energy needs are high, and they have a limited capacity for food, so they really need to eat every three to four hours.* The important thing is that you have control over the time of snacking and the type of food that is consumed.

Timing. Snacks should be offered midway between meals. They should be provided long enough after the previous meal so that your child knows he will have to go hungry for some time if he refuses the meal. This helps prevent the pattern of meal refusal followed by almost-immediate begging for food. You, too, will be much more inclined to refuse food handouts if you know that another feeding is coming up in only two or three hours.

Some parents, in their anxiety to feed their children will fall prey to this kind of tactic and end up feeding almost on demand all day. We particularly see this pattern in the child who is gaining weight slowly or growing less rapidly than average. The parent is understandably anxious about food intake and compounds the difficulty by giving in too easily to the child's food demands. In fact, these small feedings can actually decrease total calories and impair nutrient intake.

You may have to offer two snacks if you have a particularly long interval between meals. If children have an early lunch and a late dinner, it often works well to have a "heavy" snack (one with protein, fat and carbohydrate), two or three hours after lunch, and then a carbohydrate snack, such as fruit or crackers, later in the afternoon. A small amount of fruit or juice can help to tide your child over when you are dashing around getting dinner on. Some fruit or juice in the car on the way home from the day care center can prevent conflict later.

Regulation. The way to regulate snacks is to get there first. If you plan on a reasonably-consistent snack time, and get the food on the table, you will be able to manage timing, location and selection. If you feed your child before she is too hungry, she will eat a moderate amount. On the other hand, I will guarantee you a struggle if you wait until she is famished, and has already thought about what she wants to eat and where she wants to eat it. You may have to be firm about snacking either way, but at least you won't be asking for more trouble than necessary.

Selection. A snack that you want to last a while should contain some protein, some fat, and some carbohydrate, the same as a nutritious meal. It should be big and substantial enough to be filling for a hungry child. An apple or some carrots just don't do the trick when you are famished, even if they are filling for the moment; because they are only carbohydrate, they won't stay in the stomach long and your child will be hungry too soon before the next meal.

On the other hand, if it is only protein and fat, say cheese or peanut butter in celery sticks, it won't be as immediately satisfying, and may tend to be higher in calories. But if the snack contains all three major nutrients, it will be satisfying and should "stay with" the child, while still allowing her to be comfortably hungry in time for the next meal.

Figure 8-7 gives you some suggestions for nutritious snacks. However, any food that you consider appropriate for a meal is appropriate for a snack. Some parents are quite successful at sending a refused meal around again at snack time. This isn't as heartlessly sneaky as it sounds—maybe lunch has been eaten poorly because the child was tired before a nap.

Often snacktime is a good time to get the child to try new things. Maybe you can work in the servings of vegetables that are still missing in the day's food totals, particularly if you serve them raw or still-frozen. Many times children will accept as snacks foods that they ignore or refuse at meals. Experiment.

Avoid, in general, the kind of food that the advertising industry defines as snack foods. Chips, snack cakes (like Twinkies®), fruit drinks, and candies, all have very little nutritional value in relationship to the calories they contribute. In fact, nutritional surveys indicate that overall quality of the American diet is seriously diluted by snack selection. They show that meal averages look pretty good, but that when they are added in with snack patterns the quality goes down seriously. Poor-quality foods rob your child twice—once when they are eaten and a second time when the calories replace those of more nutritious food.

This is not to say that some of these questionable goodies should never be eaten. As available as they are today, it is probably wise to teach your children to manage them. Once in a while it is O.K. to make up a package of Kool-Aid® or to buy a small package of snack cakes to have along with a meal or a snack. But the trick is controlling the frequency and amount. Buy a limited quantity so it goes around once and then is gone. That way it doesn't force you to be the gatekeeper in rationing out what is left.

Even though it pains me to say this, even Kool-Aid and the snack cakes do make a nutritional contribution in the form of their calorie content. Most children are so active that they can satisfy all their nutritional requirements and still have need for more calories.

The purist in me, however, feels much more comfortable about giving sugary foods if they are hooked on to something nutritious. For a bunch of hungry and thirsty kids, I like to spike one part orange Kool-Aid with one-half to three parts orange juice. Ice cream, malts, oatmeal cookies and carrot-raisin cake are all basically nutritious foods, and they give the extra calories that most children need.

Sweets

It is valid for you to be concerned about sugar. It is not necessary to be terrified.

Americans consume a lot of sugar. Each American man, woman and child consumes on the average 130 pounds of sugar per

Figure 8-7. Nutritious Snacks

Vegetable Snacks:

Cut up fresh, raw vegetables. Serve with peanut butter, cheese, cottage cheese or milk* to get protein and fat. Add crackers or fruit juice to get carbohydrate.

Broccoli	Green beans
Carrots	Green peas
Cauliflower	Turnip sticks
Celery	Zucchini
Cucumber	

Fresh Fruit Snacks:

Slice or serve whole. Serve with peanut butter, cottage cheese, yogurt, ricotta cheese or milk to give protein and fat.

Apples	Berries	Peaches
Apricots	Grapefruit	Pears
Bananas	Grapes	Pineapple
	Melons	

Dried Fruit Snacks:

Serve with nuts, almonds, cashews, peanuts, or with seeds (pumpkin, squash, sunflower) to give protein and fat. *Be very cautious about giving seeds and nuts to young children.*

Apples	Figs	Prunes
Apricots	Peaches	Raisins
Dates	Pears	

*Use either 2% or whole milk to give fat.

Nuts and Seeds:

Peanuts, Pumpkin and squash kernels, Sunflower seeds.

Grain Products:

A. *Bread products.* Use whole wheat about half the time. Read the label to make sure the flour is enriched or whole grain. (The first listed ingredient should be *whole* wheat.) Try a variety of yeast breads and quick breads—whole wheat, rye, oatmeal, mixed grains, bran—plain or with dried fruit. Try rye crisps, whole grain flat bread, and whole grain crackers. Serve bread and crackers with cheese, peanut butter or a glass of milk to give protein and fat.

B. *Dry cereals:* Choose varieties with less than three grams of "sucrose or other sugar", *read the label*, per serving. Serve with milk to give protein and fat. Add dried fruits, nuts and seeds for variety and increased nutrients.

C. *Popcorn:* Try using grated cheese instead of salt and butter. Serve with milk or cocoa to give protein and fat.

D. *Cookies:* Bake your own, substituting ½ whole wheat flour for white flour. Try oatmeal, peanut butter or molasses cookies. Experiment with cutting down on sugar in recipes, often you can decrease sugar by ⅓ to ½. Serve cookies with milk to give protein (cookies already have fat).

Beverages:

A. Use fruit juices and vegetable juices rather than powdered or canned fruit drinks which are high in sugar and lower in vitamins.

B. Milk: Serve plain with bread, crackers, cereal, etc. Mix in blender with banana, other fruit or orange juice for a healthy milkshake. Try adding vanilla extract, honey, molasses, even a little sugar. Use chocolate and strawberry flavorings for an occasional treat.

year. That figures out to ¼ cup of sugar per person, per day. About 24% of the calories in the average diet come from sugar. Of that 24%, 14% comes from refined sugars like sucrose (table sugar), fructose, glucose, lactose and maltose. Four percent of the sugar comes from processed foods like corn syrup, corn syrup solids, maple syrup, honey and molasses. And only about six percent comes from natural sources like fruits, vegetables and milk products.

More than two-thirds of the sugar in the food supply is consumed in factory-made foods and only a quarter is in foods prepared with sugar in the home. Processors use sugar for sweetening, to help foods retain moisture, to prevent spoilage, and to improve texture and appearance.

It's very hard to avoid sugar and you needn't try. Used judiciously, sugar does improve the flavor and acceptability of some foods. Eaten along with a meal or a substantial snack, sugar won't send people off on sugar jags.

How Much Sugar. Your child does not *need* any added sugar at all in her diet. The natural foods we mentioned earlier, milk and fruit, have sugar in them. But even without these, the body can provide itself with sugar by manufacturing it from starch, protein and fat. But, whether the sweet tooth is born or made, most of us do have one. Sweet-tasting foods add considerable pleasure, as well as providing energy for our fast-growing, fast-moving children.

The U.S. dietary goals recommend that the amount of refined and processed sugar in the diet be brought down from the average level of 18% to about 10% of calories in the diet.[4] This is a pretty arbitrary figure—and a pretty drastic reduction. Short of being sure that sugar does not replace other nutritious foods in the diet, there is no real way of knowing how much sugar is "bad" for your child. But it might help you to relax about sugar intake if we are more specific, and with that in mind, I'll accept the figure of 10% as a sugar "allowance" and give you an idea of how much that is.

A child taking about 1300 calories per day, a rough guess of average calorie intake for the toddler, will have a sugar "allowance" of 130 calories per day. Each teaspoonful of table sugar gives 20 calories. You can figure a reasonable daily sugar allowance at six teaspoons or (30 grams) of sugar (or molasses, jelly, syrup or honey). A fast way of figuring a sugar "allowance," in teaspoons, for different calorie levels is to divide calories comsumed per day by 200: a person eating 1800 calories could have nine teaspoons of sugar.

Here are the amounts of sugar contained in some common foods:

Figure 8-8. Sugar Content of Common Sweet Foods

Food	Teaspoons of sugar
Candy bar, 1 ounce	7
Cookies, 1–3 inch	1–2
Brownies, 2-inch square	1–2
Frosted cake, two layer, 1/16	7
Fruit pie, 1/7 of 9 inch	6–9
Pumpkin pie, 1/7 of 9 inch	3–5
Ice cream, ½ cup	3
Chocolate milk, 1 cup	3
Milkshake, 10 ounces	9
Sweetened soda pop, 12 ounces	6–9
Kool-Aid,® 8 ounces	6

Source: U.S.D.A. Home and Garden Bulletin #72

You can figure sugar content of food by dividing the total amount of sugar in a recipe by the number of servings it makes. An apple pie recipe that serves seven and calls for ¾ cup sugar will have

36 teaspoons of sugar (3 teaspoons per tablespoon and 16 tablespoons per cup makes 48 teaspoons times ¾ = 36 teaspoons), or about five teaspoons (36 ÷ 7) per serving.

(These figures are lower than the ones you generally see in tables of "hidden sugar" in foods, although they are certainly high enough. I think other list-compilers must be figuring total carbohydrate, rather than subtracting out the starch from the sugar.)

Many nutritional labels tell the amount of sugar in an average serving of their product. Breakfast cereals do this, and declare it as grams of "sucrose and other sugars." Again, if you prefer to think in terms of teaspoons, convert by figuring five grams of sugar per teaspoon.

Having done all of this figuring, I want to put things back in perspective. I really don't want you to declare an absolute limit on your child's sweets intake, counting every cookie or glass of Kool-Aid.® I also don't want you to give free access to the candy and pop. Keep things in balance. See that your child is offered a variety of nutritious food, make most sweets nutritious, and offer the more-concentrated sweets only occasionally.

It is better to control or limit concentrated, low nutrient foods to an occasional use than it is to try to prohibit them completely. I know too many children who grew up in sugar-free households who load up on exactly this kind of food when they have a chance.

Using Sugar to Promote Nutritious Food. Good cooks use sugar to make food taste better. A teaspoon of sugar in a tomato dish takes the harsh edge off the tomato taste and makes the dish more acceptable, especially to younger tastebuds. A teaspoon of sugar in the frozen peas will give them a "just-picked" flavor.

Some desserts and sweets are very nutritious. Custards, puddings, oatmeal or peanut butter cookies, and pumpkin pie (you can skip the top crust) are all very nutritious desserts. If children like sugar on their (low-sugar) breakfast cereal, or enjoy flavoring in milk, or like jam on toast, those are valid uses of sugar. Just keep an eye on the proportion of sugar to other foods in the diet.

Desserts. Should a child be allowed to have dessert if he doesn't finish his meal? Yes! If you make dessert a reward for eating "well" (which usually means "a lot"), you will probably be encouraging your child to overeat twice: once at the meal and once when he eats dessert after he is already full. You are also teaching him that dessert is the only really-desirable part of the meal.

Make dessert something nutritious and put a serving of it at each plate at the same time as you serve the rest of the meal. So what if he eats it first. He will probably discover that he is still hungry and go on to eat the rest of his meal. If he is waiting and saving room for dessert, he will probably end up not satisfied and then harass you for more dessert.

Oral Health. Sugar promotes tooth decay by nourishing the acid-producing bacteria in the mouth. Mouth bacteria can learn to live on the sugar in milk (lactose) or the sugar in fruit (fructose) just as well as they can on table sugar.

The longer and more frequently sugar is in contact with the teeth, the more likely it is to cause tooth decay. If a child is sipping pop or fruit juice for a very long time, or fanning the refrigerator door satisfying his thirst with calorie-containing beverages, he will be bathing his teeth with sugar and promoting tooth decay.

Sugar in sticky foods will adhere to the teeth and remain in the mouth longer. Caramels and raisins, for example, stick to the teeth and also take a long time to eat, so both increase the risk of tooth decay.

Nutritional Concerns. The major nutritional problem with sugar is that it can displace other, more nutritious foods in your diet. Sugar in and of itself will not make you sick, cause insanity, or lead to any of the horrible maladies that are reported in the popular press. The only disease that we can really blame on sugar is tooth decay.*

I object to sugar-coated cereals, and their advertising, primarily because they teach kids that food has to be sweet to be good. Highly sweetened breakfast cereals dyed vivid colors disguise the delicious flavors of grains, and promote a substitute food that is more like candy than cereal. As I tell my children (and they hate it), "If you are going to eat candy, eat candy. If you are going to eat cereal, eat cereal. But don't eat that stuff and call it cereal."

We buy about two boxes of sugar-coated cereal a year for the kids to eat when we go on camping trips. They think it is a big treat and they wolf it down for snacks. They say they think I am being rigid and silly when I won't buy it all of the time. Too bad.

Too-frequent consumption of high-sugar food can send some kids and some older people on sugar jags, periodically recharging themselves with sugary foods. The body can overreact to a high sugar load and send blood sugar levels below fasting levels. This leads to more hunger and more sugar craving—and another sugar fix repeats the process.

Eating Problems

There is a mixed bag of typical eating concerns and questions that show up during the toddler period. I will lump them together in the discussion that follows.

Chewing and Swallowing Problems. An occasional child will get stuck at a developmental stage with his eating, and not move on in normal fashion to the next stage. He might insist on nursing instead of eating meals, or refuse to eat anything that is the least-bit lumpy

*Even diabetes is not "caused" by excess sugar intake.

long past the time when he should have been gumming more textured foods.

One of the causes may have been that he was not offered next-stage food when he was developmentally ready. He may have been sick or fussy when it was time to get him on table foods, or he may have had an over-developed gag response that scared his parents into backing off from teaching him to chew. For whatever reason, it is important to get the toddler on grownup type food, with only minimal modifications. That can create a problem, as the toddler can be perfectly capable of carrying on a battle over just that issue.

To get him to progress developmentally, you will have to change the texture and consistency of his food, and you will have to be firm about it. You will have to slowly introduce an increasing amount of texture and thickness into his food. If you are being slow and patient and he still refuses, you will have to tough it out. Children are capable of refusing to eat for several days before they give in and start to eat. But don't let him panhandle, and don't let him fill up on milk and juice.

If he seems like he is having particular difficulty chewing and swallowing food, or if he continues to do a lot of gagging, it is possible that he is having a real developmental problem. Talk with your pediatrician about this, and ask him to refer you to a good occupational therapist. That professional is well equipped to evaluate patterns of oral musculature, and to work, if necessary, in promoting appropriate developmental changes. An occupational therapist can also help you to know if your child is really having a problem or he is simply trying to manipulate you with food.

Overdependency on the Breast. The toddler should be eating meals rather than breastfeeding at mealtime. Breastfeeding morning and evening, or for snacks, is appropriate nutritionally, but breastmilk consumption should not interfere with the developmental and nutritional advantages of meal-eating.

If your toddler has gotten stuck on breastfeeding, you will have to be firm about refusing the breast at mealtime. It may help if mother makes herself scarce and lets someone else feed him for a while until he gets interested in table food.

Overdependency on the Bottle. If you have waited until the toddler period to wean at mealtime, that bottle is likely interfering with food consumption and you should get rid of it. You may be able to avoid a confrontation by diluting the bottle milk and giving undiluted milk in a glass. Eventually your child may begin to prefer the milk in the glass and give up the bottle voluntarily.

If that doesn't work and you can't come up with any other indirect tactic, you are simply going to have to be firm about omitting the bottle at mealtime. You are highly likely to be tested strongly—but hold firm.

Don't make the mistake of giving a bottle right after a meal or letting him run around with a bottle. A bottle must be treated as a snack, and be controlled in time and location.

Allergies. Don't put yourself through all the hassle of catering to a food allergy unless it is really necessary. Many times when children who are assumed to be allergic are challenged with an offending food, it is discovered that they aren't even sensitive to it.

Most evidence for food allergies is pretty circumstantial, and misleading. As we said earlier, perfectly healthy babies will, at times, sound congested, spit up and get gassy. About one baby in ten, through no fault of his own or his parents, is downright impossible: fussy, wakeful, irritable, sensitive to almost everything. You could begin to link a particular food with these symptoms, if you happen to provide the food just before the symptoms appear, and remove it just as symptoms disappear.

But at the same time as I encourage you not to be over ready to label your child food-allergic, I want to caution you that true food allergy can be very serious for the few children who do react significantly to certain foods. Severe allergic reactions include extreme skin rashes, pronounced breathing difficulties, marked nausea and diarrhea, and shock. For some few children, ingestion of even a small amount of an offending food can be life-threatening. Those children must be under a doctor's care and parents must know emergency procedures.

In many cases it appears that children's food allergies are transient. As they get older, the food intolerance resolves itself and the offending food may be safely reintroduced into the diet.

Sometimes children's reactions to foods are not allergies at all, but just temporary problems brought on by disease. Intestinal reactions to foods may come and go with bowel disturbances, so are really in the category of sensitivities rather than allergies. For instance, viral enteritis (viral diarrhea) will often leave a child temporarily intolerant of the lactose in milk. Occasionally someone who has had an infection will become sensitive to the protein in milk. If all goes well and these substances are removed for a few weeks, the ability to tolerate them can be regained.

The most useful tool for diagnosing food allergy is removing, then challenging, with the offending food. (Skin tests are only partially successful in diagnosis.) In most cases, you can do the challenging at home by keeping the diet constant and varying the suspected food. However, food challenge can be dangerous if the initial reaction to the food has been serious or violent. The child who has had any marked reactions to food must be under a doctor's care and any food challenging must be done with a physician *present*.

Physical symptoms of allergic reactions to foods include: abdominal pain, vomiting and diarrhea; cough, runny nose and wheezing; skin itching and rash; headache and irritability; and shock. In addition to these physical syptoms, there are a number of pseudoscientists who are selling books by saying that food allergies cause a number of behavioral problems, such as irritability, contrariness, sleeplessness, rebelliousness, and general nastiness. For the embattled parent, it is very tempting to believe that some external, definable, controllable force can be responsible for all these maddening traits.

It is extremely difficult to prove, or disprove, a food-allergy basis for a behavioral problem. (A good example is the research with hyperkinesis, which we will discuss in a subsequent section.) To prove that a particular behavior is caused by dietary intolerance, you have to keep the environment the same and change only the diet. Since behavior is so complex and changes so rapidly, it is very difficult to know whether the improvement is due to a change in diet or a change in other factors. A child may behave better after he is taken off Kool-Aid because he is sensitive to something in the Kool-Aid—or he may behave better because he is impressed by his mother's firmness in refusing to give in to his demands.

Eating and Behavior. People try to find nutritional solutions to problems such as hyperactivity, minimal brain dysfunction and learning disabilities. They aren't successful. To have a nutritional solution, you must have a nutritional problem. That is, a person can only be made better by nutritional supplementation if his symptoms are caused in the first place, by a nutritional deficiency. There is no evidence that any of these conditions is caused by nutritional deficiency. They are often *treated* with massive doses of nutrients, but the treatment doesn't work; in fact, at times it *causes* serious nutritional and physical problems.[10]

It is true that deficiency of almost any vitamin or mineral is likely to make someone behave differently, because he will be physically weak and susceptible to disease. People with iron deficiency anemia are lethargic and irritable. Some nutrients, such as niacin and thiamine, are particularly important for a steady and well-functioning nervous system. But if your child is eating a variety of foods and growing well, he is unlikely to be deficient in any nutrient.

Energy is the one nutritional factor that is likely to have an impact on your child's behavior. A child who is hungry is likely to be tired, irritable and contrary. Sometimes a hungry child is so contrary that he won't eat. The child who is very physically active and enthusiastic will often get so busy and involved that he won't notice he's getting hungry until it is too late. For a time, he will go on nerves and excitement alone, but will, eventually, collapse before your eyes into a screaming, unmanageable heap, or become even more frantically active in response to hunger.

The busy and active child is a likely candidate for a pattern of sugar jags, because he will want something he can get down in a hurry that will satisfy him in a hurry. Stand firm. Insist that he calm down and come to the table and spend some time eating. Once he gets there and finds out you mean business, he will likely eat just as enthusiastically as he plays. Be particularly careful to choose snacks for him that have a balance of protein, fat and carbohydrate.* He needs to have his food stay with him long enough so he can get some of his playing done. It's a real chore getting a person like this settled down and ready to eat. You'd better do what you can to provide food that will last him a while.

Hyperactivity. Beginning in 1973, the late Dr. Ben Feingold, a California pediatric allergist, argued that salicylates (naturally occurring compounds present in many fruits, some vegetables and a number of other foods), artificial colors and artificial flavors are causes of hyperkinesis. The Feingold diet eliminates essentially all manufactured baked goods, luncheon meats, ice cream, powdered pudding, candies, soft drinks and powdered and canned fruit drinks, as well as mouthwash, tooth paste and cough drops. The regimen also stresses includ-

---

*Look in the *Solid Foods* chapter, p. 239, for a table with protein, fat and carbohydrate content of foods, and in the *Regulation* chapter, p. 351 for a discussion on satisfaction.

ing the hyperactive child in food preparation, and encourages the entire family to participate in the diet program.

Because the Feingold regimen changes so many factors, it is hard to tell if it works and, if it does, what there is about it that helps. The child on this regimen is likely to get more attention as well as more firm limits. Because so many of the prohibited foods are high in sugar, the diet can improve nutritional status and help to prevent sugar jags.

Feingold claimed a marked improvement in over 50% of hyperactive children. Other, carefully-controlled studies have shown a much more modest response. A fraction of one percent of hyperkinetic children in controlled experiments show a mild decrease in hyperactive behavior. A very few preschool-aged hyperkinetic children appear to benefit significantly from the diet.[1,3]

Provided adequate vitamin C can be provided from "allowed" fruits and vegetables, the Feingold diet is not harmful to the child nutritionally. In fact, it may be helpful, because it strips away the high-sugar extras and forces reliance on home-prepared, basic foods. There is certainly nothing to be lost from eliminating artificial coloring and flavoring, nor is it all that difficult.

But the diet can limit a child's opportunities to eat out in many restaurants, and it will rule out the use of otherwise satisfactory convenience foods. The most serious drawback, however, may be that it could teach a child (and his parents) that his behavior is controlled by what he eats. It follows that if food controls his behavior, he (and his parents) can't, or won't have to. Thus he could be handicapped in the part of his social development that demands that he learn to curb and manage his emotional and behavioral responses.

If you are going to use this diet, I would encourage you to use it as an adjunct, not an alternative, to other behavioral and psychological counseling that you may enlist to help you evaluate and manage your family environment and your child's behavior. I would also encourage you to be subtle and matter-of-fact about your child's dietary restrictions. I don't think it's wise to emphasize any child's food intolerances or restrictions. You can be firm about food avoidance without making an issue of it.

Elevated Blood Lipids. Some few children may benefit from being started early on a special dietary regimen to control the amount of cholesterol and triglycerides in their blood.[2] These children have what we call "familial hyperlipidemia." They have inherited a marked susceptibility to heart disease, and are likely to be very sensitive to high levels of cholesterol or animal fats in their diet, and to react with elevated blood lipids. In some children this shows up as early as age two; other children don't show the family trait until they get into their twenties.

Children are at risk of having this trait if they have a close relative who has severe heart disease, particularly at a young age. Parents of this child should be tested to find out whether they have high blood cholesterol or triglyceride levels. If either or both of them do, the child should also be tested and followed to catch the trait if and when it appears.

Children who show signs of developing elevated blood lipids should be kept on a modified diet that limits saturated fats such as animal fat, coconut and palm oil, and hydrogenated shortening and margarine, and which substitutes, in moderation, polyunsaturated fats, such as safflower and corn oil. This diet also requires that use of cholesterol sources like egg yolks and liver be kept as low as possible. Get your doctor's advice about using this diet for your child, and consult with a dietitian for help in understanding and following it.

The course of action is less clear for people who do not have elevated blood lipids. Experts on heart disease have been arguing for years about whether everybody should follow a low cholesterol, modified fat diet in an attempt to lower the incidence of heart disease. Some consider the diet reasonable, moderate and desirable for everyone. Others think the changes are extreme rather than moderate, and say that such dietary intervention should be directed only to people who are clearly susceptible. I prefer to take an approach somewhere between the extremes. There are plenty of moderate and positive changes that can be made in the American way of eating that stop short of the therapeutic dieting we have talked about.

Avoidance of overeating and obesity is important.* Beyond that, Americans don't eat enough fruits and vegetables. They eat too little starch and too much meat, sugar, and fat. We could improve our diets and give our budgets a break if we would start using more meat-extender dishes like casseroles and soups, and even substituting beans for meat occasionally. We could eat a smaller portion of meat and a larger baked potato. We could choose lower fat cuts of meat and eat chicken or fish more often. We could cut down on frequency of frying. We could eat fewer sweets and drink less sugar-sweetened soft drinks.

All of these strategies would bring our diets back in better proportion to the basic-four food plan, which depends on the use, in moderation, of all types of foods to provide a healthful diet.

Vegetarianism. Children do fine on vegetarian diets as long as the diet is well-planned and includes milk, cheese and eggs. However, children on the more-restrictive vegetarian diets that omit animal protein sources may not fare as well. Some groups of vegetarian children are smaller than other children and have more problems with rickets, iron-deficiency anemia and malabsorption.[5]

For children, the major problem with the vegetarian diet is its bulk. Unless the cook makes a special effort to include fat with the meals, the vegetarian diet tends to be low in caloric density, and this makes it difficult for children to get their calorie requirement. Pro-

---

*This is not, however, the same thing as promotion of undereating and attempting to maintain excessive thinness. See the *Obesity* chapter.

tein can also be a problem. Legumes, seeds and nuts, in proper combination with grains, provide a high-quality source of the "meat and other protein" group. However, to get an adequate amount of protein from, for example, a beans and rice dish, a child would have to eat a volume of food that would be four to six times as great as if he were getting his protein from meat or cheese. Children who can't eat that much, and many don't, simply do not get enough protein.

One way in which insufficient protein limits overall nutritional status is by making the intestine less able to absorb fat. With poor fat absorption, a protein deficiency can exaggerate a calorie deficiency, and growth can fall off.

You must take some precautions if you want your child to be on a vegetarian diet.

- Continue to follow the basic-four food plan; substitute for the meat group, eggs, cheese, legumes (cooked dried beans such as kidney, lima and navy beans, or lentils) or seeds and nuts (especially peanuts). With the exception of legumes, vegetables are not good sources of protein but offer other important nutrients.
- Use vitamin D-fortified milk to provide calcium and vitamin D, as well as a concentrated source of high-quality protein and fat. If you are adamant about avoiding all animal products, substitute vitamin D and iron-fortified soy formula for the cow's milk. Do not make your own soy or nut milks or buy soy or nut milks from the health food store—these vary greatly in nutritional composition and generally do not give iron and vitamin D.
- Offer some concentrated source of animal protein at each meal, such as eggs, cheese or milk. Your child can get valuable amounts of protein from a vegetarian main dish, but he needs some help from a concentrated protein source in order to get enough total protein.
- Know what you are doing in combining vegetable protein substitutes for animal proteins. Study a reliable cookbook, such as *Laurel's Kitchen.*[11]

- Keep an eye on iron nutrition. About 3% to 8% of the iron in vegetables and grains (depending on what is in the rest of the meal) is absorbed, compared to about 20% of the iron in meat, poultry and fish. Without the well-absorbed iron and the "meat factor" from meat, poultry and fish, it will be more difficult for him to get and absorb enough iron from his diet. Be sure to keep him on iron-fortified baby cereal throughout the high-risk toddler period. Try to give a good source of vitamin C along with at least two of his meals every day to help him absorb his plant iron.
- Use whole grains only about half of the time, enriched refined grains the rest. Too much fiber in the diet can interfere with iron, copper and zinc absorption.[7] Enriched white flour, white rice and white macaroni products give some of the advantages of the grain without overloading your child with fiber.

There is nothing about the vegetarian diet that is inherently superior to the carnivorous diet. In fact, unless you have chosen to eat a vegetarian diet for philosophical or aesthetic reasons, you might consider drawing on the best features and enjoyable qualities of both. Use meat judiciously as a source of valuable trace elements, protein, iron and "meat factor." A small amount of meat in a largely legume and cereal dish can add flavor as well as nutritional value. Also learn to depend on legumes and grains as sources of protein, iron and trace elements. There are many wonderful dishes, including foods from other cultures, that are based on grain and legume combinations, such as Mexican tortillas and refried beans, Brazilian black beans and rice, and our own navy bean soup with crackers.

Fiber. For children as well as adults, it appears that a moderate amount of fiber in the diet helps good bowel function. The large intestine seems to work best when it has a certain amount of filling from a diet that has some indigestible residue of the sort that you get from whole grains, legumes, seeds and nuts and raw fruits and vegetables.

If a diet has a reasonable amount of fiber, it gives a stool that is formed, soft and somewhat bulky, and easy to pass without a lot of straining. Stools from a highly refined diet tend to be smaller, harder and more formed. If your child's stool is small and hard, it may hurt to go to the bathroom, and it could give her intestinal cramps.

To provide your child with enough fiber, offer an adequate amount of fruits and vegetables and use whole grain at least part of the time. Read the label on whole grain bread to make sure the first listed ingredient is WHOLE wheat. "Wheat flour" is not whole wheat, nor is "unbleached" wheat flour. It has to say WHOLE wheat. If your child won't eat whole wheat bread, try her out on graham crackers, brown rice or oatmeal cookies.

Don't overdo it on the whole grains, however. If she gets too much, it could backfire and give her diarrhea. Further, an extremely high-fiber diet, such as a vegetarian diet with a lot of legumes, seeds and nuts as well as whole grains, can cause nutritional problems.[7]

Looking Ahead.

Some day you will call your child to dinner and he will come willingly. Some day you will remind him to finish his dinner and it won't precipitate a major power struggle. When that day comes, your toddler will have changed to a preschooler and peace (relatively speaking) will come.

We're going to stop here in our discussion of feeding children. Although we are leaving off at the toddler stage, the nutritional and behavioral principles of feeding will remain the same as your child grows up.

Older children are easier to feed than infants and toddlers because they do not have such specialized nutritional and developmental needs. But they are also harder, because as they grow they increasingly develop their own ideas about what they want to eat and when they want to eat it.

With preadolescents, adolescents and teenagers, you will have to know when to be flexible and when to stand firm. You will likely have to loosen your controls on snack selection and eventually even meal selection. However, you will be wise to maintain consistent and reliable meals as the backbone of your family's food supply and to insist that your children, even your teenagers, show up for most meals. And it is appropriate for you to encourage snack selection that is nutritious and worthwhile. You will also be wise to insist on timing snacks so children are hungry for meals.

It is important to continue to be positive about your child's eating and food selection. You may have to overlook at lot to do that, but in the long run you will all be ahead. Children's nutritional status, at all ages, suffers from family criticism and interference.

Selected References

1. American Council on Science and Health. Diet and Hyperactivity: Is There a Relationship? 1995 Broadway, New York 10023.
2. Breslow, Jan. Pediatric aspects of hyperlipidemia. Pediatrics. 62:510–520. 1978.
3. Consensus Development Conference. Defined diets and childhood hyperactivity. National Institutes of Health. IN Journal of the American Medical Association. 248(3). 290-292. 1982.
4. Dietary Goals for the United States, prepared by the Senate Select Committee on Nutrition and Human Needs, Superintendent of Documents, U.S. Government Printing Office. Washington, D.C. 1977.
5. Dwyer, J. T., E. M. Andrew, I. Valadian and R. B. Reed. Size, obesity and leanness in vegetarian preschool children. The Journal of the American Dietetics Association. 77:434–439. 1980.
6. Gerber Products Company. Current Practices in Infant Feeding. Freemont, Michigan. 1980.

7. James, W. P. T. Dietary fiber and mineral absorption. IN Spiller, G. A. and R. M. Kay. Medical Aspects of Dietary Fiber. Plenum. New York. 1980.
8. Kinter, Martha, P. G. Boss and N. Johnson. The relationship between dysfunctional family environments and the family member food intake. Journal of Marriage and the Family. August 1981. 633–641.
9. Monson, E. R., et al. Estimation of available dietary iron. The American Journal of Clinical Nutrition. 31:134–141. 1978.
10. Pipes, Peggy L. Special concerns of dietary intake during infancy and childhood. IN Nutrition in Infancy and Childhood. C. V. Mosby. St. Louis, 1981.
11. Robertson, Laurel, Carol Flinders and Bronwen Godfrey. Laurel's Kitchen. Nilgiri Press, Petaluma, CA. 1978.

9 Diarrhea

In most cases, the condition that is loosely termed "diarrhea" isn't diarrhea at all, but is simply an increase in the frequency or liquidity of the stools. True diarrhea of the kind that should concern you is better termed acute diarrhea. *It is the sort that is caused by a virus or bacteria that makes the child truly sick—feverish or vomiting or both. With acute diarrhea you must be alert to the signs of dehydration, and vigilant about maintaining your child's fluid intake.*

The child with other forms of diarrhea is generally not sick, but has chronic diarrhea. *He has an increase in stool frequency that could be caused by any number of things—from teething to eating too much watermelon. The increased stool frequency of chronic diarrhea doesn't present the same threat of dehydration because such children remain thirsty and hungry, and their ability to absorb nutrients is not impaired.*

You will need to make some dietary modifications to help your child recover from acute diarrhea. Other dietary modifications to help decrease stool frequency associated with chronic diarrhea are optional—you would use them to help control the mess of diarrhea, not because they are necessary for the health of your child.

Why are we talking about diarrhea in a book on nutrition?—Because diarrhea can have an impact on feeding.

For one thing, an illness causing diarrhea can spoil the appetite. For another, physicians and parents often react to diarrhea by putting children on various kinds of dietary restrictions; and sometimes the dietary restrictions are so drastic, or are applied so energetically that children actually end up not growing very well. In most cases the diarrhea itself doesn't cause the growth impairment. It is the diet.[5]

Although standard treatment regimens for diarrhea are improving, some health workers are extremely tenacious at clinging to traditional though questionably-effective therapies for diarrhea, because they know diarrhea can lead to dehydration. The diarrhea of the child who is truly ill, especially if it is accompanied by vomiting, fever, or both, can take a considerable amount of water out of a child's body. An infant cannot let his adults know he is thirsty, and can actually sleep himself into dehydration. If the dehydration goes too far, the child may have to be hospitalized and put on intravenous fluids. (While this is serious, it is unusual for this dehydration to get to the point of being life-threatening.)

Health workers, like parents, are also tired of diarrhea. Small children seem to have sensitive intestines that are easily upset by a variety of physical and emotional changes, from teething to going on vacation. So health workers spend a considerable amount of contact time with parents simply doing diarrhea counseling. The counseling often doesn't help and the diarrhea often doesn't go away. When my friend Mary Ellen announced her intention to resign her position as a pediatric nurse practitioner and go off around the world, she said the main thing she would not miss about her job was talking with parents about diarrhea.

Parents do worry. To them, an increase in stool frequency and wateriness is a sign that there is something wrong with their baby. And they know that diarrhea can be dangerous. But most diarrhea does not cause dehydration, and it is not harmful nutritionally. It is a terrible nuisance. Parents of infants with diarrhea do not hand their child to doting and dressed-up godmothers. Parents of toddlers with diarrhea do not visit friends with newly-carpeted living rooms.

Normal Bowel Habits

You need to know how to identify, evaluate and respond when normal bowel habits change into diarrhea. That is not easy, because nobody really knows what are and what are not normal bowel habits.[2]

Bowel habits vary greatly from one infant to another, and from one time to another for the same individual. The normal breastfed infant at 10 days of age is likely to pass 8 to 10 stools per day, and these stools can be loose, explosive, and vary in color from yellow to brown to dark green. On the other hand, a two-month-old breastfed infant not on solids may pass only one stool in two or three days. Some older children have one stool every three or four days. Others have two or three stools a day, again varying in consistency, color, and nature of passing.

Generally the most-desirable stool from the standpoint of comfort and convenience is a soft, somewhat-formed stool, that is easily passed without apparent straining. However, many healthy children pass watery stools with no apparent discomfort. Their stools are a problem only to their parents.

Overreacting to changes in bowel habits can be simply asking for trouble. When our Kjerstin was six months old, her stools changed from their usual—a formed, even semi-solid, once-a-day pattern—to a three-times-daily pattern that was consistently softer and almost runny. I was concerned and thought there was something wrong with her. We happened to be at the doctor's office for a regular appointment, and I told the pediatrician that I thought she had diarrhea. She told me quite abruptly that it was not diarrhea, that it was simply a change in bowel habits, that my daughter was really quite normal and there was no cause for concern.

I was miffed. I thought she had dismissed my concerns in quite a cavalier fashion, and that it was abundantly clear to me that she did have diarrhea. However, having been offered nothing else to do about it, I did nothing. I continued feeding Kjerstin as I always had—and I can't remember now if the stool frequency again changed back or if I just quit paying attention to it.

I am now grateful to that doctor for dismissing my concerns, however abruptly. I have seen too many other parents in very similar circumstances, who have been advised and supervised in treating the same kind of "diarrhea," to the detriment of all concerned. I have seen children put on liquids-only diets to "rest the bowel," or taken off milk for no apparent reason. At times I have suspected that dietary manipulations actually worsened the condition, and have seen parents positively dreading each bowel movement because they felt they must react to every change in bowel habits with dietary manipulations. I have seen children irritable and restless from hunger, and be allowed only crackers and juice because they were on some sort of a diarrhea-treating dietary regimen.

Types of Diarrhea

Diarrhea may be loosely defined as the passage of frequent, unformed or watery stools. It is a term, and a definition, that means little, because as I said, many babies and toddlers have a "normal" pattern of bowel movements that look very much like diarrhea.

A change in bowel habits becomes diarrhea when you have to change the socks as well as the pants—and it bugs you.

A change in bowel habits can also begin to look like and seem like diarrhea when your baby's bottom becomes red and sore after a few minutes contact with a dirty diaper, and he cries pitifully when you clean him off. While both of these conditions are highly undesirable, they are not critical or dangerous. A better term, and one that means something in terms of taking action, is acute diarrhea.

Acute Diarrhea. Acute diarrhea goes along with an infection, generally viral enteritis.* It can also come from contamination of food or drinking water with illness-causing bacteria. A child with acute diarrhea is likely to have fever, vomiting, or both, along with his diarrhea, so he is losing fluid from more than one place. To make matters worse, when a small child is ill or feels nauseated and has a sore throat, he is likely to refuse fluids as well as foods. As he begins to be dehydrated he will sleep more and refuse more, and may eventually end up seriously dehydrated.

The other major form of diarrhea, chronic nonspecific diarrhea, rarely becomes dangerous unless the child is not eating or drinking.

Chronic Nonspecific Diarrhea. Unlike the child with acute diarrhea, the child with chronic nonspecific diarrhea (which we will call "chronic diarrhea") is not sick. He eats well, appears healthy and energetic, has a normal pattern of growth and development, and doesn't seem to have any particular food sensitivities or intolerances.

---

*This may also be called viral diarrhea. It is characterized by sudden onset and is generally accompanied by vomiting and fever. Viral enteritis is often mislabeled as flu. Flu is infiuenza, which is primarily a respiratory disease. Its symptoms are cough, respiratory congestion, fever and muscle aching.

The child with chronic diarrhea simply has a bowel pattern which someone labels excessively frequent or watery (and probably with good cause, if that someone is cleaning up after it).

Chronic diarrhea comes in many forms. It can last a day or several months, it can appear intermittently or can be consistently present from day to day. There might be five semisolid stools a day or 10 liquid stools a day. Some people will even label as diarrhea the occasional runny bowel movement. Chronic diarrhea is one of the most frequent gastrointestinal complaints in childhood, familiar to every pediatrician and to too many parents.

Chronic diarrhea is not threatening like acute diarrhea because it is not accompanied by other dehydrating stressors. The child is well and alert, so he can let you know if he is thirsty, and if he drinks something he can keep it down. Because he is not feverish he will not be sweating excessively. And he will be hungry so he will be able to get his water and other electrolytes from food. Provided he is allowed to eat appropriately, he will be able to absorb the nutrients from his food and will remain adequately nourished.

It is hard to know what causes chronic diarrhea. Babies and young children react to changes or distortions in their diets with more-frequent and watery stools. They often get diarrhea when they are teething, have a cold, or have a change in water or schedule. Antibiotics will also cause diarrhea, probably because they disrupt the bacteria in the colon. At times, chronic diarrhea may develop following an acute bowel upset, although the child is no longer ill. Many times bowel habits return to their more-usual pattern once the stress has passed. Many times they do not.

Sad to say, many infants and toddlers have intermittent diarrhea lasting in some cases as long as three years. These children seem to have a normal pattern of growth and development and don't seem to have any particular food sensitivites or intolerances. This condition is hard to treat and treatment is frequently unsuccessful. (Although we will be looking at tactics in the next section.)

Chronic Organic Diarrhea. One of the persistent forms of diarrhea, chronic organic diarrhea, is distinguished from chronic nonspecific diarrhea by the fact that it is being caused by some disease process. The child with chronic organic diarrhea will show warning signs of the disease, including growth that drops off in weight and/or height, lung problems, abdominal pain, cramps, protuberant stomach, chronic fever, and blood in the stool.

If you see these signs you should let your doctor know so he can examine your child. Don't, however, alarm yourself unnecessarily. All children show lung congestion and have stomach aches from time to time, and it is normal for the young child to have a stomach that sticks out. It is only when these signs become marked that you should be concerned.

How Do You Manage Diarrhea?

Management of diarrhea first requires some sorting out of the type of diarrhea you are dealing with. You have to watch out for acute diarrhea; specifically, you must be prepared to take firm and prompt action to prevent the dehydration of acute diarrhea. Chronic, nonspecific diarrhea really presents more social and aesthetic problems than medical ones. Your goal in treatment of chronic diarrhea is somewhat diagnostic. By changing the diet you can find out what, if anything, is causing the loose and runny bowel movements, and, with any luck, get the stools to dry up a bit.

All the types of diarrhea are not the same. It's important to separate them out in talking about treatment, even if some of the principles of treatment are somewhat similar.

Managing Acute Diarrhea. The child with acute diarrhea is genuinely sick and in danger of becoming dehydrated. Your job is to see that that doesn't happen.

The Signs of Dehydration. Your job during the acute phase of your child's illness, is to: 1) maintain an adequate fluid intake to correct the fluid loss; 2) be alert to the signs of dehydration; 3) stay in touch with the doctor.

To assess if the baby is becoming dehydrated:

- Check his skin elasticity. Pinch a fold of skin on his abdomen. Does it spring back like it should?
- Check his mouth. Is it dry?
- Check the number of wet diapers. Is he still urinating?
- Check his fontanelle (the soft spot at the top of his head). Is it sunken?
- Check his eyes. Are they sunk back into his head?

If your baby is reasonably lively, taking oral fluids, and not vomiting excessively, you should be able to look after him at home, and not have to put him in the hospital.

If the first three symptoms begin to appear, increase your efforts to get him to drink more. The last two symptoms are later signs of dehydration. If your child's eyes or soft spot begin to sink in, you definitely should get in touch with your doctor.

Providing Oral Fluids. The amount of oral fluids you should try to get into your baby depends on his body weight. A baby up to 20 pounds will require about two ounces of fluid per pound per day to keep him hydrated. If he has diarrhea, is feverish and/or is vomiting, the fluid intake should increase to about three ounces per pound.[4]

The child over 20 pounds, because she has a smaller surface area relative to the rest of her body, and is better at concentrating her urine, doesn't need so much fluid. She can probably do all right on one to one-and-one-half ounces of fluid per pound.

In order to get this amount of fluid into your baby, you will have to keep at it frequently and insistently. Even when she is vomiting, she can take tiny sips of fluids; the older child can suck on crushed ice or popsickles. Good fluid choices include water, fruit juices, soda pop or ginger ale, jello and clear broth.

Beware of arbitrary rules about how long you should wait before you start to feed your baby again after she has had acute diarrhea, or about what you feed her.

When to Feed. Feed your child when she is hungry and interested in food. There is nothing to be gained by withholding food after she starts to get better, as long as the food is properly chosen.[6]

What to Feed. Food selection for a child recovering from viral diarrhea depends on the age of the child. Generally, keep the baby under age three months off cow's milk for up to a week.* Substitute a soy formula or hypoallergenic formula during that time. You should avoid cow's milk early on because the virus can change the young infant's intestine so it lets in whole protein molecules, which, in turn can cause an allergic response.

Continue to breastfeed. The lactose in breastmilk might make the stools more watery and gassy for a couple of days, but that problem will resolve itself. It is worth tolerating that to enable you to breastfeed. There is generally no other reason to avoid breastfeeding, since breast milk protein doesn't cause sensitivites like cow's milk protein does.

Keep infants and children over age three months off large amounts of cow's milk for about 48 hours after they start feeling better. The child still taking a lot of formula should be given soy or hypo-allergenic formula during this time. The child taking a substantial amount of solid foods can probably get along without milk for a couple of days. For the older child, the milk avoidance is primarily intended to eliminate lactose.[6] A viral infection often reduces the intestine's ability to digest lactose. (This is true for people of all ages.) If children continue to get lactose during that time, it will make their

---

*This is probably longer than is absolutely necessary, but it doesn't hurt to be a little extra careful in this case.

stools watery and gassy. Losing this extra fluid is, of course, more of a stress for the younger child, who has more difficulty maintaining fluid balance.

Figure 9-1 lists foods high in lactose. Limiting lactose intake to two or three grams at each meal or snack is probably a reasonable approach for the child recovering from acute diarrhea.

Figure 9-1. Lactose Content of Common Foods

Food	Quantity	Lactose, (grams)
Milk	1 cup	12
Yogurt	1 cup	10–15
"Hard" cheeses:		
Cheddar, Swiss, American	1 oz	1
Cottage cheese	¼ cup	2
Ice cream, ice milk	½ cup	5
Sherbet	¼ cup	2

With the exception of cow's milk and other foods containing lactose, resume a normal diet. Every family has a list of foods they turn to when people are sick or convalescing, and your family is probably no different. You may give starchy foods like toast and crackers, and such foods as eggs and cheese, and meats and vegetables when she has an appetite for them. Soups are good, like chicken noodle or vegetable beef. Don't go too heavy on fruits and fruit juices at first: it appears that young children react to excessive amounts by producing loose stools. But stay away from large amounts of custards, milk toast and yogurt.

It may also be wise to stay away from large amounts of sucrose, or table sugar, during that first couple of days after your child has viral diarrhea. In about one out of three cases children's ability to digest that sugar is impaired, as well.[3]

Routine Management of Chronic Diarrhea. Don't overreact to chronic diarrhea. Remember that looseness of stools is diarrhea only by definition. In many cultures, what we define as diarrhea is a normal bowel pattern. But there are some general procedures you should use in dealing with diarrhea:

- Continue to offer a balanced diet at the usual feeding intervals.
- Wait for the stress to pass before you assume you have a stubborn or chronic form of diarrhea.
- Keep your child as comfortable as possible.

Diet. Continue to give a balanced diet, including all the foods that your child has been accustomed to having. Give the same formula, breastmilk or whole milk as always. It is only when children have had acute diarrhea that we recommend taking them off cow's milk, lactose, and sucrose for a while. Continue to give breads, cereals and crackers. Meats, fish, poultry, fat and vegetables should be given in the usual amounts. Go easy on fruits and fruit juices.

There are a few things about diet that you should check or control more carefully for the child with non-acute diarrhea:

1. Make sure the diet has enough fat in it. There is some reasonably good evidence that diarrhea of the chronic, non-specific type may be caused or prolonged by a low-fat diet.[7] Some children who were put on low-fat diets by their families in an attempt to prevent heart disease or obesity developed diarrhea, and returned to more formed stools when given high-fat diets. Other children, who were put on low-fat diets as control measures for diarrhea, continued to have diarrhea, in some cases, for two or three years. Most of them improved when they were put on high-fat diets. The speculation is that the fat helps by slowing down the activity of the stomach and intestine.

   The diet of an infant and young child should have somewhere between 30 and 55% of the calories in the form of fat. To get this adequate level of fat, make sure you give formula, breastmilk or whole milk to a child under age two. Put a little butter, or, better still, margarine* on his bread and vegetables, and use meats, poultry and fish that have moderate amounts of fat in them. Make sure that a child taking 2% milk has at least one extra teaspoon of margarine or oil* for each glass of whole milk he is drinking.

2. Limit fruit and juice intake to two or three child-sized portions per day. Kids get loose stools from too much fruit, so there's no sense aggravating things. Of course, you know that prunes and figs contain a natural laxative, so keep those away from your child. Don't forget that fig newtons contain figs.
3. Hold down on sugar. Cut out the very-sweet candies, pops and desserts. If you have dessert, make it something that is not very sweet, such as ice cream or custard, and keep the portions moderate. A little sugar on cereal is OK, and a moderate amount of syrup on pancakes is fine, but be extra-conservative about sugar in general. If you give a child too much sugar, some may slip through into the large intestine and promote the fermentation and gas we talked about earlier.
4. Avoid artificial sweeteners. Not only is there some question whether sorbitol, mannitol and saccharin are safe for children, but there is also the problem that too much of these substances can give diarrhea.

Wait for the Stress to Pass. If teething appears to be the stress, you have little choice but to wait. You can try out some of the elimination tactics we will talk about later, but you may just have to tough it out. The same thing goes for colds, sore throats and the like.

As I recall, our Curtis had diarrhea every time we went on vacation. The first few times we took our home water along, but that really didn't seem to help. If we were gone long enough, eventually his stools went back to normal, but generally we would have to get back home before things would start to dry up again.

---

*The fat in margarine and oil appears to be better-absorbed by the young child than the fat in butter.

Keep the Child as Comfortable as Possible. That means, change a dirty diaper as quickly as possible. Sometimes, however, it seems that the stools are so irritating that you just can't be fast enough—their little backsides get sore and inflamed almost immediately.

The best thing is to make sure that the whole diaper area is greased generously with zinc oxide, petroleum jelly, or some other ointment that will stick on and leave a heavy protective coat.

Dietary Treatment of Chronic Nonspecific Diarrhea. After chronic diarrhea hangs on for a while, say over two or three weeks, and it begins to look like it's not going to go away by itself, you might want to (or be driven to) see if there is anything you can do about it. There are some dietary tactics you can try out to encourage your child's stools to be less watery and less frequent. They are tactics that won't hurt him, as long as you pay attention to maintaining a basically well-balanced diet while you experiment.

It's hard to tell what might help, or even if anything will help. One approach works for one child, another for another, and nothing for a third. The important thing is to list possible causes (or remedies), then go through the list, trying out one thing at a time. Wait at least a week after initiating one change before trying another, so you can tell what, if anything, helps.

1. Try a high-fat diet. Get a dietitian's help for this one. Keep eating records on your child for three or four days, and have the dietitian analyze the amount of fat that he generally takes. (While you are at it, have her evaluate his diet for any other distortions or inadequacies.) Then make a plan for increasing the fat in his diet, up to about 50% of his daily calorie intake.

   One university pediatrician reported about an 80% success rate using this approach for treating chronic, nonspecific diarrhea.
2. Eliminate sugar. This is a cumulative approach. To start with:
   a. Eliminate table sugar as completely as practically possible.

Avoid all obviously sweet foods.

b. Eliminate citrus fruit and juice. Some children have specific intolerances to grapefruit and oranges and their juices. If that doesn't help, . . .
c. Eliminate all fruit and juice. The goal here is to complete the process of getting rid of sugar in the diet, as well as to pick up on the occasional child who gets the trots from eating fruit.

3. Vary the milk.
   a. If your child is on pasteurized milk, start out by using evaporated milk, diluted one-to-one with water. The theory here is that boiled milk is more easily digestible than pasteurized milk, and is likely to let less undigested nutrients escape into the large intestine.
   b. Use lactase-treated milk or milk that uses some other carbohydrate source instead of lactose.
   c. Avoid cow's milk altogether. The theory here is that it is not the sugar in milk but some other component that is causing a diarrhea-producing sensitivity.
4. Gradually introduce more whole grain. Start out by substituting whole grain about a quarter of the time for enriched white breads and cereals. Gradually increase to about 50%. It appears that in some cases shifting to a diet that gives more indigestible residue helps the colon to work better. It is important, however, to experiment gradually with this approach, as it can backfire. If a person gets too much fiber for his particular digestive tract, it can aggravate a case of diarrhea.
5. Include yogurt—about eight ounces per day. Use the unsweetened yogurt, and make it a little more appealing by putting in a teaspoon of sugar and a little fruit; it will still be lower in sugar than the store-bought presweetened type. Eating yogurt introduces lactobacillus bacteria into the colon. This can be helpful, providing the diarrhea is caused by overgrowth of less-helpful and diarrhea-causing colon bacteria. It is the same principle that

is used in the physician's prescription of acidolpholus culture. Some people swear by yogurt, or acidolpholus culture, as a way of controlling diarrhea caused by antibiotic therapy. Presumably, to be most helpful the yogurt "therapy" has to be instituted at the same time as the antibiotic therapy.

Keep in mind that if you are substituting yogurt for milk for an extended time, yogurt is lower than whole milk in two important nutrients: fat (if it is low-fat yogurt) and vitamin D. Both must be supplemented if low-fat yogurt is to substitute adequately for milk; and vitamin D must be supplemented with any type of yogurt substitution.*

6. If your child is developmentally ready, toilet train him. You *can* train a child who has diarrhea. They don't like being messy and will hold their stools. Then, as the stool gets to stay in the colon longer, more of the fluid may be absorbed and the stools may eventually be more formed.

I hope by the time you have gone all the way through this list that something has helped the diarrhea. Eventually your child will be toilet trained and he will be able to keep from messing. Colons, like children, grow up. Some day you will no longer know your child's bowel habits in intimate detail.

---

*Of course if you are making your own yogurt with vitamin-D fortified whole milk, it will be adequate in both nutrients.

Selected References

1. Cohen, Stanley, A., Kristy M. Hendricks, Richard K. Mathis, Susan Laramee and W. Allan Walker. Chronic nonspecific diarrhea: dietary relationships. Pediatrics 64:402–407. 1979.

2. Graham, G. G. Chronic "diarrhea" and diet. American Journal of Diseases of Childhood. 134:526. 1980.
3. Hirschhorn, Norbert. The treatment of acute diarrhea in children. An historical and physiological perspective. The American Journal of Clinical Nutrition. 33:637–663. 1980.
4. Holland, P. Diarrhea. Nursing (Oxford). 17:744–748. 1980.
5. Lloyd-Still, John D. Chronic diarrhea of childhood and the misuse of elimination diets. The Journal of Pediatrics. 95:10–13. 1979.
6. Sack, R. B., N. F. Pierce and N. Hirschhorn. The current status of oral therapy in the treatment of acute diarrheal illness. The American Journal of Clinical Nutrition 31:2251–2257. 1978.
7. ———. Role of dietary fat in chronic non-specific diarrhea in childhood. Nutrition reviews. 38:240–241. 1980.

10
Regulation of Food Intake and Body Weight

You can't control or dictate the quantity of food your child eats, and you shouldn't try. You also can't control or dictate the kind of body your child develops, and you shouldn't try. What you can *do, and it is a great deal, is set things up for your child so she, herself, can regulate her food intake as well as possible, and so she can develop a healthy body that is constitutionally right for her.*

You can do this by providing her with regular and balanced meals, and with the expectation that she come to the table and pay attention to what she is eating. You can encourage her to get an adequate amount of exercise. And you can seek the middle ground in your feeding relationship by teaching her firm expectations of appropriate eating behavior, without dominating her with your own perceptions about quantity and choice.

Years ago, when I first began consulting in pediatrics, I made up a little feeding guide for infants, a guide to be distributed to parents by the nursing staff. The guide made recommendations, by age, for solid-food additions to the child's diet and told some of the reasons for the additions. I thought it was very nice, and that it would answer most of parents' questions.

However, about two days after they began using the guide, I got a call from one of the nurses: "the mothers want to know *how much* they should feed their babies." How much? I didn't know how much. I had raised three babies and I hadn't paid much attention to how much. That question really intimidated me: how was I going to tell them how much when I didn't know myself? What kind of nutritionist and mother was I?

I thought a lot and read everything I could and I realized that I still didn't know. There was nothing consistent on which to base a recommendation. I had looked at calorie requirements for infants (which varied), food-intake studies of infants (which varied), recommendations by pediatricians, nutritionists and nurses (which varied), and I had talked with parents about how much their babies ate (which also varied).

About the only thing I could come up with that made any sense was a guide to what was the *least* amount of solid food a baby could eat and still get his nutrient requirement, and that wasn't very much—either information or food. But, as far as saying how much a child should be eating, I was really stuck. I couldn't possibly answer.

I further began to realize that for me, or even the parent, to say *how much* was inappropriate and was taking away a right that belonged to the child. It was not for me to say how much, sitting in my office miles away from where the really-important decisions were being made. It was not even the parents' right to say how much a child should be eating, because the parent cannot experience the infant's hunger and desire for food: the parent can only respond to it.

Only the child could say how much, and that information was not going to fit on my neat little feeding guide.

How much is the topic of this chapter. *How much* should a child be eating? Like all questions without easy answers, the response to this one will take a while.

Food Regulation

The way you decide how much a child should eat is different from the way you decide what a child should eat. Nutritionists can tell you types and amounts of food that will provide a nutritionally-adequate diet. But again, nutritionists can't tell you how much to feed—only your child can tell you that, through communication of his own internal cues of hunger and satiety.

Proper child-feeding depends on a division of responsibility: You are responsible for what your child is presented to eat. He is responsible for what and how much he eats.

To go into more detail, you are responsible for:

- Controlling what food comes into the house.
- Making and presenting meals.
- Insisting that children show up for meals.
- Making children behave at the table.
- Keeping kids "on task" with their eating.
- Regulating timing and food at snacks (no food right before dinner).
- And all the things your grandmother said: no fanning the refrigerator door, no candy before dinner, etc.

However, parents are NOT responsible for:

- How much a child eats.
- Whether he eats.
- How his body turns out.

You will simply have to risk it.

Predicting Calorie Requirements. The parents who asked for guides on *how much*, wanted information that I simply couldn't give and that no one else could, or should, give.

Whether people are *willing* to give it anyway is another matter. Let me give you a couple of quotes from an article on "managing feeding," written by a pediatrician who is also a university professor of medicine:[3] "Parents are not likely to look up calorie charts, so it is necessary to give them guidance as to volume needed as growth continues." He goes on to describe how he figures out how much to tell parents to feed their children, and finishes by saying that this "provides approximately the caloric intake recommended by infant nutritionists."

That pediatrician has us nutritionists all wrong. We don't say what quantity an infant *should be* eating; we ask how much a child *is* eating. Particularly when growth is taking place, I do not presume to be able to dictate to *anyone* how much they should be eating. There are too many things I don't know about and that nobody knows about: activity level, calories required for growth, and ability of the body to squander and conserve calories in response to changes in food intake, and behavioral and psychological consequences of manipulation of food intake.

Every five years a committee of the National Research Council publishes the Recommended Dietary Allowances.[10] The Committee is made up of respected nutritionists who summarize current nutritional knowledge and make estimates about levels of nutrients required for health. Over the years they have had a very hard time making recommendations for calories. In 1980 they found their way out of their dilemma by stating that "allowances must be individually adjusted," based on "observations of appetite, activity, growth and weight gain in relation to the extent of deposits of subcutaneous fat."

The table reproduced below is from the current RDA book. The committee got the energy levels from observations of the food intake of large groups of people. Notice that at every age level there are wide variations in calorie levels.

Figure 10-1. Mean Heights and Weights and Recommended Energy Intake

	Age	Weight		Height		Energy Needs (with range)		
Category	(years)	(kg)	(lb)	(cm)	(in.)	(kcal)		(MJ)
Infants	0.0–0.5	6	13	60	24	kg × 115	(95–145)	kg × 0.48
	0.5–1.0	9	20	71	28	kg × 105	(80–135)	kg × 0.44
Children	1–3	13	29	90	35	1300	(900–1800)	5.5
	4–6	20	44	112	44	1700	(1300–2300)	7.1
	7–10	28	62	132	52	2400	(1650–3300)	10.1
Males	11–14	45	99	157	62	2700	(2000–3700)	11.3
	15–18	66	145	176	69	2800	(2100–3900)	11.3
	19–22	70	154	177	70	2900	(2500–3300)	12.2
	23–50	70	154	178	70	2700	(2300–3100)	11.3
	51–75	70	154	178	70	2400	(2000–2800)	10.1
	76+	70	154	178	70	2050	(1650–2450)	8.6
Females	11–14	46	101	157	62	2200	(1500–3000)	9.2
	15–18	55	120	163	64	2100	(1200–3000)	8.8
	19–22	55	120	163	64	2100	(1700–2500)	8.8
	23–50	55	120	163	64	2000	(1600–2400)	8.4
	51–75	55	120	163	64	1800	(1400–2200)	7.6
	76+	55	120	163	64	1600	(1200–2000)	6.7
Pregnancy						+300		
Lactation						+500		

In most cases knowing the amount of calories that an infant or child is consuming is really unimportant, and just a matter of curiosity. Figuring that out for a normal child capable of making his needs known is a lot of unnecessary work, and may even be a detriment because it imposes an unnecessary element of external control. The child comes equipped with all the tools that are necessary to "individually adjust . . . energy intake on the basis of appetite, activity, growth and weight gain." Our role in that process is not to figure out and provide a carefully calibrated number of calories. Our role is to feed him and see how he grows.

Predicting Calorie Intake

About the only time that parents and health professionals should get into the business of trying to figure out and manipulate calories is when there is something that is complicating the growth process. If the child is ill or has some physical disability that makes food intake more difficult, or that distorts energy output, then it may be necessary to manipulate calories. For instance, a child with a neuromuscular disease has a hard time eating and tends to burn more calories because of spastic muscle movements. A child with heart defects uses more energy breathing and circulating blood, and also has a more difficult time taking in food. In both cases we would want to know about how much that child is eating, because it might be important to try to increase calorie intake. In a similar way, if an apparently normal child seems to be growing poorly, knowing how much he is eating will help us judge whether we have a dietary or a medical problem.

Defending Constitutional Weight

But sometimes that child's growth potential and ability to regulate overcomes even our best efforts to manipulate it. Years ago a pediatrician asked me what I would recommend to increase the growth rate in little Alice Black. Alice was six months old, a beautiful, alert little child. However, she had gained only 3 lb. and 5 inches since birth. Alice's parents had taken her for a chromosomal examination and for endocrine tests to find out if anything was wrong with her. But no one could really say. Actually, other than her size, nothing really WAS wrong with Alice. She was just tiny.

The parents, of course, were concerned. They wanted to be sure that they were doing everything they could to encourage Alice to grow. But they said that she was very emphatic about how much she wanted to eat, and cried and fussed when they tried to encourage her to take more food. We decided we would try concentrating her formula.

We knew we would have to be careful in doing this. For one thing, we knew that giving her more nutrients and less water per unit volume of formula could dehydrate her. The doctor was alert to this, and saw her frequently to watch for any signs of dehydration. We also knew that we might just make Alice fat with our extra calories, so the nurse weighed and measured and plotted her carefully to make sure that if she got an acceleration in growth rate that it would occur in both height and weight. Alice was perfectly proportioned, and we didn't want to spoil that.

Then we set about modifying the formula. Since she was taking a formula that had more protein than she really needed, the first thing we did was add a little syrup, increasing her calories by about 7%. Alice responded by decreasing her volume of intake by 7%. Since that hadn't worked, we put her back on the regular formula while we reevaluated, and she immediately increased her volume back to its previous level. We then speculated that Alice may not have liked the increased sweetness of the syrup carbohydrate, so this time we tried fat, figuring that would change the flavor less. We again increased the calories by 7% and, once again, Alice was ahead of us. She cut her intake by 7%. Back on the normal feed went Alice, and back to the previous volume went the intake.

Our last try was simply concentrating the regular formula. We carefully took out some of the water to concentrate it by 7%; and Alice again decreased her intake. At that point, we gave up. Our only other option would have been to put a tube down and force-feed her, and none of us wanted to do that.

The parents decided that they simply had to support the growth pattern that was normal for Alice. They moved away and the last time I saw them Alice was nine months old, and weighed nine pounds. She was feeding herself tiny amounts of food from the table. She was pulling herself up and walking around things and startling everyone because she looked like a newborn.

I think those parents behaved in a very moderate and responsible way: they did what they could and then they left it up to Alice. Alice's father was a nutritionist, and he was as fascinated as I was by her ability to regulate her food intake and her growth. If Alice stays that small it will be hard for her, but at least her parents won't make it harder by struggling with her over her food in attempts to change her body.

The Body's Regulation

The body will regulate if you let it—or, at least some of the time, in spite of what you do to it. Your body has powerful regulatory systems built into it which allow it to maintain a more-or-less stable pattern of weight. There are systems of regulating food intake as well as systems for conserving or squandering calories metabolically, in response to deficits or excesses in calorie intake.[5]

If you look at yourself a moment, you will realize that in the last year, in spite of all the different ways that you have lived, eaten, drunk and exercised, that your weight has probably stayed pretty stable. Regrettably, even if you have tried to lose or gain weight you probably will have found that once you relaxed your efforts to modify your food intake, your weight returned to very near its original level. Even if you are ten pounds heavier or lighter than you were a year ago you will have missed an exact balance of calorie output and input by an average of only about 100 calories per day. You can hardly call that gluttony—or starvation.

The way growing children regulate is even more remarkable. Not only do they need calories for general bodily maintenance, as do adults, they also need the right amount of calories for growth. They get taller and heavier, and usually weight increases proportionally to height. Generally once children are established on a smooth pattern of growth for height and weight they adhere to that pattern very well.

And their level of food intake will reflect their needs. As their growth velocity varies, their food intake also varies to match it. The same thing happens with a variation in exercise levels. It is all automatic; the child can do it all himself with his own feelings of hunger and satiety. All you have to do is provide the food.

This physiological reality is in marked contrast to the societal view of body weight. According to the latter view, you choose a particular body weight or physique and you work to achieve it by managing your eating and exercise.

Even this wouldn't be so bad if the societal standard for body weight were broader or more realistic. Unfortunately, the standard is *thin*, and many people have a mind set about body weight that is consistently 10 or 20 pounds less than what their body appears to want. Even the standards for children are thin, to the extent that a parent of a blocky or chubby child often feels he is doing something wrong. The aesthetic standards may have little to do with good health. Most children go through a chubby stage. For adults, body weight as much as 20% above "normal weight"* does not appear to impair health (see the discussion in the *Obesity* chapter).

Many people spend their time engaged in a struggle to force their weight below its physically preferred level, or "set point." What they don't seem to realize is that to a considerable extent body weight is constitutionally determined, that physical, behavioral and

---

*"Normal" body weight is generally accepted as that defined by the Metropolitan Life Insurance Company, Actuarial Tables, 1959.

metabolic processes tend to defend that body weight, and that achieving a different body weight will be accomplished only at considerable cost.

The chart on the next page (Figure 10-2) gives a view of the complexity of the process which maintains body weight.

Most of us are aware that eating and exercise have an impact on body weight and on each other. Most people do not know, however, that there are other, and perhaps more powerful, physical, behavioral and psychological mechanisms that defend body weight.[4]

When people undereat, they get hungry and become preoccupied with food. Conversely, when they overeat they feel full and, if pressed too much to overeat, feel a very strong aversion to food. These are behavioral reactions which exert pressure to restore "normal" food intake.[4]

Physiological mechanisms work in the same way. When people undereat they feel tired and decrease their exercise, whether they realize it or not. Their involuntary muscle activity (heart and lung action, etc.) also decreases slightly. Metabolic rate, the rate at which the body uses energy, goes down as another way of conserving calories,[4] and there is accumulating evidence that people who undereat radiate less heat from their skin and thus conserve calories.[5] When you diet you get cold more easily.

When people overeat, the converse is true. Metabolic rate increases, heat radiation increases, and energy levels increase. For some people, this increase appears to be enough to defend body weight. Others just get fat.

Some experimental volunteers who are overfed require considerably more calories than predicted to gain over their normal "set point." Once the surfeit is ended, they lose back to their previous levels, after cutting calorie intake less than would be expected. Conversely, some underfed volunteers have to establish a larger than predicted deficit in food intake to achieve weight loss, and then gain back very readily.[4]

Figure 10-2. Regulation of Body Weight.

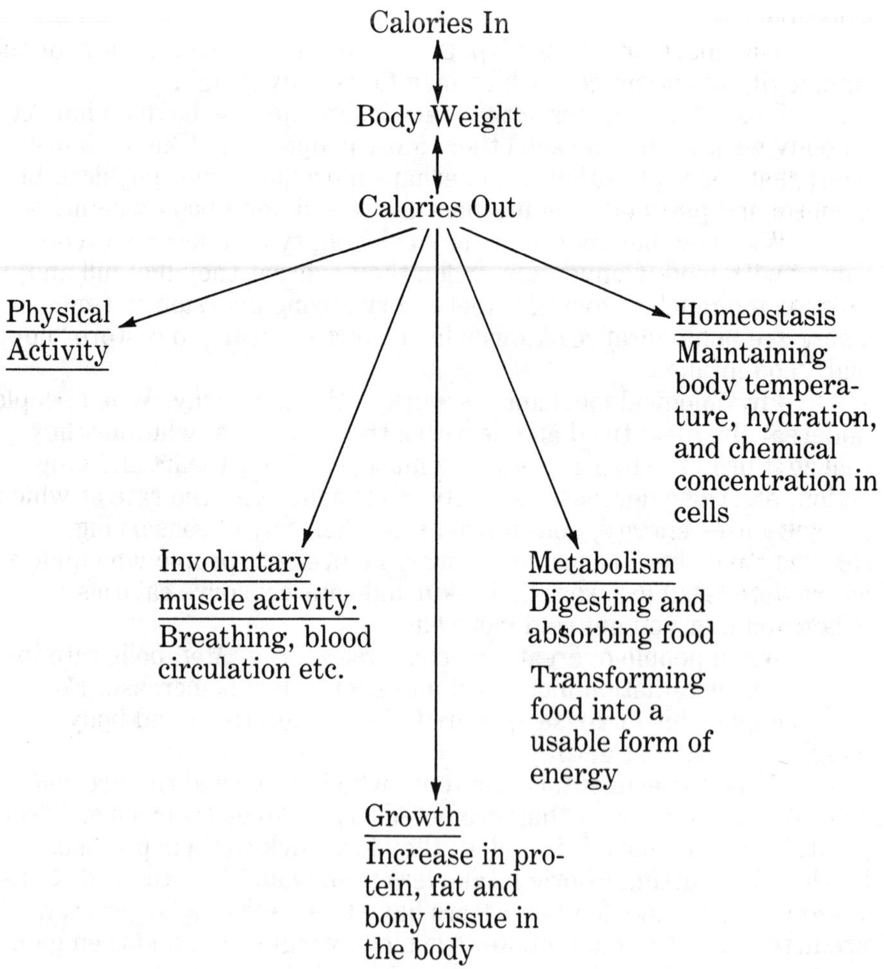

The point is that to overwhelm the tendency to regulate body weight appears to require considerable stamina. In fact, it could be that our attempts to manipulate body weight can backfire, and promote the very thing we are trying to prevent or cure. If underfed children become hungry and preoccupied with food, they will be likely to overeat when they get access to food. If overfed children become nauseous and revolted by food, they will be likely to undereat when they get a chance.

Parental Behavior and Children's Eating

Generally, children eat best when their parents are neither overmanaging or overpermissive. Mothers of small bottle-fed babies use more pressure tactics to get their babies to eat, such as pushing the nipple into the mouth, juggling it, and imposing a frequent set feeding routine. And the more active and controlling the mother, the less the baby eats.[9]

Appropriate parental attention may be a factor in obesity as well. Mothers of fatter children, ages four to eight years, talked less to their children during mealtimes, were less responsive, gave less approval, and made fewer efforts to control inappropriate behavior during mealtime.[1]

Teenaged girls, as well, showed poorer diets and higher frequency of low-quality foods when they came from families who were highly critical of their food intake.[7]

But undesirable as they are, poor eating habits may not be your worst problem if you interfere with food regulation. If the parent-child relationship about food is distorted, it is likely to distort the whole relationship. If you are attempting to manipulate or control your child's eating, it can spoil your relationship and it can have a far-reaching impact on your child.

Your attitude about your child is reflected in the way you feed your child. If you have an attitude of curiosity, relaxation and trust, you will watch for his cues and respond to them. You will depend on information coming from him and be willing to let him develop the body that's right for him. On the other hand, if your attitude is one of responsibility and control, you will not be able to be trusting. You will have to supervise eating closely, and monitor growth, being ready at all times to step in and curb or influence the growth pattern.

Your child learns about himself and about the world from the way he is fed. Can he be trusting? Is the world trustworthy? If he has to fight and struggle for every mouthful of food, then it is likely the world is not very trustworthy at all. If his needs are met, on the other hand, in a supportive and consistent fashion, then it is likely that the world is trustworthy and he can, in turn, allow himself to depend on others.

In these feeding interactions he will also learn whether or not he has the capability to influence others. If he has to fuss and fight and struggle mightily to get his needs met, or if what he gets has little or nothing to do with what he wants, then he is likely to think of himself as not having much clout in the world. On the other hand, if other people respond to him in a prompt and appropriate fashion, he learns that what he wants and needs does matter and that other people will respond to him.

The way health professionals teach you to feed your child will have an impact on your attitude about your child. If we get out our growth charts and our feeding tables that specify quantities, then we are teaching you to be controlling. If we supervise your child carefully at all times to make sure he isn't getting fat, and take preventative action at every step of the way, we are teaching you to be controlling. And, worst of all, if we encourage you to put your child on a diet, we are encouraging you to be controlling in a way that is absolutely guaranteed to disrupt the entire family. That is very serious business.

A child can outgrow a diet that is less-than optimally chosen, as long as it is offered supportively and lovingly. However, outgrowing deeply ingrained attitudes about self and the world is devilishly difficult.

It appears, then, that a child has a growth potential that he tends to maintain and defend, and that to change that or modify it requires the most persistent of efforts. Further, it appears that any sort of major effort to manage or modify food intake can backfire and promote the very things we are trying to avoid, whether it is overgrowth or undergrowth. And finally, parents who are either too over-involved or too under-involved with their children's eating appear to have children who eat less well.

The task that presents itself then, is to find the middle ground. What are the appropriate types of parental involvement and management, that are helpful and productive for children? And, further, how can parents set things up for their child so he can regulate well?

The Regulation Process

People regulate their food intake by getting hungry, by eating, by becoming full and satisfied, and by stopping eating. Your child's body will regulate if you let it. Your job is to support that process; to help set things up for your child so regulation works as well as possible.

More specifically, you need to train your child in deliberate, attentive consumption of satisfying and enjoyable food. Your key to accomplishing this goal will be your willingness and ability to tune in on and trust your child's signals of food regulation.

Make Eating Times Significant. From the very first, it is important for you to give your time and attention to feeding your child and paying attention to him, always observing and problem-solving to make sure the feeding process goes well. For the infant, that means using a system of trial and error to find out why he pulls off the nipple, or fusses, or spits up, or seemingly terminates feeding too soon. For the older child, it means paying attention to what promotes good eating, and managing him and the situation in such a way that he can eat well. We talked about this at length in the *Toddler* chapter.

Your willingness to give children the time and attention they need to allow them to eat well can have a big impact on how much they eat. As an extreme example, babies who are cared for coldly and impersonally do not thrive. Old studies from orphanages showed that babies left alone in their cribs had a higher death rate than those that were regularly fed, stimulated and cared for. The theory was that the understimulated babies died from lack of love. However, we suspect now that while the babies might indeed have died from lack of love, the major factor in their deaths was lack of food. The babies who were left alone were also fed rapidly and inattentively. The caretakers interpreted any interruption in the feeding as a sign of satiety and stopped feeding rather than soothing the baby and giving her time to go back to nursing. As the babies were fed less and less, they became less demanding, got less stimulation, and finally they became so lethargic and seriously undernourished that they became ill and died.[12]

Manage the Eating Environment. Keep food and reminders of food out of the picture until it is time to eat. You want your child to pay attention to his food and enjoy it thoroughly at eating time. Then you want him, as much as possible, to forget about it the rest of the time. If he is not thinking about food, he won't be panhandling and badgering all the time, or munching along in stomach-souring, appetite-spoiling little dibs and dabs.

I have yet to meet a child who has not been struck by a terrific hunger pang when the ice-cream truck drives up. Or one who is not immediately reminded of a cookie when he arrives at the home of the favorite aunt who always seems to have her cookie jar well-stocked. I would not for the world tell you that trips to the ice-cream truck are taboo or that the favorite aunt and the child have to be deprived of the delights of the cookie ritual. What I am saying is that there are external circumstances that remind people to eat, and that there are certain of these external circumstances that you can manipulate in regulating when and what a child eats.

If you have a cookie jar sitting on the counter and it is generally kept well-filled, it is likely that your child will have a fairly high frequency of cookie wanting. As a further example, if your child regularly eats in front of the TV set, he may set up an association between turning on the TV and wanting a snack, and may at times be reminded of eating when he really isn't hungry.

To manage the eating environment:

1. Set up the eating situation so that when he eats, he eats only. No TV, no comic book, no trucks.
2. Limit eating to one or two appropriate places in the house.
3. Keep food, as much as possible, out of sight.

Environmental control is a major tactic that is used by behaviorists to encourage and help people who want to lose weight. There, the goal is to cut down on eating. Our goal here is not to cut down on eating, but TO MAKE EATING IMPORTANT AND WORTHWHILE.

Food Distribution. You want your child to come to the table hungry, so he is interested in eating and so his appetite heightens his interest and awareness of food. We do not want him to come to the table starved, so he is either too cranky to eat or so famished that he simply wolfs down his food and gets a stomach ache. Which it is to be depends on how often he eats.

Except for the increased incidence of cavities with all-day nibbling, we really can't say much about an optimum eating pattern. The pattern of food intake that promotes the most positive comfort and energy is a pretty individual matter and one that you may more-

or-less have to explore with your child. In general, depend on three meals a day and vary the snacks according to his needs.

Select Foods that Help Regulation. A well-selected meal, with a good distribution of protein, fat and carbohydrate, can help your child regulate his food intake. Each of these nutrients has a role to play in inducing some of the many satiety factors that let your child know that he has had enough to eat.

The pattern of satisfaction you get from each when consuming each separately appears to be different from the pattern of satisfaction from all of them consumed together. To be more specific about this, using a series of graphs, we will speculate about what happens to your sensation, level, and duration of satisfaction from consuming carbohydrate, protein or fat. Generally these graphs present a simplified version of the physiological parts of satiety.* The representation ignores the psychological parts, like quality and taste, and the personal parts, like preference and emotional state. They tell you how and when the fuel from the meal becomes available, how long it is likely to last, and how the physical properties of foods are likely to affect your sense of satisfaction from eating. But before we can get to the fun part, you have to have a lesson in food composition.

Food Composition. There are three major sources of calories in the diet: protein, fat and carbohydrate (sugar and starch). The only other nutrient that gives calories is alcohol. There is a table of the protein, fat and carbohydrate content of foods in the *Solid Foods* chapter, Figure 7-4. You get protein from the meat group as well as from milk and milk products. You also get protein from cooked dried beans and peas, and in small amounts from breads and cereal products.

---

*The whole issue of satiety is extremely complex. I have purposely oversimplified, to give a general picture of how the nutritional components interact to *generally* affect satiety.

Fat is often a separate food such as butter or oil, but it is often also contained IN foods, where it may not be noticeable. Most meats have fat in them, as do many dairy products. Fat is often used in food preparation, as in frying or in buttering or creaming vegetables. Fat is also used as a spread or as a dressing on other foods.

Carbohydrate comes in two forms: the *simple*, or sugar form, and the *complex*, or starch form. (The basic chemical structure of both forms is sugar, and starches are essentially made up of dozens of molecules of sugar, linked together.) The important difference, metabolically, is that starch has to be broken down chemically before it can be made available to the body, whereas sugar is virtually ready to be absorbed, as is, from the intestine. Sugar can be transported into the blood stream very promptly with very little digestive action.

Starch is found in cereal products, like noodles, rice and breakfast cereals and anything made with flour. Starchy vegetables such as potatoes, corn and lima beans are also good sources of carbohydrate. Sugar is found in nature in fruits and honey, and in sugar cane and sugar beets. Of course, the last two are refined and used mainly as brown or white sugars. Fruits and fruit juices, as well as cookies, cakes, candies, pop and sweetened fruit-flavored beverages are all major sources of sugar in the diet.

Take a look now at the "Satisfaction" charts. Each of the charts measures "satisfaction" on the left-hand side, or vertical axis; it has no number on it because it is really a general sort of feeling that is actually made up of several factors. It is hard to calibrate because it is so subjective. On the horizontal axis is time, which is also an approximation. How quickly you feel satisfied after you eat has something to do with bodily state (including mental state), as well as with the food itself—so these lines will have to be imprecise.

Sugar. Figure 10-3 (next page) demonstrates the kind of satisfaction response a child would get if he were at a fasting or hungry level and consumed only sugar. That sugar might be fruit or fruit juice. It might also be some kind of "sweet," like jelly beans or hard candy, or pop or a sweetened fruit drink. (Many sweets, like cookies, cake or candies, have fat in them as well as sugar, so you don't get the same kind of response.)

Figure 10-3. Satisfaction from Consuming Sugar.

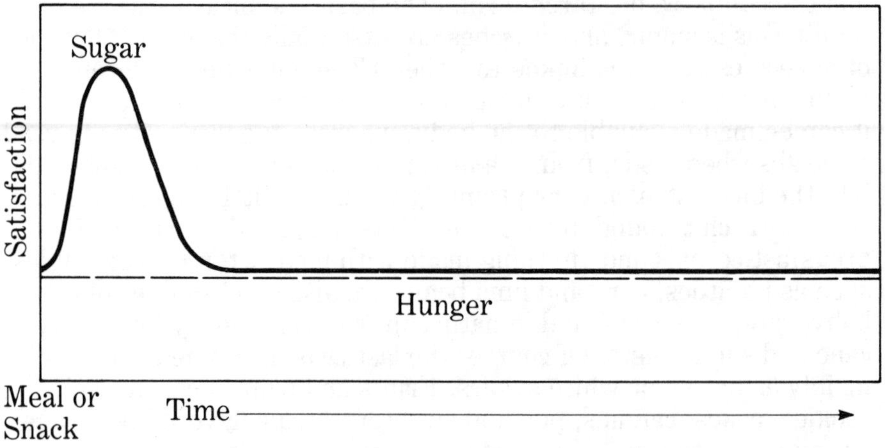

Notice that the satisfaction response to sugar is quite fast. In this case, the feeling of satisfaction probably comes from an increase in blood glucose, which is apparently one of many signals to the body that it has been fed. But the curve drops off just as fast; the sugar doesn't have much staying power. Once it is used up, the child who has had a sugar-only meal or snack will again be hungry and may even be cranky and unmanageable because of it. The sugar didn't MAKE him cranky; it just let him down before he got too far.

Starch. let's consider a sugar and starch meal, say one consisting of orange juice and dry toast. As you can see by the graph in Figure 10-4, the addition of the starch helps some in terms of extending the satisfaction period. The starch has to be disgested before it can be absorbed, and it can't be digested all at one time, so the nutrients get into the blood stream more slowly and over a more extended time.

Figure 10-4. Satisfaction from Consuming Sugar and Starch.

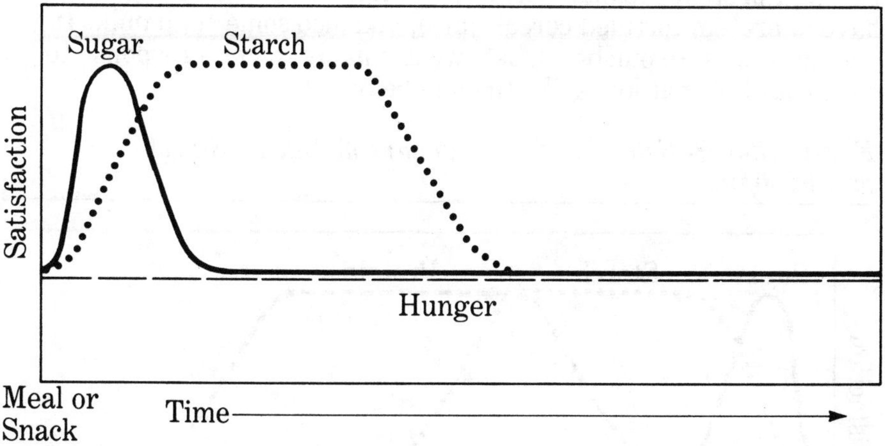

The nutrient that enters the blood is still glucose, because when starch is digested it is absorbed and carried in the blood stream as glucose. The sugar from starch is burned up by the body cells just as fast as that from refined sugar, but because it gets to the blood more slowly, it is likely to last longer.

With bread and starchy foods like cereals we are also adding other components of satisfaction: bulk and chewing. Bread is solid and it is bulky, so it gives your stomach a feeling of having something in it. Depending on the kind of bread you are eating, you are also going to do a greater or lesser amount of chewing. Some people depend heavily on chewing to let them feel that they have had enough to eat, so a tougher bread, like toast or bagels, is likely to give them a greater feeling of satisfaction than they get from squishy "sandwich bread."

Protein. But let's say we know better than to have just juice and dry toast. We have been watching TV and have seen the ad for the high-protein breakfast cereal, and that is what we are going to have: a protein-fortified cereal, juice, and also some skim milk. In adding protein to our breakfast, we are likely to get a response to our breakfast that looks like the one below.

Figure 10-5. Satisfaction from Consuming Sugar, Starch and Protein.

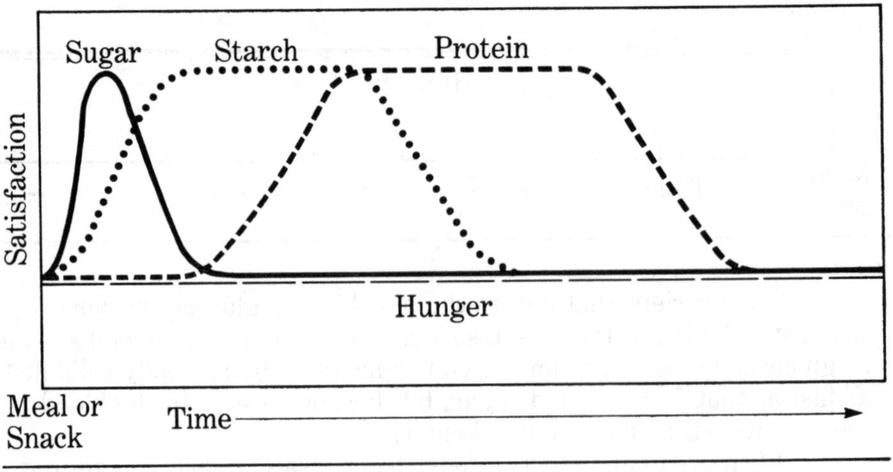

The protein helps make our breakfast last longer. It takes a while for the protein to get to you, because it has to be broken down in the intestine into amino acids before it can be absorbed into the blood stream.

Eating a source of protein adds still another component of satisfaction to the diet: that of circulating amino acids* in the blood stream. Like increases in blood sugar, it appears that the body is able to sense increases in blood amino acids, and uses that as one of the bits of information supporting a sense of satisfaction. Skim milk is one of the few sources of protein in the diet that doesn't also have some fat associated with it. Egg white is a source of fat-free protein, and some very lean fish is almost fat free, but most sources of protein come associated with varying amounts of fat.

Fat. Once you add fat to an otherwise fat-free meal, you are likely to have quite a different picture of satisfaction. Let's have our same cereal-and-milk-juice breakfast, only now let's have a source of fat with it, like 2% or whole milk on the cereal instead of skim milk.

Figure 10-6. Satisfaction from Consuming Sugar, Starch, Protein and Fat.

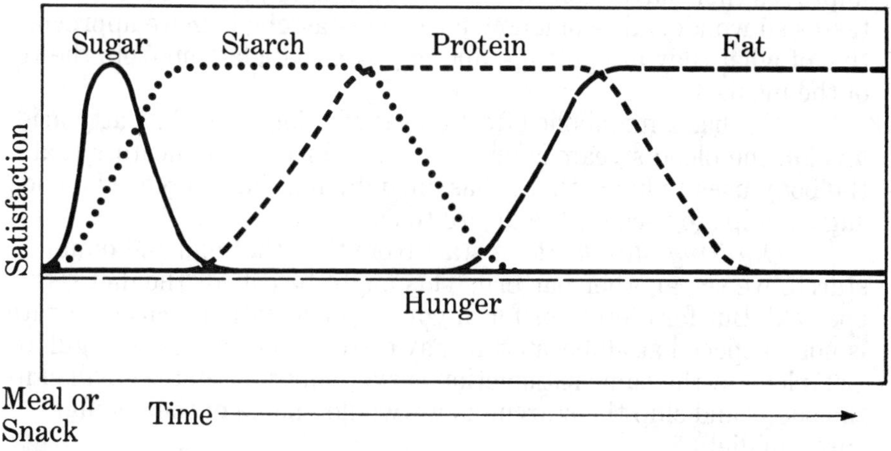

*Amino acids can also be broken down to glucose in the blood stream.

Fat is digested and absorbed slowly, so fatty acids from fat digestion get into the blood stream after sugar and amino acids, and fat is released to the blood stream over a more extended period of time than the other nutrients. But more importantly, presence of fat in the meal slows down the rate at which the whole meal is used. Fat retards the emptying time of the stomach. It keeps food in the stomach where it can be released more slowly to the intestine. Once there, it is digested and absorbed at a moderate rate, so that all accompanying carbohydrate and protein are also available to the body more slowly and over a more-extended time. So fat mixed with a meal makes the meal stay with you longer.

Also, when you include fat in the meal, you add on a couple of other components of satisfaction. One of them is just simple pleasure. Fat carries the flavor in food; addition of fat allows you to taste the food better and more acutely. You can taste the cereal when you have 2% milk rather than skim milk. A little butter on the vegetables improves their flavor considerably. And it isn't just because butter tastes so wonderful—somehow fat makes tastebuds more appreciative of what they are getting, and improves satisfaction from the rest of the meal.

Fat has a metabolic effect on satisfaction, as well. Fatty acid level in the blood stream is probably another of the indicators that the body uses to know that it has enough, and, like increased blood sugar, helps to turn off the desire to eat.

Omitting Starch. If we start from the other end and omit starch, we see another pattern. This might be called "the dieters' special." But for dieters or for anyone, a meal without carbohydrates is not so special at all because it may distort your ability to regulate. Let's look at the same satisfaction curve, only this time we will skip the sugar and skip the starch, as we would on one of the popular "protein diets."

Immediately you can see that there is an increase in the lag time before the arrival of satisfaction from this meal. Because the protein breaks down so slowly, and because the meal has fat in it, it can take quite a while before you feel satisfaction from the meal. Your body will still manufacture its essential blood glucose from protein. However, the process takes a while, and that slows down the blood glucose response. Furthermore, without the bulk of starch we will be missing the full, substantial feeling of stomach filling and comfort.

Figure 10-7. Satisfaction from Consuming Protein and Fat.

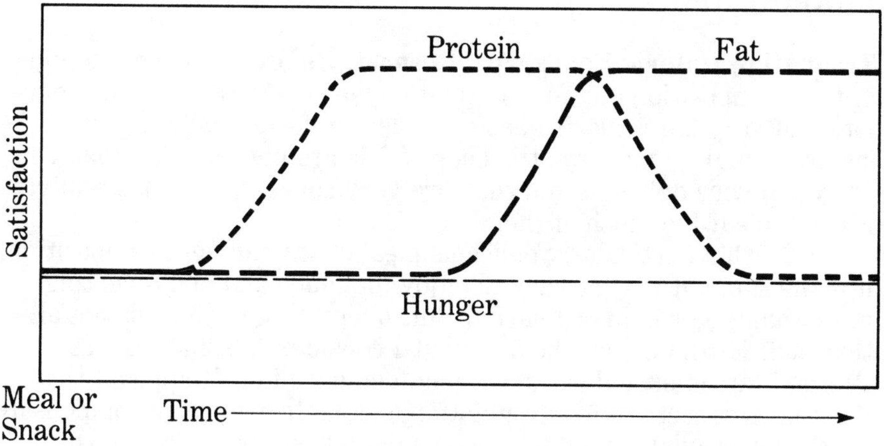

A major factor in food regulation, then, is to plan a meal to include carbohydrate, protein, and fat, because they work best nutritionally when they are consumed in combination. It is easier to regulate the amount eaten at a meal that includes all three because all the physical cues of satisfaction are present to signal you when to stop eating.

You can vary your snack selection depending on the response you want. If you want the snack to last two or three hours, choosing all three major nutrients is a good strategy. If, however, it is five o'clock and dinner is at six and your child is desperate from hunger, a glass of juice or an apple might be a better choice. The fruit sugar is quickly satisfying and has a good chance of allowing him to be hungry a short time later.

Do you get the idea? Remember, A MEAL (OR SNACK) THAT YOU WANT TO BE IMMEDIATELY SATISFYING, AND ALSO TO LAST A WHILE, MUST HAVE PROTEIN, FAT AND CARBOHYDRATE IN IT.

Treat High Calorie Foods with Respect. Before we leave the topic of food composition and food regulation we need to discuss the regulation of very high caloric density foods: the foods that are high in sugar, or high in fat, or both. These foods are harder to regulate. They are very delicious and they are very concentrated calorically; it is easy to eat too much of them.

With a particularly delicious meal of any nutrient composition, it is the same: it is very easy to enjoy too much and end up eating more than you would ordinarily. But, overeating at times is not all that bad. Even people who are what I consider "normal" eaters overdo it at times and eat until they feel quite full. It appears that the body's process of food regulation is flexible enough to compensate for this; it regulates food intake on a daily basis as well as on the basis of longer periods of time. Overeating for one day or for a period of several days is usually followed by a day or a period of undereating, as the body in some way accounts for those calorie excesses and balances the ledger.

Teach Him to Savor the Flavor. But at the same time I say this, I would also like to make the point that eating a great deal is not the only way to get full value out of a particularly delicious food or meal. There is another way that you can use, and it is a way that you can demonstrate and teach your child. That way is to be very attentive to your food—to taste and savor and expose all of your taste buds. Essentially, you can eat like a gourmet, getting all the sensations and pleasure out of the food that you possibly can. You can look at it, smell it, anticipate it, feel your teeth sinking into it, feel it in your mouth and taste it as you pay great attention to chewing it thoroughly, and generally doing as careful a job of eating as you can.

Approaching eating in this way can allow you to get a great deal more satisfaction out of the same or maybe even less food. And that is important when you are eating a food that is relatively high in calories. In fact, I would say that the higher-calorie the food you are eating, the more careful you should be to savor it. That way you won't have to overeat to enjoy it.

I am reminded of the old story of the man, finishing his lunch and asking for a second piece of pie: "This one is to taste. The other piece was so good I forgot to taste it." Too bad. The second piece never tastes as good, because part of the hunger is gone.

Make Wise Social and Emotional Use of Food. The problem is not that people eat when they are celebrating or depressed or lonely. The problem is that they do it poorly. Eating well can be wonderfully satisfying and relaxing. Many people comfort or soothe themselves with food, even though they try not to. And because they think it's wrong, they eat rapidly, or inattentively, or in some way that doesn't allow them to get the emotional solace they seek.

To allow food to be helpful for you emotionally, you have to be clear about what you are trying to do with food—and do it well. If you are depressed, it is a very good idea to take extra good care of yourself—find yourself something you really like to eat, put yourself in an environment that you find very pleasant, and be aware of letting the pleasure of the food raise your spirits. If you are uptight, food can relax you, if you will slow yourself down and concentrate, and allow the rhythm of the eating process to smooth you out.

This is not to imply that you should give your child a cookie when he scrapes his knee or is bored. It is certainly more appropriate to offer comfort or your reassurance that he can get interested in doing something. However, sooner or later he is likely to use food, to some extent, for emotional reasons. When that happens, you need to help him learn how to: first, respond appropriately to his emotional needs; and second, use food as productively as possible.

Maintain an Active Lifestyle. Getting an adequate level of exercise is essential to helping your body regulate appropriately. Exercise helps:

1. Tune the food regulation mechanism.
2. Burn off extra calories and body fat.
3. Maintain a good level of muscle tissue.

Tuning the Food Regulation Mechanism. We know very little about activity and food regulation in children, beyond knowing that children will vary their food intake to provide appropriately for their level of physical activity. We don't know whether this holds true for children, but adults must achieve a certain level of physical activity in order to regulate well.

As illustrated by Figure 10-8, when adults are at the extremes of physical activity (that is, markedly sedentary or very active), their food intake becomes disproportionate to their actual needs. A person in the sedentary range, rather than eating very small amounts of food to provide for the low requirements of the inactive lifestyle, actually tends to increase food intake above what he needs. At the other, and much less common, extreme of intense exercise, food intake tends to fall off, instead of increasing to very high levels to match the requirements of the exercise. The weight response is predictable. The sedentary, overeating person gains weight, where the exhausted, undereating person loses.*

Figure 10-8. The Relationship of Food Intake to Physical Activity.

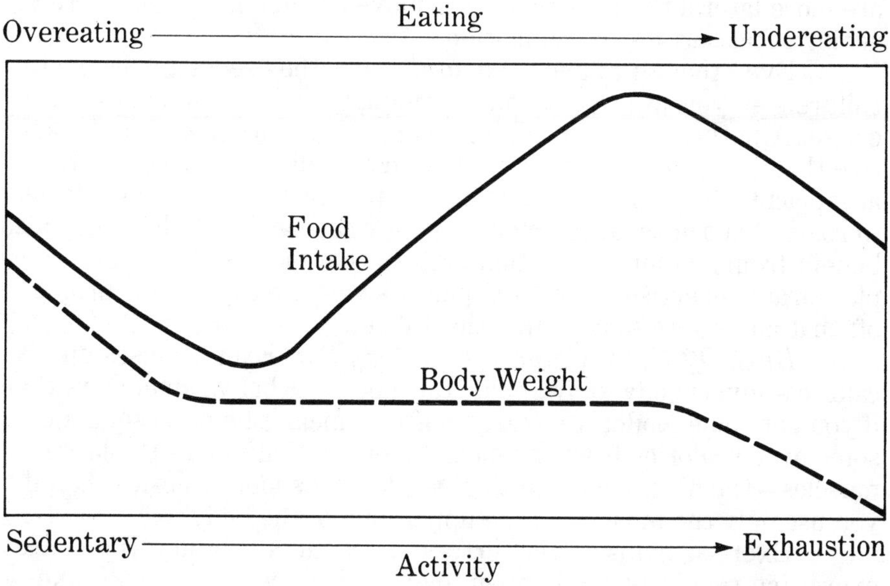

From: Mayer, Jean. Exercise and weight control. Postgraduate Medicine 25(no 3) March 1959.

Theoretically at least, you can make up for inactivity by conscious attention to regulating your food consumption at a level that will allow you to maintain your body weight. But that is going at it the hard way. It is much more functional, direct, and more likely to be successful to give your body the exercise it needs to regulate in a positive and automatic way.

The level of exercise that will allow you to accomplish automatic regulation appears to be an individual matter. The tall, thin person is likely to maintain his weight pretty well if he does little else all day but turn on the TV set. On the other hand, those of us who are more lateral than linear have to move around quite a bit more to achieve that sort of self-regulation.

Even though I have used *adult* data, they seem applicable to children—if you want your child to regulate well, let him get his exercise. A naturally placid child needs more encouragement to be active than a physically energetic child, especially if his parents are also placid. Children of all ages benefit physically from being allowed to roam about in as large an area as they can safely handle. They also benefit from a family recreation pattern that includes moderate, pleasurable exercise—and from parents who are capable of turning off that anti-exercise machine, the TV set.

Burn Off Extra Calories and Body Fat. Exercise uses up calories—everybody knows that. But not everybody remembers that if you get some moderate exercise after a meal it helps to squander some of the calories from the meal. Exercise that moves the large muscles—the hips, legs, and thighs—demands more calories than if you use only the muscles in the upper part of the body.

Exercise helps correct errors in weight regulation. If you are exercising regularly and happen to gain a little weight, it will take more energy for you to carry yourself around and you will tend to exercise that weight right off again.

Maintain Muscle Tissue. Regular exercise builds muscle tissue at the expense of fat. Since muscle tissue is more active metabolically than fat, the leaner body needs more calories to support it. Since lean tissue burns more calories than fat tissue, there is more of a margin of protection against eating too much and overshooting energy requirements.

In the whole area of food regulation we are dealing with a delicately balanced interaction of nutritional, behavioral, physical, and psychological factors, an interaction that we know little about—and even less how to manage or manipulate. Because the process is so complex, we must be extremely careful about intruding upon it. Changing or overruling the body's ability to regulate food intake and growth potential can only be done against odds, and with the possibility of unacceptable cost. We can only speculate on the consequences of intruding on weight regulation.

We have talked about social cost to the feeding relationship, and psychological cost to the infant. We can only wonder about physical and metabolic costs of producing a more-efficient body that maintains itself on less calories.

Our whole discussion of regulation supports what we have been talking about all along: Trust the child's natural growth process. Feed the child and see how he grows.

Selected References

1. Birch, L. L., D. W. Marlin, L. Kramer and C. Peyers. Mother-child interaction patterns and the degree of fatness in children. Journal of Nutrition Education 13:17–21. 1981.
2. Brazelton, T. Infants and Mothers. Delacorte, 1969.
3. Eisenberg, Bernard. Managing feeding problems in a busy pediatric practice. IN Problems Relating to Feeding in the First Two Years. Ross Laboratories, Columbus, 1977.
4. Jordan, H. A. and Levitz, L. A behavioral approach to the problem of obesity. Obesity and Bariatric Medicine 4:58–59. 1975.
5. Keesey, R. E. A set-point analysis of the regulation of body weight. IN Stunkard, A. J. OBESITY. W. B. Saunders, Philadelphia, 1980.
6. Keys, A. et al. The Biology of Human Starvation. University of Minnesota Press. Minneapolis, MN. 1950.

7. Kinter, M., P. G. Boss and N. E. Johnson. The relationship between dysfunctional family environments and family member food intake. Journal of Marriage and the Family. April, 1981.
8. Mayer, J. Exercise and weight control. Postgraduate Medicine. 25(3). March 1959.
9. Politt, E. and S. Wirtz. Mother-infant feeding interaction and weight gain in the first month of life. Journal of the American Dietetics Association. 78:596–601. 1978.
10. Recommended Dietary Allowances. The National Research Council, National Academy of Sciences, Washington, D.C. 1980.
11. Rose, H. E. and J. Mayer. Activity, calorie intake, fat storage and the energy balance of infants. Pediatrics 41:18. 1968.
12. Whitten, C. F., M. G. Pettit, and J. Fischoff. Evidence that growth failure from maternal deprivation is secondary to undereating. Journal of the American Medical Association 209:1675–1682.

11
Obesity

It is worth attempting to prevent obesity in children. While the obese infant has little increased risk of remaining obese until adulthood, the risk is greater for the fat preschooler, and greater still for the fat adolescent. Unfortunately we really don't know how to go about prevention. Dieting doesn't work, and we don't know what does.

However, despite the dismal reality of dieting failure, parents are regularly persuaded, by their own concern and by advice from others, to attempt to withhold food from their supposedly too-fat children. This often causes a struggle over food intake, with suffering and distortions on both sides.

Parents are deprived of a harmonious relationship with a contented child. The child is deprived of the security of knowing he will get enough to eat. Because he may be forced to go hungry, the child becomes preoccupied with food, prone to overeat when he gets the chance, and limited in the attention and energy he devotes to other pursuits. Dieting is generally sporadic. The pain of dieting is tolerable only for so long, and diets are abandoned, to be started another day when motivation is higher or obesity appears to be a greater threat.

It is vital that our attempts at prevention do no harm. Our tactics must be moderate, positive and permanent and our goals realistic. The essential task is to set things up for the child so his natural ability to regulate his food intake is distorted as little as possible by outside influences.

While accurate statistics on obesity are hard to find, it appears that less than 10% of infants who are obese become obese adults. The risk of developing adult obesity is increased to about 25% for the obese preschooler, and 70% for the obese adolescent.[13] The person who is obese as an adult has a considerable chance of remaining obese throughout his life.

Clearly, prevention of obesity is extremely important. The catch is being able to do it.

The Dilemma of Obesity

Here is our dilemma: We don't know how to define obesity, what causes it, how to cure it, or even how to prevent it. We have very little way of knowing what to predict or expect from a child. Some people seem to be genetically predisposed to obesity, and we have little way of knowing who they are or how to overcome that genetic tendency. We don't know if dieting helps or harms the situation or, indeed, if it has any effect at all.

We know that people who diet tend to reduce their metabolic rate, so they lose weight more slowly than predicted and regain the weight more easily. Most of the time when people lose weight they regain, and often they regain to a higher weight than before. If they manage to maintain their lowered weight, it is usually because they are able to tolerate a consistently lowered calorie intake, by accepting to some degree the symptoms of starvation, and usually, at the same time are able to maintain a consistent meticulous exercise program.

Most children lose their baby fat as they get older. We don't know if weight loss programs help or hinder this. If a program sets up struggles and anxiety around eating, it is possible that it hinders weight control.

Pressures to be Thin

Despite this sobering reality, most parents are concerned about obesity, and feel bound to intervene if their child shows signs of getting too fat. And their concern has been encouraged by health professionals. Physicians have charged themselves with the responsibility of preventing obesity in future adults by pressuring parents to keep their babies and little children slim. We nutritionists and dietitians have done our share in speaking out about the dangers of obesity and by promoting weight reduction efforts.

Like Dr. Frankenstein, I fear we have created a monster. But unlike Dr. Frankenstein, we have not done it alone. Gradually, over the last 30 years or so the national preoccupation with slenderness has increased to the point where it is now a major aesthetic concern, and even an obsession. Health issues have gotten lost as standards of appearance have become more and more narrow and unrealistic, and as people have done increasingly harmful things to themselves to lose weight.

Diet companies have become big business, many of them promoting severe, nutritionally-inadequate and expensive weight reduction regimens. To achieve weight loss, even people with a moderate or nonexistent excess in body weight are apparently willing to put up with "cures" that are physically more harmful than the condition itself. Many weight reduction regimens are so severe that they can only be justified when the obesity presents a serious health risk.

Physical Consequences

The health consequence of obesity is a very individual thing. However, it appears that at least moderate degrees of fatness are less of a health hazard than we had thought. People who are moderately overweight—up to 20% above currently-accepted standards—have been found in recent studies to reflect a health picture that is as good or better than that of thin or even normal-weight people.[7]

Above that level, obesity does appear to increase health risk. However, it is extremely difficult to sort out how much of a health risk it really presents. The obese person often has a history of erratic and poor nutrition, and fluctuation in body weight brought on by attempts to lose weight. Weight reduction diets may be severe and nutritionally inadequate. In particular, popular high-protein weight-loss diets are high in fat and often produce elevated blood lipids. Many times, rebounds from weight reduction diets are also nutritionally inadequate, and cause elevated blood lipids as people compensate with high fat foods that were previously forbidden. And even if a diet is low in fat, any weight gain causes blood lipids to increase, and may contribute to the process of heart disease.

Consequences of Chronic Dieting

In this struggle to achieve thinness there are not only physical casualties, but also emotional and social casualties. Disorders related to eating are on the increase: 1) Compulsive eating; 2) Bulimia,* which may include ritual vomiting (to compensate for eating and to

---

*Bulimia (or bulimarexia) is stuff-purge cycling. People with this disorder gorge themselves with food, and then get rid of the calories or weight by vomiting, exercising compulsively, or abusing laxatives or diuretics.

control weight); and even 3) Anorexia nervosa—self-imposed starvation. People with such eating disorders are preoccupied with food and with dieting, have distorted perceptions of their bodies, and are excessively concerned about body weight. Their struggle with eating and with body weight takes on the proportion of a major life issue, one that postpones or overshadows all other considerations. Taken to the extreme, it becomes a major disability.

Confusion about Normal Eating. Parents who are very concerned about their own weight reflect their concern in the way they feed their children. They are so preoccupied with preventing obesity that they forget about promoting normal growth. Parents who are chronic dieters have often forgotten what it is like to eat normally, as they veer between the extremes of the weight reduction diet and the compensatory eating that follows it. Because they are themselves confused about normal food regulation, they are confused about their child's food regulation. They feel constrained to manage and regulate that child's food intake.

And we health practitioners do our share—or maybe more than our share—to encourage that interference, with our willingness to weigh and measure and plot and devise strategies. At times, I am sorry to say, we get carried away by our enthusiasm, as did one of my associates when he advised a breastfeeding mother to restrict her chubby daughter to five, rather than seven feedings a day. He neglected to find out that the mother was already being careful not to overfeed her little girl. The mother tried to follow the advice, but fortunately gave up after two very trying days with her fussy infant. She was a wise mother. She acknowledged the doctor's warnings about increased risk of obesity but decided that she wasn't willing to follow the restricted regimen at the risk of losing her breastmilk or spoiling her relationship with her daughter. She was able to see that trying harder to restrict her daughter's food intake was making the situation intolerable for both of them.

That mother was right. Overenergetic attempts to regulate body weight may do more harm than good. In the first place, too little food, no matter whether it is wonderfully balanced, nutritious food, can cause nutritional deficiencies. If a person, particularly a growing person, is not allowed to eat enough, there is no way he or she can be optimally nourished. In the second place, overmanagement of the feeding process can cause distortions in self image and in the feeding relationship. Parents and children become locked in a struggle about eating, a struggle that distorts and damages not only the feeding process, but the over-all relationship. Third, overreaction to moderate degrees of overweight may, in the long run, promote more severe forms of obesity.

We discussed the hazard of too little food in the chapter on calories and normal growth, and we will deal with the third hazard later, as we discuss causes and control of obesity. Right now it is important for you to get a clear fix on the second: the impact of overmanaging on the feeding process. This is best illustrated by a horror story.

Distorted Eating—the Story of Mary. Mary was suffering from bulimia; she was obsessed with food and with dieting, disliked and distrusted her body, and ate in a bizarre and extreme fashion. She would diet severely, so severely that she virtually starved herself. Then, when she couldn't stand the pain any longer she would stuff herself, and then she would vomit.

She wouldn't just eat enough to satisfy her hunger, because as far as she was concerned an amount of food sufficient to satisfy her was extreme overeating. Once she had by her standards overeaten, she would go on an eating binge, stuffing herself in a frantic fashion, eating whole cakes and butter by the spoonful, and virtually depleting the family food supply. Then, when her stomach became so bloated and painful that she could hardly stand it, she would vomit. She used her finger, pushing it far down her throat so she could retch again and again until she had no more left to throw up. Sometimes that would be the end of it. Other times she would repeat the pattern, stuffing and purging herself repeatedly in the course of a day.

Mary perceived herself as being fat, although she was not fat. She was about 5-foot, seven inches tall. She was heavier than "model" thinness, weighing 147 lb. And she was gorgeous. She was very nicely proportioned. In fact, she was perfectly voluptuous. She had the kind of body you only see in a teenaged girl—a very womanly body with a special kind of firmness and strength and physical vitality. But Mary didn't like her body. She said she was too fat and said she was so ashamed of her size and shape that she stayed home a lot, avoiding her friends and their activities.

Part of her distress about her body came from high school standards of body shape and size, and standards of thinness. Part of her distress came from the modeling school to which her parents were sending her in hopes that it would "make her feel better about herself." (In reality it just made her feel worse to be around all those skinny women with all that emphasis on appearance.) But the most powerful pressure came from home.

Mary's mother was thin, the kind of disciplined-looking thinness you only get when you work on your weight, and work <u>hard</u>. She had the model look about her—starved. That is a different kind of look than the one people get who are constitutionally thin, because those people look for the most part like their flesh covers their bones and like they are strong and healthy. Mary's mother looked fragile, and there was a quality of being forced about her, as if she constantly had to drive herself, physically and emotionally.

Mary's father was thin, too, but not excessively so. But he was the one who voiced their concern about Mary's "overeating." He said that Mary had always eaten a lot, and wondered how much it was normal for someone of her age to eat. In fact, he said, Mary had eaten a lot ever since she was born. When she had still been in the hospital, the nurse had brought her into the room and said "Your little girl certainly eats a lot—she had two whole bottles." Of course they thought eating a lot meant Mary would get fat, so they set out to prevent that. (Actually, I wondered if Mary was hungry when she was born—had her mother gained enough weight during pregnancy?)

From that day forth, Mary and her parents engaged in a struggle over her eating. From observing other parents with their supposedly overweight babies, I can guess what that struggle was like. I would guess that Mary's parents tried to feed her less than she really wanted to have. She has a lot of spirit, and I would bet that she was not willing to go hungry without a struggle. I'll also bet that she fussed and cried until she got more to eat. How long she had to fuss probably depended on how able her parents were on any given day to tolerate her fussiness. Her crying was no doubt upsetting, and the only way they could stop it was to do the one thing they didn't want to do—feed her.

I wonder if they got support from the pediatrician for their tactics. If the concern about obesity and the approach to its prevention was as energetic as it is today, I would say that they did get support. In fact, they may have been subjected to pressure and suspicion by the doctor, because Mary managed to get the food that she needed, and to grow and stay on the chubby side despite all their efforts to keep her thin. It's possible that the doctor assumed that they were not energetic enough in their efforts to restrict Mary's food intake, and put even more pressure on them.

Mary grew into what they perceived as being a chubby toddler, and by the time she was three she was sneaking extra food from wherever she could get it. Her first memory of mealtime is of her mother dishing up her plate for her with a limited amount of carefully-selected food. And she cried at the memory of never getting enough unless she sneaked to do it. For Mary, not getting enough food felt very much like not getting enough love. Her parents said they were doing it for her own good, but I wondered how much of their own egos were involved—how important it was for them to have a thin and what they perceived as being more-beautiful daughter.

Distorted Eating Attitudes and Behavior. Mary's eating response was extreme, but it is not unusual. Many people are so upset and obsessed about their eating and body weight that they really think of little else.

Hers is a very common attitude in people who are fat and who have spent their lives trying to be thin. In most cases they speak with resentment of the struggle that they had with their parents over food and their weight, and they carry their hurt that, no matter what else they accomplished in their lives, until they lost weight it wasn't good enough. Those people have kept their fat, and have become well schooled in their negative attitudes about their bodies. And they are completely deprived in their eating—they simply don't feel entitled to eat well. Even with all their dieting, they view their eating as being shameful and out of control. They fear that if they ever stop dieting and eat what they want, they will gain terrific amounts of weight.

The people who don't come into my office are the ones who would be able to tell the success stories. These are people who were chubby children who were allowed or helped to grow up to be normal-weight adults. I know that these people exist because the great majority of obese infants do grow up to be normal-weight adults.

I do, however, see a few success stories of another type. These are fat children who grew up to be fat adults, and still maintained a good attitude about eating and about themselves.

Learning Eating Behavior

Hilde Bruch, a psychiatrist who works in the field of eating disorders, says that she sees two different types of attitudes among obese people. One fat person will see the obesity as being a part of him, a body feature, and not the most important feature at that. He will have a sense of his capabilities and opportunities, and generally get on with his life. In contrast, another fat person will see the obesity as being the absolutely most important thing about him. He will see his fatness as a complete barrier, one that absolutely has to be removed before he will be able to get any sense of achievement or satisfaction out of life. Bruch says the thing that makes the difference is parental attitude. In the growing-up years the family of the first type will have supported him and recognized his potential in many areas. They may have regretted his overweight, and have even tried to help him get rid of it, but ultimately they maintained their perspective about his real sense of worth.[1]

The parents of the immobilized type of obese person, on the other hand, are quite different. As long as their child is obese they see something as being fundamentally wrong with him, they identify it as their failure, and they devote themselves to correcting the obesity. They take the child around from one weight specialist to another, demanding that somehow the child be made thin. And the more intrusive the helpers, the poorer the outcome—the more likely that the child will see himself as a fat person who will never be successful unless he gets thin.

We must be careful that our efforts at preventing or managing obesity do not go too far. It is clear from the discussion we just had that there is very real need for caution. We are entirely too glib and too casual about interfering with the process of food regulation, both in ourselves and in our children. Intruding on balance of food and weight regulation can be tremendously disruptive. Anything that we do to intervene must be done with a real sense of our own limitations.

You must also face up to a hard truth: Despite your best efforts, in some cases a child is simply going to be fat and there won't be anything you can do to change it. Then the task will be that of raising a child who, despite a handicapping condition, can be as physically and emotionally healthy as any other child.

Trying to Understand Obesity

In the area of obesity, our limitations are very real. As I said earlier, we don't even know how to define obesity. We don't know when a child crosses the line between a normal and desirable amount of body fat, to an amount that is excessive and undesirable. We don't know what causes obesity; people who are obese seemingly do little out of the ordinary to cause them to be fat and, once fat, only the most extraordinary behavior will allow them to be thin. And, since we don't know what causes the problem, we also don't know how to treat it.

The traditional treatment of overweight has been reduction in food intake. The fact that this course, if followed, results in weight loss does not necessarily mean that obesity results from excess calorie intake. Despite our national pastime of dieting, we still are a nation of overweight people. Would the problem be worse if we didn't diet, as so many people who struggle with their eating and their weight fear, or is all of our dieting really a factor in promoting the problem? Nobody knows.

But we have to do the best we can. Right now, let's spend some time talking about what we know and what we speculate about obesity: definition, cause and cure.

Before we get into our discussion of causes of obesity, we need to have a word about vocabulary. I will refer to the physical condition of having an excessive amount of fat on the body in a number of ways. I will call it "excessively fat," "obese," (which means the same thing) and simply, "fat." My use of the word "fat" is not intended to be derogatory. If anything, it is intended to desensitize a perfectly good and descriptive word that has too-often been used in a derogatory fashion. There is a "big beautiful woman" movement starting in California that insists on the use of the word *fat* to describe themselves. They say dignifying that term is as important for them as it was for blacks to adopt a reference for themselves that was dignified. I agree. When I use the word fat, I am thinking along those lines.

"Overweight" and "heavy" are terms I have avoided. Many "heavy" people are not fat at all—their weight comes from muscle and bone, or from a broader-than-average torso.

Defining Obesity. Parents dread being told their child is fat. Not only is there social stigma attached to fatness, but most people are experienced enough about dieting and struggles to manage weight to know that it is a long-term, disruptive and discouraging process. Defining a child as obese puts pressure on parents to begin this process.

Sadly, the diagnosis of obesity is often made on the basis of the most casual of observations. A child may look fat, and, even though fatness is normal for the infant and toddler, parents will be told the fat is excessive. Some standards say a weight above the 90th percentile of weight indicates obesity, even if his height is also in the upper percentile.

Other people are more methodical and reasonable at defining obesity in children, saying that a child can be suspected of being excessively fat if he or she is in the 95th percentile, *weight for height.*[3] If you remember our discussion in Chapter 4, this refers to the plotting which tells you whether a child is proportionally thin (less than 50th percentile) or "thick" (over 50th percentile). Whether that thick child is also fat is another story. Again, a heavy child may have a barrel chest or have heavy bones or have very muscular arms and legs.

The growth charts can be particularly helpful in watching for disproportionate increases in weight. From the growth chart in the example in Figure 11-1, it is apparent that the little girl grew

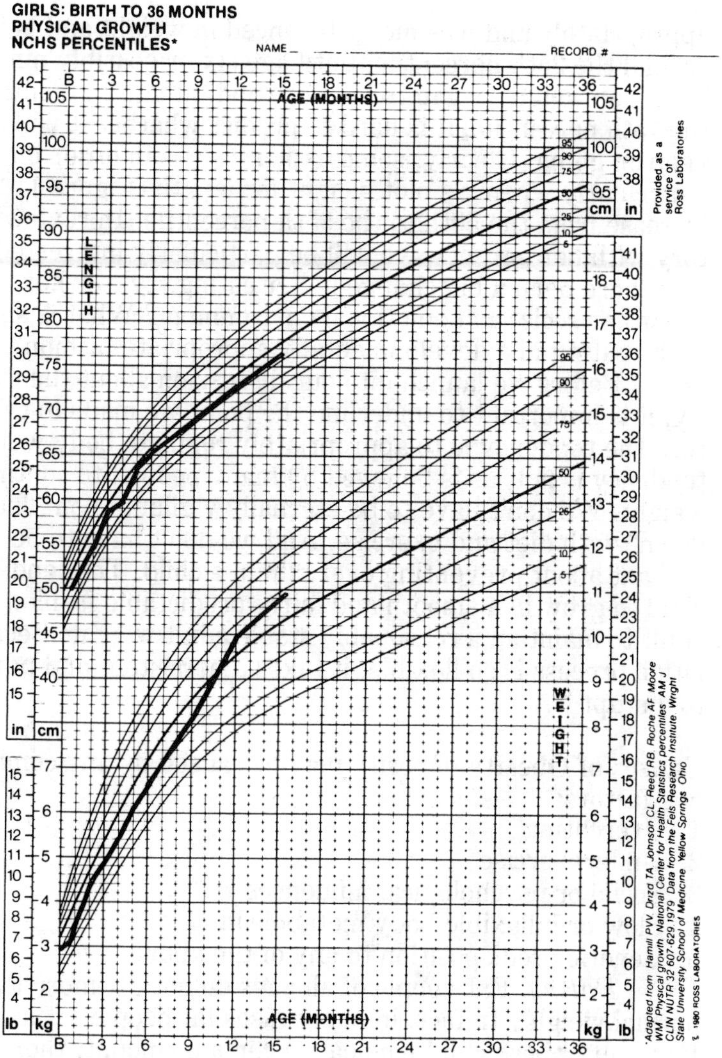

Figure 11-1. Excessive Weight Gain from 6 to 9 Months: Weight-for-age.

appropriately and was nicely balanced in weight and height, right around the 25th percentile, until age six or possibly nine months. Then her weight began to increase and, at age 15 months has reached the 75th percentile; it is hard to predict whether it will level there or keep on going. Clearly, some exploration is in order for this child, particularly when we plot weight for length (Figure 11-2) and find an increase from the 50th to the 95th percentile. In reviewing her history with her parents, we will be particularly interested in changes. Has there been a big change in her eating style or her level of activity or her social and emotional environment? What is she eating, and is she eating in a developmentally appropriate fashion?

Before we launch into our discussion about the causes of obesity, it is important to underline the point we made in the last chapter. The tendency is to appropriately regulate body weight. The tendency is not, as is believed by many people, to continually gain weight. We don't have to be eternally vigilant about "keeping it down" with diet and exercise. And we don't have to be eternally vigilant about preventing overgain in a child. The tendency is for a child to grow in a smooth and fairly-predictable fashion and for the adult to maintain a reasonably stable adult weight. Because the regulation process is so flexible, it takes a persistent and powerful force to disrupt it.

Causes of Obesity. Obesity may be caused by any combination of five factors:

1. Overeating
2. Underexercise
3. Social or psychological influences
4. Slow or inflexible body metabolism
5. Genetic predisposition to any of the above

Eating. Fat people of all ages do not eat more than people of normal weight. In fact, in many cases fat people actually eat less. For every obese child who eats a certain amount, there is a child who

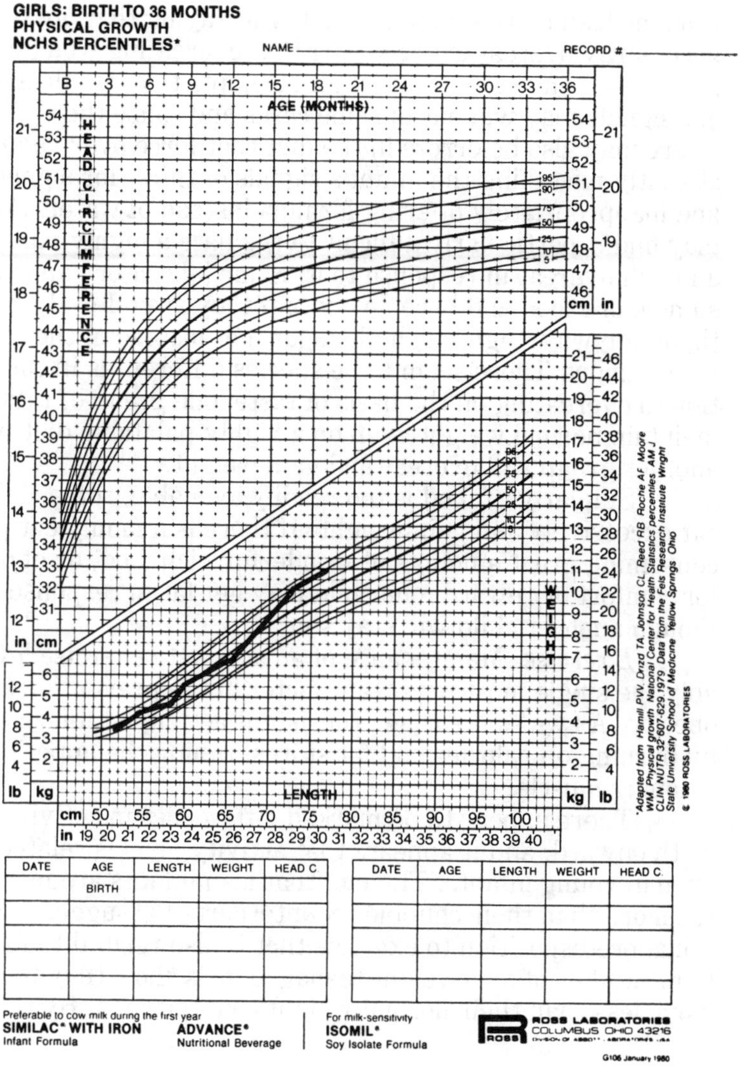

Figure 11-2. Weight-for-length Plotting of Figure 11-1.

remains lean on the same amount. But saying that obese people don't necessarily overeat is not saying that overeating won't cause obesity.

As I have said, persistent attempts to override a child's satiety signals may win out in some cases and cause the child to overeat. There may also be errors in the diet that force overfeeding, like consistently mistaking the infant's signals of thirst for signals of hunger and inappropriately offering formula instead of water. Some children may find it particularly difficult to regulate a highly-palatable diet and will overeat in response to it. Some laboratory animals will consume more food and become obese if they are offered a delicious (to them, anyway) high-fat, high-sugar diet instead of the standard laboratory chow. There seem to be species differences in this predisposition to overeating on the basis of taste; one group of rats is able to maintain normal weight even on a highly-palatable diet, whereas another group will overeat and gain weight.

Similarly, if food is too readily available, some children may eat excessively and gain weight. If there is a family eating style of consuming great amounts of wonderful, rich food, or of offering food for comfort or reward, one child may get fat in response to it, even though another child will stay slim.

Exercise. Maintenance of an adequate exercise level is probably the single most important factor in the prevention and control of obesity. As we said earlier, consistent activity stabilizes body weight by burning off calories and fat stores, tuning the appetite and developing muscle.

There appear to be marked differences in activity levels from birth onward, and it appears that activity level is related to leaness, even in young infants. The fact that lean infants are more active, and eat more than their chubbier counterparts,[10, 12] suggests a constitutional predisposition to exercise that is also related to food regulation. Studies of overweight teenaged girls show they too eat less but move less than their normal-weight counterparts. By that age it is hard to tell whether constitutional or other factors (like embarrassment or difficulty moving) promote the inactivity.

But even if exercise is constitutionally influenced, environmental influences can also have an impact. A child's level of physical activity will vary for instance, depending on whether his parents are active and responsive, or more sedentary and placid. Parents vary in their willingness to let their children take risks and explore. A very cautious or controlling parent may be less likely to allow rough playing, and thus significantly curb the child's physical activity.

Social and Emotional Factors. There are certainly social and emotional factors in overweight. People in a variety of circumstances misuse food as a way of coping with stress or resolving conflict. Carried to excess, this can cause obesity.

A child's disruption in food regulation is at times the product of a disturbed family environment. Disturbed families are rigid, have poor communication patterns, and a high level of unresolved conflict. Because of their own problems, such parents show inappropriate levels of control and concern with children. They may be so over managing that a child's failure to eat dessert provokes a family crisis, or so underinvolved that they do not even know where their children are at night.

Children in disturbed families develop patterns of coping that help them get by. They may become depressed and lethargic, or active and delinquent. They may choose overeating as a way of conforming, or gain excess weight as a way of rebelling. It appears that for a child to use food as a way of coping, rather than naughtiness or fingernail biting, eating has to be an issue in the family.[9]

Dieting appears to help set up the pattern of using food to cope. Compared with "normal" eaters, people of all weights who are chronic dieters tend to overeat rather than undereat in response to stress.[4] If a child has been raised dieting, he is likely to continue this pattern, and may also show periods of pronounced weight gain throughout his life.

Parents with hangups about their own eating send their children very mixed messages about eating. Most obese mothers are chronic dieters. (Because they are obese—not because they are mothers.) They often prefer thin babies, and can be very concerned about preventing obesity in their children. However, they tend to over-interpret hunger in their babies (they feed rather than looking for other causes of fussiness), BUT spend less time feeding. They also are more likely to use external cues for regulating feeding, such as time and quantity. To make matters worse, obese parents are prone to pressure from health professionals about preventing obesity in their children.[2, 14]

But obese mothers are not the only ones who have hangups about eating. Remember that Mary's mother was thin—but very preoccupied with eating. Slender parents who assign a lot of importance to physical fitness can have real conflict about feeding their children.

As a consequence, a child's eating experience may be inconsistent, erratic and emotionally charged. If the adult is anxious and inconsistent about feeding, the child can grow up with unreliable access to food, and having to struggle to get enough to eat. She may learn to distrust her own perception of her need for food, since it appears so often to be in conflict with her parents' ideas. On the other hand, if the parent is too ready to feed, the infant may grow up over-interpreting the need for food. She may learn the habit of using food for taking care of all kinds of discomfort, and end up eating more often than if she were depending on hunger as a cue for eating.

While we can say that many people appear to overeat, under-exercise and gain weight for social and emotional reasons, there are no consistent personality patterns in obese people. Obese people are no more depressed, dependent, anxious or uncontrolled than anybody else. They may simply have chosen a way of coping that disrupts their ability to regulate body weight.

However, even for people whose eating and weight are clearly related to psychological and emotional factors, resolving the emotional issues will not necessarily allow the person to lose weight. Psychotherapy has a very poor track record for promoting weight loss. Its benefit is in helping people feel better about themselves and improve their lives—at *any* weight level.

And finally, eating, or failing to eat, can have a major impact on people's emotions. People who are starving, whether or not the starvation is self imposed, become irritable and depressed and lose interest in other activities. They become tired and weak and think of little else but food. To function well emotionally you have to have enough to eat.

Metabolism. Body metabolic rate can have an automatic adjustment mechanism which serves to defend body weight at a preferred level. In starvation, metabolic processes slow down, muscle mass dwindles, voluntary activity decreases, and heat generation decreases.[6] These variations in metabolic efficiency can stack the deck against the person who tries to lose weight.

Dieters hit plateaus at low-calorie levels of eating, and have to restrict themselves even more severely to lose more. To maintain reduced body weight, they have to maintain continued food restriction.

A while back Erma Bombeck was lamenting confirmation of something she already knew. As she put it, thinking about food can make you fat. She had run across some research that was done at Yale showing that people who diet and are hungry and preoccupied with food may actually increase body efficiency with their preoccupation. Chronic dieters, when presented with a good-looking aromatic, sizzling steak, made more insulin in response than people who were not dieters.[11] Insulin increases body efficiency and promotes fat storage. In such cases, paradoxically, dieting may make us fat, if food deprivation makes people respond physiologically to food and less active metabolically.

The idea that there are metabolic differences that predispose to obesity has been almost totally rejected by physicians. Most doctors persist in their conviction that fatness is caused by overeating alone, and insist that the only way to control obesity is to stop overeating. Nutritionists and physiologists, who know more about metabolism, are less convinced that they know the answers. Indeed, they know it may be many years before they can be at all sure what is going on metabolically.

Until then, we know enough about metabolic responses to starvation to make us cautious. Drastic decreases in food intake, especially when they are not accompanied by increases in exercise, can shift metabolism into low gear and promote the regaining of any lost weight. Tactics for preventing or controlling obesity must therefore be selected with an eye to avoiding decreases in metabolic rate.

Genetics. Overeating and underexercise may turn some children into fat adults and have no effect on others, because of their different inherited factors.

Body build is inherited; a tendency to obesity appears to be inherited as well. Studies of identical twins who were separated early on and raised by different adoptive families found that the twins' weight resembled each other more than they did those of the adoptive families. From these studies come the often-quoted figures that if both parents are obese, the child has about an 80% chance of obesity; if one parent is obese, the odds drop to about 40%, and if neither is obese the chances drop to about 10%.

A person may be genetically programmed with respect to body composition, activity, sociability, aggressiveness, docility and even sharpness of sense of taste, all of which can in turn have an impact on energy balance. Other factors are even more clearly tied to genetics. Body build is a genetically-determined factor which has a major impact on body weight and body composition. And as much as I hate to say it, *set point* of body weight may also be largely constitutionally determined.

According to the set point theory,[6] the body works actively to defend body weight at a certain preferred level. Weight, rather than varying in response to other factors, actually is kept very stable. Appetite and calorie expenditure appear to adjust in an attempt to defend body weight.

The set point idea is worrisome because it appears so hard to influence it. What if some people simply have an inherited tendency to be fat? What is to happen to them? Do they have any chance of maintaining normal weight with that kind of genetic handicap?

Those are absolutely impossible questions. There may, however, be some room for maneuvering. Genetically-obese strains of mice don't get as fat if they are offered ample opportunity for exercise; and to turn it around, the fattening of farm animals genetically-selected for tendency toward fatness can be accelerated by penning them. That gives hope that exercise can really make a difference.

To avoid getting fat, one who is genetically predisposed to obesity will probably have to be consistently careful about both diet and exercise. In fact, it appears that a genetic predisposition to fatness is better overcome with exercise than with diet, because the metabolic slowdowns that are produced by dietary restrictions can be at least partially reversed by increasing exercise.

Perhaps the issue should be considered in terms of controlling the *degree* of fatness. It may be that the genetically obese person will be somewhat fat in any event, and that is something that he will simply have to live with. Over-reaction to moderate degrees of fatness might only make the situation worse.

Diets and Other Cures

I am not going to spend a lot of time talking about cures or controls for obesity, because as I have said, very little has worked—once people become fat, it is extremely difficult for them to become and remain thin.

Almost twenty years ago, when I first went to the University of Wisconsin hospitals, we thought that the high-protein, low carbohydrate frequent-feeding diet was the answer. It turned out not to be. About that same time there were some people who were saying that the complete starvation diet was the answer. It wasn't. Then there was the protein-modifying fast. No, again. Five years ago, we thought that the behaviorists had the answer. What they did helped, but it wasn't the answer.

All of these approaches were based on the idea that overweight people are overeaters. Or, even if they weren't really overeaters, if they were willing to cut down on calories from their present level, and were patient in waiting for change, that eventually they would lose weight. That may be the answer, but there aren't that many people who are patient enough, long enough to find out.

Even people who are able to adhere to weight reduction regimens, and lose significant amounts of weight, simply do not maintain it. Difficult as it is to lose weight, the truly difficult part seems to be maintenance of weight loss. It seems that once the active phase of the program is discontinued, people usually regain to their previous weights, and often gain more.

Those are the hard facts. I think it is unrealistic to give some sort of paternalistic peptalk about how you can and must keep your child thin. It is possible that nothing you can do will keep your child thin, and that eventually you, and your child, and I, and all the rest of your helpers may have to face up to that fact.* At that point we may all need to tell ourselves that we have been moderate and consistent in our efforts and at least we have done no harm. We might

---

*If reconciling yourself to your child's weight is very difficult for you, you might consider getting professional counseling. Your strong feelings about your child's weight are probably related to the way you feel about yourself.

even have done some good. Your child might be more slender and more healthy physically than he otherwise would have been had we not tried.

To summarize: It appears that the obese person has a predisposition to energy storage, and that once the fat is stored it is very difficult to get it out of storage. Attempting to get rid of fat by use of weight reduction diets, particularly severe ones, may only make the problem worse. Calorie deficits reduce exercise and body metabolism, and increase hunger and preoccupation with food. Rebound eating from weight reduction diets, in combination with slowed metabolism and exercise, sets the dieter up to regain the weight, and often to store even more fat, which is, again, difficult to lose.

Preventing Excessive Weight Gain

Since we are concerned about *prevention*, and since we are working with growing children, it seems to me that our task is reasonably clear. We must try to prevent the weight-gaining phase of the obesity. We must try to prevent energy intake that is in excess of the amount that the child needs for growth, maintenance and activity. We must be vigilant, and we must do it in a way that is consistent. That means that we cannot use extreme methods that we can't tolerate for long, because rebound from the extremes is likely to exaggerate fat accumulation. We cannot, as one of my neighbors said to her chubby son, give up ice cream forever.

We are not talking about supervising every bite your child eats. Children, and adults as well, vary in their hunger and appetite from day to day. Children must be allowed to eat as much as they are hungry for. It is our task to set things up for the child so that his natural ability to regulate his food intake is being distorted as little as possible by outside influences. And we have to set things up for you so you know when you have done what you can. You need to be able at some point to leave the problem, and yourself, alone. You mustn't end up feeling responsible for every bite that your child eats.

Our task is made immeasurably easier if the child is active. Activity improves his ability to regulate his eating, increases lean body mass, and helps him to use up excessive calories.

Take particular note that I do not define outcome in terms of *weight loss*. I said the goal is to *lose fat*. There is a difference. A child eating moderately and exercising well can be successful in losing fat and gaining lean, and yet not show any difference on the scale. Since fat tissue contains about five times the calories of lean tissue, he could actually be losing calories from his body and still have a stable body weight. Eating in moderation can reduce fatness while sparing the loss of lean body mass, whereas severe dieting causes the loss of much more lean (relative to fat) tissue.

Defining Goals. In order to keep yourself feeling successful, it is important to be clear about what you can expect and realistically shoot for. If you are working on obesity prevention, you should keep in mind that you are basically trying to maintain a smooth and balanced weight-to-height ratio as your child grows.

The boy in Figure 11-3, although his weight was at a higher percentile than his height, maintained his pattern until he was about six years old. Then his weight began increasing rapidly until, at age 11 years, it had reached the 90th percentile. (By that time, he was well over the 95th percentile, weight for height—Figure 11-4.) The goal for him was to get his rate of weight gain to slow down so his height could catch up to it. Figure 11-3 shows that he accomplished that by the time he was 14.

Weight loss is not desirable for a rapidly growing child. For one thing, it could impair growth. For another, it could hook you into a cycle of depriving and then compensating with food. If a child loses some weight as a fringe benefit, say, from the change of seasons or from making some changes in family food selection, that is fine. I would hope, however, that that would not be more than a pound or two a month, and the younger the child, the less the amount. Keep in

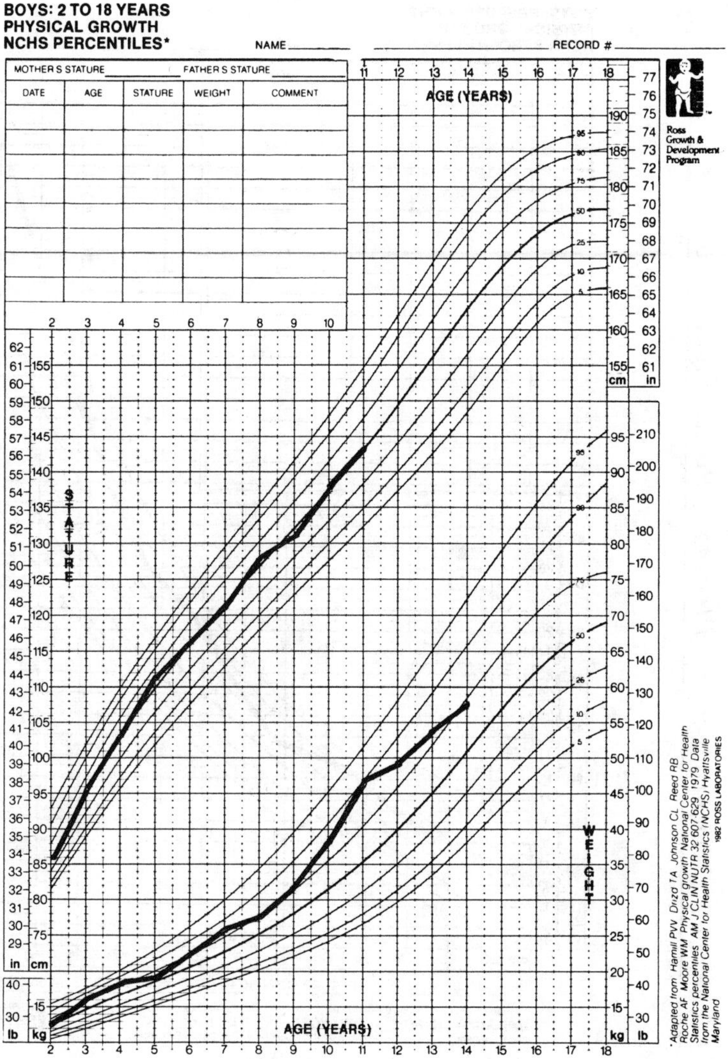

Figure 11-3. Weight Variation in Boy from 9 to 14 Years of Age.

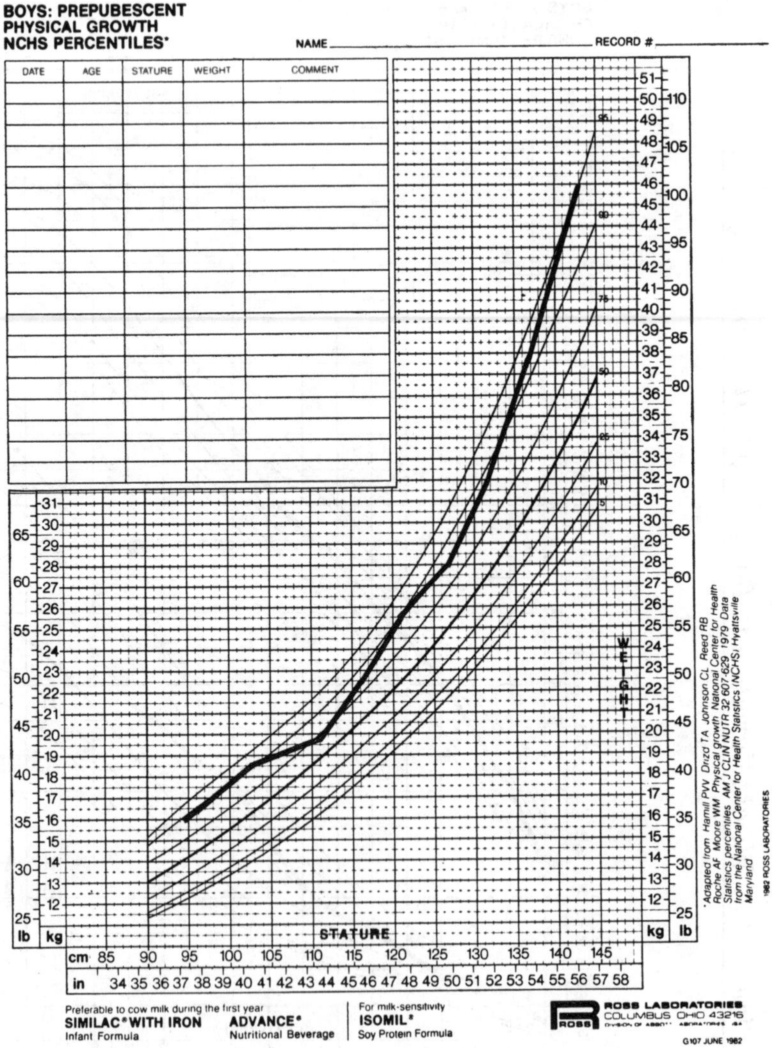

Figure 11-4. Weight-for-height Plotting of Boy in Figure 11-3.

mind that a child's weight is supposed to be increasing, and if it is instead going down, that can indicate quite a calorie deficit.

Strategy for Weight Control

The tactics that I am going to suggest now have the best chance of producing the results that we have just described, with minimal negative side effects. There are five important principles in the control and treatment of obesity in children:

1. We must prevent overeating. We must be careful to maintain sufficient but not excessive calorie intake (on the chance that we are dealing with a child who is very efficient at using his calories).
2. We must maintain a sufficient level of exercise (to maintain lean body mass, enhance food regulation and compensate for any inherited abnormalities in energy regulation).
3. We must be careful to avoid anything that will be likely to reduce metabolic rate, such as severe calorie deficits or restriction of physical activity.
4. We must be careful not to do anything that even *feels* like deprivation (as that sets up behavioral and possibly metabolic patterns, like excessive insulin production in anticipation of eating, that promote food-seeking and possible calorie storage).
5. We must select tactics that are positive enough and non-intrusive enough that they have a good chance of becoming a permanent part of life. We simply must not choose extreme methods which will be abandoned whenever the going gets tough.

In dietary management, the key strategy is prevention of overeating. Prevention of overeating is absolutely, unquestionably and emphatically NOT the same thing as promotion of under-eating. The latter is dieting, no matter how you disguise it.

As you no doubt have gathered by now, I am a real extremist about moderation. And nowhere are my views more extreme than in the area of dieting. I am unconditionally opposed to putting a child on a weight reduction diet. We just don't know how many calories are needed by any one growing child, and we don't know whether our restrictions will impair growth and development. But that is not the worst of it. I consider the outright food deprivation characteristic of some diets to be so harsh and disruptive that it extracts a great penalty from the parent, the child and the relationship. YOU MUST NOT MAKE A CHILD GO HUNGRY. Enforced hunger implants in a child the fear that she won't get enough to eat—or the feeling that she is not entitled to eat. I have pointed out that that can be very destructive, in terms of long-term attitudes toward self and about eating.

Although we are avoiding dieting, we still have some ways of modifying a child's food intake. There are many indirect, subtle and moderate approaches you can use without making a major point to the child that you are managing his eating and are concerned about preventing obesity.

Your child is entitled to learn to trust his body. If you are too intrusive, you can spoil that trust. For example, you can make a big issue out of cooking meals and avoiding desserts, and you can make your child feel singled-out and deprived. Or you can generally cook in a low-fat, low-sugar way and opt for desserts only occasionally, and your child will grow up thinking that is how people eat. The tactics I am proposing represent the kind of firm and reasonable discipline that I think is appropriate for any generally healthy child.

Eating Behavior. Teach and model for your child slow, attentive and focused eating behavior. Your aim is to get her to pay attention to her food so she can get as much satisfaction as possible whenever she eats. Part of doing this is for her to pay attention to herself while she is eating, so she can be aware of her enjoyment and can tell when she is feeling full and satisfied. Meals and snacks that are truly satisfying can help cut down on the amount of times she ends up grazing for food, perhaps searching for the satisfaction that she missed at mealtime. If she is eating slowly and in an attentive fashion, it is likely that she will feel satisfied on less food, and it is less likely that she will overeat.

The first thing to think of to encourage slow and attentive eating is to model that kind of eating yourself. If you gobble your food, chances are your child will, too. If you enjoy and savor your food, your child will get the idea.

Teach your child to eat like a gourmet, not like a gourmand. A gourmand is greedy, a glutton. A gourmet is a connoisseur of good food. She gets considerable enjoyment out of eating, and enhances that enjoyment by being very aware of the food. She looks at the food, smells it, anticipates it, and when she eats it, she does so attentively and carefully, paying attention to the textures and flavors and temperatures as she chews thoroughly before swallowing. Eating in this way, the gourmet comes to realize that it doesn't take a great deal of food, even if it is wonderful food, to be truly satisfied.

But even great gourmets have to start somewhere, and you can start with your child by helping him slow his eating rate. Encourage him to put his fork or his sandwich down between bites, and not pick it up again until his mouth is empty. Encourage him to chew thoroughly, being careful to crush all the pieces and bits of food in his mouth. Coach him in keeping the food off the back of his tongue, because if it goes back that far it gets swallowed automatically, whether he is ready or not. And remind him not to wash his food down when it is still half-chewed. Again, be a good model for all of these behaviors.

There is room for firmness in encouraging this behavior in your child. I do not consider it too harsh and intrusive for you to insist that your child chew his food well and pay attention to his eating. Some people make a game of learning this, with family members reminding each other. Sometimes a timer helps, with the condition that the first helping must last a certain amount of time. For the child who hurries through her meal so she can get back to playing, you might try requiring her to be at the table a certain amount of time, whether she is eating or not. That would be just an interim tactic, however, because if she is sitting there with all that food around she could be reminded to eat more.

Food Selection and Meal Planning. Your ability to control the source of supply is your major advantage in influencing your child's eating. You can't determine how much your child eats, but you can control, most of the time, what is presented to him to eat. There are some good strategies you can use to help your child regulate his eating.

Provide Meals and Make Your Meals Significant. Having set and reliable eating times gives a child a sense of order and predictability. This predictability seems to have an impact on perceptions about eating. It seems that people who are in the habit of eating at regular times are less likely to pick up food at odd times. Even the hungry animal will be less inclined to seek food if it is not its established time to eat.

Plan Meals that are Satisfying. You can help your child to regulate his eating appropriately by the way you plan your meals. As you recall, when we were talking about food regulation we said that the components of satisfaction are: a) the relative levels of various nutrients in the meal (glucose, amino acids, fatty acids); b) the amount of stomach filling; c) the amount of chewing involved; and d) the amount of enjoyment and appetite satisfaction from the meal. As much as possible, in planning meals, try to provide the components of satisfaction. Translated into meal planning, this means:

- Include protein, fat and carbohydrate.
- Include something of low caloric density.
- Include something chewy.
- Include one or more food items that your child is likely to enjoy.
- Be moderate in the use of high caloric-density foods.

Protein, Fat and Carbohydrate. Reread our discussion in the *Regulation* chapter (p. 350), and pay particular attention to the discussion on the "dieters special" (p. 356). Don't be tempted to omit starch; it won't work.

Low Caloric-density Food. Bulky, low-calorie foods let your child chew and fill up without adding too many calories. If you can dilute out the overall caloric density of the meal a little with some low-calorie vegetables, that makes the meal somewhat easier to regulate.

The low-calorie foods that your child is likely to enjoy the most are fresh vegetables like carrot or celery sticks. And he will be likely to continue to enjoy them as long as he doesn't get the idea that they are a form of penance, and something you have to eat when you are too fat.

The lowest caloric-density foods that I can think of are the vegetables that I have listed in Figure 11-5.

These low-calorie vegetables end up supplying a moderate number of calories overall, even with a reasonable addition of cheese sauce or some butter. But use your head. A friend gave me a recipe for a zucchini casserole that called for a stick of butter and a cup of sour cream. The recipe said it served four people, which would figure out to 300 extra calories in fat for each serving. She said the recipe was delicious, and I have no doubt that it was. If you have a passion for that particular dish, that's fine with me; enjoy yourself. But don't kid yourself that just because it has zucchini in it that it is low in calories. That is the same thing as kidding yourself that carrot cake or zucchini bread or french fried onion rings are low in calories.

Something Chewy. Chewing is important for satisfaction as well as for promoting a strong attachment of teeth to the jaws. The raw vegetables described in the previous section can do double duty as something chewy as well. Also think of bagels or other tough breads, or a piece of steak, or some nuts or crackers.

Figure 11-5. Low-calorie Vegetables.

Asparagus	Eggplant
Bean sprouts	Endive
Broccoli	Greens—beet, chard, turnip, kale, etc.
Cabbage	Lettuce
Carrots	Mushrooms
Cauliflower	Green onions
Celery	Okra
Chicory	Pea pods
Chinese cabbage	Pepper
Cucumbers	Radishes
Escarole	Summer squash
Romaine lettuce	Tomatoes or tomato juice
Sauerkraut	V8-Juice
Spinach	
String beans—green or wax	

Something Your Child Likes. If you are going to make the meal significant for your child you will need to include something that she likes. That might be something as simple as a good bread. It might be a favorite casserole or a vegetable. If you are going to allow high caloric-density foods at all, I would really encourage you to include them at mealtime—don't imprint in your child the idea that the only way to get "treat" foods is to snack.

Be Cautious about High Caloric-density Foods. Anything that is fried or prepared with a lot of additional fat is going to be high in calories. Anything that is high in sugar may be also high in fat, and the combination of both makes for particularly high-calorie food. Because these foods are so delicious, and because each mouthful carries such a caloric whallop, they merit special attention. It may be that some people, like some animals, have a particular taste for fatty or sugary foods, and will overeat and get fat if given too-free access to them. Children in general, and some children in particular seem to love sweets.

It is a good idea to limit the frequency of particularly high-calorie, low-nutrient foods, and you can develop strategies for doing so. For example, kids don't have to have candy bars all that often, and it isn't really necessary to send potato chips in the school lunch every day. Most of us probably don't have to have desserts after every meal. And even if we really do prefer fried chicken, there are other ways of preparing chicken that can be most enjoyable, that you can use every other time or so.

The more you reduce the frequency of the high-calorie foods, the more you are cutting down on calories from those foods. You don't have to cut them out altogether. Nor do you have to make your changes all at the same time. If your children are accustomed to potato chips every day, you might just plan to run out before the end of the week. You can make gradual shifts in your menu planning, and a lot of times no one will even notice.

Don't Be Afraid of Starchy Foods. It is a surprise to most people to learn that breads, potatoes and other starchy foods are really quite moderate in caloric density, especially when compared with the foods that they often accompany, such as meats and cheeses.

People worry about eating starch because they think it is fattening. I talk with a lot of mothers who won't feed their children *any* "starchy" foods. They say their children love bread, potatoes, noodles and cereal, but that they really don't dare to give them to them for fear they will get fat. They should stop reading the "diet" books and relax. The idea that starch shoots straight into fat storage in the body is largely a myth. Starchy foods are not all that concentrated in calories, and they are so filling that they are easier to regulate. And they are satisfying because they are tasty.

Watch the Beverages. Here is where you get to discover the real, true, hard-nosed rigid me, because I am extremely opinionated about beverages. I think kids should avoid almost all beverages except for water, milk and juice, and that the last two should be consumed in moderate amounts. I think that pop should be saved for special occasions only, and I think that fruit-flavored powdered or canned beverages are an abomination—although I think their occasional use is unavoidable. (Actually, powdered or liquid fruit drinks are no worse nutritionally than pop, but the way they are advertised as being so nutritious and wonderful for kids irritates the dickens out of me.) Children should not expect that everything that they drink be flavored in some way. As you can see by the table below, drinking lemonade or pop, or even juice or milk in response to thirst can provide an awful lot of excess calories, and it can kill the appetite for other nutritious food. Water is still the best thing for thirst, and children should be encouraged to drink it.

Figure 11-6. Calories in Common Beverages

	Calories in 8 ounces
Whole milk	170
2% milk	120
Chocolate milk	250
Pop	100
Kool-Aid	100
Lemonade	100
Fruit juice	80–120
Canned fruit drinks	120

If a child is drinking rather than eating his food, or if a child is overdoing on the milk and juice, you may have to impose a limit. Depending on age, children need two to four cups of milk a day and, I think should be allowed an absolute juice maximum of about 3 to 6 ounces per day.

You can make and enforce a rule in your house: no juice or milk except at meals or snacks. Imposing a limit on milk might be easier if you keep the milk carton off the table and provide a glass of water to take care of thirst.

Control the Eating Environment. Set things up for your child so that as much as possible she is encouraged to eat intentionally, in response to a deliberate decision to eat. Reminders for eating (which often lead to unintentional eating) include being in the presence of food, and being in a place where food is usually eaten. In some cases these reminders are so powerful that they overwhelm a child's attention to his own hunger and appetite as a basis for making the decision to eat. The point is that it is helpful to the child to control eating stimuli, so that as much as possible he is encouraged to eat on the basis of hunger and satiety. You can decrease eating cues and encourage a deliberate decision to eat by controlling food access, and in effect complicating eating.

Control Food Access. As much as possible keep food out of sight and make it difficult to get at. Keep cookies in an opaque container on the top shelf. Keep candy in the refrigerator, and use the candy dish for paper clips. Your child may know the foods are there but he won't think of them as often as if they were sitting right out in the open.

You can control food access at meals, too. Try not to have a laden serving platter sitting in front of the child. Anybody will eat more fried chicken if they are looking at a big mound of it directly in front of them. Anticipating the second helping also makes it more difficult to tune in on and enjoy the first. Some people have simply stopped having serving dishes on the table, and serve directly from the pans on the stove or sideboard.

The child can serve himself, but the parent can still play the role of encouraging moderation. You can reassure the child that if he wants more, he can have more, but in the meantime he can pay attention to what he has on his plate and decide later if he is still hungry.

If a child eats too fast and then wants more, you can say, "Well, you ate that pretty fast. Why don't you just sit here a couple of minutes and see if you still want it." Then, if he does, be sure you deliver, or else he won't trust you the next time.

Complicate Eating. You can set things up to make eating consume time and effort, and thus force a deliberate decision to eat. You can forbid eating in the family room and in front of the TV. You can tell a child that he can eat if he wants to, but he must be sitting at the table to do it. Of course, "sitting at the table," for children five to seven years old, has a broad definition. Kids that age wiggle, stand up with their foot on the chair seat, and rock the chair back and forth and from side to side, and turn around and swing their feet. When asked to sit still they are puzzled—as if that was what they were doing all along. But, it passes, and until then, "sitting" means being within one foot of the chair.

Encourage Exercise. Appropriate eating regulation and weight control are absolutely dependent on exercise.

For weight management, the goals in exercising are threefold: expending calories, promoting and maintaining lean body mass, and fine tuning the food regulation mechanism.

Exercise that accomplishes all three goals most effectively is that which requires movement of the whole body, but particularly of the larger muscles, like the thighs and hips. For example, comparable exertion while walking or running requires more calories than does paddling a canoe, and swimming requires more calories than either. Exercise also requires adequate time spent in motion. Sports like soccer and swimming require more sustained movement than baseball or bowling, where the activity is sporadic.

When you set out to modify exercise, just like modifying eating, it is important to be both *moderate* and *consistent*. And as with eating, setting realistic goals, and adopting positive and pleasurable ways of going about it are also essential, in order to have an exercise program that will be maintained over the years. And years it will take. It won't work to go all out and get your child involved in a high-intensity exercise program that, like the diet, will be abandoned when the going gets rough. You may well get a rebound from that just like the rebound from dieting.

There are a number of ways you can encourage an increased level of activity.

Encourage Your Child to Play Sports. If there is a choice, encourage the sports that require more energy. And be sure that you let her play the sport for fun and recreation. Watch your own competitiveness and your own ego involvement. She doesn't have to be great to get what she needs from a sport.

Encourage Children to be Mobile. Let them get around in as much space as they can handle. For the toddler that may mean the living room or the back yard. For the older child that may mean walking 12 blocks to school or riding the bike to the library a couple of miles away. It's no great kindness to lug kids around to their activities when they can make it themselves. They will kick and complain and resist, but once they have gotten themselves used to things, they feel so independent and pleased—and sure it was all their own idea.

Build in Energy-burning Habits. Take the stairs rather than the elevator and take your child along. When you are looking for a parking place, talk to yourself about how it takes no more time to park further out and walk in than to drive around looking for a closer parking place. Encourage your child to put his things away as they accumulate, rather than doing it all at one time. And if he complains about having to go ALL THE WAY UPSTAIRS, turn a deaf ear.

Develop an Active Family Recreation Style. It helps if you like biking and hiking and playing badminton. If you don't, I don't know what to recommend for you, other than to say that surely there is some kind of active recreation SOMEWHERE that you can enjoy with your child. Some families are taking up square dancing or raquetball.

Regulate Television Watching. Television entraps children in one position and keeps them passive. Television ads also remind them to eat. Some behaviorists recommend having a child earn TV time with physical activity, matching every hour of TV with an hour of physical activity. I think the idea is good, but the proportion may be way off. Physical activity is much more important for children than TV, and time spent should reflect that.

The tactics that I have suggested to you, both for diet and exercise, are all indirect, moderate and positive. They cannot, however, be utilized without effort and consistency and discipline. The problems they address won't get "solved" permanently. You will still be setting limits on your child's eating. You will still have showdowns with him about eating in front of the TV or snacking right before dinner. It may take your energy and time and commitment to be sure that your child is presented with opportunities to exercise. And you will clash when you insist on his biking or walking rather than having you drive him. As the woman advised us when we bought our shetland pony, be firm, fair, and follow through.

I wish that I could say that if you do all of this that your child will not be fat. I can't promise that. All I can say to you is that you will have done what is reasonable and moderate, and stands the best chance of helping your child to achieve normal weight. At some point you may have to decide, as did the parents of little Alice in the last chapter, that although you regret the direction that growth is taking, you simply have to support your child in the pattern that is normal for her. If your child is too fat, you will have to let yourself off the hook of feeling that you are responsible, or that you have done something wrong. Eventually your child may get thinner. The chances of that are increased if you keep your efforts moderate, consistent and positive.

If your child seems to be heading for excessive fatness, there is a great deal you can still do to help. You can define the problem in a way that permits a solution. Instead of trying to fix things by getting your child thin, you need to help your child at her elevated weight to be as physically, socially and emotionally healthy as possible. You can be clear and consistent about your love and caring. You can be understanding and supportive about the difficulties of being a fat child, but you mustn't be overprotective. That will only teach her to use her fat as an excuse for not taking risks or taking responsibility for herself.

You can dress her attractively and not settle for ugly clothing. Heavy people can look absolutely stunning if they know how to dress well, and your child can, too. You can teach her ways of being assertive and not allowing other children to hurt her or bully her. You can allow her to respect her body by encouraging her to participate in activities at which she can be successful, and by letting her feel that her eating is appropriate. Even if other people think that overweight people are overeaters, she doesn't have to think that of herself.

All of this is very difficult. The societal values and attitude are quite the opposite, and you may have feelings that get in the way of your being able to be positive and supportive. Again, if you find you are unable to accept and support your child, at *any* weight, you should consider professional counseling.

In most instances you can best help your child by supporting her as she conducts her own affairs. But in some cases you can be helpful by intervening with other adults—the teacher or gymnastics instructor or scout leader or grandparent who puts pressure on the child to lose weight. At some point it may be necessary to say to them: "Your job is not to make my child thin. Your job is to help him learn to like and accept himself as he is."

A good teacher will help a child to achieve a sense of accomplishment and status in the classroom that has nothing to do with fatness or thinness. A good gymnastics instructor will be positive and flexible in what she expects from the child, adjusting demands to fit the capability of the youngster. A good scout leader will help children to get past discrimination, and reinforce a sense of worth in individual differences. And a good grandparent will treat that child like the greatest person in the world, just like all good grandparents do.

Selected References

1. Bruch, Hilde. Eating disorders; Obesity, Anorexia Nervosa and the Person Within. New York: Basic Books, Inc. 1973.
2. Dubois, S., D. E. Hill, and G. H. Beaton. An examination of factors believed to be associated with infantile obesity. The American Journal of Clinical Nutrition. 32:1997–2004. 1979.
3. Fomon, S. J. Nutritional Disorders of Children. Prevention, Screening and Followup. DHEW Publication No. (HSA) 76-5612. 1976.
4. Herman, C. P. and J. Polivy. Restrained eating. In Stunkard, A. J. Obesity. W. B. Saunders. Philadelphia. 1980.
5. Huenemann, R. L. Environmental factors associated with preschool obesity. Part I and II. Journal of the American Dietetics Association 64:480 and 488. 1974.
6. Keesey, R. E. A set-point analysis of the regulation of body weight. In Stunkard, A. J. Obesity. W. B. Saunders, Philadelphia. 1980.
7. Keys, Ancel. W. P. Atwater memorial lecture: Overweight, obesity, coronary heart disease and mortality. Nutrition Reviews. 38:297–307. 1980.

8. Mayer, Jean. Some aspects of the problem of regulation of food intake and obesity. New England Journal of Medicine 274:610–616, 662–673, 722–731. 1960.
9. Minuchin, S., B. L. Rosman and L. Baker. Psychosomatic Families. Anorexia Nervosa in Context. Cambridge: Harvard University Press. 1978.
10. Purvis, G. A. Infant Nutrition Survey. Gerber Products Company. 1979.
11. Rodin, J. Has the distinction between internal versus external control of feeding outlived its usefulness? In G. A. Bray (ed.), Recent Advances in Obesity Research: II. London: Newman Publishing, Ltd. 1978.
12. Rose, H. E. and J. Mayer. Activity, calorie intake, fat storage and the energy balance of infants. Pediatrics 41:18. 1968.
13. Weil, W. B. Current controversies in childhood obesity. The Journal of Pediatrics 91:175–187. 1977.
14. Wooley, S. C. and Wooley, O. W. Obesity and women—I. A closer look at the facts. Women's Studies International Quarterly. 2:69–79. 1979.

12
The Feeding Relationship

The feeding relationship is all the interactions that go into working it out with your child about feeding. To be successful in feeding your child, you have to be able to share responsibility with him: You, the parent, are responsible for what he is offered to eat. But he *is responsible for how much of it he eats. To share that responsibility, you have to be accepting of your child's abilities and limitations in feeding and responsive to his messages that let you know what, when, and how much he wants to eat.*

If you establish a positive feeding relationship with your child, you increase his chances of being well nourished, and of having healthy attitudes about eating and about himself and the world. Disruptions in the feeding relationship can produce an overly finicky child or one who eats too much or too little.

You might be having trouble with feeding because you have had poor advice about food and eating, because your child has been sick and you feel like he is vulnerable, or because you are having some emotional difficulties. If feeding is a struggle that just doesn't seem to get resolved, you should get some professional help in finding a solution.

We have talked about the feeding relationship in other chapters. It is important enough to talk about it in more detail here. The relationship you establish with your child in feeding can affect his food acceptance, nutritional status, growth and the way he feels about himself and about the world.

The feeding relationship is all the interactions that go into working it out with your child about feeding.[5] Parents come equipped with their ideas and attitudes and feelings about themselves and about their child. Children bring their temperament and genetic makeup[6]. And they work it out between them. Or fail to.

Let me illustrate.

Parental Behavior and Children's Eating

Kathy and her little boy were having a difficult time with feeding. He wasn't growing very well, and she had been told by the doctor that she "had to get him to eat more." And she tried. She figured out what he generally ate and presented it to him in the ways he liked it. And sometimes he ate and sometimes he wouldn't. He was getting rather naughty at mealtimes, and she was getting angry with him and more and more desperate about his eating.

We talked some along the lines I used in the "Toddler" chapter, about how she needed to be in charge of food selection, but that she should keep the pressure off him with eating. I suggested she simply present the food to him and let him pick and choose.

That got her started thinking. As she put it, she said to herself, "I wonder what's going on here." So she observed, and thought about it and tried to figure it out. And she noticed that she *was* offering him a variety of foods from the family meal, but she was offering them *one at a time.* And he was playing the toddler's favorite game: he was saying "No" and watching her try something different. With a lovely game like that, what child would want to stop it by eating the first thing he was offered?

So *she* stopped playing. And it helped. But it also didn't help. Their meals are now more tranquil and he is developing more of an interest in his food. But he is still growing slowly and she is still worried about it, although she tries not to let him know it.

Kathy and her husband have probably done all they can at this point. They have given their son a more complete physical examination to find out if anything is the matter with him. Nothing appears to be, so they are going to have to do the most difficult thing of all—wait and see how it all turns out.

Kathy was able to change her feeding situation because she was flexible and had some energy to devote to it. Claire's parents were a different matter. Their physician encouraged them to see a dietitian because their eighteen-month-old daughter was falling off her growth curve. They were having such pitched battles with her about eating that they were "afraid the neighbors would think we were beating her." The father would hold her head and force a spoonful of food between her lips, and she would scream. They could not explain why, although she ate virtually nothing at home, she reportedly ate "very well" at the day care center.

The dietitian advised the parents to stop pressuring her about her eating, to simply present the food to her, give her some help getting started, then leave her alone to do her own eating.

The dietitian told me about it, and I called them back a few weeks later. The mother said that the advice had been helpful. She had stopped forcing her daughter, and although "Claire's eating is still the pits, I don't worry about it any more."

On the other hand, while the mother had stopped pressuring her daughter, the father was still at it. He kept a bowl of food in the living room while they watched TV, and when Claire was distracted he slipped a spoonful of food in her mouth.

I asked the mother why she didn't tell the father to stop, and she said she hadn't thought of it. I wondered afterward if she was really interested in helping her daughter, or was more concerned about allowing herself to stop feeling responsible.

There is a lot to think about in working it out with your child about feeding. Helping you to work it out with your child is the focus of this chapter.

A Division of Responsibility in Feeding

Proper feeding demands a division of responsibility. It is your basic guideline in feeding children.

The parent is responsible for what is presented to eat.
The child is responsible for how much and even whether he eats.

Children will eat—it is normal to eat and grow properly. They have their own built in hunger and appetite and their own regulators that let them know when they need to eat and when they have had enough to eat. (I talked about this in the "Calories and Normal Growth" chapter, and talked about it more in the chapter, "Regulation of Food Intake.") Parents do not have to *make* children eat. But sometimes it gets to *look* like that, because the parent gets started pushing and the child gets started resisting, like with Claire. And eating gets lost in the struggle.

Children eat best when parents recognize their needs and go along with them. Children have their own unique sense of timing and pacing in the feeding situation; they have their own food preferences and vary in their eating capabilities. You really have to assume that all those characteristics are fine, and simply take it from there. If you behave otherwise and impose your own expectations, you get in the way of eating.

Research gives guidelines for feeding relationships. People have a lot of opinions about what it takes to make a child eat well. Some opinions work, others don't. Fortunately, we have more to go on than opinion. There has been quite a bit of good research on effective feeding, and we can use it to guide us.

Mothers vary in their approach to feeding. As part of her interest in infant attachment, Mary Ainsworth observed 26 mothers and their babies in the feeding situation.[1] She noted an enormous range of behaviors.

Seven mothers were very sensitive to their babies' signals and skillful about their feeding. They presented the food so the baby could take it easily, and they enjoyed each other in the feeding situation.

Three mothers were eager to get their babies on a schedule. To achieve that, they ignored their hunger and staved them off so long that they became over-hungry and upset. As a consequence, the feedings were tense and unhappy.

Four were impatient. They said they were feeding on demand, but they seemed so eager to be finished caring for their babies that they put them down whenever they paused or smiled or fussed during the feeding. Perhaps because the mothers wanted to get the feedings over in a hurry, the nipple holes were too big so the babies choked and gagged and paused in the feeding. When they paused, the mothers assumed they were full and terminated the feedings.

Five of the the mothers overfed their babies, some to gratify them and some to fill them up so they would sleep a long time. In the latter case, the babies spit out the nipple, struggled and tried to avert their heads. But the mothers were determined to get the food in, and they did. Needless to say, the feedings were also tense and anxious.

In five of the cases, the feeding was absolutely arbitrary in timing, pacing or both. In each case, the mother was having personal problems such as depression or anxiety that made her detached and insensitive to the baby's signals. These mothers put their babies away for long periods and either tuned out the crying or failed to perceive it as a sign of hunger.

Feeding times were erratic, as were feeding styles. Sometimes the mothers forced their babies to eat long past the point where they indicated they were full, and sometimes they interpreted any pause as satiety and stopped feeding. Feeding was at their own whim, and showed little reflection of the baby's wishes. Ainsworth commented in one case that a mother's determined stuffing of her baby "had to be seen to be believed."

Although she did not measure how much the babies ate, Ainsworth did note that the overfed babies were heavier, and the babies who were fed erratically and terminated too soon were underweight.

Feeding tactics can make a child fail to thrive. A nutritionist in Texas, Ernesto Pollitt, wondered specifically if mothers' behaviors could produce underfed children. He was working with Puerto Rican children who were not growing very well. In fact they were growing so poorly that they were classified as "failure to thrive," a diagnostic term that refers to serious growth failure. Pollitt compared their mothers' feeding techniques with techniques of mothers of babies who were growing well, and observed that the mothers of the poorly-growing babies were very active during feeding. They did a lot of nipple-moving and wiping and arranging of their babies and generally disrupted the pace of the feedings.

Children's characteristics affect feeding. A researcher in England, Peter Wright[7], wondered if there were characteristics of the baby that encourage their mothers to be overactive in feeding them. Wright compared the mothers of low birth weight babies with those of normal weight babies and further subdivided the groups into bottle-fed and breast-fed babies. He found that the bottle feeding mothers were more active with low birth weight babies. And the more active they were, the less the babies ate. Mothers would ignore their babies' responses and screw the nipple into the baby's mouth whether or not he was turning toward the nipple or rooting for it.

The moderately-active bottle feeding mothers in both low and normal weight groups had babies who grew better. On the other hand, all breast-fed babies grew about the same, whether they were low or normal weight. Even the babies' smallness didn't (or couldn't) encourage overactive breastfeeding. One of the advantages of breastfeeding is that you *can't* be over managing. You have to share the responsibility for feeding whether you want to or not.

In short, Wright found that parents' concern about their child's nutrition and growth often showed up as pressure tactics in feeding. Tiffany Field[3], a specialist in developmental disabilities, observed the same thing, both with parents of premature babies and with those who were post mature (born considerably after their due date). She observed that after babies were designated as being "at nutritional risk" pressure tactics in feeding began to emerge. Parents (and health workers) did more jiggling of the bottle and pulling the nipple in and out and jostling the babies.

We can understand why they did that—when someone seems to need help it is natural to try to help. But, ironically, the "helping" tactics backfired—the children ate less, rather than more, when feeders got pushy.

How it feels to the child. It is clear from the previous discussion that good nutrition and appropriate food regulation depend on the establishment of a positive feeding relationship between parent and child. The impact of this relationship becomes more clear if we imagine what it must be like for a child who is, after all, essentially a captive audience in the feeding situation. He is absolutely in his adults' power to satisfy his needs.

Hunger is a very powerful and potentially painful drive. Whether a child learns to fear or accomodate hunger depends on his early experience with feeding. If he cries to be fed and someone shows up promptly and feeds with some sensitivity to his abilities and preferences, he associates hunger with pleasure and it makes him look forward to what happens next. But if his caretakers are slow or inconsistent about responding to his hunger cries, or forceful and insensitive about feeding, it can make him feel anxious and desperate when he gets hungry.

There are lots of feeding experiences that can frighten a child. He might have to wait a long time to eat when he is hungry—so long, in fact, that he might wonder (on whatever primitive level babies and young children wonder at) if he will *ever* get fed. He might get started eating and then have to put up with a lot of interruptions. That could be frightening again, especially if his feeder is in the habit of stopping the feeding before he really gets satisfied. He might have food forced on him when he really doesn't want it. If you have ever had to eat when you really weren't hungry, or experienced the nauseated, too-full feeling that comes from having overdone it, you know that is not a pleasant experience. Someone commented that it "feels like the food grows in your mouth."

Children need help in recognizing and sorting out what they are feeling. A sensitive caretaker can help a child differentiate hunger from loneliness from wet pants. But if a parent is insensitive and repeatedly overlooks messages coming from the child or, worse, simply ignores or overrules those cues, the child doesn't become aware of what he is feeling. He never learns to express his wishes or feels the dignity of having his needs accepted and acted on by another person.

Eventually, the child loses track of what he is feeling and simply goes along with what his grownup expects of him. He still has the feelings, but he has trouble interpreting them, or, eventually, learns to ignore them. When he gets older, he likely will be embarrassed about a hunger or desire for food that is in conflict with what his mother or father seems to think is appropriate.

A few examples of feeding relationships. Most people successfully work out the feeding relationship with their children. The relationships or solutions might not be the ones I describe in this book, but they work. A few negative experiences won't ruin feeding forever. Things can go badly for a while, and people can still work it out.

Problems with communication. A colleague told about learning with his infant son, Jerrod, to use the bottle for feedings after the boy had been breastfed for the first five months. Their problem was that in the feeding process Jerrod would suck all the air out of the bottle and the nipple would collapse. Then the father would pull the nipple out of Jerrod's mouth to let more air into the bottle, intending to resume the feeding.

But Jerrod didn't know that. To him, having the nipple removed from his mouth meant the feeding was over. And *he* was still *hungry.* So he fussed angrily whenever they paused.

Eventually Jerrod learned that the feeding would continue after the interruption. He began voluntarily letting go of the nipple, waiting a few moments (while the air bubbled back into the bottle), and then going back to feeding. They worked it out, but it took some real patience and sensitivity on the father's part.

Sometimes you have to look farther afield to find the source of a feeding difficulty. This same colleague told another feeding story about his older son, Eric. Eric, too, was breast and bottle fed. He took to the bottle quite well, but started fussing at the breast. In fact, he seemed quite angry when his mother tried to feed him, and fussed and fumed for about 20 minutes before he settled down to nurse well.

The mother was concerned enough about it to call the nurse practitioner, who did a very careful and creative job of problem solving. It turned out that when the father was feeding his son, instead of cuddling him in the crook of his arm he was stretching him out in front of him on his lap. Eric preferred that, and he was putting up a fuss to let his mother know that he wanted her to change, too. Obviously, she couldn't, so my colleague had to change. He had to feed Eric cuddled close to him. And Eric didn't like it one bit. He cried and fussed and objected for an hour that first bottle feeding before he finally settled down to eating. After that, he protested less and less and, finally, the problem was solved.

Overmanaging feeding. The research we talked about earlier demonstrated that some children do not grow very well because their caretakers don't pay enough attention to them. Sometimes that inattentiveness comes in the form of the *wrong kind* of attention. Brian's mother said she had to force in every mouthful her son ate or he wouldn't eat at all. At age three, he took an hour and lots of pressure from his mother to eat a simple meal. And he was falling off his growth curve.

Brian had been born at the 50th percentile, where he stayed for the first fourteen weeks while he was breast fed. Once solids feeding was initiated he didn't grow as fast, and his growth fell to the 10th percentile by age 18 months. Then he started to grow faster again, and returned to the 50th percentile by 26 months. But, once again, over the next ten months his growth fell, and when I saw him at 34 months it was below the fifth percentile.

The circumstantial evidence was pretty strong that the problem was Brian's mother's overbearing behavior. During the time when he was growing better, she had been ill and unable to keep her usual tight control on him. But when she got better, she went back to putting a lot of pressure on his eating. And he fell off the growth curve again.

A parent's insensitivity to a child's cues can clearly take the form of being overbearing. But not all children fight back the way Brian did. Some are docile and allow their parents to overstuff them deliberately. I was astounded to watch one example in an airport.

I heard a timer going off near me, and located the source as a woman holding a baby who looked to be about five months old. She stopped her timer, and took from her bag a jar of baby food and one of those horrid little syringe-action feeders. She loaded the syringe, and from that, loaded the baby. No other word describes it. She simply saw to it that he consumed what she wanted him to consume. When the food was gone, she returned the apparatus to her bag (I hope she at least washed it the next time she got near water) and reset her timer.

The baby was just like a little slug. He was absolutely placid and totally uninterested in what went on around him. My imagination may have been too fertile, but it seemed to me he felt very hopeless.

Withholding food from a "fat" child. If you feed (or try to feed) a child less or more than he really wants, it can produce the opposite of what you want. Children who are overfed become revolted by food and prone to undereat when they get a chance. They also become skillful at manipulating their parents to do what they want them to do by refusing to eat.

On the other hand, children who are underfed become preoccupied by food and prone to overeat when they get the chance. Recently I worked with a two year old boy, Todd, whose parents were very concerned with his "overeating." As they told it, Todd wanted second helpings even when he had eaten quite a lot. He was "always" asking for food. When they put out a plate of cheese and crackers for their company, Todd was right there, eating steadily as long as the supplies held out.

His weight fluctuated modestly, and MAY have been increasing disproportionately to his percentile curve. But to his parents, his weight pattern was beside the point. They saw his EATING as being abnormal, and that is where their major concern lay.

Mother was bulimic. She was thin, but very concerned about her weight and always putting pressure on herself to lose. She starved herself and then binged and then vomited, sometimes two or three times daily. She had absolutely no faith in her ability to automatically regulate her food intake, and was always curbing and restricting herself. Or attempting to. And she treated Todd the same way.

As I explained to the parents, the more they tried to restrict Todd's eating the more pressure he put on eating. He felt like he had to put up a struggle to get food.

To help Todd, his parents had to get the pressure off him. To do that, I treated the mother's eating to help her relax and trust her own food regulation processes. I also worked with both parents in understanding Todd's ability to regulate his own food intake and setting reasonable limits for him. It helped—Todd stopped being so demanding about food, and the last I saw them they had had company and Todd ate a couple of crackers and went off to play.

Emotional deprivation and food regulation. Sometimes children overeat because their parents are so preoccupied with their own problems that they can't provide for their childrens' emotional needs. The children try to provide for themselves instead with food and they get fat. That seemed to be what was happening with Ben. He had gained 23 pounds between his third and fourth birthday, during a time when he should have gained about seven pounds.

Ben's parents were doing what they shouldn't and failing to do what they should. Ben was very picky about what he ate and Mother short-order cooked for him. He had unlimited access to the refrigerator and made use of it a lot. But even those factors shouldn't have made him gain like that. He had been running the show with eating since he was about 18 months old, and he hadn't gained too much weight before.

In the last year Ben's family had been under a lot of pressure. They had adopted another child and they were planning a move they weren't happy about. It appeared that Ben was feeling anxious, and his anxiety was coming out in the form of extra eating. And his parents weren't good at putting limits on him. His mother said she didn't want to tell him no because she was afraid he wouldn't like her. And his father simply expected that Ben would know how to behave, and if he acted out the father would get very cold and not talk to him.

Ben was looking for limits, and no one was giving them. His eating behavior became more and more unacceptable until finally his parents took some action. Why he acted out in the area of eating I do not know. Another child might have become really naughty or wet his bed. Ben may have known that his mother couldn't take much defiance, and this was a quiet kind of defiance that she could handle.

I worked with them in setting some moderate and reasonable limits similar to those I described in the "Toddler" chapter. It seemed to be helping some, but the mother was so insecure and the father was so withdrawn that I really wonder how much they were able to do on their own. When they moved away, I suggested counseling for them, and hope they got it.

Recommendations for parents. By now, you have undoubtedly developed a bad case of medical student's hypochondria. No doubt you recognize every mistake you have ever made and have decided that you are doing a rotten job with feeding. You've undoubtedly made some mistakes; that doesn't mean you have failed as a parent. But if you are having the same struggle over and over again and can't seem to resolve it, you had better get some help. Neither you or your child is enjoying the relationship if you are struggling all the time.

Find an early childhood expert—a family counselor—and find out what makes it hard for you to be positive and sensitive with your baby. You might be worn out or overstressed or feel overly insecure. You might be getting pressure from others. You might have a difficult baby and could use some tips on being successful with him. Or all of the above. But don't assume that just because you have some struggles at times that you are doing everything all wrong.

We have all made our errors in feeding. At times we have filled a baby "too full," or have been distracted or in a hurry and not really let our baby eat until he had enough. But babies, and parents, can make up for their errors in feeding. A child who gets too full at a feeding will simply not eat as much the next time, or will wait longer before he gets hungry the next time. A baby who is underfed will get hungry sooner.

The reason the children we talked about earlier showed the effects of errors is that they were repeated, time after time. The caretakers were so inattentive to their children's needs that they just kept doing the same things over and over again. And when that happens, child and parent get caught in a downward slide and matters just get worse and worse.

Overfed children become placid and hopeless and eventually give up on having any say about their feeding. Underfed babies become less energetic and demanding. So they get less to eat the next time. In some really severe cases babies demand so little and eat so little they can't survive.

Practical Approaches to Children's Eating

In previous chapters, we have talked about practical approaches to feeding infants and toddlers. It is worth summarizing here so you can see how approaches complement and contradict as your child grows up. Some of his needs remain the same; others become different. You have to be able to adapt as he progresses.

Feeding in infancy. The infant's emotional task is to become aware of and trust both self and the world around. To do that, he needs a caretaker who is accepting of him, curious about him, and generally goes along with what he seems to want and need. The parent's task is to look for and accept information coming from him. Generally, you try to figure out the small infant, find out what he wants, what works with him, and how to make him comfortable.

Your most important tools are patience, perserverance, and a willingness to develop ways that work. To help you in your quest for effective methods, here are some nipple feeding skills that we can summarize from our earlier discussion.

Nipple feeding. During early infancy, your baby's only feeding skills are his instinctive ability to root for the nipple, to suckle and to swallow. He can't sit up and can only be held supported. It makes the greatest kind of sense with a child this age to cuddle him and feed him by nipple.

In both "The Milk Feeding" and "Breastfeeding How-to" we went into nipple feeding in some detail. Figure 12-1, Nipple Feeding Skills, summarizes effective approaches.

Figure 12-1. Nipple Feeding Skills

- Hold the baby securely but not restrictively. He needs a little room for wiggling and moving around, but not so much that he feels like he might fall.
- Hold the bottle still at an appropriate angle. Don't jiggle it. This is a place where breastfeeding has the advantage. Did you ever try to jiggle a breast? Well, you know what I mean.
- Stimulate his rooting reflex by touching his cheek. He'll turn, mouth open, toward the touch. If he's not hungry, he won't show a rooting reflex.
- Allow time and patience for learning. It takes some children, such as the premature child, a long time to really get good at sucking from a nipple. Take time to enjoy the accomplishment once you do it: don't rush right in to spoon feeding.
- Feed according to his times, or GENTLY work toward a routine. Regularity of behavior (or lack of it) is a temperamental thing[6]. If your baby is born irregular, only time will change him.

- Let him determine how much he wants to eat. It will vary from time to time and day to day. Don't withhold food or force more than he wants.
- Let him decide how fast he will eat. Get the nipple to flow at the right speed so he can handle it. You might have to hand express some breast milk if it is flowing too fast or change the nipple size in a rubber nipple.
- Talk to him in a quiet and encouraging manner while he eats, but don't overwhelm him with attention.
- Let him pause in the feeding. Give him enough time to go back to eating if he wants to.
- If he stops to fuss, soothe him and again offer the nipple. Don't force more food—you are just checking to see if he has had enough.
- Keep the feeding smooth and continuous. Avoid disrupting it with wiping, unnecessary burping, checking the amounts and arranging clothing and blankets.

Spoon feeding. Spoon feeding demands of parents much the same skills and sensitivity as nipple feeding did. Keep in mind that there is a LOT to learn in eating from the spoon. A baby has to figure out how to get the food off the spoon and into his mouth. He has to move his tongue in a different way than he does with nipple drinking, or the mush will just come right out on his chin. He has to get the food to move back in his mouth and, finally, down his throat. And to begin with, he isn't used to the feeling of the hard spoon in his mouth, and he doesn't even know that that soft stuff IS food. Very puzzling.

To help your baby learn, you need to be patient and reassuring. You need to give him the feeling that he is in control, that you are not simply going to impose something on him without his having any say in the matter.

To allow him to retain control, wait until he is developmentally ready. He should be able to sit up, open his mouth (or close it) when he sees something coming and direct his hands where he wants them to go. Sitting puts him in position to look at the food and reach out and touch it. He will be able to turn his head toward and away from the spoon, to participate in the feeding and to let you know what he wants.

Again, your instincts are the important guide to what works and what doesn't. Figure 12-2, Spoon Feeding Skills, offers some suggestions about your approach.

Figure 12-2. Spoon Feeding Skills

- Hold your baby on your lap to introduce solids. He'll be braver.
- Support him well in an upright position so he can explore his food.
- Have him sit up straight and face forward. He'll be able to swallow better and be less likely to choke.
- Wait for him to pay attention to each spoonful before you try to feed it to him.
- Let him touch his food—in the dish, on the spoon. You wouldn't eat something if you didn't know anything about it, would you?
- Feed at his tempo. Don't try to get him to go faster or slower than he wants to.
- Talk to him in a quiet and encouraging manner while he eats. Don't entertain him or overwhelm him with attention, but do keep him company.
- Allow him to feed himself with his fingers as soon as he shows an interest.
- Stop feeding when he indicates he has had enough.

You have to accept it when your child indicates he has had enough. If you try to force beyond that point you probably won't get anywhere and you may turn him off on eating. He'll show you he is full by turning his head away from the spoon, by refusing to open up for the spoon or by spitting the food back out again. Show him you trust him by stopping feeding at that point.

Feeding the toddler. Feeding the toddler and dealing with the toddler is lots different from working with an infant. The toddler has had a chance to establish trust and self awareness. Now his job is to discover and confirm that he is a person separate from his mother (or person who takes care of him the most). The only way he can do that is to explore and exert himself. He will become oppositional, because by saying "no" to other people he proves he is separate from them.

The healthy toddler is engaging, curious, energetic and recalcitrant. If you treat him like you did when he was an infant, and simply accept and support his desires, you will be failing him utterly. He needs reasonable and firm limits in order to feel secure. You don't have to make up the limits. The toddler is generally an aggressive little explorer who needs a lot of room to find out about the world. But he will go too far and he will get on your nerves and he will violate your civil rights and endanger himself and property. You will recognize it when you see it.

To help you distinguish reasonable limits from harsh intrusions, it helps to elaborate on the division of responsibility we talked about earlier. Figure 12-3, Control of Feeding in the Toddler, separates responsibilities in feeding.

Keep in mind that you are responsible for what your child is offered to eat, he is responsible for how much. In the toddler period, you add on the responsibilities of timing and location. You no longer feed the toddler on demand—you ask him to come to the table with the rest of the family. And you time his snacks so he can last until mealtime. You also have to decide if you want eating done at the table or will allow eating elsewhere.

It is important to be concerned enough about a child's eating that you plan, cook and present meals and snacks in a positive way. It

Figure 12-3. Control of Feeding in the Toddler

The parent is responsible for
- Selecting and buying food
- Making and presenting meals
- Regulating timing of meals and snacks
- Presenting food in a form a child can handle
- Allowing eating methods a child can master
- Making family mealtimes pleasant
- Helping the child to participate in family meals
- Helping the child to attend to his eating
- Maintaining standards of behavior at the table

The parent is NOT responsible for
- How much a child eats
- Whether he eats
- How his body turns out

is equally important not to get *so* concerned that you take responsibility for getting food IN to your child. Getting meals on the table regularly is difficult enough without devoting yourself to getting people to eat them.

Unacceptable mealtime behaviors include crying and whining, making a big fuss about eating generally or about particular foods, making a *provocative* mess (there will be a mess, but this kind is where the child seems to be trying to get your goat), and running back and forth from the table when parents are still eating. If your child's behavior is interfering with YOUR mealtime enjoyment, it is probably unacceptable and he should be allowed to get down. Most times, parents put up with misbehavior because they hope their child will eat a few more bites. Let him down when he loses interest in eating. There will be another snack or another meal, and he can eat then.

Hungry children are very businesslike about their eating. It's when they start to get full that they become distractible and the other behaviors start to show up.

Beyond the toddler period. Individuating was the toddler's task. Integrating is the preschooler's task. By the preschool period, a child knows who he is, he is just getting better. After the toddler period, the preschool period is EASY.

The preschooler's eating skills continue to develop and improve. He gets better at chewing and swallowing. He gets neater and more consistent at using utensils to eat and at drinking from a cup without spilling. He takes pride in his eating abilities and likes eating with the rest of the family.

Remember that. Almost everyone knows that children like to gain skills and feel pride in mastering their world. But when it comes to eating, grownups forget that important fact. For some reason we regard eating as different, and that unless we make it happen, the child will never really grow up with his eating. It's not true. At least, not to start with. You can make it true by putting a lot of pressure on eating, but without pressure it really isn't so.

Children can recognize pressure on feeding even in its most cleverly disguised forms. A child development researcher in Illinois rewarded one group of preschoolers for trying new food[2]. Another group of preschoolers was simply introduced to the foods with no kind of expectation about their eating. A few days later, they again presented the new food to the two groups of children. The rewarded preschoolers were *less* likely to go back to the new food than the ones who had been allowed to approach the food in their own way. It appears that children recognize even the most positive enticement as pressure and react negatively to it.

As children grow, their eating grows. For a couple of years now, my children have all pretty consistently been using utensils when they eat. The youngest is 13. My teenaged children accept a wider variety of foods now than they did when they were smaller, and they continue to experiment. Just the other night, Lucas, aged 15, looked at a salad I had been making for the last eight years and announced that he was going to try it. I had never noticed that he wasn't eating it. After he tried it, he allowed as how it wasn't so bad. High praise, indeed!

I would recommend that you not get too eager about having your children grow up with eating. You will have a long wait.

The feeding relationship changes as children grow up. They are always able to take the initiative with feeding, and the wise and sensitive parent supports them. But as a child progresses from infancy through preschool, school age, adolescence and the teen years and finally, (sob, hooray) leaves home, he develops more and more autonomy with his eating.

At some point you have to trust your child to make all his own eating decisions, but you will still exert an influence, for good or ill. Your child will carry with him your habits, attitudes and expectations about eating.

Selected References

1. Ainsworth, M. D. S. and S. M. Bell. Some contemporary patterns of mother-infant interaction in the feeding situation. IN Ambrose, Anthony: Stimulation in Early Infancy. New York: Academic Press, 1969.
2. Birch, L. L., D. W. Marlin and J. Rotter. Eating as the "means" activity in a contingency: effects on young children's food preference. Child Development 55(2):431–439. 1984.

3. Field, T.: Maternal stimulation during infant feeding. Developmental Psychology 13:539–540, 1977.
4. Pollitt, E. and S. Wirtz. Mother-infant feeding interaction and weight gain in the first month of life. Journal of the American Dietetic Association 78:596–601, 1981.
5. Satter, E. M.: The feeding relationship. Journal of the American Dietetic Association 86: 35–6, 1986.
6. Thomas, A. and S. Chess. Genesis and evolution of behavioral disorders: from infancy to early adult life. The American Journal of Psychiatry, 141:1–9, 1984.
7. Wright, P., J. Fawcett, and R. Crow. The development of differences in the feeding behavior of bottle and breast fed human infants from birth to two months. Behavioural Processes 5:1–20, 1980.

13
Eating Disorders

To have an eating disorder, you need two main ingredients: A disruption in eating and a significant emotional problem. Generally when we think about eating disorders, we think about anorexia nervosa and bulimia and the adolescent or adult. While these difficulties don't appear in small children, other eating problems severe enough to be called eating disorders can exist. In early childhood, an eating disorder might take the form of poor growth or excessive weight gain, severe finickiness or major battles with parents about eating.

Particularly with the young child, an eating disorder is not the child's alone—it is a disorder in the way the whole family operates. In the eating-disordered family, parents are having emotional problems that they can't explain or have great difficulty resolving. They might unconsciously distract themselves from these problems by becoming too preoccupied with their child. Or they might be so preoccupied with their own problems that they can't provide emotionally for their child, and she shows her distress with changes in her eating.

The best way to avoid eating disorders is to have a well-functioning family. If there are signs of prolonged and serious problems with eating, get an evaluation by a therapist who works with children and families. Distortions in eating can be an early warning sign of distortions in family functioning. Early correction can make a big difference in the way your family operates.

A few years ago a 16-year-old girl, we'll call her Cindy, came to my office wanting help with a weight reduction diet. She thought she was too fat and wanted to do something about it. Cindy was 5 foot, 6 inches tall and weighed 150 pounds. She had a broad, strong body, and had trouble finding clothes that fit and looked nice on her. She was an excellent basketball player, trained a lot, and was so lean that she wasn't even having her periods. She wasn't too fat, but she was very unhappy about her blocky body and had been dieting to change it.

Cindy had gone to one of the commercial weight loss organizations, paid her $500.00, and they had put her on a 800-calorie diet. She went in to be weighed every day and stuck to her eating plan religiously, but she didn't lose any weight. So the counselors in the program advised her to cut her calories down to 500 per day.

Cindy tried to do it, but at that point her will power started to slip. She no longer could stick to the diet and she began cheating—a little candy here, an extra piece of bread there. Then she began cheating a *lot.*

She went on eating binges, then suffered agonies of remorse, subsequently redoubling her efforts and then giving in again to the temptation to overeat. Almost all her thinking time was devoted to her eating and weight problem. She became preoccupied with her eating and weight and felt upset and bad about it almost all the time.

She underate at meals and nibbled at food before and afterwards. She became depressed and didn't have much energy for her friends or sports. She was crabby around home, and that didn't help her feelings about herself.

Not only was Cindy having trouble losing weight, but she also began to worry that she had an eating disorder. Just before coming to see me she had read an article in the student newspaper written by one of her classmates who was anorexic. The article described her exact symptoms—preoccupation with food and weight, lack of energy, irritability, erratic eating habits, anxiety about her physical appearance, negative feelings about herself.

Cindy *was* having some major difficulty with her eating, but she didn't have an eating disorder. She certainly wasn't anorexic: Her weight wasn't low enough. To be anorexic she would have to have lost a significant proportion of her body weight[1]. Despite all her dieting struggles, she hadn't lost anything. She didn't even qualify to be a bulimic. (That's the disorder where people starve, then binge, then purge in some way, by vomiting, starving, overexercising or abusing laxatives.)

She *was* doing that, but definitions of both anorexia nervosa and bulimia *go on to say* that the person has to have some significant emotional difficulty that is perpetuating the problem. Aside from her eating, Cindy didn't seem too upset about anything. It seemed to me that her behavior and her preoccupation with the process came more from her severe dieting than from anything else. Dieting is a form of starvation, and people who starve show exactly the symptoms that Cindy complained of.

Reactions to food deprivation. During World War II, Ancel Keys, a nutritionist from Minnesota, did a starvation experiment with 36 young men who volunteered for the study as an alternative to military service[3]. His intent was to duplicate concentration camp conditions so people who had been incarcerated during the war could be understood and cared for. During the first three months, the men ate normally while their behaviors, personalities and eating patterns were studied in detail. Then for the next six months, they were restricted to approximately half their former food. This was followed by three months of rehabilitation, during which the men were gradually refed.

During the starvation phase they lost 25% of their body weight, and eventually got to the point where their weights stabilized on the low calorie level. And they developed all the symptoms Cindy was complaining about. They thought about food a great deal, and when they did get a chance to eat, their table manners were eccentric. They hoarded food and lost interest in other activities. Because they were getting along on less calories they had a difficult time staying warm.

For the most part, the subjects became tired, depressed and hard to get along with. But their emotional responses to starvation varied widely. Some appeared to tolerate it fairly well, while others displayed severe disturbance following weight loss. They became confused and irrational, and one even had to have a psychiatric hospitalization.

At times some would lose control of their food intake and overeat, often enormously. When they did that, they were critical and disgusted with themselves.

When they went off the study and had access to food, for a time they ate a great deal. At a given feeding they would eat long past the apparent point of satiety, seemingly stuffing themselves in their attempts to get filled up. And they gained weight back to, or near to, their previous levels. But they were fatter than before: They had lost proportionately more lean tissue during their starvation and then had regained more fat.

While many of Cindy's symptoms made her look like she had an eating disorder, those symptoms may have also been coming from her severe food restriction. Keys' subjects were not eating disordered: They very easily gave up their starvation and went back to eating. People with eating disorders cling to their distorted relationship with food as if they need it.

So that became the central question in distinguishing whether Cindy had an eating disorder: How willing and able was she to give up that distortion and go back to normal eating?

I wasn't *sure* whether Cindy had an eating disorder until after we treated her eating. She was able very readily to get herself weaned off the dieting and back to eating normally again. And once her eating changed, her symptoms went away.

The deprive-overeat cycle. Cindy's cyclical eating demonstrated what Keys and his young men demonstrated: The body will defend itself against starvation. If you over-deprive yourself, you will, sooner or later, react by overeating. Because Cindy had access to food and was being deterred from eating only by her will power, her eating took on a cyclical pattern that is very typical both of the dieter and of the person suffering from an eating disorder. Table 13-1, Binge-Purge Pattern, illustrates that circular pattern.

Like Cindy, most people who come in for help see their problem as overeating, and want help controlling their chaotic eating behavior. They are surprised when I tell them the real problem is their dieting and depriving, *not* their overindulging.

They deprive themselves of food, and the symptoms accumulate. Actually, those symptoms are no more or less than the body's defenses against starvation that we talked about earlier. The symptoms increase the pressure to seek food and to eat and help insure survival. For a while dieters can stand the pain, but finally they give in to food. Since they don't give themselves any deliberate permission to eat, they figure they have blown it, so they might as well go ahead and eat a lot. And they do. They eat until they are really full.

It's interesting that often the "seasoned" dieter doesn't even actually have to GO on a diet to set off this reactive overeating. Just

Figure 13-1. Binge-Purge Pattern

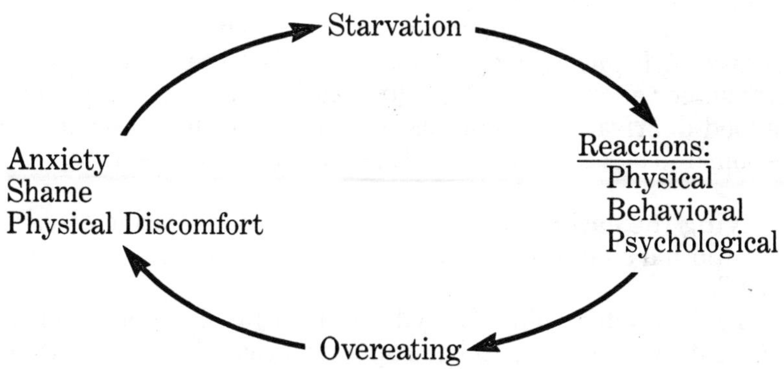

thinking about it will do it. They remind themselves that they "shouldn't" be eating something, or look at the new fashions and remind themselves to lose some weight, and off they go on an eating binge. They have gotten so sensitive to the negative feelings associated with dieting that they run away before they ever get there.

So they binge, and at first, often only momentarily, it feels like a great relief to give in to food. But as the eating progresses to *over*eating, the remorse sets in. They feel overstuffed, uncomfortable and disgusted with themselves. They are ashamed of their lack of control and anxious about not being able to manage their eating. So they purge in some way. And then they starve and start the cycle all over again.

Tolerating the reactions to starvation and holding out against hunger takes a lot of energy. That's what the weight loss "experts" are selling: A cheering section to help their clients keep going. The businesses that charge more provide a cheering section every day, along with the extra motivation tnat paying a lot of money provides. The motivation is really only some energy to help overcome all those negative symptoms of starvation.

So what happens when the dieter is tired or depressed or under stress? Right, she goes off her diet. But the reason she goes off is because her energy goes down and she can no longer overcome all those food-deprivation symptoms. It's not so much that she *over*eats in response to stress, but rather that she *stops under*eating.

Identifying the eating disorder. By definition, an eating disorder involves both a significant distortion in eating AND an emotional problem[2].

I said I didn't think Cindy had an eating disorder, and my subsequent experience with her supported that. Her frustration and concern about her eating was causing her considerable pain and was limiting her life. But she was able to give up her dieting. When she did that she became more trusting of her body's ability to regulate, and most of those negative feelings went away.

Cindy had the usual adolescent concerns about friends and boyfriends and school and parents. But she didn't seem to be in a lot of distress about her situation. Things seemed to be going reasonably well with school and friends and, particularly, she and her parents had a pretty good relationship. Things were good at home. I was surprised that her parents were willing to invest so much money in enabling their daughter to lose weight. But when we talked about it they confessed they actually were uncomfortable with the attempt, and they appreciated my helping them call a halt to it.

Cindy's parents seemed to feel that their daughter was just fine the way she was. They recognized that she didn't have a very *stylish* body, but they thought she was really very attractive and they were proud of her athletic ability. Her mother offered to go shopping with her, and she helped Cindy persist in trying on clothes until she found some that looked good on her. (As the dapper young clerk at the clothing store said. "Dressing well is the art of deception.") Cindy and her parents worked out a good solution. Even though they had momentarily gotten caught in our society's mania for thinness, they didn't have much trouble getting out of it.

Contrast Cindy with Mary, the girl with bulimia we talked about in the "Obesity" chapter. Mary's parents had "dieted" her virtually from birth because they thought she had a big appetite and they were afraid she would get too fat. Mary had struggled with her parents and with food all her growing-up years, and by age 19 had become bulimic.

When Mary and I worked on her eating, she couldn't let go of her obsession with her weight and eating. Part of the problem was that she felt so bad about herself, and she thought that if she could be thinner she would feel better. And, miserable as her bingeing and vomiting was, it had some side benefits for her.

As long as she was involved with that she didn't have the time or energy to worry about her other problems. But the real, underlying problems were her feelings about herself and her relationship with her parents. Mary had a low self esteem that reflected her parents' doubts about her. They felt uncomfortable with her weight and wanted her to get thinner. At least part of their concern was that her appearance reflected on them. They couldn't see how much pain it was causing her and how bad she felt about herself.

Mary's parents had their own problems. It was apparent to an outside observer that they weren't getting along very well with each other. But they denied it. Instead of working out their problems with each other so they could be helpful to Mary, they *distracted* themselves with concern about Mary. And she obliged with her eating disorder.

Mary's eating couldn't get any better until she felt better about herself. And she wasn't getting any help from her family. It was truly an eating disorder: Not only was her eating significantly distorted, but she was having considerable emotional difficulty.

My recommendations for her treatment included dietary management to resolve the problematic eating and psychotherapy to deal with social and emotional issues. I recommended family therapy so her parents could figure out what kind of pressure they were putting on Mary and stop it. Mary was willing, but her parents weren't. At her young age, and without their support, she wasn't able to improve very much.

The continuum of eating behavior. Eating behavior exists on a continuum, with normal balanced weight regulation on the one end and anorexia nervosa on the other. Table 13-2, Eating Behavior Continuum, illustrates that.

Normal balanced food regulation depends on internalized signals of hunger, appetite, satiety and awareness of body levels of energy and fatigue. We talked about all this in detail in the chapter, "Regulation of Food Intake."

At the other extreme, anorexia nervosa involves almost exclusively external regulation of food intake based on what the person *thinks* she should be eating, not what she *feels* like eating. In between the extremes are varying degrees of awareness and control of hunger, appetite and satiety.

Methods of regulating body weight also vary along this continuum. At the "normal" end, weight is determined largely by genetics, which influence not only body contours but also calorie need and energy level. At the other extreme, body weight is almost totally regulated externally. That is, the person chooses a particular body weight and struggles to achieve it by dietary manipulation, whether or not that weight is constitutionally appropriate. In some cases, the person imposes external control and ignores feedback from her body to the point of starvation, as in cases of anorexia nervosa.

In between the extremes there is a spectrum of eating behaviors ranging from dieting for cosmetic reasons to obsessive food managment dominated by the fear of obesity. In the category of

Table 13-2. Eating Behavior Continuum

Normal Balanced Weight Regulation	*Normal Voluntary Weight Reduction*	*Midrange Eating Disorders*	*Anorexia Nervosa*
Internal food regulation	Some external eating, weight control	Increasing external eating, weight control	External food regulation
Weight constitutionally determined	External weight regulation		

Decreasing Attention to Body Cues →

"midrange eating disorders" are the bulimics, the sports anorexics I'll talk about later, and a group of people I have come to call the "failed chronic reducers." They are the people who diet and fail at dieting repeatedly, and end up feeling intensely negative about themselves and about the process.

The farther you go along the continuum the harder it is for people to get better. Some people in the midrange category can resolve their difficulties pretty easily. Others feel so much emotional pressure that it is about as difficult for them to get better as it is for the anorexic. Cindy was probably just across the solid line from normal eating. Mary was probably off to the right very close to anorexia nervosa.

Notice that the vertical line between "normal balanced weight regulation" and "normal voluntary weight reduction" is a solid line, whereas the other vertical lines are dashed. The most major change is made in crossing that first line. Once the person crosses that solid line and initiates dieting, she begins to show the symptoms of starvation. As dieting becomes more restrictive, the symptoms become more pronounced. Further changes are subtle and simply involve more and more external control and less and less responsiveness to body cues.

When a person starts dieting, she first begins ignoring and attempting to overcome automatic food regulation processes. She has to substitute a considerably more laborious and willful process. There is a price to pay for that. She can no longer trust her body's ability to regulate. She has to ignore to some extent hunger and appetite. She has to deprive herself, either in quantity or type of food. And when she deprives she becomes preoccupied with food and with herself. Dieting makes people narcissistic.

Sports anorexia. Another eating pattern that can generally be included in the "midrange eating disorder" category is sports anorexia[6].

An increasing number of kids who are out for sports like skating, gymnastics, running and wrestling are being encouraged to lose weight as part of their training. The wrestlers diet to "make weight." (It is seen as an advantage to wrestle in lower weight categories.) In running, gymnastics and skating, correlations are being made between performance and body fatness.

Jo was a skater, doing well but perhaps not really top caliber. She worked very hard at it, and had a lot of support from her parents for her efforts: They were eager for her to excel. Her sister had been very successful at gymnastics, and they thought it had helped her be popular. Jo was having a difficult time making a particular turn, and her coach told her she thought she could do it better if she lost a little weight—maybe five pounds. So she lost her five pounds and things *might* have gone better—it was hard to tell.

So she lost another five pounds. And so on. Before long her weight had dipped into the anorexic range, she had become very preoccupied with eating and weight, she had started to cut off contacts with her friends ("all they want to do is eat"), and her skating had begun to slip.

After about six months of this, Jo's parents became concerned enough to get her into treatment. She recovered quite rapidly. Part of her treatment was working with her coach and her parents to set more realistic goals for her skating. And part of her treatment was to help her feel better about herself in general so her skating wasn't so vital to her self confidence.

She is still skating and is taking pride in her good performances, even when they are not the tops. She is enjoying it more, and enjoying her friends more. Her parents have adjusted some of their attitudes, too. They take pleasure in her accomplishments, but they aren't so determined that she take top honors. And they can see that she doesn't have to earn her way with friends.

Sports anorexia generally can be turned around much more readily than the other types. In many cases, the kids are functioning better in the first place, and the families are more positive and flexible to begin with. Plus, the disorder gets identified more quickly. In any type of eating disorder, the more quickly you can intervene the better off you are.

Eating Disturbances in Early Childhood

Disturbances in family feeding styles and attitudes about eating generally show up long before a full-blown eating disorder develops. One mother of a fourteen-year-old anorexic commented that she ". . . just knew something would go wrong with this girl's eating. From the very first, her eating was strange. I would put as much formula as she should have in the bottle, and she would just *wolf* it down and cry for more. She never seemed to be satisfied with what I gave her." It had never occurred to that mother that she wasn't giving her daughter enough food.

Some eating disturbances in early childhood are great enough to be called eating disorders in their own right, not just forerunners of a later condition[5]. The childhood eating disorder might take the form of failure to thrive, obesity, excessive finickiness, or vehement and prolonged struggles between parents and children about eating.

In the early childhood eating disorder you see a distinctively inappropriate level of parental control, a stubborn resistance to change on the part of all parties, and very intense feelings on all sides. Emotional struggles between the parents are typically so great that parents are unable to provide for childrens' emotional needs.

Let's make some distinctions between eating disordered and non-eating disordered situations using some examples from the "Feeding Relationship" chapter. You may remember Claire, the poorly-growing toddler we talked about on page 408, whose parents force-fed her until she screamed. Claire likely had an eating disorder. (For ease in writing, I'll say the *child* had an eating disorder. But, particularly with a young child, it is very apparent that the eating disorder is not the child's alone—it is a disorder in the way the whole family operates.) I didn't have a chance to test that, because I didn't get to know the parents, nor did I try to get them to change.

Five of the mothers I talked about from Ainsworth's feeding observations (p. 410) probably had eating disorders—the arbitrary mothers. They were so caught up in themselves and unaware of their babies' needs that they actually cared for them based on their own needs or convenience. Sometimes mothers would feed when babies weren't hungry; other times they failed to feed even when they screamed from hunger.

On page 415 we talked about three-year-old Brian, whose mother tried for an hour at each meal to force him to eat (as he fell from the 50th to the 10th weight percentile). On page 416 there was two-year-old Todd, who was being restrained from eating by his bulimic mother. Both of these boys had eating disorders. Parents and children were emotionally over-intense and rigid in their interactions; they were unable to resolve their difficulties on their own.

Ben gained 16 extra pounds in a year during which his parents were having a difficult time. In a short treatment centered around his eating, his parents were able to make some improvements in their dealings with Ben. But I predict relapse unless his mother can get started feeling better about herself and his father can become more warm and available to his family.

In the "Feeding Relationship" chapter I also described some relationships that were not disordered. Kathy and her little boy were not. He gained very poorly, and she just had to let him eat the way he wanted to. (She was providing appropriate food in a supportive manner and she had had him checked out medically.) And neither did my colleague who got into problems attempting to bottle feed his breast-fed sons. All of those situations could have led to horrendous misunderstandings and struggles between parent and child. But they didn't. Both parents were sensitive and flexible enough to work it out with their children.

Avoiding the Eating Disorder

We will hope that the issue of treating an eating disorder does not come up for you. If it does, acknowledge it and get in for help as quickly as you can. All families have problems. Some families, some times, get stuck and can't seem to resolve a problem. The good families are the ones who are honest with themselves about it and get help.

I hope I have made it clear that an eating disorder is not just the problem of the affected child. It is an indication that things are not going well in the family as a whole. A good counselor will understand that, help you figure out what there is about your family that isn't working and help you fix it. You may have to shop around some to find someone who is helpful, but the effort is worth it. It's very difficult to change the way you interact with other people, but if things go well in therapy, you can look forward to functioning better than you ever have before.

Enhancing emotional functioning. From the standpoint of prevention, your best chance of avoiding eating disorders is in having a well-functioning family. Parents must be helpful to each other in seeing that the family works. Fathers in the highly distorted feeding situations that Ainsworth studied should have been able to see what was going on and get help for their wives. Brian's father should have talked with his wife about the way she was handling feeding, rather than just letting her do her thing.

To function well as a couple and as parents, you need to function well as individuals. You need to feel good enough about yourself to be able to pay attention to another person and get a feeling for what it is like to be in that person's place. The mother of the anorexic I talked about earlier was so self preoccupied she couldn't make the most basic observation about her infant daughter.

When you function well as individuals and as a couple, you will have the intuition to interact positively with your child. You will be able to establish the good feeding relationship we have been talking about throughout this book. *You will be able to respect your child and depend on him, appropriately, to take the lead with feeding.*

Avoid intruding on food regulation. Resist in yourself and your child the tendency to diet, especially vehemently. We went into this at length in the *Obesity* chapter, so I will just summarize here. Trust the body's ability to regulate. Any interventions made with regulation should be made moderately and indirectly, such as changing the type or availability of food in the house or the family meal schedule. You should never impose food restriction or food excess on a child, or in any way try to manipulate his growth. Any interventions should be made with the motive of *preventing* overeating or undereating, not *promoting* it.

Eventually your child may get to the point where she wants to diet and lose weight, but you don't have to cave in to the pressure. You can let her know that you are willing to have low-calorie foods available, and that you will plan meals that generally aren't so high in sugar and fat. Don't cook "diet" meals, or you will become enraged at her when she goes out for french fries with her friends.

You can be supportive without giving in to pressure to buy a membership in an expensive weight loss business like Cindy's parents did. And you can be firm about expecting your child to attend most family meals, and steadfast in your faith that good nutritional habits are important for your child. The adolescent makes a lot of his own food choices, but parents should still function in finding out (tactfully) what those choices are, making suggestions, and encouraging her to take good care of her body. Don't preach, just express your concern.

You can get after your dieter when you see her nibbling too much between meals and remind her that she would be better off eating a little more at meal time. And, yes, you can tell her to get out of the refrigerator right before meals. Making meals important and satisfying is one helpful way of preventing being caught up in that deprive-overeat cycle we talked about earlier.

The dieting athlete. Here are some facts to help you withstand the dieting pressure on the athlete in your house.

Optimum body fat percentage for competition is higher for an adolescent than it is for an adult[4]. If your child's coach is setting body fat percentage goals, make sure the goals are appropriate for adolescents. Adolescents may do better at body fat levels 30% to 50% higher than levels established for adults.

There is nothing to be gained by severe dieting. Excessive weight loss, especially the type that is achieved by a crash program right before the competition, impairs rather than enhances performance. Wrestlers who had crash dieted just before a competition suffered in endurance and skill, even when they had gained most of their weight back after the weigh-in[8].

The best tactic is to decrease food intake moderately—say cut 500 to 1000 calories per day off normal intake. Even if she isn't eating much to begin with, no child should eat less than 1200 calories per day. Children need at least 1200 calories to cover their nutritional requirements. They should continue to follow their coaches' instructions about training. (Since gymnastics and figure skating do not expend many calories, it may be necessary for an athlete attempting to keep her weight down to to add on walking, running, biking, or another energy-expending exercise.) And whatever weight level they achieve using these modest methods should be the weight at which they compete.

If a young athlete has to use heroic methods to lose, i.e., severe dieting or exhaustive exercising, it will probably detract from fitness and performance. We are talking about the law of diminishing returns here: If children have to punish their bodies to get their weight or fat percentage down, it is likely they will impair performance. And studies have supported this conclusion[4].

As I pointed out in the "Obesity" chapter, our national attitude about weight is distorted. You will have to keep a level head not to be swept away by it. In eating for sports as well as in establishing good feeding relationships in all areas, you have to feel your way through your situation. If you and your family are functioning well, you will be doing what you can to prevent an eating disorder. A how-to book like this one is (I hope) helpful, but knowing what to do is no substitute for good instincts.

Selected References

1. American Psychiatric Association: Diagnostic and Statistical Manual of Mental Disorders, Third Edition. American Psychiatric

Association, Washington, D.C., 1980.
2. Bruch, H.: Eating Disorders: Obesity, Anorexia Nervosa and the Person Within. New York: Basic Books, 1973.
3. Keys, A. J., Brozek, A., Henschel, O., Michelsen, O., and Taylor, H. S.: The Biology of Human Starvation. Vols. 1, 2. Minneapolis: University of Minnesota Press, 1950.
4. Pipes, Peggy L. Nutrition in Infancy and Childhood. Times Mirror/Mosby. St. Louis, 1985.
5. Satter, E. M.: Childhood eating disorders. Journal of the American Dietetic Association 86: 357–61, 1986.
6. Smith, N. J. Excessive weight loss and food aversion in athletes simulating anorexia nervosa. Pediatrics 66:139–142, 1980.
7. Thomas, A. and Chess, S. Genesis and evolution of behavioral disorders: from infancy to early adult life. The American Journal of Psychiatry, 141:1–9, 1984.
8. Tipton, C. M. Consequences of rapid weight loss. IN Haskell, W., et. al. Nutrition and Athletic Performance. Proceedings of the Conference on Nutritional Determinants in Athletic Performance, San Francisco, CA, September 24–25, 1981. Bull Publishing, Palo Alto, 1982.

Appendix

Table A-1

Food and Nutrition Board, National Academy of Sciences—National Research Council Recommended Daily Dietary Allowances[a] *Revised 1980*
Designed for the maintenance of good nutrition of practically all healthy people in the U.S.A.

							Fat-Soluble Vitamins		
	Age (years)	Weight (kg)	Weight (lb)	Height (cm)	Height (in)	Protein (g)	Vitamin A (μg RE)[b]	Vitamin D (μg)[c]	Vitamin E (mg α-TE)[d]
Infants	0.0–0.5	6	13	60	24	kg × 2.2	420	10	3
	0.5–1.0	9	20	71	28	kg × 2.0	400	10	4
Children	1–3	13	29	90	35	23	400	10	5
	4–6	20	44	112	44	30	500	10	6
	7–10	28	62	132	52	34	700	10	7
Males	11–14	45	99	157	62	45	1000	10	8
	15–18	66	145	176	69	56	1000	10	10
	19–22	70	154	177	70	56	1000	7.5	10
	23–50	70	154	178	70	56	1000	5	10
	51+	70	154	178	70	56	1000	5	10
Females	11–14	46	101	157	62	46	800	10	8
	15–18	55	120	163	64	46	800	10	8
	19–22	55	120	163	64	44	800	7.5	8
	23–50	55	120	163	64	44	800	5	8
	51+	55	120	163	64	44	800	5	8
Pregnant						+30	+200	+5	+2
Lactating						+20	+400	+5	+3

[a]The allowances are intended to provide for individual variations among most normal persons as they live in the United States under usual environmental stresses. Diets should be based on a variety of common foods in order to provide other nutrients for which human requirements have been less well defined. See text for detailed discussion of allowances and of nutrients not tabulated. See Table 1 (p. 20) for

Food and Nutrition Board, National Academy of Sciences—National Research Council Recommended Daily Dietary Allowances[a] *(Continued)*

	Age (years)	Weight (kg)	Weight (lb)	Height (cm)	Height (in)	Water-Soluble Vitamins: Vitamin C (mg)	Thiamine (mg)	Riboflavin (mg)	Niacin (mg NE)[e]	Vitamin B-6 (mg)	Folacin[f] (μg)	Vitamin B-12 (μg)
Infants	0.0–0.5	6	13	60	24	35	0.3	0.4	6	0.3	30	0.5[g]
	0.5–1.0	9	20	71	28	35	0.5	0.6	8	0.6	45	1.5
Children	1–3	13	29	90	35	45	0.7	0.8	9	0.9	100	2.0
	4–6	20	44	112	44	45	0.9	1.0	11	1.3	200	2.5
	7–10	28	62	132	52	45	1.2	1.4	16	1.6	300	3.0
Males	11–14	45	99	157	62	50	1.4	1.6	18	1.8	400	3.0
	15–18	66	145	176	69	60	1.4	1.7	18	2.0	400	3.0
	19–22	70	154	177	70	60	1.5	1.7	19	2.2	400	3.0
	23–50	70	154	178	70	60	1.4	1.6	18	2.2	400	3.0
	51+	70	154	178	70	60	1.2	1.4	16	2.2	400	3.0
Females	11–14	46	101	157	62	50	1.1	1.3	15	1.8	400	3.0
	15–18	55	120	163	64	60	1.1	1.3	14	2.0	400	3.0
	19–22	55	120	163	64	60	1.1	1.3	14	2.0	400	3.0
	23–50	55	120	163	64	60	1.0	1.2	13	2.0	400	3.0
	51+	55	120	163	64	60	1.0	1.2	13	2.0	400	3.0
Pregnant						+20	+0.4	+0.3	+2	+0.6	+400	+1.0
Lactating						+40	+0.5	+0.5	+5	+0.5	+100	+1.0

weights and heights by individual year of age. See Table 3 (p. 23) for suggested average energy intakes.

[b] Retinol eqivalents. 1 retinol equivalent = 1 μg retinol or 6 μg β carotene. See text for calculation of vitamin A activity of diets as retinol equivalents.

[c] As Cholecalciferol. 10 μg cholecalciferol = 400 IU of vitamin D.

[d] α-tocopherol equivalents. 1 mg *d*-α tocopherol = 1 α-TE. See text for variation in allowances and calculation of vitamin E activity of the diet as α-tocopherol equivalents.

[e] 1 NE (niacin equivalent) is equal to 1 mg of niacin or 60 mg of dietary tryptophan.

[f] The folacin allowances refer to dietary sources as determined by *Lactobacillus casei* assay after treatment with enzymes (conjugases) to make polyglutamyl forms of the vitamin available to the test organism.

[g] The recommended dietary allowance for vitamin B-12 in infants is based on average concentration of the vitamin in human milk. The allowances after weaning are based on energy intake (as recommended by the American Academy of Pediatrics) and consideration of other factors, such as intestinal absorption; see text.

Food and Nutrition Board, National Academy of Sciences—National Research Council Recommended Daily Dietary Allowances[a] (Continued)

	Age (years)	Weight (kg)	Weight (lb)	Height (cm)	Height (in)	Minerals: Calcium (mg)	Phosphorus (mg)	Magnesium (mg)	Iron (mg)	Zinc (mg)	Iodine (μg)
Infants	0.0–0.5	6	13	60	24	360	240	50	10	3	40
	0.5–1.0	9	20	71	28	540	360	70	15	5	50
Children	1–3	13	29	90	35	800	800	150	15	10	70
	4–6	20	44	112	44	800	800	200	10	10	90
	7–10	28	62	132	52	800	800	250	10	10	120
Males	11–14	45	99	157	62	1200	1200	350	18	15	150
	15–18	66	145	176	69	1200	1200	400	18	15	150
	19–22	70	154	177	70	800	800	350	10	15	150
	23–50	70	154	178	70	800	800	350	10	15	150
	51+	70	154	178	70	800	800	350	10	15	150
Females	11–14	46	101	157	62	1200	1200	300	18	15	150
	15–18	55	120	163	64	1200	1200	300	18	15	150
	19–22	55	120	163	64	800	800	300	18	15	150
	23–50	55	120	163	64	800	800	300	18	15	150
	51+	55	120	163	64	800	800	300	10	15	150
Pregnant						+400	+400	+150	*h*	+5	+25
Lactating						+400	+400	+150	*h*	+10	+50

[h]The increased requirement during pregnancy cannot be met by the iron content of habitual American diets nor by the existing iron stores of many women; therefore the use of 30–60 mg of supplemental iron is recommended. Iron needs during lactation are not substantially different from those of nonpregnant women, but continued supplementation of the mother for 2–3 months after parturition is advisable in order to replenish stores depleted by pregnancy.

Table A-2

*Table of standard weight for height for women suggested for use by the American College of Obstetricians and Gynecologists (30)**

(Height without shoes, plus 1 inch)

	lbs.
4′-10″ =	104
4′-11″ =	107
5′-0″ =	110
5′-1″ =	113
5′-2″ =	116
5′-3″ =	118
5′-4″ =	123
5′-5″ =	128
5′-6″ =	132
5′-7″ =	136
5′-8″ =	140
5′-9″ =	144
5′-10″ =	148
5′-11″ =	152
6′-0″ =	156

*Weights were taken from Metropolitan Life Insurance Company, Actuarial Tables, 1959, for heights in inches without shoes plus one inch. For patients under age 25, one pound should be deducted for each year.

Table A-3

Nutrient content of human milk and cow's milk

Constituent (per liter)	Human milk	Cow's milk
Energy (kcal)	690	660
Protein (gm)	9	35
Fat (gm)	45	37
Lactose (gm)	68	49
Vitamins		
Vitamin A (IU)	1898	1025
Vitamin D (IU)	22	14
Vitamin E (IU)	2	0.4
Vitamin K (μg)	15	60
Thiamine (μg)	160	440
Riboflavin (μg)	360	1750
Niacin (mg)	1.5	0.9
Pyridoxine (μg)	100	640
Folic acid (μg)	52	55
Cobalamine (μg)	0.3	4
Ascorbic acid (mg)	43	11
Minerals		
Calcium (mg)	297	1170
Phosphorus (mg)	150	920
Sodium (mg)	150	506
Potassium (mg)	550	1368

Nutrient content of human milk and cow's milk (Continued)

Constituent (per liter)	Human milk	Cow's milk
Chlorine (mg)	385	1028
Magnesium (mg)	23	120
Sulfur (mg)	140	300
Iron (mg)	0.56–0.3	0.5
Iodine (mg)	30	47
Manganese (μg)	5.9–4.0	20–40
Copper (μg)	0.6–0.25	0.3
Zinc (mg)	4–.5	3–5
Selenium (μg)	20	5–50
Flouride (mg)	0.05	0.03–0.1

From Pipes, Peggy L.: Nutrition in infancy and childhood, ed. 2, St. Louis, 1981, The C. V. Mosby Co.; adapted from Hambreaus, L.: Proprietary milk versus human breast milk in infant feeding, a critical approach from the nutritional point of view. Pediatr. Clin. North Am. *24:*17, 1977; Siimes, M. A., Vuori, E., and Kuitunen, P.: Breast milk iron—a declining concentration during the course of lactation, Acta Paediatr. Scand. *68:*29, 1979; Vuori, E.: A longitudinal study of manganese in human milk, Acta Paediatr. Scand. *68:*571, 1979, Vuori, E., and Kuitunen, P.: Concentrations of copper and zinc in human milk, Acta Paediatr. Scand. *68:*33, 1978; and nayman, R., and others: Observations on the composition of milk-substitute products for the treatment of inborn errors of amino acid metabolism: comparisons with human milk, Am. J. Clin. Nutr. *32:*1279, 1979.

Table A-4

Nutrient content of commercially available milk-base formulas

Nutrient (per 100 ml)	Amount
Energy (kcal)	67
Protein (gm)	1.5–1.6
Fat (gm)	3.6–3.7
Carbohydrate (gm)	7.0–7.3
Vitamin A (IU)	165–260
Vitamin D (IU)	40–42
Vitamin E (IU)	0.9–1.5
Vitamin C (mg)	5.4–5.7
Thiamine (μg)	52–69
Riboflavin (μg)	57–100
Niacin (mg)	0.6–1.0
Pyridoxine (μg)	40–42
Vitamin B_{12} (μg)	0.1–0.2
Folic acid (μg)	5–10
Calcium (mg)	44–54
Phosphorus (mg)	33–46
Magnesium (mg)	4.1–5.2
Iron (mg)*	Trace–1.3
Zinc (mg)	0.36–0.5
Copper (mg)	.041–.062
Iodine (μg)	6.7–10

*Iron-fortified formulas contain 12 mg of iron/32 oz; others contain only a trace.

From Pipes, Peggy L.: Nutrition in infancy and childhood, ed. 2, St. Louis, 1981, The C. V. Mosby Co.

Table A-5

Nutrient content of soy formulas (soy isolates, vegetable or soy oil, corn syrup solids and/or sucrose)

Nutrient (per 100 ml)	Amount
Energy (kcal)	67
Protein (gm)	1.8–2.5
Fat (gm)	3.4–3.6
Carbohydrate (gm)	6.4–6.8
Vitamin A (IU)	167–250
Vitamin D (IU)	40–42
Vitamin E (IU)	1.0–1.5
Vitamin C (mg)	5.4–7.3
Thiamine (μg)	40–52
Riboflavin (μg)	62–104
Niacin (mg)	0.7–0.9
Pyridoxine (μg)	40–41
Vitamin B_{12} (μg)	0.21–0.30
Folic acid (μg)	5.3–10.4
Calcium (mg)	70–83
Phosphorus (mg)	50–63
Magnesium (mg)	5–7.81
Iron (mg)*	1.0–1.2
Zinc (mg)	0.3–0.5
Copper (mg)	0.04–0.06
Iodine (μg)	1.5–4.7

From Pipes, Peggy L.: Nutrition in infancy and childhood, ed. 2, St. Louis, 1981, The C. V. Mosby Co.

Table A-6

Supplemental fluoride dosage schedule (in mg F/day) according to fluoride concentration of drinking water.*

Age (Years)	Concentration of Fluoride in Water (ppm): Less Than 0.3	0.3 to 0.7	Greater Than 0.7
Birth to 2	0.25	0	0
2 to 3	0.50	0.25	0
3 to 13	1.00	0.50	0

*2.2 mg. sodium fluoride contain 1 mg fluoride.

From Council on Dental Therapeutics. In Accepted Dental Therapeutics, ed. 38 American Dental Association. Chicago, 1979.

A-7 Table of Figures

Index

GENDER
IN CROSS-CULTURAL PERSPECTIVE

second edition

GENDER IN CROSS-CULTURAL PERSPECTIVE

Edited by

Caroline B. Brettell and Carolyn F. Sargent

Southern Methodist University

Dallas, Texas

PRENTICE HALL, UPPER SADDLE RIVER, NEW JERSEY 07458

Library of Congress Cataloging-in-Publication Data

Gender in cross-cultural perspective / edited by Caroline B. Brettell and Carolyn F. Sargent.—2nd ed.
p. cm.
Filmography:
Includes bibliographical references.
ISBN 0-13-533613-9
1. Sex role—Cross-cultural studies. I. Brettell, Caroline. II. Sargent, Carolyn Fishel
GN479.65.G47 1997
305.3—dc20 96-29369
CIP

Editorial Director: Charlyce Jones Owen
Editor in Chief: Nancy Roberts
Associate Editor: Sharon Chambliss
Marketing Manager: Chaunfayta Hightower
Editorial/production supervision
and interior design: Serena Hoffman
Cover design: Bruce Kenselaar
Editorial assistant: Pat Naturale

This book was set in 10/11 Baskerville by Pine Tree Composition, Inc., and was printed and bound by Hamilton Printing Company.
The cover was printed by Phoenix Color Corp.

Printed in the United States of America

10 9 8 7 6 5

ISBN 0-13-533613-9

Prentice-Hall International (UK) Limited, *London*
Prentice-Hall of Australia Pty. Limited, *Sydney*
Prentice-Hall Canada Inc., *Toronto*
Prentice-Hall Hispanoamericana, S.A., *Mexico*
Prentice-Hall of India Private Limited, *New Delhi*
Prentice-Hall of Japan, Inc., *Tokyo*
Simon & Schuster Asia Pte. Ltd., *Singapore*
Editora Prentice-Hall do Brasil, Ltda., *Rio de Janeiro*

CONTENTS

PREFACE

The initial idea for this reader came from the experience of teaching undergraduate courses in gender and anthropology. In reviewing the textbooks available for an introductory course, we came to the conclusion that there was a need for a readable text that built on the classic contributions of the 1970s while also incorporating the more recent and diverse literature on gender roles and ideology around the world. Although a number of sophisticated theoretical works devoted to this subject existed, we felt there was a dearth of classroom material available in one volume and appropriate for less advanced students, whether undergraduates or beginning graduate students.

In selecting materials, we attempted to accomplish five goals. First, we wanted to introduce students to the most significant topics in the field of the anthropology of gender. These include the study of men and women in prehistory; the relationship between biology and culture; the cultural construction of masculinity, femininity, and sexuality; variations in the sexual division of labor and economic organization; women's involvement in ritual and religion; and the impact on gender issues of various forces of change such as colonialism, the rise of the state, and the global economy.

Second, we hoped to provide broad cross-cultural coverage to encourage comparative analysis of the themes under discussion and to encompass studies addressing issues of gender in industrial society as well as in developing societies.

Third, we wanted to complement research on women's lives with some articles that dealt with masculinity and male gender roles. Because feminist theory has only recently been applied to the study of men, a truly balanced reader is not yet possible; however, we tried to incorporate some of the most exciting new research in this domain.

Fourth, we were committed to combining theoretical and ethnographically based articles in each section of the book. We hope that we have compiled a volume that can stand alone or, if the instructor so desires, can be complemented by the use of full ethnographies.

Fifth, we wanted to include introductions to each section that would review as clearly as possible some of the significant issues debated in particular subject areas in the anthropology of gender. These introductions are intended to orient students to the articles in the section and to provide a context in which readers can more fully understand each article. Each introduction concludes with a list of references that can be used by teachers and students to examine further the questions raised in that section.

We do not expect all instructors to assign the sections in the order that they appear in the text. This order makes sense to us, but our ultimate goal is to provide for maximum flexibility in teaching. We also have no intention of imposing a particular theoretical perspective, although our own predilections may be apparent to some readers. We tried to include readings that reflect a variety of theoretical orientations to enable instructors to emphasize their own approach to the subject.

The text concludes with a list of recommended films organized by sections of this book. We have previewed many of these films, and we hope that all of them will successfully complement the readings in the text.

ACKNOWLEDGEMENTS

Many people have contributed substantially to the preparation and development of this book. For the first edition, Andrew Webb provided invaluable clerical and organizational assistance. The undergraduate students in Professor Sargent's Sex Roles course during the fall semester of 1990 and the fall semester of 1995 offered valuable criticisms of selected articles. Their opinions continue to influence us enormously in the final selection process. John Phinney acted as an invaluable library of knowledge for obscure references; Sue Linder-Linsley offered indispensible computer advice and tirelessly scanned in text to save us time in the preparation of the second edition; and Sue Racine and Scott Langley contributed clerical assistance. We also thank the reviewers of the original manuscript, and the professors around the world who have used the first edition and offered valuable suggestions for improvements to the second edition. Finally, we thank Nancy Roberts and Sharon Chambliss of Prentice Hall for their confidence in our judgment and their constant support of this project. We have a wonderful partnership!

Caroline B. Brettell
Carolyn F. Sargent

GENDER
IN CROSS-CULTURAL PERSPECTIVE

I

BIOLOGY, GENDER, AND HUMAN EVOLUTION

What is the role of biology in human behavior? To what extent are differences between men and women explained by biology, by culture, or by an interaction between the two? Is there a biological basis for the sexual division of labor? These questions are hotly debated in the United States as we struggle with such issues as why men dominate the fields of math and science, whether women are equipped for war and combat, and the implications for child development of female participation in the labor force. When issues of gender are considered in a cross-cultural context, we explore whether women are universally subordinated to men and to what extent biological differences explain the allocation of roles and responsibilities between men and women.

The relative importance of biology, or nature, versus culture, or nurture, is an enduring dilemma. This issue was addressed by Margaret Mead several decades ago. Using data drawn from her fieldwork in Samoa and New Guinea, Mead (1928, 1935) set out to establish the significance of culture or environment in molding gender differences. She wanted to offer an alternative to the powerful intellectual principles of biological determinism and eugenics (biological engineering) that dominated academic circles in the 1920s. She also hoped to demonstrate to North American women that a range of possibilities was open to them and that the social roles of housework and childrearing were not their inevitable lot. In her view, anatomy was not destiny.

Mead's work was challenged in the 1980s by Derek Freeman (1983). Freeman accused Mead of cultural determinism (that is, giving priority to culture over biology) and opened a lively debate within academic and nonacademic circles (Rensberger 1983; Scheper-Hughes 1987; Schneider 1983). For some, Freeman's book was taken (erroneously) as new support for the sociobiological approach to an understanding of human behavior, an approach formulated by Edward Wilson (1975) that contends that there is a genetic basis for all social behavior.

Although few people deny the anatomical and hormonal differences between men and women, they disagree about the importance of these differences for gender roles and personality attributes. Recent research, much of it conducted by psychologists, suggests that male and female infants cannot be significantly distinguished by their degree of dependence on parents, their visual and verbal abilities, or their aggression as measured by activity level (Bleier 1984; Fausto-Sterling 1985; Renzetti and Curran 1989). These characteristics tend to emerge later in the development process, indicating the importance of environment.

A current controversy centers on how the brain is organized and to what extent brain lateralization is related to sex differences. One position holds that women are left-brain dominant, giving them superior verbal skills, while men are right-brain dominant, giving them superior visual-spatial skills. While research on variations in the structure and development of male and female brains continues, Renzetti and Curran (1989: 33) contend that to date "there is little evidence indicating that the sexual differentiation of the brain, if it occurs in humans, consequently predisposes males and females to behave in gender-specific ways" (see also Fausto-Sterling 1985: 44–53).

Within anthropology the role of biology in explaining differences between men and women, including social behaviors such as the division of labor and the tendency for women to be subordinated to men, has been explored within an evolutionary framework. Evolutionary theories fall roughly into four categories: male strength hypotheses, male bonding hypotheses, male aggression hypotheses, and women's childbearing hypotheses. Male strength hypotheses argue that men are physically stronger than women and this gives them superiority. They are larger, and they have stronger muscles and less fat, a pelvis better adapted for sprinting, larger hearts and lungs, and so forth. These physical differences between the males and females of a species are referred to as *sexual dimorphism.*

Through comparisons drawn with nonhuman primates, Leibowitz (in this book) explores the origins of sexual dimorphism and, by analogy, sexual asymmetry and the sexual division of labor. Her discussion fits into a large body of literature that uses animals as models for understanding human behavior. She challenges the tendency to link sexual dimorphism to particular sex-role patterns by demonstrating enormous variations among different species of primates. Rather than explaining greater male size and strength solely as an adaptation to the roles of protection and provisioning associated with hunting, Leibowitz urges us to consider as well the reproductive advantage to women of the cessation of growth soon after sexual maturity is reached. In the process, she asks us to reconsider what we mean by strength.

Leibowitz particularly cautions that our stereotypes of human male attributes have been drawn from one species of primate, the plains baboon. As Sperling observed, "This use of the baboon troop as model for ancestral human populations was very influential in forming both sexist and anthropomorphic views of monkeys in popular culture" (1991: 210). Sperling, Fedigan (1986), and Leibowitz have emphasized the inappropriateness of the "baboonization" of early human life, given the distant relationship between humans and baboons. If we are going to draw comparisons with nonhuman primates, it would be preferable to draw analogies with the great apes, particularly the chimpanzees.

A second body of evolutionary theory that explains male domination emphasizes the greater ability of men to form social bonds among themselves (Tiger 1969). This ability is supposedly genetically programmed and associated with the evolutionary adaptation to hunting. Women, conversely, are thought to lack the genetic code for bonding and are therefore unsuited to the kinds of cooperative and political endeavors that give men power and prestige.

Ehrenberg (in this book) explores this bonding issue in its relation to the development of the sexual division of labor among early humans. She suggests that women were often the social center of groups. They fostered sociability and sharing. Ehrenberg also addresses a much wider debate about the relative contributions of men and women to human evolution. She provides an alternative to what has been labeled the "coattails theory" of biological evolution—"Traits are selected for in males and women evolve by clinging to the men's coattails" (Fedigan 1986: 29). The male bias reflected in this approach has been equally evident in analyses of cultural development, especially in the emphasis on hunting, a male activity, as the distinctive human activity (Lee and DeVore 1968). In her reevaluation of a discussion that essentially omitted half of humanity from the story of evolution, Ehrenberg suggests that hunting probably evolved from the physical, technological, and social innovations associated with gathering (a female activity).

A third line of argument attempts to explain male dominance with reference to the biological basis of aggression. Many studies of aggression contend that men are more aggressive than women (Wilson 1975; see Fedigan 1982: 87 for a critique of this position), and often link this difference to levels of male hormones (testosterone). According to Fausto-Sterling (1985: 126), "Many societies, including our own, have tested this belief by castrating men who have a history of violent or antisocial behavior." Scientific research has demonstrated that there is no connection between castration and aggression.

It has also been argued that male aggressive tendencies are an adaptation to the male role in defense (Martin and Voorhies 1975) among both human and nonhuman primates. The problem with any line of argument that links male dominance or male social roles to male aggression is that it ignores the wide variation in behaviors and personalities not only between the sexes, but also within them (Renzetti and Curran 1989: 38). In addition, cross-cultural data indicate that human societies differ in culturally appropriate levels of aggression expressed by men and women (Burbank 1994; Counts, Brown, and Campbell 1992).

Lee's (1979) study of conflict and violence among the !Kung San, a relatively egalitarian and peace-loving people, addresses the issue of aggression among men and women. He lends support to the argument that both men and women are aggressive in different ways. !Kung women engage in verbal abuse, but homicides are disproportionately committed by men. Lee compares trends in !Kung violence to those in several other societies. Although his statistics are from the 1950s and 1960s, more recent research indicates that the patterns remain similar. For example, although the percentage of recorded offenses of "violence against the person" committed by women in England and Wales increased by 58 percent between 1975 and 1985, the increase in such crimes by men was 40 percent; the absolute number of crimes committed by men in 1985 remained much higher than that for women, and the male-to-female ratio for violent crimes was 9:1 (Morris 1987: 35). Similarly, research on criminal activity in the United States indicates that violent offenses by women have increased but are still predominantly committed by men (Morris 1987: 35). A comparison between the !Kung and modern industrial societies suggests that the reasons for gender differences in aggressive behavior are complex. In addition to biological factors, access to weapons, culturally approved expressions of hostility, and the role of the state in the evolution of social control should also be considered.

Among the !Kung the victims of violent crimes tend to be other men, a finding that supports Maccoby and Jacklin's (1974) observation that primate males in general demonstrate more aggression against one another than against females. Dominance of men over women through aggression is thereby brought into question, as is the concept of aggression itself. As Fedigan (1982: 89) suggests, aggression "is such a heterogeneous category of behaviors and interactions that 'amount of aggression' is not a very useful concept." Fausto-Sterling (1985: 129) concurs and points to the fact that no studies on hormone levels and aggression use female subjects or compare men and women. She raises fundamental questions regarding the causal relationship between testosterone levels and aggression.

In this book, Lucinda Peach explores how the ideas about male strength, male bonding, and male aggression have shaped the debate in the United States about women in the military. Women are barred from almost all assignments involving the operation of offensive, line-of-sight weapons as well as from all positions involving ground fighting. She suggests that such exclusions are based on assumptions and stereotypes about female "nature" rather than on verifiable gender differences that clearly demonstrate women's inability to perform competently specific combat duties. Warfare is a masculine arena; women need to be protected; women lack the necessary physical strength to perform adequately; the presence of women in combat units would undermine unit cohesion by disrupting male bonding—these are some of the arguments that are put forward to justify the banishment of women from specific military activities. One result, by extension, is that women are denied certain opportunities for promotion that are predicated on active combat service.

A fourth body of theory linking biology to gender difference and gender hierarchy explains the absence of women from cooperative and political activity in the nondomestic sphere (hence their subordination) in terms of their reproductive roles. A corollary of this argument is the idea that women possess a maternal instinct. The fact that women bear children and lactate has been the basis of assertions that women innately experience an attachment to their children that forms the foundation of effective mothering, while men lack a similar capacity to nurture (Peterson 1983; Rossi 1977, 1978). This attachment may be the result of such factors as hormone levels (O'Kelly 1980: 30) or of the experiences of pregnancy, labor, and nursing (Whitbeck 1983: 186). In contrast, Collier and Rosaldo (1981: 315) argue that "there are no facts about human sexual biology that, in and of themselves, have immediate social meanings or institutional consequences. Mothering is a social relation, much like fathering, judging, or ruling, whose meaning and organization must be understood with reference to a particular configuration of relationships within a complex social whole."

The articles by Etienne and by Scheper-Hughes (in this book) illustrate this assertion. Etienne's case study focuses on the adoption of children by urban Baule women in the Ivory Coast, West Africa. Etienne shows that to be without children is considered a regrettable fate, but rights of children are not determined by reproductive capacity alone. While all women are supposed to desire children, the Baule recognize unequal distribution of talent for motherhood. Thus, some women receive many children to adopt because of their childrearing skills, while others give their children to kin because they do not like raising children. Emotional ties to adoptive parents tend to be strong, although children remain in contact with their birth parents. Etienne's research contests the assumption that paternity is inherently social, while maternity is essentially natural.

Similarly, Scheper-Hughes (1987) examines the inevitability of maternal-infant attachment among mothers in the shantytowns of northeast Brazil. In an environment of poverty, chronic hunger, and economic exploitation, Scheper-Hughes finds that mothers adopt a strategy of delayed attachment and neglect of weaker children thought unlikely to survive. Such attitudes of resignation and fatalism toward the death of children are documented in historical studies of other cultures as well; for example, Ransel's account of child abandonment in Russia relates the passive attitude toward childhood death to child death rates in the 50 percent range (1988: 273; see also Boswell 1988). Parental attitudes are reflected in an entire category of lullabies with the motif of wishing death on babies; women sang these lullabies to infants who were sickly, weak, or crippled (Ransel 1988: 273). Thus, mother love seems less a "natural and universal maternal script" than a luxury reserved for the strongest and healthiest children. In the context of frequent infant death, maternal attachment means grief, and mother love emerges as culturally and socially constructed, rather than as an innate emotion.

Hewlett (in this book) offers a somewhat different perspective on the question of maternal instinct by exploring the role of fatherhood among the Aka pygmies, a group of foragers who live in the tropical forest regions of central Africa. Aka fathers spend a significant portion of their day caring for and nurturing their children. A good father, among the Aka, is a man who stays near his children, shows them affection, and assists the mother with her work. Indeed Aka male-female relations are very egalitarian. Women and men each contribute significantly to subsistence; while Aka men hold all the named positions of status, women challenge men's authority regularly and play a decisive role in all kinds of decision making; physical violence is infrequent, and violence against women is rare (Hewlett 1991). Hewlett suggests that strong father-infant attachment among the Aka can be explained by a range of ecological, social, ideological, and demographic factors. The implications of the Aka example, especially for alternate parenting models in the United States, are clear. As Hewlett argues, "The Aka demonstrate that there are cultural systems where men can be active, intimate and nurturing caregivers" (Hewlett 1991: 171).

Research on nonhuman primates has shown that role variability and plasticity are deeply rooted in the evolutionary history of primates. Cross-cultural data suggest a similar plasticity among humans. The evidence from this section should support the argument that biology merely sets the parameters for a broad range of human behaviors. Thus, biological differences between men and women have no uniform and universal implication for social roles and relations. As Rosaldo and Lamphere (1974: 4) contend, biology, for humans, takes on meaning as it is interpreted in human culture and society.

REFERENCES

Bleier, Ruth. 1984. *Science and Gender: A Critique of Biology and its Theories on Women.* New York: Pergamon Press.

Boswell, John. 1988. *The Kindness of Strangers: The Abandonment of Children in Western Europe from Late Antiquity to the Renaissance.* New York: Pantheon Books.

Burbank, Victoria Katherine. 1994. *Fighting Women. Anger and Aggression in Aboriginal Australia.* Berkeley: University of California Press.

Collier, Jane E. and Michelle Z. Rosaldo. 1981. "The Politics of Gender in Simple Societies." In Sherry S. Ortner and Harriet Whitehead (eds.). *Sexual Meanings,* pp. 275–330. Cambridge: Cambridge University Press.

Counts, D., J. Brown, and J. Campbell (eds.). 1992. *Sanctions and Sanctuary: Cultural Perspectives on the Beating of Wives.* Boulder: Westview Press.

Fausto-Sterling, A. 1985. *Myths of Gender.* New York: Basic Books.

Fedigan, Linda Marie. 1982. *Primate Paradigms: Sex Roles and Social Bonds.* Montreal: Eden Press.

———. 1986. "The Changing Role of Women in Models of Human Evolution." *Annual Review of Anthropology* 15: 25–66.

Freeman, Derek. 1983. *Margaret Mead and Samoa: The Making and Unmaking of an Anthropological Myth.* Cambridge: Harvard University Press.

Hewlett, Barry S. 1991. *Intimate Fathers: The Nature and Context of Aka Pygmy Paternal Infant Care.* Ann Arbor: University of Michigan Press.

Lee, Richard. 1979. *The !Kung San: Men, Women, and Work in a Foraging Society.* Cambridge: Cambridge University Press.

Lee, Richard S. and Irven DeVore (eds.). 1968. *Man the Hunter.* New York: Aldine.

Maccoby, E.E. and C.N. Jacklin. 1974. *The Psychology of Sex Differences.* Stanford: Stanford University Press.

Martin, M. Kay and Barbara Voorhies. 1975. *Female of the Species.* New York: Columbia University Press.

Mead, Margaret. 1928. *Coming of Age in Samoa.* New York: Dell.

————. 1935. *Sex and Temperament in Three Primitive Societies.* New York: Dell.

Morris, Allison. 1987. *Women, Crime and Criminal Justice.* Oxford: Basil Blackwell.

O'Kelly, Charlotte. 1980. *Women and Men in Society.* New York: D. Van Nostrand Co.

Peterson, Susan Rae. 1983. "Against 'Parenting.'" In Joyce Trebilcot (ed.). *Mothering: Essays in Feminist Theory,* pp. 41–62. Totowa, NJ: Rowman and Allanheld.

Ransel, David L. 1988. *Mothers of Misery: Child Abandonment in Russia.* Princeton: Princeton University Press.

Rensberger, Boyce. 1983. "Margaret Mead: The Nature-Nurture Debate: From Samoa to Sociobiology." *Science* 83: 28–46.

Renzetti, Clair M. and Daniel J. Curran. 1989. *Women, Culture and Society.* Stanford: Stanford University Press.

Rosaldo, Michelle Z. 1974. "Theoretical Overview." In Michelle Z. Rosaldo and Louise Lamphere (eds.). *Woman, Culture, and Society,* pp. 17–48. Stanford: Stanford University Press.

Rosaldo, Michelle Z. and Louise Lamphere (eds.). 1974. *Woman, Culture, and Society.* Stanford: Stanford University Press.

Rossi, Alice. 1977. "A Biosocial Perspective on Parenting." *Daedalus* 106: 1–31.

————. 1978. "The Biosocial Side of Parenthood." *Human Nature* 1: 72–79.

Scheper-Hughes, Nancy. 1987. "The Margaret Mead Controversy: Culture, Biology and Anthropological Inquiry." In Herbert Applebaum (ed.). *Perspectives in Cultural Anthropology,* pp. 443–454. Albany: State University of New York Press.

Schneider, David. 1983. "The Coming of a Sage to Samoa." *Natural History* 92(6): 4–10.

Sperling, Susan. 1991. "Baboons with Briefcases vs. Langurs in Lipstick. Feminism and Functionalism in Primate Studies." In Micaela di Leonardo (ed.). *Gender at the Crossroads of Knowledge: Feminist Anthropology in the Postmodern Era,* pp. 204–234. Berkeley: University of California Press.

Tiger, Lionel. 1969. *Men in Groups.* New York: Random House.

Trebilcot, Joyce (ed.). 1983. *Mothering: Essays in Feminist Theory.* Totowa, NJ: Rowman and Allanheld.

Whitbeck, Caroline. 1983. "The Maternal Instinct." In Joyce Trebilcot (ed.). *Mothering: Essays in Feminist Theory,* pp. 185–192. Totowa, NJ: Rowman and Allenheld.

Wilson, Edward O. 1975. *Sociobiology: The New Synthesis.* Cambridge: Harvard University Press.

PERSPECTIVES ON THE EVOLUTION OF SEX DIFFERENCES

Lila Leibowitz

There are very real physical differences between men and women. They differ not only in the appearance of their external genitalia, but in other respects as well. Men are generally bigger, have more facial and body hair,

From Rayna R. Reiter (ed.), *Toward an Anthropology of Women* (New York: Monthly Review, 1975), pp. 20–35. Copyright © 1975 by Rayna R. Reiter. Reprinted by permission of Monthly Review Foundation. This is a revised version of a paper presented at the American Anthropological Association Meeting in New Orleans, December 1973.

narrower hips, flatter buttocks, and a tendency to greater body mass. Women generally have more fatty tissue on their breasts and buttocks. These anatomical differences were for a long time viewed as intimately related to differences in emotional and intellectual capacities, as well as to differences in physical abilities. The tasks and roles assigned to men and women in our own cultural tradition were assumed to be correlated highly with anatomically based aptitudes. It is still a commonplace belief that anatomy is destiny.

In the era between the late 1930s and the mid-1960s this notion was challenged. Research into the behavior of the sexes in other cultures forced some changes in thinking. Cross-cultural data on the sexual division of labor very quickly dispelled the idea that men (or women) are unable to do some of the tasks assigned women (or men) in our culture. Knitting, weaving, and cooking sometimes fall into the male province, while such things as pearl diving, canoe handling, and housebuilding turn out to be women's work in some settings. Mead's pioneering research on sex roles and personality styles raised some doubts about the biological basis of psychological attributes, for she reported on cultures in which men display such "feminine" emotional qualities as sensitivity, affection, and volatile emotionality, while females are aggressive and calculating. Outside of anthropology, the works of Karen Horney and Viola Klein provided support to the proposition that both men and women are behaviorally flexible, and that the way men and women behave in any particular social setting is a result of circumstances rather than anatomy. Masters and Johnson's startling studies contributed to this view and further undermined many academically propagated assumptions about the workings of the human female's body and psyche. So for a while the main thrust of the respected academic literature on human sexual behavior and social roles challenged the notion that anatomy is destiny, arguing that cultural forces work on the behavioral plasticity of both males and females, shaping their behavior and the roles they assume in society.

Despite the implications of such studies, the issue of men's and women's roles and whether or how to change them was not a significant one at the time these works were appearing. The college women who read Margaret Mead's *Male and Female* in the late 1940s and early 1950s, who admired the highly publicized Yugoslav and Russian army and guerrilla heroines, and who saw Rosie the Riveter in the United States pulling down the same pay as her male co-workers did not agitate for change. They became the ideal *McCalls* magazine mothers of the 1950s. Unaffected by their college readings, they turned to Spock's handbook on child care, gourmet cooking, and interesting arts and crafts hobbies as they pursued the traditional tasks of being wives and mothers. In the early 1960s, an attack on the "feminine mystique" (Friedan, 1963) by a housewife who felt herself cheated attracted a wide audience among them. But the issue of women's roles and whether they are based on genetic capacities or on cultural forces did not emerge onto the political and intellectual scene out of books but out of the Civil Rights struggle. From the precepts of that struggle grew the women's liberation movement and the conviction that anatomy is not destiny.

When women's liberation finally surfaced as an independent entity, it was supported by some academics (like Matina Horner) but opposed by those who felt that physical differences between the sexes are based on and lead to social-role differences. Since the mid-1960s there has been a vigorous revival of the view that social-role and intellectual differences between men and women, and girls and boys, are physiologically based, substantiated by a plethora of books and articles by psychologists and neurophysiologists. Anthropologists and sociologists have picked up on these views and tied them to renewed investigations of biosocial evolution. Interestingly, these academic investigations into sex differences come at a time of a revival of notions of innate differences in intellectual capacities between blacks and whites; both, it would seem, are reactions to efforts at implementing the liberal, nonbiogenetic social-role perspectives that gained respectability during and after World War II.

On the whole, academics no longer hold the position that particular roles or tasks universally belong to either men or women because of simple differences in bones, muscles, and sex organs. The newer arguments for a biogenetic basis in role behavior have acquired a statistical framework, an evolutionary rationale, and sophisticated physiological models of perception and behavior; researchers work with rats, apes, and babies as often as they work with adult human beings. Yet the argument still boils down to the view that because men and women are obviously different physically, they also have different intellectual and emotional capacities. Whether the traits or capacities investigated are shared by a few or many men or women is often considered "statistically insignificant," if not downright irrelevant. In overall characterizations, men, it is argued, are suitable for certain kinds of roles, women for others.

Because men are larger than the females of their species, it is held that they are naturally "dominant" over women. "Dominance," an unclear term at best, may take several forms: having priority of access to food resources, or acting as a provider; fulfilling a leadership position (among nonhuman primates, this means setting the direction and/or pace of group movement); acting as protector of the females and young; taking the initiative in sexual intercourse; or simply getting others to move out of the way. Women—smaller, softer, and fattier tissued—are supposed to be eminently better equipped to be nurturant, affective, docile followers. Dominance and large size (as well as threatening teeth, bony crests, and other male physical characteristics) supposedly go together in nonhuman dimorphised primate species. In fact, it is argued, the reason that men are larger, bonier, and more muscular than women is that these features, and "dominance" in its various expressions, are intrinsically related to one another and gave those males who had them reproductive advantage. By virtue of being leaders, providers, protectors, and sexually aggressive, larger males are more likely to father stronger babies. They are also better able to help their offspring survive than smaller and presumably less dominant males, who are therefore at a reproductive disadvantage. In short, the argument traces physical differences between the sexes (which are supposed to shape contemporary social-role differences) back to social-role differences among our supposed ancestors. Contemporary physical differences are seen as the result of ancient social-role differences, and contemporary social-role differences are treated as the result of physical differences that became established in early human and pre-human populations.

Since we have no way of observing the social arrangements of our ancestors, the social adaptations of living nonhuman primates provide the models from which this theory is drawn because what living primates do as they adapt to the various environments in which they live should, in theory, throw some light on the social behavior of our ancestors. While researchers have tended to pick the one nonhuman primate they consider to be relevant to understanding dimorphism among humans, favoring some species over others, this paper focuses on the behavior and social adaptations of several species in order to examine whether and how their social-role arrangements are related to the presence or absence of sexual dimorphism.

I will first deal briefly with a nondimorphic species, the gibbons, who are found living in the upper reaches of the forest canopies of Southeast Asia, and then touch on the social adaptations of their close neighbors, the extremely dimorphic orangutans. I will look at our closer relations, the African Great Apes: the very dimorphic gorillas and the much less sexually differentiated chimpanzees, who spend much of their time on the ground. Finally, I will examine in somewhat greater detail the adaptations of terrestrial baboons which, despite being rather distantly related to us, have been the most frequent models for speculative reconstructions of early human adaptations.

This brief overview will demonstrate that the sex-role adaptations of the sexually dimorphic nonhuman primate species do not in fact conform to the models used in current explanations of how and why dimorphism developed among humans. In fact, sexual dimorphism cannot easily be equated with sex-role patterns. The data will show, however, that dimorphic primate species do have one thing in common: they all live under environmental conditions that encourage males to range more widely than females. Thus although the data points up the inadequacy of current theory on the sources of physical sex differentiations, it suggests another.

In the closing section, I will examine the possibility that sexual dimorphism is generated not out of selection favoring animals with a predisposition to particular social-role behavior, but is the result of pressures favoring those animals that have growth and maturation rates which give them a reproductive advantage in environments which permit or encourage males to range more widely than females. Thus I am suggesting that while sexual dimorphism is the outcome of sex differences in growth and maturation rates that lead to different body conformations in adults of each sex, sexual dimorphism is at the same time perfectly compatible with a wide variety of sex-role patterns, and even compatible with the ability to adapt to a variety of social-role patterns.

Gibbons, the first of the primates we will consider, are not dimorphic. Males and females look alike; there are no significant characteristics, aside from genitals, that distinguish them. Members of both sexes take the same length of time to achieve full growth and end up in the same size range (13–16 pounds). In the wild, gibbons live in the high trees in pair groups which include an adult male, an adult female, and the immature young of one or both adults. This pair-centered group occupies a relatively fixed range from which adolescent children move off, sometimes with an opposite sexed sibling and at other times with an opposite sexed adolescent from a nearby group. A pair-centered group forages as a unit in its own arboreal niche, and intruders are driven off by either the adult male or the adult female, neither of whom travels far afield from the range the group occupies (Carpenter, 1948). Pairs mate only when females are neither pregnant or nursing, usually at two- or three-year intervals. In some pairs the male tends to give way to the female; in others the reverse is true.

Orangutans are close neighbors of the gibbons, also living in the high trees. Unlike gibbons, orangutans exhibit a marked degree of sexual dimorphism. Males weigh about 160 pounds, females 80 pounds. Males have goiterous-looking throat sacs which lend volume to their voices. They also have much larger canine teeth than do females and heavier bony prominences around their faces. Females reach sexual maturity and full growth at around age nine; males produce viable sperm at that age, but do not stop growing until several years later. An orang female and her young occupy a stable range which may overlap that of another female and her young. Where mothers and daughters with young live in adjacent areas, they sometimes join together temporarily to make a multi-female group.

Adult males travel alone, moving back and forth across a wide area that cuts across the ranges of several female groups; sometimes they visit, accompany, or follow these groups for awhile. Although these visits do not necessarily involve sexual activity, males mate when they can. Females are rarely receptive, since nursing is quite prolonged. One obvious rape episode was observed by David Horr, but uninterested females usually avoid and rarely excite males, rejecting them without difficulty. Vocalizations appear to help the animals locate one another in dense foliage and males vocalize fairly frequently. They are assiduous in avoiding one another. The large orangutan male is rarely involved in aggressive interactions and has even less opportunity to function as a leader or protector than the male gibbon, but unlike the gibbon he is a traveler and ranges much more widely than the females of his species.*

Gorillas are the largest of the apes: up to 600 pounds for males and 400 or so for females. Adult males differ from females in that they sometimes develop flaring sagital crests, have furry backs that turn silvery at maturity, and usually have larger canine teeth. Gorillas are ground-browsing vegetarians who build

* An informal presentation by David Horr to a class at Northeastern University is the source of this information on orangs.

tree nests each night, and adult females are always found in groups in which there is at least one, and usually more, silver-backed males, whose presence is a deterrent to predators. Direction-setting leadership is assumed by a silver-back. Males, especially black-backed adolescents, are not infrequently found outside such groups, evidently joining and leaving them with ease. Females never travel alone. They become pregnant almost immediately on reaching sexual maturity and are nursing an infant or pregnant nearly all their adult lives. Among female gorillas sexual receptivity is rare indeed. In a full year's observation of several groups, Schaller saw only two episodes of intercourse, and neither involved a silver-backed leader. In one case a silver-back approached a copulating pair, displacing the younger male, who ran off. The female displayed no interest whatsoever in the silver-back, who finally left the scene. The female then turned back to her preferred partner, an "outsider" who had just joined, and soon left, the group (Schaller, 1964).

Chimpanzee males weigh around 150 pounds; females weigh about 130, but there are small males as well as big females (in the 140-pound range). Aside from a tendency to larger canine teeth, males develop no marked secondary sexual characteristics, but adolescent females develop perineal sexual skins which swell and recede periodically in conjunction with the changing hormonal balance of the estrus cycle. Chimpanzees in the wild are found in several habitats: gallery forests, a mosaic of plain and forest, and on cultivated plantations or near stocked feeding stations. Although there are local variations in social organization which include troop-like arrangements, semi-stable nursery groups of mothers and children, mixed adolescent groups, all-male groups, and general assemblages, all these are essentially fluid. Groups dissolve, change personnel, and in so doing change form. The "nursery group" of mothers and their young occurs in a variety of environments, including stocked feeding station situations. Like orangutans, gibbons, and gorillas, chimpanzee females in the wild are infrequently free from pregnancy and nursing. Chimpanzee females are rather more lively than gorillas, however, when they are in estrus. Males mate with interested females wherever and whenever they find them and wait side by side, without friction or competitive scrambling (Goodall, 1965).

Before going on to describe sex differences and social behavior among baboons, let me point out how the social arrangements among gibbons, orangutans, gorillas, and chimpanzees do not confirm current popular and academic theories which associate sex-role behaviors with physical sex differences and then use these associations to account for the evolution of human sex differences. Popular notions about the kinds of sex roles that lead to dimorphism, and about how dimorphism leads to sex roles, are far too simplistic. Sex-related differences among humans, particularly the possession by females of breasts and buttocks, have been tied to pair bonding, a pair bonding in which males are protectors, aggressors, and leaders. Yet pair bonding shows up only among gibbons, who lack any significant sex differentiation either physically or with respect to social roles. Chimp, gorilla, and orangutan populations lack pair bonding but *are* dimorphic.

The sex differences typical of these species—the males are larger, stronger, hairier, and have more formidable dentition—have in turn been tied to a certain kind of social-role pattern: large males are supposed to be the protectors and leaders of the young and female members of the group, and are therefore supposed to have a sexual advantage over smaller males. Females, according to this theory, are more passive, sexually and otherwise. Similarly, the lack of dimorphism among gibbons has been attributed to an adaptation in which males do not play particularly distinctive roles as leaders, protectors, or aggressors. But orangutan males show a similar lack of leadership, and orangutans are dimorphic. And what do we find in the field? Among the dimorphic primate species, the sexes play different roles in different circumstances. Gorillas are the only dimorphic apes to live in groups stable enough to have leaders. Yet while the silver-backed males may set the direction of troop movement, they are mild mannered. Schaller's observations indicate that silver-backed males have no sexual prerogatives, have no pre-emptive rights over food, and can protect others only while they are within the safety of the group.

Further, while many reporters describe chimpanzee dominance hierarchies as being based on who "gives way" to whom, the largest male around is not necessarily dominant. In fluid chimpanzee aggregates, "leadership"—in terms of direction-setting—is temporary and unstable. There is no evidence that some males have sexual prerogatives denied others; nor does a dominant male have special access to vegetable food or in hunting small game. Even when begging meat from animals (male or female) who have taken game, a dominant male does not receive any special or exorbitant quantity of food (Teleki, 1973). Furthermore, chimpanzee and gorilla males do not go in for fights in which big canines are used. Orangutan males are neither group leaders nor protectors, for they do not live with groups. Since orangutan males generally avoid each other, they rarely get into fights. Predators are not significant threats to any of these animals as long as they can escape into trees or remain in large enough groupings to scare them off. Thus the sexual dimorphism in these primate species is not tied to the social-role arrangements that are often cited as the basis of sexual dimorphism among humans.

The physical traits discussed above continue to be attributed to such role patterns largely because of the behavior of certain baboons, who fit our cultural model of our primate past. Baboons live in the kind of terrestrial plains environment early humans apparently became adapted to. They obviously do not and did not compete directly with humans for the same econiche; if they had, they probably would not have survived. Presumably, however, they now face problems similar to those faced by our early ancestors. Baboon males are much bigger than females, and have heavier mantles and bigger canine teeth, which they display quite often. Males and females are both very volatile in temperament.

The plains-living populations of baboons first described in the anthropological literature by DeVore and Washburn (1961) are called cynocephalous baboons (Buettner-Janusch in Rowell, 1972:45). Cynocephalous baboons also live in forest and "farming" settings. The forest and farm adaptations have been described by Rowell and Maples respectively (Rowell, 1972; Maples,1971). DeVore and Washburn's early study of plains adaptations in "protected" reserves reported that baboons live in large, peaceful, and rather stable groups. Active adolescent males circulate around the periphery of the closed moving troop, while females with infants stick to the central area and cluster around subgroups of "alpha," or dominant, males. Alpha male subgroups involve alliances between several, mostly older, males, who reportedly rush to place themselves between threatening situations and the troop. Alpha males are chosen as sexual consorts by females at the height of estrus, displace other males and compete with or threaten them when they are offered delectable foods in limited quantities, and seem to set the direction of troop movements. In short, early studies of plains-living social adaptations among baboons provide a neat model which nicely correlates sex-role behavior and physical sex differences, corroborating the theory outlined above.

Forest-living cynocephalous baboons behave differently (Rowell, 1972), as do baboons who raid farms and garden plots (Maples, 1971). Groups travel in a linear pattern, with a male in the front and one at the rear. Old females "choose" and set the direction of daily movement. Adult and young males change groups rather frequently. (In at least one instance, some young adult females also changed groups.) When danger threatens males usually issue warning barks and station themselves near the threat and along an escape route; one may stay behind until the others disappear. But if danger is imminent, the first animals into the safety of the trees are those unencumbered by infants—the males. Rowell observed no patterned preferences for particular consorts by females. Females initiate intercourse, even at the height of estrus, with various males.

Hamadryas baboons live in the dry Ethiopian highlands. They congregate in large assemblages at night and disperse during the day in what has been called—erroneously—one-male groups (Kummer, 1968). Characterized by some authors as "harem" groups, one-male groups often include a junior male, as well as an older male who herds or guides one or several females with or without young. As they age, senior males spend less and less time with the group and the younger males take over herding and mating. These quasi-"family" arrangements provide substantial support for the notion that male-female role differences are related to physical sex differences; in addition, they suggest that a propensity to harem and nuclear "family" arrangements is innate.

Yet an interesting change occurred in one generation in an artificially created colony of hamadryas baboons. An elderly female took over herding-type activities when all the older males born in the wild died off and colony-reared males failed to fulfill the herder role. Behavioral plasticity and sex-role adaptability, it seems, are part of baboon behavioral capacities, since not only do we see a change of social patterning in one short generation in a group of hamadryas that was shifted from one ecological setting to another, but we encounter, as already noted, social patterns among cynocephalous baboons that vary from one setting to another.

The hamadryas one-male group pattern may not mean quite what current theorists argue for yet another reason. It is doubtful that hamadryas are a distinct species of baboon since they have mated successfully with cynocephalous types, both in the wild and in captivity (Rowell, 1972). If they are not a separate species, then their particular social adaptations may represent local adaptations, one of several alternatives available to them. In any case, when we consider all the baboon adaptations side by side—plains, forest, farm, and Ethiopian upland—we are once again left with no neat and inevitable tie between sex-role behavior and physical sex differences. The baboons join the orangutans, chimpanzees, and gorillas in what appears to be, at best, a loose correlation between sex-role behavior patterning and physical form.

Given that sex-role specializations are but weakly demonstrated in these higher primates, how can we account for the existence of such physical sex differences? Since sex dimorphism among primates is not clearly associated with or attributable to any particular set of sex-role patterns, we need another hypothesis as to the origins and functions of sexual dimorphism. The crucial physical differences boil down to elaborations of a single difference in dimorphic primate species: males continue to grow for some time past the age when females have ceased to grow and have begun to have offspring; sex differences in size and body form begin to become marked only after the age at which both males and females are reproductively mature. If differences in pubertal growth rates are the key to understanding the physical differentiation of the sexes, it seems sensible to ask what factors give a reproductive advantage to females who stop growing shortly after they achieve sexual maturity and to males who continue to grow after they develop viable sperm. In the social adaptations of orangutans, chimps, baboons, and gorillas there is one sex-differentiated behavioral common denominator: for a while males move around more actively than females. It is not that they are more aggressive—they may or may not be—but that they are more *mobile.* I therefore propose that in ecological settings in which mature males are enabled or forced to forage more widely than females, males who continue to grow after reaching sexual maturity have a reproductive advantage over males who do not.

Primate species, as species, vary in size according to the econiche to which they are adapted. For the female of any species, ceasing to grow after becoming pregnant has obvious survival advantages for the female and for her offspring. Eating for two, whether the infant is *in utero* or at breast, requires less intake and less activity for a female who stops growing than for one who continues to grow. Anything that insures a female's efficient reproductive energy allocation will be selectively favored, whether her social group is large or small, open or closed, whether she has one mate or several, or lives in the trees or on the ground.

The optimal size for females is the same as that of males in the vast majority of *arboreal* primate species, for dimorphism is rare among them. This correlates with the fact that in most arboreal primate species males and females have similar foraging patterns and are equally free from predation. Orangutans, who are unusually large when compared to other arboreal primates, also do not conform to the standard arboreal troop or pair arrangements. They are not only markedly dimorphic, but the forage ranges of males are far larger than those of females. Orangutan food resources are strained by these large animals and dispersal is a necessity. Males forage as individuals, roaming widely. A mother and her young forage together in a small area, occasionally joined by another mother and her young. Though orangutans are pre-eminently arboreal, in some ways this adaptation resembles that of ground-living primate species.

Partially or completely terrestrially adapted primates are more readily subject to predation than arboreal species, and immature animals and infant-carrying females are safe only when in a good-sized group. Mother-young groups, like those of the orangutans, simply could not survive on the ground. Ground-living species are group foragers and the core of the group is made up of immature animals and females with young. The only isolated males that are large enough to travel safely on the ground for any length of time are gorillas. Food resources at the center of a ground-foraging group are under some pressure, and there is thus an impetus for mature unencumbered animals to move toward the periphery of the group, and even to eventually leave and join another. Those males that continue to grow after reaching sexual maturity are peculiarly well adapted to foraging on the margins of a group. For one thing, they do not experience either the decline in activity level that accompanies the cessation of growth, or the decline in activity level that affects pregnant and nursing females. They tend to remain active and exploratory longer than males who stop growing, so they are ready and able to exploit resources on the margins of the group. (Sometimes they even eat foods that other members of the species don't encounter, which may explain some secondary sexual developments in the chewing equipment and head structures of males.) Furthermore, the bigger they become, the safer they are from predators in their edge locations. But most significant of all, the more mobile they become, the greater are their reproductive advantages over less mobile males.

From what does this reproductive advantage derive? Male reproductive success is linked to the number of mating opportunities a male can take advantage of. Since primate females are infrequently in estrus, males who move around on the edges of groups, and from group to group, are more likely to find fertile females than those who are bound to their own small groups all their lives, or who stay in the center with nursing mothers all the time. This means that a delayed cessation of growth can afford a male reproductive advantages whether or not he engages in active sexual competition with other males, and whether or not he becomes a leader or a protector. If he is living in a setting where predation is significant, the size he achieves may help him survive, and this of course also contributes to his reproductive success. (Since predation hardly affects orangutans at all, however, protection seems to be less a cause than a result of size increments, which are tied to mobility.)

For the mobile male the particular role he plays in the groups he encounters often changes from situation to situation. He may or may not become a dominant male capable of getting others to move out of his way, but even if he does settle down to a life of "dominance" in a particular group, the number of offspring he fathers will not be increased by his ability to displace others, since "dominance" is not particularly correlated with any special sexual prerogatives. Indeed, his reproductive success rate may be reduced as his mobility diminishes, even though he has achieved full size. If he settles down to a life of subdominance, the same holds true. The role he plays in a group seems to be less significant than how much he moves around among groups.

The hypothesis I am proposing therefore argues that in ecological settings which encourage males to forage more widely than females, reproductive advantages have fallen to those males who are active enough to move around, large enough to do so safely, and versatile enough to exploit alternative food resources and social situations. At the same time, reproductive advantage falls to those females who stop growing at pubescence and are efficient in using their limited food intakes for reproduction and nursing. This hypothesis provides a way to account for the evolution of physical differences without viewing sex roles, past or present, rigidly. (I might add, briefly and by way of support for some of the ideas incorporated into this hypothesis, that when a female baboon was prevented from becoming pregnant she continued to grow and remained active longer than her compeers.)

This hypothesis is a response to the recent spate of evolutionary theories which stress that our sex-role destiny along with our sexual anatomy, was settled a long time ago. A number of theorists have revived the view that sexual dimorphism among humans is tied to sex-role patterns that are current or idealized in our own culture. New data on nonhuman primate behavior has provided source materials for such theories: without too much difficulty, theorists have been able to find one or another population of nonhuman primates that conforms to their cultural model of how things were, are, or ought to be. Unfortunately for such theories, humans and nonhuman primates utilize a variety of social forms in which females and males play a variety of roles. Explaining human sexual dimorphism in terms which postulate that the sexes are each suited to only certain kinds of role behavior runs contrary to the accumulated evidence. Until we have an explanation that accounts both for the evolution of physical sex differences and for the existence of role plasticity, the belief that anatomy is destiny will linger on. We must familiarize ourselves with the data and deal with it in a sophisticated framework that accounts for its variability. If we don't, the growing body of evidence that role variability and role plasticity run rather deep in the primate heritage will continue to be ignored or distorted.

REFERENCES

Buettner-Janusch, J. 1966. *Folia Primatologica 4;* cited in Thelma Rowell, *Social Behavior of Monkeys.* Baltimore: Penguin Books, 1972.

Carpenter, C. R. 1948. "Life in the Trees: The Behavior and Social Relations of Man's Closest Kin." In *A Reader in General Anthropology,* edited by C. Coon. New York: Henry Holt.

DeVore, I., and Washburn, S. L. 1961. "Social Behavior of Baboons and Early Man." In *Social Life of Early Man,* edited by S. L. Washburn. Chicago: Aldine.

Freidan, Betty. 1963. *The Feminine Mystique.* New York: W. W. Norton.

Goodall, Jane Van Lawick. 1965. "Chimpanzees of the Gombe Steam Reserve." In *Primate Behavior,* edited by I. DeVore. New York: Holt, Rinehart and Winston.

Horney, Karen. 1973. "The Denial of the Vagina." In *Feminine Psychology,* edited by Harold Kelman. New York: W. W. Norton.

Kummer, Hans. 1968. *Social Organization Hamadryas Baboons.* Chicago: University of Chicago Press.

Maples, William R. 1971. "Farming Baboons." Paper presented at the 1971 Meeting of the American Association of Physical Anthropologists, Boston, Mass.

Mead, Margaret. 1950. *Male and Female: A Study of the Sexes in a Changing World.* New York: Morrow.

Rowell, Thelma. 1972. *Social Behavior of Monkeys.* Baltimore: Penguin Books.

Schaller, George B. 1964. *The Year of the Gorilla.* Chicago: University of Chicago Press.

THE ROLE OF WOMEN IN HUMAN EVOLUTION

Margaret Ehrenberg

Human evolution has traditionally been discussed in terms of the role which 'Man the Hunter' played in devising weapons and tools for catching and slaughtering animals for food, how he needed to walk upright on two feet to see his prey above the tall savanna grass, and how he was more successful than other species in his hunting exploits because he teamed up with other men and learnt the value of co-operation. And what of 'woman', meanwhile? Was she sitting at home, twiddling her thumbs, waiting for 'man' to feed her and increase his brain capacity and abilities until he became *'Homo sapiens sapiens'*? The argument went that as human evolution progressed, more and more time was needed to look after infants, so females no longer had time to hunt, and male co-operative hunting became essential in order that the men could bring enough food home to feed the family. As a result, male-female bonding in monogamous unions was an essential and a very early development. While most accounts of human evolution have assumed that all the advances in human physical and cultural development were led by men, a number of recent studies suggest alternative possibilities and have pointed out the vital role which must have been played by women.

Research into the earliest stages of human evolution is based on three strands of evidence. Physical anthropologists study the remains of early human skeletons, to assess the way in which they developed. For example, it is possible to tell from the structure of the legs and back whether an individual would have walked upright on two legs, or used the forearms for balance. Changes in the size of the skull through time give an indication of brain capacity. Secondly, the study of the behaviour of other animals, and especially primates, particularly those species closest to humans such as apes and chimpanzees, reveals some patterns which may have been shared by the earliest humans before cultural norms began to play an overriding part. For example, chimpanzees may be studied to see if males and females eat or collect different foods, or to find out whether they share any of the differences in child-care practices seen in human women and men. Thirdly, archaeological evidence for tools, settlements, environment and diet sheds light on the social and cultural development of the earliest humans.

Some scholars within all these three areas have turned away from the traditional male-dominated view of evolution and have begun to formulate an alternative model, allowing that female primates and hominids have played an important part, if not the key role, in the development of human behaviour. Different authors have stressed different factors in this development. Adrienne Zihlman[1] argues that changes in the environment were crucial in necessitating social and economic changes in human populations in order to exploit this environment efficiently. Sally Slocum[2] points out that the only division of labour by sex amongst other primates is that females take primary care of their young, while males tend to dominate in protecting the group. She argues that a division of labour in food collecting is therefore unlikely to have been a key feature of early human behaviour. Other feminist writers[3] suggest that the female's choice of a co-operative and gentle mate was a critical factor in human evolution, as the chances of survival were improved by caring more closely for near relatives; in all mammals, and especially in primates, this is much more a female task or trait.

Among the physical changes which took place in the early stages of human evolution were increases in the size of the brain and the teeth; a decrease in sexual dimorphism (difference in size between males and females); increased hairlessness over the body; and bipedalism, or walking on two feet, rather than using the forelimbs for support, as chimpanzees and apes do. While an infant chimpanzee can cling to its mother's cover of body hair, leaving her hands free for walking or carrying food, a young human or early hairless hominid would need to be carried by the mother: this seems a much more likely stimulus both to bipedalism and to the invention of tools for carrying the infant as well as food than is the need to see prey animals over tall savanna grass and to throw simple weapons at them, which has been the traditional explanation for these changes.

A key aspect of the debate about the evolution of sex-role behaviour centres on food collection, and the way in which females and males may have foraged for different foods. Many discussions, including those written by some feminist anthropologists, assume that from a very early stage in evolution females primarily gathered plant foods, while males mainly hunted animals, the pattern usual in modern hunter-gatherer societies. Many recent arguments about other aspects of the role played by females in human social and technological evolution depend on this belief, even though it is rarely argued out fully. At one end of the scale other primates show little evidence for differences in food collecting behaviour between females and males, while at the other all modern foragers apparently divide subsistence tasks on the basis of sex. The question, therefore, is when and why this difference came about, and whether looking after young offspring would have a limiting effect on hunting by females. One view[4] suggests that although males unburdened by young might have caught meat more often than females, a regular division of labour would probably have come quite late in human evolution, as the physical differences between females and males are insufficient to make one sex or the other more suitable for either task. Recent work has also questioned whether meat actually filled a significant part of the early human diet, suggesting that this would have been far more like that of other primates, based almost entirely on a wide range of plant foods. What meat was eaten in the earliest phases of the Palaeolithic was probably scavenged, rather than hunted. Both these factors are problematic for the traditional view, as they suggest that hunting was neither an important factor in physical evolution, nor in the social and economic balance between female and male activities. Both sexes would have obtained vegetable foods and occasional meat, and brought some of their day's collection back to the homebase for sharing.

If there was little division of labour in the earliest phase of human development, when and why did it become usual? Two chronological points may have provided possible contexts. Initially, hominids would have been content to catch small game or to scavenge meat caught by other animals, or to collect those that had died naturally, but perhaps around 100,000 years ago they developed suitable tools and techniques for hunting large animals. While hunting small game would not have been hazardous, big-game hunting might often have resulted in death or injury to the hunter rather than the hunted. In small societies, such as these early human groups and present-day forager societies, every unexpected death is a serious blow to the viability of the community, particularly the death of women of child-bearing age. Mobility would also have been more important in hunting large game; the hunter would have to move rapidly and quietly, with hands free to throw a spear or shoot an arrow. It would not be possible to do this while carrying a bag or basket of gathered food, nor a young child, who might cause an additional hazard by making a noise at a crucial moment. Thus gathering and hunting become incompatible as simultaneous occupations; pregnant women and those carrying very small infants would have found hunting difficult, though gathering is quite easily combined with looking after young children. It is therefore possible that at this stage women began to hunt less, until a regular pattern of dividing subsistence tasks was established.[5]

Another possible context for the origin of the division of labour[6] is the change in environment which hominids found when they first entered Europe. It is argued that this spread could not have occurred until the perceptual problems of coping with a new environment had been resolved, by splitting food foraging into separate tasks. During the Lower Palaeolithic in East Africa, plants and animals would have been abundant, so vegetable foods and small game would have provided plenty of easily obtainable food with only the occasional large game caught to supplement the diet. As the hominid population increased and went in search of new territory, some hominids moved north into Europe. There they encountered colder conditions in which plant foods were harder to come by, so meat would have formed a more significant part of their diet. If this problem was not serious enough to necessitate a solution when hominids first moved into Europe, it would have become so with the onset of the last glaciation when conditions became very much colder and vegetation more sparse (this period equates archaeologically with the Upper Palaeolithic). The time and danger involved in hunting large animals became more worthwhile, but would not have provided a regular, guaranteed source of food, and would have been more dangerous. A solution might have been for only part of the community to concentrate on hunting, while the rest continued gathering plants and small animals. It is likely that this division would usually have been on a female-male basis for the reasons already suggested.

On the other hand, more detailed studies of chimpanzee behaviour suggest that there may be slight differences in the food collecting behaviour of females and males of non-human primates, which could argue for an early gathering/hunting division.[7] Although chimpanzees eat very little animal flesh, males make nearly all the kills and eat more of the meat; however, termite fishing, involving the use of sticks as fishing rods to poke into the termite mounds, a skilled task requiring patience and simple tool use, is far more commonly carried out by females. Whether the 'changing environment' theory or the latter argument is preferred, both hypotheses suggest that a division of labour on the basis of sex would have been an early development in human history.

Tool-using was once thought to be a distinctly human attribute, but in simple form it is now known to be shared with several of the higher primates, and even other animals and birds. Most early theories suggested that tool-using by humans was intimately linked with hunting, which in turn was assumed to be a male task, and that the earliest tools would have been spears for hunting animals and stone knives or choppers for butchery. This idea was partly encouraged by the archaeological evidence of the early stone tools, most of which are thought to have had such functions. However, this is partly a circular argument, as on the one hand the function of these tools is far from certain, and many would have been just as useful for cracking nuts or digging roots, and on the other, the very earliest tools would almost certainly have been made of wood, skins or other perishable material. Artefacts such as digging sticks, skin bags, nets, clubs and spears can be made entirely of organic materials, and would not have survived, so the extant stone tools are probably quite late in the sequence of hominid tool use. The evidence of tool use by other primates and by modern foragers, combined with a more balanced theoretical view, suggests that other factors and possibilities need to be considered.

One of the most significant human tools must be the container. Whether it be a skin bag, a basket, a wooden bowl or pottery jar, it allows us to carry items around or store them safely in one place. The container may have been one of the earliest tools to be invented, though unfortunately there is little archaeological evidence to demonstrate this. Chimpanzees can carry things in the skinfold in their groin, but when hominids became bipedal this skin was stretched and the fold was lost. The use of a large leaf or an animal skin, carried over one arm or the developing shoulder, or tied to the waist, might have replicated this lost natural carrier.[8] One of the most important things that a female hominid would need to carry would be her young offspring. The complex interaction of bipedalism, food gathering, the loss of hair for the infant to cling to, and changes in the structure of the toes which made them useless for clinging to its mother would have made it necessary for the mother to carry the child. The development of a sling for supporting the infant, found in almost all modern societies, including foraging groups, is likely to have been among the earliest applications of the container.

The first tools to aid in foraging and preparing foodstuffs are perhaps more likely to have been used in connection with plant foods and small animals than in the hunting of large mammals. The tools and actions required for termite fishing, for example, are not unlike those required for digging up roots more easily. Modern foraging groups often choose a particularly suitable stone to use as an anvil for cracking nuts, which they leave under a particular tree and then return to it on subsequent occasions. Higher primates also use stones for cracking nuts, so it is very likely that early hominids would have done this even before tools were used for hunting. The role of women as tool inventors, perhaps contributing many of the major categories of tools which are most essential even today, cannot be dismissed.

The introduction of food gathering, as opposed to each individual eating what food was available where it was found, was another significant advance which would both have necessitated and been made possible by the invention of the container. More food might be gathered than was needed immediately by one individual, either for giving to someone else or for later consumption. With the exception of parents feeding very young offspring, this behaviour is unusual among other animals and presumably would not have been common amongst the very earliest hominids, but gradually developed to become a hallmark of human behaviour. Another change would have involved carrying this food to a base, which would imply both conceptual and physical changes, made possible by the use of containers, and may also have made it necessary to walk on two legs, leaving the hands free to carry the food, either directly or in containers. The development of consistent sharing, not only with offspring but with others in the group, and exchanging food brought from different environments of savanna and forest would have been a stage towards living in regular social groups.

Environmental changes would also have led to social changes within early hominid groups. In savanna grassland, as opposed to forest, it would have been more difficult to find safe places to sleep overnight, and water would have been harder to obtain. Once a suitable location was discovered, there would have been a greater tendency to remain there as long as possible rather than sleeping in a different place each night, thus introducing the idea of a homebase.

Women also played a key role in social development. A major difference between human development and that of other animals is the greater length of time during which infants need to be cared for and fed: this has probably contributed to a number of human characteristics, including food sharing and long-term male-female bonding. The sharing of food between mother and offspring would necessarily have continued for longer in early hominids than in other primates, and it is argued that when a mammal too large to be consumed by the hunters alone was killed, the males would have shared it with those who had shared with them in their youth, that is their mothers and sisters, rather than with their sexual partners. This argument is supported by a primate study[9] which shows that banana sharing almost always takes place within matrifocal groups rather than between sexual partners. This has important implications for the primacy or otherwise of monogamy and marriage. Several scholars have also pointed out that in this situation the female would choose to mate with a male who was particularly sociable and willing to share food with his partner while she was looking after a very young infant. As well as preferring those most willing to share, females would choose those males who appeared to be most friendly. Not surprisingly, female chimpanzees will not mate with males who are aggressive towards them. The more friendly-looking males would probably have been smaller, or nearer in size to the female, and would have had less pronounced teeth, and therefore have been less aggressive-looking. Over thousands of years this female sexual preference would have led to gradual evolutionary changes in favour of smaller, less aggressive, males.

The stronger tie between mother and offspring caused by the longer period of time during which human infants need to be cared for would have resulted in closer social bonds than are found in other species. The primary bond between mother and offspring would be supplemented by sibling ties between sisters and brothers growing up together. Older offspring would be encouraged or socialised to contribute towards the care of younger siblings, including grooming, sharing food, playing and helping to protect them. The natural focus of such a group would clearly be the mother rather than, as is so often supposed, any male figure. Moreover, this group behaviour would lead to increased sociability in the male as well as in the species in general. The role of the female, both in fostering this increased sociability in the species and as the primary teacher of technological innovations during this long period of caring, must be recognised.

An increase in human sociability, and particularly female sociability, would have had a number of other positive side-effects. As a result of a mutual willingness to share food and food resources, each individual would have had more access to overlapping gathering areas when a particular resource was abundant. This in turn might greatly increase the chances of the offspring being well fed and therefore surviving, and thus of the survival of the species in general. As the ability to communicate precisely increased with the development of language, it would have become possible for humans to have ordered social relationships with more individuals and other groups. This would have evolved into a pattern very similar to that found in modern foraging groups, many of which include distant relations who regularly meet up with other groups in the course of their annual movements. Males who had moved out of the matrifocal group in order to mate would have learnt a pattern of friendly contact with their ancestral females when they met them in the course of their foraging.

It can therefore be argued that the crucial steps in human development were predominantly inspired by females. These include economic and technological innovations, and the role of females as the social centre of groups. This contrasts sharply with the traditional picture of the male as protector and hunter, bringing food back to a pair-bonded female. That model treats masculine aggression as normal, assumes that long-term, one-to-one, male-female bonding was a primary development, with the male as the major food provider, and that male dominance was inherently linked to hunting skills. None of these patterns, however, accords with the behaviour of any but the traditional Western male. Other male primates do not follow this pattern, nor do non-Western human groups, in particular those foraging societies whose lifestyle in many ways accords most closely with putative early human and Palaeolithic cultural patterns.

NOTES

1. Zihlman, 1981.
2. Slocum, 1975.
3. For example, Tanner, 1981; Martin and Voorhies, 1975.
4. Zihlman, 1981; Isaac and Crader, 1981.
5. Zihlman, 1978; the same arguments are used by Friedl, 1975 and 1978, who explains in more detail than here why present-day foragers divide food collecting tasks along gender lines.
6. Dennell, 1983, 55.
7. McGrew, 1981; Goodall, 1976.
8. Tanner and Zihlman, 1976.
9. McGrew, 1981, 47.

REFERENCES

Dennell, R. 1983. *European Economic Prehistory*. London: Academic Press.

Friedl, E. 1975. *Women and Men: An Anthropologist's View*. New York: Holt, Rinehart and Winston.

———. 1978. "Society and sex roles." *Human Nature* 1: 68–75.

Goodall, J. 1986. *The Chimpanzees of Gombe: Patterns of Behavior*. Cambridge, MA: Harvard University Press.

Isaac, G. and Crader, D. 1981. "To what extent were early hominids carnivorous?" In Teleki, G. (ed.), *Omnivorous Primates: Gathering and Hunting in Human Evolution*. New York: Columbia University Press.

Martin, M. K. and Voorhies, B. 1975. *Female of the Species*. New York: Columbia University Press.

McGrew, W. 1981. "The female chimpanzee as a human evolutionary prototype." In Dahlberg, Frances (ed.). *Woman The Gatherer*. New Haven: Yale University Press.

Slocum, S. 1975. "Woman the gatherer: male bias in anthropology." In Reiter, Rayna R. (ed.), *Toward an Anthropology of Women*. New York: Monthly Review Press.

Tanner, N. 1981. *On Becoming Human*. Cambridge: Cambridge University Press.

Tanner, N. and Zihlman, A. 1976. "Woman in evolution. Part 1: Innovation and selection in human origins." *Signs* 1(3): 585–608.

Zihlman, A. 1978. "Women in evolution. Part 2: Subsistence and social organization among early hominids." *Signs* 4: 4–20.

———. 1981. "Woman as shapers of human adaptation." In Dahlberg, Frances (ed.). *Woman the Gatherer*. New Haven: Yale University Press.

GENDER AND WAR: ARE WOMEN TOUGH ENOUGH FOR MILITARY COMBAT?

Lucinda J. Peach

INTRODUCTION

Women's participation in the U.S. military was spotlighted during the Persian Gulf War. Since that time, military personnel, government officials, public policy makers, and members of the public have given increased scrutiny to the issue of whether women should participate in military combat.

A number of arguments have been made over the years to justify the exclusion of women from military combat. Although certain positions in the military designated as "combat" have been opened up to women in recent years, especially on combat aircraft and naval vessels (except for submarines), the vast majority of combat positions remain closed to them.

The definition of "direct ground combat" that was adopted in 1993 bars women from units that engage the enemy with weapons on the ground while exposed to hostile fire *and* which involve substantial probability of direct physical contact with hostile forces (see Schmitt 1994a; Schmitt 1994b: A18; Lancaster 1994: A1; Pine 1994: A5). Under the new policy, exposure to risk, *alone,* is an insufficient ground for excluding women from a particular assignment. Nevertheless, women are barred from almost all assignments that involve operating offensive, line-of-sight weapons, and from all positions involving ground fighting. This includes armor, infantry, and field artillery, the three specialities which are considered the core of combat (see Schmitt 1994b; Schmitt 1994: A7). The consequence has been that women have been excluded from certain benefits and opportunities for promotion and advancement within (and outside) the military that are available

Original material prepared for this text.

only to those with combat experience. The exclusion also functions to limit the numbers of women who can participate in military service (because of the relatively small percentage of positions that *are* available to them). In addition, the exclusion of women from combat contributes to other forms of discrimination against women, both within and outside of the military.

In this essay, I will argue that all of these arguments have been based more on "gender ideology"—that is, on assumptions, prejudices, stereotypes and myths about male and female "natures" and "natural" or "proper" sex roles and behaviors (see Code 1991: 196)—than on empirically verifiable gender differences that demonstrate women's inability to competently perform combat roles in the U.S. military.

Two ideological myths about gender in particular underlie many of the arguments against according combat positions to women. First, identification of the military as masculine makes males the standard by which females are assessed. The male standard operates, sometimes explicitly, but more often implicitly, to perpetuate the stereotype that women are out of place in the military, particularly in combat. Throughout history, war has been a theatre in which men could prove their masculinity, and in which masculinity has been deemed a necessary prerequisite to success. During his 1992 presidential election campaign, for example, Bill Clinton's lack of military experience received a lot of attention, some of it based on the view that Clinton's lack of exposure to war made him unfit for presidential leadership. The perception that the virtues of "manliness" are necessary for effective combat soldiering, and that women are incapable or ill-suited to the development of these virtues, has contributed to the maintenance of women's exclusion from most combat assignments.

The second myth used as a rationale to exclude women from combat duty suggests that the purpose for which men fight is to protect women (see Stiehm 1989: 6–7; Kornblum 1984). Women, according to the myth, are the weaker sex and need to be protected by strong men; they are victims dependent upon men rather than autonomous agents who are competent to defend themselves. Members of the military have expressed "a special regard for women who must be protected as the symbolic vessel of femininity and motherhood" (Karst 1991: 536).

These myths are supported by the argument that integrating women into combat would be deleterious to combat effectiveness and the military's ability to mobilize in time of war (Hooker 1989: 36; Kelly 1984: 103; Mitchell 1989: 159; Marlowe 1983: 194; Rogan 1981: 21). Women's supposed physical, physiological, and psychological characteristics are offered as the basis for this argument. Although none of these rationales, alone or combined, provides an adequate ethical basis for maintaining the combat restrictions for women, their popularity and prominence makes it important to note how each of them is based on ideological notions of gender that frequently are inconsistent with the realities of gender difference.

The most common arguments in support of the view that the inclusion of women would diminish combat readiness and effectiveness are that: (1) women lack the necessary physical strength to perform adequately; (2) their capacity for pregnancy and childbearing makes them inappropriate combatants; and (3) women's participation in combat units would reduce unit cohesion by disrupting male bonding and promoting sexual fraternization. Let us examine each of these arguments in greater detail.

PHYSICAL STRENGTH

Military effectiveness is often times said to be compromised by women's lack of physical strength and stamina relative to men (see, *e.g.* Mitchell 1989: 156–62; Kantrowitz 1991; Gordon and Ludvigson 1991: 20–22, D'Amico 1990: 6). Military personnel have testified before Congress that few women would meet the physical standards for combat duty (see, *e.g.,* Hackworth 1991: 25; Appropriations

Hearings 1991; Cramsie 1983: 562). Women's purported inferior physical capability is voiced especially loudly by enlisted men, who deny that women have the strength necessary for fighting on the front lines (see Kantrowitz 1991: 23). For example, one of the reasons integrated basic training was ended in the Army in 1982 was because of enlisted men's complaints that women were holding them back (see Coyle, 1989; Stiehm 1985b: 209; Rogan 1981: 27). A study of enlisted service personnel's attitudes toward women in the Army in 1975 indicated that only about 50 percent of men interviewed thought women had the physical strength for combat (see Mitchell 1989: 157–58; Stiehm 1989: 102).

There is no question that, in general, *most* men are physically stronger than *most* women. Military studies document that men have some advantages in upper body and leg strength, cardiovascular capacity, and lean muscle, which make men "more fitted for physically intense combat" (see Mitchell 1989: 157; Kelly 1984: 100–101; Marlowe 1983: 190; Hooker 1989: 44). However, these tests generally do not also indicate the fact that some women *are* capable of meeting the standards established for men. Nor do they typically take into consideration the disparities in prior physical training and physical conditioning which men and women have undergone. Army reports reveal that some women *do* have the requisite upper body strength to qualify for combat. In addition, *some* women are stronger than *some* men. Women have performed well in the limited number of combat-type situations in which they have been tested. However, because the combat exclusion has precluded the possibility of obtaining data about women's physical performance under actual combat conditions, gender-based assumptions and prejudices have dominated policy discussions.

The assumption that women lack the physical strength necessary for combat is ideological because it often persists in the face of direct evidence to the contrary. The nature of modern combat, with its emphasis on high-technology equipment, makes the issue of physical strength far less important than it was in an era when war involved primarily hand-to-hand combat. Physical size and strength are of minimal, if any, consideration, when weapons are being fired at the touch of a button from a location far removed from the combat theatre. As Judith Stiehm argues, the question should not be "how strong women are, but how strong they need to be" (1989: 219). The positive experiences with using women in traditionally all-male fields, such as police and fire fighting forces, which require similar skills to combat, support the conclusion that women are capable of performing satisfactorily in physical-defense of self and others in situations involving the use of lethal force (see McDowell 1992; Segal 1982: 286; Karst 1991: 539; Kornblum 1984: 392–93).

Nonetheless, skeptics point out that "there is no real evidence that technology has in fact reduced the need for physical strength among military men and women. What evidence there is shows that many military jobs still require more physical strength than most women possess" (Mitchell 1989: 157). To the contrary, although there are some combat positions which most women are unable to perform satisfactorily because of inadequate physical strength, there is a considerable range of combat positions that many, if not most, women *are* qualified to perform. Although sheer physical strength may occasionally be an issue when technology fails to function properly, more often than not, the physical strength issue is no longer a legitimate reason for excluding women from combat duty. In addition, physical strength is only one of many factors that needs to be assessed in determining the capability of persons for military combat.

Several proposals have been forwarded, by military personnel and others, to assign combat positions on the basis of the physical strength required to perform them, as at least one of several relevant criterion, rather than exclusively on the basis of gender (see, *e.g.* Appropriations Hearings 1991: 865; Rousch 1990: 11–12; Coyle 1989: 31; Proxmire 1986:

110; Segal 1983: 110; Segal 1982: 270–71; Nabors 1982: 51; Rogan 1981: 306).[1] Such proposals would result in a fairer and more accurate measure of "fit" between persons and assignments than the current reliance on gender difference. The main rationale used by military officers for their failure to implement such a gender neutral scheme is that it may not be "cost effective" (see Association 1991: 54; Rogan 1981: 20). However, the military's failure to demonstrate how gender neutral standards for assignments would be financially infeasible suggests that the maintenance of the combat exclusion is based more on the continuing force of gender ideology than on financial expense or damage to military effectiveness.

Sometimes the protection myth serves to reinforce the physical strength argument by portraying women as "the weaker sex" who need to be protected from the risks of being raped and physically violated in war. It is sometimes argued that the presence of women in combat would cause male soldiers to respond by becoming more concerned about protecting them than fighting the enemy, thus compromising combat effectiveness (see Barkalow 1990: 260 (quoting Colonel Houston's comment that men's emotional commitment to recapture POW women would be so intense and extreme as to cause fighting to escalate); Beecraft 1989: 43; Van Creveld 1993). Here, the protection rationale is dominant.

During the Gulf War, the press raised the argument that women soldiers would be psychologically unable to handle being taken as prisoners of war, especially because of the greater possibility that they would be raped and otherwise sexually abused (see Nabors 1982: 59; Rogan 1981: 26). Here, the assumption is that women are less stable than men emotionally, and are thus less well equipped to handle the extreme psychological stresses of combat (*e.g.*, Mitchell 1989: 7, 182–92; Marlowe 1983: 195).

There is no factual basis for the conclusion that female combatants would be any weaker or more vulnerable than men under such circumstances. To the contrary, the experience of military women such as Air Force Major Rhonda Cornum, a flight surgeon whose aircraft was shot down during the Gulf War, reveals a very matter-of-fact attitude about survival in the face of physical injury and sexual abuse at the hands of her captors. Cornum's response stands as a testament to the ability of military women to cope as POWs (see Cornum 1992).

The notion that women in the military are in *need* of protection is based on stereotypes of male machismo and female weakness and vulnerability. Further, the assumption that males are *able* to protect military women is itself a myth, since women are too integrated throughout the armed forces to be protected by their exclusion from combat. (Providing women soldiers with arms and training in self-defense would provide a measure of protection against sexual violence which they would not otherwise have.) The rationale that women need to be protected from becoming POWs because of the risk that their torture would include sexual abuse ignores the reality that men as well as women are raped in war, and that women are already subject to such sexual violence at home or by their fellow soldiers on or near the field of combat. In addition, military women are susceptible to being captured and raped during war, regardless of whether they are themselves engaged in combat.

Also related to the physical strength argument is the assumption that men are naturally more aggressive than women, and that the "natural aggressiveness" of males would be "softened" by women's participation in battle (*e.g.*, Mitchell 1989: 7; Marlowe 1983: 191; Tuten 1981: 255). More recently, some scholars have challenged the argument that women are innately less aggressive than men (see Rosoff 1991; Sunday 1991; Marquit 1991), while others observe the lack of evidence regarding women's psychological weakness (see Gordon and Ludvigson 1991; Dillingham 1990: 227–28; Kornblum 1984: 398–99).

Many of those who conclude that men are "naturally" more aggressive than women rely on incomplete studies of *primates,* not humans, conducted by anthropologist Lionel Tiger. Tiger observed that male primates in the wild spend much of their time in groups organized to fight with outsiders, whereas female primates were engaged in grooming activities in pairs. Tiger's research has since been largely discredited by further research. Subsequent studies have revealed that females also engaged in collective aggressive action to protect their young, and that both males and females spend much of their time grooming (see Appropriations Hearings 1991: 981; Holm 1982: 95).

The evidence to support the claim of women's lesser aggression is very tenuous, especially after women soldiers demonstrated their competence in performing the psychologically demanding tasks required of combat duty during the Gulf War. But even assuming that women are less aggressive than men, there is still no evidence that it stems from biological causes rather than culture and socialization, which are malleable. The military has not offered empirical evidence to demonstrate that women cannot be trained to exhibit the same degree of aggressiveness that men exhibit. Nonetheless, the assumption that women are less aggressive continues to strengthen the myth of combat as a masculine institution of which only men are capable.

PREGNANCY AND MOTHERHOOD

One specific aspect of women's physiology that some have argued disrupts unit cohesion and consequently hampers combat effectiveness is pregnancy (*e.g.* Nabors 1982: 56–58; see Barkalow 1990: 238–41; Shields 1988: 108; Stiehm 1985b: 226; Rogan 1981: 256). The Army has expressed concern with the effects of pregnancy on "readiness," "mission accomplishment," and "deployability" (Mitchell 1989: 6, 166–71; see Tuten 1982: 251; Rogan 1981: 26; Stiehm 1985a: 266). Until 1975, women were automatically discharged from the military as soon as their pregnancy was discovered. This contributed to high attrition rates for women in the armed services. In 1975, the Department of Defense (DOD) made such discharge for pregnancy voluntary (see Segal 1983: 207; Treadwell 1954: 200).

Pregnancy also arguably interferes with the ability of the armed forces to rapidly mobilize troops for combat, since it cannot be predicted in advance which women will be pregnant, and thus unavailable for deployment. Pregnancy continues to be an issue of concern, both in the military and among the public. A *Newsweek* poll conducted in 1991 revealed that 76 percent of the public is concerned about military women becoming pregnant and putting the fetus at risk (Hackworth 1991: 27). Pregnancy does account for a significant percentage of women's lost time, although military women lose *less* service time overall than do men for illness, drug and alcohol abuse, and disability (see D'Amico 1990: 8; Coyle 1989: 39; Shields 1988: 109; Kornblum 1984: 417–18).

Because of the way military units are currently structured, pregnancy does present a genuine problem to the full integration of all women into combat forces. Since military policy, at least in the Army, does not provide temporary replacements for pregnant personnel, the presence of pregnant women in a unit increases everyone else's work load, and consequently brings with it the risk of breeding resentment among co-workers. In addition, although there is no certainty that women desiring to get pregnant will be successful, some opponents of women combatants contend that enlisted women will use pregnancy as a means of avoiding combat duty.

Therefore, pregnancy may be a legitimate reason to exclude women from actually engaging in some forms of combat. However, excluding *all* women from *all* positions designated as combat is far too extreme a response. Most women are not pregnant most of the time. Only about ten percent of servicewomen are pregnant at any given time (see Gordon and Ludvigson 1991: 22–23; Hackworth 1991: 27). Further, the experience of pregnancy varies widely in affecting a woman's job performance. Some women are able to carry on their normal activities into the latter stages of pregnancy. Most logistical problems relating to pregnancy, such as deployment plans, etc., can be satisfactorily surmounted by careful planning.

The protection myth also operates here to call into question the propriety of risking the safety of the nation's child bearers by exposing them to the risks of combat. As with the lack of data on gender-integrated units, there have been no studies of the actual impact of pregnancy on military effectiveness because the combat exclusion has precluded the possibility of gathering data. Pregnancy is *one* consideration that needs to be factored into the analysis of how and whether to integrate women into certain combat roles. But it does not justify the stringency of the current restrictions.

Related to the pregnancy issue is the symbolic, if not actual, role of women as mothers. Motherhood and women's responsibilities to their families are viewed as antithetical to effective combat soldiering. The assumption underlying this view is that women's proper role is to be the center of family life. According to this perspective, women not only bear the children, but are also primarily responsible for their care and nurture (see Mitchell 1989: 6, 171–76; Rogan 1981: 26; Segal 1982: 274–75, 281–82; Costin 1983: 305). The media's promulgation of images of women soldiers kissing their infants goodbye before going off to the Gulf War, and its stories about fathers left at home to care for children emphasized the unnaturalness of female soldiers going off to combat (see Enloe 1993: 201–27).

The influence of gender ideology on this issue is evident in the view of Alexander Webster, a chaplain for the Army National Guard, who speculates about the "identity confusion that must confront any would-be woman warrior who pauses for a moment to consider her potential for motherhood." Webster also surmises that the paradigm of the citizen soldier may have been destroyed by the "social disruption and havoc among families wreaked by the mobilization and deployment of mothers of young children to the theater of operations in the Persian Gulf" (1991: 29). Webster continues: "Disturbing images on television and in the print media of mothers wrenched from their offspring may be the most enduring from the Persian Gulf War" (24–25). According to these ideological notions of gender, women need special protection because they are responsible, in turn, for protecting their children. Notably missing from this assessment is consideration of the consequences of *fathers* being "wrenched from their offspring," thus perpetuating the identification of women as the only primary parent. Such testimony assumes that mothers are more responsible for family life than are fathers, so that it is women's military involvement that is questionable, not men's, whenever families are concerned.

Such ideological assumptions about the gender of parenthood are widespread. Surveys reveal that the public continues to be more willing to send young fathers into combat than young mothers. Even supporters of combat roles for women have assumed that mothers would be more reluctant to risk their lives in combat than would men (see Campbell 1992: 18; Lieberman 1990: 219). Attrition and reenlistment data for women indicate that motherhood is a primary reason why women leave the military. And surveys indicate that the large majority of service women do want to have children (see Shields 1988: 109). Former Secretary of Defense Richard Cheney argued that exempting all single parents and dual service-career couples from deployment would weaken military capability (see Campbell 1992: 18, 20). This problem impacts more heavily on women, who comprise the larger percentage of single parents in the military. Women's family obligations may thus present a practical problem for women's ability to carry out combat assignments, particularly for single mothers.

Several other factors need to be considered, however. Many military women are not mothers, and have no plans to become mothers. Most women entering the military are not (yet) mothers. The belief that women *are* essentially mothers is an outdated ideological assumption. It leads to the irrational result that men who are fathers can be required to participate in combat whereas women who are *not* mothers cannot (see Association 1991: 25; Segal 1982: 283). Such beliefs underlie the former Army prohibition on the enlistment of women who had children in certain age groups (see Treadwell 1954: 496).[2]

Further, although most women traditionally *have* taken primary responsibility for protecting and providing for their children, not all mothers are primary caretakers. Many families include alternative arrangements for child care that do not make the mother primarily responsible. Finally, tradition should not determine who *should* be responsible for national defense in time of war. Fathers have equal responsibility for protecting and providing for their children. Yet, since the Korean War, they have not been exempted from combat duty. In addition, the legislation mandating women's exclusion from combat does not exempt them from military *service* in time of war. Children of military parents are just as much in need of care and protection during wartime, regardless of whether their mothers are assigned to combat duty or some other position. In the absence of evidence indicating that combat jobs are more incompatible with being a wife and mother than a husband and father, families should be entitled to make their own decisions about child care in the event that the mother is called to serve in combat duty. Current military policy provides that if both parents are in the services, one can claim an exemption in the event that troops are deployed. There is no rational basis for the government to preempt the parents' right to choose based on a set of assumptions about motherhood.

UNIT COHESION AND MALE BONDING

Unit or troop "cohesion" is a function of interpersonal relationships between military leaders and their troops, and the leader's ability to create and sustain "those interpersonal skills that allow him to build strong ties with his men" (Gabriel 1982: 172–73). The argument that male soldiers will lose the camaraderie and team spirit necessary for unit cohesion if they are required to share their duties with women has been advanced as a reason to exclude women from military combat. For example, former Marine Corps Commandant Robert Barrows defends the notion of male bonding as a "real . . . cohesiveness," a "mutual respect and admiration," and a "team work" that would be destroyed by the inclusion of women. "If you want to make a combat unit ineffective," he said, "assign some women to it" (Appropriations Hearings 1991: 985–96).

While the argument about the indispensability of cohesion to effectiveness is persuasive, the view that the presence of women will damage the "male bonding" linked to that cohesion is exaggerated by the influence of gender ideology. This "influence" is often supported by outdated and anecdotal evidence, such as Tiger's largely discredited research (see, *e.g.,* Mitchell 1989; Golightly 1987; Rogan 1981: 25; Hooker 1989: 45). In addition, the military has not studied the impact that integration of the forces has had on "male bonding" in actual combat for the past several years, nor has it made efforts to instill male-female or female-female bonding in its soldiers (see Stiehm 1989: 236; Stiehm 1985b:172).

The experience with female soldiers in the Persian Gulf War, as well as the limited studies that have been done in simulated combat and field conditions, indicate that the presence of women in combat units does not adversely affect combat effectiveness. The Army Research Institute conducted two of these studies, labelled "REFWAC" and "MAXWAC" (Johnson 1978; United States Army Research Institute 1977). MAXWAC results showed that female ratios varying from 0 to 35 percent had no significant effect on unit performance. REFWAC results similarly showed that the presence of 10 percent female soldiers on a REFORGER ("Return of Forces to Germany") ten day field exercise made no difference in the performance of combat support and combat service support units.

In addition, Navy Commander Barry Boyle, participating in Navy squadron preparations, Charles Moskos, observing an Army exercise in Honduras, and Constance Devilbliss, participating in rigorous Army exercises, reached similar conclusions that integrated units performed as effectively, if not more so, than all-male units (see Coyle 1989; Moskos 1985; Devilbliss 1985). Experience with women in combat in other nations, as well as the successful integration of women into police and other traditionally male-only professions, also provide useful analogies indicating that the participation of American military women in combat would not hamper unit or troop cohesion (see, *e.g.*, Association 1991; Appropriations 1991; Goldman 1982a; Goldman 1982b).

FRATERNIZATION

Women in uniform represent an anomaly to traditional social ordering based on traditional sex-gender distinctions, and thus to traditional sexual morality. Thus, in addition to their supposedly detrimental effect on male bonding, including women in combat roles is sometimes alleged to diminish troop effectiveness because of the inevitable sexual attraction and behavior that would follow from having mixed-gender units. Some express a fear that men will be preoccupied with winning the sexual favors of women rather than concentrating on their mission (see, *e.g.*, Mitchell 1989: 176–78; Golightly 1987: 46; Rogan 1981: 27).

The fraternization argument ignores the capability of the sexes to interact with one another in non-sexual ways, particularly under the exigent circumstances of combat. The limited studies that have been conducted under simulated combat conditions indicate that fraternization does not hamper combat readiness or troop effectiveness. Studies show that gender-integrated combat units are as effective as all-male units, and that members of gender-integrated units develop brother-sister bonds rather than sexual ones.

Fraternization is most likely to be a problem where there is ineffective leadership. It is likely that unit bonding depends more on shared experiences, including sharing of risks and hardships, than on gender distinctions (see Karst 1991: 537, 543; Devilbliss 1985: 519; Opinion 1988: 138). Experience has shown that actual integration diminishes prejudice and fosters group cohesiveness more effectively than any other factor. It is thus likely that women's integration into combat forces would parallel that of black men into previously all-white forces during the 1950s and 1960s (see Moskos 1990: 74; Kornblum 1984: 412, 422; Segal 1983: 203–04, 206; Holm 1982: 257).

As the discussion above reveals, none of the primary rationales that have been forwarded to exclude women from combat roles provides a legitimate basis for maintaining the current restrictions on women's participation in combat. The analysis of these rationales suggests that the resistance of Congress, the courts, the military, and the public to removing the combat restrictions results more from gender ideology than from demonstrated evidence of women's inability to perform combat roles effectively.

Once outdated stereotypes and myths about women's capabilities and deficiencies are eliminated from consideration of the ethics of women in military combat, the current restrictions on combat roles for women are revealed to lack persuasive foundations. Only when the military begins assigning women to positions on the basis of gender-neutral standards for evaluating the degree of physical strength, psychological fortitude, bonding and troop cohesiveness necessary to perform combat roles can the issue of women in combat be addressed without the undue influence of ideological notions of gender.

NOTES

1. A standard based on physical strength rather than gender could be waived in emergency situations where rapid mobilization is necessary and individual testing would be inefficient (see Segal 1982: 270–71).
2. This policy was reversed in *Crawford v. Cushman*, 531 F.2d 1114 (2d Cir. 1976).

REFERENCES

Association of the Bar of the City of New York, "The Combat Exclusion Laws: An Idea Whose Time Has Gone," *Minerva,* Vol. 9, No. 4 (Winter, 1991), pp. 1–55 (Association).

Barkalow, Carol, *In the Men's House* (New York: Poseidon Press, 1990).

———, "Women Have What It Takes," *Newsweek* (August 5, 1991), pp. 30.

Beecraft, Carolyn, "Personnel Puzzle," *Proceedings (of the U.S. Naval Institute),* Vol. 115, No. 4 (April, 1989), pp. 41–44.

Campbell, D'Ann, "Combatting the Gender Gulf," *Temple Political and Civil Rights Law Review,* Vol. 1, No. 2 (Fall, 1992), *reprinted in Minerva,* Vol. X, Nos. 3–4 (Fall/Winter 1992), pp. 13–41.

Code, Lorraine, *What Can She Know? Feminist Theory and the Construction of Knowledge* (Ithaca, NY: Cornell University Press, 1991).

Cornum, Rhonda, *She Went to War: The Rhonda Cornum Story* (Novato, CA: Presidio Press, 1992).

Costin, Lela, "Feminism, Pacifism, Nationalism, and the United Nations Decade for Women," in Judith Stiehm (ed.), *Women and Men's Wars* (Oxford: Pergamon Press, 1983), pp. 301–16.

Coyle, Commander Barry, U.S. Navy, "Women on the Front Lines," *Proceedings (of the U.S. Military Institute),* Vol. 115, No. 4 (April, 1989), pp. 37–40.

Cramsie, Jodie, "Gender Discrimination in the Military: The Unconstitutional Exclusion of Women From Combat," *Valparaiso Law Review,* Vol. 17 (1983), pp. 547–88.

D'Amico, "Women at Arms: The Combat Controversy," *Minerva,* Vol. 8, No. 2 (1990), pp. 1–19.

Devilbliss, M. C., "Gender Integration and Unit Deployment: A Study of G.I. Jo," *Armed Forces and Society,* Vol. 11, No. 3 (1985), pp. 523–52.

Dillingham, Wayne, "The Possibility of American Military Women Becoming Prisoners of War: Justification for Combat Exclusion Rules?" *Federal Bar News and Journal,* Vol. 37, No. 4 (1990), pp. 223–30.

Enloe, Cynthia, *The Morning After: Sexual Politics at the End of the Cold War* (Berkeley, CA: University of California Press, 1993).

Gabriel, Richard, *To Serve With Honor: A Treatise on Military Ethics and the Way of the Soldier* (Westport, CT: Greenwood Press, 1982).

Goldman, Nancy Loring (ed.), *Female Soldiers—Combatants or Noncombatants? Historical and Contemporary Perspectives* (Westport, CT: Greenwood Press, 1982) (Goldman 1982a).

———, *The Utilization of Women in Combat: An Historical and Social Analysis of Twentieth-Century Wartime and Peacetime Experience* (Alexandria, VA: U.S.A.R.I., 1982b).

Golightly, Lieutenant Neil L., U.S. Navy, "No Right to Fight," *Proceedings (of the U.S. Naval Institute),* Vol. 113, No. 12 (1987), pp. 46–49.

Gooch, Master Chief Sonar Technician Robert H., U.S. Navy, "The Coast Guard Example," *Proceedings (of the U.S. Naval Institute),* Vol. 114, No. 5 (May, 1988), pp. 124–33.

Gordon, Marilyn and Mary Jo Ludvigson, "A Constitutional Analysis of the Combat Exclusion for Air Force Women," *Minerva: Quarterly Report on Women and the Military,* Vol. 9, No. 2 (1991), pp. 1–34.

Hackworth, Colonel David, "War and the Second Sex," *Newsweek* (August 5, 1991), pp. 24–28.

Holm, Maj. Gen. Jeanne, U.S.A.F. (Ret.), *Women in the Military* (Novato, CA: Presidio Press, 1982).

Hooker, Richard, "Affirmative Action and Combat Exclusion: Gender Roles in the U.S. Army," *Parameters: U.S. War College Quarterly,* Vol. 19, No. 4 (1989), pp. 36–50.

Hunter, Anne E. (ed.), *Genes and Gender VI: On Peace, War, and Gender: A Challenge to Genetic Explanations* (New York: Feminist Press, 1991).

Johnson, Cecil, et al., *Women Content in the Army: REFORGER (REFWAC 77)* (Alexandria, VA: U.S.A.R.I., 1978).

Kantrowitz, Barbara, "The Right to Fight," *Newsweek* (August 5, 1991), pp. 22–23.

Karst, Kenneth, "The Pursuit of Manhood and the Desegregation of the Armed Forces," *U.C.L.A. Law Review,* Vol. 38, No. 3 (1991), pp. 499–581.

Kelly, Karla, "The Exclusion of Women From Combat: Withstanding the Challenge," *Judge Advocate General Journal,* Vol. 33, No. 1 (1984), pp. 77–108.

Kornblum, Lori, "Women Warriors in a Men's World: The Combat Exclusion," *Law and Inequality,* Vol. 2 (1984), pp. 351–445.

Lancaster, John, *Washington Post* (January 13, 1994), pp. A1, A7.

Lieberman, Jeanne, "Women in Combat," *Federal Bar News and Journal,* Vol. 37, No. 4 (1990), pp. 215–22.

Marlowe, David, "The Manning of the Force and the Structure of Battle: Part 2—Men and Women," in Robert Fullinwider (ed.), *Conscripts and Volunteers: Military Requirements, Social Justice, and the All-Volunteer Force* (Totowa, NJ: Rowman & Allanheld, 1983), pp. 189–99.

Marqit, Doris and Erwin Marquit, "Gender Differentiation, Genetic Determinism, and the Struggle for Peace," in Anne E. Hunter (ed.), *Genes and Gender VI: On Peace, War, and Gender: A Challenge to Genetic Explanations* (New York: Feminist Press, 1991), pp. 151–62.

McDowell, Jeanne, "Are Women Better Cops?" *Time* (February 17, 1992), pp. 70–72.

Mitchell, Brian, *The Weak Link: The Feminization of the American Military* (Washington, DC: Regnery Gateway, 1989).

Moskos, Charles, "Female GI's in the Field," *Society,* Vol. 22, No. 6 (1985), pp. 28–33 (Moskos 1985).

———, "Army Women," *Atlantic Monthly,* Vol. 266, No. 2 (August, 1990), pp. 70–78 (Moskos 1990).

———, "How Do They Do It? *The New Republic* (August 5, 1991), pp. 16–20 (Moskos 1991).

Nabors, Major Robert, "Women in the Army: Do They Measure Up?" *Military Review* (October, 1982), pp. 50–61.

Newsweek Staff, "Women in the Armed Forces," *Newsweek,* Vol. 95 (February 18, 1980), pp. 34–42.

"No Right to Fight?" *Proceedings (of the U.S. Naval Institute),* Vol. 114, No. 5 (May, 1988), pp. 134–39.

Pine, Art, "Women Will Get Limited Combat Roles," *Los Angeles Times* (January 14, 1994), p. A5.

Proxmire, Senator William, "Three Myths About Women and Combat," *Minerva,* Vol. 4, No. 4 (Winter, 1986), pp. 105–19.

Rogan, Helen, *Mixed Company: Women in the Modern Army* (New York: G.P. Putnams Sons, 1981).

Rosoff, Betty, "Genes, Hormones, and War," in Hunter (ed.), *Genes and Gender VI: On Peace, War, and Gender: A Challenge to Genetic Explanations* (New York: Feminist Press, 1991), pp. 39–49.

Roush, Paul, "Combat Exclusion: Military Necessity or Another Name For Bigotry?" *Minerva,* Vol. 13, No. 3 (Fall, 1990), pp. 1–15.

Schmitt, Eric, "Generals Oppose Combat by Women" *Newsweek* (June 17, 1994a) pp. A1, A18.

Schmitt, Eric, "Army Will Allow Women in 32,000 Combat Posts" *New York Times* (July 28, 1994b), p. A5.

Segal, Mady Wechsler, "The Argument for Female Combatants," in Goldman (ed.), *Female Soldiers—Combatants or Noncombatants? Historical and Contemporary Perspectives* (Westport, CT: Greenwood Press, 1982), pp. 267–90 (Segal 1982).

———, "Women's Roles in the U.S. Armed Forces: An Evaluation of Evidence and Arguments for Policy Decisions," in Robert Fullinwider (ed.), *Conscripts and Volunteers: Military Requirements, Social Justice, and the All-Volunteer Force* (Totowa, NJ: Rowman & Allanheld, 1983), pp. 200–13 (Segal 1983).

Shields, Patricia, "Sex Roles in the Military," in Charles Moskos and Frank Wood (eds.), *The Military—More Than Just a Job?* (Washington, DC: Pergamon Basseys, 1988), pp. 99–111.

Stiehm, Judith Hicks, "Women's Biology and the U.S. Military," in Virginia Sapiro (ed.), *Women, Biology, and Public Policy* (Beverly Hills: SAGE Publications, 1985), pp. 205–32 (Stiehm 1985a).

———, "Generations of U.S. Enlisted Women," *Signs: Journal of Women in Culture and Society,* Vol. 11, No. 1 (1985), pp. 155–75 (Stiehm 1985b).

———, *Arms and the Enlisted Woman* (Philadelphia: Temple University Press, 1989) (Stiehm 1989).

Sunday, Suzanne R., "Biological Theories of Animal Aggression," in Hunter (ed.), *Genes and Gender VI: On Peace, War, and Gender: A Challenge to Genetic Explanations* (New York: Feminist Press, 1991), pp. 50–63.

Treadwell, Mattie, *The Women's Army Corps,* in *World War II Special Studies,* Vol. 8 (Washington, DC: Office of the Chief of Military History of the Army, 1954).

Tuten, Jeff, "The Argument Against Female Combatants," in Goldman (ed.), *Female Soldiers—Combatants or Noncombatants? Historical and Contemporary Perspectives* (Westport, CT: Greenwood Press, 1982), pp. 237–66.

United States Army Research Institute, *Women Content in Units Force Deployment Test (MAXWAC)* (Alexandria, VA: U.S.A.R.I., 1977).

United States Senate, Hearings before the Committee on Appropriations, DOD Appropriations, 102d Cong., 1st Sess., H.R. 2521, Pts. 4 & 6, *Utilization of Women in the Military Services* (Washington, DC: Government Printing Office, 1991) (Appropriations Hearings).

Van Creveld, Martin, "Why Israel Doesn't Send Women into Combat," *Parameters,* Vol. 23, No. 1 (Spring, 1993), pp. 5–9.

Webster, Alexander, "Paradigms of the Contemporary American Soldier and Women in the Military," *Strategic Review* (Summer 1991), pp. 22–30.

THE CASE FOR SOCIAL MATERNITY: ADOPTION OF CHILDREN BY URBAN BAULE WOMEN

Mona Etienne

In interpreting the adoption of children by urban Baule women of the Ivory Coast,[1] I will focus on such transactions in parenthood as evidence that maternity, like paternity is social as well as natural.[2] In analyzing the data, I will also try to emphasize the ways in which Baule women behave as autonomous social agents, controlling their own destiny—and often determining that of others. I suggest that this autonomy, like the adoption phenomenon itself, is not specific to the contemporary postcolonial urban context, but is rooted in precolonial Baule society.

That history and structure can be summarized as follows:

Colonized in the late nineteenth century and conquered only in the early twentieth, Baule society could hardly be characterized as "egalitarian," in the reductive sense, but there was no centralized political authority and there were no clear-cut principles of stratification, certainly no class structure. Early administrators were impressed by the independent spirit of the Baule in general and by what one described as "the preponderant role of women."[3] The Baule were primarily farmers and land was accessible to all, a woman normally farming in partnership with a man, typically her husband, *and having rights to the surplus production of specific crops.*

Craft production, trade, and gold-prospecting were major sources of wealth. In all of these activities, the woman had her share, both of the labor and of the profits.[4]

Physical warfare was the province of men, but it was supported by a women's ritual that constituted magical warfare. It is said that men who went to war against the will of village women would die in combat.

Political authority was limited, only magicoreligious sanctions were in effect, but such authority as existed was vested in women as well as men; there is ample evidence that the almost total disappearance of women chiefs was due to colonization. The one clear indication of a limit on women's access to positions of authority is the principle of virilocality. A married woman normally resided in her husband's household and this prevented her from being household head or kin group elder. Baule society was not however strongly gerontocratic. There was leeway for the acquisition of wealth by all adults. Differential wealth and status were made possible both by individual enterprise and by the access an individual had to the labor of dependents—mainly children, junior kin and captives.

A head of household or kin group elder had more ready access to the labor of dependents than others. There is however clear evidence that even within her husband's household a woman could have her own dependents and profit by their labor. Besides her daughters, she could also have captives of her own, along with junior female kin living and working with her. Junior members of a woman's kin group were acquired more or less definitively by fosterage or adoption. There was in fact an established custom whereby a married woman who went to reside with her husband was accompanied by a sister, a classificatory sister or a classificatory daughter, who remained with her if she had no daughter of her own at the time of marriage.

Although this usage can be seen to reflect a concern with maintaining a married woman's kin ties, my data also suggest the

From *Dialectical Anthropology* 4:237–242, 1979. Reprinted by permission of Kluwer Academic Publishers.

concern with a woman's having her own personal dependent, a child of her own, *who is not shared with the husband,* and also a concern with maintaining precise interindividual bonds with the mother, aunt or older sister who gives her the child.

Baule marriage is marked by brideservice and symbolic gifts of consumable goods; there is no bridewealth that gives a father and paternal kin undisputed rights in children.

Descent is cognatic with matrilineal emphasis,[5] and, although there are some rules governing the relationship between a child and its maternal and paternal kin, conflicting rights in children tend to make the option of the mother herself decisive. This shows up in adoption transactions although consent of the father is required.

It is perhaps significant that in pre-colonial Baule society, where pawning of persons existed, only maternal kin, including the mother herself, could pawn a child.

Another pertinent aspect of Baule society is that, although natural maternity, like natural paternity, is highly valued, sterility does not carry with it the onus described for some other African societies and sterility does not justify divorce. To be alone, without children, without dependents, is the saddest of conditions. It is also a threat for the future, since children are a guarantee of security in old age. Rights in children, however, are not determined by reproductive capacity alone. As I shall explain, sterility can even be a positive advantage for the urban woman.

Since early colonization, Baule women have been migrating to urban centers. Although some come to town as wives of male migrants, many come as single women, on their own initiative. Their principal motivation is to seek wealth and status. For the most part, urban migrants maintain active ties with the village; and status is a function not only of wealth, but of the network of social relations wealth facilitates and is facilitated by. To return to the village well-dressed and with gifts is essential. To build a house there, even though one may never live in it, is a much sought-after goal. To leave an inheritance that will make for an important funeral and remembrance after death is an ultimate achievement. Without people, however, without dependents who will live in the house, carry out the funeral, take the inheritance, speak your name after death, wealth is futile. To fulfill these needs, children, whether natural or social are indispensable, just as they are indispensable to constitute the wealth itself and to build relationships in the present and the future.

It is necessary here to indicate the ways in which illiterate women acquire wealth in town. To a certain extent they try to appropriate the advantage of men, who have greater access to the cash economy. Baule women are rarely prostitutes in the European sense, but they may try to profit by their sexual relationships or enter into temporary marriages with a man who is at least generous enough to assume all household expenses and make occasional gifts, leaving the woman free to trade and keep her profits. A woman who has established herself in petty trade can eventually maintain both herself and dependents without a man's support. Women who are unsuccessful return to the village, often with the hope of trying again. For reasons that I shall not elaborate on here, fertility is often an obstacle to urbanization. Pregnancy favors a return to the village, that, with further pregnancy, may become definitive. It is therefore not surprising that successful urban women tend to be sterile or of low fertility.

In addition to property in the village, these women acquire their own urban compounds and can maintain dependents who consolidate their ties with the village and eventually serve their interests in many ways. They have the advantage of being able to acquire children either temporarily or permanently when the most burdensome period of motherhood is past, at an age where a child starts to become an asset rather than a liability, and at a moment in their own lives when they are economically capable of taking responsibility for a child. Sterile women are also preferential candidates as adoptive mothers because the adoptee will not be in competition with natural children.

Transfers of parental rights and obligations range from minimal to maximal and can involve children and partners of both sexes and of varying degrees of kinship, as well as non-kin and, sometimes, non-Baule. Rather than review all of these variables and the combinations in which they appear, I will describe the different forms of transfer briefly and then focus on quasi-total transfer, or *adoption*, with women as the principal participants. (Rural to urban is today the preferential direction of adoption. Although urbanization may have intensified transfers of children, it is also possible that the lower incidence of rural to rural transfers may be only a recent phenomenon, a result of the draining toward the city of children who would formerly have been transferred between rural kin.)

Clear-cut cases of temporary transfer always refer to a specific reason. A child may be sent to a guardian or foster parent for schooling or as a temporary household aid. When these transfers take place between distant kin or non-kin, the child is often treated as a servant. As in all rural-urban transfers there is nevertheless the idea that the child, even when taken on as a household aide and treated as a servant, is receiving an education in the ways of the city and thus a chance at success. Children themselves may enter into such relationships on their own initiative. Baule children, in any case, *are not forced into such fosterage situations against their will,* nor are they exploited in the sole interest of their parents. These transfers may however relieve the burden on a fertile and economically disadvantaged family and, at the same time, create ties with the city that can serve in the future.

A child may also be sent on a temporary basis to remain with an older sister or other close kin for a specified period of time or for a given task, for example to help after childbirth. This kind of transfer is, to a certain extent, part of the normal rights and obligations of close kin. If however the arrangement has not been precise enough or the foster parent begs time and again to keep the child a little longer and the child wants to remain, the ensuing relationship may be interpreted after the fact as a case of adoption, the foster mother ultimately assuming all the rights and obligations of an adoptive mother.

Cases in which the child is given simply to go with the woman, to accompany her, are the object of contradictory interpretations by informants, who refer sometimes to the closeness of kinship, sometimes to the age of the child as criteria of whether there is fosterage or adoption. Again the nature of the transfer will often be defined *a posteriori.*

In the clear-cut case of adoption, the child is given with the words "This is your own child," "Take this child for yourself," or even "Here is a child to put in your belly." Ideally the adopted is a baby and may even be promised before birth, although the actual transfer will take place only after weaning, sometimes very much later. In this type of transfer, the emphasis is on the relationship between the natural and the adoptive parent. In the case of close kin such as sisters, beyond the obligations they normally have to each other and to each other's children, the gift of a child is supposed to mark something extra, a special bond of affection. But a child can also be given to a more distant kinswoman, an affine, or even a stranger "to show that you love her." Here any suggestion that the child may be considered a burden, and given for that reason is inadmissible. When a fertile woman gives a child to a sterile woman or an older woman who has no young children, the gift is seen in terms of generosity and sharing. It would be selfish to do otherwise.

The fact remains that adoption here serves to adjust the imbalance of natural maternity. It may also serve to adjust the imbalance between natural maternity and a woman's desire to raise children, either at a given moment in her life or in general. Although all women are supposed to desire their children, the Baule recognize an unequal distribution of both the penchant, and the talent for active motherhood. Some women receive many children in adoption because they are considered to raise children well, while others systematically give their children to sisters or mothers because they simply do not like raising children.

If these cases make it appear that, in spite of the ideology, adoption serves to get rid of unwanted or excess children, many others appear to confirm the ideology and reveal the importance of the bond between natural and adoptive parents. A much-desired first-born, often promised before birth, may be given to an adoptive mother as proof of the natural mother's special affection for her. This can occur as a form of indirect exchange following a previous adoption. When a young woman has been given a younger sister to accompany her in marriage, she may later give her first-born to this adoptive daughter. Where this is not possible, because the original adoptive mother is old or sterile, one finds reinforcement and perpetuation of the original bond by duplication: An adoptee, as proof of her affection for her adoptive mother, is supposed to replace herself when she leaves to marry, ideally by the gift of her first-born. Not to offer a child to one's adoptive mother is a way of saying that the adoptee does not love her, is not happy with the way she was raised. In one case of a very old woman I found duplication of adoption over several generations.

In true adoption, life-long rights and obligations of the natural parent are transferred. An adoptive mother will assume all expenses for the child in health and in illness, perhaps send her/him to school; and she can authorize marriage without consulting the natural parents. The adult adoptee will maintain ties with the adoptive parent, returning to her in case of divorce of difficulty, caring for her in old age, eventually burying her, and possibly becoming her heir.

Ties with the natural parents are not, however, broken. A child adopted in babyhood must be taught who its natural parents are, and incest prohibitions are defined through them. They receive visits and gifts from the child, and they must be informed, if not consulted, when the child is married.[6]

It is particularly interesting, however, that, juridically at least, the bond between adoptee and adoptive parent is in some ways stronger than the bond between a child and its natural parents. As noted, Baule children have considerable autonomy and often leave home on their own. If a child insists, the natural parent cannot object. The bond between adoptee and adoptive parent, however, has the character of a sacred gift. The child must not leave, especially to return to the natural parents. If she/he does, both natural and adoptive parents must do everything possible to see that the child returns. To act otherwise would suggest that the former want to take the child back and the latter want to return it. A child will, of course, especially in cases of extreme mistreatment, sometimes return to its natural parents; but this is never accomplished easily or without conflict and bad feelings.

While there are such cases of returned children, there are also others in which women who give their first-born in adoption subsequently have no other children and are in dire straits for lack of a child helper. In such cases, the child may be sent temporarily to help the natural mother, but there can be neither a request nor an offer that she/he be given back permanently.

In another sense, the rights of an adoptive parent are stronger than those of natural parents. As suggested previously, in natural parenthood, rights in the child are considered to be shared between mother and father, although mother-right is stronger, especially in the case of girl children and babies of both sexes. The adoptive parent, however, who is most often a woman, receives the child in her name only. Her husband, if she has one, may sometimes create ties with the child by contributing to its welfare, but the transfer itself gives rights only to the woman. The adoptive mother therefore acquires, even within her husband's household, a child that is hers alone, that materializes her personal bond with the child's natural family, and, if she raises the child to successful adulthood, guarantees her future security.

Transactions involving males follow, as might be expected, similar rules.[7] Whereas a girl is traditionally considered the appropriate adoptive child for a woman because of the sexual division of labor, and women still adopt more girls for their labor value and for rights in their future children, a boy who is sent to school may become part of the urban educated elite, even the modern political power structure. If this happens, he will not forget his adoptive mother—or his natural parents. Particularly foresighted women therefore tend to give and receive a certain number of boy children as urban adoptees. Further, in spite of the generally stronger rights of mothers and maternal kin, precisely the most prestigious urban women frequently receive adoptive children both through male kin and on the initiative of fathers themselves.

These cases are important, because they show that networks constituted by urban women through adoption are not strictly female networks. Rather, while they appear to be female-dominated, they include male elements. Here the adoption data correlate with my observations of compounds, where one finds men as well as women among the urban woman's constituency of dependents.[8]

Let me note finally that further exploration of similar material will contribute to undermining the assumption that, whereas paternity is eminently social, maternity is irrevocably natural. The biological fact that only women give birth to children is seen by some as the theoretical key to male dominance—dominance that is perhaps too easily considered to be amply demonstrated by the empirical data. At the same time, the tendency of male-centered anthropology to assume that, when women's reproductive capacity is controlled or manipulated, the agents of this social action are necessarily men, is but another instance of the more general tendency to see only men as social actors. Thus the empirical data feed back into the theoretical orientation that posits the universal subordination of women.

When a contemporary theorist who has also done fieldwork in Africa—I am referring here to Meillassoux—says: "Woman, in spite of her irreplaceable function in reproduction, never intervenes as a vector of social organization. She disappears behind the man; her father, her brother, her husband"[9] we must ask ourselves to what extent the theory accounts for the reality of other societies, and its incarnation in an anthropology that makes women disappear behind fathers, brothers and husbands. I believe that only systematic attempts to make women visible, to determine whether in fact they do or do not appear as vectors of social organization, can begin to answer this question. And if they do, as among the Baule, what are the occasions for their visibility and their autonomy?

NOTES

1. This is a paper presented at the 76th annual meeting of the American Anthropological Association, Houston, Texas, 1977. An extended version of this article will be published in French: *L'Homme,* XIX (3/4, Juin/ Décembre, 1979). Data are based on 1962–63 fieldwork among rural Baule, supported by the Ivory Coast government (Ministère de Plan) in the context of the Bouaké Regional Study (Etude régionale de Bouaké), and on 1974–75 fieldwork among urban Baule of Abidjan, supported by Grant No. 3067 from the Wenner-Gren Foundation. I thank the Ivory Coast Ministère de la Recherche Scientifique and the Institut d'Ethnologie of the University of Abidjan for authorizing 1974–75 research, and the Institut de Linguistique for use of audio equipment.
2. See Nicole-Claude Mathieu, "Paternité biologique, maternité sociale," in Andrée Michel (ed.). *Femmes, sexisme et société.* (Paris: Presses universitaires de France, 1977), pp. 39–48. A critique of male bias in anthropological views of reproduction, this article strongly influenced not only the present analysis, but also my 1974–75 fieldwork. Written in 1974, it explicitly suggests adoption as one insufficiently explored object of research and as a "sign of the social manipulation of biological engendering" ("signe de la manipulation sociale de l'engendrement biologique", pp. 43–44).

3. ". . . le rôle prépondérant des femmes . . .", p. 139 in J. F. Bouet, "Quelques opérations militaires á la Côte d'Ivoire en 1909," *Revue des troupes coloniales,* IX (1910), 2ème sem., pp. 134–153. Early observers are unanimous in noting the high status of Baule women.
4. Concerning women's control of cloth, an important item in long-distance trade, see Mona Etienne. "Women and Men, Cloth and Colonization: The Transformation of Production—Distribution Relations among the Baule (Ivory Coast)", *Cahiers d'Etude Africaines,* vol. 65, XVII (1), (1977), pp. 41–64.
5. Baule kinship nomenclature is of the "generation" or "Hawaiian" type. The correlation of institutionalized adoption with this type of nomenclature and cognatic descent is frequently noted, usually with reference to non-African societies and especially Polynesia. For excellent case studies, see Vern Carroll (ed.), *Adoption in Eastern Oceania* (Hawaii: University of Hawaii Press, 1970). The only serious exploration of the subject by an Africanist is Esther Goody, "Some Theoretical and Empirical Aspects of Parenthood in West Africa," in C. Oppong, G. Adaba et al. (eds.), *Marriage, Fertility and Parenthood in West Africa* (Papers from the XVth Seminar of the International Sociological Association Committee on Family Research, Lomé, Togoland, January 1976). Changing African Family No. 4, Canberra: Australian National University; n.d., pp. 227–271.
6. An adoptee's relationship to the ancestors is determined by birth and must be maintained. In disagreement with Goody (*op. cit.*) and in accord with the Oceanists (Carroll, *op. cit.*), I use the term "adoption", in spite of its different connotations in our own society, to mark the specificity of a form of transfer significantly distinct from those that can be called "fosterage".
7. Of the three positions involved in a transfer: giver, adoptee and recipient, males appear least frequently as recipients in true adoption, although they often receive older children in fosterage, especially for schooling. The raising of young children is woman's work and creates strong emotional ties. The giver would not want such ties to develop with an unrelated woman (the wife of the recipient) and eventually cause problems in case of divorce.
8. During my 1974–75 fieldwork, the suggestions of Naomi Quinn, "Asking The Right Question: A Re-examination of Akan Residence," Wm. M. O'Barr, David H. Spain and Mark Tessler (eds.), *Survey Research in Africa* (Evanston, IL: Northwestern University Press, 1973), pp. 168–183, proved invaluable in establishing relationships of dependency in general and adoption in particular. The questions, "By whom is she/he here?" and "Who takes care of (is responsible for) her/him?" applied to all inhabitants of each compound studied, revealed relationships that genealogical and "head of household" bias would have obscured. For example, a woman residing in her brother's compound could be the autonomous head of a subgroup, a child residing in the same compound as its mother could be the adoptee of another woman.
9. ". . . la femme, malgré sa fonction irremplaçcable dans la reproduction, n'intervient jamais comme vecteur de l'organisation sociale. Elle disparait derrière l'homme: son père, son frère ou son époux." See Claude Meillassoux, *Femmes, Greniers et Capitaux* (Paris: Maspéro, 1975), p. 116. It is interesting that Meillassoux and Marvin Harris give explanations of "male dominance" that are diametrically opposed, but founded on similar assumptions. For Meillassoux (*op. cit.*), women become subordinate with the development of horticulture because their reproductive capacity is *so valuable* to societies that rely on increased population to increase production; for Harris, male dominance emerges in the first moments in human history because women's reproductive capacity is *so dangerous* to a world threatened by overpopulation. (see "Why Men Dominate Women," *The New York Times Magazine,* November 13, 1977, p. 46ss., and W. T. Divale and M. Harris, "Population, Warfare and the Male Supremacist Complex," *American Anthropologist,* vol. 78, no. 3 (1976), pp. 521–538.)

   Both theorists assume that men are the social actors, that men manipulate women's reproductive capacity but women do not (even in infanticide!). It must be noted to Meillassoux's credit that he does attempt to explain why men are the actors and women the objects in the earliest struggle to control their child-bearing potential; but his argument begs the question, reifying women to explain their reification. It belongs to the realm of anthropological mythology and, if one accepts the ground rules, could easily be converted into its opposite, an argument for matriarchy.

LIFEBOAT ETHICS: MOTHER LOVE AND CHILD DEATH IN NORTHEAST BRAZIL

Nancy Scheper–Hughes

I have seen death without weeping.
The destiny of the Northeast is death.
Cattle they kill.
To the people they do something worse.
—Anonymous Brazilian singer (1965)

"Why do the church bells ring so often?" I asked Nailza de Arruda soon after I moved into a corner of her tiny mud-walled hut near the top of the shantytown called the Alto do Cruzeiro (Crucifix Hill). I was then a Peace Corps volunteer and a community development/health worker. It was the dry and blazing hot summer of 1965, the months following the military coup in Brazil, and save for the rusty, clanging bells, of N. S. das Dores Church, an eerie quiet had settled over the market town that I call Bom Jesus da Mata. Beneath the quiet, however, there was chaos and panic. "It's nothing," replied Nailza, "just another little angel gone to heaven."

Nailza had sent more than her share of little angels to heaven, and sometimes at night I could hear her engaged in a muffled but passionate discourse with one of them, two-year-old Joana. Joana's photograph, taken as she lay propped up in her tiny cardboard coffin, her eyes open, hung on a wall next to one of Nailza and Ze Antonio taken on the day they eloped.

Nailza could barely remember the other infants and babies who came and went in close succession. Most had died unnamed and were hastily baptized in their coffins. Few lived more than a month or two. Only Joana, properly baptized in church at the close of her first year and placed under the protection of a powerful saint, Joan of Arc, had been expected to live. And Nailza had dangerously allowed herself to love the little girl.

Reprinted with permission from *Natural History* 98(10): 8–16, 1989.

In addressing the dead child, Nailza's voice would range from tearful imploring to angry recrimination: "Why did you leave me? Was your patron saint so greedy that she could not allow me one child on this earth?" Ze Antonio advised me to ignore Nailza's odd behavior, which he understood as a kind of madness that, like the birth and death of children, came and went. Indeed, the premature birth of a stillborn son some months later "cured" Nailza of her "inappropriate" grief, and the day came when she removed Joana's photo and carefully packed it away.

More than fifteen years elapsed before I returned to the Alto do Cruzeiro, and it was anthropology that provided the vehicle of my return. Since 1982 I have returned several times in order to pursue a problem that first attracted my attention in the 1960s. My involvement with the people of the Alto do Cruzeiro now spans a quarter of a century and three generations of parenting in a community where mothers and daughters are often simultaneously pregnant.

The Alto do Cruzeiro is one of three shantytowns surrounding the large market town of Bom Jesus in the sugar plantation zone of Pernambuco in Northeast Brazil, one of the many zones of neglect that have emerged in the shadow of the now tarnished economic miracle of Brazil. For the women and children of the Alto do Cruzeiro the only miracle is that some of them have managed to stay alive at all.

The Northeast is a region of vast proportions (approximately twice the size of Texas) and of equally vast social and developmental problems. The nine states that make up the region are the poorest in the country and are representative of the Third World within a dynamic and rapidly industrializing nation. Despite waves of migrations from the interior to the teeming shantytowns of coastal cities, the majority still live in rural areas on farms and ranches, sugar plantations and mills.

Life expectancy in the Northeast is only forty years, largely because of the appallingly high rate of infant and child mortality. Approximately one million children in Brazil under the age of five die each year. The children of the Northeast, especially those born in shantytowns on the periphery of urban life, are at a very high risk of death. In these areas, children are born without the traditional protection of breast-feeding, subsistence gardens, stable marriages, and multiple adult caretakers that exists in the interior. In the hillside shantytowns that spring up around cities or, in this case, interior market towns, marriages are brittle, single parenting is the norm, and women are frequently forced into the shadow economy of domestic work in the homes of the rich or into unprotected and oftentimes "scab" wage labor on the surrounding sugar plantations, where they clear land for planting and weed for a pittance, sometimes less than a dollar a day. The women of the Alto may not bring their babies with them into the homes of the wealthy, where the often-sick infants are considered sources of contamination, and they cannot carry the little ones to the riverbanks where they wash clothes because the river is heavily infested with schistosomes and other deadly parasites. Nor can they carry their young children to the plantations, which are often several miles away. At wages of a dollar a day, the women of the Alto cannot hire baby sitters. Older children who are not in school will sometimes serve as somewhat indifferent caretakers. But any child not in school is also expected to find wage work. In most cases, babies are simply left at home alone, the door securely fastened. And so many also die alone and unattended.

Bom Jesus da Mata, centrally located in the plantation zone of Pernambuco, is within commuting distance of several sugar plantations and mills. Consequently, Bom Jesus has been a magnet for rural workers forced off their small subsistence plots by large landowners wanting to use every available piece of land for sugar cultivation. Initially, the rural migrants to Bom Jesus were squatters who were given tacit approval by the mayor to put up temporary straw huts on each of the three hills overlooking the town. The Alto do Cruzeiro is the oldest, the largest, and the poorest of the shantytowns. Over the past three decades many of the original migrants have become permanent residents, and the primitive and temporary straw huts have been replaced by small homes (usually of two rooms) made of wattle and daub, sometimes covered with plaster. The more affluent residents use bricks and tiles. In most Alto homes, dangerous kerosene lamps have been replaced by light bulbs. The once tattered rural garb, often fashioned from used sugar sacking, has likewise been replaced by store-bought clothes, often castoffs from a wealthy *patrão* (boss). The trappings are modern, but the hunger, sickness, and death that they conceal are traditional, deeply rooted in a history of feudalism, exploitation, and institutionalized dependency.

My research agenda never wavered. The questions I addressed first crystallized during a veritable "die-off" of Alto babies during a severe drought in 1965. The food and water shortages and the political and economic chaos occasioned by the military coup were reflected in the handwritten entries of births and deaths in the dusty, yellowed pages of the ledger books kept at the public registry office in Bom Jesus. More than 350 babies died in the Alto during 1965 alone—this from a shantytown population of little more than 5,000. But that wasn't what surprised me. There were reasons enough for the deaths in the miserable conditions of shantytown life. What puzzled me was the seeming indifference of Alto women to the death of their infants, and their willingness to attribute to their own tiny offspring an aversion to life that made their death seem wholly natural, indeed all but anticipated.

Although I found that it was possible, and hardly difficult, to rescue infants and toddlers from death by diarrhea and dehydration with a simple sugar, salt, and water solution (even bottled Coca-Cola worked fine), it was more difficult to enlist a mother herself in the rescue of a child she perceived as ill-fated for life or better off dead, or to convince her to take back into her threatened and besieged home a baby she had already come to think of as an angel rather than as a son or daughter.

I learned that the high expectancy of death, and the ability to face child death with stoicism and equanimity, produced patterns of nurturing that differentiated between those infants thought of as thrivers and survivors and those thought of as born already "wanting to die." The survivors were nurtured, while stigmatized, doomed infants were left to die, as mothers say, *a mingua,* "of neglect." Mothers stepped back and allowed nature to take its course. This pattern, which I call mortal selective neglect, is called passive infanticide by anthropologist Marvin Harris. The Alto situation, although culturally specific in the form that it takes, is not unique to Third World shantytown communities and may have its correlates in our own impoverished urban communities in some cases of "failure to thrive" infants.

I use as an example the story of Zezinho, the thirteen-month-old toddler of one of my neighbors, Lourdes. I became involved with Zezinho when I was called in to help Lourdes in the delivery of another child, this one a fair and robust little tyke with a lusty cry. I noted that while Lourdes showed great interest in the newborn, she totally ignored Zezinho who, wasted and severely malnourished, was curled up in a fetal position on a piece of urine- and feces-soaked cardboard placed under his mother's hammock. Eyes open and vacant, mouth slack, the little boy seemed doomed.

When I carried Zezinho up to the community day-care center at the top of the hill, the Alto women who took turns caring for one another's children (in order to free themselves for part-time work in the cane fields or washing clothes) laughed at my efforts to save Ze, agreeing with Lourdes that here was a baby without a ghost of a chance. Leave him alone, they cautioned. It makes no sense to fight with death. But I did do battle with Ze, and after several weeks of force-feeding (malnourished babies lose their interest in food), Ze began to succumb to my ministrations. He acquired some flesh across his taut chest bones, learned to sit up, and even tried to smile. When he seemed well enough, I returned him to Lourdes in her miserable scrap-material lean-to, but not without guilt about what I had done. I wondered whether returning Ze was at all fair to Lourdes and to his little brother. But I was busy and washed my hands of the matter. And Lourdes did seem more interested in Ze now that he was looking more human.

When I returned in 1982, there was Lourdes among the women who formed my sample of Alto mothers—still struggling to put together some semblance of life for a now grown Ze and her five other surviving children. Much was made of my reunion with Ze in 1982, and everyone enjoyed retelling the story of Ze's rescue and of how his mother had given him up for dead. Ze would laugh the loudest when told how I had had to force-feed him like a fiesta turkey. There was no hint of guilt on the part of Lourdes and no resentment on the part of Ze. In fact, when questioned in private as to who was the best friend he ever had in life, Ze took a long drag on his cigarette and answered without a trace of irony, "Why my mother, of course!" "But of course," I replied.

Part of learning how to mother in the Alto do Cruzeiro is learning when to let go of a child who shows that it "wants" to die or that it has no "knack" or no "taste" for life. Another part is learning when it is safe to let oneself love a child. Frequent child death remains a powerful shaper of maternal thinking and practice. In the absence of firm expectation that a child will survive, mother love as we conceptualize it (whether in popular terms or in the psychobiological notion of maternal bonding) is attenuated and delayed with consequences for infant survival. In an environment already precarious to young life, the emotional detachment of mothers toward some of their babies contributes even further to the spiral of high mortality—high fertility in a kind of macabre lock-step dance to death.

The average woman of the Alto experiences 9.5 pregnancies, 3.5 child deaths, and 1.5 stillbirths. Seventy percent of all child deaths in the Alto occur in the first six months of life, and 82 percent by the end of the first year. Of all deaths in the community each year, about 45 percent are of children under the age of five.

Women of the Alto distinguish between child deaths understood as natural (caused by diarrhea and communicable diseases) and those resulting from sorcery, the evil eye, or other magical or supernatural afflictions. They also recognize a large category of infant deaths seen as fated and inevitable. These hopeless cases are classified by mothers under the folk terminology "child sickness" or "child attack." Women say that there are at least fourteen different types of hopeless child sickness, but most can be subsumed under two categories—chronic and acute. The chronic cases refer to infants who are born small and wasted. They are deathly pale, mothers say, as well as weak and passive. They demonstrate no vital force, no liveliness. They do not suck vigorously; they hardly cry. Such babies can be this way at birth or they can be born sound but soon show no resistance, no "fight" against the common crises of infancy: diarrhea, respiratory infections, tropical fevers.

The acute cases are those doomed infants who die suddenly and violently. They are taken by stealth overnight, often following convulsions that bring on head banging, shaking, grimacing, and shrieking. Women say it is horrible to look at such a baby. If the infant begins to foam at the mouth or gnash its teeth or go rigid with its eyes turned back inside its head, there is absolutely no hope. The infant is "put aside"—left alone—often on the floor in a back room, and allowed to die. These symptoms (which accompany high fevers, dehydration, third-stage malnutrition, and encephalitis) are equated by Alto women with madness, epilepsy, and worst of all, rabies, which is greatly feared and highly stigmatized.

Most of the infants presented to me as suffering from chronic child sickness were tiny, wasted famine victims, while those labeled as victims of acute child attack seemed to be infants suffering from the deliriums of high fever or the convulsions that can accompany electrolyte imbalance in dehydrated babies.

Local midwives and traditional healers, praying women, as they are called, advise Alto women on when to allow a baby to die. One midwife explained: "If I can see that a baby was born unfortuitously, I tell the mother that she need not wash the infant or give it a cleansing tea. I tell her just to dust the infant with baby powder and wait for it to die." Allowing nature to take its course is not seen as sinful by these often very devout Catholic women. Rather, it is understood as cooperating with God's plan.

Often I have been asked how consciously women of the Alto behave in this regard. I would have to say that consciousness is always shifting between allowed and disallowed levels of awareness. For example, I was awakened early one morning in 1987 by two neighborhood children who had been sent to fetch me to a hastily organized wake for a two-month-old infant whose mother I had unsuccessfully urged to breast-feed. The infant was being sustained on sugar water, which the mother referred to as *soro* (serum), using a medical term for the infant's starvation regime in light of his chronic diarrhea. I had cautioned the mother that an infant could not live on *soro* forever.

The two girls urged me to console the young mother by telling her that it was "too bad" that her infant was so weak that Jesus had to take him. They were coaching me in proper Alto etiquette. I agreed, of course, but asked, "And what do *you* think?" Xoxa, the eleven-year-old, looked down at her dusty flip-flops and blurted out, "Oh, Dona Nanci, that baby never got enough to eat, but you must never say that!" And so the death of hungry babies remains one of the best kept secrets of life in Bom Jesus da Mata.

Most victims are waked quickly and with a minimum of ceremony. No tears are shed, and the neighborhood children form a tiny procession, carrying the baby to the town graveyard where it will join a multitude of others. Although a few fresh flowers may be scattered over the tiny grave, no stone or wooden cross will mark the place, and the same spot will be reused within a few months' time. The mother will never visit the grave, which soon becomes an anonymous one.

What, then, can be said of these women? What emotions, what sentiments motivate them? How are they able to do what, in fact, must be done? What does mother love mean in this inhospitable context? Are grief, mourning, and melancholia present, although deeply repressed? If so, where shall we look for them? And if not, how are we to understand the moral visions and moral sensibilities that guide their actions?

I have been criticized more than once for presenting an unflattering portrait of poor Brazilian women, women who are, after all, themselves the victims of severe social and institutional neglect. I have described these women as allowing some of their children to die, as if this were an unnatural and inhuman act rather than, as I would assert, the way any one of us might act, reasonably and rationally, under similarly desperate conditions. Perhaps I have not emphasized enough the real pathogens in this environment of high risk: poverty, deprivation, sexism, chronic hunger, and economic exploitation. If mother love is, as many psychologists and some feminists believe, a seemingly natural and universal maternal script, what does it mean to women for whom scarcity, loss, sickness, and deprivation have made that love frantic and robbed them of their grief, seeming to turn their hearts to stone?

Throughout much of human history—as in a great deal of the impoverished Third World today—women have had to give birth and to nurture children under ecological conditions and social arrangements hostile to child survival, as well as to their own well-being. Under circumstances of high childhood mortality, patterns of selective neglect and passive infanticide may be seen as active survival strategies.

They also seem to be fairly common practices historically and across cultures. In societies characterized by high childhood mortality and by a correspondingly high (replacement) fertility, cultural practices of infant and child care tend to be organized primarily around survival goals. But what this means is a pragmatic recognition that not all of one's children can be expected to live. The nervousness about child survival in areas of northeast Brazil, northern India, or Bangladesh, where a 30 percent or 40 percent mortality rate in the first years of life is common, can lead to forms of delayed attachment and a casual or benign neglect that serves to weed out the worst bets so as to enhance the life chances of healthier siblings, including those yet to be born. Practices similar to those that I am describing have been recorded for parts of Africa, India, and Central America.

Life in the Alto do Cruzeiro resembles nothing so much as a battlefield or an emergency room in an overcrowded innercity public hospital. Consequently, morality is guided by a kind of "lifeboat ethics," the morality of triage. The seemingly studied indifference toward the suffering of some of their infants, conveyed in such sayings as "little critters have no feelings," is understandable in light of these women's obligation to carry on with their reproductive and nurturing lives.

In their slowness to anthropomorphize and personalize their infants, everything is mobilized so as to prevent maternal overattachment and, therefore, grief at death. The bereaved mother is told not to cry, that her tears will dampen the wings of her little angel so that she cannot fly up to her heavenly home. Grief at the death of an angel is not only inappropriate, it is a symptom of madness and of a profound lack of faith.

Infant death becomes routine in an environment in which death is anticipated and bets are hedged. While the routinization of death in the context of shantytown life is not hard to understand, and quite possible to empathize with, its routinization in the formal institutions of public life in Bom Jesus is not as easy to accept uncritically. Here the social production of indifference takes on a different, even a malevolent cast.

In a society where triplicates of every form are required for the most banal events (registering a car, for example), the registration of infant and child death is informal, incomplete, and rapid. It requires no documentation, takes less than five minutes, and demands no witnesses other than office clerks. No questions are asked concerning the circumstances of the death, and the cause of death is left blank, unquestioned and unexamined. A neighbor, grandmother, older sibling, or common-law husband may register the death. Since most infants die at home, there is no question of a medical record.

From the registry office, the parent proceeds to the town hall, where the mayor will give him or her a voucher for a free baby coffin. The full-time municipal coffinmaker cannot tell you exactly how many baby coffins are dispatched each week. It varies, he says, with the seasons. There are more needed during the drought months and during the big festivals of Carnaval and Christmas and São Joao's Day because people are too busy, he supposes, to take their babies to the clinic. Record keeping is sloppy.

Similarly, there is a failure on the part of city-employed doctors working at two free clinics to recognize the malnutrition of babies who are weighed, measured, and immunized without comment and as if they were not, in fact, anemic, stunted, fussy, and irritated starvation babies. At best the mothers are told to pick up free vitamins or a health "tonic" at the municipal chambers. At worst, clinic personnel will give tranquilizers and sleeping pills to quiet the hungry cries of "sick-to-death" Alto babies.

The church, too, contributes to the routinization of, and indifference toward, child death. Traditionally, the local Catholic church taught patience and resignation to domestic tragedies that were said to reveal the imponderable workings of God's will. If an infant died suddenly, it was because a particular saint had claimed the child. The infant would be an angel in the service of his or her heavenly patron. It would be wrong, a sign of a lack of faith, to weep for a child with such good fortune. The infant funeral was, in the past, an event celebrated with joy. Today, however, under the new regime of "liberation theology," the bells of N. S. das Dores parish church no longer peal for the death of Alto babies, and no priest accompanies the procession of angels to the cemetery where their bodies are disposed of casually and without ceremony. Children bury children in Bom Jesus da Mata. In this most Catholic of communities, the coffin is handed to the disabled and irritable municipal gravedigger, who often chides the children for one reason or another. It may be that the coffin is larger than expected and the gravedigger can find no appropriate space. The children do not wait for the gravedigger to complete his task. No prayers are recited and no sign of the cross made as the tiny coffin goes into its shallow grave.

When I asked the local priest, Padre Marcos, about the lack of church ceremony surrounding infant and childhood death today in Bom Jesus, he replied: "In the old days, child death was richly celebrated. But those were the baroque customs of a conservative church that wallowed in death and misery. The new church is a church of hope and joy. We no longer celebrate the death of child angels. We try to tell mothers that Jesus doesn't want all the dead babies they send him." Similarly, the new church has changed its baptismal customs, now often refusing to baptize dying babies brought to the back door of a church or rectory. The mothers are scolded by the church attendants and told to go home and take care of their sick babies. Baptism, they are told, is for the living; it is not to be confused with the sacrament of extreme unction, which is the anointing of the dying. And so it appears to the women of the Alto that even the church has turned away from them, denying the traditional comfort of folk Catholicism.

The contemporary Catholic church is caught in the clutches of a double bind. The new theology of liberation imagines a kingdom of God on earth based on justice and equality, a world without hunger, sickness, or childhood mortality. At the same time, the church has not changed its official position on sexuality and reproduction, including its sanctions against birth control, abortion, and sterilization. The padre of Bom Jesus da Mata recognizes this contradiction intuitively, although he shies away from discussions on the topic, saying that he prefers to leave questions of family planning to the discretion and the "good consciences" of his impoverished parishioners. But this, of course, sidesteps the extent to which those good consciences have been shaped by traditional church teachings in Bom Jesus, especially by his recent predecessors. Hence, we can begin to see that the seeming indifference of Alto mothers toward the death of some of their infants is but a pale reflection of the official indifference of church and state to the plight of poor women and children.

Nonetheless, the women of Bom Jesus are survivors. One woman, Biu, told me her life history, returning again and again to the themes of child death, her first husband's suicide, abandonment by her father and later by her second husband, and all the other losses and disappointments she had suffered in her long forty-five years. She concluded with great force, reflecting on the days of Carnaval '88 that were fast approaching:

> No, Dona Nanci, I won't cry, and I won't waste my life thinking about it from morning to night. . . . Can I argue with God for the state that I'm in? No! And so I'll dance and I'll jump and I'll play Carnaval! And yes, I'll laugh and people will wonder at a *pobre* like me who can have such a good time.

And no one did blame Biu for dancing in the streets during the four days of Carnaval—not even on Ash Wednesday, the day following Carnaval '88 when we all assembled hurriedly to assist in the burial of Mercea, Biu's beloved *casula,* her last-born daughter who had died at home of pneumonia during the festivities. The rest of the family barely had time to change out of their costumes. Severino, the child's uncle and godfather, sprinkled holy water over the little angel while he prayed: "Mercea, I don't know whether you were called, taken, or thrown out of this world. But look down at us from your heavenly home with tenderness, with pity, and with mercy." So be it.

THE CULTURAL NEXUS OF AKA FATHER-INFANT BONDING

Barry S. Hewlett

Despite a steady increase in the quantity and quality of studies of infants, young children and motherhood in various parts of the world (e.g., LeVine et al. 1994), we know relatively little about the nature of father-child relations outside of the U.S. and Western Europe (see Hewlett 1992 for some exceptions). In general, mother-oriented theories of infant and child development have guided cross-cultural research. The majority of these theories view the mother-infant relationship as the prototype for subsequent attachments and relationships (Ainsworth 1967, Bowlby 1969, Freud 1938, and Harlow 1961). According to Freud and Bowlby, for instance, one had to have a trusting, unconditional relationship with his or her mother in order to become a

Adapted for this text from Barry S. Hewlett, *Intimate Fathers: The Nature and Context of Aka Pygmy Paternal-Infant Care* (Ann Arbor: University of Michigan Press, 1991).

socially and emotionally adjusted adult. These influential theorists generally believed that the father's role was not a factor in the child's development until the Oedipal stage (3–5 years old). The field methods to study infancy reflected this theoretical emphasis on mother. Observations were either infant or mother-focused and conducted only during daylight hours; father-focused and evening observations were not considered. Also, standardized questionnaires and psychological tests were generally administered only to the mother. One consistent result from the cross-cultural studies was that fathers provided substantially less direct care to infants than mothers. In fact, all cross-cultural studies to date indicate that a number of other female caretakers (older female siblings, aunts, grandmothers) provide more direct care to infants than do fathers. Since fathers are not as conspicuous as mothers and other females during daylight hours researchers tend to emphasize a "deficit" model of fathers (Cole and Bruner 1974); that is, fathers are not around much and therefore do not contribute much to the child's development.

Given the paucity of systematic research outside of the U.S. on father's interactions with children, it is ironic that this variable (i.e., the degree of father vs. mother involvement with children) should be so consistently invoked as an explanatory factor in the literature. It is hypothesized to be related, for example, to gender inequality (Chodorow 1974), universal sexual asymmetry (Rosaldo and Lamphere 1974), and the origin of the human family (Lancaster 1987).

Father-Infant Bonding

Bowlby's (1969) theory, mentioned above, suggested that an early secure attachment (or "bonding") between infant and caregiver (usually mother) was crucial for normal development. Lack of bonding between mother and infant led to the infant's protest, despair, detachment, and eventual difficulty in emotional and social development. Most studies of attachment have focused on mother-infant bonding, but an increasing number of studies in the U.S. and Europe have tried to understand if and when infants become attached to fathers. Numerous psychological studies now indicate that infants are attached to their fathers and that the infants become attached to fathers at about the same age as they do to mothers (8–10 months of age) (Lamb 1981). But how does this bonding take place if infant bonding to mother is known to develop through regular, sensitive, and responsive care? American fathers are seldom around to provide this type of care. The critical factor that has emerged in over 50 studies of primarily middle-class American fathers is vigorous play. The physical style of American fathers is distinct from that of American mothers, is evident three days after birth, and continues throughout infancy. The American data have been so consistent that some researchers have indicated a biological basis (Clarke-Stewart 1980). The idea is that mother-infant bonding develops as a consequence of the frequency and intensity of the relationship, while father-infant bonding takes place because of this highly stimulating interaction. British, German, and Israeli studies generally support this hypothesis. This chapter examines the process of father-infant bonding among the Aka, a hunter-gatherer group living in the tropical forest of central Africa.

THE AKA

There are about 30,000 Aka hunter-gatherers in the tropical rain forests of southern Central African Republic and northern Congo-Brazzaville. They live in camps of 25–35 people and move camp every two weeks to two months. Each nuclear family has a hut, and each camp generally has 5–8 huts arranged in a circle. The circle of huts is about 12 meters in diameter and each hut is about 1.5 meters in diameter. Each hut has one bed of leaves or logs on which everyone in the family sleeps. The Aka have patriclans and many members of a camp belong to the same patriclan (generally a camp consists of brothers, their wives and children, and unrelated men who are doing bride service for the sisters of the men in camp). The Aka have high fertility and mortality rates: A woman generally has five to six children during her lifetime, and one-fifth of the infants die before reaching 12 months and 43 percent of children die before reaching 15 years.

Life in the camp is rather intimate. While the overall population density is quite low (less than one person per square kilometer), living space is quite dense. Three or four people sleep together on the same 4-feet-long by 2-feet-wide bed, and neighbors are just a few feet away. The 25–35 camp members live in an area about the size of a large American living room. The Aka home represents the "public" part of life, while time outside of camp tends to be relatively "private". This is the reverse of the American pattern (i.e., home is usually considered private). The camp is relatively young as half of the members of the camp are under 15 and most women have a nursing child throughout their childbearing years.

The Aka use a variety of hunting techniques, but net hunting, which involves men, women, and children, is the most important and regular hunting technique. Women generally have the role of tackling the game in the net and killing the animal. Game captured is eventually shared with everyone in camp. Some parts of the game animal are smoked and eventually traded to Bantu and Sudanic farmers for manioc or other domesticated foods. The Aka have strong economic and religious ties to the tropical forest. The forest is perceived as provider and called friend, lover, mother, or father.

Sharing and cooperation are pervasive and general tenets of Aka camp life. Food items, infant care, ideas for song and dance, and material items such as pots and pans are just some of the items that are shared daily in the camp. An Ngandu farmer describes Aka sharing:

> Pygmies [the Ngandu use the derogatory term Babinga to refer to the Aka] are people who stick together. Twenty of them are able to share one single cigarette. When a pygmy comes back with only five roots she shares them all. It is the same with forest nuts; they will give them out to everybody even if there are none left for them. They are very generous.

The Aka are also fiercely egalitarian. They have a number of mechanisms to maintain individual, intergenerational, and gender equality. The Ngandu villager mentioned above describes his concerns about Aka intergenerational egalitarianism:

> Young pygmies have no respect for their parents; they regard their fathers as their friends . . . There is no way to tell whether they are talking to their parents because they always use their first names. Once I was in a pymgy camp and several people were sitting around and a son said to his father "Etobe your balls are hanging out of your loincloth" and everyone started laughing. No respect, none, none, none. . . . It's real chaos because there is no respect between father and son, mother and son or daughter. That's why pygmies have such a bad reputation, a reputation of being backward.

Three mechanisms that promote sharing and egalitarianism are prestige avoidance, rough joking and demand sharing. The Aka try to avoid drawing attention to themselves, even if they have killed an elephant or cured someone's life-threatening illness. Individuals who boast about their abilities are likely to share less or request more from others in the belief that they are better than others. If individuals start to draw attention to themselves, others in the camp will use rough and crude jokes, often about the boastful person's genitals, in order to get the individuals to be more modest about their abilities. Demand sharing also helps to maintain egalitarianism: if individuals like or want something (cigarettes, necklace, shirt) they simply ask for it, and the person generally gives it to them. Demand sharing promotes the circulation of scarce material goods (e.g., shoes, shirt, necklaces, spear points) in the camp.

Gender egalitarianism is also important. For instance, there are male and female roles on the net hunt, but role reversals take place daily and individuals are not stigmatized for taking the roles of the opposite sex. If one does the task poorly, regardless of whether it is a masculine or feminine task, then one is open to joking and teasing by others (e.g., when the anthropologist chases the game in the wrong direction).

The rough joking mentioned above is also linked to another feature of Aka culture—playfulness. There is no clear separation between "work" and "play" time. Dances, singing, net hunting, male circumcision, sorcery accusations all include humorous mimicking, practical jokes, and exaggerated storytelling. Aka life is informal because of egalitarianism and the playful activity that occurs throughout the day by both adults and children. Play is an integral part of both adult and child life and contributes to enhanced parent-child and adult-child communication. Parents and adults have an extensive repertoire of play, and can and do communicate cultural knowledge to children through their playful repertoire.

Greater ethnographic detail on the Aka can be found in Hewlett (1991) or Bahuchet (1985).

Aka Infancy

The infant lives with a relatively small group of individuals related through his or her father (unless the infant is the first born in which case the family is likely to be in the camp of the wife for the purposes of bride service) and sleeps in the same bed as mother, father, and other brothers and sisters.

Cultural practices during infancy are quite distinct from those found in European and American cultures. Aka parents are indulgent as infants are held almost constantly, nursed on demand (breast-fed several times per hour), attended to immediately if they fuss, and are seldom, if ever, told "no! no!" if they misbehave (e.g., get into food pots, hit others, or take things from other children). An Aka father describes Aka parenting and contrasts it with parenting among his Ngandu farming neighbors:

> We, Aka look after our children with love, from the minute they are born to when they are much older. The villagers love their children only when they are babies. When they become children they get beaten up badly. With us, even if the child is older, if he is unhappy, I'll look after him, I will cuddle him.

Older infants are allowed to use and play with knives, machetes, and other "adult" items. They are allowed to crawl into a parent's lap while the parent is engaged in economic (e.g., butchering animal, repairing net) or leisure (e.g., playing a harp or drum) activity. While older infants are given considerable freedom to explore the house and camp, parents do watch infants to make sure they do not crawl into the fire.

Extensive multiple caregiving of 1–4 month-old infants (Hewlett 1989) exists, especially while the Aka are in the camp. Individuals other than mother (infant's father, brothers, sisters, aunts, uncles, grandmothers) hold the infant the majority of the time (60 percent) in this context, and the infant is moved to different people about seven times per hour. Mothers' holding increases to 85 percent and the transfer rate drops to two transfers per hour outside of the camp (i.e., on net hunt or in fields).

Infancy is very active and stimulating. Infants are taken on the hunt and are seldom laid down. They are held on the side of the caregiver rather than on the caregiver's back as in many farming communities so there are opportunities for caregiver-infant face-to-face interaction and communication. The infant can also breast feed by simply reaching for the mother's breast and can nurse while mother walks. While out on the net hunt the infant sleeps in the sling as the caregiver walks, runs, or sits.

THE STUDY

I started working with the Aka in 1973 so by the time I started the father-infant study in 1984 I was familiar with specific Aka families and Aka culture in general. Since I wanted to test some of the psychological hypotheses regarding father-infant relations, I incorporated psychological methods into my research. The quantitative psychological methods consisted of systematically observing 15 Aka families with infants from 6 A.M. to 9 P.M. (the observations focused either on the father or the infant). This enabled me to say precisely how much time Aka versus American fathers held or were near their infants and precisely describe how American versus Aka styles of interaction were similar or different. Informal discussions while on the net hunt and in camp were also utilized to develop structured interviews. Men and women, young and old, were asked about their feelings regarding relations with their mothers, fathers, and other caregivers.

The study focused on two domains important for trying to understand father-infant bonding: the degree of father involvement and mother's versus father's parenting style. For degree of father involvement I wanted to know: How often do fathers actually interact with their infants, how often are fathers available to their infants, if fathers are not involved with infants what other activities are they involved in, how do children characterize the nature of their involvement with their father? Questions regarding paternal versus maternal parenting style included: Are there distinctions between the mother's and the father's play behavior with their infants, do mothers and fathers hold their infants for different purposes, what do mothers and fathers do while they hold the infant, do infants show different types of attachment behavior to mothers and fathers, how do children view their mother's and father's parenting styles?

WHY ARE AKA FATHERS SO INVOLVED WITH THEIR INFANTS? THE CULTURAL NEXUS OF FATHER-INFANT BONDING

Although few cross-cultural studies of father-child relations have been conducted, Aka father involvement in infancy is exceptional, if not unique. Aka fathers are within an arm's reach (i.e., holding or within one meter) of their infant more than 50 percent of 24-hour periods. Table 1 demonstrates that Aka fathers hold their very young infants during the day at least five times more than fathers in other cultures, while Table 2 indicates Aka fathers are available to their infants at least three times more frequently than fathers in other cultures. American and European fathers hold their infants, on average, between 10 and 20 minutes per day (Lamb et al. 1987) while Aka fathers, on average, hold their infants about one hour during daylight hours and about 25 percent of the time after the sun goes down. At night fathers sleep with mother and infant, whereas American fathers seldom sleep with their infants. While Aka father care is extensive, it is also highly context dependent—fathers provide at least four times as much care while they are in the camp setting than they do while out of camp (e.g., out on the net hunt or in the villagers' fields). What factors influence this high level of paternal emotional and physical involvement among the Aka?

TABLE 1 Comparison of Father Holding in Selected Foraging Populations

Population	*Age of infants (mos.)*	*Father holding (percent of time)*	*Source*
Gidgingali	0–6	3.4	Hamilton (1981)
	6–18	3.1	
!Kung	0–6	1.9	West and Konner (1976)
	6–24	4.0	
Efe Pygmies	1–4	2.6	Winn et al. (1990)
Aka Pygmies	1–4	22.0	Hewlett (1991)
	8–18	14.0	

Note: All observations were made in a camp setting (Table from Hewlett 1991).

TABLE 2 Comparison of Father Presence with Infants or Children among Selected Foraging and Farming Populations

Population	*Location*	*Subsistence*	*Percent time father present/in view*	*Primary setting of observations*	*Source*
Gusii	Kenya	farming	10	house/yard & garden	1
Mixteca	Mexico	farming	9	house/yard	1
Ilocano	Philippines	farming	14	house/yard	1
Okinawan	Japan	farming	3	public places & house/yard	1
Rajput	India	farming	3	house/yard	1
!Kung	Botswana	foraging	30	camp	2
Aka Pygmies	Central African Republic	foraging	88	forest camp	3
Logoli	Kenya	farming	5	house/yard	4
Newars	Nepal	farming	7	house/yard	4
Samoans	Samoa	farming	8	house/yard	4
Carib	Belize	farming	3	house/yard	4
Ifaluk	Micronesia	farm-fish	13	house/yard	5

Sources (Table from Hewlett 1991):
1. Whiting and Whiting 1975
2. West and Konner 1976
3. Hewlett 1991
4. Munroe and Munroe 1992
5. Betzig, Harrigan, and Turke 1990

Aka father-infant bonding is embedded within a cultural nexus—it influences and is influenced by a complex cultural system. This brief overview describes some of the cultural facets linked to Aka father-infant bonding.

Like many other foragers, the Aka have few accumulable resources that are essential for survival. "Kinship resources," the number of brothers and sisters in particular, are probably the most essential "resource" for survival, but are generally established at an early age. Food resources are not stored or accumulated, and Aka males and females contribute similar percentages of calories to the diet. Cross-cultural studies have demonstrated that in societies where resources essential to survival can be accumulated or where males are the primary contributors to subsistence, fathers invest more time competing for these resources and, consequently, spend less time with their children. In contrast, where resources are not accumulable or men are not the primary contributors to subsistence, men generally spend more time in the direct care of their children. Katz and Konner (1981: 174) found that father-infant proximity (degree of emotional warmth and physical proximity) is closest in gathering-hunting populations (gathered foods by females are principal resources, meat is secondary) and most distant in cultures where herding or advanced agriculture is practiced. In the latter cultures, cattle, camels, and land are considered the essential accumulable resources necessary for survival. These findings are consistent with Whiting and Whiting's (1975) cross-cultural study of husband-wife intimacy. They found husband-wife intimacy to be greatest in cultures without accumulated resources or capital investments. While there are other factors to consider (the protection of resources and the polygyny rate), there is a strong tendency for fathers/husbands to devote more time to their children/wives if there are no accumulable resources.

Three additional factors seem to be especially influential in understanding the extraordinarily high level of Aka paternal care.

First, the nature of Aka subsistence activity is rather unique cross-culturally. Usually mens' and womens' subsistence activities take place at very different locations. The net hunt and other subsistence activities, such as caterpillar collecting, involve men, women, and children. If men are going to help with infant care on a regular basis they have to be near the infant a good part of the day. The net hunt makes this possible. The net hunt also requires that men and women walk equal distances during the day. In most foraging societies, females do not travel as far from camp as males. Older siblings are not useful for helping their mothers because of the extensive labor involved in walking long distances with an infant. If a mother is to receive help on the net hunt, it needs to come from an adult. Most of the other adult females carry baskets full of food and have their own infants or young children to carry since fertility is high. Fathers are among the few alternative caregivers regularly available on the net hunt to help mothers. While fathers do carry infants on the net hunt, especially on the return from the hunt when the mothers' baskets are full of meat, collected nuts, and fruit, father-infant caregiving is much more likely to occur in the camp.

Another influential factor is the nature of husband-wife relations. The net hunt contributes substantially to the time husband and wife spend together and patterns the nature of that time spent together. Observations in the forest and village indicate husbands and wives are within sight of each other 46.5 percent of daylight hours. This is more time together than in any other known society, and it is primarily a result of the net hunt. This percentage of course increases in the evening hours. But, husbands and wives are not only together most of the day, they are actively cooperating on the net hunt. They have to know each other well to communicate and cooperate throughout the day. They work together to set up the family net, chase game into the net, butcher and divide the game and take care of the children. Husbands and wives help each other out in a number of domains, in part because they spend so much time together. Husband-wife relations are manystranded; that is, social, economic, ritual, parenting, and leisure activities are shared and experienced in close proximity. When they return to camp the mother has a number of tasks—she collects firewood and water, and prepares the biggest meal of the day. The father has relatively few tasks to do after returning from the hunt. He may make string or repair the net, but he is available to help with infant care. He is willing to do infant care, in part, because of the many-stranded reciprocity between husband and wife. In many societies men have fewer tasks to do at the end of the day, while women have domestic tasks and prepare a meal. Men are available to help out with childcare, but seldom provide much assistance, in part, due to the more distant husband-wife relationship.

The third important factor in understanding Aka fathers' involvement with infants is father-infant bonding. Father and infant are clearly attached to each other. Fathers seek out their infants and infants seek out their fathers. Fathers end up holding their infants frequently because the infants crawl to, reach for, or fuss for their fathers. Fathers pick up their infants because they intrinsically enjoy being close to their infants. They enjoy being with them and carry them in several different contexts (e.g., out in the fields drinking palm wine with other men).

While the factors described above are especially influential, other cultural factors also play a part. Gender egalitarianism pervades cultural beliefs and practices: Men do not have physical or institutional control over women, violence against women is rare or non-existent, both women and men are valued for their different but complementary roles, there is flexibility in these gender roles, and holding infants is not perceived as being feminine or "women's work." Sharing, helping out, and generosity are central concepts in Aka life; this applies to subsistence and parenting spheres. Aka ideology of good and bad fathers reiterates the importance of father's proximity—a good father shows love for his children, stays near them, and assists mother with caregiving when her workload is heavy. A bad father abandons his children and does not share food with them. There is no organized warfare and male feuding is infrequent, so men are around camp and help with subsistence rather than being away at battle. Fertility is high, so most adult women have nursing infants and there are few other adult women around to help out. Finally, the Aka move their camps several times a year and consequently do not accumulate material goods that need to be defended.

The point here is that Aka father-infant relations have to be viewed in a complex cultural nexus. Some cultural factors are somewhat more influential than others—net hunting, husband-wife relations, for instance—but even these cultural features take place in a web of other cultural beliefs and practices that contribute to the intimate nature of Aka father-infant relations.

FATHER-INFANT BONDING IN THE AKA AND UNITED STATES

Over 50 studies of European and American fathers indicate that father's interactions with infants and young children are clearly distinguished from mother's interactions in that fathers are the vigorous rough and tumble playmates of infants and young children, while mothers are sensitive caregivers. The American literature suggests that this rough and tumble play is how infants become attached to fathers ("bond") and develop social competence (Lamb et al. 1987). The Aka father-infant study is not consistent with the American studies that emphasize the importance of father's vigorous play. Aka fathers rarely, if ever, engage in vigorous play with their infants; only one episode of vigorous play by a father was recorded during all 264 hours of systematic observation. Informal observations during more than 10 field visits over the last 20 years are also consistent with this finding. The quantitative data indicate that by comparison to mothers, Aka fathers are significantly more likely to hug, kiss, or soothe a fussy baby while they are holding the infant.

While Aka fathers do not engage in vigorous play with their infants, they are slightly more playful than mothers; fathers are somewhat more likely to engage in minor physical play (e.g., tickling) with their one- to four-month-old infants than are mothers. But characterizing the Aka father as the infant's playmate would be misleading. Other caretakers, brothers and sisters in particular, engage in play with the infant while holding much more frequently than fathers or mothers. Mothers have more episodes of play over the course of a day than fathers or other caretakers because they hold the infant most of the time. The Aka father-infant relationship might be better characterized by its intimate and affective nature. Aka fathers hold their infants more than fathers in any other human society known to anthropologists, and Aka fathers also show affection more frequently while holding than do Aka mothers.

So how can vigorous play be a significant feature in American studies of father-infant bonding, but not among the Aka? Four factors appear to be important for understanding the process of Aka father-infant bonding: familiarity with the infant; knowledge of caregiving practices (how to hold an infant, how to soothe an infant); the degree of relatedness to the infant; and cultural values and parental goals.

First, due to frequent father-holding and availability, Aka fathers know how to communicate with their infants. Fathers know the early signs of infant hunger, fatigue, and illness as well as the limits in their ability to soothe the infant. They also know how to stimulate responses from the infant without being vigorous. Unlike American fathers, Aka wait for infants to initiate interaction. Aka caregivers other than mothers and fathers are less familiar with the infants and the most physical in their play, suggesting a relationship between intimate knowledge of the infant's cues and the frequency of vigorous play while holding. Consistent with this is the finding that working mothers in the U.S. are more likely to engage in vigorous play than are stay-at-home mothers.

Second, knowledge of infant caregiving practices seems to play a role in determining how much play is exhibited in caretaker-infant interactions. Child caretakers were the most physical and the loudest (singing) in their handling of infants. Children were not restricted from holding infants, but they were closely watched by parents. While "other" caretakers were more playful than mothers or fathers, younger fathers and "other" caretakers were more physical than older ones, probably because they did not know how to handle and care for infants as well as adult caretakers.

A third factor to consider is the degree of relatedness of the caretaker to the infant. If vigorous play can assist in developing attachment, more closely related individuals may have a greater vested interest in establishing this bond than distantly related individuals. Attachment not only enhances the survival of the infant, but it can potentially increase the related caretaker's survival and fitness. Aka mothers and fathers establish attachment by their frequent caregiving; vigorous play is not necessary to establish affective saliency. Brothers and sisters, on the other hand, might establish this bond through physical play. Aka brothers and sisters, in fact, provided essentially all of the physical play the focal infants received; cousins and unrelated children were more likely to engage in face-to-face play with the infant instead of physical play.

Finally, cultural values and parental goals of infant development should be considered. American culture encourages individualistic aggressive competition; Aka culture values cooperation, nonaggression, and prestige avoidance (one does not draw attention to oneself even, for instance, if one kills an elephant). Apparently, Americans tolerate—if not actually encourage—aggressive rough-and-tumble types of play with infants. Also, due to the high infant mortality rate, the primary parental goal for Aka is the survival of their infants. The constant holding and immediate attention to fussing reflect this goal. In the United States, infant mortality rates are markedly lower and, as a result, parental concern for survival may not be as great. The Aka infant is taken away from a caretaker who plays roughly with the infant, in part because it could be seen as aggressive behavior, but also because the pervasive aim of infant care practices is survival of the infant, and rough-and-tumble play could risk the infant's safety.

These factors tentatively clarify why Aka fathers do not engage in vigorous play like American fathers, but do participate in slightly more physical play than Aka mothers (but not more than other caretakers). American fathers infrequently participate directly in infant care and consequently are not as familiar with infant cues. To stimulate interaction and (possibly) bonding, they engage in physical play. Aka brothers and sisters are also much less physical in their play with infants than America fathers (Aka never tossed infants in the air or swung them by their arms), again suggesting that Aka children know their infant brother or sister and the necessary infant caregiving skills better than American fathers. These observations are obviously speculative and need further empirical study.

Sociologists LaRossa and LaRossa (1981) also describe stylistic differences between American mothers' and fathers' interactions with their infants. They list a number of male-female role dichotomies that reflect different parenting styles. One distinction they make is role distance versus role embracement. Fathers are more likely to distance themselves from the parenting role while mothers are more likely to embrace the parenting role. American women generally want to remain in primary control of the children, and while fathers may show interest in caregiving, they are more likely to distance themselves from caregiving while embracing their roles as the breadwinners. LaRossa and LaRossa also suggest that fathers generally have low intrinsic value and relatively high extrinsic value, while mothers have the reverse.

> The intrinsic value of something or someone is the amount of sheer pleasure or enjoyment that one gets from experiencing an object or person. The extrinsic value of something or someone is the amount of social rewards (e.g., money, power, prestige) associated with having or being with the object or person. (64)

They use this dichotomy to explain why fathers are more likely to carry or hold an infant in public than in private. Fathers receive extrinsic rewards from those in public settings, while this does not happen in the home. According to LaRossa and LaRossa,

> Fathers will roughhouse with their toddlers on the living-room floor, and will blush when hugged or kissed by the one-year-olds, but when you really get down to it, they just do not have that much fun when they are with their children. If they had their druthers, they would be working at the office or drinking at the local pub. (65)

These role dichotomies may be useful for understanding American mother-father parenting styles, but they have limited value in characterizing Aka mother-father distinctions. Aka mothers and fathers embrace the parenting role. Generally, mothers and fathers want to hold their infants, and certainly they derive pleasure from infant interactions. As indicated earlier, fathers were in fact more likely to show affection while holding than mothers. Fathers also offered their nipples to infants who wanted to nurse, cleaned mucus from their infants' noses, picked lice from their infants' hair, and cleaned their infants after they urinated or defecated (often on the father). Fathers' caregiving did not appear any more or less perfunctory than mothers'. Aka fathers are not burdened with infant care; if a father does not want to hold or care for the infant he gives the infant to another person. Overall, Aka fathers embrace their parenting role as much as they embrace their hunting role.

The intrinsic-extrinsic role dichotomy does not fit well with Aka mother-father parenting styles either. Again, both Aka mothers and fathers place great intrinsic value and little extrinsic value on parenting. The fathers' intrinsic value is demonstrated above, but the lack of extrinsic value among the Aka can best be seen by comparing Aka and Ngandu fathers (the Ngandu are the horticulturalist trading partners of the Aka). When a Ngandu father holds his infant in public he is "on stage." He goes out of his way to show his infant to those who pass by, and frequently tries to stimulate the infant while holding it. He is much more vigorous in his interactions with the infant than are Aka men. The following experience exemplifies Ngandu fathers' extrinsic value towards their infants. An Ngandu friend showed me a 25-pound fish he had just caught, and I asked to take a photograph of him with his fish. He said fine, promptly picked up his nearby infant, and proudly displayed his fish and infant for the photograph. His wife was also nearby but was not invited into the photograph. Aka fathers, on the other hand, are matter-of-fact about their holding or transporting of infants in public places. They do not draw attention to their infants. Aka fathers also hold their infants in all kinds of social and economic contexts.

CONCLUSION

This paper has examined the cultural nexus of Aka father-infant bonding and has made some comparisons to middle-class American father-infant relations. American fathers are characterized by their vigorous play with infants, while Aka fathers are characterized by their affectionate and intimate relations with their infants. Aka infants bond with their fathers because they provide sensitive and regular care, whereas American infants bond to their fathers, in part, due to their vigorous play. The purpose of this paper is not to criticize American fathers for their style of interaction with their infants; physical play is important in middle-class American context because it is a means for fathers who are seldom around their infants to demonstrate their love and interest in the infant. Vigorous play may also be important to American mothers who work outside the home; studies indicate they are also more likely than stay-at-home mothers to engage in vigorous play with their infants. The Aka study does imply that father-infant bonding does not always take place through physical play, and it is necessary to explore a complex cultural nexus in order to understand the nature of father-infant relations.

Aka fathers are very close and affectionate with their infants, and their attachment processes, as defined in Western bonding theory, appear to be similar to that of mothers. While Aka mother- and father-infant relations are similar they are not the same. Fathers do spend substantially less time with infants than do mothers, and the nature of their interactions is different. Aka and American fathers bring something qualitatively different to their children; father's caregiving pattern is not simply a variation of mother's pattern. More research is needed on the unique features of father involvement so we can move away from a "deficit" model of fathering.

Finally, this paper identifies cultural factors that influence father-infant bonding; biological forces are not considered. This is unusual in that mother-infant bonding generally mentions or discusses the biological basis of mother's attachment to the infant. The release of prolactin and oxytocin with birth and lactation is said to increase affectionate feelings and actions toward the infant. These same hormones exist in men but endocrinologists generally believe they have no function in men. Is there a biology of fatherhood, or is motherhood more biological and fatherhood more cultural? This is a complex question as both men and women probably have evolved ("biological") psychological mechanisms that influence their parenting, but if one just focuses on endocrinology, few data exist on the endocrinology of fatherhood. For instance, Gubernick et al. (unpublished paper) found that men's testosterone levels decreased significantly two weeks after the birth of their children; the decrease was not linked to decline in sexual behavior, increased stress, or sleep deprivation. Another small study of American fathers indicated significant increases in plasma prolactin levels after fathers held their 3-month-old infants on their chest for 15 minutes (Hewlett and Alster, unpublished data). The few biological studies that do exist suggest that biology can and does influence fatherhood. More studies of the biocultural nexus of fatherhood are needed.

While biology probably influences both mothers' and fathers' parenting to some degree, this chapter has demonstrated that the cultural nexus is a powerful force that profoundly shapes the nature and context of father-infant bonding. Aka father-infant bonding takes place through regular and intimate (i.e., hugging, kissing, soothing) care while American father-infant bonding takes place through vigorous play. American fathers often do not know their infants very well and try to demonstrate their love and concern through vigorous play. American mothers that work outside the home also tend to be more vigorous with their infants. American fathers are not necessarily "bad" fathers because they do not do as much direct caregiving as the Aka fathers. Fathers around the world "provide" and enrich the lives of their children in diverse ways (e.g., physical and emotional security, economic well-being). The Aka data do suggest that there are alternative processes by which father-infant bonding can and does take place and that Americans and others might learn from this comparative approach as policy decisions about parental leave and other topics are considered.

REFERENCES

Ainsworth, M.D.S. 1967. *Infancy in Uganda: Infant Care and the Growth of Love.* Baltimore: Johns Hopkins Press.

Bahuchet, S. 1985. *Les Pygmees Aka et la Foret Centrafricaine.* Paris: Selaf.

Betzig, L., A. Harrigan, and P. Turke. 1990. "Childcare on Ifaluk." *Zeitscrift fur Ethnologie* 114.

Bowlby, J. 1969. *Attachment and Loss Vol. 1: Attachment.* New York: Basic Books.

Chodorow, N. 1974. "Family Structure and Feminine Personality." In *Woman, Culture, and Society,* ed. Michelle Zimbalist Rosaldo and Louise Lamphere. Stanford, CA: Stanford University Press.

Clarke-Stewart, K.A. 1980. "The Father's Contribution to Children's Cognitive and Social Development in Early Childhood." In *The Father-Infant Relationship,* ed. S.A. Pedersen. New York: Praeger.

Cole, M., and J.S. Bruner. 1974. "Cultural Differences and Inferences about Psychological Processes." In *Culture and Cognition,* ed. J.W. Berry and P.R. Dasen. London: Methuen.

Freud, S. 1938. *An Outline of Psychoanalysis.* London: Hogarth.

Gubernick, D.J., C.M. Worthman, and J.F. Stallings. "Hormonal Correlates of Fatherhood in Men." Unpublished paper.

Hamilton, A. 1981. *Nature and Nurture: Aboriginal Child-Rearing in North-Central Arnhem Land.* Canberra: Australian Institute of Aboriginal Studies.

Harlow, H.F. 1961. "The Development of Affectional Patterns in Infant Monkeys." In *Determinants of Infant Behavior,* Vol. 1, ed. B.M. Foss. London: Methuen.

Hewlett, B.S. 1989. "Multiple Caretaking Among African Pygmies. *American Anthropologist* 91: 186–191.

Hewlett, B.S. 1991. *Intimate Fathers: The Nature and Context of Aka Pygmy Paternal-Infant Care.* Ann Arbor, MI: University of Michigan Press.

———. 1992 (ed.). *Father-Child Relations: Cultural and Biosocial Perspectives.* NY: Aldine de Gruyter.

Hewlett, B.S. and D. Alster. "Prolactin and infant holding among American fathers." Unpublished manuscript.

Katz, M.M. and Melvin J. Konner. 1981. "The Role of Father: An Anthropological Perspective." In *The Role of Father in Child Development,* ed. Michael E. Lamb. New York: John Wiley and Sons.

Lamb, M.E., ed. 1981. *The Role of the Father in Child Development* 2nd Ed. New York: John Wiley & Sons.

Lamb, M.E., J.H. Pleck, E.L. Charnov, and J.A. LeVine. 1987. "A Biosocial Perspective on Paternal Behavior and Involvement." In *Parenting Across the Lifespan,* ed. J.B. Lancaster, J. Altmann, A. Rossi, L.R. Sherrod. Hawthorne, NY: Aldine.

Lancaster, J.B., and C.S. Lancaster. 1987. "The Watershed: Change in Parental-Investment and Family Formation Strategies in the Course of Human Evolution." In *Parenting Across the Life Span,* ed. J.B. Lancaster, J. Altmann, A.S. Rossi, and L.R. Sherrod. Hawthorne, NY: Aldine.

LaRossa, R., and M.M. LaRossa. 1981. *Transition to Parenthood: How Infants Change Families.* Beverly Hills: Sage Publications.

LeVine, R.A., S. Dixon, S. LeVine, A. Richman, P.H. Leiderman, C.H. Keefer, and T.B. Brazelton. 1994. *Child Care and Culture: Lessons from Africa.* NY: Cambridge University Press.

Munroe, R.H. and R.L. Munroe. 1992. "Fathers in Children's Environments: A Four Culture Study." In *Father-Child Relations: Cultural and Biosocial Contexts,* Barry S. Hewlett, ed. NY: Aldine de Gruyter.

Rosaldo, M.Z. and L. Lamphere, eds. 1974. *Woman, Culture and Society.* Stanford, CA: Stanford University Press.

West, M.M. and M.J. Konner. 1976. "The Role of Father in Anthropological Perspective." In *The Role of the Father in Child Development.* 2nd ed., M.E. Lamb, ed. NY: John Wiley and Sons.

Whiting, B.B. and J.W.M. Whiting. 1975. *Children of Six Cultures.* Cambridge, MA: Harvard University Press.

Winn, S., G.A. Morelli, and E.Z. Tronick. 1990. "The Infant in the Group: A Look at Efe Caretaking Practices." In *The Cultural Context of Infancy,* J.K. Nugent, B.M. Lester, and T.B. Brazelton, eds. NJ: Ablex.

II

GENDER AND PREHISTORY

A popular introductory archaeology text began its career 15 years ago with the title *Men of the Earth* (Fagan 1974). For the last several editions (Fagan 1977-1991) it has been called *People of the Earth.* This change is deliberate and illustrates a growing sensitivity on the part of some archaeologists to the importance of considering the contribution of women, as well as men, to the history of our species (Wylie 1991, 1992; Gero and Conkey 1991; Seifert 1991). An archaeological focus on gender provides a lens for reassessing myths about the past that glorify men as the agents of cultural change. As some archaeologists seek to reinstate women as agents and as subjects, widely held assumptions about "mankind" and "man's past" are challenged by a focus on women's involvement in production, politics, and the generation of symbol systems in past societies. In contrast to earlier archaeological orientations (see Conkey and Spector 1984 for a review of archaeological approaches), an "engendered" archaeology assumes that the process of survival throughout human history has of necessity involved a collaborative effort between men and women. Those who advocate a feminist-informed archaeology have explored such issues as women's participation in the creation of wealth (for example, women's production of textiles or ceramics), consequences of women's rule in state societies, images of powerful women in prehistoric art, and women's roles in the development of agriculture (Spielmann 1995; Simon and Ravesloot 1995).

Questions of fundamental importance regarding the sexual division of labor in past societies may benefit from an archaeological perspective that includes women's interests. Rather than assuming that "earliest human groups were conscious of and elaborated sex differences into differentially valued, gender-exclusive task groups," Spector and Whelan (1989: 73) suggest that an archaeology of gender needs to begin by raising questions about the origins of a sexual division of labor and by determining what gender differentiation might have accomplished among early human populations (Spector and Whelan 1989: 72-73; see also Ehrenberg, this book).

As Conkey (this book) suggests, in the study of gender in archaeology, we are reminded of the importance of confronting presuppositions and values that guide our work, however "scientific" we presume our methodologies to be. Conkey outlines a number of challenges for future archaeological research. First, archaeologists must recognize and eliminate biased reconstructions of past gender roles that derive from our own cultural assumptions. Second, they must pay more attention to theories about gender in analyzing their data. Third, archaeologists need to use their data to make explicit inferences about men and women in prehistory. Finally, Conkey points out biases not only in analysis but also in the very practice of archaeology. Eliminating gender bias from archaeology, as Conkey suggests, will require a major commitment to the same critical reflection that has characterized other branches of anthropology. As Nelson and Kehoe (1990: 4) observe, "disentangling our culture-bound assumptions from the actual archaeological record will be a long and wrenching procedure."

Nelson's discussion of Upper Paleolithic "Venus" figurines in archaeology textbooks (in this book) illustrates Conkey's point about the potential for distortion in the archaeological record when cultural values affect archaeological analysis. Nelson demonstrates that most textbooks convey the same ideological message in their treatment of Venus figurines—that adult male humans are fascinated by women's bodies and view them as signs of fertility. The widely held assumption that Upper Paleolithic figurines possibly depicting human females are fertility fetishes is, according to Nelson, poorly founded. Feminist analysis of the figurines suggests alternative explanations regarding their production, functions, and symbolism, and serves as a warning that "reinforcing present cultural stereotypes by projecting them into the past allows whole generations of students to believe that our present gender constructs are eternal and unchanging" (Nelson 1990: 19; see also Rice 1991).

In an effort to better explain contemporary gender relations archaeological evidence has offered a means of understanding the present by reconstructing our evolutionary past. Scholarly and public imaginations have been drawn to the possibility that archaeological data might document the existence of a matriarchal society in which women occupied a privileged position as rulers. If powerful women could be found in history or prehistory, this would serve as evidence that male dominance is not inevitable.

Images of matriarchy exist in both western and nonwestern societies. Nineteenth-century evolutionists such as J.J. Bachofen (1967) described a history of humankind that passed from a state of primitive communal marriages, through mother right, or a rule of women, to partriarchy. Similar myths of matriarchy have been recorded in several South American societies (Bamberger 1974: 266). According to Bamberger these myths share a common theme, that of women's loss of power through moral failure. The myths describe a past society in which women held power; however, through their inability to handle power when they had it, the rule of women was eventually replaced by patriarchal leadership.

Rather than representing historical events, the myths of matriarchy serve as a tool to keep woman bound to her place. They reinforce current social relations by justifying male dominance (Bamberger 1974: 280). There is no historical or archaeological evidence of matriarchal societies in which women systematically and exclusively dominated men. In spite of the absence of such evidence the idea remains popular, precisely because it conveys the possibility of a future society characterized by female dominance that is reminiscent of the matriarchal past.

Culturally based assumptions can be avoided by paying more careful attention to a range of sources at our disposal in the archaeological record. The reconstruction of gender roles and relations in past societies may be facilitated by representations of women and men in burials, images, and written texts. Literary texts pertaining to early Sumer, for instance, portray women in supportive, nurturing roles, acting to further the interests of male political rulers or heroes (Pollock 1991). In some texts, women are also described as political officeholders, or queens. Pollock concludes that some women seem to have had significant political and economic power, although few of them were written about, compared to the number of men in such positions whose lives were more fully recorded. Women also held offices in the temple hierarchy as priestesses; it is possible that these were the primary positions of power available to women. An informative example is that of the priestess Enheduanna, installed at Ur by her father King Sargon. Literary texts suggest that she acted to further her father's political ambitions as well as her own authority (Pollock 1991). These texts, as well as other representations such as burials and images, suggest that Sumerian women were not pawns to be manipulated by men, but were able to attain positions of high status and power.

Similarly, recent access to Maya history by decipherment of glyphic texts on public monuments has shown that some royal women played politically central roles in their kingdoms. Hypogamy, or the marriage of higher-status women to lower-status men, insured the alliance of these lower-status men to higher-status men of their wives' families. Hypergamy, or the marriage of lower-status women to higher-status men, also occurred. More importantly, the women involved in marriage alliance and royal politics were anything but passive pawns in the games of men. Freidel and Schele (in this book) look at the lives and exploits of powerful Maya women in two classic period kingdoms to show that generalities based on limited data often fail in the face of detailed information. They also show that royal women can emerge as extraordinarily heroic figures and great politicians when their stories are known. In the case of two important royal Maya women, whose stories are told in glyphs, Freidel and Schele explore what happened when one revived a failing kingdom and the other, whose own child was passed over for heirship to the throne, was permitted to raise a beautiful temple in her city that memorialized her in perpetuity. The various forms of power exercised by these women suggest that while there were no matriarchies in the past, women could control important resources and influence the course of public events. Little is known about the lives of commoner women, whose exploits are less visible in texts and other representations. The limited information available on commoner Maya women highlights the need for innovative conceptual and methodological approaches to the archaeological record that will help reconstruct gender roles in past societies.

Conkey and Spector discuss the general problem of the "archaeological invisibility" of women (1984: 5), which, they contend, is more the result of a false notion of objectivity and of the gender paradigms archaeologists use than of an inherent invisibility of such data (6). Questions that would elicit information about prehistoric gender behavior or organization are too infrequently asked, while researchers "bring to their work preconceived notions about what each sex ought to do, and these notions serve to structure the way artifacts are interpreted" (for example, the presumption of linkages between projectile points with men and pots with women) (Conkey and Spector 1984: 10). In contrast, goals for a feminist archaeology would include gender-inclusive reconstructions of past human behavior, the development of a specific paradigm for the study of gender, and an explicit effort to eliminate androcentrism in the content and mode of presentation of archaeological research (Conkey and Spector 1984: 15).

REFERENCES

Bachofen, Johann. 1967. *Myth, Religion and Mother Right* [Die Mutterrecht 1861 orig.]. London: Koutledge and Kegan Paul.

Bamberger, Joan. 1974. "The Myth of Matriarchy: Why Men Rule in Primitive Society." In Michelle Z. Rosaldo and Louise Lamphere (eds.). *Woman, Culture, and Society*, pp. 263–281. Stanford: Stanford University Press.

Conkey, Margaret W. and Janet Spector. 1984. "Archaeology and the Study of Gender." In

Michael B. Schiffer (ed.). *Advances in Archaeological Method and Theory,* Vol. 7, pp. 1–29. New York: Academic Press.
Fagan, Brian. 1974. *Men of the Earth.* Boston: Little, Brown and Co.
Gero, J.M. and Margaret W. Conkey (eds.). 1991. *Engendering Archaeology: Women in Preshistory.* Oxford: Basil Blackwell.
Nelson, Sarah M. 1990. "Diversity of the Upper Paleolithic Venus Figurines and Archeological Mythology." In Sarah M. Nelson and Alice B. Kehoe (eds.). *Powers of Observation: Alternative Views in Archeology,* pp. 11–23. Archeological Papers of the American Anthropological Association, Number 2.
Nelson, Sarah M. and Alice B. Kehoe. 1990. "Introduction." In Sarah M. Nelson and Alice B. Kehoe (eds.). *Powers of Observation: Alternative Views in Archeology,* pp. 1–10. Archeological Papers of the American Anthropological Association, Number 2.
Pollock, Susan. 1991. "Women in a Men's World: Images of Sumerian Women." In Joan Gero and Margaret Conkey (eds.). *Engendering Archaeology: Women and Prehistory.* Oxford: Basil Blackwell.
Rice, Patricia. 1991. "Prehistoric Venuses: Symbols of Motherhood or Womanhood?" *Journal of Anthropological Research* 37 (4): 402–414.
Seifert, Donna J. (ed.). 1991. "Gender in Historical Archaeology." *Historical Archeology* (special issue) 25 (4): 1–132.
Simon, Arleyn W. and John C. Ravesloot. 1995. "Salado Ceramic Burial Offerings: A Consideration of Gender and Social Organization." *Journal of Anthropological Research* 51 (2): 103–124.
Spector, Janet D. and Mary K. Whelan. 1989. "Incorporating Gender into Archaeology Courses." In Sandra Morgen (ed.). *Gender and Anthropology: Critical Reviews for Research and Teaching,* pp. 65–95. Washington, DC: American Anthropological Association.
Spielmann, Katherine A. 1995. "Glimpses of Gender in the Prehistoric Southwest." *Journal of Anthropological Research* 51 (2): 91–102.
Wylie, Alison, 1991. "Feminist Critiques and Archaeological Challenges." In D. Walde and N. Willows (eds.). *The Archaeology of Gender,* pp. 17–23. Calgary: The Archaeological Association of Calgary.
———. 1992. "The Interplay of Evidential Constraints and Political Interests: Recent Archaeological Research on Gender." *American Antiquity* 57 (1): 15–35.

MEN AND WOMEN IN PREHISTORY: AN ARCHAEOLOGICAL CHALLENGE

Margaret W. Conkey

> The *entire village* left the next day in about 30 canoes, leaving us alone with the *women and children* in the abandoned houses.
>
> —Levi-Strauss 1936, as cited by Michard-Marshale and Ribery 1982:7, in Eichler and Lapointe 1985:11.

When we close our eyes and think about the human societies and groups that lived thousands of years ago, what kinds of men and women do we "see"? What are they doing? What kinds of roles and relationships do we imagine? When we think about this we realize that there must have been many different roles and relationships. There must have been men of power and women of power, men with children and women as decision makers, men making pots and women making stone tools, men and women working together in the fields, men in trance and women as healers.

Yet, all too often archaeological accounts and the popular reconstructions of past societies that appear in magazines or coffeetable books suggest a much simpler picture: men hunting, women gathering plants, men mak-

Original material prepared for this text.

ing tools, women with children carrying firewood. Why do we have such simple and yet very familiar kinds of reconstructions? Certainly part of the explanation is that archaeologists have not done much that explicitly asks about gender, yet they have developed models or reconstructions that involve gender. These reconstructions derive from a variety of problematic sources: from ethnographic accounts that are gender biased (such as the previous quote from Levi-Strauss) or from the beliefs that twentieth century (mostly western, white, male) archaeologists hold about gender, about men and women, and about how prehistoric societies "worked" and changed. We are all, of course, quite susceptible to our own cultural ideas, ideals, and ideologies. Most North American archaeologists have taken somewhat longer to be as reflexive and self-critical about this than some of their anthropological colleagues.

Thus, to think about men and women in prehistoric societies and to think about their gender roles, gender ideologies, and gender relations raises several archaeological challenges. First, there is the challenge of recognizing and stripping away the biased or implied gender reconstructions. Second, there is the challenge of understanding more explicitly what gender is about so we can develop a theory of gender that is useful in archaeological research. Third, there is the challenge of making explicit inferences about gender and about men and women, using archaeological data to help answer questions concerning what might have happened in prehistory.

On one hand, archaeologists have not taken gender as an important research question; they have, in fact, come quite late to the field of gender studies or to any kind of insights from feminist theory. The first major paper that reviewed archaeology and the study of gender (Conkey and Spector 1984) came more than ten years after the first major books in sociocultural anthropology, and most archaeology in North America is housed in departments of anthropology. On the other hand, archaeology has not been silent about gender. Our accounts of prehistoric societies have been "saturated" with gender, but most of these accounts are—as we will see—male centered, or androcentric. At this point in the development of gender studies within archaeology, at least half of the task of thinking about men and women in prehistory is to question the gendered accounts that pervade our reconstructions of past societies and of how cultures have changed with time.

CHALLENGING GENDER BIAS

Although many archaeologists maintain that it is very difficult to know, or to make inferences, about gender relations or even about male and female activities in prehistoric societies, gender assertions are made regularly in interpretations. Often these assertions are so implicit that archaeologists don't really "see" them as specific ideas that need to be confirmed or tested. Most ideas about gender have come from the implicit and stereotypical gender models of our own sociopolitical lives (e.g., women at home) or from the androcentric ethnographies of sociocultural anthropology. In the early 1970s when anthropology "discovered" the widespread androcentric biases in ethnographic accounts, most of archaeology—which really *depends* on ethnographic analogies—was not paying much attention!

To take apart, or deconstruct, archaeological interpretations can be very useful, but this should not be taken as an end in itself. Rather, this critical scrutiny is part of the way in which we come to see not just *that* research and "results" can be biased, but exactly *how* they are biased and in what ways. This historical analysis of archaeological accounts is a necessary part of the process whereby we transform what we do. In reviews of the treatment of gender in the archaeological literature of the 1960s through the early 1980s, Mary Kennedy, Janet Spector, and I found some significant problems that are worth summarizing to understand how bias works (Conkey and Spector 1984).

First, we found that women—if they are present at all in reconstructions of prehistory—are usually depicted in a narrow range of passive, home-oriented tasks; they are often "exchanged" as wives, the objects of art and image making, and symbols of fertility and sexuality. In contrast prehistoric men are shown as very public, far ranging (adventurous), productive, active, and responsible for most of the significant changes in human evolution, especially technological innovations. These kinds of representations led Ruth Hubbard (1982) to write an article entitled, "Have only men evolved?"

Second, archaeologists often go through interpretive "contortions" to avoid suggesting that some prehistoric women might actually have been strong, active, or determining people in cultural life. For example one archaeological account of burials interpreted the same artifacts quite differently when they were found in a woman's grave than when found in a man's (Winters 1968). A pestle buried with a woman was there because in life she had done foodprocessing and grinding with it; the same kind of pestle in a man's grave was there because he had *made* it. If a spear-thrower (*atlatl*) was found in a man's grave, it was because he had used it; if found in a woman's grave, it was a gift to her, or, the archaeologist speculated, there really were (female) "Amazons" in this river valley. If trade goods were buried with a man, it was because he controlled the trading; if in a woman's grave, it was because she simply "had" the items. Thus, bias and differential representations of men and women can emerge in archaeological interpretations. Men, in prehistoric societies, often performed (various) "activities"; women (more passively) engaged in "tasks." Male activities are often described in more detail, and they are portrayed more frequently than female ones.

Ethnographers have noted that in many horticultural societies (those that cultivate plants with a simple technology) women do most of the field labor; they are often associated with plants. Archaeologists have long been fascinated with how and why some prehistoric people developed horticulture, which predominated over hunting-gathering-fishing as a way of life and as a subsistence system. In one study of how archaeologists account for the cultural innovation of "horticulture" (the domestication of plants) in the eastern woodlands of the United States, the analysts—Pat Watson and Mary Kennedy (1991)—show how the two major accounts have suggested some of the most obscure or contorted ways in which horticulture was developed to avoid suggesting that women might have been the innovators. One account accepts the idea that women were extremely familiar with plant resources when these societies were primarily collecting wild foods for their resources and the idea that *after* the "invention" of agriculture, women were the primary crop tenders. However, according to this account invention happened because shamans—men, of course— came to control the production and reproduction of the squashes that they used for gourd rattles in their ceremonies. Indeed, squashes were among some of the early cultivated plants in this region, but it is very difficult to link the speculative notion about shamans in one narrow context to such a major change in subsistence practices.

The other account suggests that because human occupation sites are areas of soil disturbance, this would have been a likely place for stray seeds from wild plants to have been "naturally" encouraged to the point of deliberate further modifications by humans. In other words the plants just about domesticated themselves. As Watson and Kennedy argue these two primary interpretations seem to go to considerable extremes to avoid disrupting the "sacred association" of women-passive-plants.

From this and other critiques it is clear that unexamined and present assumptions about gender have crept into archaeological interpretation. Explicit attention to women as active and as having varied roles and positions is usually absent. There is also a lack of consideration of other kinds of gender relations than those of the idealized mid-twentieth century—white, western, middle-class—with a sexual division of labor and a male-dominated, androcentric society. The reconstructions of our most ancient hominid ancestors, more than 2 million years ago, show a monogamous nuclear family unit: The male strides ahead across the savannah landscape, carrying a pointed stick as tool and/or as weapon. The female is several steps behind, carrying a young child on her hip.

The most widely touted version (Lovejoy 1981) of the social life of early hominids is that of men (mobile, risk taking, and adventurous), who "provision" the females and young with the most desirable resources (especially meat); the waiting women cluster for protection at a "home base," while making limited forays for gathered foods. Clearly, this is a familiar picture to us, not because it has been well demonstrated with archaeological (or other) data, but because it represents a culturally idealized (yet culturally limited) view of gender and socioeconomic relationships.

Such an interpretation is problematic. It invites and reifies the idea that there are deep and specific *continuities* in how men and women relate to each other in gender roles and gender positions. By suggesting that mobile men have been provisioning dependent and relatively constrained women and children for more than 2 million years, this account strongly implies that this is "natural" and therefore legitimate. Specific and narrow gender relations are universalized—"it's always been this way"—and convey the (mistaken) idea that these relationships and gender stereotypes are inevitable and immutable (unchanging and unchangeable).

The kinds of biased archaeological views I have discussed are promoted and reinforced by androcentric ethnographic and ethnoarchaeological accounts.[1] When John Yellen (1977) reported on his ethnoarchaeological studies of the !Kung people of the Kalahari desert of southern Africa, he first noted how research has shown that the female gathering of food accounts for most of the !Kung diet (60 to 80 percent). In writing about his observations based on living with and interviewing various !Kung people, however, he finds that "in practice, it is much easier to talk to the men because each day is in some way unique and stands out in the hunter's mind. Asking women where they went produces much less detailed and reliable information" (Yellen 1977:62–63).

Although this kind of reporting raises another central issue—the relationship between the observer and the people being studied—the *effects* of this kind of statement on the reader are insidious and powerful. This is particularly because ethnoarchaeological studies of contemporary people like the !Kung have been carried out specifically to build models for interpreting prehistoric hunter-gatherers. If women are never named and if they are portrayed as somehow wandering around the Kalahari with no clear recollection of what they did or where they have been, how can we avoid using these impressions in our visions of past social life?

So far we have seen how bias can creep into archaeological accounts when the analysts do not consciously reflect on their assumptions nor explicitly use some theoretical models about gender. The differential use of language to describe men and women has further contributed to problematic accounts of their activities and contributions to human societies. Further archaeology, like all other research, is influenced by and embedded in the social and political worlds within which it is practiced. At this point in the development of our field the topic with which we are concerned is just as much the gender of archaeology as the archaeology of gender.

There is now a very well established body of literature that shows how the values, cultural assumptions, and social contexts of the researchers can and do strongly affect the kind of science that is practiced.[2] *All* sciences are social; every fact has a factor, a maker, who is a person of a certain nationality, race, class, ethnicity, and gender. In many instances some of these factors do affect their research (e.g., Latour and Woolgar 1986). For example, to draw further on the !Kung case given previously, it is more likely that Yellen did not get precise information from the women because he is a western, foreign man than because they didn't know where they go and what they do. As an ethnographer Yellen was admittedly attracted to male information because !Kung men would and could speak to him and give him information in *his* terms. This needs to be recognized before an ethnographer writes in a way that creates gender differences, in this case in knowledge between !Kung men and women, that perpetuate androcentric accounts to be accepted and applied by other researchers.

In archaeology it is also true that women tend to be relegated to or take up what are considered to be more marginal positions and jobs. Usually this is the lab analysis or "housework" of archaeology (Gero 1985). In Americanist archaeology the statistics confirm that it has been predominantly a white male enterprise; Robert Ascher (citing Kidder 1949) discusses the two types of archaeologists as being either "hairy-chested" or "hairy-chinned" (Ascher 1960). *Who* the practitioners are affects the kinds of questions that are given priority in research and thus the interpretations of the past.

Gero (1991a) has shown, for example, that when archaeologists replicate various prehistoric tools and technologies through experiments, male archaeologists do all the manufacturing (and they especially manufacture the finished tools, the projectile points thought central to the hunting of wild game), and female archaeologists do much of the edge-wear or use-wear analysis. For this they study in the laboratory the polishes left on the edges of tools and used pieces from the various activities, such as hide working and plant or wood processing. Furthermore, Gero (1991b) has also shown how the studies of American Paleoindian cultures have been dominated by male archaeologists and how the primary picture of Paleoindian lifeways is one that focuses almost exclusively on activities presumed to be male, especially the hunting of big game, with all the associated tools and strategies.

The point of studies like Gero's is not merely to "expose" and critique androcentric thinking. It is a serious charge to note that the nature of archaeological knowledge about the past is directly created by the topics that are given research priority and that these are very much influenced by the gender, class, race, ethnicity, and nationality of the practitioners (and of those who fund archaeology). Rather, the point of such studies is to understand how such factors work and to ask critical questions, such as "where *do* archaeologists get the assumptions about gender and social life that underlie their interpretations?"[3]

MAKING GENDER EXPLICIT IN ARCHAEOLOGICAL RESEARCH

I have already noted how ideas about gender drawn from ethnography or ethnoarchaeology must be critically evaluated because of long-standing biases (Moore 1988). Additionally, archaeologists have been drawing primarily on specific theoretical frameworks in the last several decades that have very little to offer in terms of making inferences about social processes and social life, except in a general way. That is, the preferred—and in many ways very productive—theories have been cultural ecology (how humans relate to their environment), cultural evolution (how societies and cultures change), and systems theory (how societies and cultures "work" on a grand scale). There is very little in these theories about social *relations* and much less about gender. Even most materialist approaches have never looked at how cultural materials are part of gender relations; until recently, most material culture studies in archaeology have not viewed artifacts as active means through which social relations are produced. If archaeologists thought materials could be used to "say" something about past societies, it was usually a direct "reflection" of relatively static social phenomena, such as status (e.g., a burial item reflects the status of the deceased) or "group" (e.g., an artifact style reflects the existence of a specific "ethnic group"). When material culture and artifacts are understood as an active part of the definition and transformation of social relationships, we can then ask how the artifacts have been part of these social processes, including gender relations. For example, one ethnoarchaeological study (Braithwaite 1982) has shown how, among the Azande of the Sudan (Africa), the decorated ceramics (not the plainware) are used by women to serve food to men because this exchange and interface between men and women is considered potentially dangerous and ambiguous. The use of decorated ceramics is integral to, and signifies, the tensions and the enactments of these male/female gender relations.

However, although gender, like many other aspects of social life, was probably present in past societies (at least since the establishment of modern humans), it may not be something we can always "get at."[4] We know there were both men and women (as well as children) in prehistory, and we suspect that gender often may have been a powerful—but highly variable—dimension of social life. Just because gender inquiry is enjoying some popularity now, it should not necessarily become the goal of most archaeological research. Whether gender is considered in analyses will depend on the questions being asked, the particular archaeological contexts being studied, and the kinds of archaeological data involved. As in *all* archaeological research the kinds of questions asked successfully will be closely linked to, if not somewhat constrained by, each case. However, it is clear that by taking gender as an explicit focus, there can be important and rich insights into past human lives.

In all societies it is not just gender *per se* that is of anthropological interest, but gender relations, because gender identity, roles, and ideologies are established in relation to others of similar and different genders, roles, and classes.[5] We have seen what problems arise in archaeological interpretation when certain assumptions about gender and gender roles are not made explicit or questioned. Many archaeologists think that gender studies in archaeology are simply linking certain artifacts and activities to men or women, which is a limited view. Even then, as in the different interpretations of grave goods discussed previously, they often do not question or consider the assumptions they are making about roles and activities.

By *not* taking gender seriously archaeologists often miss powerful evidence and rich interpretations. For example, some anthropologists (e.g., Silverblatt 1987) have shown how the development of complex societies, such as the state, were often partly accomplished by a shift from societies based on kinship to relations based more on economics and politics. This means there were significant changes in gender relations. How then could archaeologists possibly explain the "rise of the state" *without* analysis of the role of gender in the successful transformations and subsequent maintenance of the state itself?

Brumfiel's (1991) recent analysis of the Aztec state in the Valley of Mexico has shown how the tribute system (the collection and redistribution of textiles), the fundamental politicoeconomic basis for state maintenance, was in large part based on female labor: Women either made textiles directly or cooked and prepared food for market "sale" to obtain the textiles for the tribute payments. How did these gender roles emerge and become established? When gender relations are viewed as one of the (many) processes "at work" in cultural change and in how humans cope and live their daily lives, we *do* get a much more human picture and a more detailed picture of the past.

There have been a number of important attempts to take gender and gender relations seriously in archaeological interpretation, and some of these are worth reviewing. For example, the traditional view on hunter-gatherers is that they lived their lives more or less dictated by their environments because they did not produce their own food. This has easily led to interpretations of hunter-gatherers either in ecological terms (focusing on such things as "resource-procurement strategies") or in biological terms (that they had to be involved in "viable mating networks"). There is little room in such characterizations for real people with social and interpersonal lives and relationships.

One archaeologist has taken a different perspective on some California hunter-gatherers (Jackson 1991). Archaeology and ethnography have shown that as a group California hunter-gatherers had much more complex social relations, alliances, and trade networks than the more "stereotypically simple" hunter-gatherer societies. Usually such phenomena as alliances and trade are viewed as ways to move resources and not to be too controlled by the environment. Although many of these people knew about the practices of agriculture (from some of their southwestern neighbors), this was not a part of their ways; however, we know that they did control the production of some resources, such as the deliberate burning of wild grasses, which could increase productivity. Often the location of their sites is described in terms of "maximizing" their access to desired or necessary resources.

But instead of thinking about these people primarily in economic terms (and terms derived from the "maximization" principles of western capitalism), we could think about them through the lens of gender. Jackson, using historic, ethnohistoric, and archaeological data on the Western Sierra Mono people, came up with a model for their food-getting and food-preparation (which are standard archaeological topics) that features women doing most of the processing of the staple crop—acorns. When he asked what the *implications* of this might be for other aspects of Mono life, he arrived at some interesting observations. For one thing much of this acorn processing (and storage) occurred in locations where outcrops of bedrock lay exposed because they created mortars, or places *in* the bedrock, for grinding acorns. Often "granaries" were built over the bedrock mortars to store the acorns. These mortars are thus "fixed" on the landscape, and it was at these locales that other activities—of men, women, and children—were often focused. Thus, these locations of women's work structured settlement patterns and social relations. In this case Jackson suggested that women's production served as an economic and social focus for Mono daily life. As a result we get a glimpse into how gender roles and relations were integral to prehistoric lifeways.

As suggested previously the many instances of large-scale cultural change, which are a favorite topic of archaeological inquiry, can be better understood if we understand how gender roles and relations were involved. Christine Hastorf (1991) studied what happened in an area of highland Peru when the Inka tried to move in and establish sociopolitical control. The study shows how changing gender relations and changes in something as mundane as food preparation and consumption have much to do with large-scale sociopolitical transformations. Hastorf's research is a powerful example, not just because it involves explicit attention to gender, but because several lines of evidence converge to reinforce the interpretation. This kind of archaeological reasoning is particularly important because one line of evidence (such as changes in location of food processing) might not be adequate to make a strong case, in this instance for shifts in gender roles and relations.

First Hastorf analyzed the pollen found in soil samples from dwelling areas or "patios," and she documented changes in the kinds of plant foods processed, including an increase in corn. Her analysis of the spatial distribution of food processing and consumption suggests that food processing, for example, was becoming more focused in certain patios. This more concentrated food production seemed to occur within individual domestic units primarily associated with women. This insight is reinforced by ethnohistoric information about sexual and spatial divisions of labor.

Second Hastorf looked at the bone chemistry of skeletons buried at different phases in the transformation to greater control by the Inka. From bone chemistry we can infer certain aspects of people's dietary intake (because the chemical composition of food leaves some "signatures" during the growth of human bone). Corn is one food product that leaves a quite distinctive signature because of its carbon content. The bone chemistry analysis showed that the diets of men and women were about the same at the beginning of the transformation, but by the time the Inka had taken over the region, there were marked differences in male and female diets. The consumption of corn in some form increased in the men. Drawing on ethnohistoric accounts of the political life of the Inkas, Hastorf suggests that men consumed corn mostly in the form of a corn-based beer, which was central to the feasting offered as tribute and as a political symbol of Inka control. The general picture of the transformation is one whereby household food production increased and men consumed increasingly more corn, probably in the form of beer.

Hastorf's study is an archaeological inquiry into what happens with the "rise of a state:" How did the Inka expand their territory and get other people to give in to them? In daily lives how does this happen? Most archaeological accounts tend to invoke large-scale processes, such as ecological pressure, warfare, and mobilization of labor for public works. Again we might ask, what happens if we inquire into how such a sociopolitical change impacts on, and was affected by, gender roles and relations? As with Brumfiel's work with the Aztecs it appears as if changing gender roles and women's labor are crucial to the establishment and maintenance of the political tributes that sustain some empires. Furthermore, archaeology performed at the level of the household—which has not been as popular as studying the big ceremonial centers and public buildings of complex societies—can be not at all marginal to answering large questions about political power and the "rise of states."

Much of the archaeological research that asks about gender and about the implications of gender for other sociocultural processes has drawn on ethnohistoric records about male and female activities and positions in society. Such data have been used to make archaeological inferences about gender more credible. It may not be possible to have such strong culturally specific starting assumptions about gender in many prehistoric situations, although as we have seen this has not always deterred archaeologists from assuming a lot about gender in prehistory. Regardless of the source or the relative strength of starting assumptions, it is, as with all archaeological interpretations, up to us to make our assumptions explicit and to make our inferences "tight." They must be as well grounded as possible.

Archaeologists may not be able to consider gender in every instance. However, the one thing to be learned from both social and gender theory and from archaeological studies in which gender has been taken seriously is that gender can be one of many powerful relations that embody the dialectics of human life. Also the one thing to be learned from studies of gender in archaeology is that the human past was also full of tensions, conflicts, and cooperation between men and women (and other possible genders). Without attention to this when possible we will have an impoverished and often mechanistic view of human lives.

We have learned in anthropology, history, archaeology, sociology, and other fields of the tremendous range and variability in gender relations, meanings, and gendered lives, even within a single society or culture. We have also learned of variations in archaeological contexts in which we are specifically inquiring into gendered social lives. It is thus increasingly unlikely that we will be able to account for hundreds of societies for long periods of time and in wide geographic areas with just one "account" or story of gender—whether that is a story of androcentric or gynecentric (women centered) social life. We are beginning to appreciate how dynamic and fluid gender relations can be and how diverse the possibilities and practices are that existed for, and were engaged in by, men and women for tens of thousands of years of past human lives.

NOTES

1. I make a distinction here between research and interpretation that is "sexist" and that which is androcentric or gynecentric. Sexism involves statements, attitudes, and theories that presuppose, assert, or imply inferiority (of one sex or the other), that accept as legitimate the subordination of one sex to the other, and that view prescriptions for defining roles on the basis of sex as legitimate and unproblematic. Androcentrism or gynecentrism is less intentional. Human life is perceived from a male (androcentrism) or female (gynecentrism) perspective without considering or describing the activity or position of the other sex or gender.
2. Within archaeology, there is an increasing amount of work being done that not only documents the different status of men and women in the field (Gero 1985; Kramer and Stark 1989; and a range of papers in Walde and Willows 1991), but also shows how the "profile of practitioners" substantively affects the kind of interpretations we develop (see also in Hastorf 1991; Trigger 1986). Also there are accounts about how the preferred topics for discussion and explanation (e.g., technological innovations as crucial to culture change) are also highly gendered (usually male) (see for example, Conkey and Williams 1991; Wylie 1991).
3. There is a rich and important literature on the concept of gender that I cannot discuss here. It is important to recognize the distinction between sex, which is biologically based, and gender. Gender is, at one level, the cultural and social construction of sex, but it is more complex than merely mapping cultural constructs onto one sex or another. There can be, for example, more than two genders, such as in the *berdache* of some native American people. Because there is often some relation between sex and whatever genders develop, some analysts have referred to this area of inquiry as the "sex/gender system" (see Fausto-Sterling 1985; Harding 1983).

   Archaeologists who wish to make inferences about gender need to consider the rich theoretical literature and understand that gender is not just another static variable for which we can find a material correlate in the archaeological record (see the critique by Stacey and Thorne 1985; Conkey 1991).
4. Archaeologists continue to debate what our "objects of knowledge" can be, especially in terms of what we call the "level of resolution." With reference to gender research there are those who are not convinced we can make inferences about individual human behavior in the past (e.g., Hayden 1991) and those who argue that "ethnographic variables" (such as gender relations) are outside the scope of a "scientifically credible" archaeology (e.g., Binford 1983, 1986; but see Wylie 1991 for a critique of these views with particular reference to gender).
5. Gender is a complex social process, involving such aspects as gender roles (what people do, what is considered appropriate), gender ideology (what meanings are assigned to male, female, or other genders; these are not universal in the sense that there are some essential, unchanging notions of male and female), and gender identity (feelings about one's own gender). Gender is, above all, highly variable; it is a social and cultural way of marking differences, and it is entangled with other social and cultural phenomena, such as (in our current western societies) ethnicity, class, and religion.

REFERENCES

Ascher, Robert. 1960. Archaeology and the public image. *American Antiquity* 25(3):402–403.

Binford, Lewis R. 1983. *Working at Archaeology.* New York: Academic Press.

———. 1986. Data, relativism, and archaeological science. *Man* (n.s.) 22:391–404.

Braithwaite, Mary. 1982. Decoration as ritual symbol: A theoretical proposal and an ethnographic study in southern Sudan. In Ian Hodder (ed.). *Symbolic and Structural Archaeology,* pp. 80–88. Cambridge, England: Cambridge University Press.

Brumfiel, Elizabeth. 1991. Weaving and cooking: Women's production in Aztec Mexico. In Joan Gero and Margaret Conkey (eds.). *Engendering Archaeology: Women and Prehistory,* pp. 224–254. Oxford: Basil Blackwell.

Conkey, Margaret W. 1991. Does it make a difference? Feminist thinking and archaeologies of gender. In Dale Walde and Noreen Willows (eds.). *The Archaeology of Gender.* Chacmool Archaeological Association. Calgary, Alberta: Department of Archaeology, University of Calgary.

Conkey, Margaret W. and Janet Spector. 1984. Archaeology and the study of gender. In Michael B. Schiffer (ed.). *Advances in Archaeological Method and Theory,* Vol. 7, pp. 1–38. New York: Academic Press.

Conkey, Margaret and Sarah H. Williams. 1991. Original narratives: The political economy of gender in archaeology. In M. DiLeonardo (ed.). *Gender at the Crossroads of Knowledge: Feminist Anthropology in the Post-Modern Era.* Berkeley and Los Angeles: University of California Press.

Eichler, Margrit and Jeanne Lapointe. 1985. *On the Treatment of the Sexes in Research.* Ottawa: Social Sciences and Humanities Research Council of Canada.

Fausto-Sterling, Anne. 1985. *Myths of Gender: Biological Theories about Women and Men.* New York: Basic Books.

Gero, Joan M. 1985. Socio-politics of archaeology and the woman-at-home ideology. *American Antiquity* 50:342–350.

———. 1991a. Genderlithics: Women's roles in stone tool production. In Joan Gero and Margaret Conkey (eds.). *Engendering Archaeology: Women and Prehistory,* pp. 163–193. Oxford: Basil Blackwell.

———. 1991b. The social world of prehistoric facts: Gender and power in knowledge construction. Paper presented at "Women in Archaeology" conference, Albury, New South Wales, Australia, February 1991. (To be published by the Australian National University, Department of Anthropology and Prehistory; Laurajane Smith and Hilary DuCros, editors.)

Harding, Sandra. 1983. Why has the sex/gender system become visible only now? In Sandra Harding and Merrill B. Hintikka (eds.). *Discovering Reality: Feminist Perspectives on Epistemology, Metaphysics, Methodology, and Philosophy,* pp. 311–324. Boston: Reidel.

Hastorf, Christine A. 1991. Gender, space, and food in prehistory. In Joan Gero and Margaret Conkey (eds.). *Engendering Archaeology: Women and Prehistory,* pp. 132–162. Oxford: Basil Blackwell.

Hayden, Brian. 1991. Observing prehistoric women. Paper presented at Anthropology and Archaeology of Women Conference, Appalachian State University, Boone, NC (May 1991).

Hubbard, Ruth. 1982. Have only men evolved? In R. Hubbard, M. S. Henfin, and B. Fried (eds.). *Biological Woman—the Convenient Myth,* pp. 17–46. Cambridge: Schenkman.

Jackson, Thomas L. 1991. Pounding acorn: Women's production as social and economic focus. In Joan Gero and Margaret Conkey (eds.). *Engendering Archaeology: Women and Prehistory,* pp. 301–328. Oxford: Basil Blackwell.

Kidder, A. V. 1949. Introduction. *Prehistoric Southwesterners from Basketmaker to Pueblo,* by Charles Amsden. Los Angeles: Southwest Museum.

Kramer, Carol and Miriam Stark. 1988. The status of women in archaeology. *Anthropology Newsletter* 29(9):11–12. Washington, DC: American Anthropological Association.

Latour, Bruno and Stephen Woolgar. 1986. *Laboratory Life: The Construction of Scientific Facts,* 2nd ed. Princeton: Princeton University Press.

Levi-Strauss, Claude. 1936. Contribution à l'étude de l'organization sociale des Indiens Bororo. *Journal de la Societe des Americanistes de Paris* 28:269–304.

Lovejoy, Owen. 1981. The origin of man. *Science* 211:341–350.

Michard-Marshale, Claire and Claudine Ribery. 1982. *Sexisme et Science Humaine.* Lille: Presses Universitaires de France.

Moore, Henrietta. 1988. *Feminism and Anthropology.* Oxford: Polity Press.

Silverblatt, Irene. 1987. *Moon, Sun, and Witches: Gender Ideologies and Class in Inca and Colonial Peru.* Princeton: Princeton University Press.

Stacey, Judith and Barrie Thorne. 1985. The missing feminist revolution in sociology. *Social Problems* 32(4):301–316.

Trigger, Bruce G. 1984. Alternative archaeologies: Nationalist, colonialist, imperialist. *Man* (n.s.) 19:355–370.

Walde, Dale and Noreen Willows (eds.). 1991. *The Archaeology of Gender.* Proceedings of the Chacmool Conference, 1989. Calgary, Alberta: Chacmool Archaeological Association, Department of Archaeology.

Watson, Patty Jo and Marcy C. Kennedy. 1991. The development of horticulture in the eastern woodlands of North America: Women's role. In Joan Gero and Margaret Conkey (eds.). *Engendering Archaeology: Women and Prehistory,* pp. 255–275. Oxford: Basil Blackwell.

Winters, Howard. 1968. Value-systems and trade cycles of the late archaic in the Midwest. In S.R. Binford and L. R. Binford (eds.). *New Perspectives in Archaeology,* pp. 175–222. Chicago: Aldine.

Wylie, M. Alison. 1991. Gender theory and the archaeological record: Why is there no archaeology of gender? In Joan Gero and Margaret Conkey (eds.). *Engendering Archaeology: Women and Prehistory,* pp. 31–54. Oxford: Basil Blackwell.

Yellen, John. 1977. *Archaeological Approaches to the Present.* New York: Academic Press.

DIVERSITY OF THE UPPER PALEOLITHIC "VENUS" FIGURINES AND ARCHEOLOGICAL MYTHOLOGY

Sarah M. Nelson

Among the earliest depictions of human beings, dating back to perhaps 30,000 years ago, are small figurines of nude females, which are found across a broad belt in Europe from the Pyrenees in southern France to the Don river in the USSR, with outliers in Siberia. Every anthropologist is familiar with these Upper Paleolithic "Venus" figurines. They are used to titillate freshman classes, and photographs or drawings, especially of the figurines from Willendorf and Dolni Vestoni e, routinely enliven introductory textbooks.

Current trends in literary criticism lean toward deconstruction of "texts," in which both words and situations may serve as the text for analysis. In this [reading], I would like to deconstruct some texts in a narrower sense, using the example of the Venus figurines to demonstrate that introductory textbooks of archeology and physical anthropology produce gender metaphors which, by ignoring much of the scholarship on the figurines, reaffirm the folk model of gender preferred by our culture.

FIGURINE DESCRIPTIONS

The figurines themselves have only gender in common. They are diverse in shape, in pose, in the somatic details depicted, and in ornamentation (Soffer 1988, Fleury 1926, Abramova 1967, Luquet 1926, Delporte 1979). They seem to represent differences in age as well (Rice 1981). Yet the textbooks tend to represent the figurines as all the same, and then to leap from this purported sameness to a supposed function for all figurines over their 3000 mile and perhaps 10,000 year spread (Soffer [1988], although Gamble [1986, 1987] asserts that most figurines fall within a 2000 year range). We need to explore this phenomenon of perceiving sameness in the diverse figurines, and ask why it occurs.

The texts our students read describe the figurines and frequently ascribe a function to them. There is little indication in the bibliographies that the authors of the texts have read any primary sources about the figurines, or that they are conversant with the rich literature which explores the variation in both the figurines themselves and the possible meanings and functions of the figurines. Rather, it seems that a kind of folklore is repeated, a folklore of the anthropology profession, too well known to require documentation.

The textbooks utilized in this study represent an unsystematic nonrandom sample—all that happen to be on my bookshelves, supplemented with those of my colleagues. Of 20 introduction to archeology or archeology and physical anthropology textbooks thus examined, eight concentrate on methodology and do not mention the figurines, while the other twelve contain cursory remarks on one to three pages. It is these twelve texts which constitute the study sample.

Table 1 shows the distribution of what is written regarding the physical characteristics of the figurines. Six of the textbooks mention exaggerated sexual characteristics as a prominent feature, whether or not they specify which traits are meant. The most common feature to be singled out is the breasts, described as "large," "generous," or "pendu-

TABLE 1 Description of Figurines

Author	*Sexual*	*Abdomen*	*Breasts*	*Buttocks*	*Hips*	*Pregnant*	*Fat*
Barnouw (1978)	×	×	×		×	×	
Campbell (1988)		×	×	×			×
Chard (1975)			×	×	×	×	×
Clark (1977)			×	×	(thighs)		×
Eddy (1984)	×		×	×			
Fagan (1986)	×		×				
Hester & Grady (1982)			×		×		
Jurmain et al. (1981)	×						
Pfeiffer (1985)	(stylized)						
Poirier (1987)		×	×	×			
Smith (1976)	×		×	×		×	
Wenke (1984)	×						

lous." All but one of the texts characterize the figurines as having either exaggerated sexual characteristics or large breasts, and four include both. Buttocks are mentioned five times, once described as "protruding," while hips, once with the adjective "broad," are specified three times. Only one author mentions both, showing that he makes a distinction between hips and buttocks. We are left to guess whether these terms are intended to refer to hindquarters in general in the other cases, or whether one set of authors indeed has protruding buttocks in mind (i.e., steatopygia), and the other really means broad hips (i.e., steatomeria) (Boule and Vallois 1957:318). In one confusing case, an illustration of Willendorf, without a trace of steatopygia but with undoubted steatomeria, is pictured side by side with a Khoi-San woman, of whom the reverse is clearly the case—that is, protruding buttocks without broad hips (Campbell 1988:508).

The assertion that pregnancy is depicted in the figurines occurs in the textbook sample three times, and one additional author points out the exaggerated "belly," allowing him the satisfying alliteration of "breasts, belly, and buttocks." Three of the authors describe the figurines as fat. The only author to refrain from asserting or implying fatness does not describe the figurines at all, but contents himself with an illustration of Willendorf (Pfeiffer 1985:203). Reading these descriptions, one would suppose that the Willendorf statuette, easily the most familiar, was typical or normal or modal. Instead, it is one of the least stylized and the most obese—referred to in another context with admiration as representing "resplendent endomorphy" (Beller 1977:78).

The generalizations in the textbooks do some violence to the facts. Few of the statuettes represent gross obesity, and some are quite slender (Fig. 1). Even the first figurines found in the 1890s were classified by Piette into svelte and obese classes (Delporte 1979:73). Half a century ago Passemard (1938) examined all the then-known figurines to see whether they were steatopygous, a description quite popular at that time, and came to the conclusion that most were not. Saccasyn Della Santa (1947:9–13) reviewed the literature on the figurines again, and also concluded that they were not meant to represent steatopygia.

An unpublished statistical study of the variation in body shapes made 22 measurements on each figurine for which both frontal and profile photographs could be found—24 measurable figurines in all. The statuettes sorted into distinct groups of 10 obese (wide hips and thick body), 3 steatopygous (protruding buttocks), and 11 normal (Nelson n.d.). Another study shows that only 39 per-

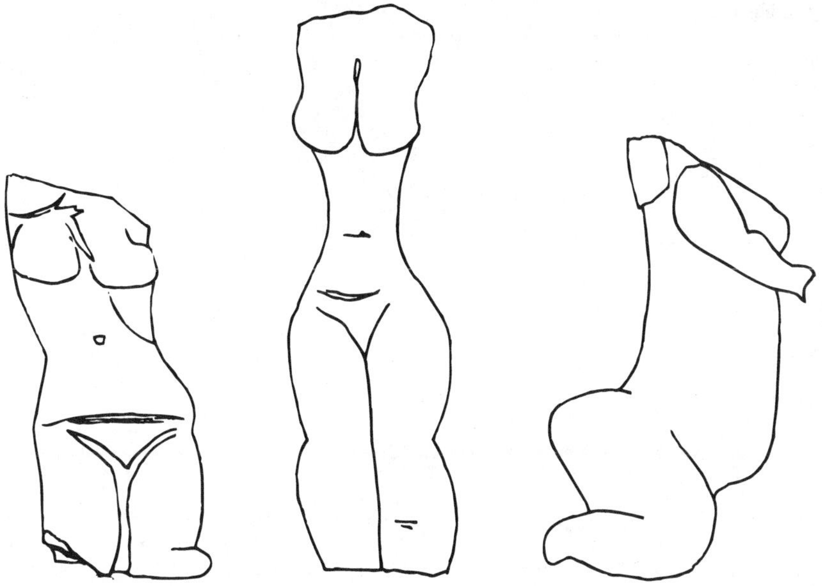

(a) (b) (c)

FIGURE 1 Slender figurines from a. Petrokovi e, Czechoslovakia; b. Elisevitchi, USSR; and c. Sireul, France.

cent of these figurines could possibly represent pregnancy, slightly over half (55 percent) have pendulous breasts, 45 percent have broad hips, and 13 percent have protruding buttocks. Twenty-two percent have none of these characteristics, (Nelson and Bibb n.d.). Bodyshapes depicted in the figurines have been divided into three or four categories by intuitive studies as well, such as those by Fleury (1926), Abramova (1967), and Luquet (1926).

Rice (1981) has suggested that this variability in body shape reflects different age groups, and has shown that different body characteristics can be so interpreted, with a high correlation between ratings. The distribution of the figurines in these age categories corresponds to the expected age pyramid for foraging societies.

Failure to acknowledge the variability of the figurines makes it easier to produce sweeping generalizations about their probable meaning or function. This is evident in the textbook interpretations. By far the most common function ascribed to the figurines is that of "fertility" (Table 2), specifically so designated in seven of the 12 texts, and called "procreation" and "maternity" by one text each. This ascription is usually not explained at all, or weakly expressed at best. For example, "It seems unlikely that Upper Paleolithic women actually looked like that, but perhaps it was an ideal type or expressed a wish for fertility" (Barnouw 1978:176). Apparently in conjunction with the fertility function is the idea of a "cult" or "Mother Goddess," since the five authors who use one or both of these expressions attach them to the fertility notion. Only one author rejects fertility as an explanation, on the grounds that hunters are not concerned with human fertility. Rather he explicitly suggests that the figurines are erotic: "Pleistocene pinup or centerfold girls" (Chard 1975:182).

TABLE 2 Functions of Figurines

Author	*Fertility*	*Goddess/Cult*	*Erotic*	*Artistic/Stylized*
Barnouw (1978)	×			
Campbell (1988)	×	×		
Chard (1975)	rejects		×	
Clark (1977)	× (maternity)			ö
Eddy (1984)	×	×	×	
Fagan (1986)	×	×		
Hester & Grady (1982)	×			×
Jurmain et al. (1981)	×	×	×	ö
Pfeiffer (1985)				×
Poirier (1987)	×	×		
Smith (1976)	×		×	×
Wenke (1984)			ö	×

HIDDEN ASSUMPTIONS

The brief descriptions and interpretations of the female figurines contain and to some extent conceal unexamined assumptions about gender. Among them are: that the figurines were made *by* men, that the figurines were made *for* men, that nakedness is necessarily associated with eroticism, and that depiction of breasts is primarily sexual.

Underlying the description of the female figurines as erotic or reproductive is a masculist construction of the world, in which females are assumed to exist primarily for the use of males, sexually or reproductively. The scholarly literature is replete with explicit examples of this worldview, which the textbooks reflect.

A few quotations from the scholarly literature will demonstrate that males are usually assumed to be the sculptors of the figurines. The italics are mine throughout. "How did the artist's vision, which reflected the ideal of *his* time, see her? For as with man, we can never know what she really looked like . . . so we have to make do with the version her comparison, man, had of her" (Berenguer 1973:48). The possibility that it was *her* version appears not to have crossed Berenguer's mind. Although this mindset focuses on males exclusively, it is not confined to males only, as shown from this quote from a woman, "He [the artist] desired only to show the female erotically and as the source of all abundance—in her he portrayed not woman but fertility" (Hawkes 1964:27). Referring to the not uncommon find of broken-off legs, Campbell (1982:410) suggests that "they may have cracked off in the baking, or when the ancient ceramicist tossed aside a work that failed to please *him*." (Most of the figurines of course are carved.) In case there is any doubt about the use of the specific rather than the generic use of the term "man", Leroi-Gourhan (1967:90) makes it crystal clear that "prehistoric man" doesn't include females, speaking of "the first figurines representing prehistoric man—or at least *his wife.*"

If the figurines are assumed to have been made by men, then it follows that they were created for male purposes. Even when they were first discovered, the Abbé Breuil (1954, cited in Ucko and Rosenfeld 1973:119) said they were for "pleasure to Paleolithic man during his meals" (do we have a euphemism here?). Berenguer (1973:52) focuses on reproductivity: "we may deduce man's obsessive need for women who would bear *him* lots of children to offset the high mortality rate caused by the harsh living conditions." Von Königswald worried about other possessions, "It certainly is an old problem: how could man protect *his* property, mark a place as 'his home', 'his living site' so that others would recognize and respect it, especially in a period where there were no houses, just *abris* and caves?" He concludes that men made the "grotesque" figurines to guard their property, and scare off intruders! Delporte (1979:308) muses more philosophically, "for [paleolithic men] as for us . . . the mother who gives and transmits life is also the woman who gives and shares pleasure: could the paleolithic have been insensitive to this novel duality?" [my translation]. Could the present be insensitive to the fact that there were paleolithic women as well as men? Are women to be denied their own sensitivity, or indeed their own existence as sentient beings?

The fact that the figurines were unclothed, or scantily clothed, for several wear belts and other decorations (a fact that is noted only by Clark [1977:105] among our textbook sample), surely has been essential to the interpretation of eroticism, in spite of the fact that there are many other possible reasons for the depiction of nudity. For example, people may have been usually unclothed inside the cave or hut, so that nakedness was not a special condition. The figurines could have been teaching devices for girls' puberty rites, as Marshack (1972:283) has suggested.

Nakedness frequently has different connotations when men rather than women are the sculptor's subject. For example, a naked male torso from Harappa is shown under the heading "Figures of Authority," in *The First Cities,* a widely used book from the Time-Life series (Hamblin 1973:133). The text tells us:

> Although male figures rarely appear among sculptures dug up at Mohenjo-Daro and Harappa, the few that do all seem to represent men of importance. In the three works reproduced here, there is a common theme, however varied the pieces themselves may be: regality or godliness.

As Conkey and Spector (1985:11) point out in another context, changing the rules of interpretation according to sex will not reveal anything about prehistoric gender roles. Rather it comforts us in supposing that things have always been the same.

In spite of being naked, however, it would seem that the fat figurines have little sex appeal to modern male scholars. This has called forth various explanations, ranging from assertions that they are stylized, to a suggestion that you cannot tell *what* might have turned on those prehistoric men (you can almost see the shrug and the wink), to a rejection of the erotic argument on the grounds that the figurines are simply too grotesque! In all of this discussion, passivity of women is assumed.

It is deserving of some comment that breasts are equated with eroticism in the textbooks, more by juxtaposition of words than by explicit statements. Sometimes, though, the equation is specified. There is one carving, referred to as the "rod with breasts," which evoked the following paean: "This statuette shows us that the artist has neglected all that did not interest *him,* stressing *his* sexual libido only where the breasts are concerned—a diluvial plastic pornography." (Absolon 1949). Surely anthropologists of all people know that exposed breasts are not at all uncommon in the warmer parts of the world, and cause little comment or excitement except for visiting tourists and perhaps a segment of the readership of *National Geographic.*

The "rod with breasts" is an interesting example of the extension of the underlying attitude toward women that is revealed in some generalizations about the figurines. Enigmatic carvings are declared to represent breasts, buttocks, or vulvae, reducing women to their "essentials" (Fig. 2). Especially the notion of the "vulvae" (some of which look rather like molar teeth), "has become an *idée fixe* and one of the most durable myths of prehistory" (Bahn 1986:99). The "rods" from Dolni Vestonice could be as easily perceived as stylized male genitalia, but if they were so described the eloquence would probably be in a different vein. It is hard to imagine exchanging the genders in the quote by Absolon above.

Alternative explanations, based on variability rather than generalizations, are not lacking in the scholarly literature. The fig-

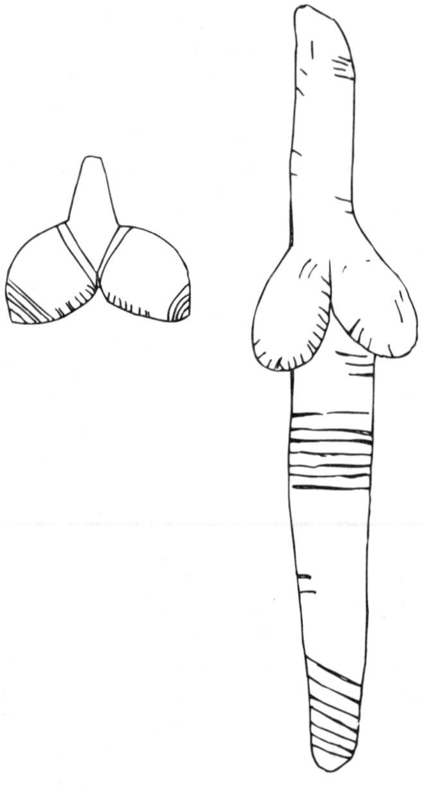

(a) (b)

FIGURE 2 "Rod with breasts" from Dolni Vestonice, Czechoslovakia.

urines have been argued to represent priests or ancestors or clan-mothers, to show women as actors with a ritual function (Klima 1962:204, Abramova 1967:83, Hancar 1940). These possibilities are not even hinted at in the texts, with one sole exception (Campbell 1988:481).

ARCHEOLOGICAL MYTHOLOGY

What are the possible reasons for the selective reporting found in the textbooks? First, to be fair, is the summary nature of the texts. Little space is given to the figurines, and it is necessary to paint a broad picture with a few strokes. But the selection of this particular way of viewing the Upper Paleolithic figures as fat, as sexual, and as representing fertility, can be linked to our own cultural stereotypes and assumptions about the nature of men, women, sexuality, and reproduction. I suggest that our own culture makes these generalizations seem so natural, so satisfying, that there is no reason to examine them. The "text" read into the figurines is ours.

Several archeologists have commented on the problems of reading our unconscious assumptions about the present into the past. "History and prehistory constitute bodies of knowledge used to legitimize social policies and to validate social trajectories" (Moore and Keene 1983:7). This tendency has been traced to the dominant paradigm in archeology: "Because of the logic of empiricist epistemology, theories rising on empiricist foundations potentially serve only to recreate in the past the dominant cultural ideologies of the present" (Saitta 1983:303). We must recognize "the importance of taking into account the conceptions we hold of our own society which inevitably mediate our understanding of the past" (Miller and Tilley 1984:2).

Recent research on gender roles in cultural anthropology proposes that "male and female, sex and reproduction, are cultural or symbolic constructs" (Ortner and Whitehead 1981:6). These constructs are often reflected in origin stories as "metaphors for sexual identity" (Sanday 1981:56), which Sanday calls "scripts." I am suggesting that culturally constructed gender roles, and our attitudes and beliefs about sex and reproduction, enter into the selectivity of reporting on the Upper Paleolithic figurines. The reading of the metaphors of the figurines derives from a masculist script.

I do not wish to impute either evil intentions or inferior scholarship to the authors of these textbooks. It is important to note the unconscious nature of the acceptance of cultural scripts. But that does not make them less pernicious. Reinforcing present cultural stereotypes by projecting them into the past allows whole generations of students to believe that our present gender constructs are eternal and unchanging. Especially those who deal in prehistory need to be alert to our cultural biases, and not imply that present gender roles are external verities.

Marvin Harris points out that "our ordinary state of mind is always a profoundly mystified consciousness. . . . To emerge from myth and legend to mature consciousness we need to compare the full range of past and present cultures" (Harris 1974:5). The trick is to examine the past without the mystification.

I am not proposing that alternative explanations are necessarily better, only that the diversity of the figurines should be taken into account. Maybe women made some of the figurines. Maybe the figurines were used for women's purposes. Maybe it isn't relevant whether men find them sexy or not. If an explanation feels intuitively right, perhaps that is the best reason to reexamine it.

REFERENCES

Abramova, Z. A. 1967. Paleolithic Art in the USSR. *Arctic Anthropology* 4(2):1–179.

Absolon, K. 1949. The Diluvial Anthropomorphic Statuettes and Drawings, Especially the So-called Venus Statuettes Discovered in Moravia. *Artibus Asiae* 12:201–220.

Bahn, P. G. 1986. No Sex Please, We're Aurignacians. *Rock Art Research* 3(2):99–105.

Barnouw, V. 1978. *Physical Anthropology and Archaeology*. 3rd ed. Homewood, IL: The Dorsey Press.

Beller, A. S. 1977. *Fat and Thin*. New York: Farrar, Strauss and Giroux.

Berenguer, M. 1973. *Prehistoric Man and His Art*. M. Heron, trans. London: Souvenir Press.

Boule, M., and H. Vallois. 1957. *Fossil Man*. New York: Dryden Press.

Campbell, B. G. 1982. *Humankind Emerging*. 3rd ed. Boston: Little, Brown.

———. 1988. *Humankind Emerging*. 5th ed. Glenview, IL: Scott, Foresman and Company.

Chard, C. 1975. *Man in Prehistory*. 2nd ed. New York: McGraw-Hill.

Clark, G. 1977. *World Prehistory in New Perspective*. 3rd ed. Cambridge: Cambridge University Press.

Conkey, M. and J. Spector. 1985. Archaeology and the Study of Gender. In *Advances in Archaeological Method and Theory*. Vol. 7. M. B. Schiffer, ed. pp. 1–38. New York: Academic Press.

Delporte, H. 1979. *l'Image de la Femme dans l'Art Préhistorique*. Paris: Picard.

Eddy, F. W. 1984. *Archaeology, A Cultural-Evolutionary Approach*. Englewood Cliffs: Prentice Hall.

Fagan, B. 1986. *People of the Earth: An Introduction to World History*. 5th ed. Boston: Little, Brown.

Fleury, C. 1926. Quelques Considerations sur la Pseudo-steatopygie des Venus Aurignaciennes. *Archives Suisses d'Anthropologie Generale* 11(1): 137–141.

Gamble, C. 1986. *The Paleolithic Settlement of Europe*. Cambridge: Cambridge University Press.

———. 1987. Interaction and Alliance in Palaeolithic Society. *Man* (n.s.) 17:92–107.

Hamblin, D. J. 1973. *The First Cities*. New York: Time-Life Books.

Hancar, F. 1940. Problem der Venus Statuetten im Eurasiatischen Jung-Palaolithikum. *Praehistorische Zeitschrift:* 30–31.

Harris, M. 1974. *Cows, Pigs, Wars and Witches: The Riddles of Culture*. New York: Random House.

Hawkes, J. 1964. The Achievements of Paleolithic Man. In *Man Before History*. C. Gabel, ed. pp. 21–35. Englewood Cliffs: Prentice Hall.

Hester, J. J. and J. Grady. 1982. *Introduction to Archaeology*, 2nd ed. New York: Holt, Rinehart and Winston.

Jurmain, R., H. Nelson, H. Kurashina, and W. Turnbaugh. 1981. *Understanding Physical Anthropology and Archaeology*. St. Paul: West Publishing Co.

Klima, B. 1962. The First Ground-Plan of an Upper Paleolithic Loess Settlement in Middle Europe and its Meaning. In *Courses Toward Urban Life*. R. Braidwood and G. Willey, eds. pp. 193–210. Chicago: Aldine.

Koenigswald, G. H. R. von. 1972. Early *Homo sapiens* as an Artist: The Meaning of Paleolithic Art. In *The Origin of Homo sapiens, Ecology and Conservation*, Vol. 3. F. Bordes, ed. pp. 133–139. Proceedings of the Paris Symposium 1969.

Laurent, P. 1965. *Heureuse Prehistoire*. Perigeux: Pierre Fanlac.

Leroi-Gourhan, André. 1967. *Treasures of Prehistoric Art*. Translated by N. Guterman. New York: Henry N. Abrams.

Luquet, G. H. 1926. *L'Art et la Religion des Hommes Fossiles*. Paris: Masson et Cie.

Marshack, A. 1972. *The Roots of Civilization*. New York: McGraw-Hill.

Miller, D. and A. Tilley. 1984. Ideology, Power and Prehistory: An Introduction. In *Ideology, Power and Prehistory*. Daniel Miller and Christopher Tilley, eds. pp. 1–15. Cambridge: Cambridge University Press.

Moore, J. A. and A. S. Keene. 1983. Archaeology and the Law of the Hammer. In *Archaeological Hammers and Theories.* J. A. Moore and A. S. Keene eds. pp. 3–13. New York: Academic Press.

Nelson, S. M. n.d. "Venus" Figurines as Evidence of Sedentism in the Upper Paleolithic. (On file, Department of Anthropology, University of Denver.)

Nelson, S. M., and L. Bibb. n.d. Notes and Statistics on Venus Figurines. (On file, Department of Anthropology, University of Denver.)

Ortner, S. B., and H. Whitehead (eds.). 1981. *Sexual Meanings: The Cultural Construction of Gender and Sexuality.* Cambridge: Cambridge University Press.

Passemard, L. 1938. *Les Statuettes Feminines Paléolithiques Dites Venus.* St. Nîmes: Libraire Teissier.

Pfeiffer, J. 1985. *The Emergence of Humankind.* 4th ed. New York: Harper and Row.

Poirier, F. E. 1987. *Understanding Human Evolution.* Englewood Cliffs, NJ: Prentice Hall.

Rice, P. C. 1981. Prehistoric Venuses: Symbols of Motherhood or Womanhood? *Journal of Anthropological Research* 37(4):402–416.

Saccasyn Della Santa, E. 1947. *Les Figures Humaines du Paléolithique Superior Eurasiatique.* Paris: Amberes.

Saitta, D. J. 1983. The Poverty of Philosophy in Archaeology. In *Archaeological Hammers and Theories.* James A. Moore and Arthur S. Keene, eds. pp. 299–304. New York: Academic Press.

Sanday, P. R. 1981. *Female Power and Male Dominance: On the Origins of Sexual Inequality.* Cambridge: Cambridge University Press.

Smith, J. W. 1976. *Foundations of Archaeology.* Beverly Hills: Glencoe Press.

Soffer, O. 1988. Upper Paleolithic Connubia, Refugia and the Archaeological Record for Eastern Europe. In *Pleistocene Old World: Regional Perspectives.* O. Soffer, ed. pp. 333–348. New York: Plenum Publishing Co.

Ucko P.J. and A. Rosenfeld. 1973. *Palaeolithic Cave Art.* New York: McGraw-Hill.

Wenke, R. 1984. *Patterns in Prehistory, Humankind's First Three Million Years.* 2nd ed. New York: Oxford University Press.

MAYA ROYAL WOMEN: A LESSON IN PRECOLUMBIAN HISTORY

David Freidel and Linda Schele

The lowland Maya civilization flourished on the Yucatan peninsula for 2,000 years before the Spanish arrived on their shores in the early sixteenth century. What particularly distinguishes the Maya civilization from the others of Mesoamerica is its literature. Some other cultures, such as the Zapotec of Oaxaca, Mixe societies of Veracruz, and the early highland Maya of Guatemala, had written scripts that approximated spoken language as did the Maya script. Yet only the lowland Maya have left posterity a sizable collection of texts. Together these texts on carved stone, painted walls, pottery vessels, and other small artifacts are a bare remnant from a civilization that mostly wrote on screen-fold books of bark paper sized with lime plaster. Nevertheless, they reveal dimensions of ancient society in the New World that are barely hinted at in other regions known primarily or exclusively through their archaeological remains.

One of the lessons from textual history is that women were much more than pawns in Maya power politics. In three cases already documented (and with the prospect of more to come with continued decipherment), the performance of royal women proved decisive to the destiny of particular late Classic period (A.D. 600 to A.D. 900) kingdoms.[1] We will briefly summarize one of these dramatic episodes in Maya history that shows how women propelled themselves to the center

Original material prepared for this text.

stage of an ancient civilization. We think there is a basic lesson to be learned by archaeologists who must deal with the remains of past complex societies without the guide of written texts detailing state politics. Despite some lip service to the contrary, current introductory archaeology texts relate the rise and fall of such ahistorical civilizations as if women did not exist and as if only men ruled and made the critical decisions guiding governments. We think, on the basis of our experience with the ancient Maya, that in some early class-structured societies with hereditary elites, such as the Maya classes of *ahaw* (supreme lord) or *sahal* (noble vassal), women ruled with men in the context of court politics revolving around family alliances and feuds. Governments ruled by royal dynasties did not merely profit by the participation of women, such participation was mandatory and necessary. The political reproduction of power required the physical reproduction of rulers, a process in which women played a clear role. Beyond this biological fact, Maya rulers inherited the social, political, and religious potential for power from their mothers and their fathers. Our cases illustrate these points.

THE GREAT CLASSIC MAYA WARS

The seventh century witnessed bloody and endemic wars of conquest between the great houses of the Maya in the interior forests of the Yucatan peninsula. On the one side were the kings of Tikal and their allies and on the other were the kings of Calakmul and theirs. Ruler 1 of Dos Pilas (Balah-Kan-K'awil)[2], a member of the Tikal royal family, established a new off-shoot capital south of Tikal in A.D. 645. He joined the Calakmul alliance, warred against Tikal, and rapidly transformed his small city into one of the great Maya conquest states. Ruler 1 consolidated his hold over the southern forest region not only through battle, but also through judicious polygamous marriage to several princesses from smaller kingdoms in the area. His ambition stretched across the vast and rich farmlands of the interior forest now called Peten in Guatemala. He engaged in the wars embroiling the Tikal and Calakmul alliances, capturing and sacrificing the contemporary king of Tikal on behalf of Calakmul.

The basic military strategy of the Calakmul alliance was to surround the centrally situated Tikal state with enemy capitals. To that end Calakmul established an alliance with the city of Naranjo, to the northeast of Tikal. The king of Naranjo, however, evidently betrayed Calakmul, so that great city and another allied city called Caracol together attacked and captured Naranjo, sacrificing its king. At the same time, the son of the Tikal king captured by Ruler 1 of Dos Pilas came to power at Tikal. He prepared to rise in vengeance against the Calakmul alliance. Calakmul needed new partners on Tikal's northeastern flank at Naranjo, ready to attack in coordination with the rest of the circle of capitals.

The Princess of Dos Pilas and the Revival of Naranjo

The Calakmul alliance then called on Ruler 1 of Dos Pilas for assistance and he sent his daughter to Naranjo to rededicate the sacred center and establish a new, loyal, dynastic family there. The new Tikal king came to the throne on May 6, A.D. 682, readying his war with his enemies. By August 30 of that same year the Dos Pilas princess had successfully crossed the forest past Tikal without being captured and had arrived at Naranjo. It takes little imagination to know the courage and resolve of this woman, riding in her sedan chair as a living declaration of war more than 100 kilometers over jungle paths through enemy territory. Every moment of that journey she faced capture and death by sacrifice at the hands of the Tikal king and his allies.

No doubt to the people of Naranjo her arrival was nothing short of miraculous, and her three-day ceremonial was precisely that. Her duty was to rededicate the sacred temple of the city. In the thinking of the Maya she reopened the Naranjo portal to the Otherworld, allowing communication and magical power to pass from the world of the ancestors to the world of the living. The usual way to accomplish this for a royal woman was to pierce her tongue in self-sacrifice with a lancet of black volcanic glass and then to pull a cord through it as she entered an ecstatic trance and brought forth the spirit of her ancestor to bless the place.

The royal princess of Dos Pilas, named Wak-Kanal-Tzuk, probably married a prince of the defeated dynasty. That man's only role was to beget a son who would take his throne and rule in the name of the Calakmul alliance. The son of the princess became king as a small child. His mother, and his mother's brother from Dos Pilas, fought wars in his name against Tikal and Tikal's allies. From the texts of this city, we know that she fought the wars and not her husband, whose name is never mentioned in the histories of Naranjo. The ignominious defeat of Naranjo by the Calakmul alliance during his early reign, or during that of his father, stripped him of the privilege of history. Without the Dos Pilas princess the kingdom of Naranjo would have slipped quietly into obscurity.

The Naranjo Wars

After her dedication of the Naranjo royal temple, the Dos Pilas princess gave birth to a royal heir, Butz-Tilwi' in ancient Mayan, nicknamed Smoking-Squirrel by scholars, on January 6, A.D. 688. There is little doubt that although her husband may have been alive, she ruled during this period, because she was the only one with a royal history from Naranjo at this time. Clearly, however, Ruler 1 of Dos Pilas was anxious to see his daughter's command of this strategic city consolidated. When the boy was only 5 years old he ascended to the throne of Naranjo on May 31, A.D. 693. Out of deference to the humiliated royal house of Naranjo, the scribes of the city never explicitly announced the parentage of the new king. But the systematic way that they linked the arrival of the princess at Naranjo, the birth of her son, and the declaration of the princesses' parentage in Ruler 1 of Dos Pilas in a single text makes it certain that she is the mother of the young king of Naranjo.

Soon after the boy became king, on June 20, A.D. 693, Naranjo went to war against the allies of Tikal to the southwest of their realm. Obviously, a 5-year-old child had little to do with this bloody work. The princess and her brother successfully prosecuted war against the kingdom of Ucanal, capturing a high lord there. On a retrospective carved stone monument celebrating this victory, the princess shows herself standing upon this prostate captive in the time honored stance of conquest taken by Maya kings. This was only the opening battle in a protracted series of campaigns by the newly refurbished dynasty of Naranjo against the Tikal state. One hundred days later Naranjo attacked Ucanal again, and on February 1, A.D. 695, Naranjo delivered a major defeat against this border kingdom ally of Tikal. This victory involved an unnamed lord from Dos Pilas, probably a relative of the princess, and it shows that Dos Pilas played an active military role in the success of Naranjo.

Naranjo continued to attack to the south and east under the aegis of Smoking-Squirrel and his mother for many years. Between them, they wreaked havoc on Tikal and other cities for two generations. The princess from Dos Pilas clearly played the key role in this success in the early and critical years of the fledgling new dynasty at Naranjo. The result of her success was a mixed blessing for her father, Ruler 1. The victories against Tikal and its allies invited counter-attacks from the city against Naranjo. Eventually, Tikal would defeat Naranjo and capture high lords there. And enemies of Dos Pilas, no doubt fueled by Tikal, would in time lay siege to the city and bring down the dynasty Ruler 1 worked so hard to establish. Still, in her lifetime the princess from Dos Pilas was a formidable leader in the great alliance wars of the ancient Maya.

The Queens of Yaxchilan

Far to the west and a few years later in the drainage of the mighty "Xokol Ha," now called the Usumacinta River, two queens nearly tore their kingdom asunder in their struggle to determine who would inherit the throne. The kingdom was Yaxchilan, its capital, a city graced with white temples, carved and terraced on a mountain facing northeast over the forested swamps of the interior. On August 24, A.D. 709, Lady Eveningstar, daughter of the royal house of Calakmul and wife to Shield-Jaguar, Holy lord of Yaxchilan, gave birth to a son named Bird-Jaguar after his illustrious grandfather. The event brought no happiness to Lady Shark, cowife to Lady Eveningstar and the senior wife of the Yaxchilan King. Lady Shark's family was local to the kingdom, a vassal lineage to the house of Yaxchilan. Lady Shark was, technically, Shield-Jaguar's mother's father's sister's daughter—or first cousin once removed. Lady Shark had every reason and precedent to support her claim to give birth to the heir to the throne, but now there was a rival claimant. The logic of Lady Eveningstar's claim no doubt derived from the powerful alliance that was sustained if the heir was from two great royal houses strategically spanning the great forest.

We don't know exactly when the old king first declared for his younger son, but we do know that the consequences were to thrust Yaxchilan to the brink of civil war. Some noble families supported the precedent that the heir should come from the union of the dynasty with a vassal noble house of Yaxchilan and others supported the king's alliance to Calakmul. Shield-Jaguar went out among his noble vassals and performed public sacrifices at their provincial capitols to cement their loyalty to him and his heir. The king attempted to settle the struggle by conceding to Lady Shark an extraordinary privilege: She was to dedicate a new royal temple in the most important location in the city. This beautiful temple contained carved stone lintels over the doorways featuring portraits of Lady Shark with Shield-Jaguar and with his ancestor. Shield-Jaguar went to war to bring back sacrificial victims to bless this temple. There was a catch, however. The text of one of the lintels celebrates a hierophany, a conjunction of planets in the sky; this conjunction occurs a magic number of days, 52, after the birth of Bird-Jaguar to Lady Eveningstar. In this indirect and discrete fashion Lady Shark was required to acknowledge through her dedication of a royal temple that the dynastic heir was to be Bird-Jaguar. In this way Lady Shark won the privilege of writing sacred history for herself in one of the most beautiful set of Maya carvings, but she had to inscribe against the starfield that her rival's son would rule the kingdom.

On the other hand, while Lady Eveningstar won the crown for her son, she forfeited her claim to history all through the lifetime of her husband. Never once in all of his inscriptions does Shield-Jaguar mention Lady Eveningstar's existence. It is only because Bird-Jaguar won his struggle for the throne and inscribed retrospective history about his mother that we know of her. It was not an easy fight. All through his waning years Shield-Jaguar worked to confirm and sanctify his son's claim to succeed him. After his death there were 10 long years before Bird-Jaguar actually acceded to the throne. We surmise that Bird-Jaguar was battling against rival claimants derived from Lady Shark and her patriline. Although he does not mention the civil wars we find him out in the provincial capitals cementing alliances with noble vassals and celebrating victory in wars by sacrificing captives. It was not until Lady Shark died on April 3, A.D. 749, and her rival Lady Eveningstar died on March 13, A.D. 751, that Bird-Jaguar could finally take his throne on February 10, A.D. 752.

Despite his success, the civil war had taught Bird-Jaguar a bitter lesson. He made sure his own heir was born to a noble woman from one of his own vassal lineages. His wife, Lady-Great-Skull, and her brother, Great-Skull, figure prominently in his official history in ceremonies carved on lintels, along with his son Chel-Te. In light of the events we can document from Bird-Jaguar's life we think his attribution by modern scholars as "Bird-Jaguar the Great" is well earned. He was clearly a charismatic and very able military and political leader. Without such skill he may have failed to repair the breach caused by his father's decision to choose him for heir. A struggle of great women underscored that the fate of major Maya kingdoms depended on them as much as their husbands and sons.

The role of Maya royal women in the history of this ancient civilization is beginning to come into focus. We have had clues for some time in the form of sumptuous tomb furniture accompanying some elite women. Slowly we have moved in our understanding of the texts from initial hypotheses that the exchange of women between dynasties strengthened alliances between their male rulers to more subtle and complicated scenarios in which Maya women have emerged as powerful personalities and active politicians. As the archaeologists continue to excavate and as the epigraphers continue to decipher texts more completely, we expect the role of royal women to become even more central in our interpretations of this New World civilization.

NOTES

1. As in any other historical inquiry, our interpretations are subject to change with new information. The present description was originally based on our book *A Forest of Kings* (Linda Schele and David Freidel, Wm Morrow & Co., Inc. 1990). Already in this outline of the complex events surrounding the life of the Dos Pilas princess, we have changed many interpretations given in our book. We are drawing on new evidence supplied by the Vanderbilt University research in the Petexbatun region and at the site of Dos Pilas. This research is directed by Arthur Demarest and Stephen Houston. We are also drawing on collaborative research by Nikolai Grube and Linda Schele and Nikolai Grube with Simon Martin. Simon Martin, in particular, is an expert on the texts of Naranjo.
2. The name given this Holy Lord, k'ul ahaw, which is what the Maya called kings, is a decipherment of the main elements of his glyphs. He is called Ruler 1 of Dos Pilas in the scholarly literature, and also Flint-Sky-God K.

III

DOMESTIC WORLDS AND PUBLIC WORLDS

In 1974, in an attempt to document a universal subordination of women, Michelle Rosaldo (1974: 18) proposed a paradigm relating "recurrent aspects of psychology and cultural and social organization to an opposition between the 'domestic' orientation of women and the extradomestic or 'public' ties, that, in most societies, are primarily available to men." The domestic-public model led Rosaldo to suggest that women's status is highest in societies in which the public and domestic spheres are only weakly differentiated, as among the Mbuti pygmies. In contrast "women's status will be lowest in those societies where there is a firm differentiation between domestic and public spheres of activity and where women are isolated from one another and placed under a single man's authority, in the home. Their position is raised when they can challenge those claims to authority . . ." (Rosaldo 1974: 36). Accordingly, women may enhance their status by creating a public world of their own or by entering the men's world. In addition, the most egalitarian societies will be those in which men participate in the domestic domain.

Correspondingly, Sanday (1974) suggests that women's involvement in domains of activity such as subsistence or defense may be curtailed because of their time and energy commitment to reproduction and mothering. Men, on the other hand, are free to form broader associations in the political, economic, and military spheres that transcend the mother-child unit. While the linkage of women with the domestic and men with the public domains may imply a biological determinism based on women's reproductive roles, Rosaldo (1974: 24) argues that the opposition between domestic and public orientations is an intelligible but not a necessary arrangement.

One aspect of women's domestic responsibilities is that it is women who primarily raise children. Nancy Chodorow (1974) develops a theory linking adult sex role behavior to the fact that children's early involvement is with their female parent. Chodorow argues that girls are integrated through ties with female kin into the world of domestic work. Age, rather than achievement, may define their status, while boys must "learn" to be men. Unlike girls, boys have few responsibilities in childhood and are free to establish peer groups that create "public" ties. To become an adult male a boy is often obliged to dissociate himself from the home and from female kin. According to Rosaldo (1974: 26), "the fact that children virtually everywhere grow up with their mothers may well account for characteristic differences in male and female psychologies" as well as setting the stage for adult organization of activities.

As scholarship devoted to an understanding of gender issues has evolved, the influential domestic-public model has been the focus of considerable controversy, revolving around three related issues: whether male domination is universal, whether male domination is explained by the domestic-public dichotomy, and whether the concept of domestic-public has relevance in all cultures.

Lamphere (in this book) reviews the formulation of the domestic-public model, and discusses the subsequent critiques of its applicability. Rosaldo herself, rethinking her original position, said that while male dominance appears widespread, it does not "in actual behavioral terms assume a universal content or a universal shape. On the contrary, women typically have power and influence in political and economic life, display autonomy from men in their pursuits, and rarely find themselves confronted or constrained by what might seem the brute fact of male strength" (1980: 394). While the domestic-public opposition has been compelling, Rosaldo suggests that the model assumes too much rather than helping to illuminate and explain.

As Lamphere observes, it has become increasingly clear that the domestic-public opposition is the heir to nineteenth-century social theory rooted in a dichotomy contrasting home and woman, with a public world of men, and reflecting an understanding of political rights based on sex. It has also been noted that conceptualizing social life as dichotomized into domestic and public domains does not make sense in societies in which management of production occurs within the household and in which household production itself involves the management of the "public" economy (Leacock 1978: 253).

In contrast, in an industrial society, where home and workplace are clearly demarcated, the domestic-public opposition may have explanatory value. For example, Murcott (in this book) analyzes one domestic task, cooking, as part of an exploration of economic relations in the family and of the division of labor between spouses. Interviews with Welsh housewives indicate that ideas about home cooking reflect understandings of the relationship between domestic and paid labor. The informants shared the view that proper eating must occur at home and that a cooked dinner is necessary to family health and well-being. Murcott suggests that the emphasis on having a proper dinner waiting for the husband when he comes in from work underscores the symbolic importance of the return home: "the cooked dinner marks the threshold between the public domains of school or work and the private sphere behind the closed front door" (Murcott, this book).

In Andalusia, in southern Spain, women are ideologically associated with the home, and men with public places (Driessen, in this book). The woman should be virtuous, docile, and devoted to husband and children; the ideal man is the head of the household, tough, but seldom at home. However, in reality, the involvement of men in the private sphere and women in the public sphere varies according to social class. Among agricultural laborers, women's labor is critical to the household economy. It is common for women to be employed, while their men are unemployed. This contradiction produces tensions that are reflected in men's sociability patterns. The bar offers men the opportunity to display their masculinity, by heavy drinking and sexual banter. Men's sociability is best understood as a response to the vulnerability of unemployed men to women who contribute substantially to the family income through wage labor. This results in blurred idealized distinctions between male and female identity.

Research on the public/private distinction has implications for the interplay among gender, status, and power. While traditional conceptions of power emphasized formal political behavior and authority associated with a status conferring the "right" to impose sanctions (Lamphere 1974: 99), informal power strategies such as manipulation and maneuvering are also important aspects of political activity. Cynthia Nelson (in this book) examines the concept of power, focusing on images of women and power in the domestic and public domains in the societies of the Middle East. Ethnographies of the Middle East have commonly differentiated two social worlds, a woman's private world and a man's public world. Women's concerns are domestic, men's political. Nelson argues that the assignment of private and public reflects the imposition of western cultural categories on the Middle East; the meaning of power is influenced by these categorizations, as well as by the limitations of data obtained by male ethnographers from male informants.

This is a point made forcefully by Annette Weiner (1976) in her reanalysis of Trobriand exchange. She argues that "we unquestioningly accept male statements about women as factual evidence for the way a society is structured. . . . Any study that does not include the role of women—as seen by women—as part of the way the society is structured remains only a partial study of that society. Whether women are publicly valued or privately secluded, whether they control politics, a range of economic commodities, or merely magic spells, they function within that society, not as objects, but as individuals with some measure of control" (228).

Similarly, Nelson argues that by asking such questions as "How do women influence men?" "Who controls whom about what?" "How is control exercised?" it becomes apparent that women exercise a greater degree of power in social life than is often appreciated. In addition, she challenges the idea that the social worlds of men and women are reducible to private and public domains, with power limited to men in the public arena. Nelson's review of ethnographies addressing the role and position of women in Middle Eastern society suggests that women play a crucial role as structural links between kinship groups in societies in which family and kinship are fundamental social institutions. Women are in a position to influence men through ritual means, to channel information to male kin, and to influence decision making about alliances; consequently, women do participate in "public" activities, and women's exclusive solidarity groups exercise considerable social control and political influence. The conceptions of power as defined by the western observer are particularly challenged by literature on women written by women who offer a perspective on the position of Middle Eastern women derived from the actors themselves.

In the course of her critique of the application of the domestic-public opposition to social organization in the Middle East, Nelson challenges longstanding assumptions regarding women's subordination and male dominance and calls into question the association between political power and a public domain that excludes women. Similarly, in studies of peasant societies Rogers (1975) and other (Friedl 1967; Reigelhaupt 1967) contend that the sector of life over which peasant women have control—the household—is in fact the key sphere of activity, socially, politically, and economically. Men occupy public and prestigious positions of authority within the village sphere, but these activities do not have the impact on daily life that household activities have. In light of these analyses demonstrating women's power and influence, we are reminded that the universality of male dominance appears untenable.

In reflecting on feminist research in anthropology, Rosaldo critiques the very tendency to look for universal truths and origins. Rather, anthropologists need to develop theoretical perspectives that analyze the relationships of men and women in a broader social context (Rosaldo 1980: 414), involving inequality and hierarchy. As Henrietta Moore emphasizes, while women in many societies share some experiences and problems, women have had very different encounters with racism, colonialism, the penetration of capitalism, and international development. We need to move from assumptions of the shared experience of "women" to a critical analysis of "concepts of difference" (1988: 9).

REFERENCES

Chodorow, Nancy. 1974. "Family Structure and Feminine Personality." In Michelle Z. Rosaldo and Louise Lamphere (eds.). *Woman, Culture, and Society*, pp. 43–67. Stanford: Stanford University Press.

Friedl, Ernestine. 1967. "The Position of Women: Appearance and Reality." *Anthropological Quarterly* 40: 97–108.

Lamphere, Louise. 1974. "Strategies, Cooperation, and Conflict Among Women in Domestic Groups." In Michelle Z. Rosaldo and Louise Lamphere, (eds.). *Woman, Culture, and Society*, pp. 97–113. Stanford: Stanford University Press.

Leacock, Eleanor. 1978. "Women's Status in Egalitarian Society. Implications for Social Evolution." *Current Anthropology* 19(2): 247–275.

Moore, Henrietta L. 1988. *Feminism and Anthropology*. Minneapolis: University of Minnesota Press.

Riegelhaupt, Joyce. 1967. "Saloio Women: An Analysis of Informal and Formal Political and Economic Roles of Portuguese Peasant Women." *Anthropological Quarterly* 40: 109–126.

Rogers, Susan Carol. 1975. "Female Forms of Power and the Myth of Male Dominance: A Model of Female/Male Interaction in Peasant Society." *American Ethnologist* 2: 727–756.

Rosaldo, Michelle Z. 1974. "Theoretical Overview." In Michelle Z. Rosaldo and Louise Lamphere (eds.). *Woman, Culture, and Society*, pp. 17–43. Stanford: Stanford University Press.

———. 1980. "The Use and Abuse of Anthropology: Reflections on Feminism and Cross-Cultural Understanding." *Signs* 5(3): 389–418.

Rosaldo, Michelle Z. and Louise Lamphere (eds.). 1974. *Woman, Culture, and Society*. Stanford: Stanford University Press.

Sanday, Peggy R. 1974. "Female Status in the Public Domain." In Michelle Z. Rosaldo and Louise Lamphere (eds.). *Woman, Culture, and Society*, pp. 189–207. Stanford: Stanford University Press.

Weiner, Annette B. 1976. *Women of Value, Men of Renown: New Perspectives in Trobriand Exchange*. Austin: University of Texas Press.

THE DOMESTIC SPHERE OF WOMEN AND THE PUBLIC WORLD OF MEN: THE STRENGTHS AND LIMITATIONS OF AN ANTHROPOLOGICAL DICHOTOMY

Louise Lamphere

Since 1974 there has been a burgeoning interest within anthropology in the study of women, sex roles, and gender. Anthropology has long been a discipline that contained important women (Elsie Clews Parsons, Ruth Benedict, and Margaret Mead among the most famous) and a field in which women have been studied as well (e.g., Kaberry 1939, 1952; Landes 1938, 1947; Leith-Ross 1939; Underhill 1936; and Paulme 1963). However, with the publication of *Woman, Culture, and Society* (Rosaldo and Lamphere 1974) and *Toward an Anthropology of Women* (Reiter 1975) women scholars, many of whom were identified as feminists, began to critique the androcentric bias in anthropology, to explore

Original material prepared for this text.

women's status in a wide variety of societies, and to provide explanatory models to understand women's position cross-culturally.

One of the most powerful and influential models was proposed by Michelle Rosaldo in her introductory essay to *Woman, Culture, and Society* (1974). Her argument began by asserting that although there is a great deal of cross-cultural variability in men's and women's roles, there is a pervasive, universal asymmetry between the sexes. "But what is perhaps most striking and surprising," Rosaldo writes, "is the fact that male, as opposed to female, activities are always recognized as predominantly important, and cultural systems give authority and value to the roles and activities of men" (Rosaldo 1974:19).

One of the quotes we chose to appear at the beginning of the book, a passage from Margaret Mead's *Male and Female,* sums up what we saw in 1974 in all the ethnographies and studies we examined. "In every known society, the male's need for achievement can be recognized. Men may cook, or weave, or dress dolls or hunt hummingbirds, but if such activities are appropriate occupations of men, then the whole society, men and women alike, votes them as important. When the same occupations are performed by women, they are regarded as less important" (Mead 1949:125). Not only were there differential evaluations of women's activities, but, Rosaldo argues, "everywhere men have some *authority* over women, that [is] they have culturally legitimated right to her subordination and compliance" (1974:21).

Having argued for a pervasive sexual asymmetry across cultures, not just in terms of cultural values, but also in terms of power and authority, Rosaldo accounted for this difference between men and women in terms of a dichotomy.[1] She argued that women are associated with a "domestic orientation," while men are primarily associated with extra domestic, political, and military spheres of activity. By "domestic" Rosaldo meant "those minimal institutions and modes of activity that are organized immediately around one or more mothers and their children." In contrast the "public" referred to "activities, institutions, and forms of association that link, rank, organize, or subsume particular mother-child groups. Put quite simply, men have no single commitment as enduring, time-consuming, and emotionally compelling—as close to seeming necessary and natural—as the relation of a woman to her infant child; and so men are free to form those broader associations that we call 'society,' universalistic systems of order, meaning, and commitment that link particular mother-child groups."

Rosaldo, along with Sherry Ortner and Nancy Chodorow who also wrote essays in *Woman, Culture, and Society,* insisted that the connection between women's role in reproduction (the fact that women everywhere lactate and give birth to children) and their domestic orientation is not a necessary one. In other words biology is not destiny. Women's domestic orientation was structurally and culturally constructed and "insofar as woman is universally defined in terms of a largely maternal and domestic role, we can account for her universal subordination" (Rosaldo 1974:7).

"Although" Rosaldo writes, "I would be the last to call this a necessary arrangement or to deny that it is far too simple as an account of any particular empirical case, I suggest that the opposition between domestic and public orientations (an opposition that must, in part, derive from the nurturant capacities of women) provides the necessary framework for an examination of male and female roles in any society" (Rosaldo 1974:24).

For Rosaldo, then, women were involved in the "messiness" of daily life; they were always available for interruption by children. Men could be more distanced and may actually have separate quarters (such as men's houses) away from women's activities. Men could thus "achieve" authority and create rank, hierarchy, and a political world away from women. The confinement of women to the domestic sphere and men's ability to create and dominate the political sphere thus accounted for men's ability to hold the greater share of power and authority in all known cultures and societies.

At the time Rosaldo wrote her overview and in the introduction we both wrote, we were faced with building a framework where none existed. Despite the number of monographs on women, Margaret Mead's work and that of Simone de Beauvoir (1953) were the most provocative, and perhaps the only, theoretical works we knew.[2] The argument for universal sexual asymmetry followed in a long tradition in anthropology where scholars have sought to look for what is broadly "human" in all cultures. In addition to language, anthropologists have discussed the universality of the incest taboo, marriage, and the family. The notion that women might be universally subordinate to men thus made sense as a first attempt at theory building in this newly revived "subfield" within anthropology.

Although Rosaldo argued for universal subordination, she was careful to make clear that women are not powerless. They exercise informal influence and power, often mitigating male authority or even rendering it trivial (Rosaldo 1974:21). In addition, there are important variations in women's roles in different cultures, and variation was discussed in most of the rest of the articles in the collection. For example, Sanday and Sacks compared women's status in a number of different societies, while Leis examined the structural reasons why women's associations are strong in one Ijaw village in Nigeria, yet absent in another. Finally, in my own article I examined the differences in women's strategies within domestic groups in a number of societies, which related to the relative integration or separation of domestic and political spheres.

Since 1974 the hypothesis of universal subordination of women and the dichotomous relationship between women in the domestic sphere and men in the public sphere have been challenged and critiqued by a number of feminist anthropologists. As appealing as this dichotomy seemed in the abstract it turned out to be difficult to apply when actually looking at examples of women's activities in different cultures. For example, in an important article written about the same time as Rosaldo's introduction, Rayna Reiter (now Rayna Rapp) described women's and men's distinct lives in a small French village in the south of France. "They inhabited different domains, one public, one private. While men fraternized with whomever they found to talk to in public places, women were much more enmeshed in their families and their kinship networks" (Reiter 1975b:253). However, two categories of public space fell into women's domain: the church and three shops, including the local bakery. Men tended to avoid women's places, entering the bakery, for example, only when several men were together and joking, "Let's attack now" (Reiter 1975b:257).

Reiter argues that men and women use public space in different ways and at different times. "The men go early to the fields, and congregate on the square or in the cafes for a social hour after work. Sometimes they also fraternize in the evenings. These are the times when women are home cooking and invisible to public view. But when the men have abandoned the village for the fields, the women come out to do their marketing in a leisurely fashion. The village is then in female hands. In the afternoon, when the men return to work, the women form gossip groups on stoops and benches or inside houses depending on the weather" (Reiter 1975b:258). Despite the powerful imagery—women associated with the private or domestic domain and men with public space—the description also shows that the dichotomy is not neat. After all women are in public a great deal; they have taken over, in some sense, the Church and the shops and even the public square in the middle of the day.

In Margery Wolf's description of women in a Taiwanese village based on data she collected in the late 1950s, she emphasizes that because researchers have focused on the dominance of patrilineal descent in the family, they have failed to see women's presence. "We have missed not only some of the system's subtleties but also its near-fatal weaknesses" (Wolf 1972:37). Women have different interests than men and build uterine families—strong ties to their daughters, but primarily to their sons who give their mothers loyalty and a place in the patrilineal extended family. Outside the family in the community women formed neighborhood groups—around a store, at a platform where women washed their clothes in the canal, or under a huge old tree. In a village strung out between a river and a canal, there was no central plaza dominated by men as in the South of France.

In Peihotien Wolf did not describe a cultural geography where women were in a private sphere and men in the public one; rather there was more of a functional separation—men and women had different activities and interests. They were often located in the same places but had a different relationship to the patrilineal extended family and the male-dominated community. Women's lack of power led them to different strategies, different tactics that often undermined male control of the household and even the community. As Sylvia Yanagisako (1987:111) has pointed out the notion of domestic-public entails both a spatial metaphor (of geographically separated or even nested spaces) and a functional metaphor (of functionally different activities or social roles) in the same conceptual dichotomy. Analysts often "mix" these different metaphors in any particular analysis—sometimes using domestic-public spatially and at other times functionally.

Even in the Middle East, the association of women with a private domain (and a lack of power) and men with a public domain (and the center of politics) was too simple, as Cynthia Nelson pointed out in her article, "Public and Private Politics: Women in the Middle Eastern World" (1974; reprinted in this book). Because they are born into one patrilineal group and marry into another, women are important structural links between social groups and often act as mediators. Because there are segregated social worlds, all-female institutions are important for enforcing social norms: Women fill powerful ritual roles as sorceresses, healers, and mediums; women are important sources of information for their male kin; and women act as "information brokers," mediating social relations within both the family and the larger society.

From Rosaldo's point of view, these aspects of women's power are primarily "informal" and very different from the public, legitimate roles of men. Nevertheless, even though Nelson affirms the separation of male and female worlds (both spatially and functionally), what is "domestic" has public ramifications (the arrangement of a marriage, the transmission of highly charged political information) and the shadow of the family and kin group (the "domestic") is present in even the most "public" of situations. What at first seemed like a simple straightforward dichotomy, in light of actual case material seems very "slippery" and complex.

Furthermore, in many cultures, particularly those with an indigenous band or tribal structure, a separation of "domestic" and "public" spheres makes no sense because household production was simultaneously public, economic, and political. Leacock pointed out the following after reviewing the literature on the Iroquois during the seventeenth and eighteenth century:

> Iroquois matrons preserved, stored, and dispensed the corn, meat, fish, berries, squashes, and fats that were buried in special pits or kept in the long house. Brown (1970:162) notes that women's control over the dispensation of the foods they produced, and meat as well, gave them de facto power to veto declarations of war and to intervene to bring about peace.... Women also guarded the "tribal public treasure" kept in the long house, the wampum quill and feather work, and furs.... The point to be stressed is that this was "household management" of an altogether different order from management of the nuclear or extended family in patriarchal societies. In the latter, women may cajole, manipulate, or browbeat men, but always behind the public facade; in the former case, "household management" was itself the management of the "public economy." (Leacock 1978:253)

Sudarkasa has made much the same point about women in West African societies such as the Yoruba. She argues that many of the political and economic activities anthropologists discuss as public are actually embedded in households (Sudarkasa 1976, as quoted in Rapp 1979:509). Furthermore, "in West Africa, the 'public domain' was not conceptualized as 'the world of men.' Rather, the public domain was one in which both sexes were recognized as having important roles to play" (Sudarkasa 1986:99).

A more appropriate conception would be to recognize two domains, "one occupied by men and another by women, both of which were internally ordered in a hierarchical fashion and both of which provided 'personnel' for domestic and extradomestic (or public) activities" (Sudarkasa 1986:94).

Furthermore, a careful examination of "domestic domain" indicates that the categories of "woman" and "mother" overlap in Western society, but the meaning of motherhood may be vastly different in another society. Women may not be exclusively defined as mothers and childrearers in terms of their status and cultural value (see Moore 1988:20–29 for a discussion of this point).

In addition to the issue of whether the domestic-public dichotomy can provide an adequate *description* of men's and women's spatial and functional relationships in our own and other societies, the model has problems as an *explanation* of women's status. One of these problems is the inherent circularity of the model. A central point is to account for the nature of these domains, yet they are already assumed to exist widely and are treated as categories in terms of which women's activities (such as food preparing, cooking, child care, washing) can be classified (as opposed to male hunting, warfare, political councils). Comaroff says that the model "can only affirm what has already been assumed—that is, that the distinction between the domestic and politico-jural is an intrinsic, if variable, fact of social existence" (Comaroff 1987:59). When the model is used to explain women's positions in different societies in relation to these two orientations, the reasoning is equally circular. To put it in the words of Yanagisako and Collier, "The claim that women become absorbed in domestic activities because of their role as mothers is tautological given the definition of 'domestic' as 'those minimal institutions and modes of activity that are organized immediately around one or more mothers and their children'" (Yanagisako and Collier 1987:19).

Finally, we have come to realize that the concepts of domestic and public were bound up in our own history and our own categories grounded particularly in a Victorian heritage. Rosaldo, in a thoughtful reevaluation of her model, came to argue this position herself.

> The turn-of-the-century social theorists whose writings are the basis of most modern social thinking tended without exception to assume that women's place was in the home. In fact, the Victorian doctrine of separate male and female spheres was, I would suggest, quite central to their sociology. Some of these thinkers recognized that modern women suffered from their association with domestic life, but none questioned the pervasiveness (or necessity) of a split between the family and society. (Rosaldo 1980:401–402)

Rosaldo traced the historical roots of domestic-public from the nineteenth century evolutionists through twentieth century structural functionalists to her own work. Instead of two opposed spheres (different and apart), Rosaldo suggested an analysis of gender relationships, an examination of inequality and hierarchy as they are created particularly through marriage (Rosaldo 1980:412–413).

The dichotomy has been usefully employed in several ways since 1974. First, several authors have shown us how it works in Western societies (e.g., France and the United States where it arose historically and still has an important ideological function) (Reiter 1975; Collier, Rosaldo, and Yanagisako 1982). In a related way analysts have explored the meanings surrounding domestic activities of women, putting together a much more complex picture of women's relation to men in this sphere (Murcott 1983; Chai 1987; both are reprinted in this book). Second, anthropological analysis has helped us to understand the historical development of domestic-public spheres in societies under colonialism. John Comaroff's analysis of the Tshidi chiefdom in South Africa during the early twentieth century is an excellent example of this approach (1987:53–85). Finally, some analysts have used the cultural concepts of other societies to critique our own model of domestic-public orientations. Sylvia Yanagisako's essay on the clear separation of "inside-outside" domains (a spatial metaphor) and "work-family" activities (a functional dichotomy) in Japanese American culture demonstrates how the anthropological model of domestic-public mixes these metaphors, which has made analysis confusing and difficult (Yanagisako 1987).

Despite these useful attempts at examining women's lives through the lens of a domestic-public opposition, many of us would agree with Rayna Rapp's 1979 summary of the problems with this dichotomy.

> We cannot write an accurate history of the West in relation to the Rest until we stop assuming that our experiences subsume everyone else's. Our public/private conflicts are not necessarily the same as those of other times and places. The specific oppression of women cannot be documented if our categories are so broad as to decontextualize what "womaness" means as we struggle to change that definition. A Tanzanian female farmer, a Mapuche woman leader, and an American working-class housewife do not live in the same domestic domain, nor will the social upheavals necessary to give them power over their lives be the same. We must simultaneously understand the differences and the similarities, but not by reducing them to one simple pattern. (Rapp 1979:511)

Thus, many of us have tired of the domestic-public dichotomy. We feel it is constraining, a "trap," while new approaches try to get away from dichotomous thinking. These approaches do one of several things. Often they take history seriously, examining women's situation as it has evolved, often in a colonial context. Furthermore, they treat women as active agents and following Collier (1974), as people who have interests, often divergent from men, and who act on them. Third, they often focus on gender relationships, rather than only on women. Finally, they do not treat all women as part of a single universal category of "woman." Rather women are usually analyzed in terms of their social location. Age, class, race, ethnicity, and kinship are all likely to divide women, so newer analyses examine women's strategies and identities as they are differently shaped. Several examples will illustrate some of the different approaches taken in recent years.

Collier's examination of Comanche, Cheyenne, and Kiowa gender relationships (1988) illustrates the recent focus on gender and on the multiple positions that men and women hold in societies in which the domestic-public dichotomy seems inappropriate. This is because these "spheres" are integrated, and there is no firm line between domestic and public space (see Lamphere 1974 and Leacock above).

The Comanche are an example of a bride service society in which, like many hunter-gatherer societies, men and women were relatively autonomous, the concept of femininity was not elaborated, and the greatest status differences were between unmarried and married men. Marriage established men as having something to achieve (e.g., a wife), leaving women without such a cultural goal. Young men, through providing meat for their in-laws (bride service), become equal adults, and older men, through egalitarian relations and generosity, become the repositories of wisdom and knowledge. Politics focused on the issue of sexuality and on male-male relationships, which often erupted in conflict and violence. Women celebrated their health and sexuality, and hence the roles of "woman the gatherer" or even "woman the mother" did not emerge as cultural themes.

Among the Cheyenne, an equal bridewealth society, and among the Kiowa, an unequal bridewealth society, marriage relationships were structured in a much different way in the nineteenth century, so gender relationships had a much different content, politics were more hierarchical, and ideology played a different role. Collier's interest is not in the subordination of women in these three societies, because in all three there are several kinds of inequality: between men and women, between older women and girls, between unmarried men and married men, and between kin and affines. An interest in "spheres" and "domains" has been replaced by an emphasis on relationships and an analysis that focuses on the ways in which inequality gets reproduced through marriage transactions, claims on the labor of others, and giving and receiving of gifts. Dominance and subordination become a much more layered, contextualized phenomenon—more interesting than the simple assertion that women are universally subordinated. The processes through which women's inequality (and that of young men) is constructed are laid bare, rather than flatly asserted.

Mary Moran's study of civilized women (1990) explores the historical beginnings and present day construction of the category "civilized," which does confine educated women among the Glebo of southeastern Liberia to a "domestic sphere." The dichotomy between "civilized" and "native" (or even tribal or country) is a result of missionization and has created a status hierarchy differentially applied to men and to women. Men, once educated and with a history of paid wage work, never lose their status as "civilized," while women, even though married to a "civilized man," may lose their status if they do not dress correctly, keep house in specific ways, and refrain from farming and marketing. Native women, who market or have farms, are more economically independent but occupy positions of lower prestige. Here we see not only the importance of historical data in examining how cultural categories evolve, but also the ways in which both civilized and native women actively manage their status positions. Civilized women, through the practice of fosterage, recruit younger women to their households to carry out the more elaborate household routines in which they must engage and to train these fostered daughters to become civilized themselves.

The civilized-native dichotomy represents the juxtaposition of two systems. One is a parallel-sex system in which native men and women are represented by their own leaders in two linked but relatively autonomous prestige hierarchies (as suggested by Sudarkasa 1986). The other is a single-sex system (based on a Western model) in which men in political positions represent both sexes, and women have little access to prestige except through their husbands. Thus, this is a much more complex system than one based on a domestic-public dichotomy. There are dichotomous categories—civilized-native, male-female—but they do not fit neatly together. Moran speaks of categories as "gender sensitive" and suggests that "The Glebo have inserted gender into the civilized/native dichotomy to the point that women's status is not only more tenuous and vulnerable than men's but also very difficult to maintain without male support." In some respects civilized women trade off dependency for prestige, but Moran provides a sympathetic picture of how both civilized and native women manage their lives.

Lila Abu-Lughod's study (1986) of Bedouin women's ritual poetry gives us further insights into the complexity of women who in 1974 we would have simply thought of as "confined to a domestic sphere." Among the Bedouin women's marriages are arranged; wives wear black veils and red belts (symbolizing their fertility); and women must behave within a code of behavior that emphasizes family honor and female modesty and shame. When confronted with loss, poor treatment, or neglect, the public discourse is one of hostility, bitterness, and anger. In the case of lost love the discourse is of militant indifference and denial of concern. In contrast, Bedouin poetry, a highly prized and formally structured art, expresses sentiments of devastating sadness, self-pity, attachment, and deep feeling (Abu-Lughod 1986:187). Although both men and women recite poetry for women it may express conflicting feelings concerning an arranged marriage, a sense of loss over a divorce, or sentiments of betrayal when a husband marries a new wife. The poems are used to elicit sympathy and get help, but they also constitute a dissident and subversive discourse. Abu-Lughod sees ritual poetry as a corrective to "an obsession with morality and an overzealous adherence to the ideology of honor. . . . Poetry reminds people of another way of being and encourages, as it reflects, another side of experience. . . . And maybe the vision [offered through poetry] is cherished because people see that the costs of this system, in the limits it places on human experiences, are just too high" (Abu-Lughod 1986:259). Bedouin women in this portrait are not simply victims of patriarchy confined to a domestic sphere; they are active individuals who use a highly valued cultural form to express their deepest sentiments, acknowledge an alternative set of values, and leave open the possibility of subverting the system in which they are embedded.

A large number of studies have been conducted in the United States that loosely focus on what used to be termed the domestic sphere and the public world of work. As in the Native American, African, and Middle Eastern cases cited previously, when one begins to examine a topic in detail, global notions like domestic-public seem too simple to deal with the complexities of women's lives. Clearly work and home are distinctly separated spheres in the United States. Women who have been employed in the paid labor force have experienced the disjunction of spending eight or more hours of the day in a place of employment where they are "female workers" and the rest of their time in the home where they are daughters, wives, and/or mothers. With this comes responsibilities for cooking, cleaning, and providing nurturance, care, and intimacy for other family members. Several recent studies have examined the contradictions women face when combining work and family, the impact of paid employment on family roles, and vice versa. I will refer to only three examples of this growing literature.

Patricia Zavella's research on Chicana cannery workers examines women's networks that link the workplace and the family (Zavella 1987). Calling these "work-related networks," Zavella describes groups of friends who saw each other outside work and who were members of a kin network employed in the same cannery. Women used work-related networks as sources of exchange for information, baby sitters, and emotional support. Networks operated in more political ways as workers organized a women's caucus and filed a complaint with the Fair Employment Practices Commission. Women's cannery work was seasonal and had relatively little impact on power relations in the family or the household division of labor. On the other hand work-related networks of friends or kin were an important "bridging mechanism" helping women to deal with the contradictions and demands that came from two different spheres.

Karen Sacks' study of hospital workers at the Duke Medical center examines the ways in which black and white women brought family notions of work, adulthood, and responsibility to work with them and used these values to organize a walk out and subsequent union drive (1988). Sacks focuses on the activities of "center women"—leaders in the union drive. Unlike the men who were often the public speakers at rallies and events, the center women organized support on an interpersonal, one-to-one basis. Rather than emphasizing the bridging aspect of women's networks, Sacks shows how the family is "brought to work" or in the old terminology how the "domestic" influences the "public."

In my own research I have traced the changes in the relationship between women, work, and family historically through the study of immigrant women in a small industrial community, Central Falls, Rhode Island (Lamphere 1987). Using the twin notions of productive and reproductive labor, I examined the rise of the textile industry in Rhode Island and the recruitment of working daughters and later of working mothers to the textile industry and to the other light industries that have replaced it since World War II. Rather than seeing production and reproduction as a rigid dichotomy (like public and domestic), I have used these categories to study relationships and to examine the kinds of strategies that immigrant women and their families forged in confronting an industrial system where wage work was a necessity and where working-class families had no control over the means of production. Such an approach revealed a great deal of variability both between and within ethnic groups—the Irish, English, French-Canadian, and Polish families who came to Central Falls between 1915 and 1984 and the more recent Colombian and Portuguese immigrants. Examination of strikes and walk outs in the 1920s and 1930s and my own experience as a sewer in an apparel plant in 1977 led me to emphasize the strategies of resistance the women workers used on the job, as well as the impact of women's paid labor on the family itself. When daughters were recruited as workers in textile mills, the internal division of labor within the household did not materially change because wives and mothers continued to do much of the reproductive labor necessary to maintain the household. Fathers, teenage sons, and daughters worked for wages. In the current period, in contrast, as more wives have become full-time workers, immigrant men have begun to do some reproductive labor, particularly child care. Immigrant couples often work different shifts and prefer to care for children themselves rather than trust baby sitters from their own ethnic group. In my study I argue that "the productive system as constituted in the workplaces has shaped the family more than issues of reproduction have shaped the workplace" (Lamphere 1987:43).

More recently Patricia Zavella, Felipe Gonzalez, and I have found that young working mothers in sunbelt industries have moved much further than Cannery women or New England industrial immigrant women in changing the nature of the household division of labor (Lamphere, Gonzalez, and Zavella nd). These new committed female workers have been employed since high school and do not drop out of the labor force for long periods of time to have children. Thus, they and their husbands construct a family life around a two-job household. Although some couples have a "traditional" division of housework (women do the cooking and the majority of the cleaning and husbands take out the garbage, do minor repairs, and fix the car), many husbands participate in "female chores" and do substantial amounts of child care (often caring for children while the wife is at work). Here we see the impact of what we used to call the "public sphere" on the domestic one, but in our analysis we have focused more on the varied ways that Anglos and Hispanics (including single mothers) have negotiated household and child-care arrangements, viewing husbands and wives as mediating contradictions. Subtle similarities and differences among and between working class Anglo and Hispanic women have emerged from this analysis, making it clear that the impact of work in the public world is not a monolithic but a variegated process.

In summary the dichotomy between the public world of men and domestic world of women was, in 1974, an important and useful starting point for thinking about women's roles in a cross-cultural perspective. As anthropologists have written more detailed and fine-grained studies of women's lives in a wide variety of other cultures and in our own society, we have gone beyond the use of dichotomies to produce analyses of the complex and layered structure of women's lives. We now treat women more historically, viewing them as social actors and examining the variability among women's situations within one culture and in their relationship to men.

NOTES

1. Rosaldo says that "the opposition does not *determine* cultural stereotypes or asymmetries in the evaluations of the sexism, but rather underlies them, to support a very general . . . identification of women with domestic life and of men with public life" (Rosaldo 1974:21–22). Thus, I would argue, Rosaldo did not attempt to *ex-*

plain women's subordination through the dichotomy, but saw it as an underlying structural framework in any society that supported subordination and that would have to be reorganized to change women's position.

2. It is interesting that we did not know of Elsie Clews Parsons' extensive feminist writing during 1910 to 1916, much of which is reminiscent of the kind of position we took in *Woman, Culture, and Society*. In another article I have noted the similarities between Shelly's prose and that of Parsons (see Lamphere 1989 and Parsons 1913, 1914, 1915).

REFERENCES

Abu-Lughod, Lila. 1986. *Veiled Sentiments: Honor and Poetry in a Bedouin Society*. Berkeley and Los Angeles: University of California Press.

Brown, Judith. 1970. Economic organization and the position of women among the Iroquois. *Ethnohistory* 17(3/4):131–167.

Chai, Alice Yun. 1987. Freed from the elders but locked into labor: Korean immigrant women in Hawaii. *Women's Studies* 13:223–234.

Collier, Jane. 1974. Women in politics. In Michelle Z. Rosaldo and Louise Lamphere (eds.). *Woman, Culture, and Society*. Stanford: Stanford University Press.

———. 1988. *Marriage and Inequality in Classless Societies*. Stanford: Stanford University Press.

Collier, Jane, Michelle Rosaldo, and Sylvia Yanagisako. 1982. Is there a family? New anthropological views. In Barrie Thorne and Marilyn Yalom (eds.). *Rethinking the Family: Some Feminist Questions*. New York and London: Longman.

Comaroff, John L. 1987. Sui genderis: Feminism, kinship theory, and structural "domains." In Jane Fishburne Collier and Sylvia Junko Yanagisako (eds.). *Gender and Kinship: Essays Toward a Unified Analysis*. Stanford: Stanford University Press.

de Beauvoir, Simone. 1953. *The Second Sex*. New York: Alfred A. Knopf. Originally published in French in 1949.

Kaberry, Phyllis M. 1939. *Aboriginal Women, Sacred and Profane*. London: G. Routledge.

———. 1952. *Women of the Grassfields*. London: H. M. Stationery Office.

Lamphere, Louise. 1974. Strategies, cooperation, and conflict among women in domestic groups. In Michelle Z. Rosaldo and Louise Lamphere (eds.). *Woman, Culture, and Society*. Stanford: Stanford University Press.

———. 1987. *From Working Daughters to Working Mothers: Immigrant Women in a New England Industrial Community*. Ithaca, NY: Cornell University Press.

———. 1989. Feminist anthropology: The legacy of Elsie Clews Parsons. *American Ethnologist* 16(3):518–533.

Lamphere, Louise, Felipe Gonzales, and Patricia Zavella. (eds.). Working Mothers and Sunbelt Industrialization: New Patterns of Work and Family. Submitted to Cornell University Press.

Landes, Ruth. 1938. *The Ojibaw Woman, Part 1: Youth*. New York: Columbia University. Contributions to Anthropology, Vol. 31.

———. 1947. *The City of Women: Negro Women Cult Leaders of Bahia, Brazil*. New York: Macmillan.

Leacock, Eleanor. 1978. Women's status in egalitarian society: Implications for social evolution. *Current Anthropology* 19(2):247–275.

Leith-Ross, Sylvia. 1939. *African Women: Study of the Ibo of Nigeria*. London: Faber and Faber.

Mead, Margaret. 1949. *Male and Female*. New York: William Morrow and Co.

Moran, Mary H. 1990. *Civilized Women: Gender and Prestige in Southeastern Liberia*. Ithaca, NY: Cornell University Press.

Moore, Henrietta L. 1988. *Feminism and Anthropology*. Minneapolis: University of Minnesota Press.

Murcott, Anne. 1983. "It's a pleasure to cook for him": Food, mealtimes and gender in some South Wales households. In Eva Gamarnikow, D. H. J. Morgan, June Purvis, and Daphne Taylorson (eds.). *The Public and the Private*. London: Heinemann Educational Books.

Nelson, Cynthia. 1974. Public and private politics: Women in the Middle East. *American Ethnologist* 1:551–563.

Parsons, Elsie Clews. 1913. *The Old Fashioned Woman*. New York: G. P. Putnam's Sons.

———. 1914. *Fear and Conventionality*. New York: G. P. Putnam's Sons.

———. 1915. *Social Freedom: A Study of the Conflicts Between Social Classifications and Personality*. New York: G. P. Putnam's Sons.

Ong, Aihwa. 1987. *Spirits of Resistance and Capitalist Discipline*. Albany, NY: State University of New York Press.

Paulme, Denise (ed.). 1963. *Women of Tropical Africa*. Berkeley: University of California Press.

Rapp, Rayna. 1979. Anthropology. *Signs* 4(3): 497–513.

Reiter, Rayna (ed.). 1975a. *Toward an Anthropology of Women*. New York: Monthly Review Press.

———. 1975b. Men and women in the South of France: Public and private domains. In Rayna Reiter (ed.). *Toward an Anthropology of Women.* New York: Monthly Review Press.

Rosaldo, Michelle. 1974. Woman, culture and society: A theoretical overview. In Michelle Z. Rosaldo and Louise Lamphere (eds.). *Woman, Culture, and Society.* Stanford: Stanford University Press.

———. 1980. The uses and abuses of anthropology. *Signs* 5(3): 389–417.

Rosaldo, Michelle Z. and Louise Lamphere (eds.). 1974. *Woman, Culture, and Society.* Stanford: Stanford University Press.

Sacks, Karen. 1988. *Caring by the Hour: Women, Work, and Organizing at the Duke Medical Center.* Urbana and Chicago: University of Illinois Press.

Sudarkasa, Niara. 1976. Female employment and family organization in West Africa. In Dorothy McGuigan (ed.). *New Research on Women and Sex Roles.* Ann Arbor: Center for Continuing Education of Women.

———. 1986. The status of women in indigenous African Societies. *Feminist Studies* 12: 91–104.

Underhill, Ruth. 1936. *Autobiography of a Papago Woman.* Supplement to *American Anthropologist* 38(3), Part II. Millwood, NY: American Anthropological Association.

Wolf, Margery. 1972. *Women and the Family in Rural Taiwan.* Stanford: Stanford University Press.

Yanagisako, Sylvia Junko. 1987. Mixed metaphors: Native and anthropological models of gender and kinship domains. In Jane Fishburne Collier and Sylvia Junko Yanagisako (eds.). *Gender and Kinship: Essays Toward a Unified Analysis.* Stanford: Stanford University Press.

Yanagisako, Sylvia Junko and Jane Fishburne Collier. 1987. Toward a unified analysis of gender and kinship. In Jane Fishburne Collier and Sylvia Junko Yanagisako (eds.). *Gender and Kinship: Essays Toward a Unified Analysis.* Stanford: Stanford University Press.

Zavella, Patricia. 1987. *Women's Work and Chicano Families: Cannery Workers of the Santa Clara Valley.* Ithaca, NY: Cornell University Press.

"IT'S A PLEASURE TO COOK FOR HIM": FOOD, MEALTIMES AND GENDER IN SOME SOUTH WALES HOUSEHOLDS

Anne Murcott

INTRODUCTION

> I think it lets him know that I am thinking about him—as if he knows that I am expecting him. But it's not as if 'oh I haven't got anything ready' . . . Fair play, he's out all day . . . he doesn't ask for that much . . . you know it's not as if he's been very demanding or—he doesn't come home and say 'oh, we've got chops again', it's really a pleasure to cook for him, because whatever you . . . oh I'll give him something and I think well, he'll like this, he'll like that. And he'll always take his plate out . . . and he'll wash the dishes without me even asking, if I'm busy with the children. Mind, perhaps his method is not mine.

Reprinted with permission from Eva Gamarnikow, David H. J. Morgan, June Purvis, and Daphne Taylorson (eds.), *The Public and the Private* (London: Heinemann Educational Books, Ltd., 1983), pp. 78–90.

Every now and then an informant puts precisely into words the results of the researcher's analytic efforts—providing in the process a quotation suitable for the title! The extract reproduced above, explaining the importance of having the meal ready when her husband arrives home, comes from one of a series of interviews on which this paper is based.[1] The discussion starts by remembering that 'everyone knows' that women do the cooking: all the women interviewed—and the few husbands/boyfriends or mothers who came in and out—took it for granted that cooking was women's work. Informants may not enjoy cooking, or claim not to be good at it; they may not like the arrangement that it is women's work, or hanker after modifying it. But all recognise that this is conventional, some volunteer a measure of approval, most appeared automatically to accept it, a few resigned themselves and got on with it.

Studies of the organisation of domestic labour and marital role relationships confirm that cooking continues to be a task done more by women than men; this is also the case cross-culturally (Stephens, 1963; Murdock and Provost, 1973). Emphasis in the literature has shifted from Young and Willmott's (1975) symmetrical view of sharing and marital democracy. Now rather more thoroughgoing empirical study suggests their assessment is little more than unwarranted optimism (Oakley, 1974a and b; Edgell, 1980; Leonard, 1980; Tolson, 1977). This work improves on earlier studies of the domestic division of labour by going beyond behaviourist enquiry about 'who does which tasks' to consider the meanings attached to them by marital partners. The distribution of work turns out not to correlate neatly with assessments of importance or allocation of responsibility. (Oakley, 1974b; Edgell, 1980).

Part of this effort (in particular, Oakley, 1974a and b) has in addition attempted to analyse domestic work as a 'job like any other', considering housewives' work satisfaction, routines, supervision and so on. While this line of enquiry has undoubtedly made visible much of women's lives conventionally rendered invisible, it has perhaps not gone far enough. The study of housework as an occupation needs to attend in addition to features such as quality control, timekeeping, client as well as worker satisfaction, and perhaps further consideration of who, if anyone, is a housewife's boss. As will be seen, each of these is implicated in the discussion that follows.

These occupational aspects of housework provide, moreover, additional means of examining the relationship of the domestic division of labour to the economic structure as a whole. Recent commentary has also proposed that the view of the family as stripped of all but the residual economic function of consumption is ill-conceived and over-simplified. Domestic labourers refresh and sustain the existing labour force and play a key part in reproducing that of the future—as well as providing a reserve of labour themselves. The precise manner in which the political economy is to be accounted continues to be debated (West, 1980; Fox, 1980; Wajcman, 1981). For the moment, however, the general drift of that discussion can be borne in mind by recalling the everyday terminology of eating; food is consumed, meals have to be produced. The language favoured in cookbooks echoes that of industry and the factory (Murcott, 1983a). Homecooking may nicely embody the terms in which the family and household's place in the division of labour has to be seen. It may also provide a convenient arena for the further exploration of the economic and labour relations in the family and the relation of the marital partners to the means of production of domestic labour (Middleton, 1974).

Examination of the household provision of meals in these terms is, however, some way in the future. This paper does no more than offer some empirical foundation on which such study might build. It brings together informants' ideas about the importance of cooking, their notions of propriety of household eating and indicates their relation to gender. It starts with views of the significance of good cooking for home life, and goes on to deal with the place of cooking in the domestic division of labour. The familiar presumption that women are the cooks is extended to show that their responsibility in this sphere is tempered with reference to their husband's, not their own, choice. The paper concludes with brief comment on possible ways these data may illuminate some of the questions already raised.

HOME COOKING

Aside from love, good food is the cornerstone of a happy household . . . (Opening lines of a 1957 cookbook called *The Well Fed Bridegroom*).

Right through the series of interviews three topics kept cropping up; the idea of a proper meal, reference to what informants call a 'cooked dinner' and the notion that somehow home is where proper eating is ensured. Moreover, mention of one like as not involved mention of another, sometimes all three. The composite picture that emerges from the whole series suggests that these are not merely related to one another in some way, but virtually equated.

It first needs to be said that informants seemed quite comfortable with a conception of a proper meal—indeed the very phrase was used spontaneously—and were able to talk about what it meant to them. Effectively a proper meal is a cooked dinner. This is one which women feel is necessary to their family's health, welfare and, indeed, happiness. It is a meal to come home to, a meal which should figure two, three or four times in the week, and especially on Sundays. A cooked dinner is easily identified—meat, potatoes, vegetables and gravy. It turns out that informants displayed considerable unanimity as to what defines such a dinner, contrasting it to, say, a 'snack' or 'fried'. In so doing they made apparent remarkably clear rules not only for its composition but also its preparation and taking. I have dealt with their detail and discussed their implications in full elsewhere (Murcott, 1982). But in essence these rules can be understood as forming part of the equation between proper eating and home cooking. And, as will be noted in the next section, they also provide for the symbolic expression of the relationship between husband and wife and for each partner's obligation to their home.

The meal for a return home is, in any case, given particular emphasis—a matter which cropped up in various contexts during the interviews. Thus, for some the very importance of cooking itself is to be expressed in terms of homecoming. Or it can provide the rationale for turning to and making a meal, one to be well cooked and substantial—not just 'beans on toast . . . thrown in front of you'.

The actual expression 'home cooking'—as distinct from 'cooking for homecoming'—received less insistent reference. Informants were straightforward, regarding it as self-evident that people preferred the food that they had at home, liked what they were used to and enjoyed what they were brought up on. Perhaps untypically nostalgic, one sums up the point:

> When my husband comes home . . . there's nothing more he likes I think than coming in the door and smelling a nice meal cooking. I think it's awful when someone doesn't make the effort . . . I think well if I was a man I'd think I'd get really fed up if my wife never bothered . . .

What was prepared at home could be trusted—one or two regarded the hygiene of restaurant kitchens with suspicion, most simply knew their chips were better than those from the local Chinese take-away or chippy. Convenience foods had their place, but were firmly outlawed when it came to a cooked dinner. In the ideal, commercially prepared items were ranged alongside snacks, and light, quick meals: lunches and suppers in contrast to proper dinners. Informants talked about home cooking, but used this or some such phrase infrequently; the following is an exception:

> I'd like to be able to make home-made soups and things, it's just finding the time and getting organised, but at the moment I'm just not organised . . . I think it would probably be more good for us than buying . . . I suppose it's only—I'd like to be—the image of the ideal housewife is somebody who cooks her own food and keeps the household clean and tidy.

The sentiments surrounding her valuation of home-made food are not, however, an exception. Time and again informants linked not only a view of a proper meal for homecoming, but a view of the proper parts husband and wife are to play on this occasion. So cooking is important when you are married.

> you must think of your husband . . . it's a long day for him at work, usually, . . . even if they have got a canteen at work, their cooking is not

> the same as coming home to your wife's cooking . . . I think every working man should have a cooked meal when he comes in from work . . .

Cooking is important—though not perhaps for everybody 'like men who don't cook'—for women whose 'place [it is] to see the family are well fed'.

In this section, I have indicated that informants virtually treat notions of proper meals, home-based eating and a cooked dinner, as equivalents. The stress laid on the homecoming not only underlines the symbolic significance attached to both the meal and the return home. It simultaneously serves as a reminder of the world beyond the home being left behind for that day. Put another way, the cooked dinner marks the threshold between the public domains of school or work and the private sphere behind the closed front door. In the process of describing these notions of the importance of cooking in the home, it becomes apparent that the familiar division of labour is assumed.

COOKING IN THE DOMESTIC DIVISION OF LABOUR

As noted in an earlier section, all those interviewed took it for granted that it is the women who cook. What they had to say refers both to conventions in general, and themselves and their circumstances in particular.[2] There are two important features of their general presumption that women are the cooks; one indicates the terms in which it is modifiable, the other locates it firmly as a matter of marital justice and obligation. The upshot of each of these is to underline the manner in which the domestic preparation of meals is securely anchored to complementary concepts of conduct proper to wife and husband.

To say that women cook is not to say that it is only women who ever do so. It is, however, to say that it is always women who daily, routinely, and as a matter of course are to do the cooking. Men neither in the conventional stereotype nor in informants' experience ever cook on a regular basis in the way women do.[3] Husband/boyfriends/fathers are 'very good really'; they help informants/their mothers with carrying the heavy shopping, preparing the vegetables, switching the oven on when told, doing the dishes afterwards (cf. Leonard, 1980). Such help may be offered on a regular enough basis, notably it is available when the women are pregnant, dealing with a very young infant, unwell or unusually tired. But none of this is regarded as men doing the cooking.

More significantly, it is not the case that men do not cook—in the strict sense of taking charge of the transformation of foodstuffs to some version of a meal. They may make breakfast on a Sunday, cook only 'bacon-y' things, can do chips or 'his' curries: all examples, incidentally, of foods that do *not* figure in the proper cooked dinner (Murcott, 1983c).

For some, however, competence in the kitchen (and at the shops) is suspect: he'll 'turn the potatoes on at such and such a time . . . but leave him he's hopeless' and another just 'bungs everything in'. For others, it is men who make better domestic cooks than women, are more methodical, less moody. Another couple jokingly disagree: she 'not taken in' by Robert Carrier on TV, he claiming that 'the best chefs are men'. The point is that either way, of course, informants do regard gender as relevant to the question of who is to cook.

It is not even the case that all men cannot cook the proper, homecoming meal. One or two, when out of work for a while, but his wife still earning (this only applied to those having a first baby) might start the meal or even have it ready for her return. But once he is employed again he does not continue to take this degree of responsibility, reverting either to 'helping' or waiting for her to do it. Now and again, wives have learned to cook not at school or from their mothers, but from their husbands. But it was still assumed that it was for the woman to learn. This was even so in one instance where the informant made a 'confession . . . my husband does the cooking'. But now that she was pregnant and had quit paid work she would take over; 'it would be a bit lazy not to'. Like others for whom the cooking may have been shared while both were employed, cooking once again became the home-based wife's task (cf. Bott, 1957, p. 225; Oakley, 1980, p. 132).

The issue is, however, more subtle than an account of who does what, or who takes over doing what. Men and women's place involve mutual obligation. 'I think a woman from the time she can remember is brought up to cook . . . Whereas most men are brought up to be the breadwinner.' The question of who does the cooking is explicitly a matter of justice and marital responsibility. A woman talks of the guilt she feels if she does not, despite the greater tiredness of late pregnancy, get up to make her husband's breakfast and something for lunch—'he's working all day'. Another insists that her husband come shopping with her so he knows the price of things—he's 'hopeless' on his own—but she has a clear idea of the limits of each person's responsibility: each should cook only if the wife *has* to earn rather than chooses to do so.

Here, then, I have sought to show that informants subscribed in one way or another to the convention that it is women who cook. In the process it transpired that it is certain sorts of cooking, i.e. routine, homecoming cooking, which are perennially women's work. The meal that typically represents 'proper' cooking is, of course, the cooked dinner. Its composition and prescribed cooking techniques involve prolonged work and attention; its timing, for homecoming, prescribes when that work shall be done. To do so demands the cook be working at it, doing wifely work, in time that corresponds to time spent by her husband earning for the family (Murcott, 1982). This is mirrored in Eric Batstone's (1983) account of the way a car worker's lunch box prepared by his wife the evening before is symbolic of the domestic relationship which constitutes the rationale for his presence in the workplace; he endures the tedium of the line in order to provide for his wife and family. It transpired also that men do cook in certain circumstances, but such modification seems to reveal more clearly the basis for accounting cooking as part of a wife's responsibility (to the family) at home corresponding to the husband's obligation (to the family) at work, i.e. their mutual responsibilities to each other as marriage partners.

WHO COOKS FOR WHOM?

At this point I introduce additional data which bear on cooking's relation to the question of marital responsibility. Repeatedly informants indicated that people do not cook for themselves; evidently it is not worth the time and effort.[4] But the data suggest implications beyond such matters of economy. Two interrelated features are involved: one is the distinction already alluded to in the previous section, between cooking in the strict sense of the word and cooking as preparation of a particular sort of meal. The other enlarges on the following nicety. To observe that people do not cook for themselves can mean two things. First it can imply that a solitary person does not prepare something for themselves to eat while on their own. But it can also imply that someone does not do the cooking on their own behalf, but in the service of some other(s). Examination of the transcripts to date suggests that not only could informants mean either or both of these, but also that each becomes elided in a way that underlines the nuances and connotations of the term cooking.

The question of a lone person not cooking themselves a meal unsurprisingly cropped up most frequently with reference to women themselves, but men, or the elderly were also thought not to bother.

Informants are clear, however, that not cooking when alone does not necessarily mean going without. Women 'pick' at something that happens to be in the house, have a bar of chocolate or packet of crisps later in the evening or a 'snack'. Men will fry something, an egg or make chips. No one said that a man would go without altogether (though they may not know), whereas for themselves—and women and girls in general—skipping a meal was thought common enough. Men—and occasionally women—on their own also go back to their mother's or over to their sister's for a meal. One informant was (the day of my interview with her) due to go to her mother's for the evening meal, but fearful of being alone in the house at night, she was also due to stay there for the next few days while her husband was away on business.

The suggestion is, then, that if a person is by themselves, but is to have a proper meal, as distinct from 'fried' or a 'snack' then they join a (close) relation's household. The point that it is women who cook such meals receives further emphasis. Indeed, when women cook this particular meal, it is expressly *for* others. In addition to the temporary lone adults just noted who return to mothers or sisters, women in turn may cook for the older generation, as well as routinely cooking for children or for men home at 'unusual' times if unemployed or temporarily of a different shift.

This conventional requirement that women cook for others is not always straightforward in practice. At certain stages in an infant's life the logistics of producing meals for husband *and* child(ren) there as well meant the woman felt difficulties in adequately meeting the obligations involved. And not all informants enjoyed cooking; most just accepted that it needed doing, though there were also those who took positive, creative pleasure in it (cf. Oakley, 1974b). Part of this is expressed in the very satisfaction of providing for others something they should be getting, and in turn will enjoy.

More generally cooking can become tiresome simply because it has to be done day-in, day-out. The pleasure in having a meal prepared for you becomes all the more pointed if routinely you are cooking for others.[5] In the absence of any data for men, it can only be a guess that going out for a meal is thus specially enjoyable for women. But for those who on occasion did eat out this clearly figures in their pleasure. Even if it rarely happened, just the idea of having it put in front of you meant a treat: 'it's nice being spoiled'.

The question 'who cooks for whom?' can now begin to be answered. Apparently it is women who cook for others—effectively, husbands and children. If husbands and children are absent, women alone will not 'cook', indeed many may not even eat. It is the others' presence which provides the rationale for women's turning to and making a proper meal—that is what the family should have and to provide it is her obligation. Men—and children—have meals made for them as a matter of routine: but for women it is a treat. That solitary men do not 'cook' for themselves either, and may go to a relative's for meals (cf. Rosser and Harris, 1965; Barker, 1972), or that a woman on her own may also do so does not detract from the main proposal that it is women who cook for others. For it is not only that informants or their husbands will go temporarily back to their mother's, not their father's, home-cooking. It is also that both men and women revert to the status of a child for whom a woman, a mother, cooks. The mother may actually be the adult's parent, but they—and I with them—may stretch the point and see that she may be mother to the adult's nieces or nephews or indeed, as in the case of cooking for the elderly, she may be mother to the adult's grandchildren.

The appreciation that it is women who cook for others elaborates the more familiar convention, discussed above, that in the domestic division of labour cooking is women's work. First of all it indicates that this work is service work. Cooking looks increasingly like a task quite particularly done for others. Second, when cooking for others women are performing a service to those who are specifically related (sic) rather than for a more generalised clientele known only by virtue of their becoming customers. The marital—and parental—relationship defines who is server, who served.

That said, there remains the question of deciding what the server shall serve. As already discussed in an earlier section, the conventional expectation shared, it seems, by both woman and man, is that meals shall be of a certain sort—a cooked dinner for a certain occasion, most commonly the return home from work, or the celebration of Sunday, a work-free day. The 'rules' involved are not entirely hard and fast, or precisely detailed. Cooked dinners are neither daily nor invariable affairs (Murcott, 1982). And the cooked dinner itself can properly comprise a number of alternative meats (and cuts) and range of different vegetables. What then, determines the choice of meat and vegetables served on any particular day? Some of the factors involved, as will be seen in the next section, once again echo ideas of responsibility and mutual obligation.

DECIDING WHAT TO HAVE

A number of factors feature in deciding what to have for a particular day's meal.[6] First, a question of cost was taken for granted. This does not necessarily mean keeping expenditure to a minimum—eating in the customary manner despite hard times was highly and expressly valued by some. Second, the conventional provision of proper dinners itself contributed to the determination of choice. These two factors present themselves as marking the limits within which the finer decisions about what the precise components of the day's dinner are to be. Here reference to their husband's—and, to a lesser extent, children's—preferences was prominent in informants' discussion of such detailed choices.

It was indicated earlier that in an important sense women's cooking is service work. This sort of work has two notable and interrelated aspects affecting decisions and choice: is it the server or served who decides what the recipient is to want? Exploring the mandate for professionals' work, Everett Hughes (1971, p. 424) highlights a key question: 'professionals do not merely serve: they define the very wants they serve'. Servants, and service workers such as waitresses (Whyte, 1948; Spradley and Mann, 1975) compliantly provide for the wants identified by the served. On the face of it, then, the professional has total and the waitress nil autonomy. Examples reflecting this sort of range occurred among informants varying from one woman apparently always deciding, through to another always making what he wants for tea. But in the same way that the maximum autonomy of the professional is continually, to a certain degree, a matter of negotiation and renegotiation with clients, and that, similarly, the apparent absence of autonomy is modified by a variety of more or less effective devices waitresses use to exert some control over customers, so a simple report of how meal decisions are reached can, I propose, either conceal negotiations already complete, or reveal their workings.

Thus informants interested in trying new recipes still ended up sticking to what they usually made because their husbands were not keen. Others reported that 'he's very good' or 'never complains' while some always asked what he wanted. A non-committal reply however did not necessarily settle the matter, for some discovered that being presented with a meal she had then decided on could provoke adverse and discouraging remarks. But it was clear that even those who claimed not to give their husbands a choice were still concerned to ensure that he agreed to her suggestion. It is almost as if they already knew what he would like, needed to check out a specific possibility every now and then but otherwise continued to prepare meals within known limits. Deciding what to have already implicitly took account of his preferences so that the day-to-day decision *seemed* to be hers.

The material presented in this section provides only a glimpse of this area of domestic decision-making. Other aspects need consideration in future work. For instance, what degree of importance do people attach to the matter (cf. Edgell, 1980, pp. 58–9)? Attention also needs to be paid to wider views of the legitimacy of choice in what one eats. In what sense do restaurant customers choose and mentally subnormal patients not? Does a child that spits out what it is fed succeed in claiming a choice or not? And in apparently acquiescing to their husband's choice, are wives circumscribing their own? But it looks as if deciding what to have is of a piece with a shared view of marital responsibility whereby he works and so deserves, somehow, the right to choose what she is to cook for him.

GENDER AND THE PRODUCTION OF MEALS

> I know a cousin of mine eats nothing but chips, in fact his mother-in-law had to cook him chips for his Christmas dinner and she went berserk . . .

This 'atrocity story' recapitulates various elements of the preceding discussion. Such unreasonableness is, no doubt, unusual but its artless reporting emphasises a number of points already made. Not only do chips break the rules of what should properly figure in a Christmas meal, superior even to the Sunday variant of a cooked dinner, but it remains, however irksome, up to the woman to prepare what a man wants. The burden of this paper, then, may be summarised as revealing allegiance to the propriety of occasion such that a certain sort of meal is to mark home (male) leisure versus (male) work-time, and that such meals are cooked by women for others, notably husbands, in deference, not to the woman's own, but to men's taste.

This examination of cooking, mealtimes and gender within the household has implications for the continuing analysis of domestic work as work. While it does not shed light on why such work is women's, only reasserting that conventionally this is so, it clearly casts the work of meal provision as service work.

The everyday way of describing dishing up a meal as serving food is embedded in a set of practices that prescribe the associated social relationships as of server and served. As already observed this involves two interrelated matters: control over the work, and decisions as to what are the 'wants' the worker shall serve, what the work shall be. Each is considered in turn.

Oakley (1974a and b) reports that one of the features of housewifery that women value is the feeling of autonomy. Care is needed, though, not to treat such attitudes as tantamount to their analysis. Just because housewives express their experiences in terms of enjoying being their own boss does not mean that their conditions of work can be analysed in terms of a high degree of autonomy. The material presented in this paper suggests that doing the cooking is not directed by the woman herself, but is subject to various sorts of control.

First of these is the prescription for certain kinds of food for certain occasions. The idea of the cooked dinner for a homecoming is just such an example of cultural propriety. Related to this is a second control, namely that the food is to be ready for a specific time. Mealtimes construed in this way may exert just the same sort of pressure on the cook as any other production deadline in industry. Third, control is also exerted via the shared understanding that it is the preferences of the consumer which are to dictate the exact variant of the dinner to be served. What he fancies for tea constrains the cook to provide it. These kinds of control in the domestic provision of meals find their counterpart in the industrial concerns of quality control, timekeeping and market satisfaction. A woman cooking at home may not have a chargehand 'breathing down her neck' which is understandably a source of relief to her. But this does not mean to say that she enjoys autonomy—simply perhaps that other controls make this sort of oversight redundant. Evidence either way is extremely sparse, but Ellis (1983) suggests that failing to cook according to her husband's wishes can contribute to a wife's battering.

Linked to the issue of control of domestic cooking is the question of decision-making. Edgell (1980) has drawn attention to the degree of importance couples attach to different aspects of family living about which decisions have to be made. He distinguishes assessments of importance from, first, whether the decision is mainly the wife's or husband's responsibility and second, from the frequency with which the decision has to be made. So, for instance, moving is the husband's decision, perceived to be very important and infrequent, a contrast to the matter of spending on food. What Edgell does not make clear, however, is quite what either his informants or he mean by 'importance'. As an analytic device, the idea does not distinguish between family matters which partners may identify as both important and somehow major or permanent such as moving, and those identified as mundane, or fleeting but important nonetheless, such as daily eating. Like refuse collection or sewage work which is regarded as vital but low status, the importance attached to meals may not be remarked in the general run of things, though noticed particularly if absent. But that does not necessarily mean that both husband and wife regard it as unimportant. And, harking back to the question of autonomy in decision-making, reports such as Edgell's that food spending, cooking or whatever is regarded as the wife's responsibility, cannot, of itself, be seen as evidence of her power and freedom from control in those areas. For as Jan Pahl (1982, p. 24) has so cogently observed, 'being able to offload certain decisions and certain money-handling chores on to the other spouse can itself be a sign of power'. The delegate may be responsible for execution of tasks, but they are answerable to the person in whom the power to delegate is originally vested.

The preliminary analysis offered in this paper has theoretical and political implications concerning power and authority in marriage and the relation between domestic and paid work. The exploration of ideas about cooking and mealtimes starts to provide additional approach to detailing the means of domestic production. And the sort of work women are to do to ensure the homecoming meal provides a critical instance of the juncture between the control of a worker and the (his) control of his wife. The meal provides one illustration not only of a point where the public world of employment and the private world of the home meet one another; it also shows how features of the public take precedence within the private. For the stress informants lay on this mealtime offers an interesting way of understanding how the industrial rhythms which circumscribe workers are linked to the rhythms which limit women's domestic work (cf. Rotenberg, 1981). And women's continual accommodation to men's taste can also be seen as a literal expression of wives' deference to husbands' authority (Bell and Newby, 1976; Edgell, 1980, p. 70). This acquiescence to his choice provides the cultural gloss to the underlying economic relationship whereby industry produces amongst other things both the wage, and the raw materials it buys, for the domestic to produce what is needed to keep the industrial worker going. Part of the conjugal contract that each in their own way provide for the other, it does indeed become 'a pleasure to cook for him'.

ACKNOWLEDGEMENTS

I am very grateful to all those necessarily anonymous people who made the research possible and who generously gave their time to answer my questions. I should like to record my appreciation of conversations with Tony Coxon, Sara Delamont, Robert Dingwall, Rhian Ellis, Bill Hudson and Phil Strong at various stages during the preparation of this paper and of the computing help and advice Martin Read provided. Only I and not they are to blame for its deficiencies. And I must thank Lindsey Nicholas, Joan Ryan, Sheila Pickard, Myrtle Robins and Margaret Simpson very much, despite flu all round, and an unusually scrawly manuscript, for their help in typing both drafts.

NOTES

1. In order to begin remedying sociology's neglect (Murcott, 1983b) of food beliefs and of the social organisation of eating, I conducted a single-handed exploratory study (supported by a grant from the SSRC) holding unstructured tape-recorded interviews with a group of 37 expectant mothers attending a health centre in a South Wales valley for antenatal care (22 pregnant for the first time), 20 of whom were interviewed again after the baby's birth. No claim is

made for their representativeness in any hard and fast sense, though they represent a cross-section of socio-economic groups. For present purposes the data are treated as providing a composite picture. The prime concern here is to indicate the range and variety of evidence gathered. An instance that occurs once only thus becomes as interesting as one occurring 30 times. This is reflected in the discussion by the deliberate use of phrases such as 'some informants' rather than '6 out of 37'. In any case reference to numbers of instances is no more exact, and risks implying a spurious representativeness.

These qualifications are most important. But for the sake of a tolerably readable account I do not hedge every other sentence with reminder of these limitations. Yet they do actively have to be taken as read.

2. Informants referred not only to themselves but also to mothers, sisters, sisters-in-law and women friends doing cooking.
3. No informant who had children old enough to cook currently shared the household with them.
4. Market researchers know how to trade on such reports. During the period of interviewing a TV commercial was running which sought to persuade busy housewives not to neglect themselves but have a frozen ready-cooked meal at lunchtime.
5. Interestingly, no one talked of hospital meals put in front of them as a treat. (None had a home delivery.) Rather it was the quality of the food provided which informants concentrated on. Institution cooking could not be home cooking.
6. It might have been expected that nutritional criteria would figure in these decisions. Analysis so far suggests that cultural prescriptions for proper eating at home override what is known about healthy eating. (Murcott, 1983d).

REFERENCES

Barker, D. L. 1972. 'Keeping close and spoiling,' *Sociological Review,* 20(4), 569–590.

Batstone, E. 1983. 'The hierarchy of maintenance and the maintenance of hierarchy: Notes on food and industry,' in A. Murcott (ed.), *The Sociology of Food and Eating,* Gower.

Bell, C. and Newby, H. 1976. 'Husbands and wives: The dynamics of deferential dialectic,' in D. L. Barker and S. Allen (eds.), *Dependence and Exploration in Work and Marriage,* Longmans.

Bott, E. 1957. *Family and Social Network,* Tavistock.

Edgell, S. 1980. *Middle Class Couples: A Study of Segregation, Domination and Inequality in Marriage,* Allen and Unwin.

Ellis, R. 1983. 'The way to a man's heart . . . ,' in A. Murcott (ed.), *The Sociology of Food and Eating,* Gower.

Fox, B. (ed.). 1980. *Hidden in the Household,* Toronto: Women's Press.

Hughes, E. C. 1971. 'The humble and the proud,' in *The Sociological Eye: Selected Papers,* Aldine-Atherton.

Leonard, D. 1980. *Sex and Generation,* Tavistock.

Middleton, C. 1974. 'Sexual inequality and stratification theory,' in E. Parkin (ed.), *The Social Analysis of Class Structure,* Tavistock.

Murcott, A. 1982a. 'On the social significance of the "cooked dinner in South Wales," *Social Science Information,* 21(4/5), 677–695.

———. 1983a. 'Women's place: Cookbook's image of technique and technology in the British Kitchen,' *Women's Studies International Forum,* 6(2) (forthcoming).

———. (ed.) 1983b. *The Sociology of Food and Eating,* Gower.

———. 1983c. 'Cooking and the cooked,' in A. Murcott (ed.), *The Sociology of Food and Eating,* Gower.

———. 1983d. 'Menus, meals and platefuls,' *International Journal of Sociology and Social Policy* (forthcoming).

Murdock, G. P. and Provost, C. 1973. 'Factors in the division of labour by sex: A cross-cultural analysis,' *Ethnology,* XII(2), 203–225.

Oakley, A. 1974a. *Housewife,* Penguin.

———. 1974b. *The Sociology of Housework,* Martin Robertson.

———. 1980. *Women Confined: Towards a 'Sociology of Childbirth',* Martin Robertson.

Pahl, J. 1982. 'The allocation of money and the structuring of inequality within marriage', *Board of Studies in Social Policy and Administration,* University of Kent, mimeo.

Rosser, C. and Harris, C. 1965. *The Family and Social Change,* Routledge and Kegan Paul.

Rotenberg, R. 1981. 'The impact of industrialisation on meal patterns in Vienna, Austria,' *Ecology of Food and Nutrition,* 11(1), 25–35.

Spradley, J. O. and Mann, B. J. 1975. *The Cocktail Waitress: Women's Work in a Man's World,* John Wiley.

Stephens, W. N. 1963. *The Family in Cross-cultural Perspective,* Holt, Rinehart and Winston.

MALE SOCIABILITY AND RITUALS OF MASCULINITY IN RURAL ANDALUSIA

Henk Driessen

In Mediterranean society the bar or café is a focal institution of public life, the stage *par excellence* of male sociability and consequently one of the main settings for doing fieldwork. Oddly enough, the bar has been left almost completely out of the ethnographic record of Southern Europe.[1] Anthropologists working in Latin Europe also haven't shown much systematic interest in the expressive culture of daily sociability.

To the casual observer the behavior of men in Andalusian bars will appear to be informal, easy-going, merry and boisterous. After prolonged participation and observation, however, the bar not only turns out to be more than a center where men congregate for recreation, but café manners also prove to be rather formal. I find it useful to employ *ritual* broadly as a pilot concept in the ethnographic description of daily male sociability.[2] When I use the phrase *rituals of masculinity* I refer to formal, repetitive, stereotyped behavior that is expressive or communicative in the sense that it carries a message about male self-perception and men's image of women. This conception of ritual has been inspired by Goffman (1967) and Leach (1968). The emphasis on expression and symbolic charge differentiates ritual from instrumental features of behavior. The symbolic and ritual dimension of sociability deserves special attention, since it yields considerable insight into the realities of domination and subordination as some recent studies on Mediterranean communities have shown (Brandes 1980; Silverman 1979, 1981).

In this essay the following questions will be dealt with: why is the bar so central a focus for Andalusian men, especially agricultural laborers and other lower-status males? Why do these men need to assert their masculinity in homosocial gatherings? In the conclusion I will briefly discuss recent explanations offered for this phenomenon in the expanding literature on gender identity in the Mediterranean area. I will argue that rituals of masculinity in bars and at festivities serve important male-identity functions in a society where the gap between the ideal and actual sexual division of space and labor is widening.

From *Anthropological Quarterly* 56 (3): 125–133, 1983. Reprinted by permission of The Catholic University of America Press.

THE SOCIO-CULTURAL SETTING

Andalusia is a region of agro-towns and latifundia. Although most of the people who live in rural towns depend on the land for a livelihood, they hate and despise the country-side which represents to them uncivilized space of hard, dirty and backbreaking work. Everything that is highly valued—ownership of land, leisure, ambiance, education, personal autonomy, cleanliness—originates in the town.[3]

The small town in the plains of Córdoba, where I conducted fieldwork, stands on a hill approximately in the center of its large municipal territory. It is made up of a higher and lower part, corresponding to two clearly defined barrios. The *plaza* lies in between. Almost three out of four employed town-dwellers work in agriculture. Ninety percent of them are dependent on casual wages. Between this large proletariat and the local elite is a growing group of hardworking, self-employed tradesmen, lower civil servants, skilled workers, and agriculturists. The opposition between town and country, educated and working class, male and female are the major divisions of local society.

Andalusia is a strongly male-dominated society, where the relationships between the sexes are ambiguous and often antagonistic. The ideal male is tough (*duro*), strong (*fuerte*), formal (*sobrio*), autonomous and undisputed head of the household. He supports his family, guards the family honor, and is seldom at home. A woman should be virtuous, competent and docile, devoting her life to her husband and children. She is the guardian of family shame. The sexual division of labor is rigid, at least in theory. Men, regardless of class and occupation, hold that their wives should not work outside their home for an income. This image corresponds to the native conceptualization of social space. The public domain (*calle*) constitutes the world of men, while the women belong to the private domain (*casa*).

However, the reality of social class and the division of labor among the sexes contradicts this image. In the middle and upper-class families men play an active part in both the private and public domain. They not only provide for the family's income, but also control the household budget, make economic decisions and participate in child-rearing. On the other hand, it is increasingly becoming respectable for middle-class women to take prestigious white-collar jobs and join their husbands at outdoor activities at festivals and on summer weekends.[4]

In the class of agricultural day-laborers, women's labor power is of paramount importance to the maintenance of a household. Female labor in agriculture is tied to the olive, cotton and grape harvests and summer crop cultivation. Although it is a generally voiced opinion that in times of unemployment men should be hired preferentially over women, in practice employers often prefer to hire women because they earn lower wages and are "easier to handle." Moreover, women have access to alternative employment, traditionally in the domestic service sector and recently in the textile and food-processing workshops. So, it is not rare to find women in casual and permanent jobs while their father, husband, brother or son are unemployed. Among the working-class families, the wife is in charge of the household finances and the socialization of children.[5] There is close cooperation between mother and daughter, who visit each other almost daily. Because of the prominence of the mother-daughter link there is a strong tendency towards matrilocality. The insecurity of the day-laborer's contribution to the household budget and his physical self-removal from the house stress female dominance in the private realm. The tension produced by the contradiction between ideology and reality plays an important role in structuring male sociability.

PLACES AND TIMES OF MALE SOCIABILITY

Cafés are focal points in the townscape. Their presence is felt to be a necessary condition for *ambiente* (ambiance), a highly important quality of community life that derives from the assemblage of large numbers of people marked by differences in age, personality and occupation. Ambiente inspires local patriotism and is one of the bases for claiming urbanity.[6] There are nine *establecimientos* in the rural town I studied, all but two located on the plaza and the main traffic artery. They mark off the social center of the town and almost exclusively belong to the male domain.

Townsfolk employ the following criteria to differentiate various types of bars: location, social class and age of the clientéle, the barowner/tender's personality and reputation and the specialities he provides, the quality of the bar's interior, and the degree to which women have access.

The *casino* is clearly set off from the others in several respects. Until recently, it acted as a center of recreation and informal politics for the landed and commercial elite. It is the center of gravity of urbanity and the local shrine of civilization. In its fashionable lounge with plush arm-chairs, carpets and engravings, the best wines and snacks are severed to gentlemen who discuss local and national politics. Workers call the casino the "fat club." It is the first establishment that opened its doors to women, though in a very restricted sense. At festivals and on summer weekends, a growing number of the local elite bring their wives to the casino to have a chat and drink in the lounge or on the pavement terrace. However, the bar and the games-room are still exclusively male realms. Adolescents rarely enter the casino.

There are two other places that stand out for quite different reasons. In the late 1970's a discothéque and a *whiskería* were established in the town's periphery. Both are closed to prevent people from looking in from the outside. The arrangement of the interior, subdued light and fancy music create a sexual atmosphere in both places. In the discothéque adolescents of both sexes can meet in relative privacy to engage in dancing and petting. The whiskey bar or night club is an expensive place where adult males can congregate with scantily-clothed waitresses. Though men maintained that these girls could be "laid," the performances taking place in the whiskería can best described as ritual seduction. After some scandals—one of them involving a group of middle-class women entering the place to fetch their husbands—the municipal council was forced to close down the whiskey bar.

A small bar attached to a grocery store on the main street is known as the snail bar for the speciality it serves. Its clientéle largely consists of young people—high school students of both sexes, engaged and newly-wed couples.

The remaining five establishments are cafés in the strict sense of the word. They all serve coffee, the usual gamut of wine, beer, *aguardiente* (cheap anisette), cognac and soft drinks and a varying number of cold and warm snacks. They all have pavement terraces from May through September. One of them is considered a traditional bar. It displays the atmosphere of a pre-Civil War *taberna* and has old-fashioned furniture. It is mainly patronized by working-class men from the lower barrio. Another accommodates the sportsclub and is the favorite café for the medium and small landowners-operators, self-employed workers, and small bureaucrats. The atmosphere of this bar is conservative. At the corner of the plaza and the main street is a large café that attracts shopkeepers, ambulant traders, skilled workers, and civil servants. The remaining two locales are typical agricultural working-class taverns. Women seldom enter these five bars.

For a man the café is both an acceptable and obligatory place to be when he is not at work. The average Andalusian male spends most of his leisure time *en la calle* (in the street), of which bar attendance is an essential part. An adult man who withdraws himself too much from the company of bar mates must have very good reasons to do so, if he is not to be accused of anti-social and anti-masculine behavior.[7] Unemployed laborers are not supposed to stay home. Drinking, smoking and sharing is a coercive script for Andalusian men. When a man gets up in the morning he immediately leaves his house and goes to a café to have a coffee and a glass of anisette or cognac. If he works in town or in the surroundings he will have some glasses of wine at one or two o'clock in the afternoon before going home for dinner. Self-employed, unemployed, retired and leisure-class men patronize the bars more frequently during the day. The high time of bar attendance is in the evening between seven and ten o'clock when the bars fill up with busily talking and gesticulating men who have returned from work. The atmosphere gets high-spirited. Wine, tall stories, horseplay, riddles, comments on diverse topics but mostly on work, sex, women and football, contribute to the ambiente.

There is some seasonal variation in this time schedule. During the annual cycle of festivals which starts with Lent and ends with the festival of the patron saint in September, bar life goes on till midnight and for a minority till one or two o'clock in the morning. November to February is a nadir in the yearly round of bar attendance. Many day-laborers march off to neighboring provinces to work in the olive harvest and people who stay go to bed early. The town turns sad (*se pone triste*) and little or nothing happens (*no pasa na'*).

Besides daily bar attendance there are two institutionalized activities in which fellowship is celebrated, the so-called *juerga* and *perol*. Both constitute a climax of male sociability. Andalusian men believe that it is necessary for their well-being to drive away daily worries through an elaborated spree. A number of bar mates agree to have a juerga. In the morning they meet in their favorite bar where they start with some drinks "in order to clean their throats." Then they travel to a neighboring town—Montilla and Puente Genil are first choice for their size and ambiance, La Carlota for its whiskerías—where they feel more free to relax and loosen up. Hopping as many bars as possible is the essence of this outing. Nostalgia for the bachelor days when they were not yet bothered by wifes, mothers-in-law, and children, sets the tone of the binge. Sometimes an interesting football match or bullfight in the cities of Córdoba and Sevilla provides an excuse for a juerga. In these cities a visit to the red-light district is often included. Wives accept these outings as an inevitable outlet for a man's nature.[8] The *perol* (literally "frying pan") differs from the juerga in various respects. It takes place in the countryside where a lamb or billy-goat is killed for a banquet prepared by the participants themselves. A larger number of men is involved and it is usually organized by the owner of a large estate. Consequently, it is often an elite affair, sometimes combined with a shooting-party.

The major communal festivities—Lent, Holy Week and the fair in honor of the patron saint—constitute another climax in male sociability. One of these festivals will be described below.

BAR ETIQUETTE

Bar attendance is a highly patterned activity and so is the behavior displayed in bars. Although on a normal day most men enter more than one café, the majority of them have a favorite which is, as a rule, close to the neighborhood where they live. A man usually starts the evening with a couple of drinks in one of the taverns but very soon finds himself in his favorite bar where he spends most of the evening with his friends and neighbors. A variation on this pattern occurs when a man happens upon an *amigo* whom he invites for some drinks in his own café. After a while the amigo attempts to persuade the host into coming along to his favorite bar. This pattern often gets more complicated because of the involvement of more than two men.

Social drinking in a bar is regulated by a strict etiquette. Though there are numerous ways in which a man may offer, accept and reciprocate a drink, there are some golden rules. A man attending his own café has a right and an obligation to invite anyone who is not a regular customer. In general, "established" men have a priority to initiate a round of drinks with entering persons. Strangers and guests are never allowed to buy a round.

The following scenario is enacted again and again, resulting in ritualized behavior. A man announces that he is going to "invite" (*invito yo*) the mates standing around him to a glass of wine. His companions protest in a roundabout way, the first man repeats his invitation for form's sake, gives the barkeeper a sign to fill the glasses, and after repeated demurrals everyone "yields" to the hospitality. Before the glasses are drained, a second man invites the group to another round, and the same performance is repeated. Cigarettes are offered, refused and accepted with similar decorum.

To cultivate friendship is a time-consuming and rather expensive but socially necessary activity. There are, of course, various strategies to limit exchanges. For instance, the frequently used expression *dame la espuela* or *penúltima* (give me the next to the last) conveys the wish to conclude a series of drinks and at the same time enables a man to reciprocate by claiming the last round. Both the refusal to allow other men to buy drinks as well as the constant acceptance without reciprocating are felt to be attacks on the code of equality and viewed as "ugly" (*feo*) behavior. Men who offend the bar etiquette are stigmatized as *sinverguenzas* (shameless ones) and treated as such. Generosity among equals is a sacred café value. Although, ultimately, exchanges should be reciprocal, Andalusians abhor the principle of "on the spot" or balanced reciprocity, sharing the costs alike or paying separately. This is also considered ugly for it offends the value of fellowship. Emigrants often refer to the instrumental behavior in city cafés to illustrate the "coldness" of industrial society, which they contrast with the "warm" social climate of rural Andalusia.

Participation in the elaborate exchange circuits of drinks, cigarettes, snacks, and small talk is a prerequisite of male adult status. Since a man's face is at stake, the politics of bar hospitality sometimes gives rise to heated arguments. It is the difficult task of the bartender to mediate and take care that none of his customers lose face.

THE MALE ETHOS AND RITUALS OF MASCULINITY

The café provides an ideal scenario for showing off masculinity. In particular men standing at the counter, which is the favorite area of the bar, stage rituals of masculinity. Basic cultural notions of manliness and womanliness model their behavior.

The native terms for masculinity are *hombría, ser hombre* or *ser macho* (in rural Andalusia the anglicism/neologism *machismo* is only used in intellectual circles), which refer first and foremost to sexually aggressive behavior. The essence of hombría is *tener cojones,* to have balls. Virility is thought to reside in the testicles.[9] Andalusians argue that it is the testicles that make the difference between a real man and a woman who acts like a man, just like they make the difference between a bull and an ox. Hence an aggressive and fearless male is called *cojonudo* (big-balled). When a man asserts himself, he so to speak extends his genital qualities. Hence men frequently touch their privy parts in public when meeting other men or entering a café, situations in which they must assert themselves. However, being a man (*todo un hombre*) means more than sexual aggression. It also involves the willpower and ability to defend one's interests and those of the family, which center upon honor. It has been argued that in Andalusia the stress on manliness is entirely upon sexual aggressiveness rather than upon physical toughness (cf. Gilmore & Gilmore 1979: 282). It is true that the actual use of violence is rare and that Andalusians strongly devalue fighting. However, this does not mean that physical strength is absent from hypermasculine behavior. In bars men are constantly showing off their *potential* for physical aggression; they show each other that they are capable of violence. While doing so, they prove their virility to their peers (cf. Brandes 1980: 126). This is apparent from the amount of force which is used when men slap each other on the shoulder, hit their coins on the counter, knock dominos on the tables, and order drinks with a sharp clap of their hands. It also appears from the muscle-tight clothes young men wear and the proofs of physical strength to which they take themselves. Behavior that communicates a man's potential for physical prowess is strongly ritualized.[10]

The celebration of manliness implies spending much time and money in bars, where one of the major topics is men's relationships with women. Their gender identity is defined by the following basic beliefs. Men are "by nature" superior to women. At the same time men are convinced of their inability to control themselves in the area of sex. They think it natural that a male is constantly on the hunt for women. It is the responsibility of females to control themselves, maintain their shame, and be aware of the social consequences of extra- or pre-marital liaisons.[11] However, men also feel that their superiority is under constant female attack. They fear women's sexuality, which they believe to be insatiable and socially disruptive. Women's seductive qualities, their power to emasculate and cuckold men, and their obstinacy are dangerous weapons in the battle between the sexes. So, men feel that they have to defend their masculinity from female incursions.

While the ideal woman is virgin and a mother, the messages men in cafés express about women is that they are whores. Many jokes, tall stories and songs reveal men's negative image of femininity.[12] In fact, mothers impress this image upon their sons when saying that they have to "beware of women, they are *astuta* (cunning) and *engañadora* (deceitful)."

The exchange of boastful stories about male sexual conquests, obscenities and jokes about female sexuality is intimately tied to social drinking in bars, and both make up the core of the masculinity cult. Although normally men do not drink to the point of losing self-control, it is considered masculine to get drunk once in a while. This socially accepted drunkenness is institutionalized in juergas, peroles and festivities.

Revels always consist of boozing and obscenities; they are charged with verbal and body-idiomatic allusions to sexual performances. At one of the peroles I attended, the owner of the estate where it was held forced one of his laborers into playing the female part in a burlesque of the coitus. He was "taken by the ass" (*tomado por culo*), an act symbolizing a double subordination, i.e., sexual in the sense of a man being feminized, and economic in the sense of an employee who has to suffer this humiliation for fear of being sacked. In fact, many practical jokes in bars, in which the victim is approached from behind, capitalize on the obsessive fear Andalusian men have for being feminized.[13]

The Holy Week is above all a high time of male sociability. The processions are prepared and staged by religious brotherhoods, which are exclusively male and organized along class lines.[14] On Ash Wednesday four of the town's seven Holy Week brotherhoods—three of working-class and one of middle-class composition—open clubhouses where in the evenings both members and non-members congregate, sharing wine and food. These clubhouses expand the bar circuit during Lent. The most important ritual object of a religious brotherhood is a saint's image. Among laborers female saints are most popular. The Good Friday procession starts at five o'clock in the morning. The great majority of the members who participate in the procession stayed up all night, drinking and eating in the clubhouses. When the procession begins most participants are already in a frantic state. Fireworks, the monotonous rolling of the drums, the excessive drinking during the procession, sleeplessness, the carrying of the heavy floats through the winding and inclined streets, hoarse competitive shouts like "long live Veronica, the prettiest of all," or "La Soledad is the best," dramatize the atmosphere. The procession ends in chaos between three and four in the afternoon. Groups of drunken boys and men sing and dance.[15]

This popular interpretation of a Holy Week procession is a reversal of the official Roman Catholic precepts. Like the revels discussed above it is also a ritual of masculinity through which men re-create their self-image. To beat the drums for hours, carry the floats, drink in excess, and go without sleep, requires toughness and endurance. Men who drop out before the ritual is completed are rebuked for being weaklings. It is highly significant that women are part of the audience, proudly watching their husbands, fathers, sons, brothers and fiancés act out their masculine role. After the procession men glory in showing each other the bruises on their shoulders from carrying the floats. They have lived up to the image of virility.

The second component of the ethos that guides male sociability is *formalidad*. This value counteracts sexual and physical aggressiveness. It means self-control, the ability to stand upon one's dignity by putting a restraint upon strong emotions. Formality is exhibited most markedly by the town's elite, who hold that the public behavior of laborers lacks this quality. However, formality has undeniably permeated the ideas and behavior of the town's proletariat. While honor and masculinity entail assertive behavior, violence is rare in Andalusian agro-towns. During my fieldwork there was only one fight among adult males in the town where I lived. This observation is confirmed for a Sevillian agro-town (Gilmore 1980: 187-88). Besides the occasions described above, I rarely saw drunks in the cafés and streets of Andalusia. Yet bar performances are a critical test for self-control. Besides competitive social drinking there is another challenge to a man's dignity.

Cachondeo, a particular type of joking, is very popular in Andalusian cafés. It is playful yet aggressive in the sense that the initiator of the joke tries to get a rise out of his victim. It is important for the victim to keep his face, withstand the jest, and strike back in a cool manner. A man who looses his temper is scorned by the audience. The following examples illustrate the mechanism at work in cachondeo:

> A group of day-laborers is engaged in a round of drinks at the counter. A landowner walks up to them and orders a glass of wine without paying attention to the laborers. One of the workers starts a cachondeo, exclaiming: "This *tio* (fellow) is a real capitalist. He owns a lot of money but pays lousy wages. Moreover he is a fascist. They should kill off fellows like him." At once he gives his victim a friendly slap on the shoulder, playing down the aggressive tone of the jest, and starts to fool around with one of the onlookers. The land-owner maintained his composure.
>
> In one of the bars a company of five men is playing a prohibited game of chance. At a given moment one of the onlookers hisses, "Look out the *cabo* (the commander of the Civil Guard)," whereupon the players stop in a fright. The audience bursts into laughter.

Since cachondeo capitalizes so heavily upon male sensibilities, there is an inherent risk that the bounds of what is acceptable are transgressed. This is apparent from the following example:

> In a café a construction worker delivers a man standing next to him a sudden push, too strong, for the victim knocks into another group and spills his glass of wine. He is furious but checks himself and does not say a word. Nobody laughs.

Andalusians call this a *broma pesa'o,* a graceless joke. This brings us to the third element of the male ethos, *gracia.* One of its meanings is the power to entertain, to evoke laughter (cf. Pitt-Rivers 1971: 189 ff.). Men have to be sociable, witty, and amusing. Metaphors, funny word games, ambiguities, riddles, tall stories, and jokes are highly praised in homosocial settings. Men with gracía are always foci of attention in bars. A carpenter, nicknamed Curro Pistola, enjoys the reputation of making even the dead laugh with his witty pranks. Jesus, a tough construction worker, has a gift of telling stories, spontaneously put into rhyme. Gracía contributes to ambiance, a quality that is warmly cherished in the cafés of Andalusian agro-towns.

CONCLUSION

So far, I have depicted the specific pattern of male sociability and shown how a strongly male ethos influences the conduct of men in cafés. The question of why masculine display is so pronounced in homosocial settings remains to be answered. One explanation in the literature on male-female relationships in the Mediterranean area focuses on male ego-formation. It is argued that a boy growing up in a household dominated by women will develop a feminine identity in the face of his father's absence. Upon reaching adolescence, the boy finds out that his early view of male and female dominance is wrong. In reaction to his primary female identity he develops hypermasculine behavior (cf. Gilmore & Gilmore 1979). The problem with this explanation is that the evidence for the link between psychodynamic and cultural processes is thin and inconclusive. Since the primary process of personality formation is largely unconscious, it can never be made perspicuous. Consequently, verification of this explanation remains highly problematic.

Another approach analyzes male sexual identity on its own terms (cf. Brandes 1981). Ignoring the socio-economic context of relationships between the sexes, this approach fails to note that there are significant differences in the degree to which Andalusian men are preoccupied with the fundamental fact that they are men. Taking male dominance for granted, it misses the all-important point that in the agricultural proletariat women do challenge the economic superiority of men. An explanation that fails to contextualize the symbolic representations of male behavior can at best be partial.

I hold that the basic characteristics of male sociability cannot be adequately comprehended except in relation to the actual division of domains, tasks and power among the sexes.[16] In a society where the notion that women are inferior to men is a cultural assumption shared by both sexes, where men's ability to provide for their family is taken as axiomatic, the position and identity of day-laborers are vulnerable. When women contribute substantially to the family income through wage labor, as is the case in the rural Andalusian working class, the dividing line between male and female identity and private and public roles tends to get blurred. To prevent this the male role and self-image are reinforced in the public domain by symbols and rituals that exclude females. Day-laborers justify their absence from the house by stressing that the "home is for women and children," for the "weak" who have to be protected from the hostile world outside. Too much involvement in the matrifocal household ruins a laborer's reputation as a *macho.*[17] The marginality of day-laborers in the private and public realm helps to explain why they engage in a more intense form of bar sociability than middle and upper-class men who hold rather firm positions of power and influence. Rituals of masculinity in cafés act to mask the reality of the day-laborer's dependence upon the female members of his household and his weak economic and political position in local society. However, I would not go to the extreme of calling male dominance in Andalusia a "myth".[18] Rituals of masculinity recreate male identity. They are forceful and efficacious in the sense that they help to keep women in a subordinate position. They really work.

NOTES

My gratitude goes to my Andalusian informants with whom I spent so much time in local bars, and to Anton Blok, Bill Christian and Willy Jansen for advice and inspiration. The generous comments of the journal's anonymous reviewers were particularly helpful.

1. Exceptions are Davis (1964), Photiadis (1965), and Brandes (1979). Hansen, who devoted a section of his monograph to bar culture, rightly suggested that the bar "would be a good place for field inquiry almost anywhere in Spain" (1977: 166).
2. The greater part of the evidence presented here has been collected from 1977–78 in a Cordobese township of 5,290 inhabitants.
3. See Driessen (1981) for an elaboration of these values and the role of an urban ethos in Andalusian agro-towns.
4. In the middle and upper-class families whose incomes are mainly derived from landownership and agriculture, domains and tasks are more strictly segregated according to sex than in families whose incomes come from professions outside agriculture. Men who rose to political and economic prominence in the Franco era hardly participate in a bar sociability; they subscribe to a very strict code of formality.
5. Also see Luque Baena (1974) and Gilmore (1980) for the organization of Andalusian households.
6. Gilmore (1980: 203) also found this to be true for an agro-town of 8,000 in the plains of Sevilla.
7. Acceptable reasons for not attending bars are illness, mourning when a close relative has died, and extreme lack of cash.
8. Also see Gilmore (1980: 190–191) for a description of juergas.
9. This is a general Mediterranean conception, cf. Blok (1981). While a man is defined as possessing "balls," a women is defined negatively, i.e., as lacking "balls."
10. More research will be needed to study the impact of state formation—the monopolization of the means of violence—on masculine behavior and the role of ritualization in the control of violent impulses.
11. Also see Aguilera (1978:29–30) on this point. Writes Press: "Backsliding or failure to meet certain expectations are almost forgivable as

'natural' consequences of being a man" (1979: 129–130).

12. There are numerous popular flamenco verses—which men sing to men—expressing the view that women are treacherous:

    El amor de la mujer
    es como el de la gallina,
    que en faltándole su gallo
    a qualquier otro se arrima.

    (A woman's love
    is like a chicken's,
    for when her cock is not around
    she gives herself to whoever she may find.)

    Quien se fía de mujeres
    muy poco del mundo sabe,
    que se fía de unas puertas
    de que todos tienen llaves.

    (He who puts faith in women
    doesn't know much of life,
    for he trusts doors
    to which everybody owns a key.)

13. In daily usage *tomar por culo* means to make a fool of a person. It clearly expresses dominance and submission. For an interesting parallel in the verbal duelling of Turkish boys see Dundes, Leach & Ozkok (1970).
14. For a useful discussion of religious brotherhoods in Andalusia see Moreno Navarro (1974). In the late 1970s one of the town's brotherhoods decided to recruit three girls to carry ritual paraphernalia in the procession. This triggered off a heated discussion since the majority of men oppose female membership in religious brotherhoods.
15. Aguilera (1978: 104-105) describes a similar procession in the Andalusian province of Huelva.
16. More than fifteen years ago the *Anthropological Quarterly* (1967) initiated a debate on the role and position of Mediterranean women from the viewpoint of women. Since then, systematic examination of female power has shown that women do participate in the public domain, that they exert considerable influence on men through their sexuality, control over channels of information, and access to the supernatural realm (cf. Nelson 1974).
17. Anthropologists working in North-American slums and in the Caribbean area have also stressed the connection between matrifocality and the cult of machismo (cf. Hannerz 1969; Wilson 1973; and Manning 1973). One is struck by the similarities in the area of male ethos and patterns of sociability.
18. See Rogers 1975 who argues that in peasant societies formal male power and prestige are balanced by informal female power and influence. This non-hierarchical power relationship is maintained by the acting of a "myth" of male dominance (Rogers 1974: 729). Her model of male-female relationships underestimates male power in the local community and in the society at large and overstresses the importance of the private domain in the power structure of peasant societies. This is not to deny that women have considerable power chances. However, the power resources controlled by men are quite different in their scope from those controlled by women, i.e., "formal" and "informal" power are not identical nor are they interchangeable.

REFERENCES

Aguilera, Francisco E. 1978. *Santa Eulalia's people. Ritual structure and process in an Andalusian multicommunity.* St. Paul (Minnesota): West Publishing Co.

Anthropological Quarterly. 1967. Appearance and reality: Status and roles of women in Mediterranean societies. 40:3 (special issue).

Blok, Anton. 1981. Rams and billy-goats: A key to the Mediterranean code of honour. *Man* 16: 427–440.

Brandes, Stanley H. 1979. Drinking patterns and alcohol control in Castilian mountain village. *Anthropology* 3: 1–16.

———. 1980. *Metaphors of masculinity: Sex and status in Andalusian folklore.* Philadelphia: University of Pennsylvania Press.

———. 1981. Wounded stags: Male sexual ideology in an Andalusian town. *In Sexual Meanings. The Cultural Construction of Gender and Sexuality.* Sherry B. Ortner & Harriet Whitehead, eds. Cambridge: Cambridge University Press, pp. 216–240.

Davis, John. 1964. Passatella: An economic game. *The British Journal of Sociology* 15: 191–207.

Driessen, Henk. 1981. *Agro-town and urban ethos in Andalusia.* Nijmegen: Centrale Reprografie Katholieke Universiteit.

Dundes, Alan, Jerry W. Leach, and Bora Ozkok. 1970. The strategy of Turkish boys' verbal duelling rhymes. *Journal of American Folklore* 83: 325–349.

Gilmore, Margaret, and David D. Gilmore. 1979.

"Machismo": A psycho-dynamic approach (Spain). *The Journal of Psychological Anthropology* 2: 281–300.
Gilmore, David D. 1980. *The people of the plain: Class and community in Lower Andalusia.* New York: Columbia University Press.
Goffman, Erving. 1967. *Interaction ritual: Essays in face-to-face behavior.* Chicago: Aldine Publishing Co.
Hannerz, Ulf. 1969. *Soulside: Inquiries into ghetto culture and community.* New York: Columbia University Press.
Hansen, Edward C. 1977. *Rural Catalonia under the Franco regime: The fate of regional culture since the Spanish Civil War.* Cambridge: Cambridge University Press.
Leach, Edmund. 1968. Ritual. *In International Encyclopedia of the Social Sciences.* Vol. 13. D. Sills, ed. New York: Macmillan and the Free Press, pp. 520–526.
Luque Baena, Enrique. 1974. *Estudio anthropológico social de un pueblo del Sur.* Madrid: Editorial Tecnos.
Manning, Frank. 1973. *Black clubs in Bermuda.* Ithaca: Cornell University Press.
Moreno Navarro, Isidoro. 1974. *Las hermandades andaluzas: Una aproximación desde la antropología.* Sevilla: Publicaciones de la Universidad de Sevilla.
Nelson, Cynthia. 1974. Public and private politics: Women in the Middle Eastern world. *American Ethnologist* 1: 551–565.
Photiadis, J. D. 1965. The position of the coffeehouse in the social life of the Greek village. *Sociologia Ruralis* 5: 45–56.
Pitt-Rivers, Julian A. 1971. *The people of the Sierra.* 2nd ed. Chicago: The University of Chicago Press.
Press, Irwin. 1979. *The city as context: Urbanism and behavioral constraints in Seville.* Urbana: University of Illinois Press.
Rogers, Susan C. 1975. Female forms of power and the myth of male dominance: A model of female/male interaction in peasant society. *American Ethnologist* 2: 727–757.
Silverman, Sydel. 1979. On the uses of history and anthropology: The palio of Sienna. *American Ethnologist* 6: 413–436.
———. 1981. Rituals of inequality: Stratification and symbol in Central Italy. *In Social Inequality: Comparative and Developmental Approaches.* Gerald D. Berreman, ed. New York: Academic Press, pp. 163–182.
Wilson, Peter. 1973. *Crab antics: The social anthropology of English-Speaking Negro societies of the Caribbean.* New Haven and London: Yale University Press.

PUBLIC AND PRIVATE POLITICS: WOMEN IN THE MIDDLE EASTERN WORLD[1]

Cynthia Nelson

THE ETHNOGRAPHIC IMAGE

One of the most commonly held assumptions found in the ethnographic literature discussing the political significance of women in the society at large is that the decisions that women make do not have repercussions on a very wide range of institutions. The general argument is most clearly stated by Mary Douglas:

Reproduced by permission of the American Anthropological Association from *American Ethnologist* 1:3, August, 1974. Not for further reproduction.

> The social division of labour involves women less deeply than their menfolk in the central institutions—political, legal, administrative, etc.—of their society. They are indeed subject to control. But the range of controls they experience is simpler, less varied. Mediated through fewer human contacts, their social responsibilities are more confined to the domestic range . . . their social relations certainly carry less weighty pressure than those which are also institutional in range. This is a social condition they share with serfs and slaves. Their place in the public structure of roles is clearly defined in relation to one or two points of reference, say in relation to husbands and fathers. As for the rest of

> their social life, it takes place at the relatively unstructured interpersonal level, with other women. . . . Of course I would be wrong to say that the network of relations a woman has with others of her sex is unstructured. A delicate patterning certainly prevails. But its significance for society at large is *less than the significance of men's relations with one another in the public role system* (1970:84).

Nowhere is this assumption more uncritically taken for granted than in the ethnographic descriptions of pastoral and sedentary societies in the Middle East in which the assertion is made that there are dual and separate worlds of men and women in which the former world is public and the latter world is private. Typical of such assertions is the following:

> The women's world is not merely more narrowly circumscribed like in most civilizations; it is also provided with a complicated system of devices for cushioning off: i.e., safeguards which provide limited access to each other's worlds. The women's world has two major manifestations: *the home* (tent) and *the private communication patterns between women of several homes.* For men there is limited access to the former and practically no access to the latter and this is paralleled by lack of interest by the men about the women's world. . . . The men's world has two major manifestations: *the sphere of earning a living and the public sphere of communications including public affairs.* Access of women to the former is limited and formally none in the latter—old grandmothers being an exception. But women are keenly interested in male affairs!!! No doubt that the two worlds have their regular meeting point in the home, for this is where a good deal of clearing goes on continuously (van Nieuwenhuijze 1965:71).

Inherent in this statement as well as most other discussions on sex roles found in the ethnographies of the Middle East, and particularly those centering on nomadic societies, is not only the commonplace notion that the human universe is segregated into two social worlds marked out by the nature of the two sexes, but also that these two social worlds are by definition characterized as being *private* (the women's) and *public* (the men's) (Asad 1970; Barth 1961; Cole 1971; Cunnison 1966; Marx 1967; Pehrson 1966; Peters 1966). The former world is invariably described as domestic, narrow, and restricted, whereas the latter is described as political, broad, and expansive. Authority is also segregated in terms of this dichotomy. The home is regarded as the woman's for all *internal purposes.* Her authority in domestic affairs is an established fact. For *external purposes,* the home is the man's, the assumption being that whatever articulates the household to the public sphere is by definition political and thereby a male concern. And the inference drawn from this assumption is that women are far more interested in men's affairs than vice versa.

Also inherent in the ethnographic accounts of these two social worlds is the notion that what is the concern of women is the domestic and not the political. This raises the whole question of the meaning of "power" and "the political" and why this should be linked to such notions as "private (domestic)" and "public (political)." By assigning private and public to the different social worlds of men and women described for certain Middle Eastern societies, I would argue that western social scientists have imposed their own cultural categories onto the experiential world of the Middle East and that the whole discussion of "power" in these societies is influenced by these categorizations.

Most anthropologists working in the Middle East tend to view power in the classic functionalist tradition. Following Radcliffe-Brown, they define the political system as the maintenance or establishment of social order within a territorial framework by the organized exercise of coercive authority through the use or possibility of use of physical force.

Barth, for example, explores the kinds of relationships that are established between persons (only males as it turns out) among the Swat Pathans and the way in which these may be systematically manipulated to build up positions of authority and the variety of political groups. The main sources of authority/power available to persons are ownership of land, the provision of hospitality, and a reputation for honor. Most statuses and rights are usually defined by contractual agreements between persons. In these circumstances, each man's aim may be seen as the adoption of the strategy that will best serve his interest. "Physical force or the threat of it is in Swat a characteristic sanction in a great many relations" (Barth 1959:53). Barth sees Swat Pathans as being driven by self-aggrandizing passion and maximizing rationale and represents the political activity of the dominant land-owning class as the foundation of social order. As Asad has so cogently pointed out, Barth's model is an anarchic, conflict-ridden, violent society which reflects Barth's Hobbesian model of human nature (Asad 1972:74–94).

Criticizing the functionalist position, Asad argues for a distinction between power and authority. For Asad, power refers to the relation between agent and an object as a means, that is, to the opposition of exploiter and exploited, whereas authority refers to the subordination of human consciousness to a legitimate rule (and contingently to those who determine the rule) (Asad 1972:86). Asad sees the problem of political domination in terms of a dialectical relationship and raises an important alternative in terms of the way ethnographers tend to look at political systems. But he, too, tends to view power and authority as the exclusive concern of men. "The overall authority of the household head is based on the fact that he has greater power and moral responsibility than any other member of the household" (Asad 1970: 100–101).

Given the fact that most ethnographers of the Middle East have been European or American males who, by virtue of their foreignness and maleness, have had limited if no access to the social world of women, we seem to be confronted with the normative image of the society as reported to male ethnographers by male informants.[2] Lienhardt expresses this dilemma cogently:

> And though the segregation of women from men not closely related to them is one of the things that must at once meet the eye of any visitor to the towns and villages of the Trucial Coast, this segregation makes it difficult for a visitor to gain any precise knowledge of the women's position. Apart from its being difficult for a man to talk to women there, it is not even proper for him to ask very much about them, particularly to ask in any detail about specific cases . . . one can easily be misled, particularly in assessing the extent of male dominance (1972:220).

From the ethnographic literature, we know precious little about how women in these societies view their situation, whether they feel they have "power" and how they wield it. If we had better knowledge of the "lived-in-world" of nomadic women, we might come up with different images of the society and the definitions of power. Also, we might ask what could the contributions to our knowledge and understanding of the relationship of women and power be, if we were to re-think the notions of "power" and recognize its special feature as a particular kind of social relation rather than as an embodied quality institutionalized in types of social structures. Some social scientists have argued along the following lines:

> The initial problem of defining social power is to recognize its special features as a particular kind of social relation, as reciprocity of influence. *Reciprocity of influence*—the defining criterion of the social itself—is never entirely destroyed in power relations, except physical violence when one treats another as object. We cannot sever power relations from their roots in social interaction. One actor controls the other with respect to particular situations and spheres of conduct—or scopes—while the other actor is regularly dominant in other areas of situated conduct (Wrong n.d.).

Olesen has suggested in an unpublished paper that the concept of "the negotiated order" is a useful idea for understanding reciprocity of influence in interactive situations (Olesen 1973). Persons in an interactive situation, she argues, negotiate the rules that define and circumscribe that relationship.

Assuming that men and women are involved in "negotiating their social order"—i.e., the rules and roles of social interaction—we must not lose sight of the fact that social action is always "situated action" and circumscribed by culturally given constructs of social reality, the social stock of knowledge at hand, as Schutz would say (1962:120–134). What becomes relevant for the purposes of our discussion is to recognize that despite the existence of segregated social worlds and the implication that there exists a differential distribution of social knowledge—the man's and the woman's—this knowledge is structured in terms of relevances, and women's relevance structures intersect with those of men at many points. Applying this to the ethnographic situation, we must ask how women can and do influence men to achieve their own objectives. The notion of power implied in the concept of the negotiated order is the potential for levying sanctions, the potential for influencing further actions of others (as well as one's own). Sanctions are not just threats of physical force but capacities for influencing the behavior (action) of others. They are ways of creating possible lines of action for others as well as for oneself.

Looking at power from this perspective, we are forced to raise a different set of ethnographic questions, questions that have been neglected perhaps due to not recognizing the ongoing dialectical process of social life in which both men and women are involved in a reciprocity of influence *vis-à-vis* each other. What are the normative constructs that facilitate, limit, and govern "negotiation"? What are the sanctions open to women? In what ways can and do women set up alternatives for men by their own action? How do women influence men? Who controls whom about what? How is control exercised? How do women control men? Other women? How conscious are women of their capacity to influence? In other words, what are women doing in this reciprocity?

In the remainder of this essay I would like to challenge the notion that the social worlds of men and women, despite the element of segregation, are reducible to spheres of private and public with power limited to males in a so-called public arena. By using data from ethnographic studies by both men and women concerning women in the Middle East, I shall suggest that women can and do exercise a greater degree of power in spheres of social life than has heretofore been appreciated.

THE ETHNOGRAPHIC EVIDENCE

The detailed and scholarly work of Ilse Lichtenstädter (1935) on *Women in the Aiyam Al-'Arab* offers an interesting analysis of the role that the Arabic women played in the warfare of her tribe and thus presents us with a view of the life and position of women in pre-Islamic Arabia.[3] Although the material deals with nomadic society during the Jahiliya, it is still informative about the manner in which women were depicted in everyday life and how they exercised political influence in the man's world.

According to the Aiyam narratives, the women's influence was felt beyond the tent. Through marriage she played an important role in Arab policy by being the link and mediator through which powerful alliances between tribes were accomplished. As matron she acted as counsellor to her son who very often submitted to the advice of his mother and, whenever it was possible, she tried to gain influence over her son in order to bring an enmity to an end. Lichstenstädter points out:

> That Fatima bint al-Khurshub tried, though unsuccessfully, to mediate between her son and Qais b. Zuhari shows that she could be sure that her opinion would at least be heard. In this case, however, the son did not accept his mother's advice; the events proved that she was right (1935:65).

In warfare the woman very often was the cause of quarrels and great feuds. She was also employed as a spy and, if captured in war, was the source of great ransoms. As the women were not far from the spot where the battle took place, they were able to watch the bustle of the fight and incite their men by acclamations. When in the greatest distress and danger, the Arabs had recourse to a device which was meant to excite their desire of fighting to the highest degree: they exposed their women, particularly noble women, to danger by forcing them to fall from their camels and litters in order to show the warriors that they must fight or die (Lichtenstädter 1935:43).

In summarizing her analysis, Lichtenstädter suggests that pre-Islamic nomadic society was a society that treated women with esteem and one in which they were allowed to take part in public life. "From the Aiyam tales pre-Islamic Arab women played a part in the life of their tribe and exercised an influence which they lost only later in the development of Islamic society" (1935:81). "But as during the time of Jahiliya women were *not* separated from men but lived in close intercourse with them they could readily get to know their plans and projects" (1935:83). "In addition the conditions of life were such that in times of distress clever advice was eagerly accepted and followed regardless whence it came, even if offered by a woman. In this sense we are justified in speaking of the 'influence' of a woman without exaggerating her importance in the public life of an Arab tribe" (1935:85).

Emrys Peters also describes the manner in which women can and do exercise influence over men in pastoral societies, for example, as mediators between natal and affinal groups in marriage alliances, as controllers of the products or the property, and as wielders of authority in the domestic sphere.

> *The pivotal points in any field of power* in this, a superficially dominant patrilineal, patrilocal and patriarchal society where the male ethos is vulgar in its brash prominence, *are the women.* What holds men together, what knots the cords of alliances are not men themselves, but the women who depart from their natal household to take up residence elsewhere with a man, and who, in this critical position communicate one group to another (Peters 1966:15).

Among the Bedouin of Cyrenaica men may boast of their dominance over women (and certainly this might be expected with male informants channeling information to male ethnographers), but they are constrained in their actions by the control women possess over the preparation of food, the provision of hospitality, the comforts of shelter, and the reputation for honor. Men may control the economic resources—land, water, animals—the durable properties, but women control the products. Utilization of the products, the dividends of their investments, are granted to women, and through these they acquire legal rights in men. Bereft of controlling rights in property, women are nevertheless critical in its manipulation. They possess the legal right to protection and support against husband as daughter or sister of the man who holds the bridewealth. Women mediate between the two, make demands on the men as a right, and are given public support (Peters 1966; Mohsen 1967).

Marx makes the same point about Bedouin of Negev—that women in multiplex role situations increase their potential for negotiation:

> A marriage link acts as a very effective communicative device between groups because the woman who conveys the communications is so intimately bound up with both her husband and sons and with her father and brothers. She has the interest of both groups at heart and would suffer most from an estrangement between the two groups. At the same time she is on the inside of both groups and *thus able to assert her influence over the sections* through the men to whom she is closely connected, as well as through women (1967:157).

Cunnison, while arguing that women occupy no formal position of power or authority among the Baggara Arabs, does suggest that:

> Women have a profound influence on politics in two respects. Firstly, they are arbiters of men's conduct, and they can make or break a man's political career. They do this by singing songs of praise or alternatively of mockery. The brave man and the cowardly man have their fame spread. The man who is undistinguished in either direction goes unsung. The songs sweep the country, and the reputations are made and broken by them. Secondly, a policy decision that the men of a camp or a *surra* (kin group) make is influenced by the kind of reactions that the women of the group are likely to have (1966:117).

In these respects, at least for the Baggara, women have a significance in the public *role* system of the society. Cunnison also points out that the Baggara ideas about the value of manliness involve the closely related aims of wealth, women, and power.

> Cattle attract women and allow a man to marry more than one wife. The possession of cattle plays an important part in the relations of men and women. It implies that a man is endowed with those qualities that Baggara men and women alike regard as most admirable. Herd building means easier access to women who play a positive part in spreading a man's virtue or challenging man's honour. Although there is often argument about amount of bridewealth to be paid, debate is not between two families; instead the men of both families agree and unite in argument to try to beat down the price. The bride's mother backed by the women of the family is demanding. Final word is that of the bride's mother. She can try to stop a marriage that she or her daughter don't want by refusing to lower the price. "Let us chase him off with our demands" (1966:116).

The Pehrsons in their study of the Marri Baluch describe the strategies used by women to achieve influence over men: (1) playing men off against each other; (2) seeking alliance and support from other women; and (3) minimizing contact with the husbands (1966:59).

In another monograph on *La Femme Chaouia de L'Aures* (1929), Gaudry draws our attention to the *power* that women can exert over men in their capacity as saints, sorceresses, magicians, and healers. The Auresian woman has, like the man, the cult of *mzara,* places sanctified by the passage of a saint, and the woman, just as the man, affiliates herself to religious organization. Gaudry describes a female Marabout, Turkeyya:

> There existed a Marabout of great virtue named Turkeyya who was most pious and exerted a great influence on her many clients and adepts. There was also a male Marabout, Sidi Moussa, seeing that his authority had diminished with a number of his followers felt peeved. He decided to put an end to this competition with his dangerous rival and he devised a simple plan to get rid of her. He appealed to one of his devouts and entrusted him to kidnap Turkeyya and marry her. As a Marabout can only enter into a family of Marabout she lost, from this mis-marriage, *all the authority she had* (1929:235).

Sorcery is another means by which women can be said to exert their influence over males in Chaouia society, and as a sorceress woman has more power over the man than as a saint because of her ability to divine the future, enhance love, deter evil, and heal illness. According to Gaudry:

> It can be said that the superstitious fear of the women which filled the Berber mind allowed the women to *impose an inferior religion of which they are the priestesses* which is a response to a collective need (1929:246).

All old women are more or less sorcerers, learning their craft from their mothers. They teach women to prepare lotions which can "tame any man." Men fear them, and some forbid their wives to receive them. A sorceress has power over the male through the women. Says a male Chaouia proverb:

> The child of male sex comes to the world with 60 *jnoun* in his body; the child of the female sex is born pure; but every year, the boy gets purified of a jinn, whereas the girl acquires one; and this is the reason that old women, 60 years and with 60 *jnoun* are sorcerers more malig-

> nant than the devil himself. Blind she sews more material, lame she jumps over rocks and deaf she knows all the news (Gaudry 1929:267).

Gaudry's work raises a fundamental issue that has *not* been the focus of much recent ethnographic field research among Middle Eastern societies; that is, the degree to which men perceive women exercising power over them through the idiom of the supernatural. Crapanzano's recent work on the Hamadsha in Morocco, however, is suggestive of the powerful significance of the "camel-footed she-demon, A'isha Qandisha" on men in the curing rituals (1972:327–348).

> Should one of A'isha's followers disobey her, he is immediately struck and suffers grave misfortune or bodily harm. The Hamadsha, her special devotees, are said to be favored by A'isha and are very proud of the intimacy of their relations with her (1972:333).

It must be noted that both Gaudry's and Crapanzano's work was conducted among Islamicized Berber cultures of North Africa among whom saint cult worship is predominant (Gellner 1969; Geertz 1968). Nevertheless, both ethnographers underscore the fear and veneration expressed by men toward these female supernatural figures and suggest lines of inquiry for further investigation. The paucity of ethnographic description surrounding the relationship of women to the religious system, in general, and the supernatural, in particular, suggests more a lack of interest on the part of ethnographers than it does a lack of concern on the part of the actors in Middle Eastern Islamic societies. This does not seem to be the case when we look at studies of women in societies of sub-Saharan Africa (Lebeuf 1971; Hofer 1972). Perhaps if we were to turn to the more recent ethnographic studies focusing specifically on women in pastoral and sedentary societies of the Middle East, we might discover evidence that suggests women do exercise control in society in a variety of ways.[4]

Farrag, in her study of social control among the Mzabite women, demonstrates convincingly how moral, social, and religious control is exercised over women by women through a specific all-female religious institution called the Azzabat. Both men and women have a very important stake in the conduct of their women in that there is a firm belief that god's anger befalls the whole community as a result of any sexual misconduct on the part of women.[5] Because of the frequent and prolonged absence of the men in the community for purposes of trade, the women have assumed an increasing importance in the mechanisms of social control over women.

> Although social changes since independence have also affected the power of the Azzabat, they still exercise a far stricter control over the women than the Ozzaba (male religious group) do over the men (Farrag 1971:318).

Yet, at the same time, increasing demands are now being made by the men for the "modernization" of the women, thus creating a situation in which certain inconsistencies and ambivalences are created. The thrust of Farrag's argument is to show how breaches of certain norms are still effectively and formally sanctioned through all-female religious institutions coupled by informal sanctions of the power of mothers-in-law, public opinion, and gossip, regardless of social status. The implications of Farrag's article to the main thesis of this paper are obvious. Instead of an image of segregated social worlds of men and women, in which women are relegated to the private domestic sphere, we find all-female institutions responsible for the sanctioning of breaches of social norms—certainly a most public concern.

Approaching her study of women from the perspective of social stratification, Vanessa Maher, in a recent study among townswomen in the Middle Atlas of Morocco, makes an exhaustive analysis of the social mechanisms, both political and ideological, by which women are confined to the traditional status-based mode of social relationship "where women are not working for wages because participation in the public sphere of the market is considered immoral" (1972:15). Given this segregation of men's and women's roles, the dependence of women on women becomes all the more necessary, especially in late pregnancy and early childbirth. These feminine links of cooperation that form are independent of those formed by the male's kindred of cooperation and operate to redress the balance of power between men and women. Maher argues that the market principles and prerogatives of kinship and status struggle for hegemony with the result that there is a structural conflict between the social necessities of marriage and the superior rewards of kinship (status-based relations), especially for women. The chief locus of conflict is marriage, and Maher argues that lacking political control over their own lives and lacking religious worth as second-rate Moslems, women are forced to turn to intrigue and witchcraft—weapons used in the power struggle between men and their wives.

Nancy Tapper (1968) explores this theme in more depth in her study of a women's sub-society among the pastoral Shahsavans in Iran. In this women's sub-society she describes how women establish among themselves a range of relationships in which *women may gain achieved status in the community* as midwives, ceremonial cooks, and religious leaders.

> In each *tira* (clan or family group) . . . were one or two women held to be knowledgeable on religious matters. Commonly, they are women who, with a male relative, have made the pilgrimage to the shrine of Imam Reza at Mashhad and are thereafter referred to by the title of *Mashadi.* In fact the position of Mashadis among women is comparable to that of a Hajji among men. The Mashadis are among the few women who pray regularly; their position is a highly conservative one and they firmly support traditional Shahsavan customs and moral attitudes, sometimes by reference to imaginary Koranic injunctions. The opinions of such a woman in matters of family law and custom are sought by both men and women and her advice is given equal weight with that of a man (Tapper 1968:17).

Al-Torki, in her pioneering study of townwomen in Jeddah, Saudi Arabia (1973a), postulates that in societies where the segregation of women prevents their participation in public affairs, elaborate networks of friendship and gift-exchange will be found. These networks are likely to enable the participants to gather vital information, which gives them considerable informal control over decisions that are nominally the exclusive prerogative of males. In Jeddah the women exercise considerable control over marriage alliances.

> This control has far-reaching consequences in a society where kinship dominates as a structural principle in local and national politics. Obviously, their influence must derive from a different source of power than control of resources. I suggest that the women's eminent control of information in matters relating to the arrangement of marriage constitutes this source. The very nature of the women's exchange networks gives them an almost exclusive access to information on which the decisions of their male relatives depend. By manipulating their knowledge to accommodate their own interests in potential marriages, the women actually manage to direct or impede the men's efforts to establish marriage alliances (1973b:5).

Lienhardt (1972) underscores this proposition in his description of marriage and the position of women in Trucial Coast society. Since shaikhs, great and small, are political personages, their marriages have a much clearer political dimension than the marriages of other people. Here some women achieve remarkable influence and power. Lienhardt suggests that the marriage of shaikhs with Bedouin women may be one of the reasons why the women of shaikhly families in general seem to lead a less secluded life than most others. When they are women of strong character, the senior women of ruling families can play an important part in affairs. One remarkable woman of the Trucial Coast, Shaikha Hussah bint al-Murr, the mother of the present ruler of Dubai and wife of his predecessor, came so far out into open public affairs as to hold her own *majlis* ('public meeting'), not for women but for men, sitting receiving visitors, as people said, like a shaikh, and when her husband ruled it is said that more men visited her *majlis* than visited his. This remarkable lady was an outstanding figure in both politics and business. On the one hand, she played a leading part in a political struggle that led to civil war and the subsequent expulsion of the reformist party. On the other, she restored her husband's family fortunes by property development, trade, and, one gathers, that profitable but risky enterprise of Dubai, smuggling with Persia and India (1972:229–230).

This may be an extreme example of the potential importance of leading women in public affairs; however, it suggests that we must re-evaluate the metaphors of private and public in terms of domestic and political. What Lienhardt's and the other ethnographic material suggest is that women do approach public affairs but they do so from private positions. In public, women are separated from men, and men mix widely in the public circle of the market. The women, on the other hand, mix in a large number of smaller groups, more exclusive than the society of men and consisting largely of closer and more distant kin affines, and other women who are friends of the women of the family, e.g., *azzabat,* female sub-societies, and kindred of cooperation as discussed above. In the societies we have been discussing, families are one of the basic groupings in its economic and political, as well as its moral aspects. Here, in some senses, the range of women is greater than that of men, and it is the very segregation of women and the impropriety of discussing them in male company that makes this so. Women, in general, are a necessary part of the network of communications that provides information for their menfolk, and at the head of the social hierarchy are some women who form a focus for the smaller groupings of women and a bridge between their concerns and the public concerns of men.

Once we begin to examine the role and position of women in Middle Eastern society from the standpoint of the woman and to describe the woman's view of the social worlds in which she lives and interacts, it becomes clear that our ethnographic imagery about domestic spheres being private and female and public spheres being political and male is misleading. This is not to argue that only women can understand or do ethnography about women, but only to suggest that by taking the standpoint of the woman, by examining her taken-for-granted assumptions about her social worlds, we discover another image of power and influence operative in society. I take the position that to place oneself imaginatively into the inner self of another (including a set of interacting "others" of which the ethnographer is one) is not only necessary, but it is the very foundation of social life (Berger and Luckman 1967; Schutz 1962; Mills 1967). Also, by re-evaluating the notion of power from the standpoint of reciprocity of influence, we can specify ethnographically those particular situations in which women can and do exercise influence over men. Based on the evidence presented, what are these situations?

One dominant theme repeated throughout the ethnographies is the crucial role women play as structural links between kinship groups in societies where family and kinship are the fundamental institutions of everyday life. Simultaneously the woman as daughter, sister, wife, and mother acts as an "information-broker," mediating social relations within the family and larger society. The implications for power (reciprocity of influence) are obvious in that by these networks of relationships, the woman is in a position to channel or withhold information to the male members of the kindred. And in this position the woman influences decision-making about alliances, actually sets up marriage relations, and informs male members of the household what is going on in other homes. But of course the "home" in question is not that of a tiny nuclear family, but of a wider family group. And this family group is one upon which many of the affairs of the society—social, economic, political—turn.

The ethnographies do support the idea of segregated social worlds but rather than seeing this as a severe limitation on women, the evidence suggests that the segregation of women can alternatively be seen as an exclusion of men from a range of contacts which women have among themselves. This emphasizes a second major theme emerging from our data, particularly from sources on women written by women, and that is that women form their own exclusive solidarity groups and that these groups exercise considerable social control (Farrag 1971; Maher 1972). Also, by seeking alliance and support from other women in the community, certain women achieve high social status in the community and consequently exercise political influence (Aswad 1967; Tapper 1968).

From the ethnographic data summarized above it is evident that women *do* participate in public activities, activities which have their reverberations and intentions in large-scale societal networks.

A third realm in which women emerge as having influence over men is through the religious or supernatural. That is, in those situations where women are publicly acknowledged as having power, it is associated with the supernatural and the fear that men have of women's sexuality or, better expressed, as the felt threat to male esteem of women's sexual misconduct. Through witchcraft, sorcery, divination, and curing, women are instrumental in influencing the lives of men.

A final point to be mentioned is the degree to which the public image of a man is influenced by the particular behavior of his women—through ridiculing, through gossip, through honor and shame (Schneider 1971; Cunnison 1966).

IMPLICATIONS FOR ETHNOGRAPHY

The main thrust of this essay has been to challenge the prevalent ethnographic image of the position of women in selected pastoral and sedentary societies of the Middle East. Specifically, it has addressed itself to the question: In what sense can we speak of women exercising power in those societies which are avowedly patrilineal, patrilocal, and patriarchal? This raised the whole issue of the conception of power as viewed by Western ethnographers in their writings about Middle Eastern society—a view that defines the sphere of masculine activity as the public—in the Greek *polis* sense, and the sphere of feminine activity as the private and domestic. What becomes defined as the public and private spheres, however, are less the categorizations of the world by the actors living in these societies than they are the metaphors of the observers who are recording the actions of men and women in these societies.[6]

The fundamental implication for ethnography emerging from this essay rests on the following question: What are the kinds of data generated in a field situation in which accessibility to the social worlds of men and women is predicated primarily on the sex role of the observer? As sex roles circumscribe the way the actors interact with each other in society, it is of fundamental importance to realize that sex roles also circumscribe the way in which actor and ethnographer interact with each other. The sex-linked aspect of social interaction places the actor and ethnographer in situations of communication in which the so-called "raw data" of ethnography are the very products of this communication. In other words, it is the interactive situation itself which produces (or generates) the data from which ethnographies are written. An awareness of this phenomenon suggests to me a quite different strategy of fieldwork than has hitherto been expressed in the ethnography of the Middle East, particularly on the important question of the position of women. What I would suggest is that we, as ethnographers, become more imaginative in the creation of our models of the activities, norms, and interpersonal linkages that make up a society's political processes. My descriptions of women as information brokers, as reputation builders and maintainers, as "power" of their own, all concern a better filling in of all the links. We must get away from the simplistic, mechanical models (either those implicit ones of the ethnographers—such as Barth's Hobbesian view of politics—or the official ones of the informants). We must become conscious that our data are not "gathered" but manufactured and grounded in the interactive foundations of the research process itself. Not being conscious of this phenomenon has led to an ethnographic image of women and power in the Middle East that is both incomplete and misleading.[7] We must ask ourselves how do we come to understand the world of the opposite sex? And as ethnographers, what are the criteria by which we have selected data to record the "true image" of society?

For most ethnographers of the Middle East, there exists an implicit assumption that "reality," the data, exist "out there" waiting to be described and that it matters little what the social position of the informant is since "as a bearer of the culture" he (or she) is as informed as anyone else. Unfortunately, this view overlooks one of the most critical problems in fieldwork—the importance of the social distribution of knowledge (Berger and Luckman 1967; Mannheim 1936; Schutz 1962). It also denies the relevance of the interactive situation as the source of our knowledge about the society and the implications of these shortcomings have been the focus of this paper.

On the one hand, I have pointed out that when we examine the literature of the Middle East on women done by women, our ethnographic image of women and power is considerably different from that of the male ethnographers. On the other hand, when I examined the literature of the male ethnographers, I discovered hints that the women in these societies are not as powerless as the ethnographer themselves had concluded. In other words, there exists internal evidence that our images are incomplete, that the dynamics of power and authority are much more subtle than we have been led to believe, and that our theoretical perspectives about the position of women in Middle Eastern society must be the common-sense world of the actors themselves.

NOTES

1. This is a much revised version of an earlier paper delivered at a symposium on nomadic-sedentary interaction in Middle Eastern societies held at the American University in Cairo, March 17–21, 1972 (Nelson 1973). The emergence of the present paper, however, is in large part due to the many stimulating and provocative discussions while on sabbatical at the Institute of International Studies, 1973–1974, with colleagues at the University of California, May N. Diaz, Lucile Newman, Elvi Whittaker, and, particularly, Virginia L. Olesen, whose incisive and critical comments forced me to sharpen my own ideas considerably. To Hildred Geertz, a note of appreciation for suggesting a closer link between the central argument of the paper and its title.
2. The argument might be made that women share the man's construction of the social world, but this seems to me more of an implicit taken-for-granted assumption than an ethnographic fact. Until we know that this is the case, based on ethnographic evidence emerging from studies of women's views about their social world, we are making generalizations from information channeled from male informants to ethnographers.
3. Although Lichtenstädter's analysis is drawn from written materials rather than from personal observations, her insights are suggestive of themes emerging from more recent ethnographic studies (Lienhardt 1972). Dr. Abdou (personal communication) of the University of Riyadh drew my attention to the fact that the Prophet Mohammed worked for a female merchant whom he later married—Khadidja. He commented that "generally speaking the Bedouin women of Saudi Arabia participate more as men in society than do their urban counterparts." Abdou attributes this to the greater Turkish influence on the seclusion of women in the urban centers. He also noted that in the Saudi Arabian town of Tadmur there are special women's markets where only women are sellers. This phenomenon is also recorded among the Berbers of the High Atlas and Rif Mountains of Morocco (Benet 1970:182, 193; Hart 1970:38).

4. Evidence that my generalizations about women and power in Arab society also held true for Arabicized Berbers in North Africa is found in several recent published and unpublished manuscripts (Alport 1970; Benet 1970; Hart 1970; Murphy 1970; Mason 1973; Joseph 1973). Subsequent to the submission of this essay, a useful exploration of this topic among pastoral nomads in the Sudan came to my attention. I wish to thank Elinor Kelly of the University of Manchester for generously sharing with me her unpublished thesis from the University of London.
5. Supporting this image of women from yet another part of Moslem Africa is the following excerpt from an *Agence France-Presse* news item quoted in the June 23, 1973 issue of the *San Francisco Chronicle:*

> Kano, Nigeria—Single women are being ordered to get married immediately or leave Northern Nigeria because religious authorities here say that the current drought in West Africa is caused by prostitution and immorality. . . . Many unmarried women are reported to have fled their homes following the get-married-or-leave order by the Emirs in the Moslem area. Landlords have been ordered not to let out rooms to single women since, according to one Emir, "because of prostitution there has been no rain."

6. One historian of the Middle East has suggested that among nomads there is no equivalent Arabic term for the concept "public" arena. The tent and the camp are not synonyms for public and private (Dols, personal communication).
7. The recent exchange between Abou Zahra (1970) and Antoun (1968) on the meaning of the modesty code in the Middle East is an excellent example of conflicting ethnographic images.

REFERENCES

Abou-Zahra, Nadia. 1979. On Modesty of Women in Arab Muslim Villages: A Reply. *American Anthropologist* 72(5):1079–1088.

Alport, E. A. 1970. The Mzab. *In Peoples and Cultures of the Middle East,* Vol. II. L. Sweet, Ed. New York: The Natural History Press, pp. 225–241.

Al-Torki, Soraya. 1973a. Religion and Social Organization of Elite Families in Urban Saudi Arabia. Unpublished Ph.D. dissertation. University of California, Berkeley.

———. 1973b. Men-Women Relationship in Arab Societies: A Study of the Economic and Political Conditions of the Status of Women. Unpublished research proposal.

Antoun, Richard. 1968. On the Modesty of Women in Arab Muslim Villages: A Study in the Accommodation of Traditions. *American Anthropologist* 70(1):671–697.

Asad, Talal. 1970. *The Kababish Arabs: Power, Authority and Consent in a Nomadic Tribe.* London: C. Hurst.

———. 1972. Market Model, Class Structure and Consent. *Man* 7(1):74–94.

Aswad, Barbara. 1967. Key and Peripheral Roles of Noble Women in a Middle East Plains Village. *Anthropological Quarterly* 40(3):139–153.

Barth, Fredrik. 1959. Political Leadership among Swat Pathans. *London School of Economics Monographs on Social Anthropology,* 19. London.

———. 1961. *Nomads of South Persia: Basseri Tribe of the Khameseh Confederacy.* Boston: Little, Brown.

Benet, Francisco. 1970. Explosive Markets: The Berber Highlands. *In Peoples and Cultures of the Middle East,* Vol. I. Louise Sweet, ed. New York: The Natural History Press, pp. 173–203.

Berger, Peter, and T. Luckman. 1967. *The Social Construction of Reality.* New York: Doubleday (Center Book).

Bujra, Abdullah. 1966. The Relationship between the Sexes amongst the Bedouin in a Town. Unpublished paper delivered at the Mediterranean Social Science Conference, Athens.

Cole, Donald. 1971. Social and Economic Structure of the Al Murrah: A Saudi Arabian Bedouin Tribe. Unpublished Ph.D. dissertation. University of California, Berkeley.

Crapanzano, Vincent. 1972. The Hamadsha. *In Scholars, Saints and Sufis: Muslim Religious Institutions Since 1500.* Nikki R. Keddie, ed. Berkeley: University of California Press, pp. 327–348.

Cunnison, Ian. 1966. *The Baggara Arabs: Power and Lineage in a Sudanese Nomad Tribe.* Oxford: Clarendon Press.

Douglas, Mary. 1970. *Natural Symbols: Explorations in Cosmology.* New York: Random House (Pantheon).

Evans-Pritchard, E. E. 1971. *The Senusi of Cyrenaica.* Oxford: Clarendon Press.

Farrag, Amina. 1971. Social Control amongst the Mzabite Women of Beni-Isguen. *Middle Eastern Studies,* Winter (3):317–327.

Gaudry, Mathea. 1929. *La Femme Chaouia de L'Aures.* Paris: Geuthner.

Geertz, Clifford. 1968. *Islam Observed.* New Haven, CT: Yale University Press.

Gellner, Ernest. 1969. *Saints of the Atlas*. Chicago: University of Chicago Press.

Hart, David M. 1970. Clan, Lineage, Local Community and the Feud in a Rifian Tribe. *In Peoples and Cultures of Middle East,* Vol. II. Louise Sweet, ed. New York: The Natural History Press, pp. 3–75.

Hofer, Carol. 1972. Mende and Sherbro Women in High Office. *Canadian Journal of African Studies* 6(2):151–164.

Joseph, Roger. 1973. Choix ou Force: Une Etude sur la Manipulation Sociale. Unpublished manuscript.

Lebeuf, Annie. 1971. The Role of Women in the Political Organization of African Societies. In *Women of Tropical Africa.* Denise Paulme, ed. Berkeley: University of California Press, pp. 93–119.

Lichtenstädter, Ilse. 1935. *Women in Aiyam al-Arab.* London: The Royal Asiatic Society.

Lienhardt, Peter A. 1972. Some Social Aspects of the Trucial States. *In The Arabian Peninsula: Society and Politics.* D. Hopwood, ed. London: Allen and Unwin, pp. 219–229.

Maher, Vanessa. 1972. Social Stratification and the Role of Women in the Middle Atlas of Morocco. Unpublished Ph.D. dissertation. Cambridge University.

Mannheim, Karl. 1936. *Ideology and Utopia.* New York: Harcourt, Brace (Harvest Books.)

Marx, Emmanuel. 1967. *Bedouin of the Negev.* New York: Praeger.

Mason, John. n.d. Sex and Symbol in a Libyan Oasis. Unpublished manuscript.

Mohsen, Safia. 1967. Legal Status of Women among the Awlad Ali. *Anthropological Quarterly* 40(3):153–166.

Mills, C. W. 1967. Situated Actions and the Vocabulary of Motives. *In Power Politics and People.* Oxford: Oxford University Press, pp. 439–452.

Murphy, Robert F. 1970. Social Distance and the Veil. *In Peoples and Cultures of the Middle East,* Vol. I. Louise Sweet, ed. New York: The Natural History Press, pp. 290–314.

Nelson, Cynthia. 1973. Women and Power in Nomadic Societies of the Middle East. *In The Desert and the Town Nomads in the Greater Society.* Cynthia Nelson, ed. Berkeley: Institute of International Studies, University of California, pp. 43–59.

Nieuwenhuijze, C. A. O. van. 1965. *Social Stratification in the Middle East.* The Hague: E. J. Brill.

Olesen, Virginia L. 1973. Notes on the Negotiation of Rules and Roles in Fieldwork Studies. Unpublished manuscript. San Francisco: Department of Social and Behavioral Sciences, University of California.

Pehrson, Robert. 1966. The Social Organization of the Marri Baluch. *Viking Fund Publications in Anthropology,* 53. New York.

Peters, Emrys. 1966. Consequences of the Segregation of the Sexes among the Arabs. Unpublished paper delivered at the Mediterranean Social Science Council Conference, Athens.

Rosenfeld, Henry. 1968. The Contradictions between Property, Kinship, and Power as Reflected in the Marriage System of an Arab Village. *In Contributions to Mediterranean Sociology.* J. Peristiany, ed. The Hague: Mouton, pp. 247–260.

San Francisco Chronicle. June 23, 1973.

Schneider, Jane. 1971. Honor, Shame and Access to Resources in Mediterranean Societies. *Ethnology* 10(1):1–24.

Schutz, Alfred. 1962. Collected Papers, Vol. II: *The Problem of Social Reality.* The Hague: Martinus Nijhof.

Sweet, Louise. 1970. *Peoples and Cultures of the Middle East,* Vols. 1 & 2. New York: The Natural History Press.

Tapper, Nancy. 1968. The Role of Women in Selected Pastoral Islamic Society. Unpublished M. A. thesis. S.O.A.S. London.

Wrong, Dennis H. n.d. Some Problems in Defining Social Power. Unpublished manuscript.

IV

THE CULTURAL CONSTRUCTION OF GENDER AND PERSONHOOD

We all live in a world of symbols that assign meaning and value to the categories of male and female. Despite several decades of consciousness raising in the United States, advertising on television and in the print media perpetuates sexual stereotypes. Although "house beautiful" ads are less prominent as women are increasingly shown in workplace contexts, "body beautiful" messages continue to be transmitted. In children's cartoons women are still the helpless victims the fearless male hero must rescue. Toys are targeted either for little boys or little girls and are packaged appropriately in colors and materials culturally defined as either masculine or feminine.

To what extent are these stereotypes of men and women and the symbols with which they are associated universal? If they are universal, to what extent are they rooted in observed differences about the biological nature of men and women that are made culturally significant? These questions have interested scholars as they have attempted to account for both similarity and difference among the people of the world.

Making the assumption that the subordination of women exists in all societies—a "true universal"—Ortner (1974: 67) sought to explain the pervasiveness of this idea not in the assignation of women to a domestic sphere of activity, but in the symbolic constructions by which women's roles are evaluated. Ortner argues that women, because of their reproductive roles, are universally viewed as being closer to nature while men are linked with culture. She defines culture as "the notion of human consciousness, or . . . the products of human consciousness (i.e., systems of thought and technology), by means of which humanity attempts to assert control over nature" (72). That which is cultural and subject to human manipulation is assigned more worth than that which is natural; hence, women and women's roles are denigrated or devalued, whether explicitly or implicitly.

The nature-culture dichotomy is a useful explanatory model in the United States where, according to Martin (1987: 17), "Women are intrinsically closely involved with the family where so many 'natural,' 'bodily' (and therefore lower) functions occur, whereas men are intrinsically closely involved with the world of work where (at least for some) 'cultural,' 'mental,' and therefore higher functions occur. It is no accident that 'natural' facts about women, in the form of claims about biology, are often used to justify social stratification based on gender."

While this model may be applicable in some cultures, its universality has been challenged not only by those who point out that nature-culture is a dichotomy of western thought in particular (Bloch and Bloch 1980; Jordanova 1980; Moore 1988), but also by those who provide ethnographic data to indicate its lack of salience in other cultures around the world (Strathern 1980). Similarly, the assumption that women are universally subordinated while men are dominant (Ortner 1974: 70) appears questionable through the lens of recent ethnographic reanalyses. The critique of the concepts of universal subordination and of the nature-culture dichotomy has stimulated significant research on how gender identity and gender roles are constructed in particular cultural contexts (Errington and Gewertz 1987; Ortner and Whitehead 1981; Weiner 1976). Whether and under what conditions social asymmetry between men and women emerges in the process of this construction is open to empirical investigation.

The cultural construction of gender in a particular society involves definitions of what it means to be masculine or feminine, and these definitions vary cross-culturally. While masculinity is thought to have a powerful biological component in the United States, among the Sambia of New Guinea it is constructed in the context of ritual. The Sambia, like many other societies in New Guinea (Brown and Buchbinder 1976; Herdt 1982; Meigs 1984), are characterized by a high degree of segregation and sexual antagonism between men and women, both of which are reinforced by powerful taboos. These taboos, and other facets of Sambian male identity including that of the warrior, are inculcated during a series of initiation rituals whereby boys are "grown" into men. As Herdt (in this book) observes, the Sambia "perceive no imminent, naturally driven fit between one's birthright sex and one's gender identity or role" (1982: 54). Indeed, Sambian boys and men engage in what some societies would label homosexual activity, yet they do it to create masculinity. It is precisely for this reason that an analytical distinction is often made between "sex" as a biological classification and "gender" as a set of learned social roles.

Through the rituals of manhood Sambian boys are progressively detached from the world of women, a world they occupied for the first six or seven years of their lives and which they must now learn to both fear and devalue. This process of detachment has been identified by Chodorow (1974) as a major phase of human male development. If it is unmarked and therefore ambiguous in most western cultures, it is marked in many nonwestern cultures and often associated with male circumcision. Among the Mende of Sierra Leone (Little 1951), for example, boy initiates are seized from their homes by the force of spirits—men wearing masks and long raffia skirts. In this act they are dramatically and suddenly separated from their childhood, carried into the bush where they will spend several weeks in seclusion and transition before they reemerge as men.

Initiation rituals that prepare girls for their roles as women and instruct them in what it means to be a woman in a particular cultural context can also be found in various societies around the world (Brown 1963; Richards 1956). However, the transition to womanhood is often part of a more subtle and continuous process of enculturation and socialization. In a description of Hausa socialization Callaway (in this book) demonstrates how girls in this society learn how to behave in culturally appropriate ways. The Hausa are an Islamic people who live in northern Nigeria. Historically, ruling class Hausa women had significant authority and social standing, but with the expansion of Islam this position was eroded and a sexually segregated society characterized by female subordination emerged. Hausa girls marry young, generally upon reaching puberty. At that time they enter *kulle* or seclusion. In seclusion, the social roles of women are specifically defined and their sexual activities are limited. Though a Hausa woman becomes part of her husband's family, her place is secured only by bearing sons, and all her children belong to her husband. Hausa women are taught the expected life course from early childhood.

In Hausa society, Callaway (1987: 22) claims, "the reproduction of 'masculine' and 'feminine' personalities generation after generation has produced psychological and value commitments to sex differences that are tenaciously maintained and so deeply ingrained as to become central to a consistent sense of self." This self is defined by reproductive roles and by deference to men; thus a good daughter-in-law gives her first-born child to her husband's mother, an act that strengthens family ties.

Conceptions of the self or personhood are, as Henrietta Moore (1988: 39) has observed, "cross-culturally as variable as the concepts of 'woman' and 'man.'" Personhood is constituted by a variety of attributes. In addition to gender, it may comprise age, status in the family and in the community, and physical appearance or impairment. In many cultures naming is also an important mechanism for constructing personhood. In the United States, for instance, the use of Ms. to replace Mrs. and Miss is an acceptable option. It is increasingly common for married women to retain the name that they were born with rather than replace it with one that only gives them an identity in relation to someone else—their husband.

Among the Chambri of New Guinea initial identity or personhood is gained through a totemic name given by a child's patrilineal and matrilateral relatives. According to Errington and Gewertz (1987: 32, 47), "these names both reflect and affect the transactions which constitute a person's fundamental social relationships and identity. . . . Totemic names allow both men and women to pursue respectively their culturally-defined preoccupations of political competition and the bearing of children. The totemic names available to men, however, convey different sorts of power and resources than do those available to women. . . . Men seek to augment their own power through gaining control of the names of others. . . . The power conveyed by [women's] names cannot shape social relationships as does the power of names men hold, but, instead, ensures reproduction."

Women's names among the Chambri work in different ways from those of men, but they nonetheless enable women to claim personhood in Chambri society. The married Chinese women described by Watson (in this book) have an entirely different experience. They are denied individuating names, and through this denial their personhood is in question. They remain, says Watson, "suspended between the anonymous world of anybodies and the more sharply defined world of somebodies." In contrast with the namelessness of Chinese women, men in Chinese culture acquire numerous names as they pass through the life cycle. Nowhere is the difference more apparent than at marriage—a time when a man acquires a name that symbolizes his new status and public roles and a woman loses her girlhood name and becomes the "inner person." Like the Hausa women who assume an identity with respect to their husbands, Chinese women begin newly married life by learning the names and kinship terms for all their husbands' ancestors and relatives. Namelessness follows them to the grave—anybodies in life, they become nobodies at death.

In many societies personhood for women is also associated with conceptions of the body and often centers on reproductive functions. One reproductive process that has particular salience is menstruation. Understandings of the symbolic meanings of menstruation influence men's and women's ideologies of gender. Buckley and Gottlieb (in this book) review symbolic analyses of menstrual taboos built on the concept of "pollution." These analyses contend that menstrual blood and menstruating women are widely viewed as dangerous; accordingly, taboos have been devised to contain women's symbolic contamination. Douglas (1966) proposes that "pollutants" represent matter out of place. Menstrual blood, for example, is out of place in that it breaches the boundaries of the body, does not issue accidentally from a wound, and is one of the rare acts in which women normatively let blood. As an anomaly, menstruation carries a certain symbolic power. Douglas also posits a close relationship between ideas about the physical and social body. Thus, menstrual blood might be seen as polluting when it reflects an underlying structural ambiguity or contradiction regarding women and women's power. Buckley and Gottlieb access the limits of these influential pollution theories, and critique the notion that women are passive recipients of male-created cultures. The treatment of pollution concepts may reflect male domination of the ethnographic record as researchers and as informants. They argue that there is a need to consult female informants before reaching conclusions about the status of menstruation as polluting in any given society.

Buckley (1982) addresses male bias and the female perspective on menstruation in his discussion of menstrual beliefs and practices among the Yurok Indians of North America. In his reanalysis of Yurok data Buckley found that while precontact Yurok men considered women, through their menstrual blood, to be dangerous, Yurok women viewed menstruation as a positive source of power. Rather than looking on the forced monthly seclusion as isolating and oppressive, women viewed it as a source of strength and sanctuary.

By contrast, among numerous groups in New Guinea, men perceive menstrual blood as dangerously polluting and engage in a range of symbolic behaviors to cleanse themselves of what they believe are the harmful effects of contact with women—for example, tongue scraping and smokehouse purification. The Mae Enga, for example, believe that "contact with [menstrual blood] or a menstruating woman will, in the absence of appropriate counter-magic, sicken a man and cause persistent vomiting, turn his blood black, corrupt his vital juices so that his skin darkens and wrinkles as his flesh wastes, permanently dull his wits, and eventually lead to a slow decline and death" (Meggitt 1964: 207).

Male beliefs about the dangers of menstrual blood can be found in a number of other cultures around the world (Buckley and Gottlieb 1988). In some contexts men appear to devalue female reproductive roles by defining menstruation as the unfortunate lot of women. For example, a creation story of a group of pastoral nomads in northern Iran goes as follows: "In the beginning men had menstruation and not women. But blood would go down their pants and it was very uncomfortable. So they went to God and complained about their situation, asking Him to give menstruation to women who had skirts. At the time of childbirth, it used to be men who had pains. Again they complained to God, and He gave the pain to women, as He had done with menstruation" (Shahshahani 1986: 87).

This creation story, like many beliefs about menstrual pollution, represents a male view that not only associates women with nature and men with culture, but also helps to explain and support sexual asymmetry in that culture. However, Rosaldo (1974: 38) and others (Gottlieb 1982; Keesing 1985; Lawrence 1988; Powers 1986) have suggested that pollution beliefs can provide a source of power and form the basis for solidarity among women. This body of work suggests that the male point of view is not wrong or unimportant, but that it is only a partial representation. Gender roles and gender identities are constructed by both men and women in any society.

REFERENCES

Ardener, Edwin. 1975. "Belief and the Problem of Women." In Shirley Ardener (ed.). *Perceiving Women,* pp. 1–18. New York: John Wiley and Sons.

Bloch, Maurice and Jean Bloch. 1980. "Women and the Dialectics of Nature in Eighteenth-Century French Thought." In Carol MacCormack and Marilyn Strathern (eds.). *Nature, Culture and Gender,* pp. 25–41. Cambridge: Cambridge University Press.

Brown, Judith K. 1963. "A Cross-Cultural Study of Female Initiation Rites Among Pre-Literate Peoples." *American Anthropologist* 65(4): 837–853.

Brown, Paula and Georgeda Buchbinder. 1976. *Man and Woman in the New Guinea Highlands.* Washington, DC: American Anthropological Association, Special Publication, number 8.

Buckley, Thomas. 1982. "Menstruation and the Power of Yurok Women: Methods in Cultural Reconstruction." *American Ethnologist* 9: 47–60.

Buckley, Thomas and Alma Gottlieb (eds.). 1988. *Blood Magic: The Anthropology of Menstruation.* Berkeley: University of California Press.

Callaway, Barbara J. 1987. *Muslim Hausa Women in Nigeria: Tradition and Change.* Syracuse: Syracuse University Press.

Chodorow, Nancy. 1974. "Family Structure and Feminine Personality." In Michele Z. Rosaldo and Louise Lamphere (eds.). *Woman, Culture, and Society,* pp. 43–67. Stanford: Stanford University Press.

Douglas, Mary. 1966. *Purity and Danger: An Analysis of Concepts of Pollution and Taboo.* London: Routledge and Kegan Paul.

Errington, Frederick and Deborah Gewertz. 1987. *Cultural Alternatives and a Feminist Anthropology: An Analysis of Culturally Constructed Gender Interests in Papua New Guinea.* Cambridge: Cambridge University Press.

Gottlieb, Alma. 1982. "Sex, Fertility and Menstruation Among the Beng of the Ivory Coast: A Symbolic Analysis." *Africa* 52(4): 34–47.

Herdt, Gilbert. 1982. *Rituals of Manhood: Male Initiation in Papua New Guinea.* Berkeley and Los Angeles: University of California Press.

Hogbin, Ian. 1970. *The Island of Menstruating Men.* Scranton, PA: Chandler.

Jordanova, L. J. 1980. "Natural Facts: A Historical Perspective on Science and Sexuality." In Carol MacCormack and Marilyn Strathern (eds.). *Nature, Culture and Gender,* pp. 42–69. Cambridge: Cambridge University Press.

Keesing, Roger. 1985. "Kwaio Women Speak: The Micropolitics of Autobiography in a Solomon Island Society." *American Anthropologist* 87: 27–39.

Lawrence, Denise. 1988. "Menstrual Politics: Women and Pigs in Rural Portugal." In Thomas Buckley and Alma Gottlieb (eds.). *The Anthropology of Menstruation,* pp. 117–136. Berkeley: University of California Press.

Little, Kenneth L. 1951. *The Mende of Sierra Leone: A West African People in Transition.* London: Routledge and Kegan Paul.

Martin, Emily. 1987. *The Woman in the Body: A Cultural Analysis of Reproduction.* Boston: Beacon Press.

Meggitt, M. J. 1964. "Male-Female Relationships in the Highlands of Australian New Guinea." *American Anthropologist* 66(4, part 2): 204–224.

Meigs, Anna S. 1984. *Food, Sex, and Pollution: A New Guinea Religion.* New Brunswick, NJ: Rutgers University Press.

Moore, Henrietta. 1988. *Feminism and Anthropology.* Minneapolis: University of Minnesota Press.

Ortner, Sherry. 1974. "Is Female to Male as Nature to Culture?" In Michelle Z. Rosaldo and Louise Lamphere (eds.). *Woman, Culture, and Society,* pp. 66–87. Stanford: Stanford University Press.

Ortner, Sherry and Harriet Whitehead. 1981. *Sexual Meanings: The Cultural Construction of Gender and Sexuality.* Cambridge: Cambridge University Press.

Powers, Marla. 1986. *Oglala Women.* Chicago: University of Chicago Press.

Richards, Audrey I. 1956. *Chisungu: A Girls' Initiation Ceremony Among the Bemba of Northern Rhodesia.* London: Faber and Faber.

Rosaldo, Michelle. 1974. "Woman, Culture, and Society: A Theoretical Overview." In Michelle Z. Rosaldo and Louise Lamphere (eds.). *Woman, Culture, and Society,* pp. 17–42. Stanford: Stanford University Press.

Shahshahani, Soheila. 1986. "Women Whisper, Men Kill: A Case Study of the Mamasani Pastoral Nomads of Iran." In Leela Dube, Eleanor Leacock, and Shirley Ardener (eds.). *Visibility and Power: Essays on Women in Society and Development,* pp. 85–97. Delhi: Oxford University Press.

Strathern, Marilyn. 1980. "No Nature, No Culture: The Hagen Case." In Carol MacCormack and Marilyn Strathern (eds.). *Nature, Culture and Gender,* pp. 174–222. Cambridge: Cambridge University Press.

Weiner, Annette. 1976. *Women of Value, Men of Renown.* Austin: University of Texas Press.

RITUALS OF MANHOOD: MALE INITIATION IN PAPUA NEW GUINEA

Gilbert H. Herdt

Sambia are a mountain-dwelling hunting and horticultural people who number some 2,000 persons and inhabit one of New Guinea's most rugged terrains. The population is dispersed through narrow river valleys over a widespread, thinly populated rain forest; rainfall is heavy; and even today the surrounding mountain ranges keep the area isolated. Sambia live on the fringes of the Highlands, but they trace their origins to the Papua hinterlands; their culture and economy thus reflect a mixture of influences from both of those areas. Hunting still predominates as a masculine activity through which most meat protein is acquired. As in the Highlands, though, sweet potatoes and taro are the staple crops, and their cultivation is for the most part women's work. Pigs are few, and they have no ceremonial or exchange significance; indigenous marsupials, such as possum and tree kangaroo, provide necessary meat prestations for all initiations and ceremonial feasts (cf. Meigs 1976).

Sambia settlements are small, well-defended, mountain clan hamlets. These communities comprise locally based descent groups organized through a strong agnatic idiom. Residence is patrivirilocal, and most men actually reside in their father's hamlets. Clans are exogamous, and one or more of them together constitute a hamlet's landowning corporate agnatic body. These men also form a localized warriorhood that is sometimes allied with other hamlets in matters of fighting, marriage, and ritual. Each hamlet contains one or two men's clubhouses, in addition to women's houses, and the men's ritual life centers on their clubhouse. Marriage is usually by sister exchange or infant betrothal, although the latter form of prearranged marriage is culturally preferred. Intrahamlet marriage is occasionally more frequent (up to 50 percent of all marriages in my own hamlet field site) than one would expect in such small segmentary groupings, an involutional pattern weakened since pacification.

Sambia male and female residential patterns differ somewhat from those of other Highlands peoples. The nuclear family is an important subunit of the hamlet-based extended family of interrelated clans. A man, his wife, and their children usually cohabit within a single, small, round hut. Children are thus reared together by their parents during the early years of life, so the nuclear family is a residential unit, an institution virtually unknown to the Highlands (Meggitt 1964; Read 1954). Sometimes this unit is expanded through polygyny, in which case a man, his cowives, and their children may occupy the single dwelling. Girls continue to reside with their parents until marriage (usually near the menarche, around fifteen to seventeen years of age). Boys, however, are removed to the men's clubhouse at seven to ten years of age, following their first-stage initiation. There they reside exclusively until marriage and cohabitation years later. Despite familial cohabitation in early childhood, strict taboos based on beliefs about menstrual pollution still separate men and women in their sleeping and eating arrangements.

Warfare used to be constant and nagging among Sambia, and it conditioned the values and masculine stereotypes surrounding the male initiatory cult. Ritualized bow fights occurred among neighboring hamlets, whose members still intermarried and usually initiated their sons together. At the same time, though, hamlets also united against enemy tribes and in staging war parties against them. Hence, warfare, marriage, and initiation were interlocking institutions; the effect of this political instability was to reinforce tough, strident masculine performance in most arenas of social life. "Strength" (*jerundu*) was—and is—a pivotal idea in this male ethos. Indeed, strength, which has both ethnobiological and behavioral aspects, could be aptly translated as "maleness" and "manliness." Strength has come to be virtually synonymous with idealized conformity to male ritual routine. Before conquest and pacification by the Australians, though, strength had its chief performative significance in one's conduct on the battlefield. Even today bitter reminders of war linger on among the Sambia; and we should not forget that it is against the harsh background of the warrior's existence that Sambia initiate their boys, whose only perceived protection against the inconstant world is their own unbending masculinity.

Initiation rests solely in the hands of the men's secret society. It is this organization that brings the collective initiatory cycle into being as jointly performed by neighboring hamlets (and as constrained by their own chronic bow fighting). The necessary feast-crop gardens, ritual leadership and knowledge, dictate that a handful of elders, war leaders, and ritual experts be in full command of the actual staging of the event. Everyone and all else are secondary.

There are six intermittent initiations from the ages of seven to ten and onward. They are, however, constituted and conceptualized as two distinct cultural systems within the male life cycle. First-stage (*moku,* at seven to ten years of age), second-stage (*imbutu,* at ten to thirteen years), and third-stage (*ipmangwi,* at thirteen to sixteen years) initiations—bachelorhood rites—are collectively performed for regional groups of boys as age-mates. The initiations are held in sequence, as age-graded advancements; the entire sequel takes months to perform. The focus of all these initiations is the construction and habitation of a great cult house (*moo-angu*) on a traditional dance ground; its ceremonialized building inaugurates the whole cycle. Fourth-stage (*nuposha:* sixteen years and onward), fifth-stage (*taiketnyi*), and sixth-stage (*moondangu*) initiations are, conversely, individually centered events not associated with the confederacy of interrelated hamlets, cult house, or dance ground. Each of these initiations, like the preceding ones, does have its own ritual status, social role, and title, as noted. The triggering event for the latter three initiations, unlike that for the bachelorhood rites, is not the building of a cult house or a political agreement of hamlets to act collectively but is rather the maturing femininity and life-crisis events of the women assigned in marriage to youths (who become the initiated novices). Therefore, fourth-stage initiation is only a semipublic activity organized by the youths' clansmen (and some male affines). Its secret purificatory and other rites are followed by the formal marriage ceremony in the hamlet. Fifth-stage initiation comes at a woman's menarche, when her husband is secretly introduced to additional purification and sexual techniques. Sixth-stage initiation issues from the birth of a man's wife's first child. This event is, de jure, the attainment of manhood. (The first birth is elaborately ritualized and celebrated; the next three births are also celebrated, but in more truncated fashion.) Two children bring full adulthood (*aatmwunu*) for husband and wife alike. Birth ceremonies are suspended after the fourth birth, since there is no reason to belabor what is by now obvious: a man has proved himself competent in reproduction. This sequence of male initiations forms the basis for male development, and it underlies the antagonistic tenor of relationships between the sexes.

It needs stating only once that men's secular rhetoric and ritual practices depict women as dangerous and polluting inferiors whom men are to distrust throughout their lives. In this regard, Sambia values and relationships pit men against women even more markedly, I think, than occurs in other Highlands communities (cf. Brown and Buchbinder 1976; Meggitt 1964; Read 1954). Men hold themselves as the superiors of women in physique, personality, and social position. And this dogma of male supremacy permeates all social relationships and institutions, likewise coloring domestic behavior among the sexes (cf. Tuzin 1980 for an important contrast). Men fear not only pollution from contact with women's vaginal fluids and menstrual blood but also the depletion of their semen, the vital spark of maleness, which women (and boys, too) inevitably extract, sapping a man's substance. These are among the main themes of male belief underlying initiation.

The ritualized simulation of maleness is the result of initiation, and men believe the process to be vital for the nature and nurture of manly growth and well-being. First-stage initiation begins the process in small boys. Over the ensuing ten to fifteen years, until marriage, cumulative initiations and residence in the men's house are said to promote biological changes that firmly cement the growth from childhood to manhood. Nature provides male genitals, it is true; but nature alone does not bestow the vital spark biologically necessary for stimulating masculine growth or demonstrating cold-blooded self-preservation.

New Guinea specialists will recognize in the Sambia belief system a theme that links it to the comparative ethnography of male initiation and masculine development: the use of ritual procedures for sparking, fostering, and maintaining manliness in males (see Berndt 1962; Meigs 1976; Newman 1964, 1965; Poole 1981; Read 1965; Salisbury 1965; Strathern 1969, 1970). Sambia themselves refer to the results of first-stage collective initiation—our main interest—as a means of "growing a boy"; and this trend of ritual belief is particularly emphatic.

Unlike ourselves, Sambia perceive no imminent, naturally driven fit between one's birthright sex and one's gender identity or role.[1] Indeed, the problem (and it is approached as a situation wanting a solution) is implicitly and explicitly understood in quite different terms. The solution is also different for the two sexes: men believe that a girl is born with all of the vital organs and fluids necessary for her to attain reproductive competence through "natural" maturation. This conviction is embodied in cultural perceptions of the girl's development beginning with the sex assignment at birth. What distinguishes a girl (*tai*) from a boy (*kwulai'u*) is obvious: "A boy has a penis, and a girl does not," men say. Underlying men's communications is a conviction that maleness, unlike femaleness, is not a biological given. It must be artificially induced through secret ritual; and that is a personal achievement.

The visible manifestations of girls' fast-growing reproductive competence, noticed first in early motor coordination and speech and then later in the rapid attainment of height and secondary sex traits (e.g., breast development), are attributed to inner biological properties. Girls possess a menstrual-blood organ, or *tingu,* said to precipitate all those events and the menarche. Boys, on the other hand, are thought to possess an inactive tingu. They do possess, however, another organ—the *kere-ku-kereku,* or semen organ—

that is thought to be the repository of semen, the very essence of maleness and masculinity; but this organ is not functional at birth, since it contains no semen naturally and can only store, never produce, any. Only oral insemination, men believe, can activate the boy's semen organ, thereby precipitating his push into adult reproductive competence. In short, femininity unfolds naturally, whereas masculinity must be achieved; and here is where the male ritual cult steps in.

Men also perceive the early socialization risks of boys and girls in quite different terms. All infants are closely bonded to their mothers. Out of a woman's contaminating, life-giving womb pours the baby, who thereafter remains tied to the woman's body, breast milk, and many ministrations. This latter contact only reinforces the femininity and female contamination in which birth involves the infant. Then, too, the father, both because of postpartum taboos and by personal choice, tends to avoid being present at the breast-feedings. Mother thus becomes the unalterable primary influence; father is a weak second. Sambia say this does not place girls at a "risk"—they simply succumb to the drives of their "natural" biology. This maternal attachment and paternal distance clearly jeopardize the boys' growth, however, since nothing innate within male maturation seems to resist the inhibiting effects of mothers' femininity. Hence boys must be traumatically separated—wiped clean of their female contaminants—so that their masculinity may develop.

Homosexual fellatio inseminations can follow this separation but cannot precede it, for otherwise they would go for naught. The accumulating semen, injected time and again for years, is believed crucial for the formation of biological maleness and masculine comportment. This native perspective is sufficiently novel to justify our using a special concept for aiding description and analysis of the data: masculinization (Herdt 1981:205 ff). Hence I shall refer to the overall process that involves separating a boy from his mother, initiating him, ritually treating his body, administering homosexual inseminations, his biological attainment of puberty, and his eventual reproductive competence as *masculinization.* (Precisely what role personal and cultural fantasy plays in the negotiation of this ritual process I have considered elsewhere: see Herdt 1981: chaps. 6, 7, and 8.)

A boy has female contaminants inside of him which not only retard physical development but, if not removed, debilitate him and eventually bring death. His body is male: his tingu contains no blood and will not activate. The achievement of puberty for boys requires semen. Breast milk "nurtures the boy," and sweet potatoes or other "female" foods provide "stomach nourishment," but these substances become only feces, not semen. Women's own bodies internally produce the menarche, the hallmark of reproductive maturity. There is no comparable mechanism active in a boy, nothing that can stimulate his secondary sex traits. Only semen can do that; only men have semen; boys have none. What is left to do, then, except initiate and masculinize boys into adulthood?

NOTE

1. I follow Stroller (1968) in adhering to the following distinctions: the term *sex traits* refers to purely biological phenomena (anatomy, hormones, genetic structure, etc.), whereas *gender* refers to those psychological and cultural attributes that compel a person (consciously or unconsciously) to sense him- or herself, and other persons, as belonging to either the male or female sex. It follows that the term *gender role* (Sears 1965), rather than the imprecise term *sex role,* refers to the normative set of expectations associated with masculine and feminine social positions.

REFERENCES

Berndt, R. M. 1962. *Excess and Restraint: Social Control among a New Guinea Mountain People.* Chicago: University of Chicago Press.

Brown, P., and G. Buchbinder (eds.). 1976. *Man and Woman in the New Guinea Highlands.* Washington, D.C.: American Anthropological Association.

Herdt, G. H. 1981. *Guardians of the Flutes: Idioms of Masculinity.* New York: McGraw-Hill.

Meggitt, M. J. 1964. Male-female relationships in the Highlands of Australian New Guinea. In *New Guinea: The Central Highlands,* ed. J. B. Watson, *American Anthropologist,* 66, pt. 2 (4):204–224.

Meigs, A. S. 1976. Male pregnancy and the reduction of sexual opposition in a New Guinea Highlands society. *Ethnology* 15 (4):393–407.

Newman, P. L. 1964. Religious belief and ritual in a New Guinea society. In *New Guinea: The Central Highlands,* ed. J. B. Watson, *American Anthropologist* 66, pt. 2 (4):257–272.

———. 1965. *Knowing the Gururumba.* New York: Holt, Rinehart and Winston.

Poole, F. J. P. 1981. Transforming "natural" woman: female ritual leaders and gender ideology among Bimin-Kuskumin. In *Sexual Meanings,* ed. S. B. Ortner and H. Whitehead. New York: Cambridge University Press.

Read, K. E. 1954. Cultures of the Central Highlands, New Guinea. *Southwestern Journal of Anthropology* 10 (1):1–43.

———. 1965. *The High Valley.* London: George Allen and Unwin.

Salisbury, R. F. 1965. The Siane of the Eastern Highlands. In *Gods, Ghosts, and Men in Melanesia,* P. Lawrence and M. J. Meggitt, pp. 50–77. Melbourne: Melbourne University Press.

Sears, R. R. 1965. Development of gender role. In *Sex and Behavior,* ed. F. A. Beach, pp. 133–163. New York: John Wiley and Sons.

Stoller, R. J. 1968. *Sex and Gender.* New York: Science House.

Strathern, A. J. 1969. Descent and alliance in the New Guinea Highlands: some problems of comparison. Royal Anthropological Institute, *Proceedings,* pp. 37–52.

———. 1970. Male initiation in the New Guinea Highlands societies. *Ethnology* 9(4):373–379.

Tuzin, D. F. 1980. *The Voice of the Tambaran: Truth and Illusion in Ilahita Arapesh Religion.* Berkeley, Los Angeles, and London: University of California Press.

HAUSA SOCIALIZATION

Barbara J. Callaway

The Hausa ethos of male domination and the Islamic emphasis on male supremacy combine to structure distinct conceptions of life for men and women. Perceptions of a woman's life cycle stress her current status in relation to men and her reproductive status as well as her approximate age—*jinjiniya* (female infant), *yarinya* (girl), *budurwa* (maiden or virgin), *mata* (woman or wife), *bazarawa* (divorced or widowed), or *tsohuwa* (old woman). The corresponding terms for males stress biological age—*jinjiri,* (infant), *yaro* (young boy), *miji* (young man), and *tsoho* (old man) (Schildkrout 1981, 96).

Married Muslim women in Hausaland live in seclusion (*kulle*). In Kano State—in contrast to other Islamic areas in West Africa—the practice appears to be increasing as the city and the countryside become more involved in the national cash economy (Abell 1962; Hill 1977; M. G. Smith 1955).

Hausa culture emphasizes siring large numbers of children, and in Kano the average number of living children per woman is seven.[1] Countries with Islamic majorities generally have the highest population growth rates in the world today. Nigeria has one of the highest (3.5 percent annually). While pronatal tendencies are strong in all Nigerian societies, they are most evident in the Islamic north, where family planning is not considered a legitimate focus of public policy. In Kano, a metropolitan area of over five million people, no family planning office or publicly available information on either planning or birth control was available as late as 1983.[2]

The number of children born to a given woman is not necessarily indicative of the number for whom she is responsible. Widespread fostering and the practice of a

Reprinted with permission from Barbara J. Callaway, *Muslim Hausa Women in Nigeria* (Syracuse, NY: Syracuse University Press, 1987), pp. 28–35 (text only).

woman's avoiding contact with her firstborn child (*kunya*) creates a great deal of fluidity in children's lives. Eighty percent of 500 Hausa children surveyed in Kano State for one study were not raised by their biological parents (Hake 1972, 23–24). Of these, 41.5 percent were raised by paternal grandmothers, 16.7 percent by stepmothers, 19.8 percent by other relatives, and 5.5 percent by "friends of the family." The giving of children for fostering indicates the strength of the bonds linking spatially dispersed kin. The firstborn child generally is given to an older woman who has no child currently living with her. A good daughter-in-law demonstrates that she is "polite" by giving her first child to her husband's mother, and in so doing strengthens ties between the two families (Interview #16, Kano, October, 1982).

Childhood is generally a mixture of good-natured freedom and harsh corporal punishment and deprivation. When 175 students at the Advanced Teachers College (male) and Women's Teachers College in Kano were asked if their childhoods had been happy or sad or both, 57.4 percent of the 102 men and 56.8 percent of the 73 women replied "both." One-third of these translated "sad" as referring to harsh punishment by parents or other adults. One-fifth complained of lack of sufficient food or clothing as children. "My brother was kind—but his wife was not good; she often gave me too little to eat." "I was not fed properly in my uncle's house where I went to live." "I lived with a stepmother, who had many children, and so I was neglected most of the time." Sixty percent of these students claimed never to have had a conversation with an adult while growing up. Eighty percent of the girls claimed to have been "often afraid" (questionnaire administered by Aisha Indo Yuguda, 1983).

While the birth of a new baby is cause for celebration in nearly all families, no matter what the economic status, the birth of a son is usually celebrated on a more lavish scale than that of a daughter. Among wealthier families, when a boy is born it is customary to slaughter *sa* or *sanuja* (a cow or an ox) for the *radin suna* (naming ceremony). When a girl is born, it is customary to slaughter a lesser animal, such as *tunkiya* (sheep) or *akuya* (goat) (Kabir 1981). In the home little girls are assigned domestic duties from about age five. By age six they are dressed in imitation of adult women and begin to be viewed as future wives. They go outside only for specific reasons, such as running errands for their mothers who cannot go out, selling food and handicrafts from bowls or baskets on top of their heads, and carrying messages; they do not go out to play. Little boys, at about age six, are sent out to play and sleep with other boys in the *zaures* or *soro* (entranceways) to their homes. They are ousted from their mother's rooms at night and virtually become visitors in her space during the day. By age ten, boys cross the line into female space less often. They eat with other boys, seldom with sisters or mothers. Boys whose fathers are artisans or traders may be apprenticed to their fathers or other adult men by age eleven or twelve. Even those going to school beyond the primary years spend little time "at home" and avoid contact with women as they approach adulthood. Adulthood means separation, even avoidance, between male and female. "The transition to manhood means moving out of the domain of female authority, into the world of men, and ultimately into marriage, where male dominance is as yet unchallenged" (Schildkrout 1978, 131).

As she grows up, a girl is made aware of her second-class status. In addition to housework, she is assigned child-care responsibilities, and she is made aware that her sex is a potential source of shame and dishonor. A girl's inferior status vis-à-vis her brothers, father, or male kin is early and constantly emphasized. She is told *ki dinga yin abu kamar mace,* "to behave like a woman." A girl should sit quietly, talk softly, cover her head, and never disagree with a male. *Ba ki ganin ke mace ce, she namiji ne,* meaning "Can't you see you are a woman while he is a man?" (and thus superior) is a refrain repeated to her from her earliest years. She will also hear *ke mace ce, gidan wani zaki,* ("after all, you are a woman and you are going to someone else's house"), or *"komai abinki, gidan wani zaki"* ("No matter what you do you are going to someone else's house") (Kabir 1981).

When a girl shows signs of independence of character, she will be snubbed by her peers and told that *tunda ke mace ce, a karkashin wani kike,* "You are a woman and you are under someone's (male) authority." The girl seeking to join boys at play may be greeted with a popular children's song:

Mai wasa da maza karya
Tunda na gan ta na rena ta.

("She who plays with boys is a bitch
When I see her, I detest her.")

Finally, girls are repeatedly admonished that *Duk mace a bayan namiji take*—"Every woman is inferior to a man" (Interviews #6, Kano, January 20, 1982; and #21, Kano, February 24, 1983).

For the overwhelming majority of girls, it is almost inconceivable to aspire to anything other than the role of wife or mother. Normally, girls are expected to be married by the time they reach puberty. The widespread introduction of Western education (*boko*) is beginning to postpone the age of marriage for girls who go to school, but even in this event, there is great pressure to marry young, before age sixteen. Girls who are not married while in secondary school (all such noncommercial schools in Kano are single sex) are viewed with suspicion and it is said that *an gama da ita,* meaning, "They have finished with her," implying that she is no longer a virgin and therefore not a good candidate for a first wife (Interviews #11 and 12, Kano, March 8 and March 12, 1982).

Although they may have heavy household responsibilities, girls are sent out to hawk wares for their mothers and are relatively free until they are abruptly married and secluded. After that, even though they are still very young, like adult women they can leave their houses only for naming ceremonies, marriages, funerals, and medical care. If they go out, it is usually at night and an older woman generally accompanies them as escorts. They must cover their heads and be accountable for their visits (Schildkrout 1979).

Since most girls are married by age twelve to fourteen, they are virtually confined to the female quarters of their compounds all their lives. If a girl is married as young as ten, she will not be expected to cook or have sexual relations with her husband until puberty begins, but she enters *kulle* and loses the freedom associated with childhood. For all practical purposes, the house or compound is a woman's world. From the time she marries and enters *kulle* until after her childbearing years, a woman has virtually no freedom of movement or association. This socialization process is pervasive and thorough. Opportunities for broadening one's experiences or raising one's expectations are few.

Unlike girls, boys do not reach adult status until they become economically productive, usually in their late twenties or early thirties, because it is one of the requirements of Islam that men do not marry until they can provide shelter, clothing, and food for their wife or wives. While in 1982, ninety percent of the 92 Muslim women students at Bayero University were married, only fifteen percent of the 2000 men students were married (Bayero University 1982).

Even in matters of religion, a woman's inferiority is underscored. While all Muslims are equal before Allah, menstruating or pregnant women are considered "religiously impure." In addition, women cannot lead the community in prayer, do not officiate at religious festivals, and rarely attend mosque. Even at the mosque on the campus at Bayero University in Kano, women may attend only by standing in a separate room out of sight of the male worshippers and may not be in public areas of the mosque during Friday prayers. Hence, the thrust of socialization through religion is to emphasize a properly subordinate place for women.

Unlike other urban settings, Kano provides no specifically female organizations for Hausa women. The one exclusively women's club in Kano, the Corona Society, a British-based international service organization for women, had no Hausa Muslim Kano women as members. The National Association of Women's Societies of Nigeria (the federally recognized umbrella organization for women's associations) had no Kano chapter, although it asked the Corona Society to help organize one; no interest in affiliation with such an organization was expressed in Kano. Although interested in the idea of women's organizations, elite Kano women preferred to avoid the visibility entailed in membership. They seemed to perceive some advantage in their current status and not many advantages in radically changing it.

At Bayero University no northern Nigerian woman holds a position of regular faculty rank (there was one female teaching assistant in sociology), nor do women generally participate in University-sponsored conferences or symposia. As of 1983, the University had never sponsored a program dealing with women's issues or concerns; no course in the curriculum deals specifically with women's history or issues.

If women are absent from the public realm, within their own restricted but private world they enjoy considerable autonomy. Houses are a woman's domain. Women can enter virtually any house, but men can enter few and then they rarely go beyond the entranceway, or, in the case of wealthier homes, the man's sitting room. Women are secluded, but men are excluded from women's space. Even kinship does not open the door, for a man would not normally enter the house of a younger married sister or the female section of his younger brother's house. He might, with the husband's permission, enter the house of an older married sister (Schildkrout, 1978a, p. 115). "It shall be no crime in them as to their fathers, or their sons, or their brothers, or their brother's sons, or their sister's sons, or their women, or the slaves which their right hands possess, if they speak with them unveiled" (*Qur'an* 3:33 and 33:55). Thus, young men and women are not thrown together in situations where they could form relationships that could lead to marriage; the system of arranged marriages, in which girls are married early and boys much later, means that relationships between unrelated young people of equal status but opposite sex are almost nonexistent. The fact that men and women live in separate and distinct worlds has profound psychological implications for women. While men's authority over women in the public domain is nearly complete, in the private domain, where interaction is highly limited and age differences between men and women are great, the differences in their interests are also great and thus the authority of men is quite precarious.

Hausa households are large and multigenerational abodes. Women are constantly surrounded by female consanguineal and affinal relatives and the children of all. The average number of persons in the households visited during the course of this study was twenty, but it was not unusual for fifty persons to be eating at a particular house or compound. Often, while fifteen to twenty people might actually be resident in a particular house, many others might be eating and sleeping there. In Kano it is exceedingly rare to visit a Hausa woman in her home and find her alone—women appear to be never alone. Thus, the large city does not provide the alleged anonymity and lower visibility attributed to urban life. Within seclusion, women maintain wide networks, through which news of the world and changing events moves in an unending flow. Marriages, naming ceremonies, and other rituals are constant. Goods, services, and money flow rapidly, and visiting of extended kin is incessant; large families ensure movement and wide-ranging networks of exchange. Nothing is as simple as it looks. Kano City, although rapidly industrializing, is nonetheless reminiscent of nonindustrial towns, where the sense of a small, face-to-face community is maintained in the midst of an urban area. When a woman leaves her compound or receives visitors to it, all her neighbors know; the many men standing outside their compounds speculate as to the identity of a stranger and the nature of his or her business.

To the casual observer, life behind the mud wall of the compound appears secure and peaceful, but time spent there brings hundreds of sad stories. Women complain of heavy labor, of marriages of young daughters against their wills, of child brides brought into the household, of forced sexual cohabitation at puberty regardless of mental or emotional development, of early motherhood and infant death. There is no sewage system, running water is unreliable, and animals roam freely. Illness, needless death, and especially female and infant mortality are commonplace. Said a mother of a twelve-year-old on her wedding day, "may the day be cursed when she was born a woman."

NOTES

1. Reproductive histories of 82 women with children in two Kano wards (Kurawa and Kofar Mazugal) were taken by Schildkrout in 1977. Of these, seventy-nine had children and three were "caregivers" (i.e., they had been given children to foster). The 79 women had given birth to a total of 164 children, or an average of 8.2 each. Women without children are assumed to be unable to conceive.
2. As of 1983, the president of the Planned Parenthood Society of Nigeria, a member of a distinguished Kano family, saw nothing disconcerting in the fact that no office of the organization existed in the city. He asserted that Kano women knew he was president of the society and were free to come to his house and request a note from him to the appropriate doctor in the city hospital if they wanted information on birth control assistance (Interview #23, 1983).

REFERENCES

Abell, H. C. 1962. "Report to the Government of Nigeria (Northern Region) on the Home Economics Aspects of the F.A.O. Socio-Economic Survey of Peasant Agriculture in Northern Nigeria: The Role of Rural Women in Farm and Home Life." Rome: F.A.O. (mimeograph).

Bayerto University, Kano. 1980–1982. *Annual Report.* Kano: Bayerto University, Office of the Registrar.

Hake, James M. 1972. *Child-Rearing Practices in Northern Nigeria.* Ibadan: Ibadan University Press.

Hill, Polly. 1977. *Population, Prosperity and Poverty: Rural Kano 1900–1970.* Cambridge: Cambridge University Press.

Kabir, Zainab sa'ad. 1981. "The Silent Oppression: Male-Female Relations in Kano." Kano: Bayerto University Faculty Seminar, Department of Sociology (May) (mimeography).

Schildkrout, Enid. 1978. "Age and Gender in Hausa Society: Socio-Economic Roles of Children in Urban Kano." In *Sex and Age as Principles of Social Differentiation.* A.S.A. Monograph 17, ed. J. S. Fontaine, 109–37. London: Academic Press.

———. 1979. "Women's Work and Children's Work: Variations among Moslems in Kano." In *Social Anthropology of Work,* A.S.A. Monograph 19, ed. S. Wallman, 69–85. London: Academic Press.

———. 1981. "The Employment of Children in Kano." In *Child Work, Poverty and Underdevelopment,* ed. Gerry Rodgers and Guy Standing, 81–112. Geneva: International Labor Office.

Smith, M. G. 1955. *The Economy of the Hausa Communities of Zaire.* Colonial Research Studies, 16. London: Her Majesty's Stationary Office.

THE NAMED AND THE NAMELESS: GENDER AND PERSON IN CHINESE SOCIETY

Rubie S. Watson

In Chinese society names classify and individuate, they have transformative powers, and they are an important form of self expression. Some names are private, some are chosen for their public effect. Many people have a confusing array of names while others are nameless. The theory and practice of personal naming in Chinese society is extremely complex and unfortunately little studied.

Reproduced by permission of the American Anthropological Association from *American Ethnologist* 13:4, November 1986. Not for further reproduction.

For the male villagers of rural Hong Kong, naming marks important social transitions: the more names a man has the more "socialized" and also, in a sense, the more "individuated" he becomes. To attain social adulthood a man must have at least two names, but most have more. By the time a male reaches middle age, he may be known by four or five names. Village women, by contrast, are essentially nameless. Like boys, infant girls are named when they are one month old, but unlike boys they lose this name when they marry. Adult women are known (in reference and address) by kinship terms, teknonyms, or category terms such as "old woman."

In Chinese society personal names constitute an integral part of the language of joking, of boasting, and of exhibiting one's education and erudition. The Chinese themselves are fascinated by personal names: village men enjoy recounting stories about humorous or clumsy names, educated men appreciate the elegance of an auspicious name, and all males worry about the quality of their own names and those of their sons. To a large extent women are excluded from this discourse. They cannot participate because in adulthood they are not named, nor do they name others. Until very recently the majority of village women were illiterate and so could not engage in the intellectual games that men play with written names. Women were not even the subjects of these conversations.

The namelessness of adult women and their inability to participate in the naming of others highlights in a dramatic way the vast gender distinctions that characterize traditional Chinese culture. The study of names gives us considerable insight into the ways in which gender and person are constructed in Chinese society. Judged against the standard of men, the evidence presented here suggests that village women do not, indeed cannot, attain full personhood. The lives of men are punctuated by the acquisition of new names, new roles, new responsibilities and new privileges; women's lives, in comparison, remain indistinct and indeterminate.

In his essay "Person, Time, and Conduct in Bali," Clifford Geertz argues that our social world "is populated not by anybodies . . . but by somebodies, concrete classes of determinate persons positively characterized and appropriately labeled" (1973:363). It is this process by which anybodies are converted into somebodies that concerns me here. Do men and women become "somebodies" in the same way? Are they made equally determinate, positively characterized and labeled?

Although this discussion is based primarily on field research carried out in the Hong Kong New Territories, examples of naming practices have been drawn from other areas of Chinese culture as well. It is difficult to determine the extent to which the patterns described in this paper are indicative of rural China in general.[1] Available evidence suggests that there is considerable overlap between Hong Kong patterns of male naming and those of preliberation Chinese society and present-day rural Taiwan (see for example Eberhard 1970; Kehl 1971; Sung 1981; Wu 1927). Unfortunately, there have been no studies that specifically examine the differences between men's and women's naming, although brief references in Martin Yang's study of a Shantung village (1945:124) and in Judith Stacey's account of women in the People's Republic (1983:43, 131) suggest that the gender differences discussed here are not unique to Hong Kong. In making these statements I do not wish to suggest that there are no substantial differences in personal naming between rural Hong Kong and other parts of China. A general survey of personal naming in China, especially one that takes the postrevolution era into account, has yet to be done.

This paper draws heavily on ethnographic evidence gathered in the village of Ha Tsuen, a single-lineage village located in the northwest corner of the New Territories. All males in Ha Tsuen share the surname Teng and trace descent to a common ancestor who settled in this region during the 12th century (see R. Watson 1985). For most villagers postmarital residence is virilocal/patrilocal.

The Ha Tsuen Teng practice surname exogamy, which in the case of a single-lineage village means that all wives come from outside the community. These women arrive in Ha Tsuen as strangers and their early years of marriage are spent accommodating to a new family and new community. The Teng find this completely natural; "daughters," they say, "are born looking out; they belong to others."

Patrilineal values dominate social life in Ha Tsuen. Women are suspect because they are outsiders. As Margery Wolf points out, Chinese women are both marginal and essential to the families into which they marry (1972:35). They are necessary because they produce the next generation, yet as outsiders their integration is never complete. Women are economically dependent on the family estate, but they do not have shareholding rights in that estate. Half the village land in Ha Tsuen is owned by the lineage (see R. Watson 1985:61–72), and the other half is owned by private (male) landlords. Women have no share in this land; they do not own immovable property nor do they have rights to inherit it. Few married women are employed in wage labor, and since the villagers gave up serious agriculture in the 1960s, most women are dependent on their husbands' paychecks for family income. At the time I conducted my research (1977–78) Ha Tsuen had a population of approximately 2500—all of whom are Cantonese speakers.

NAMING AN INFANT

Among the Cantonese a child's soul is not thought to be firmly attached until at least 30 days after its birth. During the first month of life the child and mother are secluded from all but the immediate family. After a month has passed, the child is considered less susceptible to soul loss and is introduced into village life. The infant is given a name by his or her father or grandfather at a ceremony called "full month" (*man yueh*). If the child is a son, the "full month" festivities will be as elaborate as the family can afford; if, on the other hand, a girl is born, there may be little or no celebration (except, perhaps, a special meal for family members). The naming ceremony for a boy normally involves a banquet for neighbors and village elders, along with the distribution of red eggs to members of the community. The first name a child is given is referred to as his or her *ming*.[2]

This name (*ming*) may be based on literary or classical allusions. It may express a wish for the child's or family's future, or it may enshrine some simple event that took place at or near the time of the child's birth. Examples of this kind of naming are found not only in Ha Tsuen but in other areas of China as well. Arlington, in an early paper on Chinese naming, describes how the name "sleeve" was given to a girl of his acquaintance who at the time of her birth had been wrapped in a sleeve (1923:319). In the People's Republic of China, people born during the Korean War might be called "Resist the United States" (Fan-mei) or "Aid Korea" (Pang-ch'ao). Alternatively, children may be given the name of their birthplace, for example, "Born in Anhwei" (Hui-sheng) or "Thinking of Yunnan" (Hsiang-yun). In the past girl babies might be named Nai ("To Endure"). This name was given to infant girls who survived an attempted infanticide. One way of killing an infant was to expose it to the elements. If a girl survived this ordeal, she might be allowed to live. In these cases the name Nai commemorated the child's feat of survival.[3]

A child's name may express the parents' desire for no more children. For instance, in Taiwan a fifth or sixth child may be named Beui, a Hokkien term meaning "Last Child." Alternatively, a father may try to assure that his next child will be a son by naming a newborn daughter "Joined to Brother" (Lien-ti). There are several girls with this name in Ha Tsuen. A father or grandfather might express his disappointment or disgust by naming a second or third daughter "Too Many" (A-to)[4] or "Little Mistake" (Hsiao-t'so) or "Reluctant to Feed" (Wang-shih). A sickly child might be given the name of a healthy child. My informants told me that a long-awaited son may be given a girl's name to trick the wandering ghosts into thinking the child had no value and therefore could be ignored (see also Sung 1981:81–82). For example, a Ha Tsuen villager, who was the only son of a wealthy family (born to his father's third concubine), was known by everyone as "Little Slave Girl" (in Cantonese, Mui-jai).

In most cases the infant receives a *ming* during the full month ceremony but this name is little used. For the first year or two most children are called by a family nickname ("milk name" or *nai ming*). Babies are sometimes given milk names like "Precious" (A-pao), or A-buh (mimicking the sounds infants make) or "Eldest Luck," or "Second Luck," indicating sibling order.

Some care and consideration is given to a child's *ming*, especially if it is a boy. By referring to the Confucian classics or by alluding to a famous poem, the name may express the learning and sophistication of the infant's father or grandfather. The name, as we will see, may also save the child from an inauspicious fate. Commonly girls' names (*ming*) are less distinctive and less considered than are boys' names. And, as we have seen, girls' names may also be less flattering: "Too Many" or "Little Mistake." Often a general, classificatory name is given to an infant girl; Martin Yang reports from rural Shantung that Hsiao-mei ("Little Maiden") was a "generic" girls' name in his village (1945:124).

Most Chinese personal names are composed of two characters, which follow the one character surname (for example, Mao Tse-tung or Teng Hsiao-ping). One of the characters of the *ming* may be repeated for all the children of the same sex in the family or perhaps all sons born into the lineage during one generation (for example, a generation or sibling set might have personal names like Hung-hui, Hung-chi, Hung-sheng, and so on.). Birth order may also be indicated in the child's name. In these cases part of the name indicates group affiliation and sibling order. However, one of the characters is unique to the individual and so the child is distinguished from his siblings. A variation on this theme occurs when a parent or grandparent selects a name for all sons or grandsons from a group of characters that share a single element (known as the radical—a structured component found in every Chinese character). For example, Margaret Sung (1981:80) in her survey of Chinese naming practices on Taiwan notes that in some families all son's names may be selected from characters that contain the "man" radical (for example, names like "Kind" [Jen], "Handsome" [Chun], or "Protect" [Pao]).

Individuation of the name, Sung points out, is very strong in Chinese society (1981:88). There is no category of words reserved specifically for personal names and care is taken to make names (particularly boys' names) distinct. The Chinese find the idea of sharing one's given name with millions of other people extraordinary.[5] In Taiwan, Sung notes that individuation of one's name is so important that the government has established a set of rules for name changes (1981:88). According to these regulations a name can be changed when two people with exactly the same name live in the same city or county or have the same place of work. "Inelegant" names or names shared with wanted criminals can also be changed.

In Ha Tsuen a boy might be named, in Cantonese, Teng Tim-sing, which translates Teng "To Increase Victories"; another person could be called Teng Hou-sing, "Reliably Accomplish" (Teng being the shared surname). Parents, neighbors, and older siblings will address the child or young unmarried adult (male or female) by his or her *ming* or by a nickname. Younger siblings are expected to use kin terms in addressing older siblings. It should be noted that, in contrast to personal names, Chinese surnames do not convey individual meaning. When used in a sentence or poem, the character *mao* (the same character used in Mao Tse-tung) means hair, fur, feathers, but when it is used as a surname it does not carry any of these connotations.

THE POWER OF NAMES: NAMES THAT CHANGE ONE'S LUCK

Names classify people into families, generational sets, and kin groups. Ideally, Chinese personal names also have a unique quality. Personal names carry meanings; they express wishes (for more sons or no more daughters), mark past events ("Sleeve" or "Endure"), and convey a family's learning and status. Beyond this rather restricted sense there is, however, another level of meaning. According to Chinese folk concepts each person has a unique constitution—a different balance of the five elements (fire, water, metal, earth, and wood). When the child is about one month old a family will usually have a diviner cast the child's horoscope. The horoscope consists of eight characters (*pa tzu*)—two each for the hour, day, month, and year of birth. The combination of these characters determines in part what kind of person one is (what kind of characteristics one has) and what will happen in future years. However, the *pa tzu* do not represent destiny; one is not bound to act out this fate.

By means of esoteric knowledge a person's fate can be changed. Perhaps the most common method of accomplishing such a change is through naming. For example, if one of the five elements is missing from a person's constitution or is not properly balanced with other elements, the name (*ming*) may then include a character with the radical for that element. In the event of illness the diviner may suggest that the patient suffers from an imbalance of wood and that the radical for this element be added to the child's name. In such a case the character *mei* (plum), for example, may replace one of the original characters of the *ming* and thus save the child from a bad fate, illness, or perhaps death. *Mei* achieves this astounding feat not because there is anything intrinsically wood-like about *mei* but because the written character *mei* has two major components: *mu,* the radical for wood and another symbol that is largely phonetic. It is the written form of the character that is important here; in spoken Chinese there is nothing that suggests that *mei* has within it the element wood. I will return to this point later.

Significantly, it is not only one's own horoscope that matters; one must also be in balance with the horoscopes of parents, spouses, and offspring. It is particularly important that the five elements of mother and child be properly matched to ensure mutual health.[6] If conditions of conflict arise and nothing is done to resolve this conflict, the child may become ill and even die. A name change, however, can rectify the situation. It is obvious that Chinese personal names *do* things: they not only classify and distinguish but also have an efficacy in their own right.

GENDER DIFFERENCES AND THE WRITTEN NAME

As noted above, even in childhood there are important gender distinctions in naming. Girls nearly always have less elaborate full month rituals than their brothers, and less care is taken in choosing girls' names. The greatest difference between the sexes, however, pertains not to the aesthetics of naming but to the written form of the name.

Until the 1960s in Ha Tsuen and in rural Hong Kong generally births were seldom registered with government agencies. Except in cases of a bad fate, there was no compelling reason for girls' names ever to appear in written form. There was rarely any need to attach their names to legal documents. Girls did not inherit land, they had no rights in property, and their given names were not entered in genealogies (on this point see also Hazelton 1986) or on ancestral tablets (see below). Until the 1960s girls rarely attended primary schools. Consequently, nearly all village women born prior to 1945 cannot write or recognize their own names.

Commenting on the role of nicknames, Wolfram Eberhard makes the point that in spoken Chinese with its many homonyms, a two-word combination may fail to express clearly what the speaker wants to convey. The intended meaning of a name (that is, the two-character *ming*) is only apparent when it is written. Nicknames, Eberhard notes, are not normally meant to be written and, hence, are usually longer (often three or four characters) than a person's *ming* (1970:219). Given the ambiguities, a great deal of play is possible with the spoken form of names. For example, Hsin-mei can mean "New Plum" or "Faithful Beauty" depending on the tones that one uses in pronouncing the characters. In the written form the meaning of this name is perfectly clear, but in the spoken form it can be misunderstood or misconstrued, sometimes with disastrous consequences. The Manchu (Ch'ing) authorities played the naming game when they changed the written form of one of Sun Yat-sen's many names. During Sun's long political career, he used a variety of names and aliases (see Sharman 1934), one being Sun Wen (*wen* translates as "elegant," "civil," "culture"). In Manchu attacks on Sun the character *wen* pronounced with a rising tone (elegant, culture) was replaced by another character *wen* pronounced with a falling tone (which translates as "defile"). The change was effected simply by adding the water radical to the term for elegant. *Wen* (defile), it should be noted, was also the name of a famous criminal in southern China during the last years of Manchu rule.

Upon seeing a person's written name, the beholder may comment on the beauty, the refinement, the auspicious connotations of the characters. As long as it is simply spoken, however, it is in a sense "just a name." Although women have names, these do not convey as much information as do men's names, for the obvious reason that the former were rarely written. Until recently New Territories women were not given names with a view to their written effect. The written form of "Too Many" may be offensive or unpleasant in a way that the spoken form is not.

Given that it is the written form of names that has force, that informs, that can be used to change a bad fate, there is justification for thinking that those whose names are rarely or never written are at some disadvantage. Girls, it would appear, did not have names in the same way that boys did.[7] It is also clear that girls' names are less expressive, less individuating than their brothers' names are. Fathers strove to make son's names distinctive, unique—whereas girls' names tended to classify (for example, Endure, Little Maiden) or to be used as a vehicle for changing circumstances external to the girl herself (for example, Joined to Brother). Many girls of course had names like Splendid Orchid, Morning Flower, Resembling Jade, but in general they were more likely than were their brothers to be given negative names, stereotypic names, or goal-oriented names. These gender distinctions are significant, but the contrast between men and women becomes even more dramatic when we consider adult naming practices.

MEN'S NAMING

When a Ha Tsuen man marries, he is given or takes (often he chooses the name himself) a marriage name, or *tzu*. Considering the importance of the written name it is significant that *tzu* is the same character that is commonly used for "word" or "ideograph." The marriage name is given in a ceremony called *sung tzu,* which literally means "to deliver written characters." This ceremony is an integral part of the marriage rites and is held after the main banquet on the first day of wedding festivities.

In Ha Tsuen, the marriage name (always two characters) is written on a small rectangular piece of red paper and is displayed in the main reception hall of the groom's house (alternatively, it may be hung in the groom's branch ancestral hall). This name is chosen with regard to its effect in the written form. Great care is taken in choosing the characters; they often have origins in the Confucian classics. In Ha Tsuen one of the two characters of this marriage name is usually shared by a lineage generational set. In some kin groups a respected scholar may be asked to choose a poem or aphorism to be used in generational naming. Each generation will then take in turn one character of the poem as part of their (*tzu*) name. Of course, this makes the selection of an auspicious, learned name more difficult and also more intellectually challenging. Naming at this level can become a highly complicated game.

In choosing a marriage name (*tzu*) the groom demonstrates his sophistication, learning, and goals. Among the people I studied, the possession of a marriage name is essential for the attainment of male adulthood, which gives a man the right to participate in important lineage and community rituals. In Ha Tsuen the correct way to ask whether a man has full ritual rights in the lineage is to inquire, "Does X have a *tzu?*", not "Is X married?" Marriage names are not used as terms of address; they may, however, appear in lineage genealogies and in formal documents.

By the time a man is married he will have acquired a public nickname (*wai hao,* literally an "outside name"). This is usually different from the family nickname he had in infancy or the "school name" given to him by a teacher.[8] Nicknames are widely used as terms of address and reference for males in the village; in fact, a man's birth and marriage names may be largely unknown.

In a discussion of naming among the Ilongot, Renato Rosaldo emphasizes the process by which names come into being (1984:13). Rosaldo argues that names are negotiated, and that naming, like other aspects of Ilongot social life, is a matter of give and take, challenge and response (1984:22). Rosaldo's approach is particularly useful for understanding Chinese nicknaming. *Ming* (birth names) are formally bestowed by one's seniors, one chooses the *tzu* (marriage name) and, as we will see, the *hao* (courtesy name) oneself. Nicknames (*wai hao*), however, are negotiated; both the namer and the named play the game. By setting up this dichotomy between nicknames and other given names, I do not mean to suggest that these two categories have no common features nor that *ming,* marriage names, and courtesy names are simply the consequence of a set of rigidly applied rules and structures. It is clear, however, that nicknames fit into the transactional world of local politics, friendship, and informal groups more comfortably than do formal names.

In Chinese society, one can gain a reputation for cleverness by giving nicknames that are particularly apt or make witty literary allusions. Chinese nicknames are highly personalized and often refer to idiosyncratic characteristics. They may also be derogatory or critical, whereas one's formal names would never be intentionally unflattering (especially for a man). Nicknames may refer to a physical quality (for example, "Fatty") or a personal quality ("Stares at the Sky" for someone who is a snob). Nicknames may also protect ("Little Slave Girl") or they may equalize, at least temporarily, unequal relationships. The richest and most powerful man in one New Territories village was nicknamed "Little Dog." In one respect this was a useful nickname for an extremely wealthy man whose political career depended on being accepted by everyone in the community. Rather than rejecting his derogatory nickname he embraced it.

In Ha Tsuen when a man reaches middle age or when he starts a business career, he usually takes a *hao*—"style" or "courtesy" name. A man chooses this name himself. Sung notes that such names are "usually dissyllabic or polysyllabic, and [are] selected by oneself bas[ed] upon whatever one would like to be" (1981:86). Some people have more than one courtesy name. The *hao* is a public name par excellence. Such names, Eberhard points out, are often used on occasions when a man wants "to make his personal identity clear without revealing his personal name (*ming*)" (1970:219). In the past, and to some extent today,[9] the *ming* was considered to be too intimate, too personal to be used outside a circle of close friends and kin (Eberhard 1970:218). "The Chinese I know hide their names," writes Maxine Hong Kingston in *Woman Warrior;* "sojourners take new names when their lives change and guard their real names with silence" (1977:6).

Sung notes that *hao* names are no longer popular in present-day Taiwan except among high government officials (1981:86). However, in Hong Kong *hao* are still widely used; they are commonly found, for example, on business cards, and of course many painters or writers sign their work with a *hao*.

In one sense courtesy names are different from birth and marriage names. One achieves a courtesy name. They are a mark of social and economic status, and a poor man who gives himself such a name may be accused of putting on airs. Any man may take a *hao* but if he is not a "man of substance," the *hao* is likely to remain unknown and unused. With poor men or politically insignificant men these names, if they have them at all, may appear only in genealogies or on tombstones.

Some Ha Tsuen men have posthumous names (*shih-hao*) that they take themselves or have conferred upon them by others. Among the imperial elite posthumous names or titles were given to honor special deeds. In the village, however, taking or giving a *shih-hao* is left to individual taste. The practice has declined in recent years.

The preceding discussion suggests that names mark stages in a man's social life. The possession of a birth name, school name, nickname, marriage name, courtesy name, and posthumous name attest to the fact that a man has passed through the major stages of social adulthood. By the time a man reaches middle age he has considerable control over his names and naming. He names others (his children or grandchildren, for example) and he chooses his own marriage, courtesy, and posthumous names. He also has some control over the use of these names. This is especially true of a successful businessman or politician whose business associates may only know his courtesy name, his drinking friends one of his nicknames, his lineage-mates his birth name, and so on. The use of names is situational and involves some calculation both on the part of the named and those with whom he interacts.

Beidelman, in an article on naming among the Kaguru of Tanzania, emphasizes the point that the choice of name reflects the relation between the speaker and the person to whom he speaks (1974:282; see also Willis 1982). The choice of one name or another, or the use of a kin term rather than a personal name, is a tactical decision. In Ha Tsuen the use of nicknames, pet names, birth names, courtesy names is, like the use of kin terms, highly contextual. Intimates may address each other by a nickname when they are among friends but not when strangers are present, family nicknames may be used in the household but not outside of it, birth names and surnames with titles may be used in formal introductions but not in other settings. A man might be addressed by a kin term or a nickname depending on the speaker's goals. One can give respect by using a courtesy name or claim intimacy by using a nickname. In a single lineage village like Ha Tsuen, where all males are agnatic kinsmen, the strategic use of kin terms and personal names provides a fascinating glimpse into social relationships.

Surprisingly, however, this flexibility does not continue into old age. When a man reaches elderhood at age 61, his ability to control his names diminishes just as his control over his family and corporate resources weakens. In Ha Tsuen and in China generally men often hand over headship of the family when they become elders. The village code of respect requires that male elders be addressed by a kin term (for example, in Cantonese *ah baak,* FeB, or a combination of the given name and kin term, for example, *ah Tso baak*). Only an exceptional man, a scholar or wealthy businessman, will continue to be called by one of his personal names after his 60th birthday. For example, no villager would dare refer to or address the 93-year-old patriarch of the wealthiest family in Ha Tsuen as *ah baak.* In general, however, with advancing age the playful aspects of names and naming are taken away as is a man's power to transact his name. In old age a man has little control over what he is called, and in this respect his situation is similar to that of a married woman. As with wives, old men have left (or are leaving) the world of public and financial affairs to become immersed in the world of family and kinship where they are defined not by a set of distinctive names but by their relationship to others.

"NO NAME" WOMEN

At one month a Ha Tsuen girl is given a name (*ming*); when she marries this name ceases to be used. Marriage is a critical rite of passage for both men and women, but the effect of this rite on the two sexes is very different. Just as a man's distinctiveness and public role are enhanced by his marriage and his acquisition of a marriage name, the marriage rites relegate the woman to the inner world of household, neighborhood, and family. On the one hand, the marriage rites seek to enhance the young bride's fertility, but on the other hand, and in a more negative vein, they also dramatize the bride's separation from her previous life and emphasize the prohibitions and restrictions that now confine her. When the young bride crosses her husband's threshold, what distinctiveness she had as a girl is thrust aside. It is at this point that she loses her name and becomes the "inner person" (*nei jen*), a term Chinese husbands use to refer to their wives.

While the groom is receiving his marriage name on the first day of marriage rites, his bride is being given an intensive course in kinship terminology by the elderly women of Ha Tsuen. Marriage ritual provides a number of occasions for the formal, ritualized exchange of kin terms (for a description of marriage rites in Ha Tsuen see R. Watson 1981). These exchanges, which always feature the bride, instruct the new wife and daughter-in-law in the vast array of kin terms she must use for her husband's relatives. The prevalence of virilocal/patrilocal residence means that the groom remains among the kin with whom he has always lived. It is the bride who must grasp a whole new set of kin terms and learn to attach these terms to what must seem a bewildering array of people. Two women resident in the groom's village (called in Cantonese *choi gaa*, "bride callers") act as the bride's guides and supporters during the three days of marriage rites, and it is their responsibility to instruct the bride in the kin terminology she will need in order to survive in her new environment.

These ritualized exchanges of kin terms do more, however, than serve as a pedagogic exercise; they also locate and anchor the bride in a new relational system. As the groom acquires his new marriage name—a name, it should be noted, that denotes both group or category membership *and* individual distinctiveness—the bride enters a world in which she exists only in relation to others. She is no longer "grounded" by her own special name (*ming*), however prosaic that name might have been; after marriage she exists only as someone's eBW or yBW or as Sing's mother, and so on. Eventually even these terms will be used with decreasing frequency; as she approaches old age, she will be addressed simply as "old woman" (*ah po*) by all but her close kin.

When I first moved into Ha Tsuen, I quickly learned the names of the male residents (mostly nicknames). But for the women I, like other villagers, relied on kin terms or category terms. Significantly, the rules that govern the use of these terms are not dependent on the age of the women themselves, but rather are a function of the lineage generation of their husbands. Women married to men of an ascending generation to the speaker (or the speaker's husband) may be addressed as *ah suk po* (a local expression meaning FyBW) or by the more formal *ah sam* (also meaning FyBW). For women married to men of one's own generation (male ego) the terms *ah sou* (eBW) or, if one wanted to give added respect, *ah sam* (FyBW) may be used.

A woman may also be referred to by the nickname of her husband plus "leung" (for example, ah Keung leung), or by a teknonym. For their part married women ordinarily use kin terms for their husbands' agnates and for other women in the village. I was told that a woman must use kin terms for men older in age or generation than her husband. Between husband and wife teknonyms are often used so that the father of Tim-sing might address his wife as *ah Sing nai* (*ah* is a prefix denoting familiarity, *Sing* is part of the son's *ming*, *nai* is "mother" or, literally, "milk"). In addressing their husbands, women might use nicknames; my neighbor always called her husband "Little Servant."[10]

Although there is some flexibility in deciding what to call a woman, the reference and address terms used for women in Ha Tsuen are very rigid compared to those employed for men. Furthermore, among women there is no possibility of self-naming. Men name themselves, women are named by others. Similarly, Ha Tsuen women are more restricted than their husbands in the tactical use they can make of names and kin terms. Whereas a man may refer to or address his neighbor by his nickname ("Fatty"), his *ming* (*ah Tim*), or by a kin term, decorum dictates that his wife use either a kin term appropriate to her husband's generation or one appropriate to her children. In Cantonese society, and presumably in China generally, adults often address and refer to each other by a version of the kin term their children would use for that person. I suspect, but at this point cannot document, that women are far more likely to do this than are men.

While it is true that a man has little choice in the reference or address terms he uses for women, he does have considerable freedom in distinguishing among his male acquaintances, friends, and kin. Women, as outlined above, have a restricted repertoire for both sexes. In this sense adult women may be said to carry a particularly heavy burden for guarding the kinship and sexual order. No adult woman is free to act alone or to be treated as if she were independent. The terms by which she is addressed and the terms she uses to address others serve as constant reminders of the hierarchical relations of gender, age, and generation.

As men grow older, as they become students, marry, start careers, take jobs, and eventually prepare for ancestorhood, their new names anchor them to new roles and privileges. These names are not, however, only role markers or classifiers. Ideally, they assign people to categories and at the same time declare their uniqueness. The pattern of naming in Chinese society presents an ever changing image of men. Viewed from this perspective Chinese males are always growing, becoming, accumulating new responsibilities and new rights.

Peasant women, on the other hand, experience few publicly validated life changes, and those that they do undergo link them ever more securely to stereotyped roles. Women's naming leaves little room for individuation or self-expression. Unlike males, whose changes are marked by both ascribed (for example, elderhood) *and* achieved criteria (such as student, scholar, businessman, writer, politician), a woman's changes (from unmarried virgin to married woman, from nonmother to mother, from reproducer to nonreproducer) are not related to achievement outside the home. Instead of acquiring a new name at marriage or the birth of a first child, women's changes are marked by kin terminology or category shifts. At marriage the bride loses her *ming* and becomes known by a series of kin terms. At the birth of a child she may add a teknonym ("Sing's mother"), and as she approaches and enters old age more and more people will address her simply as "old woman" (*ah po*).

The most dramatic changes that women make are the shift from named to unnamed at marriage and the gradual shift from kin term to category term as their children mature and marry.[11] It would appear that as a woman's reproductive capacity declines, she becomes less grounded in the relational system. She becomes, quite simply, an "old woman" much like any other old woman. Of course, family members continue to use kin terms for these elderly women, especially in reference and address, but gradually their anonymity increases. Unlike men, women do not become elders. There is no ceremony marking their entry into respected old age. They move from reproductively active mother to sexually inactive grandmother with no fanfare and with little public recognition of their changed status.

Even in death a woman has no personal name. On the red flag that leads the spirit of the deceased from the village to the grave is written the woman's father's surname (for example, *Lin shih,* translated "Family of Lin"); no personal name is added. For men, the deceased's surname plus his courtesy and/or posthumous name is written on the soul flag. Neither do women's personal names appear on the tombstone where, here again, only the surname of the woman's father is given ("Family of Lin"). In Ha Tsuen women do not have separate ancestral tablets; if they are commemorated at all, they appear as minor appendages on their husbands' tablets. And, once more, they are listed only under the surnames of their fathers. In subsequent generations whatever individuating characteristics a woman might have had are lost—not even a name survives as testimony of her existence as a person.

CONCLUSIONS

If one were to categorize Ha Tsuen villagers on a social continuum according to the number and quality of their names, married peasant women would stand at the extreme negative pole.[12] To my knowledge they share this dubious distinction with no other group. In the past even male slaves (*hsi min*) and household servants had nicknames (see J. Watson 1976:365). They may not have had *ming* or surnames as such but they did possess names that distinguished them from others. It is important to note that it is not only the possession of multiple names that matters but also the fact that, at one end of the continuum, people have no control over their own names while, at the other end, they name themselves and others.

At marriage women find themselves enmeshed in the world of family and kinship. It is a world, as noted in the introduction, that they belong to but do not control. In Ha Tsuen brides arrive as outsiders but quickly, one might even say brutally, they become firmly entrenched in their new environment. Village women can only be identified within the constellation of male names or within the limits of kinship terminology. Unlike their husbands and brothers, women—having no public identity outside the relational system—are defined by and through others.

In Ha Tsuen women are excluded from participation in most of the formal aspects of lineage or community life and they are not involved in decision making outside the home. Ha Tsuen women do not inherit productive resources; they are also restricted in the uses to which they can put their dowries (R. Watson 1984). Furthermore, women in Ha Tsuen cannot become household heads and, even today, they do not vote in local elections. They do not worship in ancestral halls nor do they join the cult of lineage ancestors after death. Although individual peasant women may attain considerable power within their households, they are said to have gained this power by manipulation and stealth. Women by definition cannot hold positions of authority.

In a discussion of male and female naming among the Omaha Sioux, Robert Barnes writes: "The names of Omaha males provide men with distinctive individuality, while also linking each unmistakably to a recognized collectivity. The possibility of acquiring multiple names in adulthood enhances individual prominence for men" (1982:220). Barnes goes on to say that women's names "barely rescue them from a general anonymity, neither conferring uniqueness nor indicating group membership" (1982:22). As among the Sioux, personal naming among Chinese men is a sign of both individual distinctiveness and group membership, while naming practices among village women simply confirm their marginality.

In Ha Tsuen the practice of personal naming reflects and facilitates the passage from one social level to another. Names establish people in social groups and give them certain rights within those groups. With each additional name, a man acquires new attributes.

Maybury-Lewis has argued that among many Central Brazilian societies names give humans their "social persona and link [them] to other people" (1984:5; see also Bamberger 1974). Names, Maybury-Lewis writes, "transform individuals into persons" (1984:7). Naming may not be as central to Chinese social organization and ideology as it is among the societies of Central Brazil, yet there is no doubt that, for Chinese men, names have a transformative power that binds them as individuals to society.

In Ha Tsuen the ultimate goal of all males is to produce an heir, to have a grandson at one's funeral, to leave property that guarantees the performance of one's ancestral rites. The possession of many names testifies to the fact that a man has completed the cycle of life. Full personhood is not acquired at birth, at marriage, or even at the death of one's father. It is a process that continues throughout life and is punctuated by the taking and bestowing of names. One might argue that it is a process that extends even beyond death as the named ancestor interacts with the living. If, as Grace Harris suggests, personhood involves a process of social growth "in the course of which changes [are] wrought by ceremony and ritual" (1978:49), then Chinese women never approximate the full cycle of development that their menfolk experience.[13] In stark contrast to men, women become less distinct as they age. The changes they undergo remain largely unrecognized and unnoticed.

In Chinese society, as in other societies, there is a tension between the notion of the unique individual (the individual as value) and the notion of the person tied to society.[14] In some sense the great philosophical systems of Taoism and Confucianism represent these two poles. Among men, naming involves a dual process through which they achieve personhood by being bound to society, while at the same time they acquire an enhanced sense of individuality and distinctiveness. The peasant women described in this paper seem to have been largely excluded from the individuating, individualizing world of personal naming. The situation with regard to personhood is, however, another matter. It would be wrong to say that peasant wives are nonpersons; rather, they are not persons in the same sense or to the same degree as are husbands and sons. Viewed from the perspective of names, peasant women are neither fully individuated nor "personed." In life as in death they remain suspended between the anonymous world of anybodies and the more sharply defined world of somebodies.

NOTES

Acknowledgments. The research for this study was conducted in 1977–78 and was made possible by a grant from the Social Science Research Council (Great Britain) and by the University of London Central Research Fund. An earlier version of this paper was presented at the 1984 American Anthropological Association Annual Meetings. Versions of this paper were also presented at the University of London Intercollegiate Anthropology Seminar and at the University of Rochester's Anthropology Colloquium. I thank the members of those seminars for their suggestions and criticisms. I owe a special debt to Jack Dull, Hsu Cho-yun, Sun Man-li, Roderick MacFarquhar, and James Watson, all of whom have helped in this project. Deborah Kwolek, Judy Tredway, and Martha Terry of the Asian Studies Program at the University of Pittsburgh helped in the preparation of the manuscript and I thank them for their assistance.

Cantonese terms are in Yale romanization and Mandarin terms follow the Wade-Giles system.

This paper is dedicated to the memory of my friend and fellow anthropologist Judith Strauch (1942–85).

1. There are bound to be regional, temporal, urban-rural, and class differences in Chinese naming practices. A general discussion of Chinese naming awaits further research.
2. In Taiwan the *ming* is the legal name (it appears in the official household register) and is sometimes called the *cheng ming* (correct name) (Sung 1981:70). In Hong Kong this name may or may not be the name used on legal documents.
3. I am grateful to Professor Jack Dull for pointing out to me the significance and frequency of the personal name Nai among Chinese women.

4. In a similar vein a fifth or sixth child might be named "To End" or "To Finish." One can find such names in the Hong Kong and Taipei telephone directories (see also Sung 1981:81).
5. In China there are no given names like John that are shared by millions of people; on this point see Sung 1981:85.
6. In a discussion of the cosmic relationship between mother and child Marjorie Topley writes of her Cantonese informants:

   The constitutional imbalance of a child with a queer fate may also involve other parties. First, the child may be polarized in the same direction as someone with whom it has a continuous relationship. Then both parties may suffer from continual illness. This may be corrected by adding an element to the child's name so it is compatible with that of the other party [1974:240].
7. This is changing now that girls go to school and their births are registered.
8. In the past when village boys started school at age five or six (girls did not attend school until the 1960s), the schoolmaster gave each student a school or "study name" (*hsueh-ming*). School names are no longer very important in the New Territories.
9. In the past officials' *ming* could not be used except by intimates (see Eberhard 1970 and Sung 1981).
10. After having gained some insight into the micropolitics of my neighbor's household, the name seemed well chosen.
11. Once a son marries reproduction becomes a matter for the younger generation, and in Ha Tsuen it was considered shameful for the mother of a married son to become pregnant.
12. It should be noted here that men do not constitute a uniform category in this regard. Highly literate men make up one extreme but many poorly educated or uneducated men fall somewhere between the two extremes. Like the names of their sisters, their names may be inelegant and rarely seen in written form, but unlike adult women, they do retain their names after marriage.
13. On this point see also LaFontaine 1985:131.
14. For discussions of the concept of the individual as value and the self in Chinese society see for example de Bary 1970; Shiga 1978:122; and more recently Elvin 1985; Munro 1985 (especially essays by Hansen, Yu, Munro, and de Bary).

REFERENCES

Arlington, L. C. 1923. The Chinese Female Names. China Journal of Science and Arts 1 (4):316–325.

Bamberger, Joan. 1974. Naming and the Transmission of Status in a Central Brazilian Society. Ethnology 13:363–378.

Barnes, Robert B. 1982. Personal Names and Social Classification. *In* Semantic Anthropology. David Parkin, ed. pp. 211–226. London: Academic Press.

Beidelman, T. O. 1974. Kaguru Names and Naming. Journal of Anthropological Research 30:281–293.

de Bary, William Theodore. 1970. Individualism and Humanitarianism in Late Ming Thought. *In* Self and Society in Ming Thought. Wm. Theodore de Bary, ed. pp. 145–247. New York: Columbia University Press.

Eberhard, Wolfram. 1970. A Note on Modern Chinese Nicknames. *In* Studies in Chinese Folklore and Related Essays. Wolfram Eberhard, ed. pp. 217–222. Indiana University Folklore Institute Monograph Series, Vol. 23. The Hague: Mouton.

Elvin, Mark. 1985. Between the Earth and Heaven: Conceptions of the Self in China. *In* The Category of the Person. Michael Carrithers, Steven Collins, Steven Lukes, eds. pp. 156–189. Cambridge: Cambridge University Press.

Geertz, Clifford. 1973. Person, Time, and Conduct in Bali. *In* The Interpretation of Cultures. pp. 360–411. New York: Basic Books.

Harris, Grace. 1978. Casting Out Anger: Religion among the Taita of Kenya. Cambridge: Cambridge University Press.

Hazelton, Keith. 1986. Patrilines and the Development of Localized Lineages: The Wu of Hsiu-ming City, Hui-chou, to 1528. *In* Kinship Organization in Late Imperial China. Patricia B. Ebrey and James L. Watson, eds. pp. 137–169. Berkeley: University of California Press.

Kehl, Frank. 1971. Chinese Nicknaming Behavior: A Sociolinguistic Pilot Study. Journal of Oriental Studies 9:149–172.

Kingston, Maxine Hong. 1977. The Woman Warrior: Memories of a Girlhood among Ghosts. New York: Vintage Books. (Originally published in hardcover by Alfred Knopf, 1976.)

La Fontaine, Jean. 1985. Person and Individual: Some Anthropological Reflections. *In* The Category of the Person. Michael Carrithers, Steven Collins, and Steven Lukes, eds. pp. 123–140. Cambridge: Cambridge University Press.

Maybury-Lewis, David. 1984. Name, Person, and Ideology in Central Brazil. *In* Naming Systems. Elisabeth Tooker, ed. pp. 1–10. 1980 Proceedings of the American Ethnological Society. Washington, DC: American Ethnological Society.

Munro, Donald (ed.). 1985. Individualism and Holism: Studies in Confucian and Taoist Values. Ann Arbor: University of Michigan Press.

Rosaldo, Renato. 1984. Ilongot Naming: The Play of Associations. *In* Naming Systems. Elisabeth Tooker, ed. pp. 11–24. 1980 Proceedings of the American Ethnological Society. Washington, DC: American Ethnological Society.

Sharman, Lyon. 1934. Sun Yat-sen: His Life and its Meaning. Stanford, CA: Stanford University Press.

Shiga, Shuzo. 1978. Family Property and the Law of Inheritance in Traditional China. *In* Chinese Family Law and Social Change. David Buxbaum, ed. pp. 109–150. Seattle: University of Washington Press.

Stacey, Judith. 1983. Patriarchy and Socialist Revolution in China. Berkeley: University of California Press.

Sung, Margaret M. Y. 1981. Chinese Personal Naming. Journal of the Chinese Language Teachers Association 16(2):67–90.

Topley, Marjorie. 1974. Cosmic Antagonisms: A Mother-Child Syndrome. *In* Religion and Ritual in Chinese Society. Arthur Wolf, ed. pp. 233–249. Stanford, CA: Stanford University Press.

Watson, James L. 1976. Chattel Slavery in Chinese Peasant Society: A Comparative Analysis. Ethnology 15:361–375.

Watson, Rubie S. 1981. Class Differences and Affinal Relations in South China. Man 16:593–615.

———. 1984. Women's Property in Republican China: Rights and Practice. Republican China 10(12):1–12.

———. 1985. Inequality Among Brothers: Class and Kinship in South China. Cambridge: Cambridge University Press.

Willis, Roy. 1982. On a Mental Sausage Machine and other Nominal Problems. *In* Semantic Anthropology. David Parkin, ed. pp. 227–240. London: Academic Press.

Wolf, Margery. 1972. Women and the Family in Rural Taiwan. Stanford, CA: Stanford University Press.

Wu, Ching-chao. 1927. The Chinese Family: Organization, Names, and Kinship Terms. American Anthropologist 29:316–325.

Yang, Martin C. 1945. A Chinese Village: Taitou, Shantung Province. New York: Columbia University Press.

A CRITICAL APPRAISAL OF THEORIES OF MENSTRUAL SYMBOLISM

Thomas Buckley and Alma Gottlieb

MENSTRUATION AND POLLUTION

An abundance of symbolic analyses of menstrual taboos has been built on the concept of "pollution"—symbolic contamination. These studies posit (correctly or incorrectly) that menstrual blood and menstruous women are culturally defined as dangerous to established order (in various senses)—if not universally then at least widely enough to constitute a justifiable generalization. Because menstrual blood and menstruous women are perceived as dangerous, taboos have been devised to contain their energies and keep these from spreading beyond a limited place in the order of things. Among anthropologists utilizing a pollution model in the study of menstrual customs and beliefs two lines of analysis have been followed, independently or in conjunction with each other. The first of these stresses the symbolic structures of pollu-

Reprinted with permission from Thomas Buckley and Alma Gottlieb (eds.), *Blood Magic: Explorations in the Anthropology of Menstruation* (Berkeley: University of California Press, 1988), pp. 25–40.

tion concepts in diverse cultures; the second emphasizes the sociological correlates of such symbolic structures.

Both lines of analysis have been pursued by Mary Douglas, an anthropologist perhaps best known for her work in general pollution theory. Although Douglas has written no extended work solely on the topic of menstrual pollution, her broader investigations of pollution (1966, 1972) and of body symbolism (1968, 1970) place her foremost among theoretical contributors to the comparative cultural-anthropological study of menstruation.

THE SYMBOLISM OF MENSTRUAL POLLUTION

In *Purity and Danger* (1966) Douglas proposes that the cultural coding of a substance as a pollutant is based in a shared perception of that substance as anomalous to a general symbolic, or cultural, order. Pollutants are coded as "dirt," symbolic "matter out of place." As such, pollutants are at once a product of a specific symbolic order and a danger to it. As dangers to symbolic order, pollutants are also perceived as dangers to social order given that for Douglas—following Durkheim—the symbolic system has functional goals in the maintenance of society. Hence the acknowledgment of pollutants in cultural systems is accompanied by prohibitions the intent of which is the protection of *social* order from disruptive forces symbolized by culturally defined anomalous substances.

Menstrual blood is a particularly apt candidate for analysis in terms of this theory. As blood itself, menstrual discharge is "out of place," breaching the natural bounds of the body that normally contain it. All forms of human bloodshed may be coded as polluting (and are in many cultures; see Durkheim 1897:48 ff.), but menstruation is generally found especially so. Menstrual blood does not issue randomly or accidentally, as does the blood of wounds, but from a single source and to some extent regularly and predictably (but see later discussion)—if, unlike other products of elimination, uncontrollably. Again, in flowing from the reproductive organs of women such blood, rather than signaling a threat to life, is recognized by most peoples as signaling its very possibility. Finally, in the vast majority of the world's societies men have a virtual monopoly on routine or ritual forms of bloodletting: hunting, butchering, warfare, rituals involving sacrifice, mutilation, and scarification alike (Rosaldo and Atkinson 1975). Thus the fact that menstruation may be the only act in which women normatively and routinely let blood may, depending on the culture, constitute a symbolic anomaly. In all of these senses, then, there is a compelling tendency to perceive menstrual blood as "out of place," and more so than other sorts of blood. Hence in terms of Douglas's theory, menstrual blood is perceived as a dire pollutant whose effects must be contained through stringent taboos.

In a follow-up article to *Purity and Danger,* Douglas (1972) revised her initial theory of pollution somewhat. Responding to the work of Tambiah (1969) and Bulmer (1967), Douglas argued that although all pollutants are anomalous in terms of a given symbolic order, not all symbolic anomalies must be coded as polluting. Rather, anomalies are simply "powerful," according to Douglas, their power being granted a negative or positive valence to be determined through specific cultural analysis rather than being attributed cross-culturally. An entity deemed polluting in one culture might, for example, be deemed holy in another (see our earlier discussion of Steiner).

In either case, however, the issue remains "power" and is therefore, as in Douglas's original scheme, an essentially religious matter (1966:49). Two issues are thereby addressed. First, the constitution of laws regarding pollution as supernaturally sanctioned taboos, rather than as mundane rules, becomes comprehensible through recognition of "power" as a concept grounded in spiritual notions (as, for instance, is the case in Polynesian *mana*). Second, in keeping with Durkheim's theory of the relationship between religion and society (1915), the matter of containment of extrahuman power links neatly with the social functions of taboos such as menstrual ones. For Douglas consideration of a symbolic anomaly and religious attention to it lead directly to a consideration of sociological functionality.

The Sociology of Menstrual Pollution

The social functions of religious symbolism were broadly explored early on by Durkheim (1915), and his student Marcel Mauss went on to outline a specific model for a sociological analysis of human body symbolism (1979). Mauss's premise was that symbolically elaborated body concepts mirror the society in which they occur. This insight has been further developed by investigators working on a variety of specific problems in body symbolism, including menstruation.

Other than Durkheim himself (1897), one of the first proponents of a Durkheimian perspective in menstruation studies was Meggitt (1964). Meggitt pointed out that the Mae Enga of New Guinea place unusually strong emphasis on the polluting nature of menstruation, in comparison to other nearby peoples. Meggitt proposed that menstrual pollution serves the Mae Enga as a metaphor for their distrust of outsiders, of which a man's wife is, in this virilocal society, the prototype, as the Enga "marry their enemies."

This kind of analysis, which posits a close relationship between ideas about the body social and the body physical, was greatly extended in the work of Mary Douglas (especially 1970). Pollutants such as menstrual blood that are given meanings within religious systems bespeak, for Douglas, the sociosymbolic logic primary to religion itself (1966:6 ff). By this route Douglas moves firmly back from arbitrary symbolic processes to the determination of those processes by social facts.

In particular Douglas hypothesizes that beliefs about menstrual pollution are found in a restricted number of societies and take on analogous meanings throughout these societies. Menstrual blood is seen as polluting when it symbolically encodes an underlying social-structural ambiguity regarding women and things female. On the one hand a society may have a consciously developed *ideology* of male superiority but, on the other, it may also permit women access to at least some kinds of power, thereby in a sense undermining its own ideology of male dominance. The common fact of menstruation among all women challenges the social order of a male-dominated society and defines and bounds a female subgroup within the society, thereby creating a new separate and dangerous order. Here is a social situation, then, that contains a powerful contradiction, and Douglas suggests that it is in such societies that strong concept of menstrual pollution will arise, signaling the contradiction.

Most recently Balzer (1981) has taken up Douglas's theory, documenting subtly and precisely just how this theory can be used to explain Siberian Khanty menstrual taboos in the wider context of Khanty society. Others have drawn on Douglas's central insight as well, offering variations on its theme. Raymond Kelly (cited in Ortner and Whitehead 1981:20–21) suggests that women are viewed as polluting in societies in which men are dependent on them as sources of prestige—economic, political, or social. Sanday (1981) has also been influenced by Douglas and by Meggitt as well. She proposes that a society will view menstruation as dangerous and polluting if it holds a negative view of its environment as dangerous—threatening starvation—and a concomitant negative relationship with neighboring groups in that environment. Like Meggitt, Sanday predicts that the view of menstrual blood as dangerous mirrors ideas about the outside world, with those ideas being projected onto women's bodies.

Finally, a recent book on reproductive ritual by Karen and Jeffrey Paige (1981) makes further use of Douglas's interpretation. Like Douglas, these authors seek to predict what types of social structures will generate menstrual taboos with (supposedly) concurrent notions of pollution. Paige and Paige postulate that in tribal and band societies one finds the seclusion of menstruous women when there is an unstable economy and, hence, an unstable political base. In this situation, the Paiges hypothesize, men attempt both to maintain control over and to dissociate themselves from women's reproductive cycles. These men seek to demonstrate that they have more of an interest in the society as a whole and in keeping it together in the face of economic hazard than they do in their own narrow conjugal concerns (Paige and Paige 1981:209–254).

The paired theories of menstrual pollution—symbolic and sociological—that have been summarized here have been crucial in shaping current anthropological understanding of menstrual customs and beliefs. How justified is this influence, and in what ways might anthropology now be ready to move on to new theoretical approaches to the topic?

THE LIMITS OF POLLUTION THEORY

Pollution theory, and especially Mary Douglas's initial foray into it (1966), has made notable contributions to knowledge both in anthropology and in other fields, such as the history of religions. Its usefulness, however, is not unbounded. To begin with, there is a clear limit to the fruitfulness of analyses of menstrual blood as "matter out of place," and not recognizing this leaves the replicative analyst open to the dreadful inquiry, "So what?" What, for example, lies beyond the structural grasp of symbolic grammars in the lived experiences of people, once these grammars and their anomalies have been fully explored (see Bruner and Turner 1986)?

The anomalies themselves pose further problems. Although Douglas, in her 1972 article "Self-Evidence," agreed with her critics that symbolic anomalies themselves were of neutral valence, to be "swung" either positively or negatively by the cultural system that determined their anomaly, the possibility that symbols anomalous to one subsystem within a culture could find a securely structured place within an alternate subsystem was not taken up (compare Buckley, this volume). Analyses following Douglas in finding menstrual blood, for instance, polluting because it is anomalous to *the* symbolic system can thus be both overly idealistic and simplistic.

As regards the sociological components of Douglas's overall theory of pollution, the one most frequently utilized by other investigators, there are equivalent problems. The focus on solidarity in male-dominated analytic domains of social action reflects a methodological prejudice, in classic social anthropology, for formal social structures as against informal modes of social organization. "Real" society has been located in large-scale analytic domains—politics, economics, kinship, religion—that are seen as dominated by men occupying named statuses imbued with authority. The often informal structures through which the influence of women may be exercised have customarily been disregarded as inconsequential to this "real" society, as have been formal structures dominated by women (but see, e.g., Weiner 1976). When they have been acknowledged at all, such female-dominated formal structures, and the seemingly more frequent informal ones, have usually been viewed as comprising futile "shadow" societies, generated by male domination and alienated from "real" society (e.g., Wolf 1972). In short, until recently society has been analytically treated as a result of and vehicle for male action.

This effect constitutes the sociological dimension of the cultural theory critiqued earlier: that women are the passive recipients of male-created cultures. It is this male-focal vision of culture and society that underlies analyses of pollution as an index of social-structural tension. The social vision itself, as well as the way in which pollution ideas have been related to it, may reflect the relative domination of the ethnographic record by men, to some extent as anthropologists and, even more, as informants. It is men who have by and large defined menstruation as polluting, and the typical ethnography rarely tells us what the women of the culture at hand think of their own menstrual periods, and those of other women. Thus there hardly seems much solid cross-cultural evidence to support a generalization such as the following, found in a popular text: "There is everywhere a sense that menstruation is unclean. And everywhere women seem to have internalized this attitude to feel shame or unease concerning the natural workings of their own bodies" (Hammond and Jablow 1976:7).

In two of the rare studies that do report the attitudes of individual women toward their menstrual cycles, we find much more variation than this sort of generalization indicates. The Syrian Orthodox Jewish women studied by Kharrazi (1980) express deep ambivalence, while a portion of Skultans's Welsh sample (chapter 6) apparently feel entirely positive about their periods: far from perceiving them as being polluting, these women find in their periods confirmation of their own positively valued womanhood. There is a clear need, then, to consult female informants before reaching any conclusions regarding the status of menstruation as an accepted pollutant in any given society.

However careful Mary Douglas herself may have been in attributing the notion of menstrual pollution only to certain types of societies (those in which there is evidence for strong structural ambiguity regarding women), others have not been so careful. Indeed, when one consults the index of an ethnography, if reference to menstruation is included at all, it is almost invariably included under the rubric of "menstrual pollution." One has the impression that most, if not all, societies view menstruation as a source of pollution, in extension of Douglas's general theory, and that there is no more to be said. Yet it is clear that the situation is hardly that simple, and that the very power of pollution theory, coupled with Western societies' own codings of menstrual blood as a pollutant, has perhaps created "dirt" where none previously existed, or existed only for some people and/or in some contexts in a given culture. The elegance of pollution theory itself can thus manufacture the illusion of overwhelming negativity in symbolic systems where menstruation may be coded ambiguously or even positively.

In the West we are accustomed to thinking of menstruation as largely negative. It is "the curse" or, more fully, "the curse of Eve": a part of God's punishment of women for Eve's role in the Biblical Fall (Wood 1981).[1] We are not alone in holding such a view, but it is hardly a universal one. Niangoran-Bouah (1964:52) reports, for instance, that among the Ebrié of Ivory Coast it is forbidden to collect fruits of trees protected by their owners with certain mystically powerful objects. If a man disobeys this taboo he is afflicted with impotence until he confesses to the owner; if a woman picks the fruit she is afflicted with amenorrhea—*losing* her period (rather than enduring it for eternity like the daughters of Eve) until she confesses. In this case menstruation would appear to be the female counterpart of the masculine erection: associated with fertility, not pollution; desirable, and traumatic to lose. As the Ebrié case shows, menstruation is by no means coded as a universal negative.

Moreover, the widespread exclusive use of males as ethnographic informants tends to place analytic stress on the vulnerability of men to female pollution and the consequent efforts of men to distance themselves from the sources of such pollution. Yet the consistency of reported male testimony regarding menstrual pollution disguises complexities of various kinds.

First, where there is a documented ideology of menstrual pollution, close reading often reveals that not all men are deemed vulnerable to a woman's polluting influence, but only certain classes of men—for example, husbands (e.g., Thompson 1985:706) or old men (Gottlieb, this volume). Second, women are not alone in being suspected of contaminating influence during their periods; often their husbands must share the ritual restrictions incumbent upon their menstruating wives, as among the Hadza of Tanzania (in Douglas 1968:23). The !Gwi of southern Africa, by the same token, initiate the husbands of menarcheal women together with their young wives, the two being scarified and decorated in identical manner (Silberbauer 1963:21–22). Such cases as those of the Hadza and !Gwi suggest that although pollution may be an issue in a given culture, other matters may be equally of concern. Most pertinent here is a notion of *shared substance* between husband and wife, which is quite similar to that shared substance stressed by anthropologists in analyses of the *couvade* (symbolic joint pregnancy and birth labor) which the menstrual practices of the Hadza and !Gwi resemble (see Rivière 1974–75).[2]

Both Hadza and !Gwi men (at least) do view menstruation as polluting. The meanings of menstruation cannot be exhausted in either case through a simple theory of pollution, however, for in both there is at least one other constitutent—the idea of shared substance. As we suggested for "taboo," culturally constituted symbolic anomalies such as menstrual blood may gather meaning from two directions at once to be both negative, or polluting, and positively powerful. The shortcoming of pollution theory in the analysis of menstrual meanings is that it can too easily obscure, through its own elegance, such potential multivalence. In explanations of menstrual symbolism through it, understanding too easily escapes us. We illustrate this crucial point through further ethnographic examples.

Ritual Uses of Menstrual Blood

The heuristic value of interpreting menstrual blood as an anomalous substance whose power is gained through its relationship to other items in a symbolic structure is clear (Gottlieb forthcoming); again and again menstrual discharge has indeed been granted the extraordinary powers of the anomalous, or "liminal" (Turner 1969). The symbolically constituted power of menstrual blood makes it, "naturally," in Douglas's terms (1970), a prime substance for manipulation in rituals. At the same time, its frequently multiple meanings as well as its symbolic arbitrariness suit it for use in a variety of rituals with diverse and even contradictory intent, both intra- and cross-culturally.

As a culturally specified pollutant, menstrual blood is an obvious candidate for ritual use with the negative intent of bringing harm to others, especially through witchcraft. Thus among the Mae Enga, it is held that "menstrual blood introduced into a man's food . . . quickly kills him, and young women crossed in love sometimes seek their revenge in this way" (Meggitt 1964:207). Similar alleged uses of menstrual blood may be cited for any number of cultures, in most of which—as in New Guinea—avoidance of this substance is conjoined with a fear of those who are reputed to *seek* contact with it for unscrupulous purposes. Menstrual witchcraft, where it is reported, need not necessarily be voluntary. For example, in China, according to Ahern (1975:194–195), people say that menstrual blood adheres to the ground, making it dangerous to walk on the streets. The use of menstrual blood in witchcraft thus seems to exist within a continuum of negative effects and manipulations all reflecting a clear underlying notion of pollution. Quite opposite effects and ritual manipulations have also been reported, however, that cannot be resolved through pollution theory.

Probably the most commonly reported *positive* use of menstrual blood is in the manufacture of various kinds of love charms and potions. These occur in cultures as diverse as the medieval farmers and shepherds of southwestern France (Ladurie 1979:32), the Beng of Ivory Coast (Gottlieb, 1988), and rural whites in the United States. Kirksey (1984:32) gives the following fictional but ethnographically informed rendering of a conversation in Southern Illinois:

> "You remember your Uncle Skinny and your Aunt Jac, don't you?"
>
> "Yes, ma'am," Ward said. "I remembers them pretty well."
>
> "Maybe you don't remember this, but your Uncle Skinny snuck around on your aunt a lot. That is, till she come to me, said that Skinny was stepping out on her, said she wanted to

keep him at home. So I told her to put a spoonful of her 'time of the month' in his coffee regularly. If she did, he'd never leave her. Of course, you know what happened, I'm sure. Your uncle died in your aunt's arms, loving her to the very end."

Ward was shocked to hear the tale, but he remembered his Uncle Skinny's often docile, loving manner toward Aunt Jac.

We also find accounts of *men* using menstrual blood to ensure the fidelity of their wives, as Pliny reported for Imperial Rome (in Novak 1916:273). These accounts seem better analyzed in terms of a theory of shared substance, as discussed earlier, than one of pollution. Their sense would not seem exhaustible by this or any other single cross-cultural theory, however, for the accounts themselves arise within a literature replete with positive uses of menstrual blood that cannot be explained through a notion of shared substance—such as the medicinal uses described earlier—but, rather, seem to have in common only the general theme of "power."

Such power has been specified through a variety of metaphors—"pollution," "shared substance," and others. Among such metaphors that of "life force" (Kuper 1947:107) is perhaps most striking. In this case menstrual blood is viewed as an emblem or manifestation of creative power, particularly in the sense of fertility. Thus the use of menstrual blood in fertility rituals is widespread (and, it would seem, conceptually linked to the use of this substance in love charms). The Nigerian Tiv use menstrual blood in the *imborivungu* ("owl pipe") ritual, which also involves human sacrifice (Lincoln 1975:51 ff.) Menstrual blood is mixed with that of a sacrificial child in a ritual pipe as a central act in an elaborate ritual through which the farms surrounding a ritual center are blessed, and their fertility—and that of the women who inhabit them—ensured. (For other examples see Poole 1982:105; Jetté 1911:257, 403; Yalman 1964:135.)

The use of menstrual symbols in the enhancement of life force (in the sense of fertility) seems to point in two directions at once: toward a better understanding of pollution, when it is manipulated toward the protection of life, and toward an appreciation of folk-biological components in culturally specific menstrual meanings. This complex, even dialectical, situation may again be illuminated through ethnographic examples.

Menstrual blood is often used in symbolically powerful objects the purpose of which is to keep life-threatening forces at bay. Among the Kwakiutl, for example, "the malignant power which menstrual blood was believed to have for human beings extended to monsters; therefore when women were traveling, they kept some menstrual blood in a bit of shredded bark to be used to poison a monster should one appear" (Ford 1941:35). In this instance the polluting powers of menstruation are linked with its status as a symbol of life force to be manipulated in such a way that its very negativity protects life itself.

We suspect that such a dialectical relationship between the negative and positive poles of symbolic menstrual power is found more commonly than has been remarked upon. An example is provided by the well-studied Asante of Ghana. According to Rattray (1927:74–75, 211, 234, 271), menstruating Asante women are subject to numerous taboos, some of which are kept under pain of immediate, automatic death. The strength of menstrual pollution may, however, be used by priests in assuring their own safety. Asante priests manufacture fetishes (*kunkuma*) of brooms defiled with menstrual blood, and "a priest is supposed to be safe without any other protective charm provided he has with him his *kunkuma*" (Rattray 1927:14). The logic appears simple enough: potent, negatively valued substances such as menstrual blood may be manipulated for positive ends by those who are themselves spiritually potent enough to reverse the valence and make it positive. Yet the Asante case exhibits further complications.

Although the Asante view menstrual blood as definitively polluting, subject to "one of the greatest and deadliest taboos in Ashanti"

(Rattray 1927:13), they also celebrate menarche with an elaborate ritual for individual girls in which the menarcheal girl, among other things, sits in public view beneath an umbrella (a symbol generally reserved for kings and other dignitaries), receiving gifts and congratulations and observing singing and dancing performed in her honor (Rattray 1927:69–74). Within Asante society, then, menstrual symbolism is highly complex. Menstrual blood itself causes dire pollution (especially to ancestral altars), yet menarche is celebrated with profound honors and, moreover, priests use menstrual blood toward positive ends. Among the Asante as among comparable peoples, we are in a realm far beyond the grasp of any single model of menstruation-as-pollution.

We suggest that such diversity in meaning is strongly tied to indigenous conceptions of the biological function of menstruation in the reproductive cycles of women. Though this has been symbolized in different ways among different peoples, particularly widespread conceptions focus on the symbolic role of menstruation in human fertility. When they are found these ideas further undermine the utility of a simple pollution model of menstruation.

Menstruation and Gestation

In the medieval European interpretation of Aristotle's biology, menstrual blood was held to be the "matter" to which semen supplied "form," creating the fetus (Wood 1981:715–719). In this system excess menstrual blood was retained in the womb, providing the basis for lactation at parturition (Wood 1981). The basic elements of this folk-biological theory of conception and lactation are widespread, found in many cultures that, like medieval Europe, also view menstrual blood as a pollutant.

For example, the Paiela of New Guinea have a highly elaborate theory of conception in which menstrual blood is held to be "bound" slowly by semen introduced into the womb through repeated intercourse (Biersack 1983). (Also see Evans-Pritchard 1932:407 on the Azande of the Sudan; O'Flaherty 1980:42 on fourth-century India; and Laqueur 1986 on Europe through the Renaissance.) The Mohave Indians of southern California give an added twist to this general theory, viewing the blood of parturition as "a sort of super-menstruation, expelling all at once the accumulated menstrual blood of ten missed periods" (Devereux 1950:253), and deeming this blood polluting, as they do menstrual blood.

Such folk theories—and they are both numerous and widely distributed (see Ford 1945)[3]—both complicate efforts to analyze menstrual symbolism purely in terms of a theory of pollution and, at the same time, inform that theory. The negativity of menstruation is necessarily made ambiguous by the inclusion of the menstrual cycle among the reproductive processes, which is generally viewed quite positively. Ernestine Friedl (1975:29) remarks that the very occurrence of menstruation can be interpreted as a sign of death, insofar as it is a signal that a new life has not been conceived. Friedl finds an explanation of menstrual taboos and notions of menstrual pollution in this connection between menstruation and death (but see Gottlieb 1988 for a different view).

We hypothesize that where the fetus is held to be menstrually constituted, one will find strong menstrual taboos and assertions of pollution. This is based on the supposition that such taboos and ideologies reflect a notion that the proper role of menstrual blood is in the formation of new life, and that its flow beyond the boundaries of women's bodies marks a missed opportunity for procreation. Our hypothesis would illuminate the observation of Vosselmann (1935:79) that "without a doubt this blood that is so useful . . . when it was retained in the womb lost these [useful] qualities as soon as it began to escape from it" (our translation). In this way the presence of menstrual taboos and notions of menstrual pollution, far from signaling the inherent pollution of the female principle as has so often been postulated, may instead point toward a more complex and far-reaching conceptual system that includes elements of folk-biology to constitute the basis for the meaning of the taboos themselves.

This would seem to be the case in Swazi culture, as reported by Kuper (1947; also see Wright 1982 on the Navajo): "menstrual blood is . . . considered part of the foetus that grows within the womb—its discharge is analogous to a miscarriage" (Kuper 1947:107). In keeping with our hypothesis, the Swazi say that menstrual blood can pollute crops, cattle, and men alike. However, Kuper continues (1947:107),

> In certain situations . . . menstrual blood is not destructive, but is considered a life symbol or rather a life force; thus the recurrence of menstruation after a woman gives birth "washes her" and enables her to cohabit again with her husband, and after a death in the family circle, a man should not cohabit with his wife until she has menstruated.

In this case menstruation both pollutes and purifies: "The verb (Z[ulu]) *geza,* to wash, purify after death, is a euphemism for menstruation. The flow of blood pollutes women yet also cleanses after death or bearing a child" (Kuper 1947:107). (A parallel understanding occurs in certain rabbinical commentaries among Orthodox Jews, as in this Talmudic scholar's verse: "As yeast is good for dough, / so is menstruation good for women"—cited in Vosselmann 1935:121.)

Our hypothesis may explain a certain percentage, but undoubtedly not all, of those cases in which notions of menstrual pollution are found. That is, it should explain those societies in which are found an idea both of menstrual pollution *and* of the menstrual constitution of the fetus. We hope future researchers will pursue this line of inquiry. They will need to take into account indigenous perceptions of biological processes.

NOTES

1. The Christian tradition is not entirely negative in its view of menstruation. Jesus, for example, is said to have cured a woman of the "plague" of "an issue of blood" that had lasted twelve years, making her "whole" (Mark 5:25–29). According to Mark, the incident occurred between Jesus's casting out of "unclean spirits" and "the devil" from the possessed (Mark 5:1–19), and his raising of the daughter of Jairus from death (Mark 5:23–24, 35–43). It is emphasized, however, that Jairus's daughter "was of the age of twelve years" (Mark 5:42), and the structural sense of the juxtaposition of the twelve years of dysmenorrhea, in the sick woman, and the girl's age—when coupled with other Judeo-Christian references to the age of women at menarche—is that Jesus restored the daughter of Jairus to life in the sense of full, fecund womanhood; that is, that "life" in this instance is equated positively with menarche (Jorunn Jacobsen Buckley, personal communication, 1984).

   Ambivalence may well be embedded in the very way Westerners talk about menstruation. In an early study of menstrual euphemisms in several European languages, Joffe found that such expressions fall into five general categories of metaphor: time, color, visitors, other persons, and disabilities (1948:184). Terence Hays (n.d.) is currently researching this subject, and when combined with Joffe's work, Hays's preliminary findings make it clear that in English and other European languages women express diverse perceptions of their own menstrual periods though euphemisms.
2. The notion of shared substances is not only pertinent to the analysis of some menstrual customs, such as joint husband/wife restrictions and rituals, but also to other types of beliefs regarding menstruation. The ideology that menstrual blood is inherited from the mother is widespread, especially in matrilineal societies. Mary Douglas (1969) and Wyatt MacGaffey (1969), however, have both pointed out that it is not just menstrual blood that is thought to be so inherited but veinous blood as well, and that such beliefs are not restricted to matrilineal societies. Here the topic of shared substance—an underinvestigated one, we think—connects with a wide variety of ideas regarding the composition of fetuses, examined below.
3. Ford (1945:44–46) gives nine examples of societies that hold the fetus to be composed wholly or in part from menstrual blood. Richards (1950:222–223) and M. Wilson (1957:299) both propose that such a view is found in societies in which descent is reckoned matrilin-

eally. But in accord with Douglas and MacGaffey (see note 2), we do find evidence of this notion being associated with patrilineal descent as well, as it is among the Azande of the Sudan, the Kwoma of New Guinea, and the Lepcha of Tibet and Mongolia (Ford 1945:44).

REFERENCES

Ahern, Emily Martin. 1975. "The power and pollution of Chinese Women." In *Women and the Family in Rural Taiwan,* M. Wolf and R. Witke, eds., pp. 193–214. Palo Alto: Stanford University Press.

Balzer, Majorie Mandelstam. 1981. "Rituals of gender identity: Markers of Siberian Khanty ethnicity, status and belief." *American Anthropologist* 83: 850–867.

Biersack Aletta. 1983. "Bound blood: Paiela "conception" theory interpreted." *Mankind* 14: 85–100.

Bruner, Edward M. and Victor W. Turner, eds. 1986. *The Anthropology of Experience.* Urbana: University of Illinois Press.

Buckley, Thomas. 1988. "Menstruation and the power of Yurok women." In *Blood Magic: The Anthropology of Menstruation,* Thomas Buckley and Alma Gottlieb, eds., pp. 187–209. Berkeley: University of California Press.

Bulmer, Ralph. 1967. "Why is the cassowary not a bird: A problem in zoological taxonomy among the Karam of the New Guinea Highlands." *Man* 2: 5–25.

Devereux, George. 1950. "The psychology of feminine genital bleeding." *International Journal of Psycho-Analysis* 31: 237–257.

Douglas, Mary. 1966. *Purity and Danger: An Analysis of Concepts of Pollution and Taboo.* London: Routledge & Kegan Paul.

Douglas, Mary. 1968. "The relevance of tribal studies." *Journal of Psychosomatic Research* 12: 21–28. Reprinted as "Couvade and menstruation: The relevance of tribal studies." In *Implicit Meanings,* M. Douglas, ed., pp. 60–72. London: Routledge & Kegan Paul.

Douglas, Mary. 1969. "Correspondence: Virgin Birth." *Man* 4: 133–134.

Douglas, Mary. 1970. *Natural Symbols.* London: Barrie & Rockliff.

Douglas, Mary. 1972. "Self-evidence." The Henry Myers Lecture. Proceedings of the Royal Anthropological Institute for 1972: 27–43. Reprinted in *Implicit Meanings,* M. Douglas, ed., 276–318. London: Routledge & Kegan Paul.

Durkheim, Emile. 1897. "La prohibition de l'inceste et ses origines." *L'Annee Sociologique* 1: 1–70.

Durkheim, Emile. 1915. *The elementary forms of the religious life,* trans. Joseph Ward Swain. London: George Allen & Unwin. (Original publication: *Les formes elementaires de la vie religieuse, le systeme totemique en Australie.* Paris: F. Alcan, Travaux de l'Annee Sociologique, 1911.)

Evans-Pritchard, E. E. 1932. "Heredity and gestation as the Zande see them." *Sociologus* 8: 400–413.

Ford, Clellan. 1941. *Smoke from their fires.* New Haven: Yale University Press.

Ford, Clellan. 1945. *A Comparative Study of Human Reproduction.* New Haven: Yale University Press.

Friedl, Ernestine. 1975. *Women and Men: An Anthropologist's View.* New York: Holt, Rinehart & Winston.

Gottlieb, Alma. 1988. "Menstrual cosmology among the Beng of Ivory Coast." In *Blood Magic: The Anthropology of Menstruation,* Thomas Buckley and Alma Gottlieb, eds., pp. 55–74. Berkeley: University of California Press.

Gottlieb, Alma. 1990. "Rethinking Female Pollution: The Beng Case (Cote d'Ivoire). "In *Beyond the Second Sex: Essays in the Anthropology of Gender,* Peggy Sanday, ed., pp. 113–138. Philadelphia: University of Pennsylvania Press.

Hammond, Dorothy and Alta Jablow. 1976. *Women in Cultures of the World.* Menlo Park, CA: Benjamin Cummings.

Hays, Terence E. n.d. *Menstrual Expressions and Menstrual Attitudes.* Unpublished manuscript.

Jette, A. Julius. 1911. "On the superstitions of the Ten'a Indians (middle part of the Yukon Valley, Alaska.)" *Anthropos* 6: 95–108, 241–259, 602–615, 699–723.

Joffe, Natalie F. 1948. "The Vernacular of Menstruation." *Word* 4(3): 181–186.

Kharrazi, Lily. 1980. "State of Separation: Syrian Jewish women and menstruation." *National Women's Anthropology Newsletter* 4, no. 2: 13–14, 27.

Kirksey, Matthew. 1984. "Dying." *Grassroots 1984* (Southern Illinois University at Carbondale), 32–35.

Kuper, Hilda. 1947. *An African aristocracy: Rank among the Swazi.* London: Oxford University Press for the International African Institute.

Ladurie, Emmanual Le Roy. 1979. *Montaillou: The promised land of error.* New York: Random House.

Laquer, Thomas. 1986. "Orgasm, generation, and the politics of reproductive biology." *Representations 14* (Spring) : 1–41. "Special Issue: Sexuality and the Social Body in the Nineteenth Century."

Lincoln, Bruce. 1975. "The religious significance of woman's scarification among the Tiv." *Africa* 45: 316–326.

MacGaffey, Wyatt. 1969. Correspondence: Virgin Birth. *Man* 4: 457

Mauss, Marcel. 1979. "Body techniques." In *Sociology and psychology, Essays by Marcel Mauss,* trans. Ben Brewster, 95–123. London: Routledge & Kegan Paul. (Original French publication 1935.)

Meggitt, Mervyn J. 1964. "Male-female relationships in the Highlands of Australian New Guinea." *American Anthropologist* 66, no. 4, pt. 2: 204–224.

Niangoran-Bouah, Georges. 1964. *La Division du temps et le calendrier ritual des peuples lagunaires de Cote- d'Ivoire.* Paris: Institut d'Ethnologie.

Novak, Emil, M. D. 1916. "The superstition and folklore of menstruation." *Johns Hopkins Hospital Bulletin* 27, no. 307: 270–274 (26 September).

O'Flaherty, Wendy Doniger. 1980. *Women, androgynes, and other Mythical beasts.* Chicago: University of Chicago Press.

Ortner, Sherry B. and Harriet Whitehead. 1981. "Introduction: Accounting for sexual meanings." In *Sexual Meanings,* S. B. Ortner and H. Whitehead, eds., pp. 1–27. Cambridge: Cambridge University Press.

Paige, Karen Ericksen and Jeffrey M. Paige. 1981. *The Politics of Reproductive Ritual.* Berkeley, Los Angeles, London: University of California Press.

Poole, Fitz John Porter. 1982. "The ritual forging of identity: Aspects of person and self in Bimin-Kuskusmin male initiation." In *Rituals of Manhood,* G. H. Herdt, ed., pp. 9–154. Berkeley, Los Angeles, London: University of California Press.

Rattray, R. S. 1927. *Religion and art in Ashanti.* Oxford: Clarendon Press.

Richards, Audrey I. 1950. "Some Types of Family Structure amongst the Central Bantu." In *African Systems of Kinship and Marriage,* A. R. Radcliffe-Brown and Daryll Forde, eds. London: Oxford University Press.

Riviere, Peter G. 1974–1975. "Couvade: A problem reborn." *Man* 9: 423–435; 10: 476.

Rosaldo, Michelle Zimbalist and Jane Monnig Atkinson. 1975. "Man the hunter and woman: Metaphors for the sexes in Ilongot magical spells." In *The interpretation of symbolism,* Roy Willis, ed., pp. 43–75. London: J. M. Dent & Sons, Ltd.; New York: John Wiley & Sons.

Sanday, Peggy. 1981. *Female Power and Male Dominance: On the Origins of Sexual Inequality.* Cambridge: Cambridge University Press.

Silberbauer, George B. 1963. "Marriage and the girl's puberty ceremony of the G/wi Bushmen." *Africa* 33, no. 4: 12–26.

Tambiah, S. J. 1969. "Animals are good to think and good to prohibit." *Ethnology* 8, no. 4: 423–459.

Thompson, Catherine. 1985. "The power to pollute and the power to preserve: Perceptions of female power in a Hindu village." *Social Science and Medicine* 21, no. 6: 701–711.

Turner, Victor. 1969. *The Ritual Process: Structure and Anti-Structure.* Chicago: Aldine.

Vosselmann, Fritz. 1935. "La menstruation: Legendes, coutumes et superstitions." Lyon: Faculte de Medicine et de Pharmacie de Lyon. *Annee Scolaire* 1935–1936, no. 23. These de Docteur en Medicine.

Weiner, Annette B. 1976. *Women of Value, Men of Renown: New Perspectives in Trobriand Exchange.* Austin: University of Texas Press.

Wilson, Monica. 1957. *Rituals of Kinship among the Nyakyusa.* London: Oxford University Press.

Wolf, Margery. 1972. *Women and the family in rural Taiwan.* Stanford: Stanford University Press.

Wood, Charles T. 1981. "The doctors' dilemma: Sin, salvation, and the menstrual cycle in medieval thought." *Speculum* 56: 710–727.

Wright, Anne. 1982. "Attitudes toward childbearing and menstruation among the Navajo." In *Anthropology of Human Birth,* Margarita Artschwager Kay, ed., pp. 377–394. Philadelphia: F. A. Davis Co.

Yalman, Nur. 1964. "Sinhalese healing rituals." *Journals of Asian Studies* 23: 115–150.

V

CULTURE AND SEXUALITY

The study of sexuality in anthropology is a relatively recent research emphasis. Classic anthropological monographs have reported exotic sexual practices in the course of ethnographic description (for example, we learn in Malinowski's *The Sexual Life of Savages* [1929] that the Trobriand islanders may bite each others' eyelashes in the heat of passion), but other than occasional esoterica, the naturalistic, biological bias has dominated the study of sexuality. However, as Vance observes (1984: 8), "although sexuality, like all human cultural activity, is grounded in the body, the body's structure, physiology, and functioning do not directly or simply determine the configuration or meaning of sexuality." Rather, sexuality is in large part culturally constructed. Just as we may inquire into the culturally variable meanings of masculinity and femininity, we may examine the ways in which sexuality is invested with meaning in particular societies (Ortner and Whitehead 1981: 2).

Sexuality, as a topic of analysis, links the personal and the social, the individual and society. To Americans sex may imply medical facts, Freud, and erotic techniques, but all of these aspects of sexuality are socially shaped and inevitably curbed. Within every culture there are measures for the management of sexuality and gender expression (Ortner and Whitehead 1981: 24–25) and sanctions for those who break the rules.

These sanctions may be imposed at the level of the family, the lineage, the community, or the state. Indeed, Foucault (1981) has suggested that a feature of the recent past is the increasing intervention of the state in the domain of sexuality. In this regard Ross and Rapp (1981: 71) conclude that it is not accidental that contemporary western culture conceptualizes sex as a thing in itself, isolated from social, political, and economic context: "The separation with industrial capitalism of family life from work, of consumption from production, of leisure from labour, of personal life from political life, has completely reorganized the context in which we experience sexuality. . . . Modern consciousness permits, as earlier systems of thought did not, the positing of 'sex' for perhaps the first time as having an 'independent' existence." However, Caplan (1987: 24) warns that while western culture may have a concept of sexuality divorced from reproduction, marriage, or other social domains, it is not possible to analyze sexuality without reference to the economic, political, and cultural matrix in which it is embedded.

A comparative perspective informs us that the attributes of the person seen as sexual and erotic vary cross-culturally. For example, scarification, the corsetted waist, bound feet, and the subincised penis are admired and provocative in particular cultures. Such attributes as these are not only physical symbols of sexuality, but indicators of status. Similarly, Sudanese women enforce infibulation, or pharonic circumcision, causing serious pain and health risks to young women, for the honor of the lineage. In the name of power young men applied as recruits to the palace eunuch staff in Imperial China carrying their genitals in jars (Ortner and Whitehead 1981: 24). These examples are reminders of the power of social concerns and cultural meanings in the domain of sexuality.

Abu-Lughod (in this book) explores the cultural construction of sexuality and local meanings of Islam through an analysis of wedding rituals in a Bedouin community in Egypt's Western Desert. Weddings produce and transform people's experiences of sexuality and gender relations, and serve as a marker of cultural identity. Whereas sexuality in North America is considered something essentially private, separate from society and social power, to these Bedouin the wedding involves sexuality that has a public and participatory element. Connections to kin and control of the kinship group are symbolized in wedding rites. The sexual politics of gender relations were formerly portrayed in women's wedding songs and dances. Changing power relations have led to a deemphasis of this mechanism for challenging male power. As Bedouins are drawn into the wider Egyptian state and economy, weddings increasingly are seen as entertainment and spectacle, rather than as the ritual reproduction of the social and political dynamics of the community.

Research in hunting and gathering societies also shows that sexual intercourse, while personal, can also be a political act. In such societies, claims to women are central to men's efforts to achieve equal status with others (Collier and Rosaldo 1981: 291). Through sexual relations with women, men forge relationships with one another and symbolically express claims to particular women. Shostak (in this book) presents the perspective of a !Kung woman, Nisa, on sex, marriage, and fertility in the broader context of a hunting and gathering society in which women have high status.

In !Kung society children learn about sex through observation. Boys and girls play at parenthood and marriage. If they are caught playing at sex, they are scolded but are not severely punished. No value is placed on virginity, and the female body need not be covered or hidden. A girl is not expected to have sex until the onset of menstruation, usually age 16. During adolescence, both heterosexual and homosexual sex play is permitted, and sexual liaisons outside of marriage are also permissible.

The !Kung believe that without sex, people can die, just as without food, one would starve. Shostak observes that "talk about sex seems to be of almost equal importance [to eating]. When women are in the village or out gathering, or when men and women are together, they spend hours recounting details of sexual exploits. Joking about all aspects of sexual experience is commonplace" (1983: 265). According to Nisa, "If a woman doesn't have sex . . . her thoughts get ruined and she is always angry" (Shostak 1983: 31).

From Nisa, Shostak elicits the history of her relationships with men, in particular her former husband and constant admirer, Besa, who abandons her while she is pregnant but later tries to persuade her to return and live with him as his wife. Although he seeks the intervention of the headman, Nisa refuses to return to him, and the headman supports her decision. Nisa's characterization of sexuality among the !Kung suggests that for both men and women engaging in sex is necessary to maintaining good health and is an important aspect of being human.

In contrast, for the past 150 years Anglo-American culture has defined women as less sexual than men. This represents a major shift from the widespread view prior to the seventeenth century that women were especially sexual creatures (Caplan 1987: 3). By the end of the nineteenth century the increasingly authoritative voice of male medical specialists argued that women were characterized by sexual anesthesia (Caplan 1987: 3). Victorian ideas about male sexuality emphasized the highly sexed and baser nature of men. In contrast, Muslim concepts of female sexuality (Mernissi 1987: 33) cast the woman as aggressor and the man as victim. Imam Ghazali, writing in the eleventh century, describes an active female sexuality in which the sexual demands of women appear overwhelming and the need for men to satisfy them is a social duty (Mernissi 1987: 39). Women symbolize disorder and are representative of the dangers of sexuality and its disruptive potential.

The example of the Kaulong of New Guinea further illustrates the extent to which understandings of male and female sexual natures are cultural products (Goodale 1980). Both sexes aspire to immortality through the reproduction of identity achieved through parenting. Sexual intercourse, which is considered animal-like, is sanctioned for married people. Animals are part of the forest and nature, so the gardens of married couples are in the forest. The only sanctioned purpose of sex and marriage is reproduction; sex without childbearing is viewed as shameful. Suicide was formerly considered an acceptable recourse for a childless couple. Sexual activity is thought to be dangerous to men and women in different ways: polluting for men and leading to dangers of birth for women. Goodale notes that girls are encouraged to behave aggressively toward men, to initiate sex, and to choose a husband. In contrast, men are reluctant to engage in sex, are literally "scared to death of marriage," and rarely take the dominant role in courtship (1980: 135). Thus, the Kaulong view seems to reverse the western idea of the passive woman and the active man (Moore 1988: 17).

Attempting to explain such variations in cultural constructions of sexuality, Caplan (1987) suggests that when desire for children is high, fertility and sexuality are hardly distinguished; biological sex is important and impediments to procreation (e.g., contraception, homosexuality) are viewed as wicked. Caplan shows that Hindu tradition values celibacy, although there may be a life stage in which an individual is sexually active. The spirit is valued over the flesh, and celibacy represents a purer and higher state than sexual activity. In contrast, a spirit-flesh dichotomy is less common in Africa and the Caribbean, where sexual activity is thought to be a part of healthy living (Nelson 1987: 234–235). When fertility is less valued, sexual activity is more open and less regulated, and sexuality becomes an aspect of self, not of parenthood. Thus, control of female fertility is linked to control of sexual behavior; when sexual activity is thought to be a prerequisite for good health, there tends to be greater sexual autonomy for women.

Gender, referring to sociocultural designations of behavioral and psychosocial qualities of sexes (Jacobs and Roberts 1989), is commonly contrasted with sex, or the observable biophysiological, morphological characteristics of the individual. Gilmore (in this book) examines the relationship between sex and gender in his analysis of the often dramatic ways in which cultures construct appropriate manhood. He finds a recurring notion that "real manhood is different from simple anatomical maleness, that it is not a natural condition that comes about spontaneously through biological maturation but rather is a precarious or artificial state that boys must win against powerful odds" (1990: 11).

To Gilmore the answer to the manhood puzzle lies in culture. He examines a post-Freudian understanding of masculinity as a category of self-identity, showing how boys face special problems in separating from their mother. A boy's separation and individuation is more perilous and difficult than a girl's, whose femininity is reinforced by the original unity with her mother. Thus, to become separate the boy must pass a test, breaking the chain to his mother. Ultimately, Gilmore concludes that manhood ideologies force men to shape up "on penalty of being robbed of their identity." Men are not innately different from women, but they need motivation to be assertive.

Gilmore notes that some cultures also provide for alternative gender constructs. Popular thinking in the United States dichotomizes two sexes, male and female, and corresponding gender identities, masculinity and femininity, leaving little room for culturally defined variance. Some research suggests at least three phenotypic sexes in human cultures: female, male, and androgynous or hermaphroditic people. This classification refers to characteristics observable to the naked eye rather than to medical classifications of sex types based on chromosomal evidence (Jacobs and Roberts 1989: 440). Linguistic markers for gender reveal culturally specific epistemological categories (Jacobs and Roberts 1989: 439). Accordingly, in English one may distinguish woman, lesbian, man, or gay male. The Chuckchee counted seven genders—three female and four male—while the Mohave reportedly recognize four genders—a woman, a woman who assumes the roles of men, a man, or a male who assumes the roles of women (Jacobs and Roberts 1989: 439–440). Thus, crosscultural research suggests that we need to use categories of sex and gender that reflect the evidence of diversity rather than rigid classification systems.

In any culture genders are recognized, named, and given meaning in accordance with the culture's rules or customs (Jacobs and Roberts 1989: 446). When a baby is born people generally rely on the apperance of the infant's external genitalia to determine whether that child will be treated as female or male. As a child grows, more criteria come into play, such as the phenotypic expression of sex—facial hair, voice, and breast development. In some societies spiritual development and interests may be used as criteria for gender attribution. One such example is the hijras of Indian society. The hijra role attracts people who in the West might be called eunuchs, homosexuals, transsexuals, transvestites, or hermaphrodites.

The hijra role is deeply rooted in Indian culture, and it accommodates a variety of sexual needs, gender behaviors and identities, and personalities. Nanda (in this book) shows that Hinduism encompasses ambiguities and contradictions in gender categories without trying to resolve them. In Hindu myths, rituals, and art, the theme of the powerful man-woman is significant; mythical figures who are androgynes figure in popular Indian culture. Thus the hijra represents an institutionalized third gender role.

Hinduism holds that all people contain both male and female principles, and in some sects male transvestism is used as a way of achieving salvation. There are many references in Hinduism to alternative sexes and sexual ambiguity. However, hijras are viewed ambivalently and can inspire both fear and mockery. Ancient writings indicate criticism of homosexuality, but in actuality homosexuals were tolerated, following the counsel of the classic Hindu text, the Kamasutra, that in sex one should act according to the custom of one's country and one's own inclination. Hijras see themselves as humans, neither man nor woman, calling into question basic social categories of gender. The accommodation of the hijras reflects the extent to which contradictions are embraced and tolerated in Indian culture.

Additional examples of cultures that tolerate gender ambiguity are found in Native American societies, in which a male who felt an affinity for female occupation, dress, and attributes could choose to become classified as a two-spirit, sometimes known as a berdache. Williams (in this book) discusses alternative gender identities for Native American women whom he calls amazons; others refer to them as "cross gender females" or female berdache. According to Williams' use of the term, an amazon is a woman who has manifested an unfeminine character from infancy, has shown no interest in heterosexual relations, and might have expressed a wish to become a man. Such women were known for their bravery and skill as warriors. For example, Kaska Indians would select a daughter to be a son if they had none; after a transformation ritual the daughter would dress like a man and be trained for male tasks. Ingalik Indians also recognize such a status; in this society the amazons even participated in male-only sweat baths. The woman was accepted as a man on the basis of her gender behavior (Williams, in this book).

The assignment of this changed gender "operates independently of a person's morphological sex and can determine both gender status and erotic behavior" (Williams 1986: 235). In some societies a woman could choose to be a man, as among the Kutenai Indians. The "manlike woman" was greatly respected, although the Kutenai did not recognize a similar status for men. A tribe with an alternative gender role for one sex did not necessarily have one for the other, and the roles were not seen as equivalent. The Mohave also recognized the status of amazons, subjecting these women to a ritual that authorized them to assume the clothing, sexual activity, and occupation of the opposite, self-chosen sex. It is sometimes believed that such women do not menstruate because menstruation is a crucial part of the definition of a woman. However, the category of amazon is distinct from that of men or women. It is another gender status. Thus, some Native American cultures have a flexible recognition of gender variance, and they incorporate fluidity in their world view.

Sexuality, as differentiated from sex and gender, refers to sexual behaviors, feelings, thoughts, practices, and sexually based bonding behaviors (bisexuality, heterosexuality, homosexuality) (Jacobs and Roberts 1989: 440). Sexual identity, involving an individual's self-attribution of sex preferences and practices, is both a response to and an influence on sexuality. In western culture today sexuality is thought to comprise an important part of one's identity, the core of self (Caplan 1987: 2). In the United States, where heterosexual relations are the norm, the dominant ideology suggests that heterosexuality is innate and natural. Lesbianism may be threatening to male dominance, while male homosexuality threatens male solidarity and the sense of masculine identity. In other cultures, however, gender and sexuality are conceptually separate. For example, Shepherd (1987) shows that for Swahili Muslims of Mombasa, Kenya, being in a homosexual relationship does not change one's gender, which is essentially assigned by biological sex.

In American society sexuality is an integral part of identity on a personal and a social level. Sexuality not only classifies one as male or female, but is an aspect of adult identity. In contrast, in Jamaica or parts of Africa childbirth, rather than sexuality, confers adulthood. The linkage of sexual identity and gender leads to an identification of gay men and lesbians in terms of their homosexuality, although they do not necessarily change their gender. In this culture a lack of fit between sex, gender, and sexuality causes suspicion. In addition, the conflating of sexuality and gender makes it hard to conceptualize homosexual parents. Bozett (1987) points out that there is almost no scientific literature on this subject, although there is somewhat more discussion of lesbian mothers than of gay fathers. Custodial gay fathers are less common and have been less accessible for research, although there may be as many as three million gay men who are natural fathers, not including those who adopt children, are stepfathers, or are foster parents.

Recent interest in gay families and gay parenting reflects the awareness that the "traditional" nuclear family now describes fewer than one-third of families with children (Bozett 1987: 40). Bozett's research on children of gay fathers suggests that the father-child relationship does not significantly change when the child becomes aware of the father's homosexuality. While the children may not approve, the bond to their father remains. Because of embarrassment or concern that others will think they too are gay, the children may seek to use social control strategies that will protect their public image of themselves. Gay fathers attempt to prevent homophobic harassment of their children and to prevent them from being socially marginalized. Fathers' homosexuality does not seem to influence children's sexual orientation.

The articles in this section reveal that there are a number of possible combinations of sex, gender, and sexuality, leading to different and culturally acceptable identities (Caplan 1987: 22). Although western categorizations impose a particular rigidity on gender concepts, cross-cultural data demonstrate that these identities are not fixed and unchangeable. This realization necessitates a critique of these western classifications and provokes a number of stimulating questions: Are heterosexuality and homosexuality equally socially constructed? Is there crosscultural variation in the extent to which sexuality represents a primary aspect of human identity? Is desire itself culturally constituted?

REFERENCES

Bozett, Frederick W. 1987. *Gay and Lesbian Parents.* New York: Praeger Publishers.

Caplan, Pat. 1987. "Introduction." In Pat Caplan (ed.). *The Cultural Construction of Sexuality,* pp. 1–31. London: Tavistock.

Collier, Jane E. and Michelle Z. Rosaldo. 1981. "Politics and Gender in Simple Societies." In Sherry Ortner and Harriet Whitehead (eds.). *Sexual Meanings: The Cultural Construction of Gender and Sexuality,* pp. 275–330. Cambridge: Cambridge University Press.

Foucault, Michel, 1981. *The History of Sexuality.* Harmondsworth: Penguin.

Goodale, Jane C. 1980. "Gender, Sexuality and Marriage: a Kaulong Model of Nature and Culture." In Carol P. MacCormack (ed.). *Nature, Culture and Gender,* pp. 119–143. Cambridge: Cambridge University Press.

Jacobs, Sue-Ellen and Christine Roberts. 1989. "Sex, Sexuality, Gender, and Gender Variance." In Sandra Morgen (ed.). *Gender and Anthropology: Critical Reviews for Research and Teaching,* pp. 438–462. Washington, DC: American Anthropological Association.

Malinowski, Bronislaw. 1929. *The Sexual Life of Savages in Northwestern Melanesia.* New York: Harvest Books.

Mernissi, Fatima. 1987. *Beyond the Veil: Male—Female Dynamics in Modern Muslim Society.* Bloomington and Indianapolis: Indiana University Press.

Moore, Henrietta L. 1988. *Feminism and Anthropology.* Minneapolis: University of Minnesota Press.

Nelson, Nici. 1987. "'Selling her kiosk': Kikuyu Notions of Sexuality and Sex for Sale in Mathare Valley, Kenya." In Pat Caplan (ed.). *The Cultural Construction of Sexuality,* pp. 217–240. London: Tavistock.

Ortner, Sherry B. and Harriet Whitehead. 1981. "Introduction: Accounting for Sexual Meanings." In Sherry Ortner and Harriet Whitehead (eds.). *Sexual Meanings: The Cultural Construction of Gender and Sexuality,* pp. 1–29. Cambridge: Cambridge University Press.

Ross, E. and R. Rapp. 1981. "Sex and Society: A

Research Note from Social History and Anthropology." *Comparative Studies in Society and History* 20: 51–72.

Shepherd, Gill. 1987. "Rank, Gender, and Homosexuality: Mombasa as a Key to Understanding Sexual Options." In Pat Caplan (ed.). *The Cultural Construction of Sexuality*, pp. 240–271. London: Tavistock.

Shostak, Marjorie. 1983. *Nisa: The Life and Words of a !Kung Woman.* Cambridge, MA: Harvard University Press.

Vance, Carole S. 1984. "Pleasure and Danger: Toward a Politics of Sexuality." In Carole S. Vance (ed.). *Pleasure and Danger: Exploring Female Sexuality*, pp.1–29. Boston: Routledge and Kegan Paul.

Williams, Walter L. 1986. *The Spirit and The Flesh.* Boston: Beacon Press.

IS THERE A MUSLIM SEXUALITY? CHANGING CONSTRUCTIONS OF SEXUALITY IN EGYPTIAN BEDOUIN WEDDINGS

Lila Abu-Lughod

The project of defining the nature of Muslim Arab sexuality—what it is or what it should be—has engaged many people with different stakes and interests. Western discourses have tended to contrast the negative sexuality of "the East" with the positive sexuality of the West. French colonial settlers in Algeria depicted Algerian women in pornographic postcards that suggested a fantastic Oriental world of perverse and excessive sexuality (Alloula 1986). Western feminists concerned with global issues dwell on veiling and other practices like clitoridectomy found in the Muslim Arab world as signs of the repressive control over or exploitation of women's sexuality (e.g. Daly 1978).

From the Muslim world itself come other discourses on Arab Muslim sexuality. These include religious and legal texts and pronouncements, but also, more recently, some critical studies by intellectuals and scholars. How different the understandings can be is clear from two important books. One, by a Tunisian scholar with a background in psychoanalytic thought, argues that the misogynist practices of sexuality in the Muslim world are corruptions of the ideals of the Quran and other religious texts (Bouhdiba 1985). The second, by a Moroccan sociologist, argues from a feminist perspective that the legal and sacred texts themselves, like the erotic texts that flourished in the medieval period, carry negative messages about and perpetuate certain consistent attitudes toward the bodies and behavior of Muslim women (Sabbah 1984).

What these various discourses on Arab Muslim sexuality, by outsiders and insiders, defenders and critics, share is the presumption that there is such a thing as a "Muslim sexuality." An anthropologist like myself familiar with the tremendous variety of communities to be found in the regions composing the Muslim Arab world would have to question this presumption. Neither Islam nor sexuality should be essentialzed—taken as things with intrinsic and transhistorical meanings. Rather, both the meaning of Islam and the constructions of sexuality must be understood in their specific historical and local contexts.[1]

To show why I argue this, I will analyze wedding rituals in a community of Awlad 'Ali Bedouin in Egypt's Western Dessert—a community I worked in over a period of 12 years. Weddings are the highlight of social life, awaited with anticipation and participated in

Original material prepared for this text.

with enthusiasm. Each wedding is different. And each wedding is a personal affair of great moment for the bride and groom, even if only one dramatic event in what will be their marriage, lasting for years. Yet public rituals in face-to-face societies are also arenas where people play out their social and political relations. There are other discourses and practices related to sexuality in this Bedouin community but none so powerfully seek to produce, and are now transforming, people's experiences of sexuality and gender relations as weddings. Without pretending that a symbolic analysis exhausts the meaning of weddings for the individuals involved, I would still insist that such an analysis of Awlad 'Ali weddings is useful: It reveals both how sexuality is constructed by the symbols and practices of members of particular communities and how these symbols and practices themselves are open to change and political contestation. Islam, it will be seen, figures not so much as a blueprint for sexuality as a weapon in changing relations of power.

SEXUALITY AND CULTURAL IDENTITY

In the 12 years between 1978 and 1990 that I had been regularly returning to this community of Arab Muslim sedentarized herders in Egypt, the same questions had been asked of me, sometimes even by the same people, as were asked in the first month of my stay. Usually in the context of a gathering of older women, one old woman would lean toward me and ask if I were married. After a short discussion of the fact that I was not, she or another older woman would ask me the next intense question: "Where you come from, does the bridegroom do it with the finger or with 'it'?" The first time they asked me this, I did not know what they meant by "it" and they had a good laugh. The question that followed inevitably in such conversations was, "And do they do it during the daytime or at night?" They were asking about weddings and particularly about the defloration of the virgin bride, which is for them the central moment of a wedding.[2]

In the obsessive concern with whether they do it with the finger or "it," at night or during the daytime, is a clue to one of the things the discourse on this aspect of sexuality has become as the Awlad 'Ali Bedouins have greater contact and interaction with outsiders, primarily their Egyptian peasant and urban neighbors. Whatever its former or current meaning within the community, meanings I will analyze in the following section, the central rite of weddings has now also become a marker of cultural identity—essential to the Awlad Ali's self-defining discourse on what makes them distinctive.

Individuals vary in how they evaluate their differences from their compatriots. When I met the Bedouin representative to the Egyptian Parliament, a sophisticated man in sunglasses whose long contact with other Egyptians showed in his dialect, he assured me that there were a few Bedouin practices that were wrong: One was that they used the finger in the daytime. But he defended the practice by saying that it reminded girls to be careful. Another respected man of the community explained to me that "entering" with the finger was wrong. "We're the only ones who do it this way," he noted. Then he added, "Nothing in our religion says you should." By way of excuse, though, he said, "But the faster the groom does it, the better—the more admired he is because it means he wasn't timid or cowardly." Even women occasionally complained that it was stupid how the female wedding guests waited and waited, just to see that drop of blood. But they too defended the ceremony saying that the defloration had to take place in the afternoon so that everyone could see and there would be no doubts about the reputation of the girl. Their horror at the idea that the groom would use "it" came from their fear that it would be more painful for the bride.

Besides asking whether they do it with the finger or it, day or night, the women I knew often asked whether, where I came from, there was anyone with the bride to hold her down. They were surprised to hear that she needed no one and marveled that she wasn't afraid to be alone with the man. Amongst themselves, they almost always had a few older women, usually aunts or close neighbors of the groom and bride, in the room with the bride when the groom came to her. There in theory to hold the bride, these women also end up giving advice to the groom and making sure that he knows what to do so that everything—the display of the blood on the cloth—would turn out right.

For their part, somewhat like most Europeans and Americans, non-Bedouin Egyptians and assimilated Awlad 'Ali from the agricultural areas find Bedouin weddings scandalous and distasteful. Bedouin women are not unaware of these views and the men discussed above were probably reacting defensively to them. These outsiders may laugh at some customs but they are embarrassed by others. After one wedding in the community in which I was living, the bride's aunt, who had spent most of her life in a non-Bedouin provincial town, talked about the wedding and some of the customs she had witnessed that made her laugh "until her stomach hurt." She obviously considered her new in-laws backward.[3]

What seemed to disturb her most was the public nature of what she felt should be private. She thought it humiliating, for example, that at night, the young men from the community (peers of the bridegroom) hung around the room, listening, shining a flashlight under the door and through the window, and generally being disruptive. More horrible to her was the public display of the blood-stained cloth. "It was incredible," she exclaimed. "After the defloration didn't you hear my son saying to his aunt when she went to hang the cloth on the tent ropes, 'It's shameful, my aunt, it's shameful to put the cloth out for people to see.'" Like other urban and rural Egyptians, she thought that the bride and groom should be brought together at night and left alone.

Although other Egyptians and Americans might feel that such privacy is more civilized, the Awlad 'Ali women I knew did not see it that way. Bedouin women were scandalized by the secrecy of night deflorations, the immediate and explicit link such weddings make between marriage and sexual intercourse, and what they view as either the total vulnerability of the poor bride forced to be alone with a man or, even worse, the bride's immodest desire for a man. They knew that instead of struggling, the Egyptian bride has her photo taken with her husband-to-be, she sits with him at weddings where the sexes mix, and she dresses in make-up and fancy clothes for all to see. Because poorer Bedouin men sometimes marry young women from peasant areas, whether they are of Egyptian stock or long-sedentarized Bedouin involved in agriculture, the Bedouin women also knew that unmarried sisters accompanied the bride. They interpreted this practice as a shameful attempt to display and "sell" marriageable daughters. They also knew that such brides sometimes arrived bringing a cooked duck or goose to feed a new husband; they took this as a sign of the bride's unseemly eagerness to please the groom.

Egyptian weddings, much like American ones, construct the couple as a separate unit, distinct from families or ties to members of the same gender group. At their center is a sexual joining that is private and intimate. For the Awlad 'Ali, this is a strange thing. The secrecy of private sex, in the dark, behind closed doors, and preferably in the foreign or anonymous setting (for the honeymoon) produces sexuality as something personal, intensely individual, apparently separate from society and social power. It produces sexuality as something belonging in an inviolable private sphere—the bedroom—a sphere in which others cannot interfere with whatever pleasure or violence and coercion accompanies it. One of the consequences of this construction of sexuality is that we, and perhaps Egyptians, come to think there is a part of oneself that is not social or affected by the prevailing power relations in society.[4]

The three crucial elements in the Bedouin discourse on differences between their weddings and those of other groups are (1) whether the defloration is public and participatory, (2) whether it involves sexual intercourse, and (3) whether it is seen as a contest, especially between bride and groom. These elements also had meaning within the local context. In Bedouin weddings the ways in which sexuality is related to power relations and the social order were clear. Marriages have been the occasion for people to collectively enact and reproduce this social order and the individual's place in it. And the individual's place was, until recently, very much a part of the group—whether the kin group or the group defined by gender.

WEDDINGS AS PUBLIC RITES: THE POWER OF KINSHIP AND GENDER

The participants in Awlad 'Ali Bedouin weddings instantiate, by means of a bride and groom, the relations between families or kin groups on the one hand, and the relations between men and women on the other. A symbolic analysis of the central rite, the defloration, enacted in a homologous fashion on the bodies of the bride and groom and on the collective bodies of the gathered kin and friends, reveals that it produces an understanding of sexuality as something public and focused on crossing thresholds, opening passages, and moving in and out. There are no strong messages of mingling or joining or even interchange in a private sexual act. The emphasis is on opening the bride's vagina by breaking the hymen and bringing out or making visible what was in there. And although people say that deflorations should be done during the daytime so everyone can see the cloth, the fact that in the rhythm of daily life morning and daytime generally are times of opening and going out from home or camp while evening is a time of returning inward cannot but reinforce the auspiciousness of this time for opening and taking outward.[5]

That this opening is a prelude to the insemination which should eventuate in childbirth is suggested by some practices associated with the blood-stained virginity cloth. It is taken out of the room by the groom and thrown to the women gathered just outside. It is said that if the cloth is then brought back into the room without the bride having exited first—if, as they say, the cloth enters upon her—it will block her from conceiving.[6] Young women are told to save their virginity cloths; if they have trouble conceiving they must bathe in water in which they have soaked the cloth.

Everything in the rites and the songs that accompany them suggests that the individuals engaged in this opening and being opened, taking out and showing and having something taken out and shown, embody both their kin groups and their gender groups. The connection to kin, and control by the kin group, is clear in the key role they have in arranging and negotiating marriages and is reflected in the songs the groom's female relatives sing as they go to fetch the bride from her father's household. It is also reinforced in the songs the bride's female kin sing to greet these people. Most of the songs compliment the social standing of the families of the bride and groom.

Even the practices and movements of the wedding itself perpetuate the identifications with kin groups. Most brides, even today, are brought from their fathers' households completely covered by a white woolen woven cloak (*jard*) that is the essential item of men's dress. The cloak must belong to the girl's father or some other male kinsman. So, protected and hidden by her father's cloak, she is brought out of her father's protected domain and carried to her husband's kin group's domain. There she is rushed, still hidden, into the room (or in the past, the tent) which she will share with her husband. Although nowadays the woven cloak is usually removed once she enters the room, in the past the bride remained under her father's cloak and was not revealed even to the women gathered around her until after the defloration.

The virginity of the bride is also constructed as something inseparable from her family's honor. Although one unmarred girl explained the importance of the blood-stained cloth in terms of her own reputation, she stressed the effect it would have on others.

> For us Bedouins, this is the most important moment in a girl's life. No matter what anyone says afterward, no one will pay attention as long as there was blood on the cloth. They are suspicious of her before. People talk. "She went here, she went there." "She looked at So-and-so." "She said hello to So-and-so." "She went to the orchard." But when they see this blood the talk is cut off. . . . When they see the cloth, she can come and go as she pleases. They love her and everything is fine.

The best way to get a sense of who has stakes in the girl's virginity and why is to listen to the conventional songs sung wildly outside the door of the bride's room as the defloration is underway. Unmarried girls and some young married women clap and sing rhyming songs that refer to the effect of the proof of the bride's virginity on various members of her family and community.

> Make her dear Mom happy, Lord
> Hanging up her cloth on the tent ropes
>
> O Saint 'Awwaam on high
> Don't let anyone among us be shamed

Older women sing more serious songs that take up similar themes:

> When the people have gathered
> O Generous One favor us with a happy ending
> . . .
>
> Behind us are important men
> who ask about what we are doing . . .

Relatives of the bride show their support and faith in the bride in songs like this:

> I'm confident in the loved one
> you'll find it there intact . . .

Even the groom's behavior during the defloration reflects on his relatives. One song a relative of his might sing as he arrives or is inside with the bride is the following:

> Son, be like your menfolk
> strong willed and unafraid . . .

After the virginity cloth is brought out by the groom and thrown to the women, a different set of songs is sung. These praise the cloth and the honor of the girl who had remained a virgin. The songs reflect on who is affected by her purity and who is proud. At one wedding a female relative of the bride sang to a nephew nearby:

> Go tell your father, Said
> the banner of her honor is flying high . . .

About the bride a woman might sing:

> Bravo! She was excellent
> she who didn't force down her father's
> eyelashes . . .

Given this group investment in the bride's virginity, the central rite of the wedding becomes a drama of suspense and relief that must powerfully shape people's experiences of sexuality as something that belongs to the many, and especially to one's family. The wedding is also, importantly, an occasion when families find themselves in some rivalry, the honor of each at stake. This was more apparent in the past when the young men celebrated all night on the eve of the wedding and expressed the rivalry through singing contests that sometimes broke out into actual fights between lineages.

Kinship is not the only power-laden aspect of social life that finds itself reflected and reinforced in the wedding. The second set of power relations weddings play with are those of gender. The bride and groom in the wedding rite enact the charged relations between men and women as distinct genders in a kind of battle of the sexes. Although most activities in the community are informally segregated by gender, at weddings—in part because there are non-family members present—the sexual segregation is more obvious and fixed, women and men forming highly separate collectivities for nearly all events.

Given this separation of the sexes, the defloration, taking place in the middle of the day when all are gathered in their distinct places, becomes a ritualized and extreme form of encounter between both the bride and groom and the women and men who surround each of them. The movements of the groom and his age-mates as they penetrate the crowd of women surrounding the bride mirror the groom's penetration of his bride, who forms a unit with the women in the room with her. The young men stand just outside the door, sometimes dancing and singing, ready to fire off guns in celebration when the groom emerges. They rush him back away from the women. This mirroring is expressed in the ambiguity of the term used for both moments of this event: the entrance (*khashsha*) refers both to the entry with the finger and the whole defloration process when the groom enters the bride's room, which can be thought of as his kin group's womb.

The encounter between male and female takes the form of a contest. The groom is encouraged to be fearless. He is expected to finish the deed in as short a time as possible. The bride is expected to try valiantly to fight him off. Taking the virginity she has been so careful to guard and thus opening the way for his progeny is the groom's victory; the bride doesn't give it up without a struggle. Calling this, as the literature often does, a virginity test is a misnomer in that it misses this combative dimension of the ritualized act. The way people describe what happens even on the wedding night suggests again that the groom and bride are involved in a contest. The rowdy young men who listen outside the marital chamber want to know "who won." They know this, some adolescent girls informed me, not just by whether the groom succeeds in having intercourse with his bride (a rare event), but by whether the groom succeeds in making his bride talk to him and answer his questions. This is, perhaps, another kind of opening up.

There is other evidence that weddings provoke a heightened attention to issues of gender and sexual mixing. One of the most revealing and intriguing is the spontaneous cross-dressing that sometimes happens at weddings. At several weddings I attended one woman in our community actually put on men's clothes, a fake mustache and beard, and covered her head in a man's headcloth. Amidst much hilarity she came out to dance in front of the bride. Others expressed some disapproval and called this woman a bit mad. But they laughed riotously anyway. One woman who thought it excessive described someone else who she thought was quite funny: All she did was dance in front of the bride with a shawl bunched up in front like male genitalia. Sometimes it was reported that the unmarried men and young boys had celebrated the night before the wedding by dressing up a boy with women's bracelets and a veil and dancing in front of him as if he were a bride.

SEXUAL TRANSFORMATIONS

Many Awlad 'Ali claim that their rituals are changing. In this final section, I want to explore how in these changed wedding practices we can begin to track changes in the nature of power and social relations. This is further support for my initial argument that constructions of sexuality cannot be understood apart from understandings of particular forms of social power. Most people talked about changes in weddings over the last 20 years or so in terms of what had been lost. Many said weddings were not fun any more. As far as I could determine, the main element that seems to have been lost is the celebration the night before the wedding (*saamir*). Not only do the young men no longer sing back and forth, but no longer is it even thinkable that a young woman from the community would come out to dance in front of them. This is what used to happen and the change is crucial for Bedouin gender relations.

What happened in the past was that an unmarried sister or cousin of the groom would be brought out from among the women by a young boy. She would dance amidst a semicircle of young men. Her face veiled and her waist girded with a man's white woven cloak, like the one the bride would come covered in the following day, she danced with a stick or baton in her hands. According to one man who described this to me, the young men tried to "beg" the stick from her, sometimes using subterfuges like pretending to be ill; she would often bestow the stick, he said, on someone she fancied. But according to the women I spoke with, the young men would sometimes try to grab the stick from her and she would, if they were too aggressive, get angry with them and leave. The young men took turns singing songs that welcomed the dancer and then described her every feature in flattering terms. The standard parts praised in such songs were her braids, her eyes, her eyebrows, her cheeks, her lips, her tattoos, her neck, her breasts, her arms, her hands, and her waist—most of which, it should be remembered, because of the way she was dressed were not actually visible. Thus in a sense the dancer was, through men's songs, made into the ideal woman, attractive object of men's desires.

The dancer must be seen as the bride's double or stand-in, an interpretation supported by the other occasion on which a young woman danced in front of men. In the days before cars, brides were carried from their fathers' households to their husbands' on camel-back, completely cloaked and sitting hidden inside a wooden litter (*karmuud*) covered in red woven blankets. Another woman always preceded her on foot, dancing as young men sang to her and shot off guns near her.

In both cases, the dancer as bride and as ideal womanhood went out before men who complimented and sought her. What is crucial to notice is how the women described the dancer. They attributed to her a special bravery and described her actions as a challenge to the young men. One wedding in which a young woman was accidentally wounded by a poorly aimed gun was legendary. The wedding went on, the story went, as a second dancer who had been near her merely wiped the blood from her forehead and continued to dance. More telling is the ritualized struggle over the stick, which one anthropologist who worked with a group in Libya has argued is associated with virginity (Mason 1975). A woman explained to me, "If the dancer is sharp they can't take the stick from her. They'll be coming at her from all sides but she keeps it."

But perhaps some of the short songs traditionally exchanged between the women (gathered in a tent some distance away from the young men standing in a line near the dancer) and the young men, make clearest the ways in which a challenge between the sexes was central to weddings. One especially memorable competitive exchange was the following. As her sister danced a woman sang of her:

> A bird in the hot winds glides
> and no rifle scope can capture it . . .

A man responded with the song:

> The heart would be no hunter
> if it didn't play in their feathers . . .

In the loss and delegitimation of this whole section of the wedding ritual, an important piece of the construction of Bedouin sexual relations has disappeared. Today, all that is left in a ritual that was a highly charged and evenly matched challenge between the sexes is the enactment of the men's hunt. The groom is the hunter, the bride his prey. Decked out in her make-up and white satin dress, she is brought from her father's house and her "virginity" taken by her groom in a bloody display.

Wedding songs, only sung by women now, reinforce this construction of the bride as vulnerable prey. They liken the bride to a gazelle. This is a compliment to her beauty but also suggests her innocence and defenselessness. Other songs liken the groom to a falcon or hunter. This is no longer balanced by women's former powers to create desire but elude capture.

The disappearance of the female dancer can thus be seen to have shifted the balance such that women's capacities to successfully challenge men have been de-emphasized. Although the sexes are still pitted against each other, the contest is no longer represented as even.

There is a second important point to be made about the dancer that relates to some transformations in constructions of power and sexuality. For it is not completely true that women no longer dance in front of men at Awlad 'Ali weddings. It has become unacceptable for respectable young kinswomen to dance but there are now some professional dancers. They accompany musical troupes hired to entertain at weddings of the Bedouin nouveau riche. These women may or may not be prostitutes but they are certainly not considered respectable.[7] In that sense, and in the fact that ordinary women go nowhere near the areas where these musicians and dancers perform, one cannot any longer claim that the dancer represents Women or enacts women's challenge of men. The opposite may be true. This new kind of wedding may be introducing a new view of women, one quite familiar to us in the United States but quite strange to the Awlad 'Ali: women as sexual commodities stripped of their embeddedness in their kin groups or the homosocial world of women.

The professionalization of weddings as entertainment and spectacle (if spectacles that retain vestiges of the participatory in that young men seize the microphone to sing songs) may also be signaling a fundamental shift in the relationship of the construction of sexuality and the construction of the social order. What seems to be disappearing is the participation of the whole community in the responsibility of ritually reproducing the fundamental social and political dynamics of the community. Does this indicate the emergence of a new kind of power? One that works differently? One whose nexus is perhaps the individual rather than the kin group or gender group? This new form of wedding is not being adopted universally in the Bedouin region since the poor cannot afford it and the respectable condemn it as undignified and inappropriate for pious Muslims. Nevertheless, as a public discourse it must enter and shape the field of sexuality for all.

The third and final historical shift I will discuss comes out in the comments women made about what had happened to weddings. One old woman reminisced about weddings of the past. She shook her head and laughed, "No, the things they did before you can't do anymore. Nowadays weddings are small, like a shrunken old man. People used to really celebrate, staying up all night, for days! But they have become like the Muslim Brothers now." The younger woman she was talking to had explained for me. "They say it is wrong. Now everything is forbidden. People before didn't know. They were ignorant." She used a term with connotations of the pre-Islamic era.

These women's invocations of Islam and the proper behavior of the pious in the contexts of weddings mark some significant changes in power relations. It has always been important to the Awlad 'Ali that they are Muslims and that they are good Muslims. And these two women themselves were devout. They prayed regularly and the old one had been on the pilgrimage to Mecca. Yet when they and other women brought up the religious wrongness of their traditional wedding practices, it was with some ambivalence since they were also nostalgic for the richer days of the past. After one wedding there was a hint of disapproval in women's gossip about one aunt in the community. Someone with a good voice who usually sang at weddings, she had just returned from the pilgrimage to Mecca and had refused this time. "It is wrong," she told them. They thought she was being self-righteous—and selfish.

What is really at stake comes out clearly from women's discussions of a happy wedding that had taken place in my absence. I was told that, as usual, for days before the wedding the women and girls had been celebrating by themselves every evening, drumming and singing. The older men of the community wanted them to stop and instructed them that at least once the guests (non-relatives) had begun to arrive, they would have to stop. It was shameful to sing in front of people, the men insisted. On the eve of the wedding as the women and girls gathered and began to sing and dance in celebration, the groom's father came in to greet his visiting female relatives. He also wanted to try to silence the group of women. When he entered the tent, he saw his own older sister, a dignified woman in her sixties, dancing. "Hey, what's this?" he said. "Rottenest of days, even you, Hajja?" He called her by the respectful title reserved for those who have performed the pilgrimage to Mecca. "That's right," she answered definitely, "even me!" Everyone laughed, then and each time they retold the story.

Women still refuse to be stopped from celebrating weddings. But the older men, armed with religious righteousness, are clearly trying to assert authority over them in domains that were previously inviolable. Weddings, like the discontinued sheep-shearing festivities to which they are often likened, were always before classified as occasions where young men and young women could express desires. Elder men were not to interfere. At sheep-shearing festivities young men used to sing with impunity oblique sexual songs to flirt with the women present. The songs often insulted the patriarch whose herds the young men were shearing. Similarly, at weddings young men sang to women, not just the dancer. Even more important, women sang back—songs of love and desire. Older men made sure they were not in the vicinity.[8]

Now, not only have the exchanges between young men and women stopped but older men seem to be trying to assert control over the separate women's festivities. Their motives for this intervention are irrelevant. They may genuinely believe they are encouraging their families to live up to an interpretation of Islam that denounces such frivolity as impious. The effect, however, on women and young men, is that by means of this discourse of Islamic propriety wielded by older men, they are being displaced as the prime actors in the rites that produced and reproduced Bedouin constructions of sexuality and desire.

If, as I have tried to show, in a small Bedouin community in Egypt, sexuality can come to be a crucial marker of cultural identity, and if the construction of sexuality is so closely tied to the organization of kinship and gender and changes as the community is transformed by such broad processes as its incorporation into the wider Egyptian nation and economy, then it seems impossible to assert the existence of a Muslim sexuality that can be read off texts or shared across communities with very different histories and ways of life. Instead, we need to think about specific constructions of sexuality and, in the case of the Muslim Arab world, about the variable role discourses on religion can play in those constructions.

Author's Note: Most of the research in Egypt on which this article is based was supported by an NEH Fellowship for College Teachers and a Fulbright Award under the Islamic Civilization Program. I am grateful to Samia Mehrez for inviting me to present an early version at Cornell University. I am more grateful to the women and men in the Awlad 'Ali community who shared their lives, including their weddings, with me.

NOTES

1. The literature, especially the feminist literature, on sexuality has become vast in the last decade or two. A helpful early text is Vance (1984). Anthropologists have recently begun to pay more attention to constructions of sexuality and their cross-cultural perspective should contribute to our understanding of the way that sexuality is constructed. For a good introduction to some of that work, see Caplan (1987).
2. For this reason the weddings of divorcees or widows are not celebrated with as much enthusiasm and are considered somewhat ordinary affairs.
3. For example, she described what is known as the *dayra* (the circling). On the evening of the wedding day, they had seated the bride and groom on a pillow, back to back. A neighbor carrying a lamb on his back, holding one foreleg in each of his hands, had walked around and around them—seven times. She mimicked

the audience counting: "Hey, did you count that one? One, two, three, four." "Thank God," she said at one point, "there were no outsiders (non-relatives) from back home with us. How embarrassing it would have been."

4. The theorist who has most developed this notion of the effects on subjectivity and sense of individuality of the Western discourses on sexuality is Michel Foucault (1978; 1985).
5. For an analysis of similar kinds of symbolic constructions of gender and sexuality, see Bourdieu's (1977) work on Algerian Kabyles. My analysis of the meaning of this rite differs significantly from that of Combs-Schilling (1989), who worked in Morocco.
6. For more on rituals related to fertility and infertility, see my *Writing Women's Worlds* (1993). Boddy (1989) has analyzed for Muslim Sudanese villagers the extraordinary symbolic stress on women's fertility over their sexuality.
7. As Van Nieuwkerk (1995) has documented, this is generally true about professional dancers in Egypt.
8. Peters (1990) describes a similar avoidance by elders of wedding celebrations among the Bedouin of Cyrenaica in the 1950s.

REFERENCES

Abu-Lughod, Lila. 1993. *Writing Women's Worlds: Bedouin Stories.* Berkeley and Los Angeles: University of California Press.

Alloula, Malek. 1986. *The Colonial Harem.* Myran and Wlad Godzich, trans. Minneapolis: University of Minnesota Press.

Boddy, Janice. 1989. *Wombs and Alien Spirits: Women, Men, and the Zar Cult in Northern Sudan.* Madison, WI: University of Wisconsin Press.

Bouhdiba, Abdelwahab. 1985. *Sexuality in Islam.* London and Boston: Routledge & Kegan Paul.

Bourdieu, Pierre. 1977. *Outline of a Theory of Practice.* Cambridge: Cambridge University Press.

Caplan, Patricia, ed. 1987. *The Cultural Construction of Sexuality.* London and New York: Tavistock Publications.

Combs-Schilling, M.E. 1989. *Sacred Performances: Islam, Sexuality and Sacrifice.* New York: Columbia University Press.

Daly, Mary. 1978. *Gyn/ecology, the Metaethics of Radical Feminism.* Boston: Beacon Press.

Foucault, Michel. 1978. *The History of Sexuality: Volume 1: An Introduction.* New York: Random House.

———. 1985. *The Use of Pleasure.* Vol. 2 of *The History of Sexuality.* New York: Pantheon.

Mason, John. 1975. "Sex and Symbol in the Treatment of Women: The Wedding Rite in a Libyan Oasis Community." *American Ethnologist* 2: 649–61.

Peters, Emrys. 1990. *The Bedouin of Cyrenaica.* Edited by Jack Goody and Emanuel Marx. Cambridge: Cambridge Univeristy Press.

Sabbah, Fatna A. 1984. *Woman in the Muslim Unconscious.* New York and Oxford: Pergamon Press.

Vance, Carole. 1984. *Pleasure and Danger: Exploring Female Sexuality.* Boston and London: Routledge & Kegan Paul.

Van Nieuwkerk, Karin. 1995. *"A Trade Like Any Other": Female Singers and Dancers in Egypt.* Austin, TX: University of Texas Press.

WOMEN AND MEN IN !KUNG SOCIETY

Marjorie Shostak

After Besa and I had lived together for a long time, he went to visit some people in the East. While there, he found work with a Tswana cattle herder. When he came back, he told me to pack; he wanted me to go and live with him there. So we left and took the long trip to Old Debe's village, a Zhun/twa village near a Tswana and European settlement. We lived there together for a long time.[1]

While we were there, my father died. My older brother, my younger brother, and my mother were with him when he died, but I wasn't; I was living where Besa had taken me.

Reprinted by permission of the publishers from *Nisa: The Life and Words of a !Kung Woman* by Marjorie Shostak (Cambridge, MA: Harvard University Press).

Others carried the news to me. They said that Dau had tried to cure my father, laying on hands and working hard to make him better. But God refused and Dau wasn't able to see what was causing the illness so he could heal him. Dau said, "God is refusing to give up my father."

I heard and said, "Eh, then today I'm going to see where he died." Besa and I and my children, along with a few others, left to take the long journey west. We walked the first day and slept that night. The next morning we started out and slept again that night; we slept another night on the road, as well. As we walked, I cried and thought, "Why couldn't I have been with him when he died?" I cried as we walked, one day and the next and the next.

The sun was so hot, it was burning; it was killing us. One day we rested such a long time, I thought, "Is the sun going to stop me from seeing where my father died?" When it was cooler, we started walking again and slept on the road again that night.

We arrived at the village late in the afternoon. My younger brother, Kumsa, was the first to see us. When he saw me, he came and hugged me. We started to cry and cried together for a long time. Finally, our older brother stopped us, "That's enough for now. Your tears won't make our father alive again."

We stopped crying and we all sat down. My mother was also with us. Although my father never took her back again after the time she ran away with her lover, she returned and lived near him until he died. And even though she slept alone, she still loved him.

Later, my mother and I sat together and cried together.

We stayed there for a while, then Besa and I went back again to live in the East where he had been working for the Europeans. A very long time passed. Then, my brother sent word that my mother was dying. Once again we made the journey to my family and when we arrived I saw her: she was still alive.

We stayed there and lived there. One day, a group of people were going to the bush to live. I said, "Mother, come with us. I'll take care of you and you can help me with my children." We traveled that day and slept that night; we traveled another day and slept another night. But the next night, the sickness that had been inside her grabbed her again and this time, held on. It was just as it had been with my father. The next day, she coughed up blood. I thought, "Oh, why is blood coming out like that? Is this what is going to kill her? Is this the way she's going to die? What is this sickness going to do? She's coughing blood . . . she's already dead!" Then I thought, "If only Dau were here, he would be able to cure her. He would trance for her every day." But he and my younger brother had stayed behind. Besa was with us, but he didn't have the power to cure people. There were others with us as well, but they didn't help.

We slept again that night. The next morning, the others left, as is our custom, and then it was only me, my children, my husband, and my mother; we were the only ones who remained. But her life was really over by then, even though she was still alive.

I went to get her some water and when I came back, she said, "Nisa . . . Nisa . . . I am an old person and today, my heart . . . today you and I will stay together for a while longer; we will continue to sit beside each other. But later, when the sun stands over there in the afternoon sky and when the new slim moon first strikes, I will leave you. We will separate then and I will go away."

I asked, "Mother, what are you saying?" She said, "Yes, that's what I'm saying. I am an old person. Don't deceive yourself; I am dying. When the sun moves to that spot in the sky, that will be our final separation. We will no longer be together after that. So, take good care of your children."

I said, "Why are you talking like this? If you die as you say, because that's what you're telling me, who are you going to leave in your place?" She said, "Yes, I am leaving you. Your husband will take care of you now. Besa will be with you and your children."

We remained together the rest of the day as the sun crawled slowly across the sky.

When it reached the spot she had spoken of, she said—just like a person in good health—"Mm, now . . . be well, all of you," and then she died.

That night I slept alone and cried and cried and cried. None of my family was with me[2] and I just cried the entire night. When morning came, Besa dug a grave and buried her. I said, "Let's pull our things together and go back to the village. I want to tell Dau and Kumsa that our mother has died."

We walked that day and slept that night. We walked the next day and stopped again that night. The next morning, we met my brother Kumsa. Someone had told him that his mother was sick. When he heard, he took his bow and quiver and came looking for us. He left when the sun just rose and started walking toward us, even as we were walking toward him. We met when the sun was overhead. He stood and looked at me. Then he said, "Here you are, Nisa, with your son and your daughter and your husband. But Mother isn't with you . . ."

I sat down and started to cry. He said, "Mother must have died because you're crying like this," and he started to cry, too. Besa said, "Yes, your sister left your mother behind. Two days ago was when your mother and sister separated. That is where we are coming from now. Your sister is here and will tell you about it. You will be together to share your mourning for your mother. That will be good."

We stayed there and cried and cried. Later, Kumsa took my little son and carried him on his shoulders. I carried my daughter and we walked until we arrived back at the village. My older brother came with his wife, and when he saw us he, too, started to cry.

After that, we lived together for a while. I lived and cried, lived and cried. My mother had been so beautiful . . . her face, so lovely. When she died, she caused me great pain. Only after a long time was I quiet again.

Before we returned to the East, I went with Besa to visit his family. While I was there, I became very sick. It came from having carried my mother. Because when she was sick, I carried her around on my back. After she died, my back started to hurt in the very place I had carried her. One of God's spiritual arrows must have struck me there and found its way into my chest.

I was sick for a long time and then blood started to come out of my mouth. My younger brother (he really loves me!) was visiting me at the time. When he saw how I was, he left to tell his older brother, "Nisa's dying the same way our mother died. I've come to tell you to come back with me and heal her." My older brother listened and the two of them traveled to where I was. They came when the sun was high in the afternoon sky. Dau started to trance for me. He laid on hands, healing me with his touch. He worked on me for a long time. Soon, I was able to sleep; then, the blood stopped coming from my chest and later, even if I coughed, there wasn't any more blood.

We stayed there for a few more days. Then, Dau said, "Now I'm going to take Nisa with me to my village." Besa agreed and we all left together. We stayed at my brother's village until I was completely better.

Besa and I eventually moved back East again. But after we had lived together for a long time, we no longer were getting along. One day I asked, "Besa, won't you take me back to my family's village so I can live there?" He said, "I'm no longer interested in you." I said, "What's wrong? Why do you feel that way?" But then I said, "Eh, if that's how it is, it doesn't matter."

I was working for a European woman at the time, and when I told her what Besa was saying to me, she told him, "Listen to me. You're going to chase your wife away. If you continue to speak to her like this, she'll be gone. Today, I'm pregnant. Why don't you just let her be and have her sit beside you. When I give birth, she will work for me and help me with the baby."

That's what we did. We continued to live together until she gave birth. After, I helped wash the baby's clothes and helped with other chores. I worked for her for a long time.

One day, Besa broke into a little box I had and stole the money she had paid me with. He took it and went to drink beer. I went to the European woman and told her Besa had taken five Rand[3] from me and had left with it. I asked her to help me get it back. We went to the Tswana hut where everyone was drinking and went to the door. The European woman walked in, kicked over a bucket and the beer spilled out. She kicked over another and another and the beer was spilling everywhere. The Tswanas left. She turned to Besa and said, "Why are you treating this young Zhun/twa woman like this? Stop treating her this way." She told him to give her the money and when he gave it to her, she gave it to me. I went and put the money in the box, then took it and left it in her kitchen where it stayed.

Later Besa said, "Why did you tell on me? I'm going to beat you." I said, "Go ahead. Hit me. I don't care. I won't stop you."

Soon after that, I became pregnant with Besa's child. But when it was still very tiny, when I was still carrying it way inside, he left me. I don't know what it was that made him want to leave. Did he have a lover? I don't know. He said he was afraid of a sore I had on my face where a bug had bitten me. It had become swollen, and eventually the Europeans helped to heal it. Whatever it was, his heart had changed toward me and although my heart still liked him, he only liked me a very little then. That's why he left.

It happened the day he finished working for the Europeans. He came back when the sun was low in the sky and said, "Tomorrow, I'm going to visit my younger brother. I have finished my work and have been paid. I'm going, but you'll stay here. Later, Old Debe and his wife can take you back to your brothers' village." I said, "If you are leaving, won't I go with you?" He said, "No, you won't go with me." I said, "Why are you saying you'll go without me? If I go with you and give birth there, it will be good. Don't leave me here. Let me go with you and give birth in your brother's village." But he said, "No, Old Debe will bring you back to your family."

When I saw Old Debe, he asked me what was wrong. I said, "What is Besa doing to me? If he doesn't want me, why doesn't he just end it completely? I've seen for a long time that he doesn't want me." I thought, "Besa . . . he took me to this faraway village, got me pregnant, and now, is he just going to drop me in this foreign place where none of my people live?"

Later, I said to Besa, "Why did you take me from my people? My brothers are still alive, yet you won't take me to them. You say someone else will. But, why should someone else, a near stranger, take me to my family after you've given me this stomach. I say you should take me to them, take me there and say, 'Here is your sister. Today I am separating from her.' Instead, you're saying you'll just leave me here, with these strangers? I followed you here, to where you were working, because you wanted me to. Now you're just going to leave me? Why are you doing this? Can there be any good in it?"

I continued, "You're the one who came here to work. Yet, you have no money and have no blankets. But when you had no more work and no more money, I worked. I alone, a woman. I entered the work of the European and I alone bought us blankets and a trunk. I alone bought all those things and you covered yourself with my blankets. When you weren't working, you asked people to give you things. How can you leave me here in this foreign place after all that?" He answered, "What work could I have done when there wasn't any to be had?"

I said, "It doesn't matter, because I can see that you will only be here for a few more nights, then you will go. I know that now. But, if you leave me like this today, then tomorrow, after you have gone and have lived with your brother, if you ever decide to come to where I am living, I will refuse you and will no longer be your wife. Because you are leaving me when I am pregnant."

The next morning, early, he tied up his things and left. He packed everything from inside the hut, including all our blankets, and went to his brother's village to live. I thought, "Eh, it doesn't matter, after all. I'll just sit here and let him go." He left me with nothing; the people in the village had to give me blankets to sleep with.

Besa, that man is very bad. He left me hanging like that.

Once he left, I saw that I would be staying there for a while. I thought, "Today I'm no longer going to refuse other men, but will just be with them. Then, maybe I will miscarry. Because this is Besa's child and didn't he leave it and go? I won't refuse other men and will just have them. I will drop this pregnancy; then I will go home."

That's when Numshe entered the hut with me. He spoke to me and I agreed. People said, "Yes, she will enter the hut with him. But when he tastes her,[4] the pregnancy will be ruined." Old Debe's wife said, "That won't be so bad. If her pregnancy is ruined, it won't be a bad thing. Because Besa dropped her. Therefore, I will sit here and take care of her. Later, I will bring her to her family."

I lived there for a long time. I lived alone and worked for the Europeans. Then one day, just as my heart had said, my body felt like fire and my stomach was in great pain. I told Old Debe's wife, "Eh-hey, today I'm sick." She asked, "Where does it hurt? Do you want some water? Where is the sickness hurting you." I said, "My whole body hurts, it isn't just my stomach." I lay there and felt the pains, rising again and again and again. I thought, "That man certainly has made me feel bad; even today, I'm lying here in great pain."

She looked at my stomach and saw how it was standing out. She said, "Oh, my child. Are you going to drop your pregnancy? What is going to happen? Will you be able to give birth to this child or will it be a miscarriage? Here, there are just the two of us; I don't see anyone who will bring more help to you. If you miscarry, it will be only us two." I said, "Yes, that's fine. If I drop this pregnancy, it will be good. I want to drop it, then I can leave. Because my husband certainly doesn't want it."

We stayed together all day. When the sun was late in the sky, I told her it was time and we went together to the bush. I sat down and soon the baby was born. It was already big, with a head and arms and a little penis; but it was born dead. Perhaps my heart had ruined my pregnancy. I cried, "This man almost ruined me, did he not?" Debe's wife said, "Yes, he destroyed this baby, this baby which came from God. But if God hadn't been here helping you, you also would have died. Because when a child dies in a woman's stomach, it can kill the woman. But God . . . God gave you something beautiful in giving you this baby and although it had death in it, you yourself are alive." We left and walked back to the village. Then I lay down.

After that, I just continued to live there. One day I saw people visiting from Besa's village. I told them to tell him that our marriage had ended. I said, "Tell him that he shouldn't think, even with a part of his heart, that he still has a wife here or that when we meet another time in my village that he might still want me." That's what I said and that's what I thought.

Because he left me there to die.

Soon after, a man named Twi saw me and said, "Did your husband leave you?" I said, "Yes, he left me long ago." He asked, "Then won't you stay with me?" I refused the first time he asked as well as the second and the third. But when he asked the next time, I agreed and we started to live together. I continued to work for the European woman until my work was finished and she told me I could go home. She gave us food for our trip and then all of us—Old Debe, his wife, Twi, and me—traveled the long distance back to where my family was living.

Twi and I lived together in my brothers' village for a long time. Then, one day, Besa came from wherever he had been and said, "Nisa, I've come to take you back with me." I said, "What? What am I like today? Did I suddenly become beautiful? The way I used to be is the way I am now; the way I used to be is what you left behind when you dropped me.

So what are you saying? First you drop me in the heart of where the white people live, then you come back and say I should once again be with you?" He said, "Yes, we will pick up our marriage again."

I was stunned! I said, "What are you talking about? This man, Twi, helped bring me back. He's the man who will marry me. You're the one who left me." We talked until he could say nothing more; he was humbled. Finally he said, "You're shit! That's what you are." I said, "I'm shit you say? That's what you thought about me long ago, and I knew it. That's why I told you while we were still living in the East that I wanted you to take me back to my family so we could end our marriage here. But today, I came here myself and you only came afterward. Now I refuse to have anything more to do with you."

That's when Besa brought us to the Tswana headman to ask for a tribal hearing. Once it started, the headman looked at everything. He asked me, "Among all the women who live here, among all those you see sitting around, do you see one who lives with two men?" I said, "No, the women who sit here . . . not one lives with two men; not one among them would I be able to find. I, alone, have two. But it was because this man, Besa, mistreated and hurt me. That's why I took this other man, Twi, who treats me well, who does things for me and gives me things to eat." Then I said, "He is also the man I want to marry; I want to drop the other one. Because Besa has no sense. He left me while I was pregnant and the pregnancy almost killed me. This other one is the one I want to marry."

We talked a long time. Finally, the headman told Besa, "I have questioned Nisa about what happened and she has tied you up with her talk; her talk has defeated you, without doubt. Because what she has said about her pregnancy is serious. Therefore, today she and Twi will continue to stay together. After more time passes, I will ask all of you to come back again." Later, Twi and I left and went back to my brothers' village to sleep.

The next day, my older brother saw a honey cache while walking in the bush. He came to tell us and take us back there with him; we planned to stay the night in the bush. We arrived and spent the rest of the day collecting honey. When we finished, we walked toward where we were planning to camp. That's when I saw Besa's tracks in the sand. I said, "Everyone! Come here! Besa's tracks are here! Has anyone seen them elsewhere?" One of the men said, "Nonsense! Would you know his tracks . . ." I interrupted, "My husband . . . the man who married me . . . I *know* his tracks." The man's wife came to look, "Yes, those are Besa's tracks; his wife really did see them."

The next morning, Besa walked into the camp. Besa and Twi started to fight. My older brother yelled, "Do you two want to kill Nisa? Today she is not taking another husband. Today she's just going to lie by herself." I agreed, "Eh, I don't want to marry again now."

Twi and I continued to live together after that. But later we separated. My older brother caused it, because he wanted Besa to be with me again. He liked him and didn't like Twi. That's why he forced Twi to leave. When Twi saw how much anger both Dau and Besa felt toward him, he became afraid, and finally he left.

I saw what my brother had done and was miserable; I had really liked Twi. I said, "So, this is what you wanted? Fine, but now that you have chased Twi away, I'll have nothing at all to do with Besa." That's when I began to refuse Besa completely. Besa went to the headman and said, "Nisa refuses to be with me." The headman said, "Nisa's been refusing you for a long time. What legal grounds could I possibly find for you now?"

After more time passed, a man who had been my lover years before, started with me again. Soon we were very much in love. He was so handsome! His nose . . . his eyes . . . everything was so beautiful! His skin was light and his nose was lovely. I really loved that man, even when I first saw him.

We lived together for a while, but then he died. I was miserable, "My lover has died.

Where am I going to find another like him—another as beautiful, another as good, another with a European nose and with such lovely light skin? Now he's dead. Where will I ever find another like him?"

My heart was miserable and I mourned for him. I exhausted myself with mourning and only when it was finished did I feel better again.

After years of living and having everything that happened to me happen, that's when I started with Bo, the next important man in my life and the one I am married to today.

Besa and I lived separately, but he still wanted me and stayed near me. That man, he didn't hear; he didn't understand. He was without ears, because he still said, "This woman here, Nisa, I won't be finished with her."

People told Bo, "You're going to die. This man, Besa, he's going to kill you. Now, leave Nisa." But Bo refused, "Me . . . I won't go to another hut. I'll just stay with Nisa and even if Besa tries to kill me, I'll still be here and won't leave."

At first, Bo and I sneaked off together, but Besa suspected us; he was very jealous. He accused me all the time. Even when I just went to urinate, he'd say that I had been with Bo. Or when I went for water, he'd say, "Did you just meet your lover?" But I'd say, "What makes you think you can talk to me like that?" He'd say, "Nisa, you are not still my wife? Why aren't we living together? What are you doing?" I'd say, "Don't you have other women or are they refusing you, too? You have others so why are you asking me about what I'm doing?"

One night, Bo and I were lying down inside my hut and as I looked out through the latched-branch door, I saw someone moving about. It was Besa; I was able to see his face. He wanted to catch us, hoping I would feel some remorse and perhaps return to him.

I said, "What? Besa's here! Bo . . . Bo . . . Besa's standing out there." Bo got up; Besa came and stood by the door. I got up and that's when Besa came in and grabbed me. He held onto me and threatened to throw me into the fire. I cursed him as he held me, "Besa-Big-Testicles! Long-Penis! First you left me and drank of women's genitals elsewhere. Now you come back, see me, and say I am your wife?" He pushed me toward the fire, but I twisted my body so I didn't land in it. Then he went after Bo. Bo is weaker and older than Besa, so Besa was able to grab him, pull him outside the hut, and throw him down. He bit him on the shoulder. Bo yelled out in pain.

My younger brother woke and ran to us, yelling, "Curses to your genitals!" He grabbed them and separated them. Bo cursed Besa. Besa cursed Bo, "Curses on your penis!" He yelled, "I'm going to kill you Bo, then Nisa will suffer! If I don't kill you, then maybe I'll kill her so that you will feel pain! Because what you have that is so full of pleasure, I also have. So why does her heart want you and refuse me?"

I yelled at him, "That's not it! It's you! It's who you are and the way you think! This one, Bo, his ways are good and his thoughts are good. But you, your ways are foul. Look, you just bit Bo; that, too, is part of your ways. You also left me to die. And death, that's something I'm afraid of. That's why you no longer have a hold over me. Today I have another who will take care of me well. I'm no longer married to you, Besa. I want my husband to be Bo."

Besa kept bothering me and hanging around me. He'd ask, "Why won't you come to me? Come to me, I'm a man. Why are you afraid of me?" I wouldn't answer. Once Bo answered, "I don't understand why, if you *are* a man, you keep pestering this woman? Is what you're doing going to do any good? Because I won't leave her. And even though you bit me and your marks are on me, you're the one who is going to move out of the way, not me. I intend to marry her."

Another time I told Bo, "Don't be afraid of Besa. You and I will marry; I'm not going to stay married to him. Don't let him frighten you. Because even if he comes here with arrows, he won't do anything with them." Bo said, "Even if he did, what good would that do? I am also a man and am a master of arrows. The two of us would just strike each other. That's why I keep telling him to let you go; I am the man you are with now."

The next time, Besa came with his quiver full of arrows, saying, "I'm going to get Nisa and bring her back with me." He left with another man and came to me at my village. When he arrived, the sun was high in the sky. I was resting. He said, "Nisa, come, let's go." I said, "What? Is your penis not well? Is it horny?"

People heard us fighting and soon everyone was there, my younger and older brothers as well. Besa and I kept arguing and fighting until, in a rage, I screamed, "All right! Today I'm no longer afraid!" and I pulled off all the skins that were covering me—first one, then another, and finally the leather apron that covered my genitals. I pulled them all off and laid them down on the ground. I cried, "There! There's my vagina! Look, Besa, look at me! This is what you want!"

The man he had come with said, "This woman, her heart is truly far from you. Besa, look. Nisa refuses you totally, with all her heart. She refuses to have sex with you. Your relationship with her is finished. See. She took off her clothes, put them down, and with her genitals is showing everyone how she feels about you. She doesn't want you, Besa. If I were you, I'd finish with her today." Besa finally said, "Eh, you're right. Now I am finished with her."

The two of them left. I took my leather apron, put it on, took the rest of my things and put them on.

Mother! That was just what I did.

Besa tried one last time. He went to the headman again, and when he came back he told me, "The headman wants to see you." I thought, "If he wants to see me, I won't refuse."

When I arrived, the headman said, "Besa says he still wants to continue your marriage." I said, "Continue our marriage? Why? Am I so stupid that I don't know my name? Would I stay in a marriage with a man who left me hanging in a foreign place? If Old Debe and his wife hadn't been there, I would have truly lost my way. Me, stay married to Besa? I can't make myself think of it."

I turned to Besa, "Isn't that what I told you when we were still in the East?" Besa said, "Mm, that's what you said." I said, "And, when you left, didn't I tell you that you were leaving me pregnant with your baby. Didn't I also tell you that?" He said, "Yes, that's what you said." I said, "And didn't I say that I wanted to go with you, that I wanted you to help make our pregnancy grow strong? Didn't I say that and didn't you refuse?" He said, "Yes, you said that." Then I said, "Mm. Therefore, that marriage you say today, in the lap of the headman, should be continued, that marriage no longer exists. Because I am Nisa and today, when I look at you, all I want to do is to throw up. Vomit is the only thing left in my heart for you now. As we sit together here and I see your face, that is all that rises within and grabs me."

The headman laughed, shook his head and said, "Nisa is impossible!" Then he said, "Besa, you had better listen to her. Do you hear what she is saying? She says that you left her while she was pregnant, that she miscarried and was miserable. Today she will no longer take you for her husband." Besa said, "That's because she's with Bo now and doesn't want to leave him. But I still want her and want to continue our marriage."

I said, "What? Besa, can't you see me? Can't you see that I have really found another man? Did you think, perhaps, that I was too old and wouldn't find someone else?" The headman laughed again. "Yes, I am a woman. And that which you have, a penis, I also have something of equal worth. Like the penis of a chief . . . yes, something of a chief is what I have. And its worth is like money. Therefore, the person who drinks from it . . . it's like he's getting money from me. But not you, because when you had it, you just left it to ruin."

The headman said, "Nisa is crazy; her talk is truly crazy now." Then he said, "The two of you sleep tonight and give your thoughts over to this. Nisa, think about all of it again. Tomorrow, I want both of you to come back."

Besa went and lay down. I went and lay down and thought about everything. In the morning, I went to the headman. I felt ashamed by my talk of the night before. I sat there quietly. The headman said, "Nisa, Besa says you should stay married to him." I answered, "Why should he stay married to me when yesterday I held his baby in my stomach and he dropped me. Even God doesn't want me to marry a man who leaves me, a man who takes my blankets when I have small children beside me, a man who forces other people to give me blankets to cover my children with. Tell him to find another woman to marry."

The headman turned to Besa, "Nisa has explained herself. There's nothing more I can see to say. Even you, you can hear that she has defeated you. So, leave Nisa and as I am headman, today your marriage to her is ended. She can now marry Bo."[5]

Besa went to the headman one more time. When he tried to discuss it again, saying, "Please, help me. Give Nisa back to me," the headman said, "Haven't you already talked to me about this? You talked and talked, and the words entered my ears. Are you saying that I have not already decided on this? That I am not an important person? That I am a worthless thing that you do not have to listen to? There is no reason to give Nisa back to you."

I was so thankful when I heard his words. My heart filled with happiness.

Bo and I married soon after that.[6] We lived together, sat together, and did things together. Our hearts loved each other very much and our marriage was very very strong.

Besa also married again not long after—this time to a woman much younger than me. One day he came to me and said, "Look how wrong you were to have refused me! Perhaps you thought you were the only woman. But you, Nisa, today you are old and you yourself can see that I have married a young woman, one who is beautiful!"

I said, "Good! I told you that if we separated, you'd find a young woman to marry and to sleep with. That is fine with me because there is nothing I want from you. But you know, of course, that just like me, another day she too will be old."

We lived on, but not long after, Besa came back. He said that his young wife was troubled and that he wanted me again. I refused and even told Bo about it. Bo asked me why I refused. I said, "Because I don't want him." But what he says about his wife is true. She has a terrible sickness, a type of madness. God gave it to her. She was such a beautiful woman, too. But no longer. I wonder why such a young woman has to have something like that . . .

Even today, whenever Besa sees me, he argues with me and says he still wants me. I say, "Look, we've separated. Now leave me alone." I even sometimes refuse him food. Bo tells me I shouldn't refuse, but I'm afraid he will bother me more if I give anything to him. Because his heart still cries for me.

Sometimes I do give him things to eat and he also gives things to me. Once I saw him in my village. He came over to me and said, "Nisa, give me some water to drink." I washed out a cup and poured him some water. He drank it and said, "Now, give me some tobacco." I took out some tobacco and gave it to him. Then he said, "Nisa, you really are adult; you know how to work. Today, I am married to a woman but my heart doesn't agree to her much. But you . . . you are one who makes me feel pain. Because you left me and married another man. I also married, but have made myself weary by having married something bad. You, you have hands that work and do things. With you, I could eat. You would get water for me to wash with. Today, I'm really in pain."

I said, "Why are you thinking about our dead marriage? Of course, we were married once, but we have gone our different ways. Now, I no longer want you. After all that happened when you took me East—living there, working there, my father dying, my mother dying, and all the misery you caused me—you say we should live together once again?"

He said that I wasn't telling it as it happened.

One day, he told me he wanted to take me from Bo. I said, "What? Tell me, Besa, what has been talking to you that you are saying this again?" He said, "All right, then have me as your lover. Won't you help my heart out?" I said, "Aren't there many men who could be my lover? Why should I agree to you?" He said, "Look here, Nisa . . . I'm a person who helped bring up your children, the children you and your husband gave birth to. You became pregnant again with my child and that was good. You held it inside you and lived with it until God came and killed it. That's why your heart is talking this way and refusing me."

I told him he was wrong. But he was right, too. Because, after Besa, I never had any more children. He took that away from me. With Tashay, I had children, but Besa, he ruined me. Even the one time I did conceive, I miscarried. That's because of what he did to me; that's what everyone says.

NOTES

1. This chapter covers about five years, beginning when Nisa was in her early thirties (c. the mid 1950s).
2. In fact, her husband and children were with her.
3. The Rand is a South African currency that was then legal tender in Bechuanaland (pre-independence Botswana). It was worth between \$1.20 and \$1.50. Five Rand was a very large sum of money to the !Kung at that time—perhaps as much as two months wages at a typical menial task.
4. Tastes her: A euphemism for sexual intercourse.
5. The procedure for divorce in traditional !Kung culture would have been less complicated and would have proceeded more quickly.
6. Nisa and Bo married around 1957, when Nisa was about thirty-six years old.

THE MANHOOD PUZZLE

David D. Gilmore

> There are continuities of masculinity that transcend cultural differences.
>
> —Thomas Gregor, *Anxious Pleasures*

Are there continuities of masculinity across cultural boundaries, as the anthropologist Thomas Gregor says (1985:209)? Are men everywhere alike in their concern for being "manly?" If so, why? Why is the demand made upon males to "be a man" or "act like a man" voiced in so many places? And why are boys and youths so often tested or indoctrinated before being awarded their manhood? These are questions not often asked in the growing literature on sex and gender roles. Yet given the recent interest in sexual stereotyping, they are ones that need to be considered if we are to understand both sexes and their relations.

Regardless of other normative distinctions made, all societies distinguish between male and female; all societies also provide institutionalized sex-appropriate roles for adult men and women. A very few societies recognize a third, sexually intermediary category, such as the Cheyenne *berdache,* the Omani *xanith,* and the Tahitian *mahu* . . . but even in these rare cases of androgynous genders, the individual must make a life choice of identity and abide by prescribed rules of sexual comportment. In addition, most societies hold consensual ideas—guiding or admonitory images—for conventional masculinity and femininity by which individuals are judged worthy members of one or the other sex and are

Reprinted with permission from David D. Gilmore, *Manhood in the Making* (New Haven: Yale University Press, 1990), pp. 9–29.

evaluated more generally as moral actors. Such ideal statuses and their attendant images, or models, often become psychic anchors, or psychological identities, for most individuals, serving as a basis for self-perception and self-esteem (D'Andrade 1974:36).

These gender ideals, or guiding images, differ from culture to culture. But, as Gregor and others (e.g., Brandes 1980; Lonner 1980; Raphael 1988) have argued, underlying the surface differences are some intriguing similarities among cultures that otherwise display little in common. Impressed by the statistical frequency of such regularities in sexual patterning, a number of observers have recently argued that cultures are more alike than different in this regard. For example, Gregor (1985:200) studied a primitive Amazonian tribe and compared its sex ideals to those of contemporary America. Finding many subsurface similarities in the qualities expected of men and women, he concludes that our different cultures represent only a symbolic veneer masking a bedrock of sexual thinking. In another study, the psychologist Lonner (1980:147) echoes this conclusion. He argues that culture is "only a thin veneer covering an essential universality" of gender dimorphism. In their comprehensive survey of sex images in thirty different cultures, Williams and Best (1982:30) conclude that there is "substantial similarity" to be found "panculturally in the traits ascribed to men and women."

Whether or not culture is only a thin veneer over a deep structure is a complicated question: as the rare third sexes show, we must not see in every culture "a Westerner struggling to get out" (Munroe and Munroe 1980:25). But most social scientists would agree that there do exist striking regularities in standard male and female roles across cultural boundaries regardless of other social arrangements (Archer and Lloyd 1985:283–84). The one regularity that concerns me here is the often dramatic ways in which cultures construct an appropriate manhood—the presentation or "imaging" of the male role. In particular, there is a constantly recurring notion that real manhood is different from simple anatomical maleness, that it is not a natural condition that comes about spontaneously through biological maturation but rather is a precarious or artificial state that boys must win against powerful odds. This recurrent notion that manhood is problematic, a critical threshold that boys must pass through testing, is found at all levels of sociocultural development regardless of what other alternative roles are recognized. It is found among the simplest hunters and fishermen, among peasants and sophisticated urbanized peoples; it is found in all continents and environments. It is found among both warrior peoples and those who have never killed in anger.

Moreover, this recurrent belief represents a primary and recurrent difference from parallel notions of femaleness. Although women, too, in any society are judged by sometimes stringent sexual standards, it is rare that their very status as woman forms part of the evaluation. Women who are found deficient or deviant according to these standards may be criticized as immoral, or they may be called unladylike or its equivalent and subjected to appropriate sanctions, but rarely is their right to a gender identity questioned in the same public, dramatic way that it is for men. The very paucity of linguistic labels for females echoing the epithets "effete," "unmanly," "effeminate," "emasculated," and so on, attest to this archetypical difference between sex judgments worldwide. And it is far more assaultive (and frequent) for men to be challenged in this way than for women.

Perhaps the difference between male and female should not be overstated, for "femininity" is also something achieved by women who seek social approval. But as a social icon, femininity seems to be judged differently. It usually involves questions of body ornament or sexual allure, or other essentially cosmetic behaviors that enhance, rather than create, an inherent quality of character. An authentic femininity rarely involves tests or proofs of action, or confrontations with dangerous foes: win-or-lose contests dramatically played out on the public stage. Rather than a critical threshold passed by traumatic testing, an either/or condition, femininity is more often construed as a biological given that is culturally refined or augmented.

TESTS OF MANHOOD: A SURVEY

Before going any further, let us look at a few examples of this problematic manhood. Our first stop is Truk Island, a little atoll in the South Pacific. Avid fishermen, the people of Truk have lived for ages from the sea, casting and diving in deep waters. According to the anthropologists who have lived among them, the Trukese men are obsessed with their masculinity, which they regard as chancy. To maintain a manly image, the men are encouraged to take risks with life and limb and to think "strong" or "manly" thoughts, as the natives put it (M. Marshall 1979). Accordingly, they challenge fate by going on deep-sea fishing expeditions in tiny dugouts and spearfishing with foolhardy abandon in shark-infested waters. If any men shrink from such challenges, their fellows, male and female, laugh at them, calling them effeminate and childlike. When on land, Trukese youths fight in weekend brawls, drink to excess, and seek sexual conquests to attain a manly image. Should a man fail in any of these efforts, another will taunt him: "Are you a man? Come, I will take your life now" (ibid.:92).

Far away on the Greek Aegean island of Kalymnos, the people are also stalwart seafarers, living by commercial sponge fishing (Bernard 1967). The men of Kalymnos dive into deep water without the aid of diving equipment, which they scorn. Diving is therefore a gamble because many men are stricken and crippled by the bends for life. But no matter: they have proven their precious manhood by showing their contempt for death (ibid.:119). Young divers who take precautions are effeminate, scorned and ridiculed by their fellows.

These are two seafaring peoples. Let us move elsewhere, to inland Black Africa, for example, where fishing is replaced by pastoral pursuits. In East Africa young boys from a host of cattle-herding tribes, including the Masai, Rendille, Jie, and Samburu, are taken away from their mothers and subjected at the outset of adolescence to bloody circumcision rites by which they become true men. They must submit without so much as flinching under the agony of the knife. If a boy cries out while his flesh is being cut, if he so much as blinks an eye or turns his head, he is shamed for life as unworthy of manhood, and his entire lineage is shamed as a nursery of weaklings. After this very public ordeal, the young initiates are isolated in special dormitories in the wilderness. There, thrust on their own devices, they learn the tasks of a responsible manhood: cattle rustling, raiding, killing, survival in the bush. If their long apprenticeship is successful, they return to society as men and are only then permitted to take a wife.

Another dramatic African case comes from nearby Ethiopia: the Amhara, a Semitic-speaking tribe of rural cultivators. They have a passionate belief in masculinity called *wand-nat.* This idea involves aggressiveness, stamina, and bold "courageous action" in the face of danger; it means never backing down when threatened (Levine 1966:18). To show their wand-nat, the Amhara youths are forced to engage in whipping contests called *buhe* (Reminick 1982:32). During the whipping ceremonies, in which all able-bodied male adolescents must participate for their reputations' sake, the air is filled with the cracking of whips. Faces are lacerated, ears torn open, and red and bleeding welts appear (ibid.:33). Any sign of weakness is greeted with taunts and mockery. As if this were not enough, adolescent Amhara boys are wont to prove their virility by scarring their arms with red-hot embers (Levine 1966:19). In these rough ways the boys actualize the exacting Amhara "ideals of masculinity" (Reminick 1976:760).

Significantly, this violent testing is not enough for these virile Ethiopians. Aside from showing physical hardihood and courage in the buhe matches, a young man must demonstrate his potency on his wedding night by waving a bloody sheet of marital consummation before the assembled kinsmen (ibid.:760–61). As well as demonstrating the bride's virginity, this ceremonial defloration is a talisman of masculinity for the Amhara groom. The Amhara's proof of manhood, like that of the Trukese, is both sexual and violent, and his performances both on the battlefield and in the marriage bed must be visibly displayed, recorded, and confirmed by the group; otherwise he is no man.

Halfway around the world, in the high mountains of Melanesia, young boys undergo similar trials before being admitted into the select club of manhood. In the New Guinea Highlands, boys are torn from their mothers and forced to undergo a series of brutal masculinizing rituals (Herdt 1982). These include whipping, flailing, beating, and other forms of terrorization by older men, which the boys must endure stoically and silently. As in Ethiopia, the flesh is scored and blood flows freely. These Highlanders believe that without such hazing, boys will never mature into men but will remain weak and childlike. Real men are made, they insist, not born.

PARALLELS

To be sure, there are some contextual similarities in these last few examples. The Amhara, Masai, and New Guinea Highlanders share one feature in common beyond the stress on manhood: they are fierce warrior peoples, or were in the recent past. One may argue that their bloody rites prepare young boys for the idealized life of the warrior that awaits them. So much is perhaps obvious: some Western civilizations also subject soft youths to rough hazing and initiations in order to toughen them up for a career of soldiering, as in the U.S. Marines (Raphael 1988). But these trials are by no means confined to militaristic cultures or castes. Let us take another African example.

Among the relatively peaceful !Kung Bushmen of southwest Africa (Thomas 1959; Lee 1979), manhood is also a prize to be grasped through a test. Accurately calling themselves "The Harmless People" (Thomas 1959), these nonviolent Bushmen have never fought a war in their lives. They have no military weapons, and they frown upon physical violence (which, however, sometimes does occur). Yet even here, in a culture that treasures gentleness and cooperation above all things, the boys must earn the right to be called men by a test of skill and endurance. They must single-handedly track and kill a sizable adult antelope, an act that requires courage and hardiness. Only after their first kill of such a buck are they considered fully men and permitted to marry.

Other examples of stressed manhood among gentle people can be found in the New World, in aboriginal North America. Among the nonviolent Fox tribe of Iowa, for example, "being a man" does not come easily (Gearing 1970:51). Based on stringent standards of accomplishment in tribal affairs and economic pursuits, real manhood is said to be "the Big Impossible," an exclusive status that only the nimble few can achieve (ibid.:51–52). Another American Indian example is the Tewa people of New Mexico, also known as the Pueblo Indians. These placid farmers, who are known today for their serene culture, gave up all warfare in the last century. Yet they subject their boys to a severe hazing before they can be accounted men. Between the ages of twelve and fifteen, the Tewa boys are taken away from their homes, purified by ritual means, and then whipped mercilessly by the Kachina spirits (their fathers in disguise). Each boy is stripped naked and lashed on the back four times with a crude yucca whip that draws blood and leaves permanent scars. The adolescents are expected to bear up impassively under the beating to show their fortitude. The Tewa say that this rite makes their boys into men, that otherwise manhood is doubtful. After the boys' ordeal, the Kachina spirits tell them, "You are now a man. . . . You are made a man" (Hill 1982:220). Although Tewa girls have their own (nonviolent) initiations, there is no parallel belief that girls have to be *made* women, no "big impossible" for them; for the Tewa and the Fox, as for the other people above, womanhood develops naturally, needing no cultural intervention, its predestined arrival at menarche commemorated rather than forced by ritual (ibid.:209–10).

Nor are such demanding efforts at proving oneself a man confined to primitive peoples or those on the margins of civilization. In urban Latin America, for example, as described by Oscar Lewis (1961:38), a man must prove his manhood every day by standing up to challenges and insults, even though he goes to his death "smiling." As well as being tough and brave, ready to defend his family's honor at the drop of a hat, the urban Mexican, like the Amhara man, must also perform adequately in sex and father many children. Such macho exploits are also common among many of the peasant and pastoral peoples who reside in the cradle of the ancient Mediterranean civilizations. In the Balkans, for instance, the category of "real men" is clearly defined. A real man is one who drinks heavily, spends money freely, fights bravely, and raises a large family (Simic 1969, 1983). In this way he shows an "indomitable virility" that distinguishes him from effeminate counterfeits (Denich 1974:250). In eastern Morocco, true men are distinguished from effete men on the basis of physical prowess and heroic acts of both feuding and sexual potency; their manly deeds are memorialized in verses sung before admiring crowds at festivals, making manhood a kind of communal celebration (Marcus 1987:50). Likewise, for the Bedouin of Egypt's Western Desert, "real men" are contrasted with despicable weaklings who are "no men." Real Bedouin men are bold and courageous, afraid of nothing. Such men assert their will at any cost and stand up to any challenge; their main attributes are "assertiveness and the quality of potency" (Abu-Lughod 1986:88–89). Across the sea, in Christian Crete, men in village coffee shops proudly sing paeans to their own virility, their self-promotion having been characterized as the "poetics of manhood" by Michael Herzfeld (1985a:15). These Cretans must demonstrate their "manly selfhood" by stealing sheep, procreating large families, and besting other men in games of chance and skill (ibid.).

Examples of this pressured manhood with its almost talismanic qualities could be given almost indefinitely and in all kinds of contexts. Among most of the peoples that anthropologists are familiar with, true manhood is a precious and elusive status beyond mere maleness, a hortatory image that men and boys aspire to and that their culture demands of them as a measure of belonging. Although this stressed or embattled quality varies in intensity, becoming highly marked in southern Spain, Morocco, Egypt, and some other Mediterranean-area traditions, true manhood in other cultures frequently shows an inner insecurity that needs dramatic proof. Its vindication is doubtful, resting on rigid codes of decisive action in many spheres of life: as husband, father, lover, provider, warrior. A restricted status, there are always men who fail the test. These are the negative examples, the effete men, the men-who-are-no-men, held up scornfully to inspire conformity to the glorious ideal.

Perhaps these stagy routes to manhood seem bizarre to us at first glance. But none of them should surprise most Anglophone readers, for we too have our manly traditions, both in our popular culture and in literary genres. Although we may choose less flamboyant modes of expression than the Amhara or Trukese, we too have regarded manhood as an artificial state, a challenge to be overcome, a prize to be won by fierce struggle: if not "the big impossible," then certainly doubtful.

For example, let us take a people and a social stratum far removed from those above: the gentry of modern England. There, young boys were traditionally subjected to similar trials on the road to their majority. They were torn at a tender age from mother and home, as in East Africa or in New Guinea, and sent away in age sets to distant testing grounds that sorely took their measure. These were the public boarding schools, where a cruel "trial by ordeal," including physical violence and terrorization by elder males, provided a passage to a "social state of manhood" that their parents thought could be achieved in no other way (Chandos 1984:172). Supposedly, this harsh training prepared young Oxbridge aristocrats for the self-reliance and fortitude needed to run the British Empire and thereby manufactured "a serviceable elite as stylized as Samurai" (ibid.:346). Even here, in Victorian England, a culture not given over to showy excess, manhood was an artificial product coaxed by austere training and testing.

Similar ideas motivated educators on both sides of the Atlantic, for example, the founders of the Boy Scouts. Their chartered purpose, as they put it in their pamphlets and manuals, was to "make big men of little boys" by fostering "an independent manhood," as though this were not to be expected from nature alone (cited by Hantover 1978:189). This obsessive moral masculinization in the English-speaking countries went beyond mere mortals of the day to Christ himself, who was portrayed in turn-of-the-century tracts as "the supremely manly man," athletic and aggressive when necessary, no "Prince of Peace-at-any-price" (Conant 1915:117). The English publicist Thomas Hughes dilated rhapsodically about the manliness of Christ (1879), while his colleagues strove to depict Christianity as the "muscular" or "manly" faith. Pious and articulate English Protestants loudly proclaimed their muscular religion as an antidote to what Charles Kingsley derided as the "fastidious maundering, die-away effeminacy" of the High Anglican Church (cited in Gay 1982:532). Boys, faiths, and gods had to be made masculine; otherwise there was doubt. The same theme runs through much British literature of the time, most notably in Kipling, as for example in the following lines from the poem "If":

> If you can fill the unforgiving minute
> With sixty seconds worth of distance run,
> Yours is the Earth, and everything that's in it,
> And—which is more—you'll be a Man, my son!

Consequent only to great deeds, being a Kiplingesque man is more than owning the Earth, a truly imperial masculinity consonant with empire building. The same theme of "iffy" heroism runs through many aspects of popular middle-class American culture today. Take, for example, the consistent strain in U.S. literature of masculine *Bildungsroman*—the ascension to the exalted status of manhood under the tutelage of knowledgeable elders, with the fear of failure always lurking menancingly in the background. This theme is most strongly exemplified by Ernest Hemingway, of course, notably in the Nick Adams stories, but it is also found in the work of such contemporaries as William Faulkner and John Dos Passos, and in such Hemingway epigones as Studs Terkel, Norman Mailer, James Dickey, Frederick Exley, and—the new generation—Robert Stone, Jim Harrison, and Tom McGuane. This "virility school" in American letters (Schwenger 1984:13), was sired by Papa Hemingway (if one discounts Jack London) and nurtured thereafter by his acolytes, but it is now in its third or fourth generation and going strong (for a feminist view see Fetterly 1978).

In contemporary literary America, too, manhood is often a mythic confabulation, a Holy Grail, to be seized by long and arduous testing. Take, for example, this paradigmatic statement by Norman Mailer (1968:25): "Nobody was born a man; you earned manhood provided you were good enough, bold enough." As well as echoing his spiritual forebears, both British and American, Mailer articulates here the unwritten sentiments of the Trukese, the Amhara, the Bushmen, and countless other peoples who have little else in common except this same obsessive "quest for male validation" (Raphael 1988:67). Although some of us may smile at Mailer for being so histrionic and sophomoric about it, he nevertheless touches a raw nerve that pulsates through many cultures as well as our own. Nor is Mailer's challenge representative of only a certain age or stratum of American society. As the poet Leonard Kriegel (1979:14) says in his reflective book about American manhood, "In every age, not just our own, manhood was something that had to be won."

Looking back, for instance, one is reminded of the cultural values of the antebellum American South. Southerners, whatever their class, placed great stress on a volatile manly honor as a defining feature of the southern character, a fighting principle. Indeed, Bertram Wyatt-Brown, in his book *Southern Honor* (1982), has argued convincingly that this touchy notion was a major element behind southern secessionism and thus an important and underrated political factor in U.S. history. A defense of southern "manliness" was in fact offered by Confederate writers of the time, including the South Carolina firebrand Charles C. Jones, as one justification for regional defiance, political separation, and, finally, war (cited in McPherson 1988:41). And of course similar ideals are enshrined in the frontier folklore of the American West, past and present, as exemplified in endless cowboy epics.

This heroic image of an achieved manhood is being questioned in America by feminists and by so-called liberated men themselves (Pleck 1981; Brod 1987). But for decades, it has been widely legitimized in U.S. cultural settings ranging from Italian-American gangster culture to Hollywood Westerns, private-eye tales, the current Rambo imagoes, and children's He-Man dolls and games; it is therefore deeply ingrained in the American male psyche. As the anthropologist Robert LeVine (1979:312) says, it is an organization of cultural principles that function together as a "guiding myth within the confines of our culture." But given the similarities between contemporary American notions of manliness and those of the many cultures discussed above, can we drop LeVine's qualifying phrase about "the confines of our culture"? Can we speak instead of an archetype or "deep structure" of masculinity, as Andrew Tolson (1977:56) puts it? And if so, what explains all these similarities? Why the trials and the testing and the seemingly gratuitous agonies of man-playing? Why is so much indoctrination and motivation needed in all these cultures to make real men? What is there about "official" manliness that requires such effort, such challenge, and such investment? And why should manhood be so desirable a state and at the same time be conferred so grudgingly in so many societies? These are some of the questions I want to consider here. Only a broadly comparative approach can begin to answer them.

MANHOOD AND GENDER ROLE

Let us pause at this point to take stock. What do we know so far about the origins of such gender imagery? Until very recently, studies of male and female were wedded to a persistent paradigm derived from mechanistic nineteenth-century antecedents. Most pervasive was the idea of generic types, a Universal Man counterpoised to a Universal Woman—a sexual symmetry supposedly derived from self-evident dualisms in biology and psychology (Katchadourian 1979:20). Freud, for example, held that anatomy was destiny, and Jung (1926) went so far as to develop universal principles of masculinity and femininity which he conveyed as "animus" and "anima," irreducible cores of sexual identity. Western literature and philosophy are full of such fundamental and supposedly immutable dualisms (Bakan 1966); they are also found in some Asian cosmologies, for example, the Chinese Yin and Yang, and in countless sets of binary oppositions both philosophical and scientific (e.g., Ortner 1974). What could be a neater polarity than sex? Our view of manhood in the past was often a simple reflection of these polar views of male and female "natures" or "principles." This view had some scientific support among biologists and psychologists, many of whom held that the aggressiveness of masculinity, including the testing and proving, was merely a consequence of male anatomy and hormones: men seek challenges because they are naturally aggressive. That is simply the way they are; women are the opposite. Period.

The way we look at sex roles, however, has changed drastically in the past two decades. Although appealing to many, sex dualisms and oppositions are definitely out of fashion, and so are sexual universals and biological determinisms. Part of the reason, aside from the recent movement away from static structural dualisms in the social sciences generally, lies in the feminist revolution of the past twenty years. Starting in the 1960s, the feminist attack on the bipolar mode of sexual thinking has shaken this dualistic edifice to its roots; but to be fair, it was never very sturdy to begin with. For example, both Freud and Jung accepted an inherent mixture of masculinity and femininity within each human psyche. Although he distinguished male and female principles, Jung to his credit admitted the existence of animus and anima to degrees in all people; bisexuality was in fact one of the bedrocks of Freud's psychological reasoning. In every human being, Freud (1905:220) remarks, "pure masculinity or femininity is not to be found either in a psychological or a biological sense. Every individual on the contrary displays a mixture."

Moreover, feminists of various backgrounds and persuasions (see, for example, Baker 1980; Sanday 1981; Otten 1985) have convincingly demonstrated that the conventional bipolar model based on biology is invalid and that sex (biological inheritance) and gender (cultural norms) are distinct categories that may have a relationship but not an isomorphic identity. Most observers would agree that hormones and anatomy do have an effect on our behavior. The biological anthropologist Melvin Konner has convincingly shown this in his book, *The Tangled Wing* (1982). Assessing the latest scientific and clinical literature in this highly acclaimed survey, Konner concludes that testosterone (the main male sex hormone) predisposes males to a slightly higher level of aggressivity than females (see also Archer and Lloyd 1985; 138–39). But, as Konner freely admits, biology does not determine all of our behavior, or even very much of it, and cultures do indeed vary to some degree in assigning sex roles, measured in jobs and tasks. Discrete concepts of masculinity and femininity, based on secondary sex characteristics, exist in virtually all societies, but they are not always constructed and interfaced in the same way. Gender is a symbolic category. As such, it has strong moral overtones, and therefore is ascriptive and culturally relative—potentially changeful. On the other hand, sex is rooted in anatomy and is therefore fairly constant (Stoller 1968). It is now generally accepted, even among the most traditional male researchers, that masculine and feminine principles are not inherent polarities but an "overlapping continuum" (Biller and Borstelmann 1967: 255), or, as Spence and Helmreich put it (1979:4), "orthogonal dimensions."

Still, as we have seen from the examples above, there exists a recurrent cultural tendency to distinguish and to polarize gender roles. Instead of allowing free play in sex roles and gender ideals, most societies tend to exaggerate biological potentials by clearly differentiating sex roles and by defining the proper behavior of men and women as opposite or complementary. Even where so-called "third sexes" exist, as for example the Plains Indian berdache and the Omani xanith, conventional male and female types are still strongly differentiated. So the question of continuities in gender imaging must go beyond genetic endowment to encompass cultural norms and moral scripts. If there are archetypes in the male image (as there are in femininity), they must be largely culturally constructed as symbolic systems, not simply as products of anatomy, because anatomy determines very little in those contexts where the moral imagination comes into play. The answer to the manhood puzzle must lie in culture; we must try to understand why culture uses or exaggerates biological potentials in specific ways.

PREVIOUS INTERPRETATIONS

Some feminists and other relativists have perceived the apparent contradiction between the theoretical arbitrariness of gender concepts and the empirical convergence of sex roles. Explanations have therefore been offered to account for it. The existing explanations are interesting and useful, and I do not argue against them on the grounds of logical consistency. Rather, I think that the wrong questions have been asked in this inquiry. Most explanations have been phrased in one of two ways, both ideologically satisfying depending upon one's point of view, but neither getting us very far analytically.

First, the question has been phrased by the more doctrinaire Marxists and some radical feminists in an idiom of pure conflict theory. They see gender ideology as having a purely exploitative function. Thus they ask, inevitably, cui bono? Since many male ideologies include an element of gender oppressiveness, or at least hierarchy (in the view of liberated Western intellectuals), some of these radicals regard masculine ideologies as masks or justifications for the oppression of women. They see male ideologies as mystifications of power relationships, as examples of false consciousness (see, for example, Ortner 1981; Godelier 1986). This explanation is probably true for some cases, at least as a partial explanation, especially in some extreme patriarchies where male dominance is very pronounced. But it cannot be true as a universal explanation, because it cannot account for instances in which males are tested for manhood but where there is relative sexual equality. We have seen one example of this in the African Bushmen (Thomas 1959; Lee 1979; Shostak 1981). Although these nonsexist foragers are often held up by feminists as a model of sexual egalitarianism (Shostak 1981), Bushmen boys must prove their manhood by hunting prowess. They must also undergo tests of hardiness and skill from which girls are excluded. . . . Their manhood is subject to proof and, conceptually, to diminishment or loss. The same is true of the Fox and the Tewa of North America. So if a conception of manhood has no oppressive function in these societies, what is it doing there? It seems that the conflict theorists are missing something.

The second idiom of explanation is equally reductionistic. Here, biological or psychological processes are given analytical priority. There are two forms of biopsychological reductionist argument. The first is biological/evolutionary à la Lionel Tiger in *Men in Groups* (1971). Tiger holds that men worry about manhood because evolutionary pressures have predisposed them to do so. Once we were all hunters, and our success and therefore the survival and expansion of the group depended upon our developing genetically determined "masculine tendencies," aggression and male bonding being principal among them. This sociobiological argument is useful in certain cases, again, most notably in the violent patriarchies. But it is demonstrably false as a universal explanation because there are many societies where "aggressive" hunting never played an important role, where men do not bond for economic purposes, where violence and war are devalued or unknown, and yet where men are today concerned about demonstrating manhood. Further, this argument commits the historical fallacy of proposing a historical explanation for a cultural trait that persists under changed circumstances.

The second genetic reductionism is the standard psychoanalytic one about male psychic development. It is based squarely on an orthodox reading of Freud's Oedipus complex and its derivative, castration anxiety. This orthodoxy has been challenged recently with a neo-Freudian viewpoint stressing other aspects of male development, which I find much more powerful. . . . The standard psychoanalytic view holds that men everywhere are defending against castration fears as a result of identical oedipal traumas in psychosexual development. Masculinity cults and ideals are compensations erected universally against such fears (Stephens 1967; Kline 1972).

In this view, the norms of masculinity are projected outward from the individual psyche onto the screen of culture; public culture is individual fantasy life writ large. I think this explanation is useful in some cases but supererogatory. More damaging, it fails to give proper weight to social constraints that enforce male conformity to manhood ideals; as we shall see, boys have to be encouraged—sometimes actually forced—by social sanctions to undertake efforts toward a culturally defined manhood, which by themselves they might not do. So the explanation cannot be one based solely on psychic projections. Moreover, the orthodox psychoanalytic view can also be demonstrated to be false at a universal level, for there are empirical exceptions to the culture of manhood. There are a few societies that do not place the usual stress on achieving a masculine image; in these exceptional "neuter" societies, males are freed from the need to prove themselves and are allowed a basically androgynous script, which, significantly, they find congenial. As these exceptions do exist, . . . the answer to the masculinity puzzle must have a social side to it, because formal variation cannot be explained on the basis of a psychological constant such as castration anxiety.

SOME HELP FROM THE POST-FREUDIANS

At this point we have to call upon some alternative models of male psychosexual development that accommodate social and relational factors. A psychological theory of masculinity that I find useful . . . derives in part from recent work by the post-Freudian ego psychologists. The list of relevant theorists and their works is long but may be reduced here to Erik Erikson, Ralph Greenson, Edith Jacobson, Margaret Mahler, Gregory Rochlin, Robert Stoller, and D. W. Winnicott.

The basic idea here concerns the special problems attached to the origin of masculinity as a category of self-identity distinct from femininity. The theory begins with the assumption that all infants, male and female, establish a primary identity, as well as a social bond, with the nurturing parent, the mother. This theory already departs from the classic Freudian assumption that the boy child has from the first a male identity and a natural heterosexual relationship with his mother that culminates in the oedipal conflict, that the boy's identity as male is axiomatic and unconflicted. This new theory goes on to posit an early and prolonged unity or psychic merging with the mother that Freud (1914) discussed under "primary narcissism," a period when the infant fails to distinguish between self and mother. The argument is that the physical separation of child and mother at birth does not bring with it a psychological separation of equivalent severity or finality.

As the child grows, it reaches the critical threshold that Mahler (1975) has called separation-individuation. At this juncture its growing awareness of psychic separateness from the mother combines with increased physical mobility and a motoric exercise of independent action, for example, walking, speaking, manipulating toys. These independent actions are rewarded socially both by parents and by other members of the group who want to see the child grow up (Erikson 1950). Boys and girls alike go through these same trial stages of separation, self-motivation, encouragement and reward, and proto-personhood; and both become receptive to social demands for gender-appropriate behavior. However, according to this theory, the boy child encounters special problems in the crucible of the separation-individuation stage that impede further progression toward independent selfhood.

The special liability for boys is the different fate of the primal psychic unity with the mother. The self-awareness of being a separate individual carries with it a parallel sense of a gender identity—being either a man or a woman, boy or girl. In most societies, each individual must choose one or the other unequivocally in order, also, to be a separate and autonomous person recognizable as such by peers and thus to earn acceptance. The special problem the boy faces at this point is in overcoming the previous sense of unity with the mother in order to achieve an independent identity defined by his culture as masculine—an effort functionally equivalent not only to psychic separation but also to creating an autonomous public persona. The girl does not experience this problem as acutely, according to this theory, because her femininity is reinforced by her original symbiotic unity with her mother, by the identification with her that precedes self-identity and that culminates with her own motherhood (Chodorow 1978). In most societies, the little boy's sense of self as independent must include a sense of the self as different from his mother, as separate from her both in ego-identity and in social role. Thus for the boy the task of separation and individuation carries an added burden and peril. Robert Stoller (1974:358) has stated this problem succinctly:

> While it is true the boy's first love object is heterosexual [the mother], he must perform a great deed to make this so: he must first separate his identity from hers. Thus the whole process of becoming masculine is at risk in the little boy from the day of birth on; his still-to-be-created masculinity is endangered by the primary, profound, primeval oneness with mother, a blissful experience that serves, buried but active in the core of one's identity, as a focus which, throughout life, can attract one to regress back to that primitive oneness. That is the threat latent in masculinity.

To become a separate person the boy must perform a great deed. He must pass a test; he must break the chain to his mother. He must renounce his bond to her and seek his own way in the world. His masculinity thus represents his separation from his mother and his entry into a new and independent social status recognized as distinct and opposite from hers. In this view the main threat to the boy's growth is not only, or even primarily, castration anxiety. The principal danger to the boy is not a unidimensional fear of the punishing father but a more ambivalent fantasy-fear about the mother. The ineradicable fantasy is to return to the primal maternal symbiosis. The inseparable fear is that restoring the oneness with the mother will overwhelm one's independent selfhood.

Recently, armed with these new ideas, some neo-Freudians have begun to focus more specifically on the puzzle of masculine role modeling cults. They have been less concerned with the questions of gender identity and castration anxiety than with the related questions of regression and its relation to social role. In a recent symposium on the subject, the psychoanalyst Gerald Fogel (1986:10) argues that the boy's dilemma goes "beyond castration anxiety" to a conflicted effort to give up the anaclitic unity with the mother, which robs him of his independence. In the same symposium, another psychoanalyst (Cooper 1986:128) refers to the comforting sense of omnipotence that this symbiotic unity with the mother affords. This sense of omnipotence, of narcissistic completeness, sensed and retained in fantasy as a blissful experience of oneness with the mother, he argues, is what draws the boy back so powerfully toward childhood and away from the challenge of an autonomous manhood. In this view, the struggle for masculinity is a battle against these regressive wishes and fantasies, a hard-fought renunciation of the longings for the prelapsarian idyll of childhood.

From this perspective, then, the manhood equation is a "revolt against boyishness" (Schafer 1986:100). The struggle is specifically "against regression" (ibid.). This revisionist theory provides us with a psychological key to the puzzle of manhood norms and ideals. Obviously, castration fear is also important from an individual point of view. But manhood ideologies are not only intrapsychic; they are also collective representations that are institutionalized as guiding images in most societies. To understand the meaning of manhood from a sociological point of view, to appreciate its social rather than individual functions and causes, regression is the more important variable to consider. The reason for this is that, in aggregate, regression poses a more serious threat to society as a whole. As we shall see, regression is unacceptable not only to the individual but also to his society as a functioning mechanism, because most societies demand renunciation of escapist wishes in favor of a participating, contributing adulthood. Castration anxiety, though something that all men may also need to resolve, poses no such aggregate threat to social continuity. In sum, manhood imagery can be interpreted from this post-Freudian perspective as a defense against the eternal child within, against puerility, against what is sometimes called the Peter Pan complex (Hallman 1969).

REFERENCES

Abu-Lughod, Lila. 1986. *Veiled Sentiments: Honor and Poetry in a Bedouin Society.* Berkeley: University of California Press.

Archer, John, and Barbara Lloyd. 1985. *Sex and Gender.* Cambridge: Cambridge University Press.

Bakan, David. 1966. *The Duality of Human Existence.* Chicago: University of Chicago Press.

Baker, Susan W. 1980. Biological influences on human sex and gender. *Signs* 6:80–96.

Bernard, H. Russell. 1967. Kalymnian sponge diving. *Human Biology* 39:103–30.

Biller, Henry B., and Lloyd Borstelmann. 1967. Masculine development: An integrative view. *Merrill-Palmer Quarterly* 13:253–94.

Brandes, Stanley H. 1980. *Metaphors of Masculinity: Sex and Status in Andalusian Folklore.* Philadelphia: University of Pennsylvania Press.

Brod, Harry (ed.). 1987. *The Making of Masculinities: The New Men's Studies.* Boston: Allen and Unwin.

Chandos, John. 1984. *Boys Together: English Public Schools, 1800–1864.* New Haven: Yale University Press.

Chodorow, Nancy. 1978. *The Reproduction of Mothering.* Berkeley: University of California Press.

Conant, Robert W. 1915. *The Virility of Christ.* Chicago: no publisher.

Cooper, Arnold M. 1986. What men fear: The facade of castration anxiety. In *The Psychology of Men: New Psychoanalytic Perspective,* ed. Gerald Fogel, F. M. Lane, and R. S. Liebert, pp. 113–30. New York: Basic Books.

D'Andrade, Roy G. 1974. Sex differences and cultural institutions. In *Culture and Personality: Contemporary Readings,* ed. Robert A. LeVine, pp. 16–39. Chicago: Aldine.

Denich, Bette. 1974. Sex and power in the Balkans. In *Women, Culture, and Society,* ed. Michelle Rosaldo and Louise Lamphere, pp. 243–62. Stanford: Stanford University Press.

Erikson, Erik. 1950. *Childhood and Society.* New York: Norton.

Fetterly, Judith. 1978. *The Resisting Reader: A Feminist Approach to American Fiction.* Bloomington, Ind.: Indiana University Press.

Fogel, Gerald I. 1986. Introduction: Being a man. In *The Psychology of Men: New Psychoanalytic Perspectives,* ed. Gerald Fogel, F. M. Lane, and R. S. Liebert, pp. 3–22. New York: Basic Books.

Freud, Sigmund. 1905. Three Essays on the Theory of Sexuality, III: The Transformations of Puberty. *Standard Edition,* ed. James Strachey 7:207–30. London: Hogarth Press (1975).

———. 1914. On narcissism. *Standard Edition,* ed. James Strachey, 14:67–102. London: Hogarth Press (1975).

Gay, Peter, 1982. Liberalism and regression. *Psychoanalytic Study of the Child* 37:523–45. New Haven: Yale University Press.

Gearing, Frederick O. 1970. *The Face of the Fox.* Chicago: Aldine.

Godelier, Maurice. 1986. *The Making of Great Men.* Cambridge: Cambridge University Press.

Gregor, Thomas. 1985. *Anxious Pleasures: The Sexual Life of an Amazonian People.* Chicago: University of Chicago Press.

Hallman, Ralph, 1969. The archetypes in Peter Pan. *Journal of Analytic Psychology* 14:65–73.

Hantover, Jeffrey P. 1978. The Boy Scouts and the validation of masculinity. *Journal of Social Issues* 34:184–95.

Herdt, Gilbert H. 1982. Fetish and fantasy in Sambia initiation. In *Rituals of Manhood,* ed. Gilbert H. Herdt, pp. 44–98. Berkeley: University of California Press.

Hertzfeld, Michael. 1985. *Gender pragmatics: agency, speech and bride-theft in a Cretan mountain village.* Anthropology 9:25–44.

Hill, W. W. 1982. *An Ethnography of Santa Clara Pueblo, New Mexico,* ed. and annotated by Charles H. Lange, Albuquerque, N. Mex.: University of New Mexico Press.

Hughes, Thomas. 1879. *The Manliness of Christ.* London: Macmillan.

Jung, Carl. 1926. *Psychological Types.* New York: Harcourt, Brace and Co.

Katchadourian, Herant A. 1979. The terminology of sex and gender. In *Human Sexuality: Comparative and Developmental Perspectives,* ed. Herant A. Katchadourian, pp. 8–34. Berkeley: University of California Press.

Kline, Paul. 1972. *Fact and Fantasy in Freudian Theory.* London: Methuen.

Konner, Melvin. 1982. *The Tangled Wing: Biological Constraints on the Human Spirit.* New York: Harper Colophon Books.

Kriegel, Leonard, 1979. *On Men and Manhood.* New York: Hawthorn Books.

Lee, Richard B. 1979. *The !Kung San: Men, Women, and Work in a Foraging Society.* Cambridge: Cambridge University Press.

Levine, Donald N. 1966. The concept of masculinity in Ethiopian culture. *International Journal of Social Psychiatry* 12:17–23.

Levine, Robert A. 1979. Anthropology and sex: Developmental aspects. In *Human Sexuality: Comparative and Developmental Perspectives,* ed. Herant A. Katchadourian, pp. 309–31. Berkeley: University of California Press.

Lewis, Oscar. 1961. *The Children of Sanchez.* New York: Random House.

Lonner, Walter J. 1980. The search for psychological universals. In *Handbook of Cross-Cultural Psychology,* ed. Harry C. Triandis and William W. Lambert, 1:143–204. Boston: Allyn & Bacon.

McPherson, James M. 1988. *Battle Cry of Freedom: The Civil War Era.* New York: Oxford University Press.

Mahler, Margaret, et al. 1975. *The Psychological Birth of the Human Infant.* New York: Basic Books.

Mailer, Norman. 1968. *Armies of the Night.* New York: New American Library.

Marcus, Michael. 1987. "Horsemen are the fence of the land": Honor and history among the Ghiyata of eastern Morocco. In *Honor and Shame and the Unity of the Mediterranean,* ed. David D. Gilmore, pp. 49–60. Washington, D.C.: American Anthropological Association, Special Pub. no. 22.

Marshall, Mac. 1979. *Weekend Warriors.* Palo Alto, CA: Mayfield.

Munroe, Robert L. and Ruth H. Munroe. 1980. Perspectives suggested by anthropological data. In *Handbook of Cross-Cultural Psychology,* ed. Harry C. Triandis and William W. Lambert 1:253–317. Boston: Allyn and Bacon.

Ortner, Sherry B. 1974. Is female to male as nature is to culture? In *Woman, Culture, and Society,* ed. Michelle Z. Rosaldo and Louise Lamphere, pp. 67–88. Stanford: Stanford University Press.

———. 1981. Gender and sexuality in hierarchical societies: The case of Polynesia and some comparative implications. In *Sexual Meanings,* ed. Sherry B. Ortner and Harriet Whitehead, pp. 359–409. Cambridge: Cambridge University Press.

Otten, Charlotte M. 1985. Genetic effects on male and female development and on the sex ratio. In *Male-Female Differences: A Bio-Cultural Perspective,* ed, Roberta L. Hall, pp. 155–217. New York: Praeger.

Pleck, Joseph. 1981. *The Myth of Masculinity.* Cambridge, Mass.: MIT Press.

Raphael, Ray. 1988. *The Men from the Boys: Rites of Passage in Male America.* Lincoln, Nebr.: University of Nebraska Press.

Reminick, Ronald A. 1976. The symbolic significance of ceremonial defloration among the Amhara of Ethiopia. *American Ethnologist* 3:751–63.

———. 1982. The sport of warriors on the wane: a case of cultural endurance in the face of social change. In *Sport and the Humanities,* ed. William H. Morgan, pp. 31–36. Knoxville, Tenn.: Bureau of Educational Research and Service, University of Tennessee Press.

Sanday, Peggy R. 1981. *Female Power and Male Dominance: On the Origins of Sexual Inequality.* Cambridge: Cambridge University Press.

Schafer, Roy. 1986. Men who struggle against sentimentality. In *The Psychology of Men: New Psychoanalytic Perspectives,* ed. Gerald I. Fogel, L. M. Lane, and R. S. Liebert, pp. 95–110. New York: Basic Books.

Schwenger, Peter. 1984. *Phallic Critiques: Masculinity and Twentieth-Century Literature.* London: Routledge and Kegan Paul.

Shostak, Marjorie. 1981. *Nisa: The Life and Words of a !Kung Woman.* Cambridge, Mass.: Harvard University Press.

Simic, Andrei. 1989. *Management of the male image in Yugoslavia.* Anthropological Quarterly 42: 89–101.

Spence, Janet, and Robert L. Helmreich. 1979. *Masculinity and Femininity: Their Psychological Dimensions, Correlates and Antecedents.* Austin, Tex.: University of Texas Press.

Stephens, William N. 1967. A cross-cultural study of menstrual taboos. In *Cross-Cultural Approaches,* ed. Clellan S. Ford, pp. 67–94. New Haven: HRAF Press.

Stoller, Robert. 1968. *Sex and Gender.* New York: Science House.

———. 1974. Facts and fancies: An examination of Freud's concept of bisexuality. In *Women and Analysis,* ed. Jean Strousse, pp. 343–64. New York: Dell.

Thomas, Elizabeth Marshall. 1959. *The Harmless People.* New York: Vintage Books.

Tiger, Lionel. 1971. *Men in Groups.* New York; Random House.

Tolson, Andrew. 1977. *The Limits of Masculinity: Male Identity and the Liberated Woman.* New York: Harper and Row.

Williams, John E., and Deborah L. Best. 1982. *Measuring Sex Stereotypes: A Thirty-Nation Study.* Beverly Hills: Sage Publs.

Wyatt-Brown, Bertram. 1982. *Southern Honor: Ethics and Behavior in the Old South.* New York: Oxford University Press.

NEITHER MAN NOR WOMAN: THE HIJRAS OF INDIA

Serena Nanda

The hijra role is a magnet that attracts people with many different kinds of cross-gender identities, attributes, and behaviors—people whom we in the West would differentiate as eunuchs, homosexuals, transsexuals, hermaphrodites, and transvestites. Such individuals, of course, exist in our own and perhaps all societies. What is noteworthy about the hijras is that the role is so deeply rooted in Indian culture that it can accommodate a wide variety of temperaments, personalities, sexual needs, gender identities, cross-gender behaviors, and levels of commitment without losing its cultural meaning. The ability of the hijra role to succeed as a symbolic reference point giving significant meaning to the lives of the many different kinds of people who make up the hijra community, is undoubtedly related to the variety and significance of alternative gender roles and gender transformations in Indian mythology and traditional culture.

Whereas Westerners feel uncomfortable with the ambiguities and contradictions inherent in such in-between categories as transvestism, homosexuality, hermaphroditism, and transgenderism, and make strenuous attempts to resolve them, Hinduism not only accommodates such ambiguities, but also views them as meaningful and even powerful.

In Hindu mythology, ritual, and art—important vehicles for transmitting the Hindu world view—the power of the combined man/woman is a frequent and significant theme. Indian mythology contains numerous examples of androgynes, impersonators of the opposite sex, and individuals who undergo sex changes, both among deities and humans. These mythical figures are well known as part of Indian popular culture, which helps explain the ability of the hijras to maintain a meaningful place for themselves within Indian society in an institutionalized third gender role.

One of the most important sexually ambivalent figures in Hinduism with whom hijras identify is Shiva, a deity who incorporates both male and female characteristics.[1] Shiva is an ascetic—one who renounces sex—and yet he appears in many erotic and procreative roles. His most powerful symbol and object of worship is the phallus—but the phallus is almost always set in the *yoni,* the symbol of the female genitals. One of the most popular forms of Shiva is that of *Ardhanarisvara,* or half-man/half-woman, which represents Shiva united with his shakti (female creative power). Hijras say that worshipers of Shiva give them special respect because of this close identification, and hijras often worship at Shiva temples. In the next chapter, I look more closely at the identification of the hijras with Shiva, particularly in connection with the ritual of emasculation.

Other deities also take on sexually ambiguous or dual gender manifestations. Vishnu and Krishna (an *avatar,* or incarnation, of Vishnu) are sometimes pictured in androgynous ways. In one myth, Vishnu transforms himself into Mohini, the most beautiful woman in the world, in order to take back the sacred nectar from the demons who have stolen it. In another well-known myth, Krishna takes on the form of a female to destroy a demon called Araka. Araka's strength came from his chasteness. He had never set eyes on a woman, so Krishna took on the form of a beautiful woman and married him. After 3 days of the marriage, there was a battle and Krishna killed the demon. He then revealed himself to the other gods in his true form. Hijras, when they tell this story, say that when Krishna revealed himself he told the other gods that "there will be more like me, neither man nor woman, and whatever words come from the mouths of these people, whether good [blessings] or bad [curses], will come true."

In Tamil Nadu, in South India, an important festival takes place in which hijras, identifying with Krishna, become wives, and then widows, of the male deity Koothandavar. The story behind this festival is that there were once two warring kingdoms. To avert defeat, one of the kings agreed to sacrifice his eldest son to the gods, asking only that he first be allowed to arrange his son's marriage. Because no woman could be found who would marry a man about to be sacrificed, Krishna came to earth as a woman to marry the king's son, and the king won the battle as the gods promised.

For this festival, men who have made vows to Koothandavar dress as women and go through a marriage ceremony with him. The priest performs the marriage, tying on the traditional wedding necklace. After 1 day, the deity is carried to a burial ground. There, all of those who have "married" him remove their wedding necklaces, cry and beat their breasts, and remove the flowers from their hair, as a widow does in mourning for her husband. Hijras participate by the thousands in this festival, coming from all over India. They dress in their best clothes and jewelry and ritually reaffirm their identification with Krishna, who changes his form from male to female.

Several esoteric Hindu ritual practices involve male transvestism as a form of devotion. Among the Sakhibhava (a sect that worships Vishnu) Krishna may not be worshiped directly. The devotees in this sect worship Radha, Krishna's beloved, with the aim of becoming her attendant: It is through her, as Krishna's consort, that Krishna is indirectly worshiped. The male devotees imitate feminine behavior, including simulated menstruation; they also may engage in sexual acts with men as acts of devotion, and some devotees even castrate themselves in order to more nearly approximate a female identification with Radha (Bullough, 1976:267–268; Kakar, 1981; Spratt, 1966:315).

Hinduism in general holds that all persons contain within themselves both male and female principles. In the Tantric school of Hinduism, the Supreme Being is conceptualized as one complete sex containing male and female sexual organs. Hermaphroditism is the ideal. In some of these sects, male (never female) transvestism is used as a way of transcending one's own sex, a prerequisite to achieving salvation. In other Tantric sects, religious exercises involve the male devotee imitating a woman in order to realize the woman in himself: Only in this way do they believe that true love can be realized (Bullough, 1976:260).

Traditional Hinduism makes many specific references to alternative sexes and sexual ambiguity among humans as well as among gods. Ancient Hinduism, for example, taught that there was a third sex, which itself was divided into four categories: the male eunuch, called the "waterless" because he had desiccated testes; the "testicle voided," so called because he had been castrated; the hermaphrodite; and the "not woman," or female eunuch (which usually refers to a woman who does not menstruate). Those who were more feminine (whether males or females) wore false breasts and imitated the voice, gestures, dress, delicacy, and timidity of women (Bullough, 1976:268). All of these categories of persons had the function of providing alternative techniques of sexual gratification, some of which are mentioned in the classical Hindu sex manual, the Kamasutra.

Another ancient reference to a third sex, one that sounds similar to the hijras, is a prostitute named Sukumarika ("good little girl"), who appears in a Sanskrit play. Sukumarika is accused of being sexually insatiable. As a third sex, she has some characteristics advantageous in her profession: "She has no breasts to get in the way of a tight embrace, no monthly period to interrupt the enjoyment of passion, and no pregnancy to mar her beauty" (O'Flaherty, 1980:299).

As just suggested, ancient Hindus, like contemporary ones, appeared to be ambivalent about such third gender roles and the associated alternative sexual practices. The figure of Sukumarika, for example, was considered inauspicious to look upon and, not coincidentally, similar to the hijras today, inspired both fear and mockery. Historically, both eunuchism and castration were looked down on in ancient India, and armed women and old men were preferred to eunuchs for guarding court ladies (Basham, 1954:172). Whereas homosexuality was generally not highly regarded in ancient India, such classic texts as the Kamasutra, however, did describe, even prescribe, sexual practices for eunuchs, for example, "mouth congress."[2]

Homosexuality was condemned in the ancient lawbooks. The Laws of Manu, the first formulation of the Hindu moral code, held that men who engaged in anal sex lost their caste. Other medieval writers held that men who engaged in oral sex with other men were reborn impotent. But homosexuals were apparently tolerated in reality. Consistent with the generally "sex positive" attitude of Hinduism, Vatsyayana, author of the Kamasutra, responded to critics of oral and anal sex by saying that "in all things connected with love, everybody should act according to the custom of his country, and his own inclination," asking a man to consider only whether the act "is agreeable to his nature and himself" (Burton, 1964:127).

Even the gods were implicated in such activities: Krishna's son Samba was notorious for his homosexuality and dressed as female, often a pregnant woman. As Sambali, Samba's name became a synonym for eunuch (Bullough, 1976:267). An important ritual at the Jagannatha temple in Orissa involves a sequence in which Balabhadra, the ascetic elder brother of the deity Jagannatha, who is identified with Shiva, is homosexually seduced by a transvestite (a young man dressed as a female temple dancer) (Marglin, 1985:53). In some Hindu myths a male deity takes on a female form specifically to experience sexual relations with another male deity.

Islam also provides a model of an in-between gender—not a mythological one, but a true historical figure—in the traditional role of the eunuch who guarded the ladies of the harem, under Moghul rule. Hijras often mention this role as the source of their prestige in Indian society. In spite of the clear connection of hijras with Hinduism, Islam not only provides a powerful positive model of an alternative gender, but also contributes many elements to the social organization of the hijra community. Hijras today make many references to the glorious, preindependence Indian past when the Muslim rulers of princely states were exceedingly generous and reknowned for their patronage of the hijras (see Lynton & Rajan, 1974).

Today the religious role of the hijras, derived from Hinduism, and the historical role of the eunuchs in the Muslim courts have become inextricably entwined in spite of the differences between them. Hijras are distinguished from the eunuchs in Muslim courts by their transvestism and their association with men. Muslim eunuchs dressed as males and associated with women and, unlike the hijras, were sexually inactive. More importantly, the role of hijras as ritual performers is linked to their sexual ambiguity as this incorporates the elements of the erotic and the ascetic; Muslim eunuchs had no such powers or roles. Today, the collapsing of the role of the hijra and that of the Muslim eunuchs leads to certain contradictions, but these seem easily incorporated into the hijra culture by hijras themselves; only the Western observer seems to feel the need to separate them conceptually.

The hijras, as human beings who are neither man nor woman, call into question the basic social categories of gender on which Indian society is built. This makes the hijras objects of fear, abuse, ridicule, and sometimes pity. But hijras are not merely ordinary human beings; . . . they are also conceptualized as special, sacred beings, through a ritual transformation. The many examples that I have cited above indicate that both Indian society and Hindu mythology provide some positive, or at least accommodating, roles for such sexually ambiguous figures. Within the context of Indian social roles, sexually ambiguous figures are associated with sexual specializations; in myth and through ritual, such figures become powerful symbols of the divine and of generativity.

Thus, where Western culture strenuously attempts to resolve sexual contradictions and ambiguities, by denial or segregation, Hinduism appears content to allow opposites to confront each other without resolution, "celebrating the idea that the universe is boundlessly various, and . . . that all possibilities may exist without excluding each other" (O'Flaherty, 1973:318). It is this characteristically Indian ability to tolerate, even embrace, contradictions and variation at the social, cultural, and personality levels that provides the context in which the hijras cannot only be accommodated, but even granted a measure of power.

NOTES

1. The Hindu Triad, or Trinity, is made up of Brahma, the creator; Vishnu, the preserver (protector and sustainer of the world); and Shiva, the destroyer. Brahma is the Supreme Being and the creator of all creatures. Vishnu is believed to descend into the world in many different forms (*avataras,* or incarnations) and is worshiped throughout India. One of Vishnu's incarnations is Ram. Krishna is sometimes considered an aspect or incarnation of Vishnu but more commonly is worshiped as a god in his own right. Shiva is the god of destruction or absorption, but he also creates and sustains life. In addition to the Triad Hinduism includes a large number of deities, both male and female, all of whom are aspects of the Absolute. This concept of the Absolute Reality also includes matter and finite spirits as its integral parts; the divine spirit is embodied in the self and the world, as well as in more specifically religious figures. The religious concepts of Hinduism are expressed in the two great Hindu epics, the Mahabharata and the Ramayana, both of which are familiar to every Hindu and many non-Hindus as well. These epics, along with other chronicles of the gods and goddesses, are frequently enacted in all forms of popular and elite culture. Thus, for the hijras, particularly the Hindu hijras, the incorporation of these divine models of behavior into their own world view and community image is in no way unusual.
2. In an editor's note Burton (1962:124) suggests that this practice is no longer common in India and has been replaced by sodomy, which was introduced after the Muslim period began in the tenth century. In a later chapter (Nanda 1990) we will see that Meera, a hijra elder, specifically says that oral sex is "not a good thing and goes against the wishes of the hijra goddess" and that it brings all kinds of problems for those who practice it.

REFERENCES

Basham, A. I. 1954. *The Wonder That Was India.* New York: Grove Press, p. 172.

Bullough, V. 1976. *Sexual Variance in Society and History.* Chicago: University of Chicago Press, pp. 260, 267–268.

Burton, R. F. (Trans.) 1962. *The Kama Sutra of Vatsyayana.* New York: E. P. Dutton, p. 127.

Kakar, Sudhir. 1981. *The Inner World: A Psychoanalytic Study of Childhood and Society in India.* Delhi: Oxford University Press.

Lynton, H. and Rajan, M. 1974. *Days of the Beloved.* Berkeley: University of California Press.

Marglin, Frederique Apffel. 1985. Female Sexuality in the Hindu World. In Clarissa Atkinson, Constance H. Buchanan, and Margaret R. Miles (Eds.), *The Immaculate and the Powerful.* Boston: Beacon Press, pp. 39–59.

Nanda, Serena. 1990. Neither Man Nor Woman: The Hijras of India. Belmont, California: Wadsworth Publishing Co.

O'Flaherty, Wendy Doniger. 1973. *Siva: The Erotic Ascetic.* New York: Oxford University Press, p. 318.

———. 1980. *Women, Androgynes, and Other Mythical Beasts.* Chicago: University of Chicago Press, p. 299.

Spratt, Philip. 1966. *Hindu Culture and Personality: A Psychoanalytic Study.* Bombay: Manaktalas.

AMAZONS OF AMERICA: FEMALE GENDER VARIANCE

Walter L. Williams

When Pedro de Magalhães de Gandavo explored northeastern Brazil in 1576, he visited the Tupinamba Indians and reported on a remarkable group of female warriors.

> There are some Indian women who determine to remain chaste: these have no commerce with men in any manner, nor would they consent to it even if refusal meant death. They give up all the duties of women and imitate men, and follow men's pursuits as if they were not women. They wear the hair cut in the same way as the men, and go to war with bows and arrows and pursue game, always in company with men; each has a woman to serve her, to whom she says she is married, and they treat each other and speak with each other as man and wife.[1]

Gandavo and other explorers like Orellana were evidently so impressed with this group of women that they named the river which flowed through that area the River of the Amazons, after the ancient Greek legend of women warriors.

To what extent did this recognized status for women exist among Native Americans? The sources are few, since European male explorers dealt almost entirely with aboriginal men. Most documents are unclear about anything to do with women, and as a result it is difficult to make conclusions about those females who took up a role similar to that of the Tupinamba Amazons. But we can begin by making it clear that this institution was not the same as berdache. As specified earlier, the term *berdache* clearly originated as a word applying to males. Anthropologist Evelyn Blackwood has done a thorough search of the ethnographic literature and found mention of a recognized female status in thirty-three North American groups. Because she sees it as distinct from berdachism, she does not use the term "female berdache" but instead calls this role "cross-gender female." She notes that it was most common in California, the Southwest, the Northwest, and the Great Basin, but she also notes a few instances among peoples of the Subarctic and the northern Plains.[2]

Because I have some disagreement with the concept of gender crossing, and also because "cross-gender female" is linguistically awkward, I prefer the word *amazon*. This term is parallel to berdache, but it is a status specific to women that is not subservient to male definitions. American Indian worldviews almost always recognize major differences between amazons and berdaches. With the single exception of the Navajo, those cultures that recognize alternative roles for both females and males, have distinct terminologies in their languages that are different for each sex. The Papago word translates as "Light Woman," and such women even up to the 1940s were considered simply socially tolerated variations from the norm.[3] Among the Yumas of the Southwest, berdaches are called *elxa'*, while amazons are called *kwe'rhame*. They are defined as "women who passed for men, dressed like men and married women." There is no ceremony marking their assumption of the role, as there is for the *elxa'*.[4]

The parents of a *kwe'rhame* might try to push her into feminine pursuits, but such a child manifested an unfeminine character from infancy. She was seen as having gone through a change of spirit as a result of dreams. In growing up she was observed to hunt and play with boys, but she had no interest in heterosexual relations with them. According to Yuman informants in the 1920s, a *kwe'rhame* "wished only to become a man." Typical of amazons in several cultures, she was said to have a muscular build and to desire to dress like a man, and it was also claimed that she did not menstruate. A Yuman *kwe'rhame* married a woman and established a household with herself as husband. She was known for bravery and for skillful fighting in battle.[5]

RAISING A FEMALE HUNTER

While there are parallels between berdaches and amazons, female amazons are also very different from male berdaches. Among the Kaska Indians of the Subarctic, having a son was extremely important because the family depended heavily on big-game hunting for food. If a couple had too many female children and desired a son to hunt for them in their old age, they would simply select a daughter to "be like a man." When the youngest daughter was about five years old, and it was obvious that the mother was not going to produce a son, the parents performed a transformation ceremony. They tied the dried ovaries of a bear to a belt which she always wore. That was believed to prevent menstruation, to protect her from pregnancy, and to give her luck on the hunt. According to Kaska informants, she was dressed like a male and trained to do male tasks, "often developing great strength and usually becoming an outstanding hunter."[6]

The Ingalik Indians of Alaska, closely related to the Kaska as part of the Dene culture, also recognized a similar status for females. Such a female even participated in the male-only activities of the *kashim,* which involved sweat baths. The men ignored her morphological sex in this nude bathing, and accepted her as a man on the basis of her gender behavior.[7] Other notable Subarctic amazons from the eighteenth century included the leader of the eastern Kutchin band from Arctic Red River, and a Yellowknife Chipewayan who worked for peace between the various peoples of the central Subarctic.[8]

Among the Kaskas, if a boy made sexual advances to such a female, she reacted violently. Kaska people explained her reaction thus: "She knows that if he gets her then her luck with game will be broken." She would have relationships only with women, achieving sexual pleasure through clitoral friction, "by getting on top of each other."[9] This changed-gender demonstrates the extreme malleability of people with respect to gender roles. Such assignment operates independently of a person's morphological sex and can determine both gender status and erotic behavior.

TRANSFORMATION INTO A MAN

In other areas, becoming an amazon was seen to be a choice of the female herself. Among the Kutenai Indians of the Plateau, for example, in what is now southern British Columbia, such a female became famous as a prophet and shaman. She is remembered in Kutenai oral tradition as being quite large and heavy boned. About 1808 she left Kutenai to go with a group of white fur traders, and married one of them. A year later, however, she returned to her people and claimed that her husband had operated on her and transformed her into a man. Kutenai informants from the 1930s told ethnographer Claude Schaeffer that when she returned she said: "I'm a man now. We Indians did not believe the white people possessed such power from the supernaturals. I can tell you that they do, greater power than we have. They changed my sex while I was with them. No Indian is able to do that." She changed her name to Gone-To-The-Spirits, and claimed great spiritual power. Whenever she met people she performed a dance as a symbol of her transformation.[10]

Following her return, she began to dress in men's clothes, and to carry a gun. She also began to court young women. After several rebuffs she met a divorced woman who agreed to marry her. "The two were now to be seen constantly together. The curious attempted to learn things from the consort, but the latter only laughed at their efforts." A rumor began that Gone-To-The-Spirits, for the pleasure of her wife, had fashioned an artificial phallus made of leather. But whatever their sexual technique, the wife later moved out because of Gone-To-The-Spirits's losses in gambling. Thereafter, Gone-To-The-Spirits changed wives frequently.

Meanwhile, she began to have an interest in warfare and was accepted as a warrior on a raid. Upon coming to a stream, Kutenai oral tradition recalled, the raiders would undress and wade across together but she delayed so as to cross alone. On one of these crossings, her brother doubled back to observe her. He saw her nude and realized that her sex had not been changed at all. Seeing him, she sat down in the water and pretended that her foot was injured. Later, trying to protect her reputation, she told the others that she was injured in the stream and had to sit. She declared that she hereafter wished to be called *Qa'nqon ka'mek klau'la* (Sitting-In-The-Water-Grizzly).

Her brother did not tell what he saw, but refused to call her by her new name. Later, she took still another wife, and as she had done with previous wives eventually began accusing her of infidelity. Qa'nqon was of a violent temper, and when she began to beat this wife, the brother intervened. He yelled out angrily, in the hearing of the entire camp: "You are hurting your woman friend. You have hurt other friends in the same way. You know that I saw you standing naked in the stream, where you tried to conceal your sex. That's why I never call you by your new name."[11]

After this, according to Kutenai informants, all the people knew that Qa'nqon had not really changed sex. It is conceivable that the community already knew about her sex before this pronouncement since Qa'nqon's ex-wives must have spread the truth. The oral tradition does not explain why women continued to marry the temperamental Qa'nqon. Soon after this incident, evidently, she and a wife (whether the same woman or another is unknown) left to serve as guides for white traders. The couple seemed to get along fine once they arrived at Fort Astoria on the Columbia River in 1811.

One trader named Alexander Ross characterized them as "two strange Indians, in the character of man and wife." "The husband," he said, "was a very shrewd and intelligent Indian" who gave them much information about the interior. Later, this trader learned that "instead of being man and wife, as they at first gave us to understand, they were in fact both women—and bold adventurous amazons they were." Qa'nqon served as guide for Ross's party on a trip up the Columbia to the Rocky Mountains. Ross recounted that "the man woman" spread a prophesy among the tribes they passed, saying that the Indians were soon going to be supplied with all the trading goods they desired.

> These stories, so agreeable to the Indian ear, were circulated far and wide; and not only received as truths, but procured so much celebrity for the two cheats, that they were the objects of attraction at every village and camp on the way; nor could we, for a long time, account for the cordial reception they met with from the natives, who loaded them for their good tidings with the most valuable articles they possessed—horses, robes, leather, and higuas [?]; so that, on our arrival at Oakinacken [Okanagon, near the present-day border of British Columbia and Washington State], they had no less than twenty-six horses, many of them loaded with the fruits of their false reports.[12]

Another white traveler in the area nearly a decade later heard the Indians still talking about Qa'nqon, whom they referred to as "Manlike Woman." She had acquired a widespread reputation as having supernatural powers and a gift of prophesy. Her most important prediction was that there would soon be a complete change in the land, with "fertility and plenty" for all tribes. According to this traveler, writing in 1823, she had predicted that the whites would be removed and a different race of traders would arrive "who would supply their wants in every possible manner. The poor deluded wretches, imagining that they would hasten this happy change by destroying their present traders, of whose submission there was no prospect, threatened to extirpate them."[13] What we can see from these stories is that Qa'nqon sparked a cultural movement similar to "cargo-cults" that twentieth-century anthropologists have observed among Melanesians and other tribal peoples coming in close contact with Western trade cargo goods. This movement also reflected the dissatisfaction the Indians felt with the white traders.

After establishing her fame, Qa'nqon returned to settle with the Kutenai and became noted as a shamanistic healer among her people. A twentieth-century elderly headman named Chief Paul remembered his father telling stories of her curing him of illnesses when he was a child. In 1825 she accompanied a Kutenai chief to the Hudson's Bay Company post among the Flathead Indians, taking the role of interpreter. The company trader described her as "a woman who goes in men's clothes and is a leading character among them. . . . [She] assumes a masculine character and is of some note among them."[14]

In 1837 she was traveling with some Flatheads when a Blackfoot raiding party surrounded them. Through her resourcefulness the Flatheads made an escape while she deceived the attackers. The Blackfeet were so angry that they tried to kill her, but after several shots she was still not seriously wounded. They then slashed her with their knives. But according to Kutenai oral tradition, "Immediately afterwards the cuts thus made were said to have healed themselves. . . . One of the warriors then opened up her chest to get at her heart and cut off the lower portion. This last wound she was unable to heal. It was thus *Qa'nqon* died." Afterward, the story goes, no wild animals disturbed her body.[15]

This story, which was passed down among the Kutenai for over a century, signifies the respect the Indians had for the shamanistic power of the "Manlike Woman." Even the animals recognized this power and respected it. It should be noted that the Kutenai did not recognize a berdache status for males. A tribe that had an alternative gender role for one sex did not necessarily have another role for the other sex. Native Americans did not see the two roles as synonymous so equating amazons with berdaches does not clarify the matter.

MANLIKE WOMAN

The Mohaves, like other cultures, have different words for berdaches and amazons. *Hwame* girls are known to throw away their dolls and refuse to perform feminine tasks. It is said that they dreamed about their role while still in the womb. Adults recognize this pattern and, according to ethnographer George Devereux, make "occasional half-hearted and not very hopeful attempts to discourage them from becoming inverts. When these efforts fail, they are subjected to a ritual, which is half 'test' of their true proclivities and half 'transition rite' and which authorizes them to assume the clothing and to engage in the occupations and sexual activities of their self-chosen sex." Adults then help the *hwame* to learn the same skills that boys are taught.[16]

Mohaves believe that such females do not menstruate. In the worldview of many American Indians, menstruation is a crucial part of defining a person as a woman. Some amazons may have in fact been nonmenstruating, or, since they wished to be seen as men, if they did menstruate they would hide any evidence of menses. The other Indians simply ignored any menstrual indicators out of deference to their desire to be treated like men.[17]

Mohaves also accept the fact that a *hwame* would marry a woman. There is even a way to incorporate children into these female relationships. If a woman becomes impregnated by a man, but later takes another lover, it is believed that the paternity of the child changes. This idea helps to prevent family friction in a society where relationships often change. So, if a pregnant woman later takes a *hwame* as a spouse, the *hwame* is considered the real father of the child.[18]

George Devereux, who lived among the Mohaves in the 1930s, was told about a famous late nineteenth-century *hwame* named Sahaykwisa. Her name was a masculine one, indicating that she had gone through the initiation rite for *hwames*. Nevertheless, she dressed more like a woman than a man, proving that cross-dressing is not a requirement for assuming amazon status. While she was feminine in appearance and had large breasts, Mohaves said that she (typical of others like her) did not menstruate. As evidence of this, they pointed out that she never got pregnant, despite the fact that she hired herself out as a prostitute for white men.

Sahaykwisa used the money that she received from this heterosexual activity to bestow gifts on women to whom she was attracted. With her industriousness as a farmer (a woman's occupation) and as a hunter (a man's occupation), she became relatively prosperous. She was also noted for her shamanistic ability to cure venereal diseases. Shamans who treated venereal diseases were regarded as lucky in love. This fame, plus her reputation as a good provider, led women to be attracted to her.

Sahaykwisa's first wife was a very pretty young woman, whom many men tried to lure away from her. Motivated by jealousy, they began teasing her, "Why do you want a *hwame* for a husband? A *hwame* has no penis; she only pokes you with her finger." The wife brushed off the remark saying "That is alright for me." But then later the wife eloped with a man. Such a breakup was not unusual, given the fact that heterosexual marriages among Mohaves were equally subject to change. After a time the wife returned to Sahaykwisa, having found the man less satisfying. People referred to Sahaykwisa by the name Hithpan Kudhape, which means split vulvae, denoting how the *hwame* would spread the genitals during sex. This part of the oral tradition indicates that the Mohaves were well aware that an amazon role involved sexual behavior with women.

While accepting these relationships, Mohaves nevertheless teased Sahaykwisa's wife unmercifully. While teasing is quite common in American Indian cultures generally, in this case it was done so much that the woman left a second time. Sahaykwisa then began to flirt with other women at social dances, soon easily attracting another wife, and then a third one later on. Mohaves explained this by the fact that Sahaykwisa was, after all, lucky in love. Her reputation as a good provider was also an obvious factor. But after the third woman left her, and returned to the man from whom Sahaykwisa stole her, the man attacked the *hwame* and raped her. Rape was extremely uncommon among the Mohaves, so this incident had a major impact on her life.

Sahaykwisa became demoralized and an alcoholic, and ironically began having wanton sex with men. She claimed to have bewitched one man who rejected her advances, and when he died in the late 1890s she boasted about having killed him. The man's son was so enraged by this that he threw her into the Colorado River, where she drowned. In telling this story Devereux's Mohave informants were convinced that Sahaykwisa claimed witchcraft intentionally so that someone would kill her. They explained that she wanted to die and join the spirits of those she had earlier loved.[19]

While this story does not have a happy ending, it does nevertheless point out that female-female relationships were recognized. Sahaykwisa was killed because it was believed that she had killed another person by witchcraft, not because of her gender status or her sexual relations with women.

While the social role of the *hwame* was in some ways like that of men, the story of Sahaykwisa does not support Blackwood's view of gender *crossing*. The Mohaves did not in fact accept Sahaykwisa as a full-fledged man, and the wife was teased on that regard. She was regarded as a *hwame*, having a distinct gender status that was different than men, women, or *alyha*. Mohaves thus had four genders in their society.

To what extent an amazon was accepted as a man is unclear. The variation that existed among Indians of the Far West typifies this matter. The Cocopa *warrhameh* cut her hair and had her nose pierced as men did, and did not get tattooed as women did.[20] Among the late nineteenth-century Klamath a woman named Co'pak "lived like a man.... She tried to talk like a man and invariably referred to herself as one." Co'pak had a wife, with whom she lived for many years, and when the wife died Co'pak "observed the usual mourning, wearing a bark belt as a man does at this time." Nevertheless, this mourning may have been the standard for a "husband" rather than for a "man," and we do not know if Klamath custom made a distinction between the two categories. Co'pak also retained woman's dress, which certainly implies a less than total crossover. Other Klamaths continued to see her as a manlike woman rather than as a man.[21]

A survey of California Indian groups that recognized amazon status revealed that in half of the groups amazons performed both men's and women's work, while in the other half they did only men's work.[22] No doubt this variation of roles is typical of cultural diversity in aboriginal America generally.

Unlike Western culture, which tries to place all humans into strict conformist definitions of masculinity and femininity, some Native American cultures have a more flexible recognition of gender variance. They are able to incorporate such fluidity into their worldview by recognizing a special place for berdaches and another one for amazons. "Manlike Woman" is how Indians described the Kutenai female, and that phrase recurs in anthropological literature when direct translations are given. By paying more attention to words used by Indians themselves, we can make more precise definitions. Gender theory is now beginning to make such distinctions. Terms like gender crossing imply that there are only two genders, and one must "cross" from one to the other. As with the male berdache, most recent theorists argue, the amazon is either a distinct gender role, or is a gender-mixing status, rather than a complete changeover to an opposite sex role.[23]

WARRIOR WOMEN IN THE GREAT PLAINS

When we turn to the nomadic Plains cultures, the picture becomes even more complex. Here, an accepted amazon status was generally lacking. Female divergence into male activity was not recognized as a distinct gender comparable to the institutionalized berdache role. Women could participate in male occupations on the hunt or in warfare, but this did not imply an alternative gender role. Precisely because they had various activities open to them on a casual and sporadic basis, there was not as much need to recognize a specific role for females behaving in a masculine way. For example, they could become "Warrior Women." Such a woman might join a war party for a specific occasion, like a retribution raid for the death of a relative. She might even accumulate war honors, called *coup*. But since it did not affect her status as a woman, she should not be confused with an amazon. Male warriors simply accepted female fighters as acting within the parameters of womanhood, without considering them a threat to their masculinity.[24]

Warrior women were not the same as amazons partly because their menstruation continued to define them as women. Among Plains peoples, as among many other American Indians, blood was seen as an important and powerful spiritual essence. An individual who bled would not be able to control the power of this bleeding, so if a person bled it might disrupt any important activity that depended on spiritual help, like a hunt or a raid. Consequently, if a woman began her period, the raid would have to be delayed while the spirits were placated. As a result of this belief, the "manly hearted women" who sometimes participated in warfare were almost always postmenopausal.[25]

This belief was not just a restriction on women; a male who bled from an accident or a wound had to go through the same efforts to placate the spirits. The matter was more a question of power than of restriction. Menstruation "was not something unclean or to be ashamed of," according to the Lakota shaman Lame Deer, but was sacred. A girl's first period was cause for great celebration. Still, Lame Deer concluded, "menstruation had a strange power that could bring harm under some circumstances."[26] Paula Gunn Allen explains: "Women are perceived to be possessed of a singular power, most vital during menstruation. . . . Indians do not perceive signs of womanness as contamination; rather they view them as so powerful that other 'medicines' may be cancelled by the very presence of that power." American Indians thought of power not so much in terms of political or economic power, but as supernatural power. Being a matter of spirituality, woman's power comes partly by her close association with the magical properties of blood.[27]

Another possible factor inhibiting the development of amazon status among Plains women had to do with the economic need for their labor and procreation. Women were responsible for the preparation of buffalo meat. Since a successful hunter could kill more bison than one woman could dress and preserve for food or trade, every available woman was needed to do this work. This economic system limited women's choice of occupation and put more pressure on them to marry than in other North American cultures. Furthermore, with the loss of men from warfare, there was the expectation that every woman would marry and have children.[28]

There was such a strong need for female labor that Plains men began taking multiple wives. A typical pattern was for an overworked wife to encourage her husband to take a second wife. The first wife now had higher status, as a senior wife who directed younger women, and the family as a whole benefited from the extra output of the additional wife. Quite often it would be the younger sisters of the first wife who were later brought in as co-wives. This pattern gave advantages to women. It kept female siblings together, giving them support and strength throughout their lives. In contrast to Western culture, which keeps women separated by promoting competition among them for men, Plains polygyny meant that wives were added to the family rather than replaced by divorce and serial monogamy.[29]

Despite these pressures on women to marry and procreate, even in the Plains culture there were exceptions. An amazon role was followed by a few females, with the most famous example being Woman Chief of the Crows. She was originally a Gros Ventre Indian who had been captured by Crow raiders when she was ten years old. She was adopted by a Crow warrior, who observed her inclination for masculine pursuits. He allowed her to follow her proclivities, and in time she became a fearless horseback rider and skilled rifle shooter. Edward Denig, a white frontiersman who lived with the Crows in the early nineteenth century, knew Woman Chief for twelve years. He wrote that when she was still a young woman she "was equal if not superior to any of the men in hunting both on horseback and foot. . . . [She] would spend most of her time in killing deer and bighorn, which she butchered and carried home on her back when hunting on foot. At other times she joined in the surround on horse, could kill four or five buffalo at a race, cut up the animals without assistance, and bring the meat and hides home."[30]

After the death of the widowed man who adopted her, she assumed control of his lodge, "performing the double duty of father and mother to his children." She continued to dress like other women, but Denig, writing in 1855, remembered her as "taller and stronger than most women—her pursuits no doubt tending to develop strength of nerve and muscle." She became famous for standing off an attack from Blackfoot Indians, in which she killed three warriors while remaining unharmed herself: "This daring act stamped her character as a brave. It was sung by the rest of the camp, and in time was made known to the whole nation."[31]

A year later she organized her first raid and easily attracted a group of warriors to follow her. She stole seventy horses from a Blackfoot camp, and in the ensuing skirmish killed and scalped two enemies. For these acts of bravery she was awarded *coups,* and by her subsequent successful raids she built up a large herd of horses. As a successful hunter, she shared her meat freely with others. But it was as a warrior, Denig concluded, that her fame was most notable. In every engagement with enemy tribes, including raids on enemy camps, she distinguished herself by her bravery. Crows began to believe she had "a charmed life which, with her daring feats, elevated her to a point of honor and respect not often reached by male warriors." The Crows were proud of her, composing special songs to commemorate her gallantry. When the tribal council was held and all the chiefs assembled, she took her place among them, as the third-highest-ranked person in the tribe.[32]

Woman Chief's position shows the Crows' ability to judge individuals by their accomplishments rather than by their sex. Their accepting attitude also included Woman Chief's taking a wife. She went through the usual procedure of giving horses to the parents of her intended spouse. A few years later, she took three more wives. This plurality of women added also to her prestige as a chief. Denig concluded, "Strange country this, where [berdache] males assume the dress and perform the duties of females, while women turn men and mate with their own sex!"[33]

Denig's amazement did not denote any condemnation on his part, for individual traders on the frontier often accepted Indian ways of doing things. Rather, he respected his friend as a "singular and resolute woman.... She had fame, standing, honor, riches, and as much influence over the band as anyone except two or three leading chiefs.... For 20 years she conducted herself well in all things." In 1854 Woman Chief led a Crow peacekeeping mission to her native Gros Ventre tribe. Resentful because of her previous raids against them, some Gros Ventres trapped her and killed her. Denig concluded sadly, "This closed the earthly career of this singular woman." Her death so enraged the Crows that they refused to make peace with the Gros Ventres for many years.[34] Woman Chief's exceptionally high status was rather unique on the Plains; stories that were passed down made her a hero in the classic Plains mode. Even her death, at enemy hands, was typical of the pattern for the honored male warrior.

WIVES OF AMAZONS

What about the wives of the amazon? Woman Chief, like the other amazons, evidently had no difficulty finding women to marry. Yet, these women did not identify as lesbian in the Western sense of the word. American Indian women were not divided into separate categories of persons as is the case with Anglo-American homosexual and heterosexual women. The white lesbian often sees herself as a member of a minority group, distinct from and alienated from general society. She is seen as "abnormal," the opposite of "normal" women, and often suffers great anguish about these supposed differences. Paula Gunn Allen writes, "We are not in the position of our American Indian fore-sister who could find safety and security in her bond with another woman because it was perceived to be destined and nurtured by non-human entities, and was therefore acceptable and respectable."[35]

With the exception of the amazon, women involved in a relationship with another female did not see themselves as a separate minority or a special category of person, or indeed as different in any important way from other women. Yet, they were involved in loving and sexual relationships with their female mates. If their marriage to an amazon ended, then they could easily marry heterosexually without carrying with them any stigma as having been "homosexual." The important consideration in the Indian view is that they were still fulfilling the standard role of "mother and wife" within their culture. The traditional gender role for women did not restrict their choice of sexual partners. Gender identity (woman or amazon) was important, but sexual identity (heterosexual or homosexual) was not.[36]

WOMEN-IDENTIFIED WOMEN

Socially recognized marriages between an amazon and her wife only tell part of the story. Relationships between two women-identified women were probably more common. American Indians, while not looking down on sex as evil or dirty, generally see it as something private. Consequently, it is not something that is talked about to outsiders, and there is not much information on sexual practices. It is most important for a woman to have children, but in many tribes a woman's sexual exclusiveness to the child's father is not crucial. Thus, a woman might be sexually active with others without worrying that she or her children would be looked down on. In many Native American societies, a woman has the right to control her own body, rather than it being the exclusive property of her husband. As long as she produces children at some point in her life, what she does in terms of sexual behavior is her own private business.[37]

Individual inclinations, after all, are usually seen as due to a direction from the spirits. This spiritual justification means that another person's interference might be seen as a dangerous intrusion into the supernatural. "In this context," writes Paula Gunn Allen, "it is quite possible that Lesbianism was practiced rather commonly, as long as the individuals cooperated with the larger social customs." Allen wrote a poem to native "Beloved Women" which expresses this attitude of noninterference:

> It is not known if those
> who warred and hunted on the plains . . .
> were Lesbians
> It is never known
> if any woman was a lesbian
> so who can say. . . .
> And perhaps the portents are better
> left written only in the stars. . . .
> Perhaps
> all they signify is best left
> unsaid.[38]

It is precisely this attitude, that sexual relations were not anyone else's business, that has made Indian women's casual homosexuality so invisible to outsiders. Except for some female anthropologists, most white observers of native societies have been males. These observers knew few women, other than exceptional females who acted as guides or go-betweens for whites and Indians. Most writers expressed little interest in the usual female lifestyle. Yet even if they did, their access to accurate information would be limited to bits that they could learn from Indian males. Given the segregation of the sexes in native society, women would not open up to a male outsider about their personal lives. Even Indian men would not be told much about what went on among the women.[39]

Given these circumstances, it is all the more necessary for women researchers to pursue this topic. Openly lesbian ethnographers would have a distinct advantage. In contrast to institutionalized male homosexuality, female sexual variance seems more likely to express itself informally. Again, enough cross-cultural fieldwork has not been done to come to definite conclusions. However, Blackwood suggests that female-female erotic relationships may be most commonly expressed as informal pairings within the kin group or between close friends.[40]

GENDER AND SEXUAL VARIANCE AMONG CONTEMPORARY INDIAN WOMEN

In what ways do these patterns continue today? An idea of the type of data that might be gathered by contemporary fieldworkers is contained in a report by Beverely Chiñas, who has been conducting research among the Isthmus Zapotecs of southern Mexico since 1966. While she details an accepted berdache status for males, among females the picture is somewhat different. In two decades of fieldwork she has observed several instances of women with children leaving their husbands to live with female lovers. She sees these relationships as lesbian: "People talk about this for a few weeks but get used to it. There is no ostracism. In the case of the lesbians, they continued to appear at fiestas, now as a couple rather than as wives in heterosexual marriages." At religious festivals, she points out, such female couples do not stand out, since every woman pairs up with another woman to dance together as a couple. There is virtually no male-female couple activity in religious contexts. The sexes are always separated in ceremonies, with different roles and duties.[41]

The only negative reaction that Chiñas reports concerned an unmarried daughter of a close friend and informant who "left her mother's home and went to another barrio to live with her lesbian lover. The daughter was only 25 years old, not beyond the expected age of heterosexual marriage. The mother was very upset and relations between mother-daughter broke off for a time but were patched up a year later although the daughter continued to live with her lesbian partner."[42]

The Zapotec mother's anger at her daughter was due to the latter's evident decision not to have children. By refusing to take a husband at least temporarily, the daughter violated the cultural dictate that females should be mothers. It was thus not lesbianism per se that caused the mother-daughter conflict. It would be interesting to know if the mother was reconciled by the daughter's promise that she would get pregnant later. If so, it would fit into the traditional pattern for American Indian women. The importance of offspring in small-scale societies cannot be ignored; female homosexual behavior has to accommodate to society's need to reproduce the population.

Chiñas explains that in such *marimacha* couples, "one will be the *macho* or masculine partner in the eyes of the community, i.e., the 'dominant' one, but they still dress as women and do women's work. Most of the lesbian couples I have known have been married heterosexually and raised families. In 1982 there were rumors of a suspected lesbian relationship developing between neighbor women, one of whom was married with husband and small child present, the other having been abandoned by her husband and left with children several years previously."[43]

These data offer an example of the kind of valuable findings that direct fieldwork experience can uncover. The fact that one of the women was looked on as the macho one, even though she did not cross-dress, points up the relative *un*importance of cross-dressing in a same-sex relationship. An uninformed outsider might have no idea that these roles and relationships exist, and might assume that the practice had died out among the modern Zapotecs.

Since the field research that could answer these questions has not yet been done with enough Native American societies, I am reluctant to agree with Evelyn Blackwood's statement that by the end of the nineteenth century "the last cross-gender females seem to have disappeared."[44] Such a statement does not take into account the less formalized expressions of gender and sexual variance. If I had trusted such statements about the supposed disappearance of the male berdache tradition, I never would have carried out the fieldwork to disprove such a claim.

As also occurs with the berdaches, contemporary Indians perceive similarities with a Western gay identity. A Micmac berdache, whose niece recently came out publicly as gay, reports that the whole community accepts her: "The family members felt that if she is that way, then that's her own business. A lot of married Indian women approach her for sex. A male friend of mine knows that she has sex with his wife, and he jokes about it. There is no animosity. There might be some talking about her, a little joking, but it is no big deal as far as people on the reserve are concerned. There is never any condemnation or threats about it. When she brought a French woman to the community as her lover, everyone welcomed her. They accept her as she is."[45]

Despite the value of such reports, it is clear that a male cannot get very complete information on women's sexuality. I hope that the data presented here will inspire women ethnographers to pursue this topic in the future.

Paula Gunn Allen, who is familiar with Native American women from many reservations, states that there is cultural continuity.

She wrote me that "There are amazon women, recognized as such, *today* in a number of tribes—young, alive, and kicking!"[46] They may now identify as gay or lesbian, but past amazon identities, claims Beth Brant (Mohawk), "have everything to do with who we are now. As gay Indians, we feel that connection with our ancestors." Erna Pahe (Navajo), cochair of Gay American Indians, adds that this connection gives advantages: "In our culture [and] in our gay world, anybody can do anything. We can sympathize, we can really feel how the other sex feels. [We are] the one group of people that can really understand both cultures. We are special." Paula Gunn Allen also emphasizes this specialness, which she sees as applying to non-Indian gay people as well. "It all has to do with spirit, with restoring an awareness of our spirituality as gay people."[47] As with the berdache tradition for males, modern Indian women's roles retain a connection with past traditions of gender and sexual variance. There is strong evidence of cultural revitalization and persistance among contemporary American Indians.

NOTES

1. Pedro de Magalhães de Gandavo, "History of the Province of Santa Cruz," ed. John Stetson, *Documents and Narratives Concerning the Discovery and Conquest of Latin America: The Histories of Brazil* 2 (1922): 89.
2. Evelyn Blackwood, "Sexuality and Gender in Certain Native American Tribes: The Case of Cross-Gender Females," *Signs: Journal of Women in Culture and Society* 10 (1984): 27–42. These tribes are listed on p. 29: California (Achomawi, Atsugewi, Klamath, Shasta, Wintu, Wiyot, Yokuts, Yuki), Southwest (Apache, Cocopa, Maricopa, Mohave, Navajo, Papago, Pima, Yuma), Northwest (Bella Coola, Haisla, Kutenai, Lillooet, Nootka, Okanagon, Queets, Quinault), Great Basin (Shoshoni, Ute, Southern Ute, Southern and Nothern Paiute), Subarctic (Ingalik, Kaska), and northern Plains (Blackfoot, Crow).
3. Alice Joseph, et al., *The Desert People* (Chicago: University of Chicago Press, 1949), p. 227.
4. C. Caryll Forde, "Ethnography of the Yuma Indians," *University of California Publications in American Archeology and Ethnology* 28 (1931): 157; Leslie Spier, *Yuman Tribes of the Gila River* (Chicago: University of Chicago Press, 1933), p. 243.
5. Forde, "Ethnography of the Yuma," p. 157. E. W. Gifford, "The Cocopa," *University of California Publications in American Archeology and Ethnology* 31 (1933): 294.
6. John J. Honigmann, *The Kaska Indians: An Ethnographic Reconstruction* (New Haven: Yale University Press, 1964), pp. 129–30.
7. Cornelius Osgood, *Ingalik Social Culture* (New Haven: Yale University Press, 1958); commented on in Blackwood, "Sexuality and Gender," p. 32.
8. K. J. Crowe, *A History of the Original Peoples of Northern Canada* (Montreal: McGill-Queen's University Press, 1974), pp. 77–78, 90.
9. Honigmann, *Kaska*, pp. 129–30.
10. Claude Schaeffer, "The Kutenai Female Berdache: Courier, Guide, Prophetess, and Warrior," *Ethnohistory* 12 (1965): 195–216.
11. Quoted in ibid.
12. Alexander Ross, *Adventures of the First Settlers on the Oregon or Columbia River* (London: Smith and Elder, 1849), pp. 85, 144–49; quoted in Schaeffer, "Kutenai Female."
13. John Franklin, *Narrative of a Journey to the Shores of the Polar Seas* (London: J. Murray, 1823), p. 152; quoted in Schaeffer, "Kutenai Female."
14. T. C. Elliott, ed. "John Work's Journal," *Washington Historical Quarterly* 5 (1914): 190; quoted in Schaeffer, "Kutenai Female."
15. Quoted in Schaeffer, "Kutenai Female," pp. 215–16.
16. George Devereux, "Institutionalized Homosexuality of the Mohave Indians," *Human Biology* 9 (1937): 503. George Devereux, *Mohave Ethnopsychiatry* (Washington, D.C.: Smithsonian Institution, 1969), p. 262.
17. Devereux, *Mohave Ethnopsychiatry*, pp. 416–17.
18. Ibid., p. 262.
19. Ibid., pp. 416–420.
20. E. W. Gifford, "The Cocopa," *University of California Publications in American Archeology and Ethnology* 31 (1933): 257–94.
21. Leslie Spier, *Klamath Ethnography* (Berkeley: University of California Press, 1930), p. 53.
22. Erminie Voegelin, *Culture Element Distribution: Northeast California* (Berkeley: University of California Press, 1942), vol. 20, pp. 134–35.
23. Charles Callender and Lee Kochems, "Men

and Not-Men: Male Gender-Mixing Statuses and Homosexuality," *Journal of Homosexuality* II (1985); and by the same authors, "The North American Berdache," *Current Anthropology* 24 (1983): 443–56. See also Harriet Whitehead, "The Bow and the Burden Strap: A New Look at Institutionalized Homosexuality in Native North America" in *Sexual Meanings,* ed. Sherry Ortner and Harriet Whitehead (Cambridge: Cambridge University Press, 1981), pp. 80–115. The beginnings of a sophisticated approach, recognizing cultural variation in the number and statuses of genders, are suggested in M. Kay Martin and Barbara Voorhies, *Female of the Species* (New York: Columbia University Press, 1975), chap. 4.

24. Beatrice Medicine, "'Warrior Women'—Sex Role Alternatives for Plains Indian Women," in *The Hidden Half: Studies of Plains Indian Women,* ed. Patricia Albers and Beatrice Medicine (Washington, D.C.: University Press of America, 1983), p. 269. Though Medicine criticizes Sue-Ellen Jacobs for suggesting that Plains Warrior Women were parallel to berdachism, Jacobs has clarified that "they should not be confused with transsexuals, third gender people, homosexuals or others." Sue-Ellen Jacobs, personal communication, 17 May 1983. See also Whitehead, "Bow and Burden Strap," pp. 86, 90–93; Donald Forgey, "The Institution of Berdache among the North American Plains Indians," *Journal of Sex Research* II (1975): I; and Ruth Landes, *The Mystic Lake Sioux* (Madison: University of Wisconsin Press, 1968).
25. Ibid., pp. 92–93; Oscar Lewis, "The Manly-Hearted Women among the Northern Piegan," *American Anthropologist* 43 (1941): 173–87.
26. John Fire and Richard Erdoes, *Lame Deer, Seeker of Visions* (New York: Simon and Schuster, 1972), pp. 148–49.
27. Paula Gunn Allen, "Lesbians in American Indian Cultures," *Conditions* 7 (1981): 76.
28. Blackwood, "Sexuality and Gender," p. 39; Jeannette Mirsky, "The Dakota," in *Cooperation and Competition among Primitive Peoples,* ed. Margaret Mead (Boston: Beacon Press, 1961), p. 417.
29. The best recent works on the position of Plains women are the essays in Albers and Medicine, *Hidden Half.*
30. Edwin Thompson Denig, *Five Indian Tribes of the Upper Missouri,* ed. John Ewers (Norman: University of Oklahoma Press, 1961), pp. 195–200.
31. Ibid.
32. Ibid.
33. Ibid.
34. Ibid.
35. Allen, "Lesbians," pp. 68, 78–79.
36. Blackwood, "Sexuality and Gender," pp. 35–36.
37. Allen, "Lesbians," pp. 65–66, 73.
38. Ibid.
39. Blackwood, "Sexuality and Gender," p. 38; Allen, "Lesbians," pp. 79–80; Albers and Medicine, *Hidden Half,* pp. 53–73.
40. Evelyn Blackwood, "Some Comments on the Study of Homosexuality Cross-Culturally," *Anthropological Research Group on Homosexuality Newsletter* (3 (Fall 1981): 8–9. Important source material on female homosexual behavior is in the classic study by Ferdinand Karsch-Haack, *Das Gleichgeschlechtliche Leben der Naturvölker* (The same-sex life of nature peoples) (Munich: Verlag von Ernst Reinhardt, 1911). It and July Grahn, *Another Mother Tongue: Gay Words, Gay Worlds* (Boston: Beacon Press, 1984), are the starting points for future cross-cultural research on lesbianism. Just two examples of female-female relationships which bear further investigation include groups of women silk weavers, "spinsters," in China—see Agnes Smedley, *Portraits of Chinese Women in Revolution* (Old Westbury, N.Y.: Feminist Press, 1976)—and female marriages in Africa—see Denise O'Brian, "Female Husbands in Southern Bantu Societies," in *Sexual Stratification,* ed. Alice Schlegel (New York: Columbia University Press, 1977).
41. Beverly Chiñas, "Isthmus Zapotec 'Berdaches,'" *Newsletter of the Anthropological Research Group on Homosexuality* 7 (May 1985): 3–4.
42. Ibid.
43. Ibid.
44. Blackwood, "Sexuality and Gender," p. 38.
45. Joseph Sandpiper, Micmac informant I, September 1985.
46. Paula Gunn Allen, personal communication, 6 September 1985.
47. Quoted in Will Roscoe, "Gay American Indians: Creating an Identity from Past Traditions," *The Advocate,* 29 October 1985, pp. 45–48.

VI

EQUALITY AND INEQUALITY: THE SEXUAL DIVISION OF LABOR AND GENDER STRATIFICATION

In most societies certain tasks are predominantly assigned to men while others are assigned to women. In European and American cultures it used to be considered "natural" for men to be the family breadwinners; women were expected to take care of the home and raise the children. An underlying assumption of this division of labor was that men were dominant because their contribution to the material well-being of the family was more significant than that of women. Women were dependent on men and therefore automatically subordinate to them.

The "naturalness" of this division of labor has been called into question as women increasingly enter the labor force. However, has this significantly altered the status of women within their families and in the wider society? Or has it simply meant that women are now working a double day, performing domestic tasks that are negatively valued and not considered work once they get home from their "real" day's work? If employment enhances the social position of women, why is it that women still earn only 70 percent of what men earn for the same work? Why is there still a high degree of occupational segregation by gender?

What precisely is the relationship between the economic roles of women and gender stratification? Cross-cultural research on the sexual division of labor attempts not only to describe the range of women's productive activities in societies with different modes of subsistence, but also to assess the implications of these activities for the status of women.

In many parts of the world women contribute significantly, if not predominantly, to subsistence. This is perhaps most apparent among hunting and gathering or foraging populations, and for this reason such groups have been labeled the most egalitarian of human societies. Hunters and gatherers used to form the bulk of the human population, but today only a small number remain. They are found in relatively isolated regions; they possess simple technology and therefore make little effort to alter the environment in which they live. They tend to be characterized by a division of labor whereby men hunt and women gather. Friedl (1975: 18) outlines four reasons for this division: the variability in the supply of game, the different skills required for hunting and gathering, the incompatibility between carrying burdens and hunting, and the small size of seminomadic foraging populations. Friedl (1975) further argues that in foraging societies in which gathering contributes more to the daily diet than hunting, women and men share equal status (see also Lee 1979; Martin and Voorhies 1975). Conversely, in societies in which hunting and fishing predominate (such as among the Eskimos), the status of women is lower. It seems that female productive activities enhance the social position of women in society, but Sanday (1974) cautions that participation in production is a necessary but not sufficient precondition. Control over the fruits of their labor and a positive valuation of this labor are other factors to consider, as is the extent to which women are involved in at least some political activities. In addition, the absence of a sharp differentiation between public and private domains (Draper 1975) and the fact that there is no economic class structure and no well-defined male-held political offices (Leacock 1975) have been cited as explanations for the relative egalitarianism in foraging societies compared to more complex societies.

Despite the common assumption that men hunt and women gather, in some foraging societies the division of labor is not sharply defined. This often provides the basis for the highest degree of egalitarianism. Among the Tiwi, Australian aborigines who live on Melville Island off the coast of northern Australia, both men and women hunt and gather. Goodale (1971) demonstrates that resources and technology, rather than activities, are divided into male domains and female domains. Although the big game that Tiwi men hunt provides most of the meat to the group and therefore gives them a dominant position in the society, Tiwi women, who hunt and gather, provide more than half of the food consumed; they share in both the comradery and the spoils of their endeavors. As major provisioners, women are economic assets and a source of wealth and prestige for men in this polygynous society. Despite the fact that their opportunities for self-expression may be more limited than those of men, with age women acquire social status and can be politically influential. In general Goodale suggests that Tiwi culture emphasizes the equality of men and women in society.

Among the Agta, women enjoy even greater social equality with their men than among the Tiwi. This is a society in which the division of labor and the battle of the sexes appear to be virtually absent. Agta women hunt game animals and fish just as men do. Not only do they make significant contributions to the daily food supply, but they also control the distribution of the foods they acquire, sharing them with their families and trading them in the broader community. The Griffins (in this book) argue that these roles are clearly the basis for female authority in decision-making within families and residential groups.

The Agta case challenges the widely held notion that in foraging societies pregnancy and child care are incompatible with hunting (Friedl 1978: 72). Agta women have developed methods of contraception and abortion to aid them in childspacing. After becoming pregnant, they continue hunting until late in the pregnancy and resume hunting for several months after the birth of the child. There are always some women available to hunt, during which time children may be cared for by older siblings, grandparents, or other relatives. Reproduction is clearly not a constraint on women's economic roles in this society.

In horticultural societies, in which cultivation is carried out with simple hand-tool technology and slash and burn methods of farming, women also play important roles in production (Boserup 1970). One theory argues that the economic importance of female production in horticultural societies emerged from women's gathering activities in foraging groups. Horticultural societies vary in the degree to which men participate in crop cultivation as well as whether this cultivation is supplemented by hunting, fishing, and raising livestock. In addition, many horticultural societies are matrilineal (reckoning descent through the female line), and in these societies women tend to have higher status than in patrilineal societies.

Despite descent systems and economic roles that enhance the status of women among horticulturalists, Friedl (1975) cautions that male control of valued property and male involvement in warfare (an endemic feature in many of these societies) can be mitigating factors that provide the basis for male dominance over women. For example, among horticulturalists in highland New Guinea, women raise staple crops but men raise prestige crops that are the focus of social exchange. This cultural valuation is the foundation for gender stratification.

Murphy and Murphy (in this book) take us through the active day of a woman among the Mundurucú Indians, a group of people who live in the Amazon region of Brazil. The Mundurucú are a sexually segregated society. Men sleep in a men's house, and women and children share other dwellings. Men hunt, fish, and fell the forest area for gardens. Women plant, harvest, and process manioc. In their daily tasks women form cooperative work groups, have authority, and are the equals of men. To the extent that their work "draws women together and isolates them from the immediate supervision and control of the men, it is also a badge of their independence" (Murphy and Murphy 1985: 237)

However, according to a male-dominated ideology, women are subservient to men. Despite the contributions that Mundurucú women make to subsistence, what men do is assigned more value. As Murphy and Murphy state, "Male ascendancy does not wholly derive from masculine activities but is to a considerable degree prior to them" (234). Male domination among the traditional Mundurucú is symbolic. As the Mundurucú become increasingly drawn into a commercial economy based on the rubber trade, men, with their rights to rubber trees and to trading, may gain a more complete upper hand. "The women may well discover that they have traded the symbolic domination of the men, as a group, over the women, as a group, for the very real domination of husbands over wives" (238).

While women's labor is clearly important in horticultural societies, it has been argued that it becomes increasingly insignificant relative to that of men with the development of intensive agriculture. Intensive agriculture is based on the use of the plow, draft animals, fertilizers, and irrigation systems. In a survey of 93 agricultural societies, Martin and Voorhies (1975: 283) demonstrate that 81 percent delegate farming to men who then achieve primacy in productive activities. One explanation for the decline in female participation in agriculture is that the female domestic workload tends to increase when root crops are replaced by cereal crops and when animal labor replaces manual labor (Martin and Voorhies 1975). Cereal crops require more extensive processing, and field animals must be cared for. Both these activities fall to women. In addition, the kin-based units of production and consumption become smaller, and this too adds to the burdens on individual women.

Concomitant with the presumably declining importance of women in agricultural activities is a supposed decline in social status (Boserup 1970). Women's value is defined by their reproductive abilities rather than by their productive activities. It has been suggested that the lesser status of women in some agricultural societies, particularly those of Eurasia, compared to some horticultural societies, as in sub-Saharan Africa, is reflected in the contrast between systems of bridewealth and systems of dowry (Goody 1976). Bridewealth is a compensation to the bride's parents or her kin for the productive and reproductive rights of the bride; dowry, as a form of inheritance, provides a bride with land and other wealth and helps her to attract a husband (see Stone and James, this volume).

Despite arguments describing a decline in women's status and their relegation to the domestic sphere in association with the emergence of intensive agriculture, cross-cultural data indicate that women in agricultural societies lead much more diverse and complex lives than some theories suggest. In northwestern Portugal women do most of the agricultural activity, inherit property equally, and are often the recipients of a major inheritance that generally includes the parental household (Brettell 1986). This division of labor has emerged because men have been assigned the role of emigrants. Another exception is rural Taiwan, where, despite the patriarchal and patrilineal character of Chinese society, women construct a familial network that gives them a good deal of power and influence in later life (Wolf 1972).

Japanese women have traditionally played an important role in farming, but today these activities are often combined with wage employment. Haruko, a farm woman who lives just outside the town of Unomachi in Ehime Prefecture in western Japan (Bernstein, this book), is the busiest member of her family. Like many urban western women, she juggles wage-paying work with household chores and community responsibilities. She does not define what she does at home, or the assistance that she gives her husband in the rice fields, as real work. Her real work is her job in construction—"man's work" for which she gets paid. Haruko regrets that all these responsibilities have to be carried out at the expense of her children who, she says, "raised themselves" (Bernstein 1983: 47).

Haruko perceives of her work not only as a necessary supplement to the family income, but also as a means to the end of a middle-class lifestyle. In Haruko's eyes the money she earns does not have meaning as a symbol of independence. Her status, she claims, comes from feeling that she is needed. Her desire to become just a housewife with time to spare is one expressed by other women in agricultural societies around the world, especially those who have entered the cash economy on a part-time or temporary basis (Brettell 1995).

A final economic adaptation is that of pastoralism or herding. Some pastoralists are fully nomadic, moving their entire communities in accordance with the demands of the herd. Others are involved in cultivation and are therefore transhumant. They engage in seasonal migration. Among pastoralists the ownership, care, and management of herds are generally in the hands of men. Though there are exceptions, male domination of herding tends to be reflected in other aspects of social organization—the near universality of patrilineal descent and widespread patrilocal residence. Pastoral societies are also generally characterized by patriarchy and a dichotomization of the sexes, both symbolically and socially. Segregation of the sexes and gender stratification, in other words, are fundamental attributes of many pastoral people.

The symbolic opposition between men and women is apparent among the Sarakatsani, a group of transhumant shepherds who live in the mountainous regions of the province of Epirus in Greece. According to Campbell (1964) the life of pastoral Sarakatsani revolves around three things: sheep, children (particularly sons), and honor. "The sheep support the life and prestige of the family, the sons serve the flocks and protect the honour of their parents and sisters, and the notion of honour presupposes physical and moral capacities that fit the shepherds for the hard and sometimes dangerous work of following and protecting their animals" (18). Gender ideology is embedded in these three valued items, especially in the parallel oppositions between sheep and goats on the one hand and men and women on the other. The practical division of labor parallels this symbolic opposition. Women give assistance in the care of animals and make major contributions to their families. The economic roles of husband and wife are complementary. Nevertheless, Sarakatsani husbands have ultimate authority over their wives; obedience to a husband is a moral imperative for a wife. As among the Mundurucú, ideology assigns women to a lesser status, in spite of their economic complementarity.

Men and women are also symbolically and economically complementary among the seminomadic and polygynous WoDaaBe Bororo (Fulani) of Niger, West Africa, described by Dupire (in this book). The WoDaaBe Bororo are characterized by a dramatic spatial and conceptual segregation of the sexes. Each camp is divided into an eastern women's domain and a western men's domain. Herding activities provide about 85 percent of the Bororo subsistence and are dominated by men. Women, however, are involved in the care and milking of cattle, as well as the care of other animals such as sheep and goats. These economic responsibilities, certain rights of ownership, and the fact that they head matricentric units when their husbands are absent give Bororo women a good deal of autonomy.

Generalizations are often made about the status of women according to different modes of adaptation. However, these readings demonstrate that there is a great deal of diversity within each subsistence strategy. For example, in foraging societies women may hunt as well as gather; in intensive agricultural societies not all women are powerless, dependent, and relegated to the domestic sphere.

While women's contributions to subsistence are important to gender stratification, a number of other factors need to be considered. These include leadership roles in family and kinship units and in the wider community; inheritance of property; control of the distribution and exchange of valued goods; authority in childrearing; and participation in ritual activities. In addition, the ideological definitions of women's roles and valuations of their economic activities are often powerful determinants of status.

To fully understand gender stratification both ideology and participation in production must be taken into account. As Atkinson (1982: 248) states, "It is too facile to deny the significance of sexual stereotypes or to presume that women's influence in one context cancels out their degradation in another. Just as we know that women's status is not a unitary phenomenon across cultures, we need to be reminded that the intracultural picture is equally complex."

REFERENCES

Atkinson, Jane. 1982. "Review: Anthropology." *Signs* 8: 236–258.

Bernstein, Gail. 1983. *Haruko's World: A Japanese Farm Woman and Her Community.* Stanford: Stanford University Press.

Boserup, Esther. 1970. *Women's Role in Economic Development.* London: G. Allen and Unwin.

Brettell, Caroline B. 1986. *Men Who Migrate, Women Who Wait: Population and History in a Portuguese Parish.* Princeton: Princeton University Press.

———. 1995. *We Have Already Cried Many Tears: The Stories of Three Portuguese Migrant Women.* Prospect Heights, IL: Waveland Press.

Campbell, John K. 1964. *Honour, Family and Patronage.* Oxford: Oxford University Press.

Draper, Patricia. 1975. "!Kung Women: Contrasts in Sexual Egalitarianism in Foraging and Sedentary Contexts." In Rayna Reiter (ed.). *Toward an Anthropology of Women,* pp. 77–109. New York: Monthly Review Press.

Friedl, Ernestine. 1975. *Women and Men: An Anthropologist's View.* New York: Holt, Rinehart and Winston.

———. 1978. "Society and Sex Roles." *Human Nature* April: 68–75.

Goodale, Jane C. 1971. *Tiwi Wives: A Study of the Women of Melville Island, North Australia.* Seattle: University of Washington Press.

Goody, Jack. 1976. *Production and Reproduction.* Cambridge: Cambridge University Press.

Leacock, Eleanor. 1975. "Class, Commodity, and the Status of Women." In Ruby Rohrlich-Leavitt (ed.). *Women Cross-culturally: Change and Challenge*, pp. 601–616. The Hague: Mouton.

———. 1978. "Women's Status in Egalitarian Society: Implications for Social Evolution." *Current Anthropology* 19(2): 247–275.

Lee, Richard. 1979. *The !Kung San*. Cambridge: Cambridge University Press.

Martin, M. Kay and Barbara Voorhies. 1975. *Female of the Species*. New York: Columbia University Press.

Murphy, Yolanda and Robert F. Murphy. 1985. *Women of the Forest*. New York: Columbia University Press.

Sanday, Peggy Reeves. 1974. "Female Status in the Public Domain." In Michelle Z. Rosaldo and Louise Lamphere (eds.). *Woman, Culture, and Society*, pp. 189–206. Stanford: Stanford University Press.

Wolf, Margery. 1972. *Women and the Family in Rural Taiwan*. Stanford: Stanford University Press.

WOMAN THE HUNTER: THE AGTA

Agnes Estioko-Griffin and P. Bion Griffin

Among Agta Negritos of northeastern Luzon, the Philippines, women are of special interest to anthropology because of their position in the organization of subsistence. They are substantial contributors to the daily subsistence of their families and have considerable authority in decision making in the family and in residential groups. In addition, and in contradiction to one of the sacred canons of anthropology, women in one area frequently hunt game animals. They also fish in the rivers with men and barter with lowland Filipinos for goods and services.[1]

In this chapter, we describe women's roles in Agta subsistence economy and discuss the relationship of subsistence activities,authority allocation, and egalitarianism. With this may come an indication of the importance of the Agta research to the anthropology of women and of hunter-gatherers in general. . . .

Women, especially women in hunting-gathering societies, have been a neglected domain of anthropological research. The recent volume edited by Richard Lee and Irven DeVore (1976) and the *!Kung of Nyae Nyae* (Marshall 1976) begin to remedy the lack but focus solely on the !Kung San of southern Africa. Other works are either general or synthetic (Friedl 1975; Martin and Voorhies 1975), or report narrowly bounded topics (Rosaldo and Lamphere 1974). Sally Slocum, writing in *Toward an Anthropology of Women* (Reiter 1975), has provided impetus for the Agta study. Slocum points out a male bias in studying hunter-gatherers, showing how approaching subsistence from a female view gives a new picture. From the insights of Slocum we have sought to focus on Agta women, to compare the several dialect groups, and to begin investigating the nature and implications of women as not "merely" gatherers but also hunters.

THE AGTA

The Agta are Negrito peoples found throughout eastern Luzon, generally along the Pacific coast and up rivers into the Sierra Madre interior. . . . Although perhaps fewer in numbers, they are also located on the western side of the mountains, especially on the tributary rivers feeding the Cagayan. In general terms, the Agta of Isabela and Cagayan provinces are not dissimilar to other present and past Philippine Negritos. (See Vanoverbergh 1925, 1929–30, 1937–38; Fox 1952; Garvan 1964; and Maceda 1964 for information on Negritos outside the present study area.) In the more remote locales, hunting forest

Abridged with permission from Frances Dahlberg (ed.), *Woman the Gatherer* (New Haven: Yale University Press, 1981), pp. 121–140.

game, especially wild pig, deer, and monkey, is still important. Everywhere, collection of forest plant foods has been eclipsed by exchange of meat for corn, rice, and cultivated root crops. Fishing is usually important throughout the dry season, while collection of the starch of the caryota palm (*Caryota cumingii*) is common in the rainy season. An earlier paper (Estioko and Griffin 1975) gives some detail concerning the less settled Agta; both Bennagen (1976) and Peterson (1974, 1978*a,b,* n.d.) closely examine aspects of subsistence among Agta in the municipality of Palanan.

A brief review of Agta economic organization will be sufficient for later discussion of women's activities. Centuries ago all Agta may have been strictly hunter-gatherers. Since at least A.D. 1900 the groups near the towns of Casiguran (Headland and Headland 1974) and Palanan have been sporadic, part-time horticulturalists, supplementing wild plant foods with sweet potatoes, corn, cassava, and rice. The more remote, interior Agta, sometimes referred to as *ebuked* (Estioko and Griffin 1975), plant small plots of roots, a few square meters of corn, and a banana stalk or two. They usually plant only in the wet season, harvesting an almost immature crop when staples are difficult to obtain by trade. *Ebuked* neglect crop production, preferring to trade meat for grains and roots.

Lee and DeVore (1968:7) argue that women produce much of the typical hunter-gatherers' diet and that in the tropics vegetable foods far outweigh meat in reliability and frequency of consumption. The Dipagsanghang and Dianggu-Malibu Agta strikingly contradict this idea. They are superb hunters, eat animal protein almost daily, and, as noted above, may have both men and women hunting. (The Tasaday, to the south in Mindanao, may represent an extreme nonhunting adaptation, one in which plant food collection is very dominant [Yen 1976].) Hunting varies seasonally and by techniques used among various groups, but is basically a bow and arrow technology for killing wild pig and deer, the only large game in the Luzon dipterocarp forests. Monkey, although not large, is a reliable rainy season prey. Among Agta close to Palanan and Casiguran, hunting is a male domain. Many hunters pride themselves on skill with bow and arrow; less able hunters may use traps. Dogs to drive game are very desirable in the dry season when the forest is too noisy for daylight stalking of animals.

The collecting of wild plant food is not a daily task. Most Agta prefer to eat corn, cassava, and sweet potatoes, and neglect the several varieties of roots, palm hearts, and greens procurable in the forest. . . . Forest foods are difficult to collect, necessitate residence moves over long distances, and do not taste as good as cultivated foods. Emphasis of trade networks with lowland farmers favors deemphasis of forest exploitation of plants. Only in the rainy season do Agta actively process a traditional resource, the sago-like caryota palm. Fruits are often picked on the spur of the moment; seldom do parties leave camp solely for their collection.

Trade with farmers is practiced by all Agta known to us. Rumors of Agta "farther into the mountains" who never trade (or cultivate) seem to be without substance. In the report of the Philippine Commission (1908:334), evidence of lowland-Agta trade around 1900 indicates the *ibay* trade partner relationship to have some antiquity. As the lowlander population has increased since World War II, trade has also increased. Agta are more and more dependent on goods and foodstuffs gained from farmers; adjustments of Agta economic behavior continue to be made, with labor on farms being one aspect of change. Agta formerly simply traded meat for carbohydrates. Around Palanan they may now work for cash or kind when residing close to farmers' settlements. Hunting decreases as the demands of cultivation are met. A cycle is created, and further withdrawal from forest subsistence occurs. Farmers live in areas once solely owned by Agta. Debts to farmers increase with economic dependence; freedom of mobility and choice of activity decrease; and Agta in farming areas become landless laborers.

At the same time, Agta seek to get out of the cycle by emulating the farmers. Many Agta within ten kilometers of Palanan Centro are attempting to become farmers themselves. While the success rate is slow, the attempt is real. Again, when questioned by an early American anthropologist, Agta close to Palanan Centro claimed to be planting small rainy season plots with corn, roots, and upland rice (Worcester 1912:841). Living informants confirm the long practice of cultivation, but suggest a recent expansion of Agta fields and commitment to abandoning forest nomadism (especially over the last fifteen years). Around the areas of Disuked-Dilaknadinum and Kahanayan-Diabut in Palanan, Agta are well known for their interest in swidden cultivation. Even the most unsettled Agta farther upriver claim small fields and sporadically plant along the rivers well upstream of lowland farmsteads.

The horticultural efforts of the Agta appear less than is the case, since the social organization and settlement patterns are very different from those of the farmers. Agta throughout Isabela and Cagayan are loosely organized into extended family residential groups. A group, called a *pisan,* is seldom less than two nuclear families and very rarely more than five (in the dry season—perhaps slightly higher average during the wet season). The nuclear family is the basic unit of Agta society, being potentially self-sufficient under usual circumstances. The residential group is organized as a cluster of nuclear families united either through a common parent or by sibling ties. Non-kin friends may be visitors for several weeks, and any nuclear family is able to leave and join another group of relatives at will.

As is typical of hunting-gathering societies, no formal, institutionalized authority base exists. The nuclear family is the decision maker concerning residence, work, and relations with other people. Older, respected individuals, often parents and grandparents of group members, may be consulted, but their opinions are not binding. Often group consensus is desired; people who disagree are free to grumble or to leave.

The settlement pattern is determined, in part, by the seasonal cycle of rains and sunny weather, and by these influences on the flora and fauna exploited for food. Rainy season flooding restricts forest travel, brings hardships in exchange, but is compensated by good condition of the game animals. The dry season permits travel over greater distances and into the remote mountains. Predictable fish resources enhance the advantages of human dispersal; only the need to carry trade meats to farmers inhibits distant residence placement.

WOMEN'S ACTIVITIES

Women participate in all the subsistence activities that men do. Women trade with farmers, fish in the rivers, collect forest plant foods, and may even hunt game animals. Tasks are not identical, however; a modest sexual division of labor does exist. Furthermore, considerable variation is found among the groups of Agta of Isabella and Cagayan provinces. These differences may possibly be ascribed to degree of adjustment of Agta to lowland Filipino culture. Some differences may be due to unique culture histories and to little contact.

Although in Isabela most Agta women do not hunt with bow and arrows, with machetes, or by use of traps, most are willing to assist men in the hunt. Not uncommonly, women help carry game out of the forest. Since mature pig and deer are heavy and the terrain is difficult, this is no small accomplishment. Even in areas around Palanan and Casiguran, women are known to accompany men and dogs into the forest and to guide the dogs in the game drive. Some women are famous for their abilities to handle dogs; one informant, a girl about fifteen years of age, was especially skilled. In Palanan and Casiguran, women and men laugh at the idea of women hunting. Such a practice would be a custom of wild, uncivilized Agta (*ebuked*) far in the mountains, they say. Many of the attributes of *ebuked* seem to be old-fashioned customs still practiced by interior groups.

Two groups studied as part of the present research do have women who hunt. Among the Dipagsanghang Agta, several mature women claim to have hunting skills; they learned these in their unmarried teen years. They only hunt under extreme circumstances, such as low food supplies or great distances from farmers and a supply of corn. All these Agta are found in southern Isabela between Dipagsanghang and Dinapiqui.

In the northernmost section of Isabela and well into Cagayan province, women are active and proficient hunters. While we have termed the Agta here as the Dianggu-Malibu group, we are actually referring to speakers of the southeast Cagayan dialect who live on the river drainage areas of the Dianggu and Malibu rivers.[2] Both the dialect and women who hunt are found over a considerably greater territory, according to informants, reaching north to Baggao, Cagayan, and at least to the Taboan River.

Among the Dianggu-Malibu women some variation, perhaps localized, perhaps personal, is found. On the Dianggu, some of the women questioned, and observed hunting, carried machetes and were accompanied by dogs. They claim to prefer the machete to the bow and arrow, allowing dogs to corner and hold pigs for sticking with the knife. Our sample of actual observations is too small to argue that only immature pigs are killed, but we do know that in the dry season adult male pigs are dangerous in the extreme. Dogs may be killed during hunts. Since Agta dogs are seldom strong animals, we wonder if mature pigs are acquired only occasionally. On the other hand, so many dogs are owned by these Agta that sheer numbers may favor large kills. We have observed two Agta women with as many as fifteen dogs. Other Dianggu women prefer the bow.

On the Malibu River, Agta women are expert bow and arrow hunters. On both of our brief visits to this group, women were observed hunting. They claim to use bows always, and they seek the full range of prey animals. Wild pig is most desired, while deer are often killed. Future work must quantify the hunting details, but women seem to vary slightly from men in their hunting strategies. Informants say they hunt only with dogs. On closer questioning they admit to knowing techniques that do not involve dogs—for example, they may climb trees and lie in wait for an animal to approach to feed on fallen fruit. Among all Agta, hunting practices vary considerably between the rainy and dry seasons. Our fieldwork in Malibu has been confined to the dry season, when dogs are important. In the rainy season solitary stalking is practiced. Field observations should eventually provide quantitative data on women hunting in this season; we must stress that our data are primarily from interview and brief observation. We have not resided among Cagayan Agta long enough to advance quantitatively based generalizations.

Women not only hunt but appear to hunt frequently. Like men, some enjoy hunting more than others. The more remotely located Agta seem most to favor hunting. Even among Agta certain males and females are considered lacking in initiative, a fault that may not be confined to hunting.

Informant data indicate that while women may make their own arrows, the actual blacksmithing of the metal projectile points is a male activity. More field research is necessary to confirm the universality of this detail. Other items of interest pertain to the composition of hunting parties. Most people in any one residence group are consanguineally or affinely related. We have observed several combinations of hunting parties. Men and women hunt together or among themselves. Often sisters, or mother and daughter, or aunt and niece hunt together. At Malibu, two sisters, co-wives of one male, hunt together, and either or both sisters join the husband to hunt. When young children exist, one of the two wives may stay at the residence while the husband and the other wife hunt and fish. Also, sisters and brothers cooperate on the hunt. A woman would not hunt with, for example, a cousin's husband unless the cousin were along.

The only real argument, in our opinion, that has been advanced to support the contention that women must gather and men hunt relates to childbearing and nurture. Among the Agta, during late pregnancy and for the first few months of nursing, a woman will not hunt. In spite of the small size of each residential group, however, some females seem always to be around to hunt, although one or more may be temporarily withdrawn from the activity. Women with young children hunt less than teenagers and older women. On the occasion of brief hunts—part of one day—children are cared for by older siblings, by grandparents, and by other relatives. Occasionally a father will tend a child. Only infants are closely tied to mothers.

Girls start hunting shortly after puberty. Before then they are gaining forest knowledge but are not strong. Boys are no different. We have no menopause data, but at least one woman known to us as a hunter must have passed childbearing age. She is considered an older woman, but since she is strong, she hunts. The pattern is typical of men also. As long as strength to travel and to carry game is retained, people hunt. Our best informant, a young grandmother, hunts several times a week.

Both Agta men and women fish. In fact, from early childhood until the infirmity of old age all Agta fish. If most adults are gone on a hunting trip for several days, the remaining adults and children must obtain animal protein by themselves. Only women in late pregnancy, with young infants, or into old age, withdraw from fishing, which makes considerable demands of endurance as well as skill. Some men excel at working in rough, deep, and cold waters. The everyday techniques for fishing are limited to underwater spear fishing. Glass-lensed wooden goggles, a heavy wire spear or rod varying according to size of fish sought, and an inner-tube rubber band complete the equipment. To fish, people simply swim underwater, seeking fish in the various aquatic environments known for each species. Girls in their teens are very capable at fishing. When fishing individually, women may be major contributors to the daily catch.

When group fishing is undertaken, a drive is conducted. In this operation, a long vine is prepared by attaching stones and banners of wild banana stalks. Two people drag the vine, one on each end and on opposite sides of the river, while the people in the water spear fish startled by the stones and stalks. Women join men in the drives, with older men and women dragging the vine while all able-bodied youths and adults work in the water.

Difficulty of fishing may be characterized as a gradient upon which men and women become less and less able as age and debilities increase. The elderly, when mobile, may still be productive, but instead of true fishing, their activities may be termed collecting. Both the coastal reef areas and freshwater rivers and streams have abundant shellfish, shrimp, and amphibians that may be caught by hand. Elderly women and grandchildren are especially eager to harvest these resources. Older men are not ashamed to follow suit, although the enthusiasm of others for the task seldom gives old men incentive. Men are much less eager to give up riverine fishing after middle age than are women. Clearly some emphasis on males securing protein is found among Agta. Women, however, seem to have traditionally been active in fishing. Interestingly, as a few Agta adopt lowland fishing technology, especially nets, women seldom participate. Like their female counterparts in lowland society, women are deemed not appropriate in net fishing.

One might expect that, on the basis of worldwide comparison, tropic hunters would really be gatherers, and that women would be the steady and substantial providers. Agta do not fit the generalizations now accepted. Few Agta women regularly dig roots, gather palm hearts, seek fruit, or pick greens. Most Agta daily consume domesticated staples grown by the farmers. Women are, however, very knowledgeable concerning flora and its use, and among the less settled Agta, young girls are still taught all traditional forest lore. Brides-to-be among these Agta are partially evaluated on the basis of their knowledge, skill, and endurance in collecting jungle plant foods.

Roots are collected by women whenever more desirable food is unobtainable, when several wild pigs have been killed and the men want to eat "forest food" with pig fat, or when a visit to relatives or friends calls for a special treat. The interior groups may actually combine meat and wild roots for weeks when camped so far from farmers that exchange for corn is impossible. Downriver Agta consider such a practice a real hardship, not to be willingly endured. Men are known to dig roots, even though they say it is women's work. On long-distance hunts men do not as a rule carry food, and they may occasionally dig roots to alleviate the all meat-fish diet.

As hunting is thought of as a "sort of" male activity among many Agta (in Isabela), processing the starch of the caryota palm is a female activity. Women cruise the forest searching for trees containing masses of the starch; they also chop down the trees, split the trunks, adze out the pith, and extract the flour. Often parties of women and girls work together, speeding up the laborious task. On occasion, men will assist. Extracting the flour starch is moderately heavy work, and tiring. Husbands may help when wives have a pressing need to complete a task quickly. Since much of the final product is given in gift form, the need for haste occurs frequently. Perhaps most important to note is the male participation. Sexual division of labor is tenuously bounded among all Agta. Emphases may exist, but a man can even build a house (i.e., tie the fronds to the frame—a female task).

As noted at the beginning, trade, exchange, and horticulture are not new to Agta. Informants, early photographs, and writings indicate that all but the most remote Agta were not "pure" hunter-gatherers after about A.D. 1900. Since the mountains have been a final retreat—from the earliest Spanish attempts to conquer the Cagayan Valley until the present—Agta must have been in contact with former farmers/revolutionaries in hiding. Keesing (1962), summarizing the peoples of northern Luzon, documents several societies of pagan swiddeners adjacent to or in Negrito territory. The Palanan River drainage area was inhabited by farmers before Spanish contact in the sixteenth century. Doubtless, Agta have participated in economic exchange and social intercourse for centuries. Agta now have institutionalized trade partnerships, at least in Palanan and Casiguran municipalities. Trade partners are called *ibay* (Peterson [1978*a,b*] discussed the *ibay* relationship in detail), and partnerships may last between two families over two or more generations. *Ibay* exchange meat for grains and roots, or meat for cloth, metal, tobacco, beads, and other goods. Services may be exchanged, especially in downriver areas. Fields may be worked by Agta, who then borrow a carabao, receive corn or rice, and satisfy any of a number of needs. What is important in relation to this chapter is that Agta women may engage in *ibay* partnerships. Among the lowland farmers almost all *ibay* are males. An Agta woman may be an *ibay* with a lowland man. According to our data, an Agta husband often is not also *ibay* with his wife's *ibay,* but he must treat the farmer as he would his own *ibay.* Of course Agta men and women trade with any farmer they choose, but such exchange is without the consideration given to an *ibay.* (Considerations include credit, acts of friendship, and first choice/best deal on goods.) Not only do women have *ibay,* but they very frequently are the most active agents of exchange. In areas where the trade rests mostly on meat and where men do most of the hunting, women are likely to carry out the dried meat and bring back the staple. They therefore gain experience in dealing with the farmers. We should note that many farmers attempt to cheat the Agta by shortchanging them on counts or weights, but they do so on the basis of gullibility or naiveté of the Agta, not on the basis of sex. Agta women are actually more aggressive traders than are men, who do not like confrontation.

Among the Dipagsanghang Agta, women seldom hunt today, and infrequently dig roots. They do carry out meat to trade. They seem to have an easier life, with emphasis on corn, rice, and roots instead of gathering wild foods. However, downriver, close to farmers, Agta women have reversed this trend, and are working harder and longer hours.[3] Intensification of the *ibay* relationship and need to own and cultivate land has forced women to become horticulturalists and wage laborers for farmers. On their own family plots (family-owned, not male- or female-owned) they, together with adult males and youths, clear land, break soil, plant, weed, and harvest. When clearing virgin forest of large trees, women do not participate. They do clear secondary growth in fallowed fields.

In the families that reside close to Palanan . . . men and women work almost daily in the fields of farmers. Women go to the forest to collect the lighter raw materials for house construction, mats, betel chews, medicines, and so on. Men follow a similar pattern, giving up hunting for field labor and a corn and sweet potato diet supplemented by small fish. Again we see a remarkable parallel in the activities of males and females.

Looking more closely at specialized women's activities, one may suggest increasing importance in downriver areas. Women have several domains that they use to gain cash or kind income. As just stated, income from labor in fields adds to the economic power of women. A small-scale traditional pursuit, shared by men and women, is the gathering of copal, a tree resin common to trees (*Agathis philippinensis*) found scattered in the Sierra Madre. Women often collect and carry the resin out to lowland "middlemen," who sell it to the depot in town. While corn and cash may be sought in exchange, cloth is desired in order to make skirts. Medicine and medical treatments for ailing children may be paid for by copal collection. Another example of entrepreneurship by females is a small-scale mobile variety store effort. After working in fields for cash and building a surplus, families may cross the Sierra Madre to the towns of San Mariano, Cauayan, and Ilagan. There Agta, often women, purchase in markets and stores goods for use and resale in Palanan. Palanan Centro itself has no real market, only several small general stores selling goods at highly marked up prices. Since no road reaches Palanan, all manufactured supplies must enter town by airplane from Cauayan or boat from Baler. Freight costs are high. Some Agta women are very eager to hike outside to get tobacco, which always commands a high price and a ready market.

DISCUSSION

The role of women in Agta economic activities has been reviewed. Assessment of an hypothesized egalitarian position of women may be more difficult, and rests on assertions and interpretations drawn from the economic roles. First, drawing in part from Friedl (1975), an argument can be made that women in Agta society have equality with men because they have similar authority in decision making. The authority could be based on the equal contribution to the subsistence resources. Working back, we see that among many Agta, women do contribute heavily to the daily food supply, do perform maintenance tasks with men, and may initiate food acquisition efforts through their own skills. They do control the distribution of their acquired food, sharing first with their own nuclear family and extended family, then trading as they see fit. They may procure nonfood goods as they desire. Men may do the same; generally spouses discuss what work to do, what needs should be satisfied, and who will do what. Whole residential groups frequently together decide courses of action. Women are as vocal and as critical in reaching decisions as are men. Further examples could strongly validate the hypothesis that women do supply a substantial portion of foods, and the assertion that women have authority in major decision making. Two questions arise. May we accept a causal relationship between percentage of food production and equality? Certainly there are cases to the contrary. According to Richard A. Gould (personal communication), Australian Aboriginal women in various areas collected the bulk of the food, yet remained less than equal (as we will define equality). Second, we may ask if Agta males and females are actually "equal."

Two avenues may suffice in answering this question. First, one might explore a definition of equality, surely a culturally loaded concept. Since Agta women have authority or control of the economic gain of their own labor, they may be equal in this critical domain. Equality must surely be equated with decision-making power and control of one's own production. The second avenue of equality validation by the scientist may be to examine the female's control over herself in noneconomic matters. These could include selection of marriage partner, lack of premarital sexual intercourse proscription, spacing of children, ease of divorce, and polygyny rules.

In marriage, two forms are typical of Agta. One, the less common, is elopement by young lovers. While such marriages admittedly are fragile, elopement is not uncommon. In this case both partners must be willing. Rape and abduction are rare. Rape by Agta men is not known to the authors. Abduction must involve a slightly willing female, and is not done by young people. A mature man might abduct a married woman, crossing the mountains to a safe locale. To abduct a young girl would be difficult. Parents of eloping couples may be enraged, but usually reconcile themselves to the marriage. If the newlyweds stay together, no more is made of it.

The proper form of marriage is one arranged by customary meetings and discussions, as well as exchange of goods between two families. Often neither the bride nor the groom has had much say in the matter, although serious dislike by either would probably kill the negotiations before the marriage. Mothers are the most important in choosing who will marry whom. Even when their children are young, they are looking about for good partners. Word filters around when a young girl is marriageable, and efforts are made to get the appropriate young man and his family into negotiations before an undesirable family appears. Once any family with a prospective groom formally asks, a rejection is given only for strong and good reasons, since the denied family loses considerable face and may be angry enough to seek revenge.[4]

Criteria for choice of a marriage partner are varied. Often a young man in his early twenties marries a girl about fifteen. Girls entering marriage before puberty are not uncommon. In such cases the husband may help raise the girl until the time the marriage is consummated and full wifehood is recognized. Other combinations are seen. One much discussed case was the marriage of a woman in her forties to a man in his mid-twenties. The couple seemed very happy, with the wife paying rather special attention to her husband. The man's mother, a friend of the wife's, decided that the marriage was peculiar but acceptable.

Premarital female chastity is not an idea of much currency. Agta close to farmers will pay lip service to the idea, but should a girl become pregnant she will take a husband. There are no illegitimate Agta children, although an occasional rape of an Agta by a lowland male may produce a child. Since by the time a girl is fertile she likely will be married, illegitimacy is not the issue. Although some data are difficult to collect concerning sex, almost certainly girls are able to engage in sexual activity with relative ease; promiscuity is not favored in any circumstance. Males may have as little or great difficulty in engaging in sex as females. The Agta are widely dispersed in extended family groups; hence appropriate sexual partners are seldom seen. No homosexuality is known to exist.

Agta gossip suggests that many Agta, male and female, married and unmarried, constantly carry on extramarital sexual relations. This may be a function of gossip, and a gross exaggeration. Whatever reality, neither males nor females seem to be especially singled out for criticism.

Women say they space their children. The practice certainly varies hugely from person to person, as does fecundity and luck in keeping children alive. The Agta use various herbal concoctions that supposedly prevent conception, cause abortions shortly after conception, and have several functions related to menstruation. These medicines are known to all Agta and are frequently used. Our census data indicate that some women seem to be successful in spacing births. Other cases note high infant mortality yet no infanticide, female or male. All Agta abhor the idea.

Divorce is infrequent among Agta, with elopement being more prone to failure than are arranged marriages. Divorce does happen often enough, however, for us to look at the causes and relate them to an inquiry into female equality. First, either sex may divorce the other with equal ease. Agta have no possessions. Some gift giving between the two families establishes the marriage, but most of the gifts are food. Cloth, kettles, and minor items make up the rest. Return of marriage gifts is unlikely. Spouses simply take their personal possessions and return to the residential group of close relatives.

Causes for divorce are mainly laziness or improvidence, excessive adultery, or personality clashes and incompatibility, usually caused by a combination of the first two conditions. Skill and success in subsistence activities is of primary importance to marriage. While some Agta are less industrious and less skilled than others, all Agta expect a mate to work hard at all appropriate tasks. Should a male fail, divorce is likely. Occasionally, very young couples experience extra difficulties. These may be accentuated by displeased parents of either party.

Polygamy is not found in most of Isabela. Census data collected to date reveal only monogamy or serial monogamy. That is, spouses may be divorced or widow(er)ed several times in a lifetime. In Cagayan the data are incomplete but startling. Probably some of the strongest support for the equality of women hypothesis, when added to the facts of women as hunters, comes from a study of Agta polygamy. We noted earlier that two co-wives, sisters, hunted together in Malibu. South of Malibu at Blos, another husband and two sisters/co-wives arrangement was found. In the same residential unit we recorded a woman residing with her two co-husbands. They were not brothers; one was older than the wife, one younger. The other women considered this arrangement as humorous, but acceptable. An insight into the male sexual jealousy found in many societies worldwide is the comment of a Palanan Agta man. This old man, when told of the polyandrous marriage to the north, thought for a moment and commented, "Well, perhaps one man with two wives is OK, but a woman with two husbands? I find that totally bad." The women laughed at him.

NOTES

1. Although the authors have worked among the Agta about fourteen months, visits to the northerly group in the Dianggu-Malibu area have been brief. The practice of women hunting was first observed during a survey trip in 1972. We again visited the Dianggu group in 1975. In August 1978 we returned for one week to Dianggu and Malibu, where we verified in greater detail the subsistence activities of women. Data were collected using the Palanan Agta dialect and Ilokano.
2. Dianggu and Malibu are river names used by Agta and nearby Malay Filipinos. On the Board of Technical Surveys and Maps (Lobod Point, Philippines), the Dianggu is named the Lobod and the Malibu is named the Ilang.
3. Peterson (n.d.) argues that "downriver" Agta women are highly variable in their devotion to labor, older women being hardworking and young mothers not at all industrious.
4. Thomas Headland tells us that rejection of a prospective spouse may be a less serious matter among Casiguran Agta than among those we know.

REFERENCES

Bennagen, Ponciano. 1976. Kultura at Kapaligiran: Pangkulturang Pagbabago at Kapanatagan ng mga Agta sa Palanan, Isabela. M. A. thesis, Department of Anthropology, University of the Philippines, Diliman, Quezon City.

Briggs, Jean L. 1974. Eskimo women: makers of men. In *Many sisters: women in cross-cultural perspective,* ed. Carolyn J. Matthiasson, pp. 261–304. New York: Free Press.

Estioko, Agnes A., and P. Bion Griffin. 1975. The *Ebuked* Agta of northeastern Luzon. *Philippines Quarterly of Culture and Society* 3(4):237–44.

Flannery, Regina. 1932. The position of women among the Mescalero-Apache. *Primitive Man* 10:26–32.

———. 1935. The position of women among the eastern Cree. *Primitive Man* 12:81–86.

Fox, Robert B. 1952. The Pinatubo Negritos, their useful plants and material culture. *Philippine Journal of Science* 81:113–414.

Friedl, Ernestine. 1975. *Women and men: an anthropologist's view.* New York: Holt, Rinehart and Winston.

Garvan, John M. 1964. *The Negritos of the Philippines,* ed. Hermann Hochegger, Weiner beitrage zur kulturgeschichte und linguistik, vol. 14. Horn: F. Berger.

Goodale, Jane C. 1971. *Tiwi wives: a study of the women of Melville Island, north Australia.* Seattle, Wash.: University of Washington Press.

Gough, Kathleen. 1975. The origin of the family. In *Toward an anthropology of women,* ed. Rayna R. Reiter, pp. 51–76. New York: Monthly Review Press.

Hammond, Dorothy, and Alta Jablow. 1976. *Women in cultures of the world.* Menlo Park, Calif.: Benjamin/Cummings.

Harako, Reizo. 1976. The Mbuti as hunters—a study of ecological anthropology of the Mbuti pygmies. *Kyoto University African Studies* 10:37–99.

Headland, Thomas, and Janet D. Headland. 1974. *A Dumagat (Casiguran)–English dictionary.* Pacific Linguistics Series C. No. 28. Australian National University, Canberra: Linguistics Circle of Canberra.

Howell, F. Clark. 1973. *Early man,* rev. ed. New York: Time-Life Books.

Isaac, Glynn L. 1969. Studies of early culture in East Africa. *World Archaeology* 1:1–27.

———. 1971. The diet of early man: aspects of archaeological evidence from lower and middle Pleistocene sites in Africa. *World Archaeology* 2: 278–98.

———. 1978. The food-sharing behavior of protohuman hominids. *Scientific American* 238(4): 90–109.

Jenness, Diamond. 1922. *The Life of the Copper Eskimos. Report of the Canadian Arctic Expedition 1913–1918,* vol. XII, pt. 9. Ottawa: Acland.

Keesing, Felix. 1962. *The ethnohistory of northern Luzon.* Stanford, Calif.: Stanford University Press.

Lancaster, Jane B. 1978. Carrying and sharing in-human evolution. *Human Nature* 1(2):82–89.

Landes, Ruth. 1938. *The Ojibwa Woman.* New York: Columbia University Press.

Lee, Richard B. and Irven DeVore. 1968. Problems in the study of hunters and gatherers. In *Man the hunter,* ed. Lee and DeVore. Chicago: Aldine.

———. 1976. *Kalahari hunter-gatherers: studies of the !Kung San and their neighbors.* Cambridge, Mass.: Harvard University Press.

Maceda, Marcelino M. 1964. *The culture of the mamanuas (northeast Mindanao) as compared with that of the other Negritos of Southeast Asia.* Manila: Catholic Trade School.

Marshall, Lorna. 1976. *The !Kung of Nyae Nyae.* Cambridge, Mass.: Harvard University Press.

Martin, M. Kay, and Barbara Voorhies. 1975. *Female of the species.* New York: Columbia University Press.

Peterson, Jean Treloggen. 1974. An ecological perspective on the economic and social behavior of Agta hunter-gatherers, northeastern Luzon, Philippines. Ph.D. dissertation, University of Hawaii at Manoa.

———. 1978*a.* Hunter-gatherer farmer exchange. *American Anthropologist* 80:335–51.

———. 1978*b.* The ecology of social boundaries: Agta foragers of the Philippines. *Illinois Studies in Anthropology No. 11.* University of Illinois, Urbana-Champaign, Ill.

———. n.d. Hunter mobility, family organization and change. In *Circulation in the Third World,* ed. Murray Chapman and Ralph Mansell Prothero. London: Routledge & Kegan Paul.

Philippine Commission. 1908. *8th Annual Report of the Philippine Commission: 1907.* Bureau of Insular Affairs, War Department. Washington, D.C.: Government Printing Office.

Quinn, Naomi. 1977. Anthropological studies on women's status. In *Annual review of anthropology,* ed. Bernard J. Siegel, pp. 181–225. Palo Alto, Calif.: Annual Reviews.

Reiter, Rayna R., ed. 1975. *Toward an anthropology of women.* New York:Monthly Review Press.

Rosaldo, Michelle Zimbalist, and Louise Lamphere, eds. 1974. *Woman, culture and society.* Stanford, Calif.: Stanford University Press.

Slocum, Sally. 1975. Woman the gatherer: male bias in anthropology. In *Toward an anthropology of women,* ed. Rayna R. Reiter, pp. 36–50. New York: Monthly Review Press.

Tanner, Nancy, and Adrienne Zihlman. 1976. Women in evolution. Part I: Innovations and

selection in human origins. *Signs: Journal of Women in Culture and Society* 1:585–608.
Tanno, Tadashi. 1976. The Mbuti net-hunters in the Ituri Forest, Eastern Zaire—their hunting activities and band composition. *Kyoto University African Studies* 10:101–35.
Turnbull, Colin M. 1965. *Wayward servants: the two worlds of the African pygmies.* Garden City, NY: Natural History Press.
Vanoverberg, Maurice. 1925. Negritos of northern Luzon. *Anthropos* 20:148–99.
———. 1929–30. Negritos of northern Luzon again. *Anthropos* 24:1–75, 897–911; 25:25–71, 527–656.
———. 1937–38. Negritos of eastern Luzon. *Anthropos* 32:905–28; 33:119–64.
Washburn, Sherwood L., and C. S. Lancaster. 1968. The evolution of hunting. In *Man the hunter,* ed. Richard B. Lee and Irven DeVore, pp. 293–303. Chicago: Aldine.
Worcester, Dean C. 1912. Head-hunters of northern Luzon. *National Geographic* 23(9):833–930.
Yen, D. E. 1976. The ethnobotany of the Tasaday: III. Note on the subsistence system. In *Further studies on the Tasaday,* ed. D. E. Yen and John Nance. Makati, Rizal: PANAMIN Foundation Research Series No. 2.

WOMAN'S DAY AMONG THE MUNDURUCÚ

Robert Murphy and Yolanda Murphy

Dawn came first as a shift of light and shadow in the eastern sky, etching out of the blackness of the night the outline of the hills on the watershed of the rivers. With it, the forest fell silent, the raucous noises of the night creatures faded, and the great quietude separating the life of the night from that of the day reached its brief ascendancy. As the eastern sky turned a dark, then a lighter, gray, the houses of the Mundurucú village of Cabruá began to emerge from shadows into pale images, and the first stirring of the people was heard.

Borai tossed in her hammock, wrapped it tightly around and snuggled her baby closely against the chill dawn. The child began to whimper, and she took a breast from under her worn dress and placed it by his mouth. While he suckled, Borai lay half-asleep, gazing out through the space between the walls and roof of the house, watching the light strengthen in the east. The eight-month-old baby finished feeding, fell back to sleep, and Borai gently disengaged herself from it and eased out of her warm cocoon into the cold of the wakening house. She yawned and stretched, scratched herself luxuriantly, and then kicked at the dogs nestled around the smoldering household fire.

Reprinted with permission from Robert Murphy and Yolanda Murphy, *Women of the Forest* (New York: Columbia University Press, 1985), pp. 1–20.

The earth around the hearth was still warm, and she stood close to it, warming the bottoms of her feet. Borai then took some kindling and placing it next to the fire, took a still glowing end of a piece of wood from last night's fire and blew it into flame. She placed the kindling carefully around the small flame, like spokes about a hub, and when the fire crackled into life, brought over larger pieces of firewood to prepare for the day's cooking. She swung rather halfheartedly with a piece of firewood at the lingering dogs, chasing them out of the house, and then went to stand at the back door, pensively watching the breaking day.

The sky in the east had by then turned to delicate and striated bands of mauve and pink, and the land in the valley below was beginning to appear from the gloom. The hills beyond the headwaters of the river could now be seen in sharp relief, and the islands of forest in the rolling savannah appeared as dark blotches, their trees gaining distinction as the light grew stronger. The valleys were still covered with the mist of the dawn, and small pockets of fog moved slowly across the faces of the hills. It was a calm and serene period, and the other women of the house only spoke to each other in whispers, lest the stillness of the natural world be torn by human beings.

The life of the village gained momentum as the natural order of the day asserted itself. Before the sun had edged over the horizon, a rooster crowed from somewhere in the underbrush bordering the village, another in the brush near the *farinha*-making shed answered, and the morning litany of cock-crowing was joined by the first snarling fight of dogs competing for a shred of tapir intestine outside the village. In the men's house many of the men were stirring, though a few were still lying in their hammocks, their feet dangling over the small fires they had built beneath. Most of them planned to hunt that day, and they were already testing bow strings and sighting down arrow shafts for straightness. Others squatted by a fire to discuss where to hunt, passing from one to another the single cigarette one of them had rolled.

Borai's husband, Kaba, broke away from the group of men and came to the house. He sat on a log that served as a seat, and Borai brought him a half gourd of farinha, flour made from bitter manioc, mixed with water. He tilted the container back, pushing the farinha toward his mouth with a hunting knife, and passed it back to her when he had finished. Borai had warmed up, over the fire, two monkey legs left from the previous night's dinner, and she passed one of the legs over to him with a small gourd of salt. He dipped the scrawny and heat-shriveled meat in the salt between each bite, washed it down with water, and went back to join the gathering hunting party. Few words had been exchanged. The baby had a slight cold; Kaba asked how he had spent the night, and he played with the child for a short time before leaving.

Borai's older son by a previous marriage, a boy of twelve, arrived from the men's house for food and water, but left quickly to join the other boys, who were planning a day of stalking fish with bow and arrow in a nearby stream. The boys would roast the small fish near the stream and eat palm fruits, so she did not expect to see him again until the men began to return from the hunt, bringing the boys out of the forest to examine the day's kill. The baby having begun to cry, she picked him out of the hammock and gave him the breast again, then passed the child to her sister's ten-year-old daughter, who put the now squalling baby in a carrying sling passed around her shoulder, forming a seat for the baby on her narrow hip. Freed of her burden, Borai gnawed on monkey bones, took some farinha and water, and then went off some 200 feet from the village to relieve herself. Three thin and mangy dogs, not suited for hunting and thus reduced to scavenging garbage and human waste, followed her, sat patiently on their haunches, and waited.

The sun had cleared the hills and the house was in full motion when Borai returned. Children were laughing, crying, and shouting, emerging from their houses to wander through the village and explore the other four dwellings. Wherever the little ones went, they were offered a bit of food and fondled, for in this village of ninety people, every child was well known to each adult, and most of them were related in ways that people could not quite specify, however much they categorized their kinship ties. The men by this time had left the village, winding single file down the path that led from the grass-covered hill into the still mist-shrouded forests bordering the stream below. The column of hunters passed out of sight, but the women and children could still hear the barks of the hunting dogs and the deep sounds of the horns of the hunters signaling to each other, ever more faintly until only the low murmur of village life broke the calm that had settled on the community.

As the sun rose, it evaporated the mists, driving away the cool of the dawn and touching the village with a promise of the oppressive heat of midday. It was May, and though the worst of the rains had passed from the uplifted drainage south of the Amazon River, the air remained humid, and afternoon thunderstorms were still frequent. But the streams had receded to the confines of their banks, their waters had cleared, and the small rivulets of the high savannahs flowed cool through the tunnels of forest they watered. The women of Borai's house—her mother, two sisters, the wife of one of her brothers, and a maternal cousin of her mother—gathered up their gourd water containers and, bidding the children to follow, went down to the stream below. As the procession wound through the village and past the back doors of other houses, more women joined them, calling out to each other, while the little children ran down the grassy hill, playing as they went; the boys were empty-handed, but their small sisters carried their own little gourds. As they neared the stream, the older boys finished their morning swim and began to work their way downstream to one of the better fishing holes.

The smallest children, who were naked, ran into the water with shrieks of glee, while their older sisters shucked off their thin dresses and followed them. The older women eased into the stream, taking off their clothes as the water rose higher on their bodies. The water was stinging cold at first, but they soon became accustomed to it, ducking under the surface and splashing each other happily. The women rubbed their bodies with the water and scrubbed the backsides of the smallest children to clean them. They splashed about for another half hour and then slipped on their cotton Mother Hubbard dresses and sat in the sun to warm and dry.

Their ablutions done, the women filled the water gourds, and most started back up the hill to the village. A few stayed behind to wash clothes, dipping them in the water, rubbing their folds against each other, and smacking the wet clothing against flat rocks. Last week, the village had run out of the soap they had gotten from the trader, but most of the dirt was washed out without it. Borai had only two dresses, the one she was wearing and the one being washed; Kaba had promised her another after he had sold some rubber to the trader during the coming months of the dry season.

The washing done, the remainder of the women returned to the village together. Both propriety and fear of lone and wandering males kept any from remaining behind, forcing them to stay in small groups on almost any venture beyond the immediate vicinity of the village. Back at the house, Borai hung her tattered wash on a small cotton bush near the back door and began to clean up garbage, which she simply threw in the underbrush, from the cleared area around the house. She started to sweep out the house with a broom improvised from a few branches, but the baby began to cry in earnest, and she took him from her niece. This time, however, instead of offering the breast to the child, she mashed up a piece of banana with a chunk of boiled sweet manioc and spooned it into his mouth. She then put the baby in its carrying sling and swept the floor in a rather desultory way with one hand, while stroking the baby with the other. One of her sisters joined in the housecleaning, and they swept the remains out the door, where a tame parrot and two hens immediately began to pick through the trash for pieces of grain and fruit. The women watched in amusement as the hens tried unsuccessfully to drive off the parrot, who reared back in outrage and squawked at the menacing fowl. The sisters then sat in their hammocks and talked to their mother about the day's work ahead; housekeeping in the large, uncompartmented, and dirt-floored dwellings was the least of their chores.

The sun had risen full into the morning sky, but the peak of the day's heat was still four hours away, making most of the women anxious to get their garden work done. The supply of manioc flour in the house had already been eaten, and for the last two days the women of Borai's house had been drawing on the larders of their neighbors. Borai's mother went to the open-walled shed in the middle of the village where manioc flour was made, and began to build a fire in the large earth-walled oven on which the farinha was toasted. She directed her three daughters to fetch tubers from the stream, where they had been soaking in water for the past three days, and sent her daughter-in-law for more firewood. The daughter-in-law put an axe in her carrying basket, which she carried on her back with a bark-cloth tump-line hung across her forehead, and went through the village to ask her cousin to come help her. Borai and her sister stopped at another house to tell the women where they were going and enlisted the support of two of the occupants. The four then set out for the stream on a path which took them well below the area where they bathed and drew water, and they began to load their baskets with the softened, almost crumbling, manoic tubers. The children had been left with their grandmother, allowing the women to take another, more leisurely, bath and to discuss some of the shortcomings of their sister-in-law.

The carrying baskets were heavy with the water-laden manioc, and they squatted in a genuflecting position with their backs to the baskets, passed the tumplines across their foreheads, and slowly stood up, using the full strength of their torsos and necks to lift the burdens. The sun was beating down on the path as they made their way laboriously back up the hill to the village, walking in silence to conserve their strength. Arriving at the farinha shed, they gratefully dropped their loads into a long hollowed-out log used as a tub and sat down in the shade to rest. Borai's baby began crying as soon as he saw her, quickly escaping from his older cousin to crawl through the dirt to his mother. She nursed him, more for comfort than food, and then let him crawl back and forth across her lap. The sister-in-law and her helper returned from the garden, where they had gathered felled, but unburned, wood and chopped it into stove lengths, and dumped the contents of their baskets next to the farinha oven. They too sat in the shade against one of the shed uprights and joined the conversation. Three other women drifted across the weed-choked village plaza to help, and to tell of their own plans to make farinha in two days' time.

The work party having increased to eight, the women decided that the dull and laborious chore could be put off no longer. Borai and her mother stepped into the trough filled with soft manioc and began to walk back and forth, working their feet up and down, to break up the tubers and separate the pulp from the skins. As they worked, the water oozed out of the broken tubers, mixed with the pulp into a thick mass, and squished rather pleasurably between their toes. Another woman began picking out the skins and throwing them to one side. The sister-in-law and her cousin went off to the old garden for more firewood, and three of the other women went down to the stream to get more manioc. One woman remained seated in the shade, helping Borai's niece in keeping the children from underfoot.

Despite the tedium of the work, the conversation in the farinha shed never slowed. Borai's mother brought up the possibility that the trader might pay a visit to the village in the near future, a story she had heard from the wife of a young man who had been visiting on the Tapajós River. One woman added that is seemed to make little difference whether he arrived or not, as he rarely brought very much desirable merchandise. Another commented that on his last visit the trader had brought nothing but *cachaça,* the regional cane rum, and that the men had exhausted all their credit in becoming thoroughly drunk. Borai's mother reminded the critic that she, too, had drunk her fair share of the trader's rum on that occasion, and the onlookers dissolved in laughter. Given the fact that many of the women had drunk as much as the men would let them have, the subject was quickly turned to the men. One of the chief topics of conversation at the time was the visit in the village of a young man, who was in a late stage of courtship of one of the village's girls. The progress of the romance was carefully examined by the group in the farinha shed, and the young man's merits mercilessly evaluated. One of the women noted that the suitor had a small penis, bringing forth the sour remark that he was not much different from the other men. At least, said another, his penis showed more life than those of most of the other men. The women laughed and all looked over with amusement toward the men's house, where two or three occupants still lingered. The men, aware of the derision, became furiously intent on whatever they were doing, their eyes turned carefully away from the farinha shed.

In the meantime, the work was progressing at a slow and steady pace. Large wads of wet pulp were taken from the trough and placed in the open end of a *tipití*. The tipití was a long tube made of loosely woven palm leaves, with an open mouth at the top and closed at the bottom. The top end was suspended from a rafter, and a long pole was placed through a loop at the bottom. Two of the women sat on the end of the pole, the other end of which was secured near the ground, and the resultant lever pulled powerfully downward on the tipití. This caused it to elongate and constrict, squeezing out the water from the pulp and leaving the contents still moist, ready to be sieved. When only a dribble of water came from the tipití, the women emptied the pulp into a large sieve placed over a shallow basin and gently worked it through the mesh with their fingers. It dropped into the receptacle as a coarse, damp cereal, and the pieces that did not go through were taken by another of the women and pounded with a wooden mortar and pestle.

The day's production of farinha would not last the household much more than a week, and the women agreed that they should put more tubers in the water to soak. Borai and three of the other women took their carrying baskets and machetes and headed out of the village to the gardens. They followed a path from the village plaza that passed in back of one of the houses. The path narrowed through the dense underbrush surrounding the village and emerged suddenly into the open savannah. The land ahead rolled gently. The sandy soil was covered with clumps of short grass and small flowering shrubs, and here and there were small islands of trees, some of which marked the sites of old and abandoned villages. These were easily identified by the scattered fruit palms in their midsts, the end products of palm pits thrown away decades ago. As the women walked single file along the narrow path worn through the grasses, they commented on almost everything they saw—a pair of doves cooing in a distant grove, a parrot flying from one tree clump to another, the activity around a termite hill, a curious cloud formation.

The trail entered suddenly into the forest and dropped to a small stream that bubbled among rocks. A log served as a bridge across the water, but the women stopped to bathe before going on to the garden. The path wound for a while among very tall trees, whose leafy branches almost 100 feet above kept out the sunlight and left the forest floor clear of underbrush. As the trail rose, it became lighter and the underbrush became thicker, for they were entering a tract that had been farmed many years ago and was still under the cover of lower, secondary forest. Shadow gave way to brightness, dark greens to light hues, and coolness to heat as the women broke out of the forest and into the garden.

The garden was no more than two acres in extent, and along with two other producing gardens provided the main source of vegetable food for the household. This garden had been cleared two years earlier and was yielding only manioc on its second planting. One of the women, however, spotted a pineapple growing among the weeds and picked it for her children to eat. The garden was rank with weeds and, since no further planting would be done in it, nobody bothered any longer to keep it cleared. To the women, it looked like any other garden, though an outsider would see nothing more than stumps, felled and charred tree trunks lying at various angles, and a clutter of undergrowth. Most of the higher vegetation, however, was bitter manioc, the tall stalks of which had grown to six feet and over.

The women set to their harvest work, taking the machetes from their baskets and cutting the manioc stalks near their bases. They put the stalks aside, and then proceeded to dig out the tubers clustered at the base of each stalk, like fingers from a hand, with the machetes. Each plant yielded two to five tubers, ranging in size from six inches to over a foot in length; if the manioc had been left in the ground to grow for a few months longer, some would reach a length of two feet or so. After knocking the dirt from the manioc, the tubers were put in the baskets. Before going back, the women made a brief reconnoiter of the garden in search of more pineapples or an unharvested squash. Unsuccessful, they took up their burdens and, with another stopover for a drink of water, went directly to the stream near the village where they put the manioc in a quiet pool to soak.

By the time this chore was done, the sun was almost directly overhead, and the morning breezes had died completely. The village lay beaten down by the sun, quiet and somnolent under the noonday heat. The roosters and chickens were not to be seen, and the few dogs remaining in the village were lying in the shade. One of the men in the men's house was still working on a basket, but the other two had retired to their hammocks in its shady recesses. Borai and her companions went to the farinha shed, where she found her baby crying lustily from hunger. She sat in the shade to nurse him, while watching her mother and another woman slowly turning and stirring the manioc flour, which was being toasted on a copper griddle above the furnace. The women each had a canoe paddle which they used as a spatula to prevent the manioc from burning on the pan and to turn under the flour on top to expose it again to the heat. It would take well over an hour for each panful to become dry and toasted brown, and other women took up the task at intervals of about fifteen minutes to relieve the heat-parched workers.

As the work dragged on, most of its preliminary phases, such as bringing in the manioc, mashing it, running the pulp through the tipití, and sieving the resulting mash, were already largely completed, and many of the helpers from the other houses had drifted away to escape the heat of the oven. Borai was hungry after her morning's work and she went to the dwelling, where she put the baby in her hammock. One of her sisters had cooked some plantains in the coals of the fire and offered her some, and Borai rounded out the meal with manioc mixed with a drink made of palm fruit. She then lay down in the hammock to rest with her child and almost immediately fell into a light sleep.

Borai drowsed in the heavy heat of the afternoon and finally awakened after the baby's fitfulness had turned into crying. She fed him and then went out to the farinha shed, where she gave the baby to one of the young girls and took a turn at toasting the manioc flour. The rest of the farinha-making process was now completed, but two five-gallon cans filled with damp sieved pulp remained to be put on the griddle, and it would be almost dark before they were finally done. Though only one or two women at a time were required for the work, others drifted out from the houses to join in the conversation. The sun was already halfway between its zenith and the horizon, and dark cumulus clouds were beginning to build up in the west. The breezes freshened as the storm approached, dispelling the heat and lifting everybody from their afternoon torpor. One of the women suggested that it was time to get water for the evening meal, and the group scattered to their houses to gather up gourds and children. Some twenty of them trooped down to the stream to bathe off the day's sweat and to immerse themselves in the cold stream, lolling in it until their teeth chattered and they had to seek the warmth of a sun-bathed rock.

From the distance, still deep back in the forest, the faint sound of a horn was heard, followed a short time later by another, somewhat closer. The women quickly filled the water containers and shooed the children ahead of them as they hurried to get back to the village before the hunting party. The storm, too, was approaching, and the silence of the forest and savannahs was broken by still remote rumbles of thunder. Borai went to her house and placed more wood on the fire, put the baby in the hammock, and waited for the return of her husband.

The hunters split up just outside the village and took the separate paths that led to the back entrances of their houses. Borai was waiting there when Kaba walked through the door carrying a wild pig, weighing about 100 pounds, across his shoulders. He dropped the pig to the floor, put his bow and arrow on a platform under the rafters, and sat to wait for Borai to bring him a half gourd of water and manioc. She commented on the fatness of the wild pig, asking her husband where he had taken it. "We cornered the herd at a crossing of the River of the Wild Turkey, not far from the Cabruá River and at a place where there are still ripe *buriti* palm fruit," he replied. "The arrow of my brother Warú hit this one in the flank, and I brought him down with another over the heart." He went on to tell Borai that four pigs had been killed before the herd broke and ran, and individual hunters had also taken two monkeys, an agouti, and a paca. One of the dogs had been gashed by a boar, but the wound would probably heal. It had been a good hunt.

Kaba saw two men leave the men's house for the stream and hurried after them to take a bath before the storm hit. The other women of Borai's house joined with her in butchering the wild pig. They took long knives, finely honed on smooth rocks, and drew incisions down the stomach and along the legs. Two of them then carefully pulled back the hide, cutting the gristle at points where it stuck the flesh. The skin was stretched out with sticks and hung up outside to dry and cure for later sale to the trader. The pig was then sliced through the ventral section to the viscera, the intestines removed and thrown outside to the ravenously hungry dogs. They fell on it ferociously, snarling and fighting while they gulped down whole chunks of the offal. The rest of the pig was quartered, the head and neck put aside as a fifth portion. Pieces of meat were then taken by the women to all the houses in the village, and by the time the usual reciprocity had been observed, almost a whole wild pig was ready for cooking in each dwelling.

The fire was now burning strongly, and Borai half filled a bell-bottomed ceramic pot with water and placed it in the center of the hearth, the flames licking up its sides. As the water heated, she cut a hind quarter of pig into chunks, which she placed in the pot for the evening meal. When the water came toward a boil, she threw in several pinches of salt. Her mother and one of the young girls, in the meanwhile, were cracking Brazil nuts and grating their meats, throwing the fragrant and milky pulp into the pot. The women then sat by the fire, stirring the pot, savoring the smells, and talking happily about the excellence of the meat. The men had by this time returned from their baths and were resting in their hammocks in the men's house, recalling events in the day's hunt, and laughing at some of their misadventures.

The sky had now turned completely dark, though there was still an hour and a half before the sun would set, and a cool breeze blew in advance of the storm. Suddenly the storm struck, with brilliant flashes of lightning and sharp claps of thunder which reverberated off the hills across the valley. The rain fell in sheets, the wind driving it into the open sides of the men's house, forcing some of the occupants to move further into the back and others to run for the walled dwelling houses. The roofs all leaked in places, but the residents had already arranged their hammocks and belongings in dry locations, and nobody paid much attention to the puddles forming on the floor. Borai's mother, nonetheless, took the occasion to ask her sons-in-law when they were going to build a new village. "The roofs are old and leak, the house poles creak in the wind, and one of the children was almost bitten by a scorpion in the underbrush," she said. "Do we have to wait until our gardens are a half-day's walk away before you men decide to move?" Kaba stared intently at his toes and muttered that they were talking about building another village during the next rainy season. There was no time now, for soon after the next full moon most of the people would be leaving to collect rubber on the larger rivers. Enjoying his discomfiture, the old woman reminded him that this is what the men had said last year and then went back to stirring the pot.

The front of the storm had passed, the wind died down, and the rain became lighter. Several of the men wandered back from the dwellings of the women to the men's house and climbed into their hammocks under the shelter of the overhanging roof. Many of the little boys trailed after them to play among the hammocks, and one three-year-old girl toddled along, too; her father took her into his hammock and played with her while talking to the other men. Everybody was in good spirits. There was enough food in the village for at least two days, the rain had made the day's end cool, and the smells of cooking wild pig occasionally wafted over from the houses. The men chatted with each other from their hammocks, and, in one, three teenage boys were rolling about in obvious sex play, unnoted by the adults.

In the houses, the boiled meat was now cooked, and Borai took a large gourd, filled it with meat and broth, while one of her sisters filled another with freshly made farinha. They brought them across the plaza to the cleared area in front of the men's house, where Kaba took them and called to the other men. Other women were bringing food to their husbands, too, and the men, with most of the boys squatting around them, sat on their haunches in a ring about the bowls. The men took spoons and scooped up meat and broth from the common bowls, occasionally dipping their hands into the farinha bowls and throwing the manioc flour into their mouths with quick tosses. The hunters were hungry after a long day with little more than farinha and water and ate steadily, but quietly and soberly; boisterous and noisy behavior while eating would offend the spirit protectors of the game animals. Other spirits had to be appeased, too, and one of the men took a gourd of meat into the closed chamber adjoining the men's house, where he offered the meat to the ancestral spirits, saying, "Eat grandfathers, and make me lucky in the hunt." The offering made, he brought the bowl of meat back out and placed it with the others.

After the meal had been cooked, the women of Borai's house placed a babricot over the fire. This consisted of a tripod with a horizontal rack of green wood strips running across it a foot from the base. The remaining meat was placed on the babricot, where it would slowly roast and smoke until bedtime. The meat would then be removed, but it would be placed over a low fire again in the morning to complete the cooking process and prevent rotting. One of the women stayed by the fire to turn the meat occasionally and to hit any dogs that approached it. The other women, and the girls and little boys, sat around the pot of boiled meat, filling little half gourds with the stew and eating. The meat was tender, and the sauce of broth and Brazil nut milk delicious. There had been little meat in the village for the past few days, and they all gorged themselves. They also knew that by the third day, the remaining meat would be tough and barely chewable.

Dusk is very brief in the tropics, and the sunset glowed brilliantly against the broken clouds in the clearing western sky. The colors shifted, modulated, changed, and were suddenly gone. Night rapidly enfolded the village, and the people who were watching the setting sun remained a moment in silence and reentered their dwellings. In each house, the women lit small kerosene lamps which cast a flickering glow over the interiors, supplementing the flames of the fires. Borai sat in her hammock, talking with her mother about plans for the next day's work, while her baby sat in the sling on her hip and nursed, more for solace than for food. A few of the children of the house were playing with a puppy, pulling its tail, twisting its legs, and preventing it from running away from them.

Borai and her mother went back to the farinha shed in the middle of the village to finish toasting the manioc flour. They stoked the fire back to life and after letting the oven warm up, poured in the remaining pulp. The glow from the open front of the oven cast a dim and flickering light over their work as they slowly turned and stirred the flour. Other women wandered from their houses to join the group, though the women of the chief's house, who were miffed because they felt they were being gossiped against, stayed home. Finally, unable to bear the thought that the farinha-shed group really was talking about them, two of the chief's daughters joined them. Everybody took a turn at stirring the farinha, but interest centered on a plan to gather *assaí* palm fruits the next morning at a grove a few miles away. The fruit drink, and the abundance of roast meat, would make the day a festive one, and they would hold a dance in the evening.

Across the village plaza, a small fire was burning in front of the men's house. A poorly played guitar was trying to pick out the strain of a Brazilian song heard at a trader's post, and another man was softly playing one of their own songs on a traditional flute. The conversation of the men drifted across as a low murmur, broken occasionally by a raucous cry from one of the boys. After a while, the music stopped, but the silence was soon broken by a deep vibrant note from one of the karökö, the long tubular musical instruments which contained the ancestral spirits and which the women were forbidden even to see. The first notes were joined by the second and then the third karökö, playing in counterpoint to each other, slowly, repetitively, and in measured cadence. The men fell silent for a moment, then the conversation picked up again, the guitarist tried futilely to catch the elusive melody, and one of the boys dumped another from his hammock. But the mournful notes of the karökö dominated the village, shut out the night noises, accentuated the calm.

"There they go again," said Borai, as the first sounds of the karökö reached the farinha shed. The women listened for a moment, trying to identify the players by style and skill, laughing at an off-note played by one of the younger men. They then turned back to their conversation and the work of farinha toasting. Many of the little ones were becoming cranky from tiredness, and their mothers caressed them, or nursed the infants. One five-year-old climbed onto his mother's lap to nurse, but giggles from the older girls made him give up after a few minutes. The farinha was finally finished, scooped out of the pan with the paddles into loosely woven baskets lined with palm leaves, and placed on a storage rack in the house. A large bowl of the freshly made flour was kept in the shed, and the women occasionally dipped their fingers into it, enjoying the tanginess of the still hot grains. Some of the women brought their children back to their hammocks and remained in the houses; the rest of the group lingered a while and then went home, two by two, leaving the farinha shed to a few dogs huddled near the warmth of the oven.

The men's house had grown quiet as people drifted off to sleep, and finally the last sounds of the karökö faded. The players emerged from the enclosed sacred chamber, climbed into their hammocks, talked a while, and then fell asleep. One of the men drowsily told the boys to be quiet, and they, too, rolled up inside their hammocks, still whispering to each other. The dying fire cast in flickering outline the arching, open-ended roof of the men's house and the two rows of hammocks.

Borai took the meat off the babricot, placing it in a covered basket, which she put on a storage rack. She threw a bit of dirt on the fire to bank it for the night, removed the babricot, and then slid gently into her hammock so as not to waken the already sleeping baby. Two of the other women went outside to urinate, but they stayed near the house, as the underbrush in the night was a hiding place of the *Yurupari* and other evil spirits. They reentered, blew out the kerosene lamp, and the house fell into silence.

The hills in the east began to emerge from the total blackness as a three-quarter moon rose, bathing the countryside and the village in pale light. The circle of houses around the village plaza could now be clearly seen; yet nothing moved, and the only sounds were an occasional cough or a baby's whimper. Traces of smoke from the smoldering fires were picked up by the moonlight, and the inside of the farinha shed was tinged with orange by the glowing embers of the dying fire. The village was silent, but the forests were not. From far off in the distance, a band of howler monkeys made an ululating uproar, and the noise of tree frogs near the stream was a steady backdrop of tone, broken by the cries of night birds and the chirping of crickets in the brush around the village. Borai listened for a very short while before tiredness overtook her; her last thought before drifting into full sleep was a hope that her husband would not decide to pay a night visit. A woman's day had ended.

HARUKO'S WORK

Gail Lee Bernstein

"I lead a relatively relaxed life," Haruko told me, kneeling on the floor, folding the laundry, a few days after my arrival in Bessho. "I have a circle of four or five close friends who are, like myself, only housewives. Most other women in this area work outside in factories or stores. I prefer not to work, because I don't need the money that much and would rather have free time. Working women are so busy they don't have time to help their husbands." I gradually discovered that in reality she had very little free time; in fact she had stayed home from work only to help me get settled.

During the first weeks of my stay, the pace of Haruko's daily routine quickened noticeably. It soon became evident that she was more than just "a housewife." Although machinery had freed both women and men from most of the arduous work of rice cultivation, many other farming chores remained, and they usually fell to the women. In addition, once the harvest season was over, Haruko, like most other women in Bessho, sought part-time wage-paying work nearby.

Reprinted from *Haruko's World: A Japanese Farm Woman and Her Community* by Gail Lee Bernstein with the permission of the publishers, Stanford University Press. © 1983 by the Board of Trustees of the Leland Stanford Junior University.

Watching her daily activities over several months, I concluded that Haruko was the busiest member of her family.

Yet it was not always easy to ascertain exactly what work Haruko and other farm women performed. For one thing, farm women did not consider their round of household chores to be work, and they viewed vegetable farming as merely an extension of their domestic sphere of activity—a part of cooking. Nor did they define rice cultivation as work. Even though they had labored side by side with men in the paddies, transplanting rice seedlings in late spring or early summer, weeding together with other women during the remainder of the summer, and again working with their menfolk during the harvest in early fall, farm women referred to such labor as "helping my husband." Only wage labor constituted work. Thus to rely on simple questions like, "What work do you do?" was to invite deceptive answers, because even women who farmed almost entirely on their own but were not employed "outside" for pay, might reply, "I do not work; I stay at home."

In addition, women's work included numerous separate, discrete tasks that varied according to the season of the year and the time of day, and that were performed in countless different places inside and outside the house, the shed, and other farm buildings and on various plots of land scattered throughout the hamlet. Every day I had to ask Haruko where she would be working, and even after she told me, "I'll be hoeing in the vegetable field," I often could not find her, because the family farmed several vegetable fields in different places. By the time I did locate her, she might be finished with the hoeing and on to another task, such as separating out the weeds from the edible grasses she had picked the day before.

Equally difficult to study was the diversity of part-time, wage-paying jobs women performed. Their jobs in factories, shops, and offices or as orderlies in hospitals and as day laborers on other farmers' land took them out of the hamlet during the day. To observe such work required trailing after each hamlet woman and gaining entry into half a dozen different work sites. Also, the work was often temporary: small factories hiring only a few women might close down for several months during an economic slump, and women working as agricultural hired hands might be laid off after the harvest was over.

By tagging after Haruko for several months, I was eventually able to compile a list—by no means complete—of her work responsibilities. They fell broadly into three categories: homemaking, farming, and wage earning.

As a homemaker, Haruko had more extensive responsibilities than ever before: not only was she in charge of such traditional domestic work as cooking, cleaning, sewing, and participating in communal functions, but in recent years she had assumed the newer tasks of shopping, paying the bills, and guiding her children's education. Except in matters relating to the children, Shō-ichi, like most Japanese men, removed himself altogether from these domestic concerns.

Haruko's daily round of household chores began at six o'clock, when recorded Westminster chimes, broadcast from the loudspeaker installed on the roof of the hamlet social hall, awakened the farmers of Bessho and set her scurrying around the house. Every morning she prepared a breakfast of *misoshiru* (bean-paste soup enriched with white cubes of bean curd, an egg, and a few garden greens), boiled rice, and green tea. The children, who needed to be coaxed awake, ate toasted white bread. Before sitting down to breakfast at seven o'clock, Haruko placed six cups of green tea as offerings on the Buddhist altar in the bedroom. Whenever she made special food, such as rice balls, she also offered some to *hotoke-sama,* the spirits of the ancestors of Shō-ichi's family.

After sending the children off to school at eight o'clock in a flurry of last-minute searches for clothing and books and hastily delivered instructions, Haruko ran a load of wash in the washing machine and hung it out to dry. She also aired the heavy mattresses and quilts to prevent mildew, a perennial problem in Japan's humid climate. These two tasks were part of her morning routine on every clear day, but regardless of the weather, at five o'clock every single evening, just before starting dinner, she filled the deep bath tub with hot water for the family's bath. Going without the daily bath was unthinkable; and if Haruko was detained, Obāsan or Yōko did this chore in her place. Her routine did not include housecleaning, however. There were neither windows to wash nor furniture to dust, and since shoes were removed at the door, the tatami-covered floor remained clean and required only sweeping. Such cleaning as was necessary was relegated to rainy days, when farmers do not work in the fields.

Lunch was a simply prepared meal of rice, processed or raw fish, and leftovers. For dinner, taken punctually at six o'clock, Haruko again made boiled rice, this time served with numerous side dishes, each on its own little plate, such as raw tuna or mackerel, boiled octopus, sliced vinegared cucumbers, noodles, seaweed, or spinach sprinkled with sesame seeds, and green tea. Thanks to Shō-ichi's pig business the family enjoyed more meat than other farm families, and occasionally they also ate small cubes of fried chicken bought at the Agricultural Cooperative supermarket in Unomachi.

As the woman of the house, Haruko also had several traditional community obligations that were impossible to shirk. Custom demands that all the women in a *kumi* (a grouping of several neighboring households) help prepare food for receptions following the funerals or weddings of member families. Furthermore, each household sends one woman to attend regular meetings of the Women's Guild of the Agricultural Cooperative Association. Haruko and other Bessho farm wives took turns serving in administrative capacities within the guild. They also participated in the cooking classes sponsored by the guild, as well as in meetings of the Parent-Teacher Association.

In addition to being a homemaker, Haruko was the family's chief farm worker. She grew the fruits and vegetables consumed by the household almost entirely on her own: carrots, peppers, Chinese cabbage, spinach, strawberries, broccoli, corn, onions, and a small scallion called *nira*. In the summertime, after the rice crop was planted, she prepared year-long supplies of staple food items such as pickled vegetables and bean paste for *misoshiru,* and she further supplemented the family diet with wild grasses picked in the hills surrounding the rice plain or along the road. Once, when Haruko was not feeling well, Shō-ichi offered to plant the onions, but she had to tell him what to do.

Since the money for modernizing agriculture had been diverted primarily to the rice paddies, vegetables were still grown in tiny, scattered fields. Haruko's garden was actually four different plots of land: a vegetable patch in front of the house, another one across the road from the house, a cabbage patch down the road toward town, and a potato field about a half mile away in the opposite direction. While the men were learning to use the new rice-transplanting machines and the combines, Haruko worked with an old iron grubbing fork and a scythe. To enrich the soil, she relied on organic materials: chicken manure for fertilizer, and chicken feathers and rice husks for mulch. To irrigate a nearby vegetable field, she drew water from a spigot in front of the goldfish pond and carried it in a watering can.

Haruko did not always farm alone. For one week in autumn, for example, she worked with Obāsan and Shō-ichi harvesting potatoes, which were grown on a quarter-acre plot and fed to the pigs. (Farmers who ate mainly potatoes during the war do not care for them now, though their children have developed a taste for them.) The three worked silently in the fields from ten o'clock in the morning until five at night, stopping only for one hour at noon, when a siren announced the lunch break, and again at three o'clock, when they took a snack of green tea, tangerines, and a sweet cake. The women's work consisted of cutting the potato vines with a scythe, arranging them in piles, and tying them together. Then they put the potatoes in sacks for Shō-ichi to load onto his truck. Shō-ichi also operated a small, motor-driven plow that turned over the soil after the potatoes were harvested. Neighbors carted away the vines and fed them to their cows.

Haruko also worked with her mother-in-law and husband on a neighborhood team husking rice. The group, which included Obā-san's sister and the sister's husband, son, and daughter-in-law, together with two neighbors, had collectively purchased a wooden husking machine in the early 1960's. It was run by a generator. Before purchasing the husker, they had paid a husking company to do the job for them, and before that, when Obāsan came to Bessho as a bride, a hand-operated device had been used to turn the rice around for hours at a time. The fall of 1974 was the last time the husking group would work together; beginning with the next harvest, all the rice would be husked mechanically in a large machine operated by the Agricultural Cooperative.

Members of the husking group took turns husking rice at each other's houses, and the host family was expected to provide refreshments. On the morning when it was their turn to use the machine, Obāsan and Haruko were up early getting the house in order and preparing the food. While Obāsan raked a gravel area in front of the house, where the gangling wooden contraption would be set up, Haruko turned on the rice steamer, made a swipe at the cobweb strung from the overhead lampshade in the living room to the side wall, climbed the persimmon tree for some fruit, leaped on her scooter for a quick errand to town, and, upon returning, set out the straw baskets used to carry the family's rice kernels from the storage shed to the husker. Shō-ichi telephoned to town for an order of beer.

Once the work team assembled (all but one worker arrived at exactly eight o'clock), the women and the men worked separately on each side of the husker. There was no need to delineate chores or to explain how the work would be done: everyone knew exactly what to do. The women filled the straw baskets with rice, hauled them to the machine, and poured in the rice, while the men weighed the husked rice as it flowed out of the machine, recorded the amount, and sacked and hauled the rice back to the storage shed.

Two hours later, the work was done and a mid-morning feast was served. Mats were spread out between the machine and the side of the road. The workers gathered in a circle, the women on one side, kneeling, and the men on the other, sitting cross-legged. An abundance of food was pressed on the guests, who ritually refused once or twice before accepting rice cakes, raw fish, assorted vegetables, hardboiled eggs, fruit, tea, beer, and *sake.* Haruko peeled persimmons, cut them into four slices each, and handed them around. Sitting on dust and gravel by the side of the road, after two hours of labor, it was nevertheless possible at that moment to feel like royalty being wined and dined, filling one's belly, laughing and joking, indulged by the host and hostess, whose turn to be served would come the following day, when the wooden husker would be wheeled down the road to work at another house.

One of Haruko's principal farm chores was feeding the pigs, which were housed in a wooden structure several hundred yards behind the house. More than half of the Utsunomiyas' annual income came from the pig business. Twice a day, once in the morning and once at night, the couple fed the ninety pigs and cleaned the pigsty. There were about twelve pens, with seven or eight pigs in each. Haruko poured feed into the trough and mixed water in with it, while her husband cleaned the pens one by one, shoveling out the dung. They worked quickly and in silence. The stench and the flies seemed not to trouble either of them.

"Which of your tasks do you least like?" I asked Haruko one day, emerging from the pigsty to take a deep breath of fresh air. The air inside the sty was suffocating, and the pink, flesh-colored pigs, crowded into their stalls, were loudly squealing for food. Haruko was pouring feed from a tank into a wheelbarrow. Without looking up, she answered, "If you farm, you can't say you hate any work."

Shō-ichi operated a larger pig business in the mountains about twenty minutes' drive from the house. He and five other men raised one thousand pigs and took turns staying overnight to feed the animals, clean the pens, and tend to any emergencies.

Occasionally Haruko went along to help Shō-ichi and the other men at the pig farm. Neither she nor her husband showed any sentimentality toward the animals. A mother pig, too exhausted after giving birth to move into the warmer quarters prepared for her and her piglets, and uncomfortable with a stillborn infant inside her, was first punched and then prodded with a hog catcher that was attached to her snout. Dead piglets from other litters lay in the aisle between the pens. Frightened pigs being weighed for market were kicked in the face, pulled by the ears or tails, or punched on their backs to make them heed. Haruko seemed unperturbed by the din of grunts and squeals, and while some of the men loaded pigs in a basket onto a truck, she calmly swept one of the sties. When the truck drove off, she put down her broom and stood on the pig scale to weigh herself.

An important part of pig farming was mating the pigs. As soon as the male was led into the female's pen, he became aroused, but he could not perform without assistance. Shōichi helped guide the penis, and if the pig failed to penetrate, he punched him as a reminder to try again. It took about ten to fifteen minutes to align a pair; copulation itself took only a few seconds. Meanwhile, Haruko stood ready to help, opening the gates to the pen or simply standing on the sidelines cheering and offering advice, like a third-base coach at the world series. "A little higher," she would yell, or "Oh, oh, too bad. OK now, off to the right a bit," alternately laughing at and sympathizing with the efforts of both pig and husband. She shared fully in her husband's work—it was equally her work—and the two performed their tasks like partners.

By early November, Haruko usually looked for part-time, wage-paying jobs. In previous years, she had worked in a small textile factory in Bessho. She had also commuted by bus to Akehama township to pick tangerines as a day laborer, earning four dollars a day (at a time when a tube of lipstick cost five dollars), but since she had returned home from that job too late to prepare the bath and fix dinner, she decided to look for work closer to home. Her options were limited, however.

The local economy offered various small jobs that called for manual dexterity, such as scraping barnacles off oyster shells, wrapping pastry in leaves, or planting tobacco seedlings with chopsticks. This work was often unappealing, however: it usually required either sitting or hunkering for hours at a time, and in such jobs as tobacco planting one was not paid until the crop was harvested and sold.

A few women from Bessho had found office or sales positions in Unomachi, but these positions required special training. When I asked Haruko whether she could get an office job in town, perhaps at the telephone company, where a younger hamlet woman worked, she replied tersely, "I don't have the qualifications." Besides, some of these jobs required a full-time commitment. The best-paying jobs for women, she added, were jobs as schoolteachers, clerks in government offices, shopkeepers, and factory workers. Her own opportunities were confined largely to manual labor.

When day laborers were needed during the reorganization of the rice paddies, Haruko was taken on as a *dokata,* or construction worker (literally, a "mud person"), and she worked on a team with two other women and three men. In most other wage-paying jobs women and men worked apart, at distinct kinds of work, but on the construction teams they worked side by side. The women were paid about $6.65 a day for eight hours' work, and the men were paid about $11.65.[1] They took one hour for lunch and two additional breaks of one-half hour each.

The female *dokata*'s work was physically demanding: women hauled heavy boulders, climbed down into trenches to lay irrigation pipes, constructed bridges over irrigation ditches, and shoveled snow from steep mountain slopes. Though they feminized their work outfits with aprons and bonnets, some were embarrassed when I asked them what work they did, and one female *dokata* replied indirectly, "I do the same work as Haruko."

The *dokata*'s work could be hazardous, too, especially for women unaccustomed to it. In early January, after two months on the construction crew, Haruko was hit on the side of the head by a falling rock. Although her employer had distributed helmets to all workers, Haruko did not like to wear hers. By a freak coincidence, her head was hit by another falling rock the very next day; she was wearing only her bonnet. This time she began to suffer fainting spells, dizziness, and headaches that prevented her from riding her motor scooter. X-rays did not reveal any bone damage, but the doctor decided that her "nerves" had been affected and prescribed one month's bed rest and a daily dose of eighteen tablets. She was also instructed not to take baths or wash her hair until she recovered. By the end of the month she was feeling better, though a brain scan now showed some abnormality and she had recurrent attacks of asthma. Daily injections at the hospital helped control the asthma; but whenever she tried to work in the fields, the headaches returned. National health insurance and her employee's insurance covered both the bulk of her medical expenses and her loss of income.

Haruko much preferred farming to construction work, she said. She was not thinking of hazards, however, or of physical demands; it was simply that she favored farming over any kind of wage labor. As a farmer, she could see the results of her endeavors. "The greatest pleasure of farming is the autumn harvest," she commented, and on more than one occasion she spoke of the "joy of producing one's own food," and of her "pride" in being the wife of a farmer. She also liked being able to work alongside her husband. Another advantage of farming was that "the farmer is master of himself; he can do whatever he chooses to do." In contrast, outside labor meant "you are used by others." When Haruko had worked in the Bessho knitting mill, she had always been watching the clock, "driven by time," because wages were determined by the worker's productivity—the number of finished goods she produced. Women stood hour after tedious hour in front of the machines, pushing a bobbin from right to left.

Not all farm women shared Haruko's views. Five women working in the Bessho mill, a one-room operation owned by a man in Yawatahama, said they enjoyed the piecework he sent them to do. "Paddy work is hard labor," said one woman. "This is easy." Another said, "We all live in Bessho. We are like relatives. It's pleasant here. Sometimes we sing songs." They worked their own hours, after the farm season was over. From late November they spent most of their time in the factory; in December, however, the factory abruptly closed down, a victim of market fluctuations caused by the oil scarcity in late 1974.

Women working in larger, more impersonal factories echoed some of Haruko's sentiments about factory work. In *Minori* (Harvest) magazine, published by the Women's Guild of Uwa township, one woman voiced her complaints: "When I first started working, I felt uneasy about leaving the housework and the children, but there was no other way to pick up ready cash. Under today's completely changed work conditions, nerve fatigue, more than physical labor, is what quickly gets to you. You have to learn your work. You have to think about dealing with people you are working with in the organization. You have a lot of different feelings when you go out working. And you think: Aren't you taking money but making plainer meals? Can you really manage the household? Are you really taking care of your children's and your husband's health if you come home tired? By working [outside the home] won't you make your family unhappy?"

Factory work in Higashiuwa county consisted primarily of making blue jeans (called g-pants) and canning and packing *mikan* (Japanese tangerines). Women working in blue-jeans factories could earn between $5.60 and $6.60 a day, depending on their experience and the number of jeans they completed. In one factory in Nomura township, women worked from eight in the morning until five at night, with one hour for lunch. Each woman received a flat wage for working on one part of the pants and a bonus depending on the group's productivity as a whole. In a *mikan*-packing plant operated by the Agricultural Cooperative in Unomachi, the women earned $5.10 for eight hours of work; in Yawatahama, about thirty minutes away by train, similar work paid between $7.14 and $8.50. Daily wages in the cooperative's plant were supplemented by a bonus, however, and by disability insurance like the *dokata's* wages, which meant that the workers' real income in effect compared respectably with that of other non-salaried workers in the county (see the accompanying table), and was actually greater than that of a *dokata*, who did not work on rainy days.

Whereas the canning plant's equipment for folding and stapling cartons and sending fruit speeding along the conveyor belts was both modern and efficient, conditions of work were neither: some women knelt on

TABLE 1. Sample Daily Wages Paid to Female Workers in Higashiuwa County in 1975 (U.S. dollar equivalent)[a]

Job	*Women's Wages*	*Men's Wages*
Dokata in Bessho	6.80 + disability insurance	11.90
Jeans factory in Nomura	5.60–6.60 + bonus	
Mikan-packing plant in Unomachi	5.10 + disability insurance + bonus	
Mikan-packing plant in Yawatahama	7.14–8.50	
Piecework at home	1.20	
Silkworm cultivation in Nomura	7.82	
Textile factory in Nomura	5.10–5.80	11.90
Tobacco planting in nursery beds in Bessho[b]	7.82	9.52
Construction work in cities		16.00–20.00 after room and board
Pruning trees in commonly held forest in Bessho	70% of men's wages	
Rice transplanting in Bessho	equal wages with men	
Public works projects in Bessho	equal wages with men if woman is single head of household	

Note: A blank entry indicates that the information in question was either unavailable or inapplicable.
[a]Computed from the 1975 rate of 294 yen = U.S. $1.00. Some wages had recently been raised by 300–500 yen.
[b]The women placed tobacco seedlings into containers; the men did the planning, organizing, and record keeping. The women were paid their wages only after the crop was sold.

cushions in a dimly lit, unheated building placing fruit into cartons, and others stood under a bare electric lightbulb separating out damaged fruit. Factory work was sought after because it paid a wage, but as a contributor to *Minori* wrote, the poor air, the indoor environment, the long work day, and the clatter of the machines could not compare with "farming under the endless blue sky, in clean air, doing the work as you want to do it."

It was difficult to determine what portion of the women's income went toward household expenditures. For one thing, farm women, especially farm women of Haruko's generation, who were unaccustomed to having large sums of money at their disposal, tended not to keep a budget or records of their daily household expenses. As more and more farmers took wage-paying jobs, however, some kind of record keeping was becoming necessary. Since the practice in the countryside, following urban customs, was for men to turn over all of their money to their wives to manage, the Women's Guild of the Cooperative had recently begun to distribute record ledgers to teach farm women how to maintain household budgets separate from the family's farm records. At a meeting of the Uwa branch of the Women's Guild, a guild leader lectured on the virtues of frugality and disciplined spending. "If you follow a budget," she said, "you will not buy merely what your neighbor buys. Also, if you don't go shopping every day, but only every three or five days, you won't buy so much." Similarly, during the cooking class sponsored by the guild, the instructor slipped in words of advice on budgeting. Women were told first to estimate their income for the coming year and then to apportion their spending as follows: thirty percent for farm equipment, fertilizer, and other farming needs; fifty percent for food, clothing, electricity, telephone, and other household expenses; ten percent for taxes; and the remaining ten percent for savings. If the women followed this advice, said the teacher, they would not overspend. "Budget yourselves," she urged. "Write it down."

Haruko asked the instructor to repeat the numbers and hastily scribbled them down, but then forgot what each referred to. "I'm no good at budgeting," she muttered.

The Utsunomiyas were an exception in the sense that Shō-ichi handled money matters: when the family needed money, Shō-ichi withdrew cash from his savings account at the Agricultural Cooperative. He kept most of the vital figures in his head. Writing on the back of a napkin, he estimated that the family's annual income was a little over $10,000—about the average for farmers in Japan. The income from rice was $4,500 and the income from the pig business, in a good year, was $5,600. Government statistics for 1971 showed that, like Shō-ichi, other farmers in the prefecture typically derived sixty to eighty percent of their incomes from nonfarm sources or supplementary farm occupations, such as animal husbandry.[2]

Shō-ichi's estimate did not include Haruko's earnings, which varied from year to year with the availability of part-time and seasonal work. I calculated that in a good year Haruko might earn as much as $700 to $800, which was in keeping with the average earnings of other farm women. A government survey conducted in 1973 showed that forty percent of all farm women took on outside work, and they earned between $330 and $660 annually.[3] My own survey in Higashiuwa county, distributed in the spring of 1975, set the average at about $700, and the head of the local Agricultural Cooperative estimated it to be close to $800.

Why were farm women taking outside jobs? Or, to put it another way, how were their additional earnings used? In the 1973 government survey, sixty percent of the farm women who reported taking on outside work said that they did so in order to pay for the "basic necessities" of life. In my survey of women in the country, fifty percent said they spent most of their earnings on such essentials as food, and another twenty percent said they spent them on clothing for family members and on their children's education. Haruko believed that Bessho women worked not so much to eat as to make extra cash: "Even the wife of the head of Uwa township works."

When I asked Haruko how she spent her own earnings, however, and whether it was really necessary for her to work, I received conflicting responses. "If I had my choice," Haruko said, "I would rather spend every day knitting sweaters for the children and straightening up the house." Yet although Shō-ichi said she did not have to take part-time jobs, she would not stay at home. She admitted that she liked having the extra spending money, even if earning it meant exhausting herself and, as she once remarked, not being able to complain, because Shō-ichi had not asked her to do it. It is also true that she worried about having to draw on their savings to pay for the machinery. On several occasions, she even implied that her wage-paying jobs were necessary to cover the cost of the new farm equipment, and Obāsan, sharing this view, commented privately about how sad it was that Haruko had to work.

When I pressed the matter further, I hit a sensitive nerve. Shō-ichi claimed that even without Haruko's earnings their income could cover the monthly payments of about eighty dollars for the machines. "Haruko is a worrier," he said. Haruko retorted that I could not be expected to understand the problem, and Shō-ichi countered, "There is no problem!" Later, however, he modified his position, saying that unless the price of rice increased, women's work would still be necessary to supplement farm income.

It is likely that Haruko worked for a variety of reasons. Her earnings, like those of other farm women, helped the family keep pace with inflation, contributed to mechanization efforts, and also satisfied new consumer desires. It was difficult for anyone to determine in exactly which of these areas expenditure was or was not "necessary." Shō-ichi and Haruko incurred many expenses that reflected the steady erosion of the Japanese farmer's traditional sense of self-sufficiency. Fertilizers, chemical sprays, and electricity and the telephone had become virtual necessities. Gasoline and animal feed, both imported, were among the family's greatest expenses, and these costs were tied to fluctuations in world politics and international trade, so that from one year to the next their incomes rose and fell with little predictability. Shō-ichi had a bad year in 1974, when the American corn crop was damaged and the Middle East oil embargo was imposed. The family's expenses thus varied from year to year, making outside sources of cash imperative.

In addition, the desire for ready-made western-style clothing and for packaged food also drove the Utsunomiyas and other farm families in the area to supplement their farm incomes, making them dependent on the wider economy. Farm women everywhere in Japan, exposed to urban goods and life-styles on television screens, expected more out of their life than their parents' generation did. Haruko was no exception, and her greatest pleasure was shopping for western-style clothing. Yōko wanted the fashionable blue jeans, whose popularity was sweeping the countryside and created jobs for women in blue-jeans factories. Hisashi asked for a record player. Both children preferred packaged white bread to boiled rice for breakfast, and they toasted the bread in a new red electric toaster. The children also expected to go beyond the free junior high school level of education to the high school level, for which tuition fees were charged. Haruko's wages, in other words, went toward attaining a middle-class life-style for her farm family.

Even Obāsan entered the paid labor market, working for a pittance in order to accumulate ready cash of her own. The piecework she did at home for a local factory paid her only one dollar a day for seven or eight hours of knitting pocketbooks. Still, the money enabled her to give cash as birthday gifts to her grandchildren.

In their search for wage-paying jobs, residents of Bessho commuted to Unomachi, if they were lucky enough to find employment there, or they traveled by train to Uwajima, Yawatahama, or even Matsuyama. Almost every women in Bessho, except those above the age of sixty and mothers of pre-school children, held some kind of part-time job. As a result of this daily exodus, Bessho by day was a ghost town, a bedroom community whose population of children, men, and women emptied into Unomachi early in the morning and headed for schools, jobs, or the railroad station, leaving behind only children under six years of age tended by their grandparents or even great-grandparents, and dogs, caged or tied up outside.

Unlike younger farm women in their late twenties and early thirties, Haruko did not view her income as a passport to independence. It is true she squirreled away her earnings, saving some for old age, spending the rest as she pleased. But for younger women still living in the shadow of their mothers-in-law, possession of one's own money implied something more. One of Haruko's neighbors, who worked part time as a store clerk and lived with her husband's parents, described how she had deliberately lied to her mother-in-law about the sum she had spent on groceries for the household. She told the older woman she had spent less than she actually had, because she did not want to be fully reimbursed from her mother-in-law's purse. That extra amount represented her small measure of economic independence. Other women hearing the story laughed in agreement.

Haruko viewed her position in the family as depending more on her labor than on her wage earnings. Indeed, work itself, rather than her separate though modest pin money, was Haruko's way of ensuring that her voice would be heard. "Do you want to know why I have a say in this family?" she asked one day, angrily interrupting a conversation I was having with one of her friends about the position of Japanese women. "I'll tell you why. Because I work harder than anybody else. It's for that reason that we've been able to increase our landholdings. You saw how my husband was dressed today to attend Yōko's graduation: in a white shirt, a silk tie, and a brown suit. That's the way it's always been. I've done all the work."

Any discussion of Haruko's household work provoked a similar emotional response. Although she felt angry about the way she had been worked in her husband's household, her belief that her status depended on her labor value made her reluctant to allow her mother-in-law to undertake too many household tasks; she seemed to fear that if she were no longer indispensable, her worth might be diminished. Was it perhaps this fear that also made her less than enthusiastic about her husband's mechanization project, even though it promised to free her from some of the most tiring aspects of rice farming? Haruko needed to be needed.

Haruko's anxiety about further investment in machinery, and her resistance to it, also reflected the more general confusion felt in the farming community over the future role of farm women. Would machinery eliminate altogether the need for female labor in the fields or would it simply tie women to other crops, while removing their husbands from the farm? Over one-third of farm women already farmed on their own. Again, would farm households become dependent on the wage labor of women as well as men, and would enough nonagricultural jobs be available?

In the face of these uncertainties, numerous suggestions from various sources floated around the countryside. A speaker addressing the Agricultural Cooperative in Uwa advised women to make more of their own food, as they did in the self-sufficient economy of the past, but then to sell it. And Shōichi, who thought it might be profitable for women to stick with farming, suggested that after the harvest they plant rice paddies with cash crops such as tobacco and wheat.

What such proposals had in common was the idea of added reliance on women's work of one sort or another; for during the transitional period at least—while the machines were still new and their efficacy uncertain—women were actually being called upon to perform more functions, rather than fewer. It is not surprising that the almost universal complaint of farm women was lack of sufficient time for rest, for domestic work, and for child care. Moreover, mechanization did not necessarily promise the economic security that would ease the demands on women in the near future. "We have put in machines to do our work," wrote one contributor to *Minori,* "and now we must work to pay for the machines. No sooner do we repay our loans than we have to buy machines. We want binders and automobiles. Our ideals are high, our income is low."

It was understandable that most farm wives envied the comparative leisure enjoyed by their middle-class counterparts in the towns, in their more secure roles as the wives of white-collar salaried men. Even Haruko, though she was perhaps too restless and ambitious to enjoy being anything but busy, nevertheless aspired to the kind of life-style such women represented. Many of her friends were affluent town women whose sole responsibility was homemaking, and perhaps she hoped that by her labor, in farming and in part-time work, she too might one day become, literally, just a housewife.

Haruko's town friends, cheerful and girlish, with graceful, refined manners, seemed to belong to a social class that set them apart from Haruko, who was accustomed to strenuous manual labor and blunt, direct communication. Their fashionable dress (skirts with dainty blouses and cardigan sweaters), their curler-set hairstyles, and their hobbies (raising parakeets and growing prize-winning chrysanthemums) gave evidence of their leisure and affluence. Their lives were so comfortable, in fact, that at least one of the women, in her late thirties, had begun jogging to keep her weight down. All of them wore face cream and powder and had beautiful teeth. (They all used dental floss, whereas Haruko was often too tired at night to give her teeth even a perfunctory brushing.) Because they had no need to take jobs, they had withdrawn into their homes, where they concentrated on being attentive mothers and attractive wives.

One day, one of Haruko's town friends bicycled out to the farm, her skirt gently billowing in the breeze, to get cabbage for her son's pet rabbits. Haruko, dressed in her ankle-high boots, baggy pantaloons, and apron, looked more than ever like a gnome, standing next to her elegant friend and loading the homegrown cabbage heads onto the back of the bicycle. The two women, who lived less than one mile apart, were a study in contrasts, and watching them, it was easier to understand why most farm women, inspired by the middle-class feminine ideal of the housewife, wished they were the wives of salaried men and wanted their own daughters to marry one.

NOTES

1. Money values have been calculated from the fall 1974 exchange rate of 300 yen = U.S. $1.00.
2. I am grateful to Ms. Miho Nagata of the Uwa branch of the Farmers Extension Bureau (Nōkyō Kairyō Fukyūshō) for providing this figure.
3. Fujin ni kansuru shomondai chōsa kaigi (Conference for investigating various problems concerning women), ed., *Gendai Nihon josei no ishiki to kōdō* (Contemporary Japanese women's attitudes and behavior) (Okurashō [Ministry of Finance]: Tokyo, 1974), p. 267.

THE POSITION OF WOMEN IN PASTORAL SOCIETY (THE FULANI WODAABE, NOMADS OF THE NIGER)

Marguerite Dupire

In Bororo beliefs, the sexes are opposite and complementary, but belong to one and the same human category which is totally different from, and excludes, all other categories. Here it should be briefly mentioned that in the Fulani language masculine and feminine genders do not exist, but nouns are arranged in a number of classes which indisputably indicate a manner of conceiving the universe which is both qualitative (classes of plants, trees, insects, birds, antelopes and the like, liquids, bounded objects) and geometrical or quantitative (plurals, length and duration, small quantities, parts of a whole, diminutives, augmentatives). Among these classes, the ones which appear to us Europeans as the strangest are probably the most important, or at least were so for a pastoralist society.

Reprinted with permission from Denise Paulme (ed.), *Women of Tropical Africa* (Berkeley and Los Angeles: University of California Press, 1963), pp. 43–53, 75–85. Originally published as *Femmes d'Afrique Noir* by Mouton & Co. in 1960.

The first of these is the human class, to which belong both sexes of human beings and a certain number of abstract nouns. With domestic animals, however, males and females belong to different categories (class *ndi* comprising most male domestic animals, castrated and uncastrated; class *nge,* cows). The term used as the generic term for the species is sometimes the one that designates the female of the species (as in the case of the goat, the ass, the cow, the sheep) and sometimes the male (the dog, the horse), the reason for this probably being the importance ascribed, in the cases where the female term is employed, to the producer of milk, an important feature in the pastoral economy.

The second important class presents a most fascinating riddle to which so far no answer has been found. This is the class *nge,* which includes, as well as the cow (female and generic), also fire and sun. Although no discoverable common element exists between these three things, one must suppose that whatever people it was (the Fulani?) that originally invented this class must have done so in virtue of some essential value shared by all the things assigned to it, and this might also mean that a ritual meaning was attached to them.

Thus, linguistically speaking, while the class of things human is asexual, with domestic animals the males belong to a different class from the females. But there are constant similarities and interrelations between the three orders of animate objects, human, animal and vegetable, all of which depend, for the maintenance of the species, on the same basic principle—prolificacy. Procreative power is thought of as being transferable from one order to the other, evidence for this belief being provided by numerous magic recipes, particularly those concerning the increase of the herd. However, although stress on this common factor is carried to great lengths in the universe of magic, where like is called upon to produce like in a different but parallel order (without any conscious appeal to a superior power), that does not mean that the human order is regarded as sharing anything except this one common factor with the other two orders. Thus the human species, male and female, is on a different level from the animal and vegetable kingdoms.

If we leave linguistics and the philosophical concepts they imply and turn to every day life, we find that it is characterized by a cleavage between the sexes, whose contrasted roles are expressed either directly, by the activities each engage in and by the behaviour manifested, or symbolically, by the difference between the male and the female manner of arranging material objects, or by the ritual distribution of meat at ceremonies, to mention only the more obvious instances.

Man and woman complete each other like the prow and poop of a ship, the west and east of a line on the horizon, the head and hindquarters of an animal, the blood and the milk of a living creature. The man precedes and the woman follows, as is indicated by the word for woman, *debbo,* from the root *rew,* to follow. In contrast to what has often been observed in societies of hunters or farmers, it is the man, the herdsman, who, when camp is struck, goes on ahead, with his herd following him, to spy out the grazing lands in advance, while the women, in Indian file behind the pack oxen which are in their charge, follow at the tail-end of the procession, carrying on their heads the household calabashes filled with goods. If the pack ox is primarily a pack animal for the women which a man would scorn to ride, a woman for her part never uses a camel saddle, for when she rides with her husband she sits behind him, astride against the hump.

Within the camp, the arrangement of the women's huts, of the cattle enclosures, and of all material objects always follows the principle of sex differentiation. When the members of an extended family live together, the eldest of the heads of the component individual families—the father or the eldest brother—takes up the position furthest to the south, with his juniors following in order of seniority. But within each separate polygynous group, each man's wives will arrange their huts in hierarchical order in the opposite direction, that is, from north to south. The eastern part of the camp is the women's domain, and the western the men's. Behind each hut (to the east of it), the woman washes her cooking utensils, and also herself. Here she can be metaphorically protected from view, if not actually so, since the hut is no more than a simple screen of thorn, unroofed. This is also the place where she will be buried. The man, on the other hand, does his work on the other side of the hut, for the cattle corral is to the west, near the entrance to the hut, and it is in this corral, or a little beyond it, that his grave will be dug. Because they come under the sphere of masculine activities, the calves are tethered in a row running in the masculine direction, from south to north, arranged according to age, from the oldest to the youngest; while the calabashes belonging to the women are arranged on a raised table in order of decreasing size running in the feminine direction from north to south. In the foreground, then, are the men and the goods that belong specifically to them, while behind are the women with their property arranged in a hierarchy like the men's and according to the same principle, the essential difference between them being expressed by an inversion of orientation: to the women belong the east, and the direction north-south; to the men, the west, and the direction south-north.

In all ceremonies in which the women take part along with the men, they have a customary right to certain portions of the meat. Normally the portions are distributed to groups, according to age-grade, and there are only two occasions when an individual receives a portion: at a betrothal ceremony, when the wife of the paternal uncle of the fiancé (this uncle having directed the distribution of the animal offered up by his brother) and a cross-cousin of the fiancée each receives an individual portion; and at a ceremony for naming a child, when the mother receives a portion of the sacrificial animal. When specially reserved parts such as these, as well as portions assigned to men who have played certain designated roles in the ceremony, have been set aside, the following groups receive collective portions: adults (*ndotti'en:* old men and adult men who have reached the age when they can direct public affairs), young men, young girls, married women and their children, old women. This distribution underlines differences in sex, age, and role, and does so not only quantatively, but also qualitatively, because a particular portion of the animal is assigned to each of these groups in accordance with the idea that certain qualities are shared in magical participation by the human and the bovine species. According to this principle, women

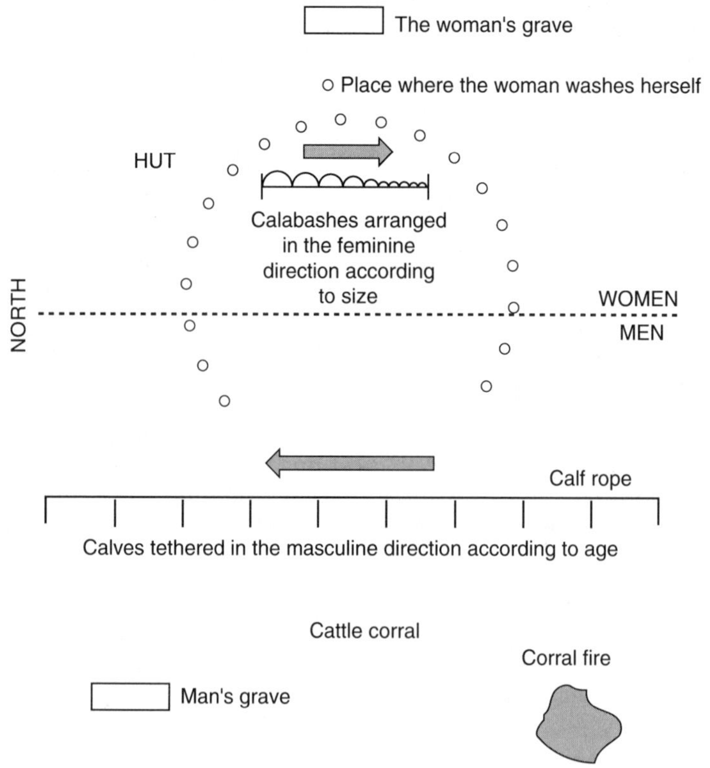

FIGURE 1

have a prior claim not only to the intestines (*reedu,* the belly, comprising the first stomach, the uterus, and the large intestines), which are regarded as the seat of procreation, but also to the hind quarters, including the hinder end of the vertebral column: "Is it not natural that the women should have the hindquarters? Is it not they who follow the men?" So, whether it be the assignment of hindquarters "because they follow" or of the intestines because of their procreative capacities, the distribution of meat to women differentiates not only between age-grades, but also between social roles. Just as the portion assigned to married women is in contrast to that assigned to adult men, so that assigned to young girls is in contrast to that assigned to young men: they receive the heart, the centre of the feelings, while the young men receive the *biol,* a piece of the breast regarded as the organ of potency. The group of senior members on either side (maternal and paternal) of the family each receives one of the two sides of free ribs. As for the cross cousins of the fiancée, young or old they all fight tooth and nail, along with the full cousins who have cut up the animal, for the half of the skin which is their due and from which each individual attempts to cut off a piece to make sandals from. Neither age nor sex counts, and a brutal free-for-all momentarily abolishes all the usual rules of the code of politeness. A young man will jostle his mother-in-law, who may be a cross-cousin with the same rights as he has, and will only say with a laugh: "Too bad! It is my mother-in-law," knowing that she will make a scene when she gets home because he has prevented her from bringing back anything from the slaughter. Everything will calm down later, but on this unique occasion, and in public, the differences of role and of sex are abolished.

At these ceremonies which bring together the kin on both sides as well as the neighbours, the distribution of meat seems to express symbolically a recognition of the various social roles. The women figure as companions of the men, whom they have to follow; as mothers, whose warm flow of affection makes them the paramount representatives of that "kinship through the milk" that characterizes uterine descent; as old women, who have the right to certain special marks of respect; and as cross cousins—and in this capacity they have to compete on the same level as their masculine counterparts, beyond all the rules of kinship, sex, age and status which ordinarily regulate social relations.

DIVISION OF LABOUR

The characteristic association: man-cattle, as against woman-household, is a feature that has already been stressed. The basis of the differences in rights between the sexes must be sought in a division of labour which has the characteristic features common to most cattle-keeping peoples, in Africa at least.[1] To look after the humped cattle, which are only semi-domesticated, demands activities of which a woman is physically incapable. It would be beyond a woman's strength to draw water for the herd in the dry season, to go on long marches to reconnoitre for grazing-lands, to protect the herd against wild animals and thieves, to hold her own with a buyer at the market, to castrate bulls, or to train the pack oxen. This hard, dangerous life, full of uncertainty and of prolonged absences from the camp, would be incompatible with the duties of motherhood, which require a more sedentary and more regular life.

Thus among the activities required for the care of the herd, only those that are compatible with staying at home are assigned to her: those of milking and of making butter. She also looks after the minor ailments of the animals under her care, and has a direct interest in doing so; but for anything requiring more forceful treatment (blood-letting, yoking . . .) she passes all responsibility over to the head cattlekeeper. Among the Bororo it is inconceivable that a woman should be *jom-na'i,* master of the herd.

It should be noted that this division of labour is not in any way a hard and fast affair. Apart from the period of married life preceding the birth of the first child and the month or two following upon each time she gives birth, there is no period in a woman's life when she may not do the milking. However, although the reason why Bororo men do not undertake this task is because they have never learnt to do so, should the necessity arise, they would not hesitate to assume this feminine role. Thus it is the very conditions of existence that have determined cultural choice. This is proved by the fact that among the semi-nomad Fulani of the Niger it is the men who practise the technique of milking, while the women are unversed in it. The reason why, in this society, it is the herdsmen who have learnt how to milk, is because they spend half the year, parted from the women, looking after the cattle in the bush at some distance from the village. The few milch cows left behind in the village are milked by the older men, while the butter is churned by the women.[2] It is obvious therefore how much these habits, which sometimes persist long after there has been a change in the mode of life, are functional in origin, and not based on any magico-philosophical concepts of irreducible differences between the sexes. In any case, a man sometimes has to intervene when things go wrong with the milking, for if the cow is restive, or if her milk does not flow after the first calving, she has, in the first case, to be controlled by tying her up, or, in the second, to be treated by blowing air into the vagina or, in the last resort, by appealing to a specialist in incantations.

Women also do the milking of the smaller livestock, and here their responsibilities have a wider range (including looking after the animals and negotiating sales), due to the fact that these smaller animals are more amenable to treatment which requires less physical strength. Normally, small flocks of sheep and goats belong to women rather than to men. Being a form of capital that is easily convertible, they provide women with the same kind of "savings bank" as castrated cattle do for men.

Women also undertake all the tasks concerned with the house. As soon as the head of a camp has decided upon the place where they will stay for several days or several weeks, it is the women who build the huts from the thorn branches they have gathered, while their husbands busy themselves with tethering their calves and taking the herd to graze. It is also they who decorate the calabashes, fabricate the mats made out of bark, weave the winnowing fans. They look after the fires belonging to the hut, while the men look after those for the cattle—a task which requires knowledge of the magic talismans associated with it. The women plait the light ropes that are all that is required for their own use, while the men plait the heavy ones needed for drawing water or for tethering the calves; but it is the men who collect the bark used in making them. Helped by her children, the mistress of the house fetches water from the well for domestic purposes, while it is the man's job to draw water for watering the livestock. At the market which both attend, the wife sells her milk and her butter, while the husband buys salt, millet when necessary, and tobacco, sugar and tea for himself, as well as haggling over prices for the sale of cattle.

Both men and women know how to ply a needle for sewing or repairing their own clothes. Nor do men despise doing some cooking, although they usually leave this task to the women. When a man is on his own, or when he is taking part in a ceremony, he cooks meat by grilling it on a skewer, while women boil it in one of the pots they have made.[3]

In this allocation of work between the sexes there is no idea whatsoever of inferiority of status being associated with those tasks normally assigned to women. But it is obvious that in a pastoralist society, in which it is the man who undertakes the heavy work and the responsibilities involved in looking after the cattle, that he, as master of the herd, will achieve social and economic superiority over the woman, whose tasks are confined to managing household affairs and looking after her sheep and goats.

The few fields cultivated by some families at the beginning of the winter season do not employ more than one or two men; and as soon as the crops are sown, these men hasten to rejoin the other members of the camp who are on the move with their herds. Here again it is considerations of a practical order which determine the arrangement, and this is particularly the case with the WoDaaBe, among whom the men are responsible for providing the supply of millet for the family, while the women supply the milk. The Bororo, however, are not unaware of the magical associations which link woman with the fertility of the soil, for one of their recipes for the fertility of the herd includes some seeds from a field belonging to a female sedentary farmer, which are called *umma* (meaning "arise!" in their language).

In the Niger region, WoDaaBe women do not either spin cotton or know how to make cheese, in contrast to their Fulani sisters belonging to tribes that practice sedentary farming.

From this picture it can be seen that upon women fall the less strenuous tasks, but also those which are the most monotonous and which take up the most time. In the dry seasons, they often walk a distance of 20 to 30 kilometers to sell one or two litres of milk in the village. It is the woman who is the first to get up in the morning, at dawn, to pound the grain, when the air is still chilly. But her night will have been undisturbed, unless her baby has wakened her; whereas her husband may have had to stay up half the night getting his herd watered; or he may have had to get up in the middle of the night because a jackal was prowling round the camp.

PROPERTY BELONGING TO WOMEN

From their earliest years, children enjoy undisputed rights of possession over their personal belongings. No mother will give away or exchange her little girl's doll without first asking her permission. With stock, however, the situation is different, for, although both boys and girls are indeed the owners of the cattle given to them by their father, mother, or other relatives, and refer to them in the possessive, yet they have no active control over this property so long as they remain members of the paternal household. The father looks after the cattle, while the mother does the milking and uses the dairy products to supply the needs of the household. If the father's herd is failing to produce enough to support the family, the children cannot raise any objection if the cattle-keeper finds himself forced to sell one of their animals which had been given to them in front of witnesses. It will be accepted philosophically as "God's will," in the same way as nobody will be held responsible for the good or ill luck that may attend the first heifers given to them by their parents. At birth and as the children grow up, portions of the herd are allotted to them which cannot then be re-allotted or compensated for (in principle, at least). These allotted portions remain under the exclusive control of the father until his children marry, or more precisely, until they leave the paternal camp. This economic dependence acts as a stimulus to married sons to set up on their own as soon as possible. When a daughter gets married, the care of her cattle passes from her father to her husband, who is then responsible for their well-being in the interests of his wife and her children. That women consider this question of control to be a delicate one is proved by the fact that young wives are in the habit of leaving their stock with their father until they can feel sure of the integrity of their husbands, preferring to be temporarily deprived of the dairy products of their herd. Some of them even leave them there for good. When the husband becomes cattle-keeper, he keeps his wife's animals along with his own, but is aware that they do not belong to him.

If a woman wants to sell one of her animals, she must first ask the consent of her husband, and he in turn, should he find himself in difficulties, may not sell one of his wife's animals without her consent. Any sharp practice concerning the cattle will immediately bring complaints on the part of the wife and departure to her family. But if husband and wife get on well together and the husband has shown himself to be trustworthy, his wife is not likely to refuse him one of her animals in order to pay tax or, as is more often the case, to make up the *sadaaki* to be given by one of their sons to his fiancée. In such an event, the combined wealth of husband and wife provides for the maintenance or for the future of their children, thus playing the normal role for which the double contribution of cattle was intended.

Astonishing though it may seem, a wife maintains a much stricter supervision over the *sadaaki,* of which she is only co-owner with her husband, than she does over her own stock given to her by her family. To a woman, keeping the *sadaaki* intact is equivalent to preserving a tangible symbol of her matrimonial rights while also safeguarding the future of her children. For this reason, it is the most socially sacrosanct part of the herd, and the one which must remain the last to be depleted. A wife will as little pardon her husband for having misappropriated their *sadaaki,* especially if he has done so for the children of another wife, as she will be willing to distribute it during her lifetime among her children when they get married. This prevents further quarrels with her husband on the subject without entirely depriving her of her rights to the dairy products, for a mother can easily go to live with one of her sons. Thus a married woman as often as not prefers to hand over her stock to her family or to her children rather than to her husband.

A second way in which women play an important role in the transmission of cattle derives from the manner in which the herd belonging to the father of the family is divided out.

To his chief wife a husband entrusts, in addition to the *sadaaki,* a certain number of milch cows (*darnaaji*), the milk of which will belong to her personally, and which immediately become part of the stock which her children alone will inherit together with the dairy rights. His other wives, with whom he is united by the *teegal* form of marriage, do not receive any *sadaaki,* but he assigns to them a certain number of animals (*senndereeji*) on a scale comparable, in so far as is possible, with the combined *sadaaki* and *darnaaji* of the chief wife. In addition to those cows which have been divided out, the head of the family may possess others which he can entrust to anyone he pleases for varying lengths of time. He is free to dispose of these animals and their progeny as he wishes. Along with the steers and bulls which do not come from the *sadaaki* or *darnaaji* they will form part of the common inheritance of all his children.

This manner of dividing out the herd accentuates the economic basis of the group of full brothers, who share common interests with their mother. Their calves are tethered in front of their hut, and the children get to know them and are aware that they can be certain of inheriting some of them, to the exclusion of their half-brothers and sisters. They understand, too, that the well-being of the animals depends on the care their mother bestows on them and on her firmness in preventing any depredations. In this way, the mother, without herself being its source, is the channel through which a large part of the father's stock is transferred to his children.

A woman enjoys much greater economic independence with regard to the small livestock which she acquires out of her personal savings. She can in fact do what she likes with it. She is free to a considerable degree to put to use the results of her labours. The milk from her cows belongs to her, but out of the income derived from this she must contribute towards the household needs. In principle, the husband is responsible for expenditure required for the cattle (natron, taxes . . .), and for clothing and the supply of millet, while the woman's share of the budget covers expenditure on daily requirements such as cereals, cooking salt, and condiments (which are however a luxury). But actually, in the dry season it is customary to barter milk for millet, and during the winter season the WoDaaBe do not eat cereals. There remains the difficult period before the harvest, at the end of the dry season, when the milk yield is low and there is no surplus for exchange. The husband is then often obliged to sell one of his sheep, or even a bullock, although this is an extreme measure to which he is loath to resort. It is in fact also in the wife's interests to safeguard the family capital, and in the dry season it is much more sensible to exchange milk, which is scarce, for millet, than to sell a skinny animal at a low price. Milk and butter are the basis of the household economy. Particularly during the winter season, the women manage to accumulate large quantities of butter stored in calabashes, which, already rancid, is sold in the villages on return from winter quarters. This provides pocket money for buying, for themselves and their children, extra gowns, trinkets, and even sheep. It is astonishing what a Bororo woman manages to do with the small savings from the "butter money," which gradually mount up. During the worst time of the year, four cows give a daily yield of a pat of butter weighing about 250 grammes (costing 15 C.F.A. francs in 1951). This butter is exchanged in the villages or sold on the market, and the women spend quite a lot of their time on these petty commercial transactions.

They may also mend calabashes for village women, or, when food is very scarce, offer to pound grain for a slight payment in cereals or bran. But a young and active Bororo woman will avoid such menial tasks. Similarly, it is only young men who have no cattle of their own who will offer themselves as herdsmen in a locality where they are not known, where they will be less likely to feel ashamed. None of the other articles which women make, such as mats, winnowing fans, or ropes, are saleable.

Occupied as she is with her house and her children, a woman is nevertheless just as much sentimentally attached to the cattle as the men are. In her earliest years she was accustomed to stroke gently the ears or the vagina of the cow her mother was milking. She has to keep constant watch over the calves entrusted to her, and like her husband and her children, she knows the history of every single animal. When she has to part with a cow that is ill or too old and that has to be killed, it is like parting from a human being, and her sorrow speaks volumes for the attachment she feels for these companions in good times and bad.

It goes without saying that for men as for women the expression *miin-jei,* "I possess," covers various methods of appropriation entailing varying rights: of alienation, of administration, of usufruct. A woman will say of the pack ox that forms part of her *sadaaki* "my pack ox," and it is true that she has exclusive use of it so long as she remains with her husband; but she can neither sell it without her husband's consent, nor take it with her should her marriage be dissolved (this at least is the case among the WoDaaBe groups of the western Niger region).

If a woman's rights over the large livestock are restricted owing to the fact that she is considered incapable of looking after it, those of a married man over the herd of which he is nominally "master" are no less so, (1) by his wife's co-ownership of the *sadaaki,* (2) by each wife's ownership of the cattle given to her by her family, (3) by the wives' exclusive rights over the milk of certain animals, (4) by his children's rights of ownership and of inheritance over the stock divided out during his lifetime.

A glance at the following table in which the various types of ownership are listed will show that a wife not only has exclusive rights to the use of the milk from the animals in one category or another (*darnaaji* and *sadaaki* for the chief wife, *senndereeji* for the others, as well as the *sukaaji* of their children and their own *sukaaji*), but also enjoys co-ownership of her *sadaaki* with her husband and exclusive rights of ownership over the animals given to her by her family, although the care of them is entrusted to her husband, the master of the herd. The restrictions on the rights of the father of the family over his cattle are connected with his children's future. As for the wives, their rights to the use of the milk and the co-ownership of the *sadaaki* act as a guarantee for the services they render their husband.

TABLE 1. Rights of Ownership Held by the Nominal Master of the Herd over His Cattle

Category of cattle	*Description and source*	*Looked after by . . .*	*Alienation rights held by . . .*	*Rights to use the milk held by . . .*	*Inheritance rights held by . . .*
birnaaji	Stock held by the head of the family. Acquired through inheritance, gifts, purchases, or *nannga na'i* loans . . .	Father of the family.	Father of the family.	*All the wives alike* as required.	The children of all the wives.
darnaaji	Portion of the stock of the head of the family entrusted to the chief wife, *koowaaDo* (same sources as *birnaaji*).	Father of the family.	Father of the family.	*Only* the wife to whom they have been entrusted.	Only the children of the wife who has rights to the milk.
sadaaki (Western Niger region).	Stock given to the *koowaaDo* wife.	Father of the family even after divorce or repudiation.	*Husband or wife* with the consent of spouse.	*Only* the wife who is co-owner.	Only the children of the wife who is co-owner.
sadaaki (Islamized Eastern Niger region).	Stock given to the *koowaaDo* wife.	Father of the family except in cases of repudiation.	*Husband or wife* with the consent of spouse.	*Only* the wife who is co-owner	Only the children of the wife who is co-owner.
senndereeji	Portion of the stock of the head of the family entrusted to secondary wives (in place of *sadaaki* and *darnaaji*).	Father of the family.	Father of the family.	*Only* the wife to whom they have been entrusted.	Only the children of the wife who has rights to the milk.
sukaaji of the children.	Gifts received by the children	Father during their minority, sons after setting up households, husband of married daughters.	Father of the family during their minority, sons on on coming of age.	Usually *the wife who is the mother of the children who own the stock.*	This is an inheritance in advance of each child in question.
sukaaji of the wives.	Gifts received by each wife from her family.	Father of the family.	*The wife with the consent of her husband.*	*Only* the wife who is the owner	Only the children of the wife who is the owner.

These rights of ownership, co-ownership or merely of use of the milk which a wife enjoys over certain animals are connected with the fact that the capital which these animals represent is inalterably destined to be transmitted to her own children (Table 1, col. 6). A mother not only transmits to her children life and "milk," but also channels to them the cattle belonging to their father, simply in virtue of being married to him.

The ownership of all other goods belonging to husband and wife (clothes, furniture and other articles) remains completely separate throughout their married life. When a wife leaves her husband or is repudiated by him, she leaves the hut, people say, with "nothing but the dust" in it, and perhaps also the old blackened cooking pot which would be too cumbersome to take away. She removes all her possessions, including her own livestock and the dowry given to her by her parents. But the presents given to her by her husband's family are left behind: the *sadaaki* and the furniture lent to her by her mother-in-law. Clothes, furniture, and other articles down to sewing needles, are individually acquired either by the husband or by the wife. Marriage does not entail any sharing of such belongings by the couple.

Thus the only rights of ownership that marriage brings to a woman are her rights of co-ownership or of usufruct in cattle belonging to her husband, while her husband only has the use of his wife's possessions (dowry and stock) for as long as she remains with him. Whatever the reasons for the dissolution of a marriage (separation, repudiation, death), the sharing of goods in common ceases with the physical separation of the couple.

The belongings over which a woman possesses permanent rights of alienation or usufruct are, in fact, not those which come from her husband, but those which come from her own family or which have been acquired as a result of her own work under her husband's roof: the gifts of cattle and the dowry given to her by her parents, and the livestock bought with her "butter money."

She is, however, complete mistress of those belongings which do not fall within the large number of restricted categories. But a BoDaaDo woman possesses little enough stock: a few cattle calved by the heifer given to her by her parents, supposing it has survived, and a small flock of goats and sheep. It is usually childless women that have the flocks of sheep, because otherwise a married woman finds that most of her slender income goes on necessary household expenses. Among the WoDaaBe there are no much-sought-after widows whose personally owned cattle and *sadaaki* make them wealthy, such as can be found among the sedentary Fulani, because when a husband dies it is the children and not the wife who inherit the stock. I only came across one widow possessing a small herd of cattle, who was married to an old man without any property at all, and lazy into the bargain. This man who allowed himself to be kept by his wife soon became the laughing-stock of his neighbours. The widow lived with her son, the future inheritor, who threatened to go away, taking the herd with him, if she did not get rid of her good-for-nothing spouse. Even if a widow has no son, her property is controlled by the consanguineous kin who will inherit it, directly if she has made a leviratic marriage with her husband's brother, indirectly if she has opted for some other arrangement.

The Bororo maintain that women are thus incapacitated both because of their lack of physical strength and because of their marital instability. But it is clear that the situation arises from the very nature of the structure of inheritance in this thoroughly patrilineal society.

Since among pastoralists women are usually not owners of capital, that is to say, of cattle, which belong to the men, their economic position would appear to be less favourable than it is in some agriculturalist societies in Africa. There it is land, inalienable in the traditional context, that represents capital, but capital that is less valuable because it is neither mobile nor easily convertible. Hence the position of the women, who are the direct producers, should be, by comparison, higher in relation to the men of the lineage, who own the land that they cultivate. But this would appear to be too summary a generalization, because in some pastoralist societies women do have the right to manage the herd. J. H. Driberg reports that among the Lango a man may not dispose of his property without the permission of his wife, who is co-owner of the property which the children will inherit. She even has sole rights of administration over the property of her husband during the minority of the inheritors. In this society a woman also enjoys far greater political rights than is the case with a BoDaaDo woman, for the widow of a village head may even govern a village during the minority of her son. Thus there is considerable variation in the economic and legal rights of women in African pastoralist societies, whether of Nilotics, Nilo-Hamitics, or Fulani, in spite of the fact that in all of them it is the men who deal with the cattle.

The prestige which her wealth confers upon a woman is similar to that which a man derives from his cattle. At the ceremonies that take place when the lineage segment gathers together in the winter season, the heads of families who are celebrating the marriage of a son parade the herds of the extended family to display in public how many of them there are, and how strong and beautiful they are. The women have their own display, exhibiting their possessions in their huts: calabashes and polished-up spoons from their dowry stores, gourds and countless straw hats from the *kaakol* bags. . . . The whole display bears witness for all to see of feminine wealth, which gives personal prestige to the woman who owns it.

NOTES

1. J. H. Driberg, "The status of women among the Nilotics and Nilo-Hamitics," *Africa,* V, 5, 1932.
2. J. H. Driberg, *op. cit.;* among the Nilotics, the milking is done by the men, but by the women among the Nilo-Hamitics.
3. Driberg (*op. cit.*) has already recorded this difference.

VII

GENDER, PROPERTY, AND THE STATE

The relationship between sexual inequality, the emergence of class structures, and the rise of the state has been an enduring interest in anthropological studies of gender. The subordination of women appears to emerge as an aspect of state formation. According to Gailey (1987: 6), "Institutionalized gender hierarchy . . . is created historically with class relations and state formative processes, whether these emerge independently, through colonization, or indirectly through capital penetration." We are led to ask what relationship class and state formation have with the oppression of women and, when gender hierarchy occurs, why women are the dominated gender. How does the state have power to penetrate and reorganize the lives of its members, whether in Sumerian legal codes declaring monogamy for women or in welfare laws in the United States that influence household composition? Eventually, studying state formation may help us understand the origins and interrelationships of class and patriarchy, and the social reproduction of inequality.

Much discussion of this subject has centered on Engels' book *The Origin of the Family, Private Property, and the State,* a nineteenth-century text in which Engels argues that the emergence of the concept of private property and its ownership by men, as well as the development of a monogamous family, led to the subordination of women. In Engels' scheme, prior to this gender relations were characterized as egalitarian and complementary. All production was for use, and people worked together for the communal household. Thus, changes in gender relations were linked to changes in material conditions because the ownership of productive property (initially domestic animals) was concentrated in the hands of men. This thesis has been influential in many Marxist and feminist analyses of women's subordination. For example, Leacock notes, "There is sufficient evidence at hand to support in its broad outlines Engels' argument that the position of women relative to men deteriorated with the advent of class society" (1973: 30).

Following Engels, Leacock observes that in early communal society the division of labor between the sexes was reciprocal, and a wife and her children were not dependent on the husband. Further, "The distinction did not exist between a public world of men's work and a private world of women's household service. The large collective household was the community, and within it both sexes worked to produce the goods necessary for livelihood" (1973: 33). In this view the oppression of women was built on the transformation of goods for use into commodities for exchange; the exploitation of workers and of women was generated by this process, which involved the emergence of the individual family as an isolated unit, economically responsible for its members, and of women's labor as a private service in the context of the family. This led to the "world historical defeat of the female sex" (Engels 1973: 120; Silverblatt 1988: 430).

In a reanalysis of Engels, Sacks agrees that women's position declined with the elaboration of social classes but disputes Engels' emphasis on the role of private property in this process (Silverblatt 1988: 435). Rather, Sacks links state formation and the decline in the centrality of kinship groups to the deterioration in women's status. She delineates two relationships defining women in noncapitalist societies: sisterhood and wifehood. "Sister" refers to women's access to resources based on membership in a kin group. This relation implies autonomy, adulthood, and possible gender symmetry. "Wife," on the other hand, refers to a relationship of dependency on the husband and his kin. Sacks suggests that the development of states undermined women's status by dismantling the kin group corporations that formed the basis for sister relations (Sacks 1982).

However, critics of Sacks' position have argued that the process of state formation may involve uneven and contradictory developments. For example, elite women in the Kingdom of Dahomey, West Africa, challenged state imperatives by means of control of marketing associations. Thus, Silverblatt rebuts Sacks' evolutionary paradigm, suggesting the inevitability of the decline in women's status with state formation; instead, she suggests that we acknowledge the complex history of the emergence of elite privilege in the rise of the state. In addition, elite women such as the royalty of Dahomey may or may not share the goals of peasant women. They may instead join with the male elite in suppressing the authority and power of peasant market women. This illustrates the potential contradictions of gender affiliation on one hand, and class position on the other.

Several anthropologists have observed that Engels lacked reliable ethnographic information and oversimplified the complexities of gender relations in kinship societies and in precapitalist states (Gailey 1987: 15). In a critique of Engels, Moore argues against his essentialist assumption that there is a "natural" division of labor in which men are concerned with productive tasks and women with domestic ones. She also disagrees that an inevitable relationship will transpire between property, paternity, and legitimacy, in which men "naturally" want to transmit property to genetic offspring (1988: 47–48).

While Rapp (in this book) agrees with these criticisms, she points out that Engels addresses many current concerns, such as the relationship between women's participation in production and female status, and the implications of the separation of the domestic-public domains for women's roles in society (see also Silverblatt 1988: 432).

She warns against overgeneralizing when trying to understand the origins of the state and ignoring the history and context in which political formations change. In her view we must examine kinship structures that were supplanted with the rise of the state and replaced by territorial and class-specific politics. Kinship domains, formerly autonomous, were subjugated to the demands of emergent elites with repercussions for gender roles and relations.

Among the processes that we need to examine are the politics of kinship, the intensification of military complexes, the impact of trade on social stratification, and the changing content and role of cosmology. For example, in stratified societies the establishment of long-distance trade and tribute systems may affect elite marriage patterns, leading to the emergence of dowry and the exchange of women to cement male political alliances. Similar alliances are forged in societies that have experienced a rise in militarism. When economies change and demand increases for a traded commodity, exploitation of labor to produce it may also increase, and marriage systems that expand trading relations may be solidified through the exchange of women. Women themselves may be important figures in trading networks, as in West Africa and in Mesoamerica, where women are active in the marketplace.

Alternatively, the extension of the state into localized communities can significantly influence gender roles and relations. This occurs, for example, by undermining women's ritual responsibilities or by generating conflict between government policy and the respective interests of men and women (see Browner, this book). Finally, changes in political hierarchies were legitimated by cosmological explanations in early states such as those of the Inca and the Maya. For example, as Maya society became increasingly stratified, a category of elite rulers known as *ahaw* emerged. These rulers were legitimized by myths that established them as mediators between the natural and supernatural worlds and as protectors of the people. State ideology involved the celebration of both male and female forces, and the elite contained both men and women. Mothers of kings were always members of the high elite, and this class affiliation was also validated in myth (Schele and Freidel 1990, Freidel and Schele, this book).

Ortner examines the process of state formation, with particular regard to its effect on gender ideology (1978). She analyzes the widespread ideology that associates the purity of women with the honor and status of their families. This pattern is evident in Latin America and the Mediterranean, and in societies of the Middle East, India, and China. Broad similarities exist in these varied societies. Ortner questions why the control of female sexual purity is such a ubiquitous and important phenomenon. She notes that all modern cases of societies concerned with female purity occur in states or systems with highly developed stratification, and they bear the cultural ideologies and religions that were part of the emergence of these states. She argues that no prestate societies manifest the pattern linking female virginity and chastity to the social honor of the group. Thus, concern with the purity of women was, in Ortner's view, structurally, functionally, and symbolically linked to the historical emergence of state structures.

The rise of the state heralds a radical shift in ideology and practice, with the emergence of the patriarchal extended family in which the senior man has absolute authority over everyone in the household. Women are brought under direct control of men in their natal families and later by their husbands and affinal kin. Ideologically women are thought to be in danger, requiring male protection; they are idealized as mothers and for their purity.

One of the central questions in the analysis of the impact of state formation is the role of hypergamy (up-status marriage, usually between higher-status men and lower-status women). Ortner (1978) suggests that a significant development in stratified society involves the transformation of marriage from an essentially equal transaction to a potentially vertical one, where one's sister or daughter could presumably marry into a higher strata (wife of a nobleman, consort of a king). Hypergamy may help explain the ideal of female purity because concepts of purity and virginity may symbolize the value of a girl for a higher-status spouse. Thus "a virgin is an elite female among females, withheld, untouched, exclusive" (Ortner 1981: 32).

Hypergamous marriages often involve the exchange of significant amounts of property, particularly in the form of dowry. The relationship between dowry, inheritance, and female status has been explored in a number of societies with varying marriage patterns. Dowry has been described as a form of premortem inheritance, parallel to men's rights in property accrued through inheritance after death of parents or other legators. However, considering dowry as a form of inheritance prior to death and as part of a woman's property complex obscures an important difference between the clear legal inheritance rights that men possess and the dowry that women may or may not receive (McCreery 1976; see also Stone and James in this book). Women obtain dowry at the discretion of their parents or brothers, and dowry is not based on the same rights as other forms of inheritance to which men have access.

While dowry has been viewed as a form of inheritance for women, the dowry system in northern India has taken a pernicious turn as brides are burned to death, poisoned, or otherwise "accidentally" killed by husbands and in-laws who believe that the women have brought inadequate dowries. Conservative estimates are that at least 2,000 women die each year as a result of dowry murders (Stone and James in this book). Legislation enacted in 1961 banning dowries, and in 1986 amending the penal code to introduce a new offense, now known as dowry death, has been ineffective, and the dowry system continues to be deeply embedded in local culture (Koman 1996). Although the bestowing of dowry in India is centuries old, dowry murders are a recent social problem. Stone and James argue that dowry deaths represent a response to a growing materialist consumerism sweeping India that has stimulated demands for larger and ever-increasing dowries. They analyze these murders in the context of a patrilineal and patrilocal society with strongly prescribed subservience of wives to husbands and in-laws, in which parents prefer to see a daughter dead, rather than divorced. Women's fertility, which may once have been a source of power, is increasingly less valued. Even a woman who gives birth to sons is not protected from the risk of wife-burning. Thus women's relative lack of economic power and the loss of their one traditional source of leverage, their fertility, have heightened their vulnerability to violence.

While the status of Indian women as reflected in the exchange of property at marriage appears to be deteriorating, in other parts of the world women's legal status and property rights have improved through state-sponsored changes in the judicial system. For example, Starr (in this book) examines how in Turkey the impact of capitalistic agriculture and settled village life profoundly affected gender relations and women's access to property. These changes occurred in the cultural context of Islamic notions of male dominance and female submission and legislation giving equal rights to women.

Ottoman family law gave women rights to divorce and some protection against polygamous marriage, but inheritance practices remained constrained by Islamic law, in which women were under the authority of their husbands, had the status of a minor, received half the share of the patrimony obtained by their brothers, and had no rights to children of a marriage. According to Ataturk's secular reforms in the 1920s, women's rights were expanded to full adult status, women received equal rights to paternal inheritance, protection was granted to widows, and other legislation was enacted promoting equality for women. At first these state-initiated rights were incongruent with cultural practices, but by the late 1960s women had begun to use the courts to protect their rights to property and their reputation. Starr points out that while Engels emphasized the negative impact of private ownership on women's status, in this case law and culture played a positive counterbalancing role resulting in women's emancipation.

If the state shapes family and gender relations directly through legislation such as that determining rights to property, it may also have more indirect impact. Allison (in this book) argues that in Japan, boxed lunches (*obento*), prepared by mothers for their children, are invested with a gendered state ideology. The state manipulates the ideological and gendered meanings associated with the box lunch as an important component of nursery school culture. Nursery schools, under state supervision, not only socialize children and mothers into the gendered roles they are expected to assume but also introduce small children to the attitudes and structures of Japanese education. The *obento,* elaborately and artistically arranged, is intended to allow the mother to produce something of home and family to accompany the child into this new and threatening outside world. Embedded in the school's close scrutiny of *obento* production and consumption is a message to obey rules and accept the authority of the school, and by extension, of the state. The *obento's* message is also that mothers sustain their children through food and support state ideology as well.

In all the works included in this chapter we see the enduring influence of the issues raised by Engels with regard to the relationship between gender, property rights, and state structures. However, cross-cultural data demonstrate that this relationship is much more complex and varied than Engels' original formulation. Equally, universal evolutionary paradigms that posit a uniform impact of the rise of the state on gender roles cannot do justice to the myriad ways in which specific cultural histories, diverse social hierarchies, and systems of stratification affect gender relations and ideology. Thus, Silverblatt (1988: 448) asks, "What of the challenges that women and men, caught in their society's contradictions, bring to the dominant order of chiefs and castes, an order they contour and subvert, even as they are contained by it? And what of the other voices, the voices that chiefs and rulers do not (or cannot or will not) express?" The complex histories of the relationship between any particular state and gender relations in it show that while state formation has contributed to the definition of womanhood, women have also contributed to the definition of states (Silverblatt 1988: 452).

REFERENCES

Engels, Frederick. 1973. *The Origin of the Family, Private Property and the State.* New York: International Publishers.

Gailey, Christine Ward. 1987. *Kinship to Kingship: Gender Hierarchy and State Formation in the Tongan Islands.* Austin: University of Texas Press.

Koman, Kathleen. 1996. "India's Burning Brides." *Harvard Magazine* 98 (3): 18–19.

Leacock, Eleanor Burke. 1973. "Introduction." In Frederick Engels (ed.). *The Origin of the Family, Private Property and the State,* pp. 7–57. New York: International Publishers.

McCreery, John L. 1976. "Women's Property Rights and Dowry in China and South Asia." *Ethnology* 15: 163–174.

Moore, Henrietta L. 1988. *Feminism and Anthropology.* Minneapolis: University of Minnesota Press.

Ortner, Sherry. 1978. "The Virgin and the State." *Feminist Studies* 4 (3): 19–35.

———1981. "Gender and Sexuality in Hierarchical Societies: The Case of Polynesia and Some Comparative Implications." In Sherry B. Ortner and Harriet Whitehead (eds.). *Sexual Meanings: The Cultural Construction of Gender and Sexuality,* pp. 359–410. Cambridge: Cambridge University Press.

Sacks, Karen. 1982. *Sisters and Wives: The Past and Future of Sexual Equality.* Urbana: University of Illinois Press.

Schele, Linda and David Freidel. 1990. *A Forest of Kings.* New York: William Morrow.

Silverblatt, Irene. 1988. "Women in States." *Annual Review of Anthropology* 17: 427–461.

THINKING ABOUT WOMEN AND THE ORIGIN OF THE STATE

Rayna Rapp

While anthropologists vary widely in their assessment of the autonomy of women in prestate societies, there seems to be a general consensus that with the rise of civilization, women as a social category were increasingly subjugated to the male heads of their households (Gailey 1987; Leacock 1978; Rohrlich 1980; Sacks 1982; Sanday 1981; Silverblatt 1988). This consensus is based, implicitly or explicitly, on a formulation developed by Frederick Engels in *The Origin of the Family, Private Property, and the State.* Engels linked the growth of private productive property to the dismantling of a system of communal kinship that existed in prestate societies. In this process, he argued, marriage grows more restrictive, legitimacy of heirs more important, and wives generally become means of reproduction to their husbands. At the same time, reciprocal relations among kin are curtailed, unequal access to strategic productive resources gradually develops, and estates or classes arise out of formerly kin-based social organizations. In this analysis, the creation of a class hierarchy is intimately linked to the creation of the patriarchal family and to restrictions on women's autonomy.

Engels' analysis provides the foundation for many themes concerning women that are currently being investigated: the relation between the economic roles of women, their control of resources, and their social status; the relation between the mode of production and the mode of reproduction;[1] and the effects of the separation or merger of domestic and public spheres of activity on the lives of women.[2] However, a thesis central to Engels' analysis—the link between class oppression and gender oppression—has remained less well examined. Drawing on a growing body of theory and data concerning state formation that has been amassed in recent years by twentieth-century archaeologists,[3] this article examines Engels' theory about the relationship between the subjugation of women, social stratification, and the rise of the state.

Most of the early theoretical work on emergence of state society was reductive, and it often condensed a multiplicity of processes into overly simplistic models. These theories ranged from a concentration on the extraction of social surplus (surplus material resources or labor beyond that needed for subsistence) via increasing division of labor and more productive technology (Childe 1950, 1952); to a focus on the emergence of central political authority to administer irrigation-based societies (Wittfogel 1955, 1957); to the effects of population pressure and warfare within circumscribed environments (Carneiro 1970, Harner 1970).

All of these theories tend to see the state as an inevitable and efficient solution to a particular set of problems. They ignore the specific historical, political, and economic contexts in which societies change.[4] Finally, they underplay the importance of kinship as a domain within which resistance to state formation is situated.[5] Not uncoincidentally, it is within the kinship domain that women's subordination appears to occur.

In recent years, a new set of theoretical formulations that are more processual and systemic have been developed. Such formulations offer fascinating hints about the role of kinship structure, and possibly women, in

Revised by the editors with the permission and approval of the author.

stratification. Some of the processes examined in state formation—the politics of kinship, the changing content and role of religious systems, the intensification of military complexes, and the role of trade in stimulating or increasing social stratification—are most pertinent to our interests here. I will discuss each of these briefly, suggesting some of the lines of inquiry they direct us to pursue.

THE POLITICS OF KINSHIP

Many anthropologists have examined the internal tensions of ranked kinship systems (Kirchoff 1959; Sahlins 1958; Fried 1967). In highly ranked kinship systems, the role of women is of crucial importance. Women not only transmit status, but may be contenders for leadership positions, either directly or through their children. This seems to be the case in Polynesia and in parts of Africa. As Gailey (1987) shows for Tonga, the existence of elite, ranked women became more problematic as stratification increased.

We need to know more about marriage patterns in such systems. In archaeology, ethnology, and Western history, we find that elite marriages may be implicated in the politics of establishing and maintaining long-distance trade and tribute systems.[6] Dowry is associated with highly stratified systems and dowered, elite women may appear as pawns in a classic case of male alliances formed via their exchange.[7] Ortner (1978) suggests that in state-organized systems, marriage may shift from horizontal alliances between individuals of similar social and economic backgrounds to vertical alliances between individuals of different backgrounds. In the latter situation there is a marked tendency toward hypergamy whereby lower-status women marry upper-status men. Ortner links these structural properties of the marriage system with ideologies requiring sexual purity and the protection of women (but not of men).

Silverblatt (1987), in a study of the Inca elite, suggests that as the Incas extended their rule, they required conquered communities to send women to Cuzco to serve in the temples, courts, and as noblemen's wives. For the conquered communities, this practice represented a loss of autonomy in marriage patterns, and a burden. At the same time, it made possible upward mobility to the specific males who sent sisters and daughters to Cuzco. The women themselves gained a great deal of prestige, but lost any control they might have had in arranging their own marriages and living within their natal communities.

CHANGING COSMOLOGIES

Both Silverblatt and Ortner draw our attention to the relationship between women and the religious systems in early states. They remind us that religious systems were the glue that cemented social relations in archaic societies. Such systems were used, as in the Inca case, to underwrite and justify changes in political hierarchies.

Tension about female status is often found within these religious systems. Eliade (1960) claims that the ritual expression of sexual antagonism and the existence of bisexual and/or androgynous gods accompanies the social organizational changes associated with the neolithic period. Male gods are often superimposed on female and androgynous gods. Evidence for this layering over of female and/or androgynous figures comes from Mesoamerica (Nash 1980), Peru (Silverblatt 1987), and is, of course, a favorite theme of classicists for early Greek society (Arthur 1976; Pomeroy 1975).

Pagels (1976), working with second-century A.D. Gnostic texts, analyzes the symbol system of sects in which the early Christian god was bisexual, and the Holy Family consisted of mother, father, and son. Such sects were organized into non-hierarchical religious communities, in which offices were rotated, and women participated in both teaching and preaching—a far cry from the ascendant

Christian cosmology and practice which became the mainstream tradition. Cosmological changes are ideological precipitates of structural tensions; it is clear that their form and content have a great deal to tell us about class and gender.

INTENSIFICATION OF WARFARE

As early states became increasingly militaristic, social organization was transformed.[8] Several case histories lead us to believe that under conditions of intense warfare, men were not only burdened by conscription, but were blessed with increasing power as household heads (Muller 1987; Rohrlich 1980). Elite males may gain land, political domains, and alliance-forming wives in the process. Yet, sweeping statements about male supremacy and warfare (Divale and Harris 1976) are overgeneralized, and some evidence seems to contradict the association of warfare and an elevation of male status at the expense of female autonomy.

In the ancient West, for example, the correlation often works the other way: Spartan women held offices, controlled their own property, and had a great deal of sexual freedom, allegedly because they kept society functioning while the men were at war. Moreover, producing soldiers was considered as important as training them. In Athens, women's access to public places and roles seems to have increased a great deal during times of warfare. In Rome, during the Second Punic War, women gained in inheritance settlements and held public offices formerly closed to them (Pomeroy 1975). In the medieval Franco-Germanic world, noblewomen attained approximate parity in politics and property-management during the years of the most brutal military crisis (McNamara and Wemple 1973).

All these examples concern elite women only; we know very little about the effects of warfare on laboring women, who probably suffered then, as they do now. Nonetheless, it is not clear that warfare degrades women's status; the specific context within which military organization and practice occurs must be taken into account. Blood and gore clearly are not universal variables in theorizing about women's subordination.

TRADE

The role of trade in increasing and/or spreading stratification is an intriguing one.[9] Foreign-trade goods may be spread in many ways: by middlemen, via migrations, through central trading centers, and in marriage exchanges, to name but a few. Several studies suggest that the social relationships that surround production and distribution, and which undergird trade, may generate class and gender inequality (Adams 1974; Kohl 1975; Wiley 1974; Gailey and Patterson 1987). We need to know who produces goods, who appropriates them, and who distributes them. As demand for a trade commodity increases, exploitation of labor to produce it may arise. Marriage systems may also be intensified to expand the reproduction of trading alliances. Certainly there are numerous ethnographic examples of polygyny as a means to increase access to goods that wives produce. There are also many instances of increasing class division linked to increasing bridewealth.

But the control, ownership, and distribution of valued resources after they are produced is not exclusively a male function. In Mesoamerica and the Andes, to this day, women are active in the marketplace. Silverblatt (1978) suggests that they were important traders in early Incan times. Adams (1966) records their existence in Mesopotamia. And of course, their presence is felt in stratified groups throughout Africa and the Caribbean as well (Mintz 1971). Under what conditions does long-distance trade pass into the hands of men, and when is it possible for women to continue to perform it? When women are traders, do they constitute an elite, class-stratified group? To the extent that trade is implicated in the intensification of production for exchange, women as producers, reproducers, and traders must be implicated too.

CONCLUSION: COLONIALISM, CAPITALIST PENETRATION, AND THE "THIRD WORLD"

As we come to identify the factors in state formation as they affect women, we must be careful to think in probabilistic rather than deterministic terms. We need to better understand the relative power of kinship and class, the interplay of household and public economic functions, the flexibility within religious systems, and the relative autonomy or subordination of women, in light of the possibilities open to each society. We should expect to find variations within state-making (and unmaking) societies over time, and between such societies, rather than one simple pattern.

Nowhere is this more evident than in analysis of the process of rapid penetration by patriarchal national states into the so-called Third World. While the history of such penetration varies from place to place and must be taken into account, certain patterns affecting the ways of life of women can be traced at a general level. Wherever women have been active horticulturalists of collective lands, the imposition of private property, taxation, labor migration, and cash cropping has had devastating effects. Their realm of productivity and expertise has been deformed and often destroyed (Blumberg 1976; Boserup 1970; Tinker 1976). Depending upon context, they may become either super-exploited, or underemployed, but always more dependent upon men.

The evidence also suggests a general pattern concerning political organization. Prior to colonial penetration, gender relations in indigenous cultures appear to have been organized along essentially parallel and complementary lines. Men and women had distinct but equally significant roles in production, distribution, and ritual activities.[10] Case histories from Africa, Asia, and the Americas suggest that patriarchal, colonizing powers rather effectively dismantled native work organizations, political structures, and ritual contexts. Leadership and authority were assigned to male activities, while female tasks and roles were devalued or obliterated. The complementary and parallel gender relations that characterized indigenous societies were destroyed. Several authors have gone so far as to argue that women, thus divested of their social organization and collective roles, have become like underdeveloped, monocrop regions. Once they lived in a diversified world; now they have been reduced to the role of reproducing and exporting labor power for the needs of the international world economy (Bossen 1973; Boulding 1975; Deere 1976).

State formation and penetration occurs over time; its form and force are highly variable, both within and between societies. Yet it is important to remember that the processes which began millennia ago are ongoing. Cumulatively, they continue to transform the lives of the masses of people who exist under their structures. It is a long way from the Sumerian law codes declaring monogamy for women to the welfare laws of the United States which affect parental relations and household structure. But in both cases, the power of the state to penetrate and reorganize the lives of its members is clear. As we seek to understand the complex, stratified societies in which we now operate, we are led to reflect on archaic societies in which the dual and intertwined processes of hierarchy we now retrospectively label "class" and "patriarchy" took their origins.

NOTES

1. Productive activities are those that generate income in cash, or other valued resources. Reproduction refers, broadly, to the set of activities encompassing domestic chores and other household activities such as childbearing, childrearing, and cooking.

2. For analyses implicitly or explicitly influenced by *Origins* see Brown 1975; Meillassoux 1975; Reiter 1975; Rubin 1975; Sacks 1974; Sanday 1974.
3. Summaries of the state formation literature may be found in Flannery 1972; Krader 1968; Service 1975; Webb 1975.
4. A less determinant and more processual perspective on stratification and state formation is set forth in Flannery 1972; Sabloff and Lamberg-Karlovsky 1975; and Tilly 1975. Such thinking also informs the corpus of Marxist historiography.
5. This has been a major thrust in Stanley Diamond's work (1951, 1974).
6. Such links are suggested in Flannery 1972; Wiley and Shimkin 1971; and by much of the literature on stratified chiefdoms (Sahlins 1958; Kirchoff 1959; and Fried 1967). In European history, we find instances in the international royal marriage patterns. See McNamara and Wemple (1973) for some of the implications of feudal marriage patterns.
7. See Arthur 1976; Ortner 1978; Goody and Tambiah 1973.
8. The temple and military complexes figure in the state formation schemes of Adams 1966; Steward 1955; and Wiley 1974 to name but a few.
9. The archaeology of trade is discussed in Sabloff and Lamberg-Karlovsky 1975, and is critically summarized in Adams 1974 and Kohl 1975. See also Wiley 1974.
10. Parallel and interarticulating forms of gender social organization are analyzed by Brown 1970; Silverblatt 1978; Siskind 1978; and Van Allen 1972.

REFERENCES

Adams, R. M. 1966. *The Evolution of Urban Society.* Chicago. Aldine

———. 1974. "Anthropological Perspectives on Ancient Trade." *Current Anthropology* 15: 239–258.

Arthur, M. 1976. "Liberated Women: The Classical Era." In R. Bridenthal and C. Koontz (eds.). *Becoming Visible: Women in European History.* New York: Houghton and Mifflin.

Blumberg, R. 1976. "Fairy Tales and Facts: Economy, Fertility, Family and the Female." Unpublished paper.

Boserup, E. 1970. *Women's Role in Economic Development.* London: George Allen and Unwin.

Bossen, L. 1973. "Women in Modernizing Societies." *American Ethnologist* 2: 587–601.

Boulding, E. 1975. *Women, Bread and Babies.* University of Colorado, Institute of Behavioral Sciences, Program on Research of General Social and Economic Development.

Brown, J. 1970. "A Note on the Economic Division of Labor by Sex." *American Anthropologist* 72: 1073–1078.

Brown, J. 1975. "Iroquois Women." In R. Reiter (ed.). *Toward an Anthropology of Women.* New York: Monthly Review Press.

Carneiro, R. J. 1970. "A Theory of the Origin of the State." *Science* 169: 733–738.

Childe, G. 1950. "The Urban Revolution." *Town Planning Review* 21 (3): 3–17.

Childe, G. 1952. "The Birth of Civilization." *Past and Present* 2: 1–10.

Deere, C. 1976. "Rural Women's Subsistence Production in the Capitalist Periphery." *Review of Radical Political Economics* 8: 9–18.

Diamond, S. 1951. *Dahomey: A Protostate in West Africa.* Ann Arbor: University of Michigan Press.

Diamond, S. 1974. *In Search of the Primitive: A Critique of Civilization.* New Brunswick NJ: Transaction Books.

Divale, W. and M. Harris. 1976. "Population Warfare and the Male Supremacist Complex." *American Anthropologist* 78: 521–538.

Eliade, M. 1960. "Structures and Changes in the History of Religions." In C. Kraeling and R. Adams (eds.). *City Invincible.* Chicago: University of Chicago Press.

Flannery, K. 1972. "The Cultural Evolution of Civilizations." *Annual Review of Ecology and Systematics* 3: 399–426.

Fried, M. 1960. "On the Evolution of Social Stratification and the State." In S. Diamond (ed.). *Culture and History.* New York: Columbia University Press.

———. 1967. *The Evolution of Political Society.* New York: Random House.

Gailey, Christine Ward. 1987. *Kinship to Kingship: Gender Hierarchy and State Formation in the Tongan Islands.* Austin: University of Texas Press.

Gailey, Christine Ward and Thomas C. Patterson. 1987. "Power Relations and State Formation." In Thomas C. Patterson and Christine W. Gailey (eds.). *Power Relations and State Formation,* pp. 1–26. Washington, DC: American Anthropological Association.

Goody, J. and S. Tambiah. 1973. *Bridewealth and Dowry.* Cambridge: Cambridge University Press.

Harner, M. 1970. "Population Pressure and Social Evolution of Agriculturalists." *Southwestern Journal of Anthropology* 26: 67–86.

Kirchoff, P. 1959. "The Principles of Clanship in Human Society." In M. Fried (ed.). *Readings in Anthropology* (Vol. 2). New York: Thomas Crowell.

Kohl, P. 1975. "The Archaeology of Trade." *Dialectical Anthropology* 1: 43–50.

Krader, L. 1968. *Formation of the State.* Englewood Cliffs: Prentice Hall.

Leacock, Eleanor. 1978. "Women's Status in Egalitarian Society: Implications for Social Evolution." *Current Anthropology* 19: 247–275.

McNamara, J. and S. Wemple. 1973. "The Power of Women through the Family in Medieval Europe: 500–1100." *Feminist Studies* 1: 126–141.

Meillassoux, C. 1975. *Femmes, greniers et capitaux.* Paris: Maspero.

Mintz, S. 1971. "Men, Women and Trade." *Comparative Studies in Society and History* 13: 247–269.

Muller, Viana. 1987. "Kin Reproduction and Elite Accumulation in the Archaic States of Northwest Europe." In Thomas C. Patterson and Christine W. Gailey (eds.). *Power Relations and State Formation.* pp. 81–97. Washington, DC: American Anthropological Association.

Nash, J. 1980. "Aztec Women: The Transition from Status to Class in Empire and Colony." In M. Etienne and E. Leacock (eds.). *Women and Colonization.* New York: Praeger.

Ortner, S. 1978. "The Virgin and the State." *Feminist Studies* 4 (3): 19–35.

Pagels, E. 1976. "What Became of God the Mother? Conflicting Images of God in Early Christianity" *Signs* 2: 293–303.

Pomeroy, S. 1975. *Goddesses, Whores, Wives and Slaves.* New York: Schoken Books.

Reiter, R. 1975. "Men and Women in the South of France." In R. Reiter (ed.). *Toward an Anthropology of Women.* New York: Monthly Review Press.

Rohrlich, Ruby. 1980. "State Formation in Sumer and the Subjugation of Women." *Feminist Studies* 6: 76–102.

Rubin, G. 1975. "The Traffic in Women." In R. Reiter (ed.). *Toward an Anthropology of Women.* New York: Monthly Review Press.

Sabloff, J. and C.C. Lamberg-Karlovsky. 1975. *Ancient Civilizations and Trade.* Albuquerque: University of New Mexico Press.

Sacks, K. 1974. "Engels Revisited." In Michelle Rosaldo and Louise Lamphere (eds.). *Woman, Culture and Society.* Stanford: Stanford University Press.

———. 1982. *Sisters and Wives: The Past and Future of Sexual Equality.* Urbana: University of Illinois Press.

Sahlins, M. 1958. *Social Stratification in Polynesia.* Seattle: University of Washington Press.

Sanday, Peggy. 1974. "Toward a Theory of the Status of Women." In Michelle Rosaldo and Louise Lamphere (eds.). *Woman, Culture and Society.* Stanford: Stanford University Press.

———. 1981. *Female Power and Male Dominance: On the Origins of Sexual Inequality.* Cambridge: Cambridge University Press.

Service, E. 1975. *Origins of the State and Civilization.* New York: Norton.

Silverblatt, Irene. 1978. "Andean Women in Inca Society." *Feminist Studies* 4 (3): 37–61.

———. 1987. *Moon, Sun, and Witches: Gender Ideologies and Class in Inca and colonial Peru.* Princeton: Princeton University Press.

———. 1988. "Women in States." *Annual Review of Anthropology* 17: 427–461.

Siskind, J. 1978. "Kinship and Mode of Production." *American Anthropologist* 80: 860–872.

Steward, J. 1955. *The Theory of Culture Change.* Urbana: University of Illinois Press.

Tilly, C. 1975. "Reflections on the History of European State-Making." In C. Tilly (ed.). *The Formation of National States in Western Europe.* Princeton: Princeton University Press.

Tinker, I. 1976. "The Adverse Impact of Development on Women." In I. Tinker and M. Bramsen (eds.). *Women and World Development.* Washington, DC: Overseas Development Council.

Van Allen, J. 1972. "Sitting on a Man: Colonialism and the Lost Political Institutions of Igbo Women." *Canadian Journal of African Studies* 6: 165–181.

Webb, M. 1975. "The Flag Follows Trade." In J. Sabloff and C.C. Lamberg-Karlovsky (eds.). *Ancient Civilizations and Trade.* Albuquerque: University of New Mexico Press.

Wiley, G. 1974. "Precolumbian Urbanism." In J. Sabloff and C.C. Lamberg-Karlovsky (eds.). *Ancient Civilizations and Trade.* Albuquerque: University of New Mexico Press.

Wiley, G. and D. Shimkin. 1971. "The Collapse of the Classic Maya Civilization in the Southern Lowlands." *Southwestern Journal of Anthropology* 27: 1–18.

Wittfogel, K. 1955. "Oriental Society in Transition." *Far Eastern Quarterly* 14: 469–478.

———. 1957. *Oriental Despotism.* New Haven: Yale University Press.

DOWRY, BRIDE-BURNING, AND FEMALE POWER IN INDIA

Linda Stone and Caroline James

Synopsis—An increasing number of bride-burnings or dowry murders have been reported from India. These are cases of married women being murdered, usually burned to death, by husbands or in-laws whose demands for more dowry from the bride's family remain unmet. Using published accounts of these incidents along with interview material from one woman who escaped burning, this article examines the problem in terms of recent changes in women's roles and sources of female power. It is tentatively suggested that bride-burnings not only reflect women's relative lack of economic power in modern India, but might also reflect a diminishing of the power Indian women traditionally exercised through their fertility.

Over the last two decades, the reports from India have shocked the world: married women murdered (usually burned to death) by their husbands and/or in-laws over the issue of inadequate dowry. These recent incidents of bride-burning are a shocking example of the new forms of violence against women which are arising in modern, or modernizing, settings in many areas of the world. In India, these events are occurring alongside the growth of feminist organizations, the expansion of educational and economic opportunities for women, and some societal questioning of traditional gender roles.

This article examines the bride-burning problem in India by looking at recent changes which have occurred not only with respect to dowry transactions, but also with respect to more traditional sources of female domestic power. It is not possible here to consider all of the complex factors which are contributing to the dowry murders in India, but we suggest, though necessarily tentatively, that along with the traditional lack of female control over family property and marriage arrangements, the problem may be further compounded by a new loss of female power in another important sphere, namely the power women could traditionally exercise through their fertility.

The article draws upon published accounts of bride-burning combined with material from interviews with a bride-burning survivor carried out by one of the authors (James). This case emerged not from research focused on bride-burning, but rather as part of a larger study of literacy programs in adult education centers in Madhya Pradesh. In this study James (1988) found that many of the women who came to the adult education centers were fleeing dowry harassment or attempted burnings. The case we present here was selected for the depth and detail of information provided by the woman involved.

Before examining dowry murders, we offer some comments on dowry in India to place the issue in a broader cross-cultural perspective.

DOWRY IN INDIA

One feature of dowry systems in general which applies strongly to India is their association with socioeconomic stratification and the concerns of kin groups with maintaining or enhancing social status through marriage. In an historical treatment of dowry, Goody (1971, 1973, 1976) argued that in Eurasia, in contrast to Africa, intensive plow agriculture created differential wealth, promoting divisions between status groups. It then became important to perpetuate these divisions over the generations to insure that control over

Reprinted with permission from *Women's Studies International Forum* 18 (2): 125–135, by Linda Stone and Caroline James. (Oxford, England: Elsevier Science Ltd., Pergamon Imprint, 1995.)

property remained within the status group. This was achieved in part by instituting "status group endogamy" through the mechanism of dowry marriage. Thus, "status group endogamy"

> . . . is not simply a question of the absence of marriage between groups . . . but of matching like for like, or getting an even better bargain. And the usual mechanism by which this is achieved is the matching of property, often by means of the dowry. . . . (Goody, 1973, p. 593)

Dowry, then, goes hand-in hand with a class system and with maintenance of the superiority of higher groups over lower. Here marriages, at least among the upper classes, must be well-controlled and, by extension, so must courtship. The roles of matchmaker and chaperone become important in this Eurasian context, along with a high value placed on female virginity at marriage (Goody, 1976, p. 17). Women must be endowed with property in order to attract husbands of equal or higher rank, and their sexuality must be controlled in order to limit ". . . the possibility of conflicting claims on the estate in which a woman has rights" (Goody, 1976, p. 14). Schlegel (1991) has more recently confirmed the strong association between dowry transactions and cultural concerns with female premarital virginity, which, she argues, helps to prevent lower class males from claiming wealth through impregnating higher class females. Ultimately the whole complex of cultural values centering on female "purity" and the notion that the honor of male kin groups rests on the seclusion and sexual purity of its women (see Mandelbaum, 1988) is related to the institution of dowry as an instrument in preserving and perpetuating socioeconomic classes. As we shall see, both the themes of social status and female chastity recur through accounts of dowry murders.

There is, however, another common idea about dowry systems which does not apply well in India. This is the idea that dowry is a form of female property or wealth. Thus, Goody (1973) and others (e.g., Tambiah, 1973) have seen Eurasian dowry universally as "female inheritance"—women receive a portion of the family estate at marriage, rather than upon the death of the father or mother. This portion they receive as movable property rather than land which is left to sons. But many working in India, such as Miller (1981) and Sharma (1984), have convincingly shown that whereas this may be true in many areas of the world, in India dowry is property which passes from the bride's family to that of the groom, and that even if perceived to be "women's property" (*stridhan*) by some Indians themselves, in fact a bride does not have (and historically never had) genuine control over the use and distribution of this property. Women in the Indian dowry system should be seen as vehicles of property transmission rather than as true inheritors.

Madhu Kishwar (1986), who has written several articles on dowry for the Indian feminist magazine *Manushi,* has argued that Indian dowry effectively functions to disinherit women and promote their economic dependency on men, which in her view is the real crux of the modern problem of dowry murders. Although current law permits daughters to inherit from the father's estate, more often women are upon marriage made to sign over these rights to their brothers. As for the dowry itself, Kishwar (1986) writes:

> In actuality, a woman is seldom allowed to have control even over things that are supposedly for her personal use. Gold and other jewelry are traditionally supposed to be a woman's personal security, but, in practice, the gold usually stays in the custody of her mother-in-law or husband. It is up to them to give her what they wish for her personal use and daily wear . . . It is fairly common for certain items of her jewelry to be incorporated into her husband's sister's dowry. (pp. 6–7)

Moreover, Kishwar points out that were the point of Indian dowry to provide a daughter with some financial security, parents would give her productive assets such as land or a shop, rather than clothing and household goods, which depreciate in value.

Defining dowry as female inheritance, Goody (1976) saw it as a kind of economic "gain" for women. But the irony, to him, was that the system also entails a "loss" of women's control over their marriages or their sexual behavior:

> The positive control of marriage arrangements . . . is stricter where property is transmitted to women. It is a commentary on their lot that where they are more propertied they are initially less free as far as marital arrangements go. (Goody, 1976, p. 21)

But in the Indian context, it would appear that women lose on all counts. This context (and the whole question of sources, or lack of sources, of female power) is important to bear in mind in any discussion of dowry murders. In India dowry not only serves to promote status group endogamy (hypergamy) to maintain a class system, but it is now actively manipulated to serve new ends of status-seeking among individual families. In this modern context, women as vehicles of property transmission not only lack control over both property and marriage arrangements, as was largely the case previously, but may in fact suffer considerable harassment, physical abuse, and even murder in connection with their roles as bringers of dowry.

DOWRY MURDERS

From what is known about dowry deaths, it is possible to see some patterns, although exceptions exist in every case. They appear to be largely, though not exclusively, occurring in Northwest India, and they are largely, though no longer exclusively, among Hindu groups. They occur most often in cases of arranged marriages (the most common form of marriage in India) but have occurred in cases of a "love match," and they occur predominantly among the urban middle-class (Kumari, 1989; van Willigen & Channa, 1991). It is difficult to know how widespread the problem is, but most conservative estimates are that at least 2000 women are victims of dowry deaths per year in India (Chhabra, 1986, pp. 12–13). The area showing the greatest problem is New Delhi, with an estimated two dowry deaths per day (Bordewich, 1986, p. 21). The number of reported cases increases yearly. It is not known to what extent the increase reflects an increase in reporting rather than an increase in the crime. However, it may be that the crime is still underreported since the number of hospital cases of severe burns in young married women exceeds reports of violence against women by burning (Kumari, 1989, p. 24).

The preponderance of cases of bride-burning in North India is significant. This is also the area in which Miller (1981) finds significantly more males than females in juvenile age groups. This she attributes to neglect of female children, who are an economic liability relative to males. In the Northern region, too, dowry marriages are more common. The expense of providing dowry for daughters is one reason which Miller finds for the relatively intense preference for sons and relative neglect of female children in the North.

Sharma suggests that North Indian dowry has dramatically inflated as India has shifted to a market, cash economy over the last 50 years: ". . . dowry used to be more or less conventionally determined and many items could be made in whole or part by members of the bride's family themselves (e.g. rugs, clothing, bedding)" (Sharma, 1984, p. 70). But now, especially among the urban middle classes, expectations of televisions, motor scooters, refrigerators, large sums of cash, and so on are usual. Many observers related modern dowry and dowry deaths to the frustration of the urban middle class, caught in a new consumerism, status-seeking, and rising expectations of a life style they cannot on their own earning power quite afford (Bordewich, 1986, pp. 24–25).

Sharma's (1984) work on dowry has also cleared up one confusion, namely how it is that marriageable women appear to be in great supply (everyone is anxious to marry off a daughter and even accused dowry murderers manage to secure new brides!) even though there are far more males than females in the marriageable age groups in the North. Hypergamy (marriage of women upward into higher status groups) was traditionally common in the North and with modern dowry is becoming more so. In addition, lessening of caste restrictions in modern marriages promotes more hypergamous competition. Dowry givers are thus competing upwards for scarce grooms at the top (Sharma, 1984, p. 72).

Dowry and dowry murders continue despite the fact that dowry transactions have been illegal in India since the Dowry Prohibition Act of 1961.[1] As a result of pressure by women's organizations, subsequent amendments to the Act have even strengthened the laws against dowry and dowry harassment (Ghadially & Kumar, 1988, pp. 175–176). However, what is actually dowry can be legally claimed as "voluntary gifts" at marriage. Dowry persists not only because the law is ineffective or difficult to enforce, nor because of the pressures and demands of the groom's family, but also because the families of brides, in spite of growing public awareness of the tragic consequences, continue to give dowry. This may be due to concerns that otherwise a daughter could not be married at all (universally considered and undesirable event in India), or that the family could not secure an appropriate match. Also, parents of the bride may continue to believe that a lavish dowry will help to secure their daughter's favorable treatment in her in-laws' home, after which they may "yield to extortion out of fear for their daughter's safety . . ." (Bordewich, 1986, p. 24). Stein (1988) reports that many Indian women "still believe . . . that not only can dowry be used to overcome disadvantages in the marriage market, such as dark skin color, but it gives them dignity and status" (p. 485).

From the reported cases of dowry murders, it appears that the difficulties usually start early in the marriage. A new bride is harassed and criticized for the pitiful dowry she has brought. She is encouraged to wrangle more and more from her family, yet her in-laws remain unsatisfied until, at some point, the situation explodes into an attempt on her life. One woman ("Sita") whose husband attempted to burn her, reported the following:

> I got married when I was 23 years old to a person whose family was not as wealthy as our family. My father [a businessman] gave $8,000 cash as dowry. [He] gave me expensive clothes like 500 saris, 10 golden jewelry sets and one diamond set, all the pots and pans necessary for the house, a television set, wardrobe, freezer, cooler fan, double bed, furniture and other things he thought would be useful in the house. More than that, he used to send things from time to time, like on festivals. One year of my marriage has not passed when my in-laws and husband started giving me trouble every day for more dowry. My mother-in-law started telling my husband, "Leave this woman and we will get you another one, at least the other party will give us more and better dowry than what these people have given us. What her parents have given us is nothing. Moreover, this girl is ugly and she is dark."

Sita's reference to the relative wealth of her family and her detailed description of her lavish dowry appear to reinforce the same materialistic values which evidently lie behind dowry harassment and murders. Later she spoke with bitter resentment about her husband's new wife who ". . . is using all my things, like all my expensive saris, jewelry and other things." Her account also suggests a blatant economic motive for dowry murder—that it frees the woman's in-laws to get a new bride and an additional dowry. A similar idea reported in an article by Bordewich (1986) is expressed by the father of an allegedly murdered bride:

> . . . as soon as we agreed on the marriage they started troubling us. First they told us to buy diamond rings instead of mere gold ones . . . Then they insisted on a sofa bed for fifteen thousand rupees, but I could only afford one that cost seven thousand. Whatever was in my means I did, but they were always displeased . . . they demanded a stereo and tape-cassette system, and then they asked for saris for the boy's sisters . . .

and then for a gas stove. I gave them . . . I had read that there were so many tortures and murders of young women over dowry and I was afraid of what might happen to [my daughter]. I told them I would pay whatever I could . . . But they didn't even wait for the money to come. They probably realized they had gotten all they could from us. A few days later [my daughter] was dead . . . There has never been an investigation . . . Now they can marry their son to another girl and get another dowry. (p. 25)

The most common means of murder is soaking the bride in kerosene and setting her aflame, with a report to the police of a suicide or an accident in the kitchen. Sita describes how this was attempted on her:

[The winter my son was born] my mother-in-law started telling me not to wear so much gold jewelry at home, to remove it at night and keep it in the wardrobe. I did not understand why she was telling me this when she had not done so before. But I did what she asked. [Then] one evening my husband went into the kitchen and asked for a match box. My mother-in-law's sister-in-law gave him a match box which my husband then kept in the wardrobe very close to our bed. Then he left the house, saying he would be coming in late that night. That same evening, the electricity went off and my mother-in-law's sister-in-law came to get the match box to light a lamp. She found the match box in the wardrobe and took it. My husband came in very late that night when my son and I were sound asleep. Due to the cold, I had pulled the covers up over our heads. Suddenly I felt that the quilt was wet and cold, but I thought it was just due to being cold at night. But when I removed the quilt from my face, there was a strong smell of kerosene. I got up quickly and saw my husband getting into bed and covering himself, pretending he was sound asleep . . . he had been looking for the match box which he could not find. You can imagine that if he could have found the match box, my son and I would not have survived. We would have been burned to ashes.

One theme recurrent in many dowry murder cases is the issue of the bride's "reputation" and sexual "purity," which, as we saw in Goody's (1976) discussions of dowry, serves as a link between the institution of dowry, family concerns with status, and the perpetuation of socio-economic classes. With respect to this issue, a woman facing dowry harassment is truly vulnerable as any suggestion of her "loose" character is an easy defense for her husband or in-laws. In the case above Sita reports that after fleeing from the bed,

I started crying loudly, then my husband and mother-in-law came and started telling me to leave the house. I told them I would not step out of the house until my parents came, because if I would have left the house, they would have told the police and everybody that I was the one who wanted to leave the husband and the house, that it was my fault and not anyone else's in the family. They would have cooked up another story that I am a bad character and that that is why I left the house at that hour of the night (3:00 a.m.).

In a dowry murder case discussed by Kumari (1989), the husband accused of burning his young wife claimed that she had committed suicide because she could not forget her own "murky past" involving previous sexual activity (p. 64). Similarly, in newspaper accounts of dowry deaths it is common to find some innuendo of lapsed sexual behavior on the part of the victim.[2] Also illustrative is the following account, taken down by Bordewich (1986), from a woman who virtually sees a dowry murder:

. . . In the house across the street we could see a man beating his wife. I went out onto the balcony and saw that the neighbors had gathered in the street to watch . . . A moment later I heard a scream . . . and there in front of me was the woman, burning in the window. She tried to wrap herself in the curtains, but they went up in flames. I ran into the street, but none of the neighbors seemed disturbed. People were saying it was "just a domestic issue" or that the woman must have had "a loose moral character." The woman died soon afterward in the hospital. The husband was never charged. (p. 26)

DOWRY, FERTILITY, AND FEMALE POWER

Dowry murders must be viewed within the context of Indian culture, which is characterized by patrilineal descent, patrilocality, the joint family, and strongly prescribed subservience of wives to husbands and in-laws. In both the popular press and scholarly literature, discussions of dowry murders incorporate these and other elements of Indian cultural traditions and women's roles within them. Certainly the association of death, fire, and female chastity or purity has caught the attention of writers who have drawn parallels between modern bride-burning and the ancient upper caste custom of *sati,* or the burning of a widow alive on her husband's funeral pyre. This was considered a (theoretically self-willed) act of great religious merit, only to be performed by a chaste wife in a state of ritual purity (Stein, 1988, p. 464). Again, in Hindu mythology, Sita must prove her chastity to her husband, Rama, through passing unburned through fire, and in another myth Sati Devi proves her loyalty to her husband, Shiva, by leaping to her death into the ceremonial fire of her father who insulted him.

Whatever deeper meaning all this may have within the Indian consciousness, Stein (1988) rightly points out that both the ancient sati and modern bride-burning reflect one clear fact of Indian life: the unacceptability of the unmarried adult woman. Thus sati was a way to dispose of the widow, who in earlier times among high castes, could not remarry, but who could, if alive, remain in society as a threatening, uncontrolled sexual woman. In the modern context, the existence of an unmarried adult daughter, with all the same connotations of uncontrolled, dangerous sexuality, brings shame and dishonor to her parents whose duty it is to marry her off, and who receive religious merit for doing so. So great is the pressure to marry the daughter (and keep her married, a divorced woman being equally unacceptable and threatening in Indian society) that a woman's parents remain in a weak and vulnerable position with respect to dowry harassment. Stein (1988) concludes:

> . . . marriage is still seen as the only way in which Indian women can be part of their own society, can function as social beings, even at the expense of their own personalities, and occasionally their lives. (p. 485)

The situation is compounded by another deep-rooted Indian tradition: the religious and social inferiority of the bride's family to that of the groom. In Hindu tradition a bride is a religious gift (*kanyadan,* gift of the virgin) and, as such, can only be given upward to those of higher rank, those to whom one must show perpetual deference and respect. The inferior and subservient position of a wife to her husband is on another level shared by the family who gives her. Thus "the subordination and frequently oppressed position of the daughter-in-law is exacerbated by the exclusion and deference of her own kin" (Stein, 1988, p. 476).

Kishwar (1986) also refers to these relationships in her discussions of dowry deaths, highlighting the powerless position of a bride and her parents. For her, dowry harassment is but one of many techniques by which a groom and his family can humiliate a bride to "accept a subordinate position within the family and feel grateful for being allowed to survive at all in the marital home" (p. 4). She also affirms that marriage of the daughter and dowry are matters of status and family honor, so that ". . . most parents would rather see their daughters dead than have them get a divorce and return permanently to the parental home" (p. 5).

Chhabra (1986), noting the many cases of dowry deaths which involve the mother-in-law, discusses the role of the traditionally problematic relationship between a woman and her daughter-in-law in India in terms of modern dowry harassment. Participating in or encouraging dowry harassment is the mother-in-law's way of rejecting the new bride, whom she perceives as a threat to her son's support and loyalty to herself (pp. 6–10).

All of these socio-cultural factors and many more are fundamental to accounting for dowry deaths and, along with the inability of police and the courts to alleviate the problem, go a long way toward explaining why these deaths persist. However, most of these cultural traditions, which have in various ways, degrees, and combinations deeply shaped Indian women's lives, have been around for centuries, whereas dowry murders are apparently quite new, becoming a recognized social issue in India in the 1970s (Kumari, 1989). The concept of "dowry death" was only legally established in India in the 1980s (van Willigen & Channa, 1991, p. 371).

What has changed in Indian society to bring about this form of violence against women? Along with the new socioeconomic issues already referred to, it is important to ask also whether women in this modern context have lost sources of power which previously gave them some leverage. Despite all the constraints on women and the general sense of powerlessness which any account of the traditional Hindu woman's life will give, it was still the case that a new bride did not endlessly suffer ill-treatment from and subservience to in-laws, but gradually transformed herself from lowly bride to respected mother, perhaps eventually to become a powerful mother-in-law herself.[3] Regardless of however lowly the position of the affinal women in this strongly patrilineal society, she was, at worst, a necessary evil since she alone held the power to reproduce the husband's lineage. In a more traditional scenario, the adept Hindu woman tried to please her husband not only to express a culturally required subservience but also in order to become pregnant, as this would ultimately be her way out of misery and toward a rising status within the husband's household. With each sign of successful fertility, and particularly with the birth of sons, her position improved. As with many areas of Asia, sons were desired to continue the patrilineage, serve as heirs, perform important funeral rituals for parents, and to provide security in old age. Economically they contributed to home-based production or could bring in cash income.

A woman's fertility was the key to what can be considered a "great transition" in her status and identity. Summarizing this for the whole of India, Mandelbaum (1970) wrote of the bride that

> . . . the real relief comes when she becomes pregnant. Her mother-in-law can afford to relax a bit in her role as taskmistress; her husband is pleased; the men of the household are glad; there is an awakened interest in seeing that she eats well and rests easily. This first burgeoning also marks her first upward move in the family status hierarchy. . . .[then with childbirth] She is no longer the lowly probationer she was at first. If the child is a son, she has proved herself in the most important way of all and her confidence is the more secure. The son is her social redeemer and thenceforth her importance in the family tends gradually to increase. (pp. 88–89)

Raising this issue shifts the focus somewhat away from dowry, over which women evidently never had much control, and toward other sources of female power which may be changing, at least among the urban middle classes of the North. In a sense, female fertility, or the high value placed on women's successful reproduction, may have served as a "safety valve" for women in the past. But once this fertility value diminishes, women's position is indeed insecure. One startling feature of the dowry murder cases is the high number of women murdered who had already produced children, even sons. In one study 36% of the dowry murder cases involved women who had already produced children; another 11% of the women were pregnant at the time of death (Ghadially & Kumar, 1988, p. 168). Although she does not give numbers, Stein (1988) notes of dowry murder victims that ". . . a surprising number of them are pregnant when they die" (pp. 474–475).

Even victims of dowry harassment seem surprised to realize that childbirth and particularly the birth of a son does not alleviate their situation. Sita, in the case discussed earlier, remarked that after being harassed over dowry, "I gave birth to a male child. [But even with this] they did not want to keep me or the child either. They cared only for the dowry." Similarly in the case of Suman, described in the Indian feminist magazine *Manushi,* it was reported that

> ... [The husband's] maltreatment of Suman continued to escalate. He pawned all her jewelry. Even the birth of her son did not improve the situation. When the son was a year old, Suman was once more beaten and thrown out of the house in the hope of pressuring her parents to give more dowry. (Kishwar, 1986, p. 8)

Demographic data from India supports the suggestion that the country's traditional strong value on high fertility may be changing. Fertility rates are declining and have been since the mid-1960s. An analysis of the 1981 census produced the following report:

> India, the second most populous country in the world, is experiencing the early stages of fertility transition. The unprecedented acceleration in the rate of growth of India's population, sparked off by declining mortality as early as 1921, has finally been arrested ... It is beyond doubt that a significant contribution to this phenomenon lately has been from declining fertility, of which there is ample cumulative evidence. (Rele, 1987, p. 513)

One reason for the decline is undoubtedly urbanization, which tends to dampen fertility since the "cost" of children increases while their economic benefits decline. The above report also shows that the pace of decline is accelerating and that although the decline is occurring in both rural and urban areas, urban fertility remains much lower than rural fertility. Other studies show that fertility rates are lower and declining faster among wealthier and more educated groups (Goyal, 1989). Along with fertility declines, some studies show declines in desired number of children, again most notable among urban, educated, and wealthier groups (Jejeebhoy & Kulkarni, 1989).

Could it be that changes in fertility values are taking place and that, however advantageous this may be for India's population problems, it may be a contributing factor to dowry murders? Demonstrating a significant change in fertility values (beyond merely showing a decline in fertility levels) and a definite connection with dowry murders would, of course, require much further research. Nevertheless, our inquiry into dowry murders, and discussion of the problem within the context of more traditional ways in which women acquired some domestic leverage, is suggestive. Previously through much of India a large joint family and the production of many sons was itself a source of prestige. Through successful reproduction, women could gain respect and greater security in the husband's household. In today's context, children and grandchildren, though undoubtedly still desired for all the same cultural reasons as before, become economically less important. At the same time a new urban consumerism and concern with material displays of wealth is widely reported in India and is directly referred to in all studies of dowry deaths. We suggest that insofar as these shifts in values may be occurring, they may diminish the domestic leverage women once exercised through reproduction.

WOMEN IN PRODUCTION AND REPRODUCTION

In his study of dowry systems, Goody (1976) incorporated the work of Boserup (1970), who distinguished systems of "female farming" (shifting cultivation), where women perform the major part of agricultural work, from "male farming" (plow agriculture) where male labor predominates. The latter is associated with private land ownership, a landless class of laborers, and dowry, as opposed to bridewealth marriages. Boserup saw the development of male farming in Asia, and the later shift to male farming in Africa, as detrimental to women since the diminution of their roles in production increased their economic and social marginalization.[4]

Boserup (1970) made the important point that in regions of female farming, women are valued both as workers and as child bearers, whereas in systems of male farming, they are valued as mothers only (p. 51). Applying these ideas to modern, urban India (where the valued economic activity is income-earning), it appears that a new problem facing women, at least among the middle classes, may be that women lack value, and therefore power, either as workers or as mothers. Of course middle class Indian women can and do make important contributions to household income, increasingly so in the modern context. But, as Sharma (1984) points out, we need to look at women's work in relation to the proportion of their economic potential relative to that of men:

> It might be possible to show that the expansion of dowry has been accompanied by a decline in women's capacity to contribute household income *compared with that of men,* even though there has been no absolute diminution of women's economic activity. New opportunities to earn cash wages in factories, in government employment and white collar occupations have expanded far more rapidly for men than for women . . . .(pp. 67–68)

Boserup's critics (Beneria & Sen, 1981) claim that one problem with her analysis is that she ignored women's roles in reproduction. Their point is that women's reproductive roles in many cases hinder their full or equal participation in wage labor or other socially valued economic activities, whereas Boserup laid the blame on sexually biased cultural values and changes in technology. In fact, however, Boserup did address women's roles in reproduction, though not quite in the way her critics would have liked to have seen. Writing before 1970, she seems to have foreseen that changes in fertility values could occur and could negatively impact women. Speaking in general of societies with male farming systems, where women have been devalued as workers but are still valued as mothers, she wrote: "There is a danger in such a community that the propaganda for birth control, if successful, may further lower the status of women both in the eyes of men and in their own eyes" (Boserup, 1970, p. 51). Whereas it is unlikely that "propaganda for birth control" alone would have this effect, it may be that in India, urbanization and the growth of the consumer economy are bringing about the same result.

CONCLUSION

Many observers of the problem of dowry murders in India have contributed to showing a powerful link between this form of violence against women and women's relative lack of economic power. With the urbanization and consumerism characterizing India today, women have not shared in access to new economic opportunities with men. We suggest that at the same time, their one traditional source of leverage, their fertility, has possibly diminished in value. Regrettably, women are valued for the dowry they will bring; but so long as their valuation rests primarily in their being vehicles of property transmission, they will remain vulnerable to dowry harassment and murder.

NOTES

1. In India there has been a long history of anti-dowry movements, and only recently have they concerned dowry harassment and murder issues. For discussion see Kumari (1989).
2. This observation was made by Frank Myka (personal communication) in his review of cases of dowry murders in the *Hindustan Times* during 1989.
3. For discussion of these aspects of women's lives in Hindu Nepal see Bennett (1983).
4. Boserup's work was an early contribution to what has become a vast literature that links female subordination to women's roles in production and women's access to property. Many of the arguments put forth in this line of research follow, with modification, Engels' (1884) treatise on the origin of the family. Important current studies can be found in Leacock and Safa (1986). Modern studies have in

general emphasized that both the development of the world capitalist system and international development projects in the Third World have had adverse consequences for women. Today, different positions are taken within this framework. For a review of the literature see Tiano (1987).

REFERENCES

Beneria, Lourdes, & Sen, Gita. (1981). "Accumulation, Reproduction and Women's Role in Economic Development: Boserup Revisited." *Signs,* 7, 279–298.

Bennett, Lynn. (1983). *Dangerous Wives and Sacred Sisters: Social and Religious Roles of High Caste Women in Nepal.* New York: Columbia University Press.

Bordewich, Fergus M. (1986. July). "Dowry Murders." *Atlantic Magazine,* pp. 21–27.

Boserup, Ester. (1970). *Women's Role in Economic Development.* London: George Allen & Unwin, Ltd.

Chhabra, Sagari. (1986). *Dowry Deaths in India: A Double Bind Perspective.* Unpublished master's thesis, Washington State University, Pullman.

Engels, Fredrich. (1884). *The Origin of the Family, Private Property and the State.* New York: International.

Ghadially, Rehana, & Kumar, Promod. (1988). "Bride-burning: The psycho-social dynamics of dowry deaths." In Rehana Ghadially (Ed.), *Women in Indian Society* (pp. 167–177). New Delhi: Sage Publications.

Goody, Jack. (1971). "Class and Marriage in Africa and Eurasia." *American Journal of Sociology.* 76, 585–603.

Goody, Jack. (1973). "Bridewealth and Dowry in Africa and Eurasia." Jack Goody & S. J. Tambiah (Eds.), *Bridewealth and Dowry* (pp. 1–58). Cambridge: Cambridge University Press.

Goody, Jack. (1976). *Production and Reproduction.* Cambridge: Cambridge University Press.

Goyal, R. S. (1989). "Social Inequalities and Fertility Behavior." In S. N. Singh, M. K. Premi, P. S. Bhatia, & Ashish Bose (Eds.) *Population Transition in India* (Vol. 2, pp. 153–161). New Delhi: B. R. Publishing Corporation.

James, Caroline. (1988). *People and Projects in Development Anthropology: A Literacy Project in Madhya Pradesh, India.* Unpublished PhD dissertation, Washington State University, Pullman.

Jejeebhoy, Shireen J., & Sumati, Kulkami. (1989). "Demand for Children and Reproductive Motivation: Empirical Observations from Rural Maharashtra." In Singh, M. K. Premi, P. S. Bhatia, & Ashish Bose (Eds.), *Population Transition in India* (Vol. 2; pp. 107–121). New Delhi: B. R. Publishing Corporation.

Kishwar, Madhu. (1986). Dowry: "To Ensure her Happiness or to Disinherit her?" *Manushi,* 34, 2–13.

Kumari, Rajana. (1989). *Brides are not for Burning: Dowry Victims in India.* London: Sangam Books Ltd.

Leacock, Eleanor, Safa, Helen, & Contributors. (1986). *Women's Work, Development and the Division of Labor by Gender.* Boston: Bergin and Garvey Publishers, Inc.

Mandelbaum, David, (1970). "Society in India," Vol 1: *Continuity and Change.* Berkeley: University of California Press.

Mandelbaum, David, (1988). *Women's Seclusion and Men's Honor.* Tuscon: University of Arizona Press.

Miller, Barbara. (1981). *The Endangered Sex.* Ithaca: Cornell University Press.

Rele, J. R. (1987). "Fertility Levels and Trends in India." *Population and Development Review,* 13, 513–530.

Schlegel, Alice. (1991). "Status, Property and the Value on Virginity." *American Ethnologist,* 18, 719–734.

Sharma, Ursula. (1984). "Dowry in North India: Its Consequences for Women." Renee Hirschon (Ed.). *Women and Property—Women as Property* (pp. 62–73). New York: St. Martin's Press.

Stein, Dorothy. (1988). "Burning Widows, Burning Brides: The Perils of Daughterhood in India." *Pacific Affairs,* 61, 465–485.

Tambiah, S. J. (1973). "Dowry and Bridewealth and the Property Rights of Women in South Asia." In Jack Goody & S. J. Tambiah (Eds.), *Bridewealth and Dowry* (pp. 59–169). Cambridge, MA: Cambridge University Press.

Tiano, Susan. (1987). "Gender, Work and World Capitalism: Third World Women's Role in Development." In Beth B. Hess & Myra Marx Ferree (Eds.), *Analyzing Gender: A Handbook of Social Science Research* (pp. 216–243) Newbury Park: Sage Publications.

van Willigen, John, & Channa, V.C. (1991). "Law, Custom, and Crimes Against Women: The problem of Dowry Death in India." *Human Organization,* 50, 369–376.

THE LEGAL AND SOCIAL TRANSFORMATION OF RURAL WOMEN IN AEGEAN TURKEY

June Starr

INTRODUCTION

This paper links three independent ideas. First, it provides an alternative model to Engels' provocative theory, expounded in *The Origin of the Family, Private Property and the State* (first published in 1884).[1] Engels suggested that women lose out in the historical process at exactly the point in time that capitalist enterprise develops in each society. Not only do women get squeezed out of the right to claim property for themselves and their children, but as marriage systems change from plural spouses to monogamy, women themselves become a kind of property for men. Monogamous marriage, according to Engels, makes women dependent on men for economic support. Thus men become dominant and women become subordinate and submissive to protect themselves and their young.[2]

Second, it asserts—contrary to much existing theory—that both written and unwritten law is never neutral on the issue of the relationship between the sexes. When law is silent, it supports the dominant power structure and cultural values of a society. The power structure is almost always controlled by adult males (sometimes with a few token women). When written laws specifically promote norms of equality, however, as in the case of Turkey, they provide a useful option for overturning the cultural bias which favours male dominance.

Third, it builds on the Ardeners' suggestive notion that women's models of the world may be quite different from men's, because the men have generated the norms for the arenas of *reasoned public argument.* Women thus may not be as good as men at articulating their unverbalised thoughts because they have not been socialised into modes of 'public discourse' which is characteristically male-dominated (S. Ardener, 1975: xi–xvii).

Although Engels foresaw that women would be excluded from owning land as the economic system evolved from transhumance to settled capital intensive agriculture, he foresaw neither how the legal system nor how specific cultural systems would interact with the changing productive and marketing systems. This essay argues that the penetration of capitalist agriculture into the Bodrum region produced a class system which made marriages within a village an advantageous way of consolidating landholdings. Such marriages aid women in two ways. First, it keeps females in close proximity to their mothers, mother's sisters, and own siblings who provide a daily work and supportive group. This prevents young, impressionable brides from being psychologically intimidated into submission by a husband and his kin. Second, a wife's legal right to her share of the patrimony provides a powerful sanction to make a husband treat her well, because the new laws also allow a comparatively easy divorce[3] for mistreatment. I argue that the gradual exposure of females to the law system in Bodrum allows them to learn the necessary forms of behaviour to use the law courts to their advantage. Finally, I suggest that laws providing female access to land, in combination with judicial willingness to enforce these laws, is a powerful mechanism for female emancipation in Aegean Turkey.

Reprinted from Renée Hirschon (ed.), *Women and Property: Women As Property* (New York: St. Martin's Press, 1984), pp. 92–116.

BODRUM: A CHANGING REGION

Many feminist scholars consider the modernisation process[4] as always adversely affecting the position of women.[5] Islam, too, is commonly thought to provide a cultural system in which women for the most part are totally subordinate to men, have few legal rights and little or no autonomy.[6] Turkey thus provides a unique situation in which to study problems of development relating to women because ninety per cent of its population are Moslem, and European legal codes were introduced in the 1920s. Furthermore, it is geographically, culturally and historically diverse. This diversity allows female/male relations to be contrasted across temporal, spatial, and cultural dimensions.

The particular focus of this paper is in the southwestern part of Turkey where the region takes its name from the town of Bodrum. In this essay we examine how male and female relationships are mediated by rights to property. In western countries property is identified with valuable resources such as land, houses, jewels and other highly-valued material goods which can be converted into saleable items on the market. In the Turkish region where I lived, orchards, houses, and productive fields were considered valuable property, as were cows, donkeys, camels, bicycles, jeeps, trucks and boats. Because women did not ride bicycles and were not taught to drive other vehicles, jeeps, trucks, bicycles and boats were owned and used only by men and do not figure further in this discussion.

In addition to material property, in Middle Eastern and Mediterranean cultures there is another valued resource, albeit intangible. This is honour. This essay argues that honour or reputation is also a valued possession, that is worth protecting and that it is as valuable to women as to men.[7] Furthermore, how a woman behaves affects the honour of her husband if she is married, and always that of her father and her brothers. This gives males social control over females, lessening women's autonomy. Much of female behaviour in the village intensively studied and in nearby Bodrum town only becomes understandable by knowing that honour and shame play a significant part in daily affairs. Like property, honour or reputation can be accumulated and can be lost.[8] It is a scarce resource.

Questions raised in the paper are: how does access to property and other resources defined as scarce by the society, affect male/female relationships? Under what conditions do women begin to assert their legally granted but customarily withheld rights to land, houses and other inheritance? Does a woman's changing relationship to property facilitate her emergence as an independent person with a growing ability to assert control over certain aspects of her life?

Turkey today is a complex nation-state involved economically with the European Common Market, Nato, and with its eastern neighbours.[9] It has a small but growing industrial sector which was hard hit by the oil crisis of 1973–74. Close to 65 per cent of the country is still agricultural. Poverty and lack of opportunities in rural areas led hundreds of thousands of migrant workers between 1960 and 1974 to seek employment in European countries.[10]

Turkey is divided into sixty-seven different administrative provinces (*il, vilayet*). There are strong class divisions, sharp cleavages between urban and rural dwellers (although migrant workers begin to blur these distinctions among the poor) and at least seven historic, cultural and geographic areas with rich distinctiveness.[11] Differences exist between the two religious groups: the dominant *Sunni* and the minority *Alevi* (or *Shi'ites,* some of them remarkably heterodox). Throughout the 1970s tremendous political instability occurred, caused by violence among rival political groups. In September 1980 a military junta took over in a bloodless coup, ostensibly to restore order and to return to the principles of Atatürk.

Answers to questions concerning gender relationships and property need to be regionally, culturally and historically specific. Within the context of a changing social order this essay examines data collected from a village, Mandalinci, (cf. *mandalina,* 'tangerines') (population 1,000) and a district town, Bodrum (population 5,200) from December 1966 through August 1968.[12]

Bodrum region (*kaza*) is 66,000 hectares[13] of which 22,614 hectares or just over one-third is farmed land. Bodrum town[14] is the administrative centre for the thirty surrounding villages which vary in size from 293 to 2,000 people. In 1966 tangerines were grown in walled irrigated fields in Bodrum and the villages to its west, while animals, tobacco, and wheat were cash crops grown in villages on the Mumcular plateau to Bodrum's east.

Geopolitics and Economics

This section of the essay argues that marriage patterns changed with the changing economic, legal and social order. For centuries the Bodrum coastal region was inhabited by two ethnic groups: Christian Orthodox, Greek-speaking townspeople who inhabited harbour areas and Sunni Moslem, Turkish-speaking *Yörük* sheep herders who practised transhumance (cf. Ramsay, 1917, pp. 31, 83). The Greeks farmed coastal valleys around harbours on the Ottoman mainland and were good sailors. The Turkish transhumants migrated between summer pastures near the sea and winter grazing areas further inland on the Bodrum peninsula.

A second Turkish-speaking ethnic group, remnants of the once powerful Turcoman confederacy,[15] occupied an ecological niche on the higher, inland plain commencing about 25 miles east of Bodrum town. These pastoral nomads had migrated over several centuries down to the region from the Anatolian plateau. They gradually settled into eight villages on the Mumcular plain about 125 years ago.[16] For cultural and religious reasons none of these three groups inter-married.

Between 1900 and 1919 the Greek and Turkish populations were on friendly terms. The Greek population farmed figs, olives, and wheat, and were the craftsmen of the region. They were carpenters, lime-makers, and house builders.[17] The area now known as Mandalinci village was a summer camp ground (*yayla*) for Turkish-speaking *Yörük* transhumants. Their winter quarters (*kisla*) were more protected. The Greek population also was larger in summer than in winter as attested to by ruins of houses and cafes along Mandalinci's deep water harbour (Starr, 1978, pp. 23–4).[18] The population in the entire Bodrum region was in 1912, 8,817 Turkish people and 5,060 Greeks (Soteriadis, 1918, p. 9).[19]

In this period Turkish women from nearby islands were considered the most beautiful and were desired as wives by Turkish-speaking men.[20] Thus marriage practices reveal special socio-economic concerns: far-flung networks, embedded in transhumance, provided pastoral households access to diverse pastures, lands, brides, and information. For women, outward stretching networks meant that after marriage at the age of twelve to fourteen a girl was separated from her natal household for much of the year, because the groom was obligated to give labour to his father who had provided the bridewealth for his marriage. This created a virilocal post-marital residence pattern. But, groups moved with flocks between traditional camp grounds, population pressure was not considerable, land was not scarce, and mostly the Greeks owned private farmlands.

The increasing animosity between the Ottoman homeland and Greece from 1919 onward changed the situation. As news of the fighting between Greek and Turkish peoples in the Izmir area spread southward, Greek-speaking families fled from their Mandalinci seaside farmlands and cafes, abandoning the entire area to Turkish transhumant households. During the population exchanges of 1923 between Greece and Turkey, the Turkish government took an interest in Greek landholdings in the village area. Several elite Turkish households were granted farmlands in Mandalinci for their role in the war of 1919–1922 (Starr, 1978, pp. 23–27). Moslem Turkish-speaking people from Crete were moved into '*Rum*' ward in Bodrum, now called *Kumbahçe* (in Turkish *Rum* means Greek).[21]

In the early 1930s tangerine agriculture was introduced from Rhodes into Betes, a seaside hamlet near Bodrum town.[22] The first orchard of tangerines in Mandalinci dates from 1940. To grow tangerines required a capital investment in three year old trees, as well as in a deep water well or overland cement waterways. It meant that soil had to be checked during dry months of summer (from mid-May until mid-October) to determine when the orchard should be flooded with irrigation water. Such water is raised from ground wells by mechanical lifts or motorised pumps.

Capital for intensive cultivation could be obtained through a bank loan, but to negotiate one, a person needed a *legal* title (*tapu*) and not merely usufruct rights to land. Elite families, of course, already had ties to banking personnel and they obtained much of the best farmland at valley level. Other villagers did obtain legal titles, while others still continued with traditional use rights to grazing lands or fields. There were recognised under village customary law-ways, but they had marginal status under state law until converted through the state legal system into a legally recognised form of ownership.[23] Households owning a tangerine orchard (the only crop raised on irrigated land) tended to invest profits into building a house at the edge of their orchard.

The transformation to single Turkish occupancy of the region and to cash-cropping agriculture led to settled village life. This made privately-owned orchards a prime resource. Marriage between children of orchard-owning families developed, creating both dense kin ties within each seaside village, and an incipient class structure.

The impact of capitalistic agriculture, settled village life and an emergent class structure had profound effects on female/male relations and on females' access to property. But to comprehend fully these changes, we need to consider the third variable, the cultural system.

The Cultural Framework

In this essay culture has an ideological, institutional and behavioural component. It is viewed as the product of specific historical processes. But, cultural codes of behaviour, developed to cope with particular stresses in a certain historic period, may live on into a new era. Thus they can be viewed as transcending one productive system to emerge side-by-side with more adaptive forms of behaviour exhibited by some members of the group.

The value systems of the Turkish ethnic groups were based on male control of females and a rather loose adherence to Islamic religion. Islamic attitudes toward women had comingled for centuries with Hellenistic attitudes in the Bodrum region.[24] Moreover, transhumant populations by and large are not known for their religious ardour.[25] A daughter was under her father's control until marriage. After that her husband had strict control and responsibility for her behaviour. Like most transhumant people in Western Turkey, veiling was not practised. Bridewealth was given by the fiance to the girl's father in the form of sheep, and some gold coins were given to the girl. Lineages were shallow and blood feuding did not develop. The ideology of honour and shame, however, tended to keep males watchful of female actions.

The transition from transhumance to settled village life did not undercut the ideology of honour and shame, despite the pragmatic views of an emerging entrepreneurial class. Thus the Islamic notions of male dominance/female submission became pitted against the secular notions of the Turkish state which had enacted legislation giving equal rights to women.

Three Types of Marriage. The increase of capitalist agriculture and the involvement with the market prompted marriages to be arranged within the village between orchard-owning households. Marriages within the village consolidated property and focused, mobilised and united resources. The effect for women was to forge dense kin networks within a community. Keeping a young bride near (or in the same village as) the parental household gave her some protection from an aggressive or cruel husband and some leverage against a demanding domineering mother-in-law.

Villagers distinguish three marriage modes: marriage by engagement negotiations, marriage by connivance and marriage by abduction.

Marriages arranged by negotiation (*nikah*) are never handled directly by the boy or girl. A mother first makes casual enquiries of her relatives and friends as to the whereabouts of a suitable mate for her child. Then a series of negotiations is carried out first by the boy's father or father's brother on behalf of the youth, and at a later stage by the boy's father and mother with the father and mother of the bride-to-be.

During these negotiations what is discussed is the amount and kind of land and houses each spouse is due to inherit at the division of the patrimony. Types of land include a house and lot, irrigated orchards, fields and woodlands or grazing pastures. Discussions also include the amount and kinds of gifts the groom will give his bride in the bridewealth.

In Mandalinci the groom gives the gifts to the bride at the time the actual engagement (*nisan*) is celebrated. He cannot go with his parents when they carry his gifts to his fiance. The bridewealth for a middle class agricultural family customarily includes four or more gold bracelets, some gold coins for the girl to wear around her neck or forehead, a watch, head scarves, some cloth for dresses for the bride, her mother and her sisters. Shoes are given to the girl's father, and socks and handkerchiefs to her brothers. The cost of such gifts in 1967 ran from seven hundred to three thousand Turkish lira ($700 to $3,000). In one instance, a 28 year old Mandalinci man and his father mortgaged the first good crop of their newly planted tangerine orchard to the man who lent them money to buy the engagement gifts so the youth could marry.

It is normal to wait at least three months between the giving of engagement gifts and the village wedding (*düğün*). But in Mandalinci the engagement often lasts much longer, because the groom may need to be away for military service, or the girl is not yet ready to leave home, or all the bridewealth has not yet been accumulated and given.

There are two modes of engagement and marriage in Mandalinci—early and later—reflecting economic differences, and especially the difficulties of poor households to accumulate the cash necessary for the bridewealth. The most approved form of marriage (and the only marriage mode available to the wealthy) is for the groom to marry when he is eighteen or nineteen a female of about fourteen or fifteen. The marriage is celebrated and consummated before the groom leaves the village for two years of compulsory military service. In this case the new bride is brought to live at the parental house of the groom where a room or even a house is provided for the couple (the word for bride, *gelin,* also means daughter-in-law and is from *gel*—'to come').

Most households cannot amass sufficient capital for early male marriages. Youths from impoverished families earn their own bridewealth which means they marry much later, around 26 to 30 years of age. They work in the village as day labourers and tenant-farmers or outside the village as more job opportunities occurred with the expanding Turkish road system of the 1950s. The improved transportation also allowed more production of perishables and with it developed a prosperous fishing trade. Jobs were also available in sponge-diving and boat-building industries of Bodrum town.

The breakdown in obligations across the father/son generation in combination with tangerine agriculture has meant that virilocal residence patterns are giving way towards more neolocal households (compare Stirling, 1974). A newly married couple still may begin with virilocal residence (depending on the marriage mode and who provided the bridewealth), but many develop their own home separate from the groom's family. Ritual and emotional ties to both sets of parents are maintained, however.

A girl who did not wish to accept a proposal or whose parents were arranging a marriage not to her liking needed to convince her parents why that union was unacceptable. She might threaten suicide if they persisted. More usually, however, she found a youth she liked better and persuaded him to elope with her. A boy had many more options for avoiding a marriage not to his liking, thus underlining once again the gender asymmetry of rural Turkish society.

The second type of marriage is by connivance, or elopement (*kiz kaçirma*).

The advantages of elopement is that the groom does not have to give any bridewealth. It also allows both males and females to marry the person of their own choosing. The girl often is the one to suggest it. The usual pattern is for the couple to flee in the night, have sexual relations and then go to the house of a friendly relative who will plead their cause to the girl's parents.

When the girl's parents notice her absence, they immediately report it to the nearest police station. The police will search for the couple. Once apprehended, they bring them back and formal charges are brought against the youth. Or the couple will reappear on their own and plead with the girl's family that they be allowed to marry. Because everyone assumes they have had sexual relations (whether they have or not), the girl is no longer desirable as a local bride, since virginity is a prime requirement. Thus, unless the parents are vindictive they allow them to marry. The fate of a girl who has eloped and not married is a worse shame to a family than a less wealthy bridegroom.

Whether they are apprehended or reappear on their own, a criminal case would be opened against the boy by the Public Prosecutor in Bodrum. Charges would be dropped when they produced a marriage licence for the court to see. The girl's active role in marriage by connivance challenges western stereotypes about submissive Turkish women.

The third marriage type is by abduction (*zorla kiz kaçirma*). Turkish villagers and Turkish criminal law distinguish between elopement by mutual consent (*kiz kaçirma*) and forcible abduction (*zorla kiz kaçirma*). The Bodrum court and written law recognise a number of different actions and degrees of guilt, each carrying more severe penalties. Thus, rape of a virgin who is a minor is more severe than rape of a virgin of legal age to marry. Kidnapping and rape of a married woman also carried severe penalties.

A girl who has been forcibly abducted, kept against her will, and forced to have sexual intercourse, after a time may agree to marry her abductor as the only solution to her future. It is the major way she can be reunited with her family and be re-admitted to local community life, albeit now as a married woman. Because of the norms regarding virginity in a bride (which are supported by the pervasive notions of honour and shame) the girl may realise that if she wishes to marry at all, she must agree to marry her abductor. Here is one victim's story:

> I was on my way to school when he came with two friends and put me into his car and carried me off. He was a driver of a jeep between Milas and Bodrum and had noticed me. I was just a small girl. I didn't know about men. I didn't think about marriage. I was only twelve. He forced me to have sex with him . . . My father didn't open a court case against him because by the time they found us I was pregnant. . . . It was hard at first, but now I am more used to him.[26]

By the summer of 1968, after five years of marriage, they had two small children and had moved to a neighbourhood of Bodrum, near the girl's parents.

In the three year period 1965 through 1967 the Bodrum Middle Criminal Court (*Asliye Ceza*) processed 29 cases ranging from voluntary elopement to forcible abduction and rape (see Table 1). In 17 of these cases the couple married, so charges against the youth were dropped. We can assume that most of these were voluntary elopements on

TABLE 1 Cases Ranging from Voluntary Elopement to Forcible Abduction and Rape (1965–1967 inclusive)

Married	17
Charges dropped	3
Innocent of Charges	1
Unfinished	5
Fine and Prison Sentence	3
Total	29

the girl's part. In three cases, each boy was sentenced to large fines and prison which suggests forcible abduction. (We can draw no conclusions from the five cases which had not finished by the time court records were copied, nor from the three cases where charges were dropped for insufficient evidence.) Thus 3 of 20 cases or 15 per cent were clear instances of violence against women.

Two of the five cases I witnessed were noteworthy. In one a girl changed her testimony. At the police station she had said she had gone willingly; in court she said it was under duress. Whether the police forced her to say she was willing to protect the lad, or whether her father forced her in court to say it was by force is unclear. In another case a girl said she loved the youth and they had eloped at her suggestion. When asked if they would marry, she looked downcast while her father stated, 'I have already married her to another'.[27] There was nothing the judge could do to save the ill-starred romance. Paternal control had overpowered female autonomy and independence, and this father had outwitted the legal norms promoting female rights.

Post-Marital Residence and Social Class. Although Bodrum people still affirm the virilocal residence ideal, actual post-marital residence is linked to class, mode of production, resources and bridewealth. By the late 1960s an emerging pattern of class structure had developed, based on intermarriage of landowning households in the village. The strata were:

1. Absentee landowning households, which controlled citrus orchards, which were farmed by tenant farmers (*ortakçi*);
2. Resident orchard-owning households, who did their own farming, hiring day labourers as needed, or had an *ortakçi*;
3. Resident field-owning households with no hired labourers;
4. Landless households, whose heads are tenant farmers or day labourers for others.

With capitalist agriculture came absentee landowners and tenant farming. Tenant farmers were provided a small rent-free cottage for their services, which for women from poorer strata meant their own home, separated from their mother-in-law. Wives of day labourers often worked in the fields or orchards for wages themselves in order to add to the household income. In this stratum newly-married couples lived in whatever accommodation could be provided for them by either family.

It was the wealthier households who could demand virilocal residence, because the father had the resources to build a room for the newly-wedded couple adjoining his house, and to provide the bridewealth which obligated the son to work his farmlands. Yet, some wealthier patriarchs chose to set up their older sons in small businesses in Izmir or Aydin. In two cases they married their younger daughters to village men with whom they established tenant farming arrangements. Such a son-in-law is called an *iç güvey* (literally the groom who marries in). This allowed a young girl to stay in close contact with her natal household and provided a father with an assistant who may be more docile than his own sons. It also assured the girl's parents that they could mediate to a great extent the ways their daughter's husband behaved toward her.

Female kin living in adjoining households co-operated in food preparation, fieldwork, childcare, and sometimes in gathering vegetables and cutting tangerines. Mutual cooperation among female kin occurred even when sisters and mothers lived in separate parts of the village. Socialisation of village girls and also Bodrum women de-emphasised female rivalry and emphasised warm, mutually supportive relationships. Most girls thought it was a great advantage to remain near their mothers and sisters after marriage. The most adventurous village girls, however, dreamed of being married to a youth in Izmir or at least in Bodrum.

Mothers were also glad not to be separated from their daughters. Even more important, it meant they would be taken care of in their old age.

The Legal Framework

Islamic Law of the Ottoman Empire. During the 19th century several reforms in Ottoman Law affected the legal and social status of women. The major Ottoman innovation, however, its civil code, affected women only tangentially. Known as the *Mecelle,* it was simply a modern-looking codification of pure Hanafi law. The committee prepared the code between 1869 and 1888, and published it sequentially between 1870 and 1877. The project was abandoned in 1888 when it proved politically unwise to produce a modern codification of Islamic family law (Onar, 1955, p. 295). Thus it left untouched the *Seriat,* the core of Islamic family law which governed all aspects of family life and personal status including marriage, renunciation of wives, inheritance, and adoption of children.

Other Ottoman reforms affected women directly. For example, the old Ottoman *tax* on brides (*arus resmi*)—of 60 aspers for girls and 40 or 30 for widows and divorcees—was replaced by a *fee* for permission to marry, given to the local Islamic judge (*kadi*). The new fee charged 10 piastres for girls and 5 for widows. Under the old Ottoman tax the amount and destination of payment was determined by the status of a bride's father. For widows' remarriage, however, the tax was paid where she resided or married (B. Lewis, 1960, p. 679). The significance of the new fee was its implicit recognition of a relationship between an unmarried female and the place she lived. Atatürk's secular laws continued the payment of a fee for marriage, which became a fee paid to a secular civil servant for a licence to marry.

Ottoman domestic legislation limited the bridewealth to a maximum of 1,000 piastres and specified that no gifts might be exchanged among the relatives of the bride and groom, nor brought by the wedding guests. The bridal dinner was limited to soup, wedding cake, and five other dishes. The bride was to buy her own cosmetics, but the groom was to pay for her use of the public baths (Young, 1905, vol. II, pp. 209–10).[28]

Attempts to limit the amount of bridewealth and of gifts exchanged among relatives of the bride and groom again appear in the reformist Ottoman Family Laws of 1915 and 1917. But, the importance of the law of 1917, called the Ottoman Law of Family Rights, was its expanded application of the *Seriat.* It allowed whatever school of Islamic law couples wished to use to be applied. This meant that the most flexible rule of any school, *Hanafi,* might be used. It also allowed a woman to have written into her marriage contract her right to annulment should her husband take a second wife. This was a major concession to those Europeanised reformers who were pushing for a monogamous marriage law in Turkey.[29]

The Ottoman Family Law of 1917 gave women rights to divorce on grounds such as impotence, insanity or abandonment. If a woman wished to divorce her husband on grounds of extreme cruelty or incompatibility, the law provided that three male family members must first attempt reconciliation of the couple before divorce was possible. Age limits were set, for the first time in Ottoman history, below which females and males could not marry.[30]

But, inheritance practices continued as they had under the *Seriat.* When a man died his widow had the right to one-eighth of his estate, and the remainder was to be divided among all his children (one-quarter if there were no children); each female share was to be half that of a male's. In practice in rural Turkey women rarely obtained their land in

Ottoman times, and in Anatolian and Southeastern Turkey even in the early 1950s and 1960s women were denied access to the patrimony (Stirling, 1965, pp. 121–2; Aswad, 1978, p. 475).[31]

In conclusion, despite the contractual nature of Moslem marriages, women suffered a number of disabilities under Islamic law. Girls moved from control by their father to the authority of their husbands. They had the status of a minor and could not act as independent persons. Women's share of the patrimony was half that of their brothers', and the widow's one-eighth share of the husband's estate was not much reward for a lifetime of service. Furthermore, according to the law, a husband could turn a wife out at will by renouncing her in front of three witnesses; he had rights to the children produced by their marriage, she did not. Culture and circumstances may make this right of males under Islam less absolute than the law provides, but strict application means children always belong to the agnatic line.

Secular Law Reforms of Atatürk. Under Atatürk's revolutionary vision of the early 1920s, women's rights in Turkey were brought closer to men's. The new Turkish Civil Code, adapted in 1926 from the Swiss Civil Code, abolished male's right to divorce by renunciation and his right to plural wives. Monogamous marriage was established as the only form recognised by the State. A civil certificate, obtainable from a town clerk was the necessary prerequisite for registering a marriage with the state. To obtain a divorce, each party had to apply to the new secular law courts. Polygamy and bigamy were both made punishable by law, and children of polygamous unions were only given legitimate status by a series of separate legislative Acts.[32] Women's rights to their paternal inheritance were now legally recognised as equal to their brothers'. A widow's share was increased to one-fourth the estate, and she got the first choice.

Age limits for marriages were again set; this time males were allowed to marry at eighteen, females at seventeen, and in exceptional cases both could marry at fifteen. The Turkish legislature in 1938 reduced the ages of marriage to seventeen for males and fifteen for females, and in exceptional circumstances with a judge's permission to fourteen for females and fifteen for males (Velidedeoğlu, 1957, p. 63).

Atatürk's policies strongly opposed social and cultural symbols, such as the male *fez* and the female veil (*carsaf*). Turkish friends remember their mothers' stories of walking in city streets in the early 1930s and seeing soldiers rip veils off women. In rural areas of western Turkey, however, agricultural and nomadic women rarely were veiled as it was a hindrance during work in the fields or with animals.

These new policies, codes and legislation promoting equality for women were put in place by a small western-oriented elite. They did not occur in response to demands of a large segment of society, mobilised for action if rights were not granted. In 1934 this small elite even obtained by legislative act the right of Turkish women to vote in all elections (G. Lewis, personal communication).

Sir Henry Maine once remarked that law is always out of step with society; there is always a gap between the legal rules and the existing social reality (Maine, 1861, p. 69). Thus, it is an empirical matter to establish the extent to which cultural practices changed under the impact of the new legislation. The remainder of the paper uses data from fieldwork in 1966 through 1968 to assess the consequences of these new rights for women, especially the ways women's rights to property are changing their relationships to men in rural areas of the Bodrum region.

WOMEN'S ACCESS TO VALUABLES

Earlier we defined property as bridewealth, land, and houses. Reputation is also a valuable resource. It is hoarded in the required virginity of a bride, and in the care with which wives present a modest public demeanour. It is lost through careless and unchaste behaviour of women. A great compliment to a rural Turkish woman is to call her *temiz,* which means clean, virtuous.

Under the new codes a woman can defend her honour and reputation at court in lawsuits against men who attempt to seduce her, who solicit her favours, or who abduct and rape her. She can bring suit against other women and men for spreading rumours and slander about her, and for bearing false witness. She can oppose her husband's attempt to divorce her to marry a new wife and she can sue him if he takes a common-law wife. In other words, she has become a legal person with full adult status to act on her own behalf with legal rights that no Islamic law system ever gave her.

The extent to which she is using these rights is explored, in a preliminary way, below. But, first we discuss tangible property because it is an implicit premises of this paper that access to self-sufficiency through owning fields, the means of food production, is an important value.

Through Her Life Cycle

Women's access to valuable property in Mandalinci combines both traditional practices and the growing penetration of the market into everyday life. The significant markers in the female life cycle which mediate her access to property are:

1. Engagement, when she is given the bridewealth;
2. Marriage at about fifteen years of age when the moveable trousseau which she prepared is transferred to her new home;
3. The death of her father, when the patrimony is divided;
4. Widowhood, when the patrimony of her husband is divided, and;
5. Old age (which may occur with (4) above), when she becomes a dependent person in the home usually of a married daughter, but sometimes of a married son.

From the ages of eleven to fourteen a girl will begin to embroider pillow cases, bed sheets, curtains and hand towels in anticipation of her marriage. The sheeting is bought for her by her parents.

During the bridewealth negotiations prior to marriage, she will have learned how much land, houses and family heirlooms (e.g. old pots, kilims, carpets, and some painted pottery) she will inherit when her father dies and his estate is divided. At the celebration of the engagement (*nikah*) she will be given the bridewealth, her fiance's gifts to her. In middle strata households these include gold bracelets, gold coins, perhaps a watch and cloth for dresses.

At the celebration of the village wedding, a bride will be given a small amount of cash by her parents and close relatives at the moment she is ready to leave her parent's house and mount the horse to be carried to the groom's house (or enter the hired jeep to travel to a village further away). Her parents also give her a winter coat, guests bring cooking pots, cooking utensils, towels, plates, cups and other useful household items as gifts.

Bridewealth: Broken Engagements and Divorce.[33] When an engagement is broken, no matter who is at fault all the gold and all the other gifts are returned to the fiance. If the cloth has already been made into dresses then the dresses themselves are returned. The candies and Turkish delights are the only things not returned, because they would no longer be fresh or might already have been eaten.

At divorce, however, none of the gold or presents are returned no matter if the woman is at fault. The bridewealth is considered 'the price of her virginity'. Only if a man married a woman to discover on her wedding night that she is not a virgin can he obtain the return of his bridewealth. But, a provident mother has probably tucked into the bosom of her daughter's wedding dress a handkerchief dipped in chicken blood. Not only is the nuptial room a traumatic occasion for the couple, but they must produce a bloodied handkerchief for the ritual benefit of the groom's sisters waiting outside the door. At divorce all the 'things of the house,' the blankets, quilts, bedding, kilim, rugs, cooking utensils, pottery, heirlooms and sewing machine if there is one, belong to the woman. The house itself belongs to the spouse whose family provided it.

Orchards and Houses. Generally, the first opportunity a village woman has to own land is when her father dies. However, I have documented one situation in which a married woman sued her brother for her share of the patrimony and won rights to a house and grounds while her father was still alive (Starr, 1978, pp. 213–23). This was accomplished with her husband's help. He not only acted as her legal representative (*vekil*) in the lawsuit, but quietened her down during the court's visit to the disputed house and house lot in the village, when she began shouting at her brother (Star, 1978, pp. 216–7). As the angry woman and her husband already owned a house in which they lived, this represents a clear example of accumulation of property by asserting a woman's rights to her father's estate.

This contrasts sharply with Anatolia in the late 1940s where 'a simple division of land between sons seems to have been the normal customary procedure' (Stirling, 1965, p. 122). It differs also from the Hatay region of south-eastern Turkey in 1965, where 'women are also denied access to land through inheritance unless they are brotherless' (Aswad, 1971; 1978, p. 475). In the Bodrum region by the mid-1960s husbands were realising they could markedly increase their household's prosperity by utilising the wife's legal rights to land. Furthermore, during a year's observation of the Bodrum courts I saw numerous cases of division of patrimony in which female siblings actually appeared in court. Inheritance cases (*veraset*) and land division cases (*taksim*) which represented 'routine' (as opposed to disputed) land cases made up the vast majority of the caseload in the High Court in Bodrum (*Asliye Hukuk*).[34]

Land at Divorce. In the three year period 1965 through 1967, 138 divorce cases were heard, and half were brought by wives. The usual grounds were incompatibility and hence most divorces were uncontested. The person who became complainant usually lived nearer the court or desired the divorce more avidly. No stigma was attached to being either defendant or complainant.

Division of land is comparatively easy at divorce, according to the judge interviewed, because each spouse keeps control of her/his orchard during the marriage. If a woman inherited an orchard from her father, the husband merely worked in it. If he bought a motorised pump for the orchard, he could take the pump out of the orchard at divorce. But, if the husband bought the fruit trees while the wife owned the land, the trees belong to the orchard, based on the legal principle 'the person who owns the land owns the trees' (*toprak kimin, ağaç onun*). If the husband built a house on her land, and there was no contract, the house belonged to the person who owned the land. If there was a contract, the person who owned the more expensive thing, would buy the other out. (For a more detailed discussion of divorce cases, cf. Starr, 1983.)

Land at Widowhood. An estate is divided at the death of the patriarch. The legal principle is that the widow gets first choice of one-fourth of the estate, and the remaining parts are divided among all his legitimate heirs equally, regardless of gender. If the wife took the house and remarried, she could live there with her new husband. If the house was given to a child and she remarried , the child could ask her to leave when he/she was of legal age. If a man and woman had no children when he died, the wife still got one-fourth his estate and the rest was divided equally between the dead man's mother and father. But, if there was even one child, the wife still got one-fourth and the child the remainder. His parents then got no part of his estate. Property only went to the deceased's brothers and sisters if he had no children and his parents were not living.

When women were widowed after thirty or forty years of age they may have chosen not to remarry but to live near a married child. They then helped with cooking and child-care, and when they were too old to work they would be looked after by their children till they died.

Women's Use of the Courts

Women's interaction with the Bodrum courts is in part a function of their position in the life cycle and in part a reflection of their growing sophistication in defending their position in society. A young female is slowly socialised into viewing the courts as an institution capable of helping her in a crisis. As a child she may have watched the judge and court recorder come to their village to hold a court hearing to award title to land or to view the place of a serious crime or of a land dispute. Perhaps she had to apply to a judge to have her age raised as her father registered her birth several years after the fact, and without proper age she is too young to marry. Or she may need to waive the required fifteen day period between obtaining a state licence to marry and celebration of the wedding. If she has eloped, she will have to appear in court to clear her husband of charges of abduction. If she was abducted, her testimony in court will determine his freedom or prison sentence. Later she may be called as a witness to a crime or to a neighbour's application for land title. She and her brothers may need judicial advice about how to divide their father's property. The largest number of civil cases in the Bodrum court concerns land division (*taksim* and *veraset* cases).

Thus in mid-life she is prepared to view the court as a major resource when her husband or brothers fail her.[35] For example, in August 1967, a woman entered the Bodrum judge's office and requested that the judge appoint her as guardian for her mother, who was 'insane'. 'She is giving land to all my brothers and sisters, but not to me' she said. The judge accepted the case and asked that the mother have a doctor's evaluation.[36]

In a different case, Ayse, a fifty year old woman went to the Director of Bodrum (*Kaymakam*) to ask his intervention in a dispute with her neighbour, Hasan. The fifty year old man had built a wall for his orchard on Ayse's field. After viewing the disputed ground, the Director gave a verdict that Hasan must take the wall down from Ayse's land. When he didn't remove the wall, Ayse opened a criminal lawsuit against him in court. She paid for witnesses to appear and eventually she won her case.[37]

In a third case, Zehra, a forty-five year old woman asked the *kaymakam* to prohibit Mehmet's farming of land she had bought. After reviewing the title and the site, the *Kaymakam* made judgment in her favour. But, Mehmet refused to leave. Zehra then opened a lawsuit claiming. 'I just bought this land a year ago, and I find him still farming it.'

Mehmet answered, 'We have been farming this land for thirty years now.'

The judge asked, 'Who has the title?' Zehra responded that she did. 'But', the defendant said, 'It is not her land. She went to the *Kaymakam* and he stopped my farming of it.'

Eventually, Zehra won.[38] Here we see a woman who not only knows about farm titles but actively opposed a man who had usufruct land rights only. This case demonstrates a situation where usufruct was predominant but is now being replaced by notions of private ownership and a woman is able to take advantage of these changing conceptions of property rights.

Women are using the courts not only to gain and keep their property, but also to protect that intangible valuable, reputation.

For example, Hafise, a widow of sixty-five years, had lived in her house for thirty-seven years, raising eight children there. A civil servant inherited (from his mother) the house next door to Hafise. Although Turkish law specifies that windows cannot be put into a side of a house overlooking someone else's walled courtyard, he had built a window in the back of his house, overlooking Hafise's backyard. In making the extension on his home, he had also cut down most of Hafise's almond tree. In the summer of 1968 I went to Hafise's neighbourhood to find out how that case had ended. The following is part of an extended interview I had with Hafise:

Hafise said:

> The cases are not finished and I have been in court for one year and three months now. I have hired a legal representative (*vekil*) so that I don't have to go every week to court. The case about cutting down the tree was decided in his favour, but we sent it to Appeal court in Ankara.

I asked if Hafise had opened a case to gain restitution for the destruction of the tree. Hafise answered:

> No. I sent the dossier to the Appeal Court. I want to wait and see what they will do first. Maybe they will send him to jail. . . . He wanted to buy my wall. Do you remember that 'viewing' the court had of my garden and wall? Well, that 'viewing' determined the wall was mine. I said I'd sell the wall to him for 26,000 Turkish lira, but he offered me only 24,000 T.L. We then opened a different court case to determine the value of the wall. In this 'viewing' the judge only looked at the wall. They established that the wall was worth 1,300 T.L., but they neglected to look at the land it stood on. We are waiting for a viewing of the ground . . . I'll only sell if he pays my price . . . But, I still don't want his window open. Look, I wash in that garden. My toilet is there. I bathe there. I am an old lady. Sometimes I go out in my *don* (baggy pants). Can he be always looking at me? I saw apartment buildings in Ankara; they are all open, but this isn't Ankara. Bodrum is a small, old town. We are not so modern here. He should have his window on a street or in his garden. . . .[39]

Thus Hafise used the court to protect her modesty and her property. She had never been to court before this dispute. Nevertheless she pursued the restitution for her almond tree and the issue of his window through three different cases against her male neighbour, and when too many court hearings and postponements taxed her energies, she hired a local legal expert (*vekil*) for legal advice and court appearances.

In a final example, a twenty-two year old married woman, named Sevcihan, from Saz village (to Bodrum's east, adjoining the government forest) brought criminal charges at court. She accused a forest ranger, Mehmet, of molesting her after drinking with her husband while spending the night in their house. In court she told how two other forest rangers had offered her 500 T.L. to drop charges against their friend. Nevertheless, she pursued her grievance through five separate hearings over a five month time period. For each hearing she needed to travel twenty-five miles over rough terrain to court. On at least two occasions she had to bring witnesses and pay their expenses. On three different occasions she had had to retell the events of that night:

> The woman, Sevcihan, in court: That night the forest ranger and my husband came. They had been drinking at the coffee-house. They brought another bottle of *raki* to our house, and my husband told me to make some food ready. And then my husband became drunk and he fell asleep. I went to my husband's father, and I called him. He came to the house for a while and then he left. I went to bed next to my husband. I went to sleep. Someone is touching me and I woke up.
>
> Judge: How is he touching you? Where is he touching you?
>
> Sevcihan: He is stroking my neck, my breasts, my arms, my hands. I ran outside. He followed me. I came back again. I went to the room where my husband was sleeping and I locked the door. He knocked at the window, saying, 'Come. I am waiting for you.' I went again to bed next to my husband.
>
> Mehmet's version: I went home with her husband. We had been drinking at the coffee-house, and we had a bottle of *raki* with us. And then her husband got drunk. He went to sleep. Later his father came and I offered him some *raki*, but he said, 'I do not drink.' When he left I went to the bed they gave me. When I woke up in the morning I went to wash my face. She came to me, and I asked where her husband was. She said, 'He went. He went to the coffee-house.' (He is the proprietor.) She gave me a cup of water. I drank it and then said, 'Say good-bye to your husband for me.'

Judge: Do you go to their house often?

Mehmet: This is the first time.

Lawyer for Mehmet: That girl and her husband made a plan to get 500 T.L. from my client.

Judge: Do you have proof? What kind is it?

Lawyer: Witnesses. Next time I will give a list of witnesses.

Sevcihan: That's not true. The next day two forest rangers came to me by Jeep. They said if you will give up this court case, we will give you 500 T.L. But, I didn't want to give up this case.

The testimony of the witnesses can be summarised as follows:

One witness had said, 'I drive a jeep for hire. The day after that event I carried two forest rangers to her village, and they went to her house, but I didn't overhear the conversation there.' Another witness had testified that he saw two forest rangers going to her village, and had seen the defendant and her husband drinking in the village coffee-house the night of the alleged event. A third witness, a twenty-three year old woman, testifying for Sevcihan said:

> About a month ago we were stringing tobacco leaves onto thread. This man comes up to Sevcihan and said, 'My dear, Sevcihan, why do you not come to me? Are you angry with me?' She didn't go to him. . . . No, I didn't see him touching her.[40]

Eventually, the charges against the forester were dismissed for insufficient evidence, despite the female witness' testimony which implied that Mehmet was aggressively pursuing Sevcihan.

From a different perspective Sevcihan can be seen to have won her goal. Her ardent pursuit of justice through the court made Mehmet's actions public—his co-workers, her villagers, and even her debauched husband must now recognise his lecherous inclinations toward her. After five months of fearing a large fine and jail sentence (which would have meant loss of his job), Mehmet's lusts were probably tempered by prudence. Sevcihan's use of a district level court thus provided her the opportunity to vindicate her honour and safeguard her reputation.

BROADER IMPLICATIONS

In the Bodrum region factors which allowed women to develop more self-sufficient lives were: changing land-use patterns which constructed the daily work routines for both females and males; a change in post-marital residence in response to the emergence of a new class structure, which occurred as a result of the penetration of capitalist agriculture. And third, the law. Judges' willingness to enforce legislation promoting norms of equality in union with women's growing knowledge of how to activate the official law system were emancipating mechanisms in western Turkey. In central and eastern Anatolia women's independence is apparently less advanced.[41] I would argue this is due to differences in the agrarian hierarchy, land use patterns, culture, historic conditions, and type of integration into the world market.

An explanation of Bodrum's successful acceptance of the new Civil Code may lie in several directions. Bodrum has a unique geographic and political position as a frontier of Turkish-Greek contact, and it was early pacified by the new Republic of Turkey. With good reason officials in Ankara would have wanted to keep Aegean Turkey pacified, economically productive and indoctrinated into the values of nation-statehood. Bodrum is much too accessible to the Greek Islands to let it remain a backwater, illustrating the failure of the nation to maintain a western democratic outlook. Furthermore, it is an area of increasing productivity since the 1940s, and since 1968 Bodrum town has had a huge economic boom in summer months due to tourism. The winter population of the town has doubled between 1965 and 1980.[42]

Earlier I suggested that in Aegean Turkey, Hellenistic and Islamic attitudes toward women had long co-existed as Turkish-speaking nomads over a period of several hundred years migrated into and settled in the region now called Bodrum. The ecology of transhumance required far-flung networks for the Yörük sheep herders to gain access to diverse pastures in this multi-ethnic region. Marrying daughters to Turkish-speaking transhumants of different camps within the same ethnic group cemented pastoral relations. The Islamic ideology concerning male dominance and the required submission of females was supported by the institutions of bridewealth, post-marital virilocal residence, divorce by renunciation and the ideology of honour and shame.

Yet, despite the change from pastoral life to settled capitalist agriculture, cultural institutions such as bridewealth and virilocal post-marital residence remained as 'ideal forms'. Writing about European manners and cultural change in the emerging Renaissance Europe, Elias (1939) demonstrated that two or three hundred years may be necessary for ideas, etiquette, and new cultural practices to diffuse throughout a society. Yet, in the Bodrum region, work routines changed rapidly in response to new crops and a new productive system. Marriage patterns changed, too, as cash-cropping agriculture and the transformation of the class structure made marriages within the village a way to consolidate land holdings for middle and upper strata peasants. And third, the norms of sexual equality promoted by the secular legal system through both written law and judicial decisions, provided a way for females to gain control of resources, especially productive land, which for women (as for anyone), are a bridge to autonomous personage.

Thus, Engels', dynamic theory of the process of change from pre-capitalist social formations to capitalist relations neglected the positive role law and culture play. In the region of Bodrum law balanced the disruptive effect that capitalist agriculture and the emergence of private ownership had on women's lives. With increasing scarcity of land for intensive agriculture, the norms of equal division of patrimony had become salient to husbands as a way to increase household land holdings. Elsewhere I noted that tangerine cultivation promotes nuclear households because two adults and two teenage children can provide all the needed labour from within (see Starr, 1978, pp. 38–42). Mastery of the economic processes behind tangerine marketing is information easily accessible to any female who keeps her ears open.

Thus, I can unequivocally state that less than fifty years after the introduction of European Civil and Criminal codes in Turkey, women in the Bodrum region were reaping the benefits of laws of equality. They were able to hold titles to land in their own names. Some women successfully opposed husbands' attempts to usurp their economic resources during marriage and at divorce, and many women went to court to protect their landed interests and their reputations.

Some might argue that under the older system women were protected by fathers, husbands, and brothers; that going to court clearly indicates the breakdown of the older protective system.[43] Didn't women lead better lives, they ask, in a material, social and qualitative sense in the past? I answer, that depends upon your goals for women. Data presented here clearly indicate, I think, that husbands, brothers and fathers do not always look out for a wife's, sister's or daughter's best interests. They may not even know them (even if they wished to) because some women may not be sure what their best interests are, while others may not be able to develop a plan which they can communicate by reasoned argument (cf. S. Ardener, 1975, pp. xi–xviii; E. Ardener, 1975). Given these facts it is better that women have ways to look out for their own interests, that they judge for themselves what these interests are, and that they develop habitual modes of thought and action which allow them to do so.

Therefore, the Bodrum example suggests that several factors need to intersect for women's emergence as more autonomous adults. The implication for policy makers is that legal rights and economic opportunities for women and for men must go hand in hand. The Bodrum study also suggests that we need to take a longer time span than twenty-five years[44] in deciding whether the results of change have improved women's lives. Of course we need to study the processes along the way. But, fifty years after the introduction of new secular codes, and twenty or more years after the gradual emergence of settled village life, we can see ways that women's access to valuables—land, houses, and reputation—are changing their relations to men, allowing them to become fully responsible persons.

NOTES

Acknowledgements. I owe a debt of gratitude to Dr. Geoffrey Lewis, Oriental Institute, Oxford, for taking the time to read critically this manuscript, although I take responsibility for its remaining faults. I also acknowledge with pleasure conversations and careful readings of the essay by Helen Callaway, Shirley Ardener, and especially Renée Hirschon.

1. Engels, of course, was not the only nineteenth century anthropologist to discuss woman's position in society in an evolutionary framework. But, precisely because his writing is the culmination of an anthropological perspective beginning with Maine, and developed by Bachofen, McLennan, Lubbock and Morgan, I choose to confront Engels's theories. Two recent critiques of Engels (1884) are Leacock (1981) and Sacks (1974).
2. See Engels (1981, pp. 120–21, 142–44).
3. Divorce is now easier for women and harder for men than it had been under the previous Islamic law system of the 20th century Ottoman Empire. Divorce was now accessible under the new Civil Code of 1926 by a spouse applying to the nearest secular district court on one of the six grounds: adultery, dishonourable life of the spouse, desertion, mental infirmity, or incompatibility (Ansay and Wallace, 1966, p. 122). For a more detailed discussion Starr (1978).
4. Modernisation is here roughly defined as integration of the group into a nation-state. The linkages between the group and the state may, of course, be imperfectly achieved, e.g., the Kurds in Turkey.
5. See Boserup (1970), Bossen (1975), Papanek (1977), and Nelson (1981).
6. Even those sympathetic to the cultural system of Islam and who advocate reform within Islamic law rather than a complete break, acknowledge Islamic law provides few rights for women and many disabilities when women's rights are compared to men's. See, for example, Coulson and Hinchcliffe (1978) and White (1978, pp. 52–3).
7. The organising force of codes of honour and shame in Mediterranean countries has been argued by Campbell (1964), Davis (1977), Peristiany (1965), Schneider (1971), Schneider and Schneider (1976, p. 2) and others.
8. See Stirling (1955, pp. 98, 168, 230–3); Starr (1978, p. 56); Abel (1979).
9. Approximately half of Turkey's trade in 1982 has been with Islamic countries (*The Guardian,* 12th May, 1982) and in the same year Turkey signed a major Trade Pact with Russia for 600 million lira (*New York Times,* 20th January, 1982, p. a7).
10. In 1960, 22,700 workers left Turkey (Abadan-Unat, 1981, p. 2). The figure continued to rise each year until the oil crisis of 1973–4. In 1980 the combined figure of Turkish residents in France, Germany, the Netherlands, Sweden and Switzerland was 1,762.9 thousand (SOPEMI, 1981, p. 3).
11. Fisher (1963, pp. 293–338) divides Turkey into five geographic regions, the Anatolian plateau, the Black sea coast, eastern Turkey, the Mediterranean, and the Aegean coast, but I suggest six. European Turkey ought to be separated from Aegean and Mediterranean Turkey at the Meander River.
12. The field research between 1966–68 was financed by a United States National Institute of Mental Health Predoctoral Fellowship and Grant and I gratefully acknowledge this support.
13. A hectare is 100 ares or 2.471 acres.
14. For a very interesting study of Bodrum town, see Mansur (1972).
15. Fieldwork revealed cultural differences between villagers on the Bodrum peninsula to Bodrum's west, and those on the Mumcular plain to Bodrum's east which villagers themselves recognise saying 'They are very different from us'. Identifying which villagers were Yurük and which Turcoman was harder and is the topic of current research. But see Field (1881, pp. 62–3), De Planhol (1958, pp. 526, 528, 531) and Ramsay (1897, pp. 100–1; 1917, pp. 31, 83).
16. The transition from pastoralism to settled village life and the identity of these villages was first suggested to me by Osman Nuri Bilgin,

Director of the Primary School in Bodrum, and a historian of the Bodrum region.
17. Interview with the Director of Rural Agriculture, Bodrum.
18. In the later 19th century the Turkish population was losing control of the Aegean areas to Greek-speaking farmers and shepherds. (Ramsay, 1897, pp. 130–31, 133). See also Starr (1978, pp. 23–5).
19. The population from the 1965 Census lists Bodrum town as having 5,136 while the surrounding villages are placed at 20,675 (*Genel Nüfus Sayimi* 1965, p. 483).
20. Most women fifty years or older also remember Greek, for they came from islands of Kos and Kalimnos as brides.
21. See note 17.
22. Marketing tangerines only became feasible with the completion of a dirt road linking Bodrum to Milas in 1927, because tangerines ripen between December and March, the period of sudden, violent storms on the Aegean. This makes sea transport particularly precarious at this season.
23. The procedure of converting usufruct rights to a state recognised legal title (*tapu*) involved going to court and applying under Art. 639 of the Turkish Civil Code. 'If the land is not previously registered in the Land Registry and if the person occupies and uses the land as if he were the real owner for 20 years without interruption and dispute, he may request a court to order the registration of the land in his name.' (Letter from Prof. T. Ansay, Dean of Ankara University Law Faculty. 14 December 1980.)
24. Cosar (1978, p. 131) astutely observes that as one moves from east to west in Turkey the 'situation of women improves with the general socio-economic situation'.
25. The lack of religious behaviour among Turkish-speaking transhumants has been noted by Barth for the Basseri, (1961, p. 135) and by R. Tapper for the Shahsevan (1975, pp. 2, 155, 158, 164). But, see Beck for women's religious and ritual practices among the Turkish-speaking *Qashqa'i* (1978, pp. 363–5).
26. Interview with Ayhan A., concerning Bodrum Court Case, B.C. 62. Bodrum *Court Cases File.* Also see Case 11 on film, '*Adliye*: An Ethnography of a Turkish Rural Court,' 1968.
27. Fieldnotes, filed under *Kiz Kaçirma* (Elopement) Cases, 1967.
28. This is interesting as an attempt to use legislation to regulate custom and tradition.
29. See Allen (1935, pp. 137–9), Coulson (1964, p. 184), Starr (1978, ftn.2, pp. 1–2).
30. See B. Lewis (1961, pp. 225–6).
31. Maher (1978, p. 102) makes the same point for rural Moroccan women. The male lineage members justify this deprivation of inheritance by saying that if daughters were given their land, it would be transferred to another lineage when they married.
32. The Turkish National Assembly enacted laws legitimising children of irregular marriages in 1932, 1934, 1945, 1950, 1955, 1965 and 1974.
33. The following is a summary of two days of discussions I had in August 1967 with the senior court judge and the Public Prosecutor concerning female and male property rights and bridewealth, at critical times in the life cycle or when engagements were broken or marriages were dissolved.
34. See, Starr and Pool (1974, pp. 552–54) for an analysis of women and men's use of the courts in Bodrum. Also Starr (1983) for women versus men in divorce suits.
35. Additional confirmation of this assertion is available. Female complainants against male defendants as a total of all cases processed in the Bodrum Middle Criminal Court rose from 14 per cent in 1950 to 28 per cent in 1967 (Starr and Pool, 1974, p. 353).
36. Witnessed by me 7 August 1967. Filed under Conversations with Bodrum judges and Public Prosecutor, p. 33, titled, 'Opening a Case, *Sulh Hukuk* (Lower Civil Court).'
37. Bodrum Court Cases, File. *Sulh Ceza* (Lower Criminal Court), B.C. 23, 1967.
38. Bodrum Court Cass, File. *Sulh Hukuk* (Lower Civil Court), B.C. 78.
39. Bodrum Court Cases, File. *Asliye Hukuk* (Higher Civil Court) B.C. 72 and *Asliye Ceza* (Middle Criminal Court) B.C. 85.
40. Bodrum Court Cases, File. *Sulh Ceza* (Lower Criminal Court) B.. 41B.
41. For overviews and comparative statements about women in Turkey, see Abadan-Unat (1963, 1978 and 1981), Cosar (1978), and Kandiyoti (1977, 1980). For ethnographic accounts of women's position, see Aswad (1967, 1974, 1978).
42. Winter population figures for 1980 were: Bodrum town—10,000 people; Bodrum district (*kaza*) including the town and all the villages had 38,000 people. (Personal communication, Mrs. Emine Cam, Director of Tourism Bureau in Bodrum.

43. Nader (1964, 1965) hypothesized that women in Oaxaca, Mexico used the court only when they did not have a husband, father or brother to protect their interests. In Turkey, however, family structures, law and the market interact so that it is frequently a *brother* or husband who has usurped the women's resources (see Stirling, 1957, p. 27); or a *father* may exploit his daughter for his own financial gain (see Stirling, 1957, p. 31). Even in areas of strong kin group control, 'the "protection" of the lineage which had previously been to the economic advantage of the woman is turning increasingly into dominance and exploitation' (Aswad, 1978, p. 475).
44. Twenty-five years was the time period of the evaluative conference in Istanbul, entitled the 'Reception of Foreign Law in Turkey,' which essentially was pessimistic (see Stirling, 1957, and Velidedeoğlu, 1957).

REFERENCES

Abadan-Unat, Nermin, 1963. *Social Change and Turkish Women.* Publication of the Faculty of Political Science, University of Ankara, No. 17.

———. 1978. The Modernization of Turkish Women. *The Middle East Journal* 32: 291–306.

———. ed. 1981. *Women in Turkish Society.* Leiden: E. J. Brill.

Abel, R. 1979. The Rise of Capitalism and the Transformation of Disputing: From Confrontation over Honor to Competition for Property. *UCLA Law Review* 27(1): 223–255.

Ansay, T. and Wallace, Jr. 1966. *Introduction to Turkish Law.* Ankara: Guzel Instanbul Matbaasi.

Ardener, E. 1975. Belief and the Problem of Women. In J. La Fontaine, ed. *The Interpretation of Ritual.* London: Tavistock Press.

Ardener, S. 1975. Introductory Essay. In S. Ardener, ed. *Perceiving Women.* New York: Halsted.

Aswad, Barbara. 1967. Key and Peripheral Roles of Noblewomen in a Middle Eastern Plains Village. *Anthropological Quarterly* 40: 139–152.

———. 1971. Property Control and Social Strategies: Settlers on a Middle Eastern Plain. *Anthropological Papers No. 44.* Ann Arbor, Michigan: University of Michigan.

———. 1974. Visiting Patterns Among Women of the Elite in a Small Turkish City. *Anthropological Quarterly* 47: 9–27.

———. 1978. Women, Class and Power: Examples from the Hatay, Turkey. In Lois Beck and Nikki Keddie, eds., pp. 473–481. *Women in the Muslim World.* Cambridge: Harvard University Press.

Boserup, Ester. 1970. *Woman's Role in Economic Development.* New York: St. Martin's Press.

Bossen, Laurel. 1975. Women in Modernizing Societies. American *Ethnologist* 2(4): 587–601.

Campbell, John K. 1964. *Honour, Family, and Patronage.* Oxford: Clarendon Press.

Cosar, Fatna Mansur. 1978. Women in Turkish Society. In Lois Beck and Nikki Keddie, eds., pp. 124–140. *Women in the Muslim World.* Cambridge: Harvard University Press.

Coulson, Noel and Doreen Hinchcliffe. 1978. Women and Law Reform in Contemporary Islam. In Lois Beck and Nikki Keddie, eds. *Women in the Muslim World,* pp. 37–52. Cambridge: Harvard University Press.

Davis, John. 1977. *People of the Mediterranean: An Essay in Comparative Social Anthropology.* London: Routledge and Kegan Paul.

Elias, N. 1982. *The Civilizing Process, Vol 1. The History of Manners.* Oxford: Blackwell. Originally published as Uber den Prozess der Zivilisation, 1939.

Engels, F. 1981. *The Origin of the Family, Private Property and the State.* Edited with an introduction by E. B. Leacock. London: Lawrence and Wishart.

Kandiyoti, D. 1977. Sex Roles and Social Change: A Comparative Appraisal of Turkey's Women. *Signs* 3(1): 57–73.

———. ed. 1980. *Major Issues on the Status of Women in Turkey: Approaches and Priorities.* Ankara: Cag Matbaasi.

Leacock, Eleanor B. 1981a. *Myths of Male Dominance.* London: Monthly Review Press.

Leacock, Eleanor B. 1981b. Introduction to Engels' *The Origin of the Family, Private Property and the State.* London: Lawrence and Wishart.

Lewis, B. 1961. Arus Resmi. In *Encyclopedia of Islam,* Vol. 1, p. 697.

Maine, H. S. 1861. *Ancient Law: Its Connection with the Early History of Society and its Relation to Modern Ideas.* London: John Murray.

Nelson, N. 1981. Introduction to African Women in the Development Process. *Journal of Development Studies* 17(3): 1–8.

Onar, S. S. 1955. The Magalla. *Law in the Middle East* 1: 292–308.

Papanek, Helen. 1977. Development Planning for Women. *Signs* 31: 14–22.

Peristiany, John G., ed. 1965. *Honour and Shame: The Values of Mediterranean Society.* London: Weidenfeld and Nicolson.

Ramsay, W. M. 1917. *The Intermixture of Races in*

Asia Minor, Some of its Causes and Effects. Proceedings of the British Academy, Vol. 7, pp. 31, 83. London: Oxford University Press.

Sacks, Karen. 1974. Engels Revisited: Women, The Organization of Production and Private Property. In Michelle Rosaldo and Louise Lamphere, eds. *Woman, Culture and Society,* pp. 207–220. Stanford: Stanford University Press.

Schneider, Jane. 1971. Of Vigilance and Virgins: Honor, Shame and Access to Resources in Mediterranean Societies. *Ethnology* 10(1): 1–24.

Schneider, Jane and Peter Schneider. 1976. *Culture and Political Economy in Western Sicily.* New York: Academic Press.

Soteriadis, G. 1918. *An Ethnological Map Illustrating Hellenism in the Balkans Peninsula and Asia Minor.* London: Edward Stanford.

Starr, J. 1978. *Dispute and Settlement in Rural Turkey: An Ethnography of Law.* Leiden: E. J. Brill.

Stirling, Paul. 1957. Land, Marriage and the Law in Turkish Villages. *International Social Science Bulletin* 9: 21–33.

———. 1965. *Turkish Village.* London: Weidenfeld and Nicolson.

———. 1974. Cause, Knowledge and Change: Turkish Village Revisited. In J. Davis, ed. *Choice and Change: Essays in Honour of Lucy Mair.* London: Athlone Press.

Velidedeoğlu, H. V. 1957. The Reception of the Swiss Civil Code in Turkey. *International Social Science Bulletin* 9: 60–65.

White, Elizabeth H. 1978. Legal Reform as an Indicator of Women's Status in Muslim Nations. In Lois Beck and Nikki Keddie, eds., *Women in the Muslim World,* pp. 52–68. Cambridge: Harvard University Press.

Young, G. 1905. *Corps de Droit Ottoman.* Vol. II. Oxford: Clarendon Press.

JAPANESE MOTHERS AND *OBENTŌS*: THE LUNCH-BOX AS IDEOLOGICAL STATE APPARATUS

Anne Allison

Obentōs are boxed lunches Japanese mothers make for their nursery school children. Following Japanese codes for food preparation—multiple courses that are aesthetically arranged—these lunches have a cultural order and meaning. Using the *obentō* as a school ritual and chore—it must be consumed in its entirety in the company of all the children—the nursery school also endows the *obentō* with ideological meanings. The child must eat the *obentō*; the mother must make an *obentō* the child will eat. Both mother and child are being judged; the subjectivities of both are being guided by the nursery school as an institution. It is up to the mother to make the ideological operation entrusted to the *obentō* by the state-linked institution of the nursery school, palatable and pleasant for her child, and appealing and pleasurable for her as a mother. [food, mother, Japan, education, ideology]

Reprinted with permission from *Anthropological Quarterly* 64: 195–208, 1991.

INTRODUCTION

Japanese nursery school children, going off to school for the first time, carry with them a boxed lunch (*obentō*) prepared by their mothers at home. Customarily these *obentōs* are highly crafted elaborations of food: a multitude of miniature portions, artistically designed and precisely arranged, in a container that is sturdy and cute. Mothers tend to expend inordinate time and attention on these *obentōs* in efforts both to please their children and to affirm that they are good mothers. Children at nursery school are taught in turn that they must consume their entire meal according to school rituals.

Food in an *obentō* is an everyday practice of Japanese life. While its adoption at the nursery school level may seem only natural to Japanese and unremarkable to outsiders, I will argue in this article that the *obentō* is invested with a gendered state ideology. Overseen by the authorities of the nursery school, an institution which is linked to, if not directly monitored by, the state, the practice of the *obentō* situates the producer as a woman and mother, and the consumer, as a child of a mother and a student of a school. Food in this context is neither casual nor arbitrary. Eaten quickly in its entirety by the student, the *obentō* must be fashioned by the mother so as to expedite this chore for the child. Both mother and child are being watched, judged, and constructed; and it is only through their joint effort that the goal can be accomplished.

I use Althusser's concept of the Ideological State Apparatus (1971) to frame my argument. I will briefly describe how food is coded as a cultural and aesthetic apparatus in Japan, and what authority the state holds over school in Japanese society. Thus situating the parameters within which the *obentō* is regulated and structured in the nursery school setting, I will examine the practice both of making and eating *obentō* within the context of one nursery school in Tokyo. As an anthropologist and mother of a child who attended this school for fifteen months, my analysis is based on my observations, on discussions with other mothers, daily conversations and an interview with my son's teacher, examination of *obentō* magazines and cookbooks, participation in school rituals, outings, and Mothers' Association meetings, and the multifarious experiences of my son and myself as we faced the *obentō* process every day.

I conclude that *obentōs* as a routine, task, and art form of nursery school culture are endowed with ideological and gendered meanings that the state indirectly manipulates. The manipulation is neither total nor totally coercive, however, and I argue that pleasure and creativity for both mother and child are also products of the *obentō*.

CULTURAL RITUAL AND STATE IDEOLOGY

As anthropologists have long understood, not only are the worlds we inhabit symbolically constructed, but also the constructions of our cultural symbols are endowed with, or have the potential for, power. How we see reality, in other words, is also how we live it. So the conventions by which we recognize our universe are also those by which each of us assumes our place and behavior within that universe. Culture is, in this sense, doubly constructive: constructing both the world for people and people for specific worlds.

The fact that culture is not necessarily innocent, and power not necessarily transparent, has been revealed by much theoretical work conducted both inside and outside the discipline of anthropology. The scholarship of the neo-Marxist Louis Althusser (1971), for example, has encouraged the conceptualization of power as a force which operates in ways that are subtle, disguised, and accepted as everyday social practice. Althusser differentiated between two major structures of power in modern capitalist societies. The first, he called, (Repressive) State Apparatus (SA), which is power that the state wields and manages primarily through the threat of force. Here the state sanctions the usage of power and repression through such legitimized mechanisms as the law and police (1971: 143–5).

Contrasted with this is a second structure of power—Ideological State Apparatus(es) (ISA). These are institutions which have some overt function other than a political and/or administrative one: mass media, education, health and welfare, for example. More numerous, disparate, and functionally polymorphous than the SA, the ISA exert power not primarily through repression but through ideology. Designed and accepted as practices with another purpose—to educate (the school system), entertain (film industry), inform (news media), the ISA serve not only their stated objective but also an unstated one—that of indoctrinating people into seeing the world a certain way and of accepting certain identities as their own within that world (1971: 143–7).

While both structures of power operate simultaneously and complementarily, it is the ISA, according to Althusser, which in capitalist societies is the more influential of the two. Disguised and screened by another operation, the power of ideology in ISA can be both more far-reaching and insidious than the SA's power of coercion. Hidden in the movies we watch, the music we hear, the liquor we drink, the textbooks we read, it is overlooked because it is protected and its protection—or its alibi (Barthes 1957: 109–111)—allows the terms and relations of ideology to spill into and infiltrate our everyday lives.

A world of commodities, gender inequalities, and power differentials is seen not therefore in these terms but as a naturalized environment, one that makes sense because it has become our experience to live it and accept it in precisely this way. This commonsense acceptance of a particular world is the work of ideology, and it works by concealing the coercive and repressive elements of our everyday routines but also by making those routines of the everyday familiar, desirable, and simply our own. This is the critical element of Althusser's notion of ideological power: ideology is so potent because it becomes not only ours but us—the terms and machinery by which we structure ourselves and identify who we are.

JAPANESE FOOD AS CULTURAL MYTH

An author in one *obentō* magazine, the type of medium-sized publication that, filled with glossy pictures of *obentō*s and ideas and recipes for successfully recreating them, sells in the bookstores across Japan, declares, ". . . the making of the *obentō* is the one most worrisome concern facing the mother of a child going off to school for the first time (*Shufunotomo* 1980: inside cover). Another *obentō* journal, this one heftier and packaged in the encyclopedic series of the prolific women's publishing firm, *Shufunotomo*, articulates the same social fact: "first-time *obentō*s are a strain on both parent and child" (*"hajimete no obentō wa, oya mo ko mo kinchōshimasu"*) (*Shufunotomo* 1981: 55).

An outside observer might ask: What is the real source of worry over *obentō*? Is it the food itself or the entrance of the young child into school for the first time? Yet, as one look at a typical child's *obentō*—a small box packaged with a five or six-course miniaturized meal whose pieces and parts are artistically arranged, perfectly cut, and neatly arranged—would immediately reveal, no food is "just" food in Japan. What is not so immediately apparent, however, is why a small child with limited appetite and perhaps scant interest in food is the recipient of a meal as elaborate and as elaborately prepared as any made for an entire family or invited guests?

Certainly, in Japan much attention is focussed on the *obentō*, investing it with a significance far beyond that of the merely pragmatic, functional one of sustaining a child with nutritional foodstuffs. Since this investment beyond the pragmatic is true of any food prepared in Japan, it is helpful to examine culinary codes for food preparation that operate generally in the society before focussing on children's *obentō*s.

As has been remarked often about Japanese food, the key element is appearance. Food must be organized, re-organized, arranged, re-arranged, stylized, and re-stylized to appear in a design that is visually attractive. Presentation is critical: not to the extent that taste and nutrition are displaced, as has been sometimes attributed to Japanese food, but to the degree that how food looks is at least as important as how it tastes and how good and sustaining it is for one's body.

As Donald Richie has pointed out in his eloquent and informative book *A Taste of Japan* (1985), presentational style is the guiding principle by which food is prepared in Japan, and the style is conditioned by a number of codes. One code is for smallness, separation, and fragmentation. Nothing large is allowed, so portions are all cut to be bite sized, served in small amounts on tiny individual dishes, and are arranged on a table (or on a tray, or in an *obentō* box) in an array of small, separate containers.[1] There is no one big dinner plate with three large portions of vegetable, starch, and meat as in American cuisine. Consequently the eye is pulled not toward one totalizing center but away to a multiplicity of de-centered parts.[2]

Visually, food substances are presented according to a structural principle not only of segmentation but also of opposition. Foods are broken or cut to make contrasts of color, texture, and shape. Foods are meant to oppose one another and clash: pink against green, roundish foods against angular ones, smooth substances next to rough ones. This oppositional code operates not only within and between the foodstuffs themselves, but also between the attributes of the food and those of the containers in or on which they are placed: a circular mound in a square dish, a bland colored food set against a bright plate, a translucent sweet in a heavily textured bowl (Richie 1985: 40–1).

The container is as important as what is contained in Japanese cuisine, but it is really the containment that is stressed, that is, how food has been (re)constructed and (re)arranged from nature to appear, in both beauty and freshness, perfectly natural. This stylizing of nature is a third code by which presentation is directed; the injunction is not only to retain, as much as possible, the innate naturalness of ingredients—shopping daily so food is fresh and leaving much of it either raw or only minimally cooked—but also to recreate in prepared food the promise and appearance of being "natural." As Richie writes, ". . . the emphasis is on presentation of the natural rather than the natural itself. It is not what nature has wrought that excites admiration but what man has wrought with what nature has wrought" (1985: 11).

This naturalization of food is rendered through two main devices. One is by constantly hinting at and appropriating the nature that comes from outside—decorating food with seasonal reminders, such as a maple leaf in the fall or a flower in the spring, serving in-season fruits and vegetables, and using season-coordinated dishes such as glassware in the summer and heavy pottery in the winter. The other device, to some degree the inverse of the first, is to accentuate and perfect the preparation process to such an extent that the food appears not only to be natural, but more nearly perfect than nature without human intervention ever could be. This is nature made artificial. Thus, by naturalization, nature is not only taken in by Japanese cuisine, but taken over.

It is this ability both to appropriate "real" nature (the maple leaf on the tray) and to stamp the human reconstruction of that nature as "natural" that lends Japanese food its potential for cultural and ideological manipulation. It is what Barthes calls a second order myth (1957: 114–7): a language which has a function people accept as only pragmatic—the sending of roses to lovers, the consumption of wine with one's dinner, the cleaning up a mother does for her child—which is taken over by some interest or agenda to serve a different end—florists who can sell roses, liquor companies who can market wine, conservative politicians who campaign for a gendered division of labor with women kept at home. The first order of language ("language-object"), thus emptied of its original meaning, is converted into an empty form by which it can assume a new, additional, second order of signification ("metalanguage" or "second-order semiological system"). As Barthes points out however, the primary meaning is never lost. Rather, it remains and stands as an alibi, the cover under which the second, politicized meaning can hide. Roses sell better, for example, when lovers view them as a vehicle to express love rather than the means by which a company stays in business.

At one level, food is just food in Japan—the medium by which humans sustain their nature and health. Yet under and through this code of pragmatics, Japanese cuisine carries other meanings that in Barthes' terms are mythological. One of these is national identity: food being appropriated as a sign of the culture. To be Japanese is to eat Japanese food, as so many Japanese confirm when they travel to other countries and cite the greatest problem they encounter to be the absence of "real" Japanese food. Stated the other way around, rice is so symbolically central to Japanese culture (meals and *obentōs* often being assembled with rice as the core and all other dishes, multifarious as they may be, as mere compliments or side dishes) that Japanese say they can never feel full until they have consumed their rice at a particular meal or at least once during the day.[3]

Embedded within this insistence on eating Japanese food, thereby reconfirming one as a member of the culture, are the principles by which Japanese food is customarily prepared: perfection, labor, small distinguishable parts, opposing segments, beauty, and the stamp of nature. Overarching all these more detailed codings are two that guide the making and ideological appropriation of the nursery school *obentōs* most directly: 1) there is an order to the food: a right way to do things, with everything in its place and each place coordinated with every other, and 2) the one who prepares the food takes on the responsibility of producing food to the standards of perfection and exactness that Japanese cuisine demands. Food may not be casual, in other words, nor the producer casual in her production. In these two rules is a message both about social order and the role gender plays in sustaining and nourishing that order.

SCHOOL, STATE, AND SUBJECTIVITY

In addition to language and second order meanings I suggest that the rituals and routines surrounding *obentōs* in Japanese nursery schools present, as it were, a third order, manipulation. This order is a use of a currency already established—one that has already appropriated a language of utility (food feeds hunger) to express and implant cultural behaviors. State-guided schools borrow this coded apparatus: using the natural convenience and cover of food not only to code a cultural order, but also to socialize children and mothers into the gendered roles and subjectivities they are expected to assume in a political order desired and directed by the state.

In modern capitalist societies such as Japan, it is the school, according to Althusser, which assumes the primary role of ideological state apparatus. A greater segment of the population spends longer hours and more years here than in previous historical periods. Also education has not taken over from other institutions, such as religion, the pedagogical function of being the major shaper and inculcator of knowledge for the society. Concurrently, as Althusser has pointed out for capitalist modernism (1971: 152, 156), there is the gradual replacement of repression by ideology as the prime mechanism for behavior enforcement. Influenced less by the threat of force and more by the devices that present and inform us of the world we live in and the subjectivities that world demands, knowledge and ideology become fused, and education emerges as the apparatus for pedagogical and ideological indoctrination.

In practice, as school teaches children how and what to think, it also shapes them for the roles and positions they will later assume as adult members of the society. How the social order is organized through vectors of gender, power, labor, and/or class, in other words, is not only as important a lesson as the basics of reading and writing, but is transmitted through and embedded in those classroom lessons. Knowledge thus is not only socially constructed, but also differentially acquired according to who one is or will be in the political society one will enter in later years. What precisely society requires in the way of workers, citizens, and parents will be the condition determining or influencing instruction in the schools.

This latter equation, of course, depends on two factors: 1) the convergence or divergence of different interests in what is desired as subjectivities, and 2) the power any particular interest, including that of the state, has in exerting its desires for subjects on or through the system of education. In the case of Japan, the state wields enormous control over the systematization of education. Through its Ministry of Education (Monbushō), one of the most powerful and influential ministries in the government, education is centralized and managed by a state bureaucracy that regulates almost every aspect of the educational process. On any given day, for example, what is taught in every public school follows the same curriculum, adheres to the same structure, and is informed by textbooks from the prescribed list. Teachers are nationally screened, school boards uniformly appointed (rather than elected), and students institutionally exhorted to obey teachers given their legal authority, for example, to write secret reports (*naishinsho*), that may obstruct a student's entrance into high school.[4]

The role of the state in Japanese education is not limited, however, to such extensive but codified authorities granted to the Ministry of Education. Even more powerful is the principle of the *"gakureki shakkai"* (lit. academic pedigree society) by which careers of adults are determined by the schools they attend as youth. A reflection and construction of the new economic order of post-war Japan,[5] school attendance has become the single most important determinant of who will achieve the most desirable positions in industry, government, and the professions. School attendance is itself based on a single criterion: a system of entrance exams which determines entrance selection and it is to this end—preparation for exams—that school, even at the nursery school level, is increasingly oriented. Learning to follow directions, do as one is told, and *"ganbaru"* (Asanuma 1987) are social imperatives, sanctioned by the state, and taught in the schools.

NURSERY SCHOOL AND IDEOLOGICAL APPROPRIATION OF THE *OBENTŌ*

The nursery school stands outside the structure of compulsory education in Japan. Most nursery schools are private; and, though not compelled by the state, a greater proportion of the three to six-year old population of Japan attends preschool than in any other industrialized nation (Tobin 1989; Hendry 1986; Boocock 1989).

Differentiated from the *hoikuen,* another pre-school institution with longer hours which is more like daycare than school,[6] the *yochien* (nursery school) is widely perceived as instructional, not necessarily in a formal curriculum but more in indoctrination to attitudes and structure of Japanese schooling. Children learn less about reading and writing than they do about how to become a Japanese student, and both parts of this formula—Japanese and student—are equally stressed. As Rohlen has written, "social order is generated" in the nursery school, first and foremost, by a system of routines (1989: 10, 21). Educational routines and rituals are therefore of heightened importance in *yochien,* for whereas these routines and rituals may be the format through which subjects are taught in higher grades, they are both form and subject in the *yochien.*

While the state (through its agency, the Ministry of Education) has no direct mandate over nursery school attendance, its influence is nevertheless significant. First, authority over how the *yochien* is run is in the hands of the Ministry of Education. Second, most parents and teachers see the *yochien* as the first step to the system of compulsory education that starts in the first grade and is closely controlled by Monbushō. The principal of the *yochien* my son attended, for example, stated that he saw his main duty to be preparing children to enter more easily the rigors of public education soon to come. Third, the rules and patterns of "group living" (shūdanseikatsu), a Japanese social ideal that is reiterated nationwide by political leaders, corporate management, and marriage counselors, is first introduced to the child in nursery school.[7]

The entry into nursery school marks a transition both away from home and into the "real world," which is generally judged to be difficult, even traumatic, for the Japanese child (Peak 1989). The *obentō* is intended to ease a child's discomfiture and to allow a child's mother to manufacture something of herself and the home to accompany the child as s/he moves into the potentially threatening outside world. Japanese use the cultural categories of *soto* and *uchi; soto* connotes the outside, which in being distanced and other, is dirty and hostile; and *uchi,* identifies as clean and comfortable what is inside and familiar. The school falls initially and, to some degree, perpetually, into a category of *soto.* What is ultimately the definition and location of *uchi,* by contrast, is the home, where family and mother reside.[8] By producing something from the home, a mother both girds and goads her child to face what is inevitable in the world that lies beyond. This is the mother's role and her gift; by giving of herself and the home (which she both symbolically represents and in reality manages[9]), the *soto* of the school is, if not transformed into the *uchi* of home, made more bearable by this sign of domestic and maternal hearth a child can bring to it.

The *obentō* is filled with the meaning of mother and home in a number of ways. The first is by sheer labor. Women spend what seems to be an inordinate amount of time on the production of this one item. As an experienced *obentō* maker, I can attest to the intense attention and energy devoted to this one chore. On the average, mothers spend 20–45 minutes every morning cooking, preparing, and assembling the contents of one *obentō* for one nursery school-aged child. In addition, the previous day they have planned, shopped, and often organized a supper meal with leftovers in mind for the next day's *obentō.* Frequently women[10] discuss *obentō* ideas with other mothers, scan *obentō* cookbooks or magazines for recipes, buy or make objects with which to decorate or contain (part of) the *obentō,* and perhaps make small food portions to freeze and retrieve for future *obentō.*[11]

Of course, effort alone does not necessarily produce a successful *obentō.* Casualness was never indulged, I observed, and even mothers with children who would eat anything prepared *obentō*s as elaborate as anyone else's. Such labor is intended for the child but also the mother: it is a sign of a woman's commitment as a mother and her inspiring her child to being similarly committed as a student. The *obentō* is thus a representation of what the mother is and what the child should become. A model for school is added to what is gift and reminder from home.

This equation is spelled out more precisely in a nursery school rule—all of the *obentō* must be eaten. Though on the face of it this is petty and mundane, the injunction is taken very seriously by nursery school teachers and is one not easily realized by very small children. The logic is that it is time for the child to meet certain expectations. One of the main agendas of the nursery school, after all, is to introduce and indoctrinate children into the patterns and rigors of Japanese education (Rohlen 1989; Sano 1989; Lewis 1989). And Japanese education, by all accounts, is not about fun (Duke 1986).

Learning is hard work with few choices or pleasures. Even *obentō*s from home stop once the child enters first grade.[12] The meals there are institutional: largely bland, unappealing, and prepared with only nutrition in mind. To ease a youngster into these upcoming (educational, social, disciplinary, culinary) routines, *yochien obentō*s are designed to be pleasing and personal. The *obentō* is also designed, however, as a test for the child. And the double meaning is not unintentional. A structure already filled with a signification of mother and home is then emptied to provide a new form: one now also written with the ideological demands of being a member of Japanese culture as well as a viable and successful Japanese in the realms of school and later work.

The exhortation to consume one's entire *obentō*[13] is articulated and enforced by the nursery school teacher. Making high drama out of eating by, for example, singing a song; collectively thanking Buddha (in the case of Buddhist nursery schools), one's mother for making the *obentō,* and one's father for providing the means to make the *obentō;* having two assigned class helpers pour the tea, the class eats together until everyone has finished. The teacher examines the children's *obentōs*, making sure the food is all consumed, and encouraging, sometimes scolding, children who are taking too long. Slow eaters do not fare well in this ritual, because they hold up the other students, who as a peer group also monitor a child's eating. My son often complained about a child whose slowness over food meant that the others were kept inside (rather than being allowed to play on the playground) for much of the lunch period.

Ultimately and officially, it is the teacher, however, whose role and authority it is to watch over food consumption and to judge the person consuming food. Her surveillance covers both the student and the mother, who in the matter of the *obentō*, must work together. The child's job is to eat the food and the mother's to prepare it. Hence, the responsibility and execution of one's task is not only shared but conditioned by the other. My son's teacher would talk with me daily about the progress he was making finishing his *obentōs*. Although the overt subject of discussion was my child, most of what was said was directed to me; what I could do in order to get David to consume his lunch more easily.

The intensity of these talks struck me at the time as curious. We had just settled in Japan and David, a highly verbal child, was attending a foreign school in a foreign language he had not yet mastered; he was the only non-Japanese child in the school. Many of his behaviors during this time were disruptive: for example, he went up and down the line of children during morning exercises hitting each child on the head. Hamada-sensei (the teacher), however, chose to discuss the *obentōs*. I thought surely David's survival in and adjustment to this environment depended much more on other factors, such as learning Japanese. Yet it was the *obentō* that was discussed with such recall of detail ("David ate all his peas today, but not a single carrot until I asked him to do so three times") and seriousness that I assumed her attention was being misplaced. The manifest reference was to boxlunches, but was not the latent reference to something else?[14]

Of course, there was another message, for me and my child. It was an injunction to follow directions, obey rules, and accept the authority of the school system. All of the latter were embedded in and inculcated through certain rituals: the nursery school, as any school (except such non-conventional ones as Waldorf and Montessori) and practically any social or institutional practice in Japan, was so heavily ritualized and ritualistic that the very form of ritual took on a meaning and value in and of itself (Rohlen 1989: 21, 27–8). Both the school day and school year of the nursery school were organized by these rituals. The day, apart from two free periods, for example, was broken by discrete routines—morning exercises, arts and crafts, gym instruction, singing—most of which were named and scheduled. The school year was also segmented into and marked by three annual events—sports day (*undōkai*) in the fall, winter assembly (*seikatsu happyōkai*) in December, and dance festival (*bon odori*) in the summer. Energy was galvanized by these rituals, which demanded a degree of order as well as a discipline and self-control that non-Japanese would find remarkable.

Significantly, David's teacher marked his successful integration into the school system by his mastery not of the language or other cultural skills, but of the school's daily routines—walking in line, brushing his teeth after eating, arriving at school early, eagerly participating in greeting and departure ceremonies, and completing all of his *obentō* on time. Not only had he adjusted to the school structure, but he had also become assimilated to the other children. Or restated, what once had been externally enforced now became ideologically desirable; the everyday practices had moved from being alien (soto) to familiar (uchi) to him, from, that is, being someone else's to his own. My American child had to become, in some sense, Japanese, and where his teacher recognized this Japaneseness was in the daily routines such as finishing his *obentō*. The lesson learned early, which

David learned as well, is that not adhering to routines such as completing one's *obentō* on time leads to not only admonishment from the teacher, but rejection from the other students.

The nursery school system differentiates between the child who does and the child who does not manage the multifarious and constant rituals of nursery school. And for those who do not manage there is a penalty which the child learns either to avoid or wish to avoid. Seeking the acceptance of his peers, the student develops the aptitude, willingness, and in the case of my son—whose outspokenness and individuality were the characteristics most noted in this culture—even the desire to conform to the highly ordered and structured practices of nursery school life. As Althusser (1971) wrote about ideology: the mechanism works when and because ideas about the world and particular roles in that world that serve other (social, political, economic, state) agendas become familiar and one's own.

Rohlen makes a similar point: that what is taught and learned in nursery school is social order. Called *shūdanseikatsu* or group life, it means organization into a group where a person's subjectivity is determined by a group membership and not "the assumption of choice and rational self-interest" (1989: 30). A child learns in nursery school to be with others, think like others, and act in tandem with others. This lesson is taught primarily through the precision and constancy of basic routines: "Order is shaped gradually by repeated practice of selected daily tasks . . . that socialize the children to high degrees of neatness and uniformity" (p. 21). Yet a feeling of coerciveness is rarely experienced by the child when three principles of nursery school instruction are in place: 1) school routines are made "desirable and pleasant" (p. 30), 2) the teacher disguises her authority by trying to make the group the voice and unit of authority, and 3) the regimentation of the school is administered by an attitude of "intimacy" on the part of the teachers and administrators (p. 30). In short, when the desires and routines of the school are made into the desires and routines of the child, they are made acceptable.

MOTHERING AS GENDERED IDEOLOGICAL STATE APPARATUS

The rituals surrounding the *obentō*s consumption in the school situate what ideological meanings the *obentō* transmits to the child. The process of production within the home, by contrast, organizes its somewhat different ideological package for the mother. While the two sets of meanings are intertwined, the mother is faced with different expectations in the preparation of the *obentō* than the child is in its consumption. At a pragmatic level the child must simply eat the lunch box, whereas the mother's job is far more complicated. The onus for her is getting the child to consume what she has made, and the general attitude is that this is far more the mother's responsibility (at this nursery school, transitional stage) than the child's. And this is no simple or easy task.

Much of what is written, advised, and discussed about the *obentō* has this aim explicitly in mind: that is making food in such a way as to facilitate the child's duty to eat it. One magazine advises:

> The first day of taking *obentō* is a worrisome thing for mother and "*boku*" (child[15]) too. Put in easy-to-eat foods that your child likes and is already used to and prepare this food in small portions (*Shufunotomo* 1980: 28).

Filled with pages of recipes, hints, pictures, and ideas, the magazine codes each page with "helpful" headings:

- First off, easy-to-eat is step one.
- Next is being able to consume the *obentō* without leaving anything behind.
- Make it in such a way for the child to become proficient in the use of chopsticks.
- Decorate and fill it with cute dreams *(kawairashi yume)*.
- For older classes (*nenchō*), make *obentō* filled with variety.

- Once he's become used to it, balance foods your child likes with those he dislikes.
- For kids who hate vegetables. . . .
- For kids who hate fish. . . .
- For kids who hate meat . . . (pp. 28–53).

Laced throughout cookbooks and other magazines devoted to *obentō*, the *obentō* guidelines issued by the school and sent home in the school flier every two weeks, and the words of Japanese mothers and teachers discussing *obentō*, are a number of principles: 1) food should be made easy to eat: portions cut or made small and manipulable with fingers or chopsticks, (child-size) spoons and forks, skewers, toothpicks, muffin tins, containers, 2) portions should be kept small so the *obentō* can be consumed quickly and without any left-overs, 3) food that a child does not yet like should be eventually added so as to remove fussiness (*sukikirai*) in food habits, 4) make the *obentō* pretty, cute, and visually changeable by presenting the food attractively and by adding non-food objects such as silver paper, foil, toothpick flags, paper napkins, cute handkerchiefs, and variously shaped containers for soy sauce and ketchup, and 5) design *obentō*-related items as much as possible by the mother's own hands including the *obentō* bag (*obentōfukuro*) in which the *obentō* is carried.

The strictures propounded by publications seem to be endless. In practice I found that visual appearance and appeal were stressed by the mothers. By contrast, the directive to use *obentō* as a training process—adding new foods and getting older children to use chopsticks and learn to tie the *furoshiki*[16]—was emphasized by those judging the *obentō* at the school. Where these two sets of concerns met was, of course, in the child's success or failure completing the *obentō*. Ultimately this outcome and the mother's role in it, was how the *obentō* was judged in my experience.

The aestheticization of the *obentō* is by far its most intriguing aspect for a cultural anthropologist. Aesthetic categories and codes that operate generally for Japanese cuisine are applied, though adjusted, to the nursery school format. Substances are many but petite, kept segmented and opposed, and manipulated intensively to achieve an appearance that often changes or disguises the food. As a mother insisted to me, the creation of a bear out of miniature hamburgers and rice, or a flower from an apple or peach, is meant to sustain a child's interest in the underlying food. Yet my child, at least, rarely noticed or appreciated the art I had so laboriously contrived. As for other children, I observed that even for those who ate with no obvious "fussiness," mothers' efforts to create food as style continued all year long.

Thus much of a woman's labor over *obentō* stems from some agenda other than that of getting the child to eat an entire lunch-box. The latter is certainly a consideration and it is the rationale as well as cover for women being scrutinized by the school's authority figure—the teacher. Yet two other factors are important. One is that the *obentō* is but one aspect of the far more expansive and continuous commitment a mother is expected to make for and to her child. "*Kyōiku mama*" (education mother) is the term given to a mother who executes her responsibility to oversee and manage the education of her children with excessive vigor. And yet this excess is not only demanded by the state even at the level of the nursery school; it is conventionally given by mothers. Mothers who manage the home and children, often in virtual absence of a husband/father, are considered the factor that may make or break a child as s/he advances towards that pivotal point of the entrance examinations.[17]

In this sense, just as the *obentō* is meant as a device to assist a child in the struggles of first adjusting to school, the mother's role generally is perceived as being the support, goad, and cushion for the child. She will perform endless tasks to assist in her child's study: sharpen pencils and make midnight snacks as the child studies, attend cram schools to verse herself in subjects her child is weak in, make inquiries as to what school is most appropriate for her child, and consult with her child's teachers. If the child succeeds, a mother is complimented; if the child fails, a mother is blamed.

Thus at the nursery school level, the mother starts her own preparation for this upcoming role. Yet the jobs and energies demanded of a nursery school mother are, in themselves, surprisingly consuming. Just as the mother of an entering student is given a book listing all the pre-entry tasks she must complete, for example, making various bags and containers, affixing labels to all clothes in precisely the right place and with the size exactly right, she will be continually expected therafter to attend Mothers' Association meetings, accompany children on fieldtrips, wash the clothes and indoor shoes of her child every week, add required items to a child's bag on a day's notice, and generally be available. Few mothers at the school my son attended could afford to work in even part-time or temporary jobs. Those women who did tended either to keep their outside work a secret or be reprimanded by a teacher for insufficient devotion to their child. Motherhood, in other words, is institutionalized through the child's school and such routines as making the *obentō* as a full-time, kept-at-home job.[18]

The second factor in a woman's devotion to over-elaborating her child's lunch-box is that her experience doing this becomes a part of her and a statement, in some sense, of who she is. Marx writes that labor is the most "essential" aspect to our species-being and that the products we produce are the encapsulation of us and therefore our productivity (1970: 71–76). Likewise, women are what they are through the products they produce. An *obentō* therefore is not only a gift or test for a child, but a representation and product of the woman herself. Of course, the two ideologically converge, as has been stated already, but I would also suggest that there is a potential disjoining. I sensed that the women were laboring for themselves apart from the agenda the *obentō* was expected to fill at school. Or stated alternatively, in the role that females in Japan are highly pressured and encouraged to assume as domestic manager, mother, and wife, there is, besides the endless and onerous responsibilities, also an opportunity for play. Significantly, women find play and creativity not outside their social roles but within them.

Saying this is not to deny the constraints and surveillance under which Japanese women labor at their *obentō*. Like their children at school, they are watched by not only the teacher but each other, and perfect what they create, partially at least, so as to be confirmed as a good and dutiful mother in the eyes of other mothers. The enthusiasm with which they absorb this task then is like my son's acceptance and internalization of the nursery school routines; no longer enforced from outside it becomes adopted as one's own.

The making of the *obentō* is, I would thus argue, a double-edged sword for women. By relishing its creation (for all the intense labor expended, only once or twice did I hear a mother voice any complaint about this task), a woman is ensconcing herself in the ritualization and subjectivity (subjection) of being a mother in Japan. She is alienated in the sense that others will dictate, inspect, and manage her work. On the reverse side, however, it is precisely through this work that the woman expresses, identifies, and constitutes herself. As Althusser pointed out, ideology can never be totally abolished (1971: 170); the elaborations that women work on "natural" food produce an *obentō* which is creative and, to some degree, a fulfilling and personal statement of themselves.

Minami, an informant, revealed how both restrictive and pleasurable the daily rituals of motherhood can be. The mother of two children—one, aged three and one, a nursery school student, Minami had been a professional opera singer before marrying at the relatively late age of 32. Now, her daily schedule was organized by routines associated with her child's nursery school: for example, making the *obentō*, taking her daughter to school and picking her up, attending Mothers' Association meetings, arranging daily play dates, and keeping the school uniform clean. While

Minami wished to return to singing, if only on a part-time basis, she said that the demands of motherhood, particularly those imposed by her child's attendance at nursery school, frustrated this desire. Secretly snatching only minutes out of any day to practice, Minami missed singing and told me that being a mother in Japan means the exclusion of almost anything else.[19]

Despite this frustration, however, Minami did not behave like a frustrated woman. Rather she devoted to her mothering an energy, creativity, and intelligence I found to be standard in the Japanese mothers I knew. She planned special outings for her children at least two or three times a week, organized games that she knew they would like and would teach them cognitive skills, created her own stories and designed costumes for afternoon play, and shopped daily for the meals she prepared with her children's favorite foods in mind. Minami told me often that she wished she could sing more, but never once did she complain about her children, the chores of child-raising, or being a mother. The attentiveness displayed otherwise in her mothering was exemplified most fully in Minami's *obentōs*. No two were ever alike, each had at least four or five parts, and she kept trying out new ideas for both new foods and new designs. She took pride as well as pleasure in her *obentō* handicraft; but while Minami's *obentō* creativity was impressive, it was not unusual.

Examples of such extraordinary *obentō* creations from an *obentō* magazine include: 1) ("donut *obentō*"): two donuts, two wieners cut to look like a worm, two cut pieces of apple, two small cheese rolls, one hard-boiled egg made to look like a rabbit with leaf ears and pickle eyes and set in an aluminum muffin tin, cute paper napkin added, 2) (wiener doll *obentō*): a bed of rice with two doll creations made out of wiener parts (each consists of eight pieces comprising hat, hair, head, arms, body, legs), a line of pink ginger, a line of green parsley, paper flag of France added, 3) (vegetable flower and tulip *obentō*): a bed of rice laced with chopped hard-boiled egg, three tulip flowers made out of cut wieners with spinach precisely arranged as stem and leaves, a fruit salad with two raisins, three cooked peaches, three pieces of cooked apple, 4) (sweetheart doll *obentō—abekku ningyō* no *obentō*): in a two-section *obentō* box there are four rice balls on one side, each with a different center, on the other side are two dolls made of quail's eggs for heads, eyes and mouth added, bodies of cucumber, arranged as if lying down with two raw carrots for the pillow, covers made of one flower—cut cooked carrot, two pieces of ham, pieces of cooked spinach, and with different colored plastic skewers holding the dolls together (*Shufunotomo* 1980: 27, 30).

The impulse to work and re-work nature in these *obentō* is most obvious perhaps in the strategies used to transform, shape, and/or disguise foods. Every mother I knew came up with her own repertoire of such techniques, and every *obentō* magazine or cookbook I examined offered a special section on these devices. It is important to keep in mind that these are treated as only flourishes: embellishments added to parts of an *obentō* composed of many parts. The following is a list from one magazine: lemon pieces made into butterflies, hard boiled eggs into *daruma* (popular Japenese legendary figure of a monk without his eyes), sausage cut into flowers, a hard-boiled egg decorated as a baby, an apple piece cut into a leaf, a radish flaked into a flower, a cucumber cut like a flower, a *mikan* (nectarine orange) piece arranged into a basket, a boat with a sail made from a cucumber, skewered sausage, radish shaped like a mushroom, a quail egg flaked into a cherry, twisted *mikan* piece, sausage cut to become a crab, a patterned cucumber, a ribboned carrot, a flowered tomato, cabbage leaf flower, a potato cut to be a worm, a carrot designed as a red shoe, an apple cut to simulate a pineapple (pp. 57–60).

Nature is not only transformed but also supplemented by store-bought or mother-made objects which are precisely arranged in the *obentō*. The former come from an entire industry and commodification of the *obentō* process: complete racks or sections in stores selling *obentō* boxes, additional small containers, *obentō* bags, cups, chopstick and utensil containers (all these with various cute characters or designs on the front), cloth and paper napkins, foil, aluminum tins, colored ribbon or string, plastic skewers, toothpicks with paper flags, and paper dividers. The latter are the objects mothers are encouraged and praised for making themselves: *obentō* bags, napkins, and handkerchiefs with appliqued designs or the child's name embroidered. These supplements to the food, the arrangement of the food, and the *obentō* box's dividing walls (removable and adjustable) furnish the order of the *obentō*. Everything appears crisp and neat with each part kept in its own place: two tiny hamburgers set firmly atop a bed of rice; vegetables in a separate compartment in the box; fruit arranged in a muffin tin.

How the specific forms of *obentō* artistry—for example, a wiener cut to look like a worm and set within a muffin tin—are encoded symbolically is a fascinating subject. Limited here by space, however, I will only offer initial suggestions. Arranging food into a scene recognizable by the child was an ideal mentioned by many mothers and cookbooks. Why those of animals, human beings, and other food forms (making a pineapple out of an apple, for example) predominate may have no other rationale than being familiar to children and easily re-produced by mothers. Yet it is also true that this tendency to use a trope of realism—casting food into realistic figures—is most prevalent in the meals Japanese prepare for their children. Mothers I knew created animals and faces in supper meals and/or *obentō*s made for other outings, yet their impulse to do this seemed not only heightened in the *obentō* that were sent to school but also played down in food prepared for other age groups.

What is consistent in Japanese cooking generally, as stated earlier, are the dual principles of manipulation and order. Food is manipulated into some other form than it assumes either naturally or upon being cooked: lines are put into mashed potatoes, carrots are flaked, wieners are twisted and sliced. Also, food is ordered by some human rather than natural principle; everything must have neat boundaries and be placed precisely so those boundaries do not merge. These two structures are the ones most important in shaping the nursery school *obentō* as well, and the inclination to design realistic imagery is primarily a means by which these other culinary codes are learned by and made pleasurable for the child. The simulacrum of a pineapple recreated from an apple therefore is less about seeing the pineapple in an apple (a particular form) and more about reconstructing the apple into something else (the process of transformation).

The intense labor, management, commodification, and attentiveness that goes into the making of an *obentō* laces it, however, with many and various meanings. Overarching all is the potential to aestheticize a certain social order, a social order which is coded (in cultural and culinary terms) as Japanese. Not only is a mother making food more palatable to her nursery school child, but she is creating food as a more aesthetic and pleasing social structure. The *obentō*'s message is that the world is constructed very precisely and that the role of any single Japanese in that world must be carried out with the same degree of precision. Production is demanding; and the producer must both keep within the borders of her/his role and work hard.

The message is also that it is women, not men, who are not only sustaining a child through food but carrying the ideological support of the culture that this food embeds. No Japanese man I spoke with had or desired the experience of making a nursery school *obentō* even once, and few were more than peripherally engaged in their children's education. The male is assigned a position in the outside world where he labors at a job for money and is expected to be primarily identified by and committed to his place of work.[20] Helping in the management of home and raising of children has not become an obvious male concern or interest in Japan, even as more and more women enter what was previously the male domain of work. Females have remained at and as the center of home in Japan and this message too is explicitly transmitted in both the production and consumption of entirely female-produced *obentō*.

The state accrues benefits from this arrangement. With children depending on the labor women devote to their mothering to such a degree, and women being pressured as well as pleasurized in such routine maternal productions as making the *obentō*—both effects encouraged and promoted by institutional features of the educational system heavily state-run and at least ideologically guided at even the nursery school level—a gendered division of labor is firmly set in place. Labor from males, socialized to be compliant and hard-working, is more extractable when they have wives to rely on for almost all domestic and familial management. And females become a source of cheap labor, as they are increasingly forced to enter the labor market to pay domestic costs (including those vast debts incurred in educating children) yet are increasingly constrained to low-paying part-time jobs because of the domestic duties they must also bear almost totally as mothers.

Hence, not only do females, as mothers operate within the ideological state apparatus of Japan's school system that starts semi-officially, with the nursery school, they also operate as an ideological state apparatus unto themselves. Motherhood is state ideology, working through children at home and at school and through such mother-imprinted labor that a child carries from home to school as with the *obentō*. Hence the post-World War II conception of Japanese education as being egalitarian, democratic, and with no agenda of or for gender differentiation, does not in practice stand up. Concealed within such cultural practices as culinary style and child-focussed mothering, is a worldview in which the position and behavior an adult will assume has everything to do with the anatomy she/he was born with.

At the end, however, I am left with one question. If motherhood is not only watched and manipulated by the state but made by it into a conduit for ideological indoctrination, could not women subvert the political order by redesigning *obentō*? Asking this question, a Japanese friend, upon reading this paper, recalled her own experiences. Though her mother had been conventional in most other respects, she made her children *obentōs* that did not conform to the prevailing conventions. Basic, simple, and rarely artistic, Sawa also noted, in this connection, that the lines of these *obentōs* resembled those by which she was generally raised: as gender-neutral, treated as a person not "just as a girl," and being allowed a margin to think for herself. Today she is an exceptionally independent woman who has created a life for herself in America, away from homeland and parents, almost entirely on her own. She loves Japanese food, but the plain *obentōs* her mother made for her as a child, she is newly appreciative of now, as an adult. The *obentōs* fed her, but did not keep her culturally or ideologically attached. For this, Sawa says today, she is glad.

NOTES

Acknowledgments The fieldwork on which this article is based was supported by a Japan Foundation Postdoctoral Fellowship. I am grateful to Charles Piot for a thoughtful reading and useful suggestions for revision and to Jennifer Robertson for inviting my contribution to this issue. I would also like to thank Sawa Kurotani for her many ethnographic stories and input, and Phyllis Chock and two anonymous readers for the valuable contributions they made to revision of the manuscript.

1. As Dorinne Kondo has pointed out, however, these cuisinal principles may be conditioned by factors of both class and circumstance. Her *shitamachi* (more traditional area of Tokyo) informants, for example, adhered only casually to this coding and other Japanese she knew followed them more carefully when preparing food for guests rather than family and when eating outside rather than inside the home (Kondo 1990: 61–2).
2. Rice is often, if not always, included in a meal: and it may substantially as well as symbolically

constitute the core of the meal. When served at a table it is put in a large pot or electric rice maker and will be spooned into a bowl, still no bigger or predominant than the many other containers from which a person eats. In an *obentō* rice may be in one, perhaps the largest, section of a multi-sectioned *obentō* box, yet it will be arranged with a variety of other foods. In a sense rice provides the syntactic and substantial center to a meal yet the presentation of the food rarely emphasizes this core. The rice bowl is refilled rather than heaped as in the preformed *obentō* box, and in the *obentō* rice is often embroidered, supplemented, and/or covered with other foodstuffs.

3. Japanese will both endure a high price for rice at home and resist American attempts to export rice to Japan in order to stay domestically self-sufficient in this national food *qua* cultural symbol. Rice is the only foodstuff in which the Japanese have retained self-sufficient production.
4. The primary sources on education used are Horio 1988; Duke 1986; Rohlen 1983; Cummings 1980.
5. Neither the state's role in overseeing education nor a system of standardized tests is a new development in post-World War II Japan. What is new is the national standardization of tests and, in this sense, the intensified role the state has thus assumed in overseeing them. See Dore (1965) and Horio (1988).
6. Boocock (1989) differs from Tobin et al. (1989) on this point and asserts that the institutional differences are insignificant. She describes extensively how both *yōchien* and *hoikuen* are administered (*yōchien* are under the authority of Monbushō and *hoikuen* are under the authority of the Kōseishō, the Ministry of Health and Welfare) and how both feed into the larger system of education. She emphasizes diversity: though certain trends are common amongst preschools, differences in teaching styles and philosophies are plentiful as well.
7. According to Rohlen (1989), families are incapable of indoctrinating the child into this social pattern of *shūndanseikatsu* by their very structure and particularly by the relationship (of indulgence and dependence) between mother and child. For this reason and the importance placed on group structures in Japan, the nursery school's primary objective, argues Rohlen, is teaching children how to assimilate into groups. For further discussion of this point see also Peak 1989; Lewis 1989; Sano 1989; and the *Journal of Japanese Studies* issue [15(1)] devoted to Japanese preschool education in which these articles, including Boocock's, are published.
8. For a succinct anthropological discussion of these concepts, see Hendry (1987: 39–41). For an architectural study of Japan's management and organization of space in terms of such cultural categories as *uchi* and *soto,* see Greenbie (1988).
9. Endless studies, reports, surveys, and narratives document the close tie between women and home; domesticity and femininity in Japan. A recent international survey conducted for a Japanese housing construction firm, for example, polled couples with working wives in three cities, finding that 97% (of those polled) in Tokyo prepared breakfast for their families almost daily (compared with 43% in New York and 34% in London); 70% shopped for groceries on a daily basis (3% in New York, 14% in London), and that only 22% of them had husbands who assisted or were willing to assist with housework (62% in New York, 77% in London) (quoted in *Chicago Tribune* 1991). For a recent anthropological study of Japanese housewives in English, see Imamura (1987). Japanese sources include *Juristo zōkan sōgō tokushu* 1985; *Mirai shakan* 1979; *Ohirasōri no seifu kenkyūkai* 3.
10. My comments pertain directly, of course, to only the women I observed, interviewed, and interacted with at the one private nursery school serving middle-class families in urban Tokyo. The profusion of *obentō*-related materials in the press plus the revelations made to me by Japanese and observations made by other researchers in Japan (for example, Tobin 1989; Fallows (1990), however, substantiate this as a more general phenomenon.
11. To illustrate this preoccupation and consciousness: during the time my son was not eating all his *obentō* many fellow mothers gave me suggestions, one mother lent me a magazine, his teacher gave me a full set of *obentō* cookbooks (one per season), and another mother gave me a set of small frozen food portions she had made in advance for future *obentō*s.
12. My son's teacher, Hamada-sensei, cited this explicitly as one of the reasons why the *obentō* was such an important training device for

nursery school children. "Once they become *ichinensei* (first-graders) they'll be faced with a variety of food, prepared without elaboration or much spice, and will need to eat it within a delimited time period."

13. An anonymous reviewer questioned whether such emphasis placed on consumption of food in nursery school leads to food problems and anxieties in later years. Although I have heard that anorexia is a phenomenon now in Japan, I question its connection to nursery school *obentōs*. Much of the meaning of the latter practice, as I interpret it, has to do with the interface between production and consumption, and its gender linkage comes from the production end (mothers making it) rather than the consumption end (children eating it). Hence while control is taught through food, it is not a control linked primarily to females or bodily appearance, as anorexia may tend to be in this culture.
14. Fujita argues, from her experience as a working mother of a daycare (*hoikuen*) child, that the substance of these daily talks between teacher and mother is intentionally insignificant. Her interpretation is that the mother is not to be overly involved in nor too informed about matters of the school (1989).
15. "*Boku*" is a personal pronoun that males in Japan use as a familiar reference to themselves. Those in close relationships with males—mothers and wives, for example—can use *boku* to refer to their sons or husbands. Its use in this context is telling.
16. In the upper third grade of the nursery school (*nenchō* class; children aged five to six) my son attended, children were ordered to bring their *obentō* with chopsticks and not forks and spoons (considered easier to use) and in the traditional *furoshiki* (piece of cloth which enwraps items and is double tied to close it) instead of the easier-to-manage *obentō* bags with drawstrings. Both *furoshiki* and chopsticks (*o-hashi*) are considered traditionally Japanese and their usage marks not only greater effort and skills on the part of the children but their enculturation into being Japanese.
17. For the mother's role in the education of her child, see, for example, White (1987). For an analysis, by a Japanese of the intense dependence on the mother that is created and cultivated in a child, see Doi (1971). For Japanese sources on the mother-child relationship and ideology (some say pathology) of Japanese motherhood, see Yamamura (1971); *Kawai* (1976); Kyūtoku (1981); *Sorifu seihonen taisaku honbuhen* (1981); *Kadeshobo shinsha* (1981). Fujita's account of the ideology of motherhood at the nursery school level is particularly interesting in this connection (1989).
18. Women are entering the labor market in increasing numbers yet the proportion to do so in the capacity of part-time workers (legally constituting as much as thirty-five hours per week but without the benefits accorded to full-time workers) has also increased. The choice of part-time over full-time employment has much to do with a woman's simultaneous and almost total responsibility for the domestic realm (Juristo 1985: see also Kondo 1990).
19. As Fujita (1989: 72–79) points out, working mothers are treated as a separate category of mothers, and non-working mothers are expected, by definition, to be mothers full time.
20. Nakane's much quoted text on Japanese society states this male position in structuralist terms (1970). Though dated, see also Vogel (1963) and Rohlen (1974) for descriptions of the social roles for middle-class, urban Japanese males. For a succinct recent discussion of gender roles within the family, see Lock (1990).

REFERENCES

Althusser, Louis, 1971. *Ideology and Ideological State Apparatuses (Notes toward an investigation in Lenin and philosophy and other essays).* New York: Monthly Review.

Asanuma, Kaoru. 1987. *"Ganbari" no Kozo (Structure of "Ganbari").* Tokyo: Kikkawa Kobunkan.

Barthes, Roland. 1957. *Mythologies.* Trans. by Annette Lavers. New York: Noonday Press.

Boocock, Sarane Spence. 1989. Controlled diversity: An overview of the Japanese preschool system. *The Journal of Japanese Studies* 15(1): 41–65.

Chicago Tribune. 1991. Burdens of Working Wives Weigh Heavily in Japan. January 27, Section 6, p. 7.

Cummings, William K. 1980. *Education and Equality in Japan.* Princeton NJ; Princeton University Press.

Doi, Takeo, 1971. *The Anatomy of Dependence: The Key Analysis of Japanese Behavior.* Trans. by John Becker. Tokyo: Kodansha Int'l. Ltd.

Dore, Ronald P. 1965. *Education in Tokugawa Japan.* London: Routledge and Kegan Paul.

Duke, Benjamin. 1986. *The Japanese School: Lessons for Industrial America.* New York: Praeger.

Fallows, Deborah. 1990. "Japanese Women." *National Geographic* 177(4): 52–83.

Fujita, Mariko. 1989. "It's All Mother's Fault": Childcare and the Socialization of Working Mothers in Japan. *The Journal of Japanese Studies* 15(1): 67–91.

Greenbie, Barrie B. 1988. *Space and Spirit in Modern Japan.* New Haven, CT: Yale University Press.

Hendry, Joy. 1986. *Becoming Japanese: The World of the Pre-School Child.* Honolulu: University of Hawaii Press.

———. 1987. *Understanding Japanese Society.* London: Croom Helm.

Horio, Teruhisa. 1988. *Educational Thought and Ideology in Modern Japan: State Authority and Intellectual Freedom.* Trans. by Steven Platzer. Tokyo: University of Tokyo Press.

Imamura, Anne E. 1987. *Urban Japanese Housewives: At Home and in the Community.* Honolulu: University of Hawaii Press.

Juristo zōkan Sōgōtokushu. 1985. Josei no Gensai to Mirai (The present and future of women). 39.

Kadeshobo shinsha. 1981. *Hahaoya (Mother).* Tokyo: Kadeshobo shinsha.

Kawai, Hayao. 1976. *Bosei shakai nihon no Byōri (The Pathology of the Mother Society—Japan).* Tokyo: Chuo Koronsha.

Kondo, Dorinne K. 1990. *Crafting Selves: Power, Gender, and Discourses of Identity in a Japanese Workplace.* Chicago, IL: University of Chicago Press.

Kyūtoku, Shigemori. 1981. *Bogenbyō (Disease Rooted in Motherhood).* Vol. II. Tokyo: Sanma Kushuppan.

Lewis, Catherine C. 1989. From Indulgence to Internalization: Social Control in the Early School Years. *Journal of Japanese Studies* 15(1): 139–157.

Lock, Margaret. 1990. Restoring Order to the House of Japan. *The Wilson Quarterly* 14(4): 42–49.

Marx, Karl and Frederick Engels. 1970 (1947). *Economic and Philosophic Manuscripts,* ed. C.J. Arthur. New York: International Publishers

Mirai shakan. 1979. Shufu to onna (Housewives and Women). Kunitachishi Komininkan Shimindaigaku Semina - no Kiroku. Tokyo: Miraisha.

Mouer, Ross and Yoshio Sugimoto. 1986. *Images of Japanese Society: A Study in the Social Construction of Reality.* London: Routledge and Kegan.

Nakane, Chie, 1970. *Japanese Society.* Berkeley: University of California Press.

Ohirasōri no Seifu kenkyūkai. 1980. Katei Kiban no Jujitsu (The Fullness of Family Foundations). (Ohirasōri no Seifu Kenkyūkai - 3). Tokyo: Okurashō Insatsukyōku.

Peak, Lois. 1989. "Learning to Become Part of the Group: The Japanese Child's Transition to Preschool Life." *The Journal of Japanese Studies* 15(1): 93–123.

Ritchie, Donald. 1985. *A Taste of Japan: Food Fact and Fable, Customs and Etiquette, What the People Eat.* Tokyo: Kodansha International Ltd.

Rohlen, Thomas P. 1974. *The Harmony and Strength: Japanese White-Collar Organization in Anthropological Perspective.* Berkeley: University of California Press.

———. 1983. *Japan's High Schools.* Berkeley: University of California Press.

———. 1989. "Order in Japanese Society: Attachment, Authority and Routine." *The Journal of Japanese Studies* 15(1): 5–40.

Sano, Toshiyuki. 1989. "Methods of Social Control and Socialization in Japanese Day-Care Centers. *The Journal of Japanese Studies* 15(1):125–138.

Shufunotomo Besutoserekushon shiri-zu. 1980. Obentō 500 sen. Tokyo: Shufunotomo Co., Ltd.

Shufunotomohyakka shiri-zu. 1981. 365 nichi no obentō hyakka. Tokyo: Shufunotomo Co.

Sōrifu Seihonen Taisaku Honbuhen, 1981. Nihon no kodomo to hahaoya (Japenese mothers and chldren): Kokusaihikaku (international comparisons). Tokyo: Sōrifu Seishonen Taisaku Honbuhen.

Tobin, Joseph J., David Y. H. Wu, and Dana H. Davidson. 1989. *Preschool in Three Cultures: Japan, China, and the United States.* New Haven, CT: Yale University Press.

Vogel, Erza. 1963. *Japan's New Middle Class: The Salary Man and his Family in a Tokyo Suburb.* Berkeley: University of California Press.

White, Merry. 1987. *The Japanese Educational Challenge: A Commitment to Children.* New York: Free Press.

Yamamura, Yoshiaki. 1971. *Nihonjin to Haha: Bunka Toshite No Haha no Kannen Ni Tsuite no Kenkyu (The Japanese and Mother: Research on the Conceptualization of Mother as Culture).* Tokyo: Toyo-shuppansha.

VIII

GENDER, HOUSEHOLD, AND KINSHIP

The study of kinship has been central to cross-cultural research. Marriage customs, systems of descent, and patterns of residence have been described and compared in a range of societies around the world. At the heart of traditional studies of kinship is the opposition between the domestic domain on the one hand and the public, political, and jural domain on the other. Anthropologists, particularly those working in Africa, studied kinship in this latter domain. They delineated large corporate descent groups called lineages that managed property and resources and that were the basic building blocks of political organization (Fortes 1949, 1953). Marriage, for some kinship theorists, is a political transaction, involving the exchange of women between men who wish to form alliances (Levi-Strauss 1969; see also Ortner 1978). A woman, from this perspective, is a passive pawn with little influence over kinship transactions. She is viewed "in terms of the rights her kin have to her domestic labor, to the property she might acquire, to her children, and to her sexuality" (Lamphere 1974: 98). The dynamic, affective, and even interest-oriented aspects of women's kinship are essentially ignored in an approach that is rooted in androcentric principles: Women have the children; men impregnate the women; and men usually exercise control (Fox 1967).

Recent critiques of the traditional study of kinship have pointed out that it is "no longer adequate to view women as bringing to kinship primarily a capacity for bearing children while men bring primarily a capacity for participation in public life" (Collier and Yanagisako 1987: 7). A gendered approach to kinship takes a number of different directions but focuses on the status of men and women in different kinship systems and on the power (defined as the ability to make others conform to one's desires and wishes) that accrues to women through their manipulation of social relations (Maynes et al 1996). Cross-cultural variations in the status of men and women have been examined in relation to rules of descent and postmarital residence (Martin and Voorhies 1975; Friedl 1975). Among horticuturalists, for example, women have higher status in societies characterized by matrilineal descent (descent through the female line from a common female ancestor) and matrilocal residence (living with the wife and her kin after marriage) than in societies characterized by patrilineal descent (descent through the male line from a common male ancestor) and patrilocal residence (living with the husband and his kin after marriage). In matrilineal systems descent group membership, social identity, rights to land, and succession to political office are all inherited through one's mother.

When matrilineality is combined with matrilocal residence, a husband marries into a household in which a long-standing domestic coalition exists between his wife and her mother, sisters, and broader kin relations (Friedl 1975). These women cooperate with one another in work endeavors and provide mutual support. Although in a matrilineal system a man retains authority over his sisters and her children, the coalitions formed by kin-related women can provide them with power and influence both within and beyond the household (Brown 1970; Lamphere 1974) and also with a degree of sexual freedom. The important issue for women's status, as Schlegel (1972: 96) has argued, is not the descent system per se but the organization of the domestic group.

In contrast to matrilineal and matrilocal systems, in patrilineal and patrilocal societies women do not have their own kin nearby. A woman enters her husband's household as a stranger. Separated from her own kin, she cannot forge lateral alliances easily. However, other opportunities are open to women that enhance their power and status in patrilineal and patrilocal societies. Taiwanese women, for example, marry into the households of their husbands (Wolf 1972). A Taiwanese wife must pay homage to her husband's ancestors, obey her husband and mother-in-law, and bear children for her husband's patrilineage. According to Wolf (1972: 32), "A woman can and, if she is ever to have any economic security, must provide the links in the male chain of descent, but she will never appear in anyone's genealogy as that all-important name connecting the past to the future."

After a Taiwanese wife gives birth to a son, her status in the household begins to change, and it improves during her life course as she forges what Wolf calls a uterine family—a family based on the powerful relationship between mothers and sons. The subordination of conjugal to intergenerational relationships that is exemplified by the Taiwanese case, as well as the opportune ways in which women take advantage of filial ties to achieve political power within and beyond the household, are apparent in other societies around the world—for example, in sub-Saharan Africa (Potash 1986).

When a Taiwanese wife becomes a mother-in-law she achieves the greatest power and status within her husband's household. Wolf (1972: 37) concludes that "the uterine family has no ideology, no formal structure, and no public existence. It is built out of sentiments and loyalties that die with its members, but it is no less real for all that. The descent lines of men are born and nourished in the uterine families of women, and it is here that a male ideology that excludes women makes its accommodations with reality." Similarly, Hausa trading women are able to compensate for an ideology that keeps them in residential seclusion by depending on their children to distribute their goods, provide information on the world outside the household, and help with child care and cooking (Schildkrout 1983).

Wolf's research on Taiwanese women substantiates Lamphere's (1974: 99) observation that "the distribution of power and authority in the family, the developmental cycle of the domestic group, and women's strategies are all related." By strategies Lamphere is referring to the active ways in which women use and manipulate kinship to their own advantage. The strategic use of kinship is a mechanism for economic survival among the African-American families of a Midwestern town described by Stack (in this book). The households of these families are flexible and fluid; they are tied together by complex networks of female kinship and friendship. If the boundaries of the household are elastic, the ties that unite kin and friends are long-lasting. Through these domestic networks, women exchange a range of goods and services including child care. They rely on one another and through collective efforts keep one another afloat. When one member of the network achieves a degree of economic success she can choose to withdraw from kin cooperation to conserve resources. However, by reinitiating gift-giving and exchange, at some point she can easily reenter the system. Stack's research shows one example of a strategy pursued by many families in the United States who must cope with urban poverty and the constant threat of unemployment.

A similar approach is shown in research on Afro-Caribbean families, who also live in conditions of economic uncertainty and stress. This research has generated a vigorous debate about a complex of characteristics, including female-headed households, women's control of household earnings and decision making, kinship networks linked through women, and the absence of resident men. This complex of characteristics has been referred to as matrifocality. Drawing on data from her research in Jamaica, Prior (in this book) reviews the concept of matrifocality, a concept first introduced by Raymond Smith in 1956 to describe the central position and power of the mother within the household. Rather than viewing these households as disorganized or pathological results of slavery and colonialism, anthropologists recently have stressed their adaptive advantages (Bolles and Samuels 1989) for women who are both mothers and economic providers. Furthermore, as Prior suggests, the composition of households in the Caribbean is fluid; they can be female-headed at one point in time and nuclear at another. Arguing against a widely held conception within anthropology, Prior suggests that fathers and male partners are by no means marginal to the household.

Prior points out that very little work has been done on the relations between men and women in such households because men were always assumed to be absent. One neglected aspect of male-female household relations is domestic violence. Such violence often emerges because the expectations that women hold for men, whether they are monetary contributions to the household or fidelity, are not fulfilled. The potential for violence that can erupt when women challenge men about these unfulfilled obligations can undercut the power that women otherwise maintain within the household.

Women-centered families like those of African-Americans and Afro-Caribbeans have been described for other parts of the world (Tanner 1974). Cole (in this book) introduces us to Maria, a fisherwoman who lives in a small town on the northern coast of Portugal. Forced into productive activity because her husband emigrated to Brazil and abandoned her for many years, Maria has taken control of her life and her personhood. Like Taiwanese women, she has invested in her relationship with her children rather than in the conjugal tie with her husband, although in this case the significant children are daughters rather than sons. Children, says Cole, are a resource for women. This is most evident in the high rates of illegitimacy that have characterized this town, and northern Portugal in general, until fairly recently. Also characteristic of the region are the significant inheritance of property by women and the tendency for matrilocal residence or neolocal residence near the wife's kin. These women-centered patterns are, as Cole and others (Brettell 1986) stress, closely linked to a longstanding pattern of male emigration. Whether in agriculture or in fishing, many women in northern Portugal must fulfill both male and female roles within the household.

The matrilateral bias in kinship described by Cole for northern Portugal is also apparent among Japanese-American immigrants in the urban United States (Yanagisako 1977). Manifested in women-centered kin networks, this bias influences patterns of co-residence, residential proximity, mutual aid, and affective ties.

Rather than stressing the economic reasons for the maintenance of kinship ties, Yanagisako draws attention to the role of women as kin keepers who foster and perpetuate channels of communication and who plan and stage elaborate family rituals.

The social and ritual importance of kinship is precisely what di Leonardo (in this book) focuses on in her discussion of the female world of cards and holidays. The Italian-American women she describes work in the labor market and at home, but they are also engaged in "kin work." Kin work is women's work and involves maintaining contact through all kinds of mechanisms with family members who are deemed important. Unlike child care and house cleaning, it is a task that has to be carried out by the woman herself. Though it is often burdensome work women undertake kin work, according to di Leonardo, because through it they can set up a chain of valuable and long-term obligations within a wide circle of social relations.

Although di Leonardo identifies other parts of the developed world in which women have greater kin knowledge than men and work hard at maintaining kinship networks (for example, Lomnitz and Perez-Lizaur 1987), several questions are open to further empirical investigation. For example, why does kin work take on ritual significance in some societies, and why is it culturally assigned to women in some contexts and to men in others? Di Leonardo interprets the emergence of gendered kin work in association with a relative decline in importance of the domain of public male kinship that is found, for example, in African societies characterized by a powerful principle of descent. The shift, she suggests, is part of the process of capitalist development. Enloe (1990) has taken these arguments much further by demonstrating how both global politics and global economics are engendered. Without kin work, for example, Hallmark (the card manufacturer) would be out of business.

Collier and Yanagisako (1987) have argued that gender and kinship are mutually constructed and should be brought together into one analytic field. Kinship and gender are closely allied because they are both based in, but not exclusively determined by, biology and because what it means to be a man or a woman is directly linked to the rules of marriage and sexuality that a culture constructs. As Lindenbaum (1987: 221) has observed, "Relations of kinship are in certain societies, relations of production. If kinship is understood as a system that organizes the liens we hold on the emotions and labors of others, then it must be studied in relation to gender ideologies that enmesh men and women in diverse relations of productive and reproductive work. The variable constructions of male and female that emerge in different times and places are central to an understanding of the character of kinship."

REFERENCES

Bolles, A. Lynn and Deborah d'Amico Samuels. 1989. "Anthropological Scholarship on Gender in the English-speaking Caribbean." In Sandra Morgen (ed.). *Gender and Anthropology*, pp. 171–188. Washington, DC: American Anthropological Association.

Brettell, Caroline B. 1986. *Men Who Migrate, Women Who Wait: Population and History in a Portuguese Parish.* Princeton: Princeton University Press.

Brown, Judith K. 1970. "Economic Organization and the Position of Women Among the Iroquois." *Ethnohistory* 17: 151–167.

Collier, Jane Fishburne and Sylvia Junko Yanagisako. 1987. *Gender and Kinship: Essays Toward a Unified Analysis.* Stanford: Stanford University Press.

Enloe, Cynthia. 1990. *Bananas, Beaches and Bases: Making Feminist Sense of International Politics.* Berkeley: University of California Press.

Fortes, Meyer. 1949. *The Web of Kinship Among the*

Tallensi. London: International African Institute, Oxford University Press.
———. 1953. "The Structure of Unilineal Descent Groups." *American Anthropologist* 55: 25–39.
Fox, Robin. 1967. *Kinship and Marriage: An Anthropological Perspective.* Harmondsworth: Penguin.
Friedl, Ernestine. 1975. *Women and Men: An Anthropologist's View.* New York: Holt, Rinehart and Winston.
Lamphere, Louise. 1974. "Strategies, Cooperation, and Conflict Among Women in Domestic Groups." In Michelle Z. Rosaldo and Louise Lamphere (eds.). *Woman, Culture, and Society,* pp. 97–112. Stanford: Stanford University Press.
Levi-Strauss, Claude. 1969. *The Elementary Structures of Kinship.* Boston: Beacon Press.
Lindenbaum, Shirley, 1987. "The Mystification of Female Labors." In Jane Fishburne Collier and Sylvia Junko Yanagisako (eds.). *Gender and Kinship: Essays Toward a Unified Analysis.* Stanford: Stanford University Press.
Lomnitz, Larissa and Marisol Perez-Lizaur. 1987. *A Mexican Elite Family, 1820–1980.* Princeton: Princeton University Press.
Martin, M. Kay and Barbara Voorhies. 1975. *Female of the Species.* New York: Columbia University Press.
Maynes, Mary Jo, Ann Waltner, Birgitte Soland, and Ulrike Strasser. 1996. *Gender, Kinship, Power: A Comparative and Interdisciplinary History.* New York: Routledge.
Ortner, Sherry. 1978. "The Virgin and the State." *Feminist Studies* 4 (3): 19–35.
Potash, Betty (ed.). 1986. *Widows in African Societies.* Stanford: Stanford University Press.
Schildkrout, Enid. 1983. "Dependence and Autonomy: The Economic Activities of Secluded Hausa Women in Kano." In Christine Oppong (ed.). *Female and Male in West Africa.* Winchester, MA: Allen and Unwin.
Schlegel, Alice. 1972. *Male Dominance and Female Autonomy: Domestic Authority in Matrilineal Societies.* New Haven: Human Relations Area Files.
Smith, Raymond. 1956. *The Negro Family in British Guiana: Family Structure and Social Status in the Villages.* London: Routledge and Kegan Paul.
Tanner, Nancy. 1974. "Matrifocality in Indonesia and Africa and Among Black Americans." In Michelle Z. Rosaldo and Louise Lamphere (eds.). *Woman, Culture, and Society,* pp. 129–156. Stanford: Stanford University Press.
Wolf, Margery. 1972. *Women and the Family in Rural Taiwan.* Stanford: Stanford University Press.
Yanagisako, Sylvia Junko. 1977. "Women-centered Kin Networks in Urban Bilateral Kinship." *American Ethnologist* 2: 207–226.

DOMESTIC NETWORKS: "THOSE YOU COUNT ON"

Carol Stack

In The Flats the responsibility for providing food, care, clothing, and shelter and for socializing children within domestic networks may be spread over several households. Which household a given individual belongs to is not a particularly meaningful question, as we have seen that daily domestic organization depends on several things: where people sleep, where they eat, and where they offer their time and money. Although those who eat together and contribute toward the rent are generally considered by Flat's residents to form minimal domestic units, household changes rarely affect the exchanges and daily dependencies of those who take part in common activity.

The residence patterns and cooperative organization of people linked in domestic networks demonstrate the stability and collective power of family life in The Flats. Michael Lee grew up in The Flats and now has a job in Chicago. On a visit to The Flats, Michael described the residence and domestic organization of his kin. "Most of my kin in The Flats lived right here on Cricket Street, numbers sixteen, eighteen, and twenty-two, in these three apartment buildings joined together. My mama decided it would be best for me and my three brothers and sister to be on Cricket Street too. My daddy's mother had a small apartment in this building, her sister had one in the basement, and another brother and his family took a larger apartment upstairs. My uncle was really good to us. He got us things we wanted and he controlled us. All the women kept the younger kids together during the day. They cooked together too. It was good living."

Yvonne Diamond, a forty-year-old Chicago woman, moved to The Flats from Chicago with her four children. Soon afterwards they were evicted. "The landlord said he was going to build a parking lot there, but he never did. The old place is still standing and has folks in it today. My husband's mother and father took me and the kids in and watched over them while I had my baby. We stayed on after my husband's mother died, and my husband joined us when he got a job in The Flats."

When families or individuals in The Flats are evicted, other kinsmen usually take them in. Households in The Flats expand or contract with the loss of a job, a death in the family, the beginning or end of a sexual partnership, or the end of a friendship. Welfare workers, researchers, and landlords have long known that the poor must move frequently. What is much less understood is the relationship between residence and domestic organization in the black community.

The spectrum of economic and legal pressures that act upon ghetto residents, requiring them to move—unemployment, welfare requirements, housing shortages, high rents, eviction—are clear-cut examples of external pressures affecting the daily lives of the poor. Flats' residents are evicted from their dwellings by landlords who want to raise rents, tear the building down, or rid themselves of tenants who complain about rats, roaches, and the plumbing. Houses get condemned by the city on landlords' requests so that they can force tenants to move. After an eviction, a landlord can rent to a family in such great need of housing that they will not complain for a while.

Poor housing conditions and unenforced housing standards coupled with overcrowding, unemployment, and poverty produce hazardous living conditions and residence changes. "Our whole family had to move when the gas lines sprung a leak in our apartment and my son set the place on fire by accident," Sam Summer told me. "The place belonged to my sister-in-law's grandfather. We had been living there with my mother, my brother's eight children, and our eight children. My father lived in the basement apartment 'cause he and my mother were separated. After the fire burned the whole place down, we all moved to two places down the street near my cousin's house."

When people are unable to pay their rent because they have been temporarily "cut off aid," because the welfare office is suspicious of their eligibility, because they gave their rent money to a kinsman to help him through a crisis or illness, or because they were laid off from their job, they receive eviction notices almost immediately. Lydia Watson describes a chain of events starting with the welfare office stopping her sister's welfare checks, leading to an eviction, co-residence, overcrowding, and eventually murder. Lydia sadly related the story to me. "My oldest sister was cut off aid the day her husband got out of jail. She and her husband and their three children were evicted from their apartment and they came to live with us. We were in crowded conditions already. I had my son, my other sister was there with her two kids, and my mother was about going crazy. My mother put my sister's husband out 'cause she found out he was a dope addict. He came back one night soon after that and murdered my sister. After my sister's death my mother couldn't face living in Chicago any longer. One of my other sisters who had been adopted and raised by my mother's paternal grandmother visited us and persuaded us to move to The Flats, where she was staying. All of us moved there—my mother, my two sisters and their children, my two baby sisters, and my dead sister's children. My sister who had been staying in The Flats found us a house across the street from her own."

Overcrowded dwellings and the impossibility of finding adequate housing in The Flats have many long-term consequences regarding where and with whom children live. Terence Platt described where and with whom his kin lived when he was a child. "My brother stayed with my aunt, my mother's sister, and her husband until he was ten, 'cause he was the oldest in our family and we didn't have enough room—but he stayed with us most every weekend. Finally my aunt moved into the house behind ours with her husband, her brother, and my brother; my sisters and brothers and I lived up front with my mother and her old man."

KIN-STRUCTURED LOCAL NETWORKS

The material and cultural support needed to absorb, sustain, and socialize community members in The Flats is provided by networks of cooperating kinsmen. Local coalitions formed from these networks of kin and friends are mobilized within domestic networks; domestic organization is diffused over many kin-based households which themselves have elastic boundaries.

People in The Flats are immersed in a domestic web of a large number of kin and friends whom they can count on. From a social viewpoint, relationships within the community are "organized on the model of kin relationships" (Goodenough 1970, p. 49). Kin-constructs such as the perception of parenthood, the culturally determined criteria which affect the shape of personal kindreds, and the idiom of kinship, prescribe kin who can be recruited into domestic networks.

There are similarities in function between domestic networks and domestic groups which Fortes (1962, p. 2) characterizes as "workshops of social reproduction." Both domains include three generations of members linked collaterally or otherwise. Kinship, jural and affectional bonds, and economic factors affect the composition of both domains and residential alignments within them. There are two striking differences between domestic networks and domestic groups. Domestic networks are not visible groups, because they do not have an obvious nucleus or defined boundary. But since a primary focus of domestic networks is child-care arrangements, the cooperation of a cluster of adult females is apparent. Participants in domestic networks are recruited from personal kindreds and friendships, but the personnel changes with fluctuating economic needs, changing life styles, and vacillating personal relationships.

In some loosely and complexly structured cognatic systems, kin-structured local networks (not groups) emerge. Localized coalitions of persons drawn from personal kindreds can be organized as networks of kinsmen. Goodenough (1970, p. 49) correctly points out that anthropologists frequently describe "localized kin groups," but rarely describe kin-structured local groups (Goodenough 1962; Helm 1965). The localized, kin-based, cooperative coalitions of people described in this chapter are organized as kin-structured domestic networks. For brevity, I refer to them as domestic networks.

RESIDENCE AND DOMESTIC ORGANIZATION

The connection between households and domestic life can be illustrated by examples taken from cooperating kinsmen and friends mobilized within domestic networks in The Flats. Domestic networks are, of course, not centered around one individual, but for simplicity the domestic network in the following example is named for the key participants in the network, Magnolia and Calvin Waters. The description is confined to four months between April and July 1969. Even within this short time span, individuals moved and joined other households within the domestic network.

THE DOMESTIC NETWORK OF MAGNOLIA AND CALVIN WATERS

Magnolia Waters is forty-one years old and has eleven children. At sixteen she moved from the South with her parents, four sisters (Augusta, Carrie, Lydia, and Olive), and two brothers (Pennington and Oscar). Soon after this she gave birth to her oldest daughter, Ruby. At twenty-three Ruby Banks had two daughters and a son, each by a different father.

When Magnolia was twenty-five she met Calvin, who was forty-seven years old. They lived together and had six children. Calvin is now sixty-three years old; Calvin and Magnolia plan to marry soon so that Magnolia will receive Calvin's insurance benefits. Calvin has two other daughters, who are thirty-eight and forty, by an early marriage in Mississippi. Calvin still has close ties with his daughters and their mother who all live near one another with their families in Chicago.

Magnolia's oldest sister, Augusta, is childless and has not been married. Augusta has maintained long-term "housekeeping" partnerships with four different men over the past twenty years, and each of them has helped her raise her sisters' children. These men have maintained close, affectional ties with the family over the years. Magnolia's youngest sister, Carrie, married Lazar, twenty-five years her senior, when she was just fifteen. They stayed together for about five years. After they separated Carrie married Kermit, separated from him, and became an alcoholic. She lives with different men from time to time, but in between men, or when things are at loose ends, she stays with Lazar, who has become a participating member of the family. Lazar usually resides near Augusta and Augusta's "old man," and Augusta generally prepares Lazar's meals. Ever since Carrie became ill, Augusta has been raising Carrie's son.

Magnolia's sister Lydia had two daughters, Lottie and Georgia, by two different fathers, before she married Mike and gave birth to his son. After Lydia married Mike, she no longer received AFDC benefits for her children. Lydia and Mike acquired steady jobs, bought a house and furniture, and were doing very well. For at least ten years they purposely removed themselves from the network of kin cooperation, preventing their kin from draining their resources. They refused to participate in the network of exchanges which Lydia had formerly depended upon; whenever possible they refused to trade clothes or lend money, or if they gave something, they did not ask for anything in return. During this period they were not participants in the domestic network. About a year ago Lydia and Mike separated over accusations and gossip that each of them had established another sexual relationship. During the five-month-period when the marriage was ending, Lydia began giving some of her nice clothes away to her sisters and nieces. She gave a couch to her brother and a TV to a niece. Anticipating her coming needs, Lydia attempted to reobligate her kin by carrying out the pattern which had been a part of her daily life before her marriage. After Lydia separated from her husband, her two younger children once again received AFDC. Lydia's oldest daughter, Lottie, is over eighteen and too old to receive AFDC, but Lottie has a three-year-old daughter who has received AFDC benefits since birth.

Eloise has been Magnolia's closest friend for many years. Eloise is Magnolia's first son's father's sister. This son moved into his father's household by his own choice when he was about twelve years old. Magnolia and Eloise have maintained a close, sisterly friendship. Eloise lives with her husband, her four children, and the infant son of her oldest daughter, who is seventeen. Eloise's husband's brother's daughter, Lily, who is twenty, and her young daughter recently joined the household. Eloise's husband's youngest brother is the father of her sister's child. When the child was an infant, that sister stayed with Eloise and her husband.

Billy Jones lives in the basement in the same apartment house as Augusta, Magnolia's sister. A temperamental woman with three sons, Billy has become Augusta's closest friend. Billy once ran a brothel in The Flats, but she has worked as a cook, has written songs, and has attended college from time to time. Augusta keeps Billy's sons whenever Billy leaves town, has periods of depression, or beats the children too severely.

Another active participant in the network is Willa Mae. Willa Mae's younger brother, James, is Ruby's daughter's father. Even though James does not visit the child and has not assumed any parental duties toward the child, Willa Mae and Ruby, who are the same age, help each other out with their young children.

Calvin's closest friend, Cecil, died several years ago. Cecil was Violet's husband. Violet, Cecil, and Calvin came from the same town in Mississippi and their families have been very close. Calvin boarded with Violet's family for five years or so before he met Magnolia. Violet is now seventy years old. She lives with her daughter, Odessa, who is thirty-seven, her two sons, Josh, who is thirty-five and John, who is forty, and Odessa's three sons and daughter. Odessa's husband was killed in a fight several years ago and ever since then she and her family have shared a household with Violet and her two grown sons. Violet's sons Josh and John are good friends with Magnolia, Ruby, and Augusta and visit them frequently. About five years ago John brought one of his daughters to live with his mother and sister because his family thought that the mother was not taking proper care of the child; the mother had several other children and did not object. The girl is now ten years old and is an accepted member of the family and the network.

Chart 1 shows the spatial relations of the households in Magnolia and Calvin's domestic network in April 1969. The houses are scattered within The Flats, but none of them is more than three miles apart. Cab fare, up to two dollars per trip, is spent practically every day, and sometimes twice a day, as individuals visit, trade, and exchange services. Chart 2 shows how individuals are brought into the domestic network.

The following outline shows residential changes which occurred in several of the households within the network between April and June 1969.

APRIL 1969

Household Domestic Arrangement

1. Magnolia (38) and Calvin (60) live in a common-law relationship with their eight children (ages 4 to 18).
2. Magnolia's sister Augusta and Augusta's "old man," Herman, share a two-bedroom house with Magnolia's daughter Ruby (22) and Ruby's three children. Augusta and Herman have one bedroom, the three children sleep in the second bedroom, and Ruby sleeps downstairs in the living room. Ruby's boyfriend, Art, stays with Ruby many evenings.
3. Augusta's girlfriend Billy and Billy's three sons live on the first floor of the house. Lazar, Magnolia's and Augusta's ex-brother-in-law, lives in the basement alone, or from time to time, with his ex-wife Carrie. Lazar eats the evening meal, which Augusta prepares for him, at household #2.
4. Magnolia's sister Lydia, Lydia's "old man," Lydia's two daughters, Georgia and Lottie, Lydia's son, and Lottie's three-year-old daughter live in Lydia's house.
5. Willa Mae (26), her husband, her son, her sister Claudia (32), and her brother James (father of Ruby's daughter) share a household.
6. Eloise (37), her husband Jessie, their four children, their oldest daughter's (17) son, and Jessie's brother's daughter Lily (20), and Lily's baby all live together.
7. Violet (70), her two sons, Josh (35) and John (40), her daughter Odessa (37), and Odessa's three sons and one daughter live together. Five years ago John's daughter (10) joined the household.

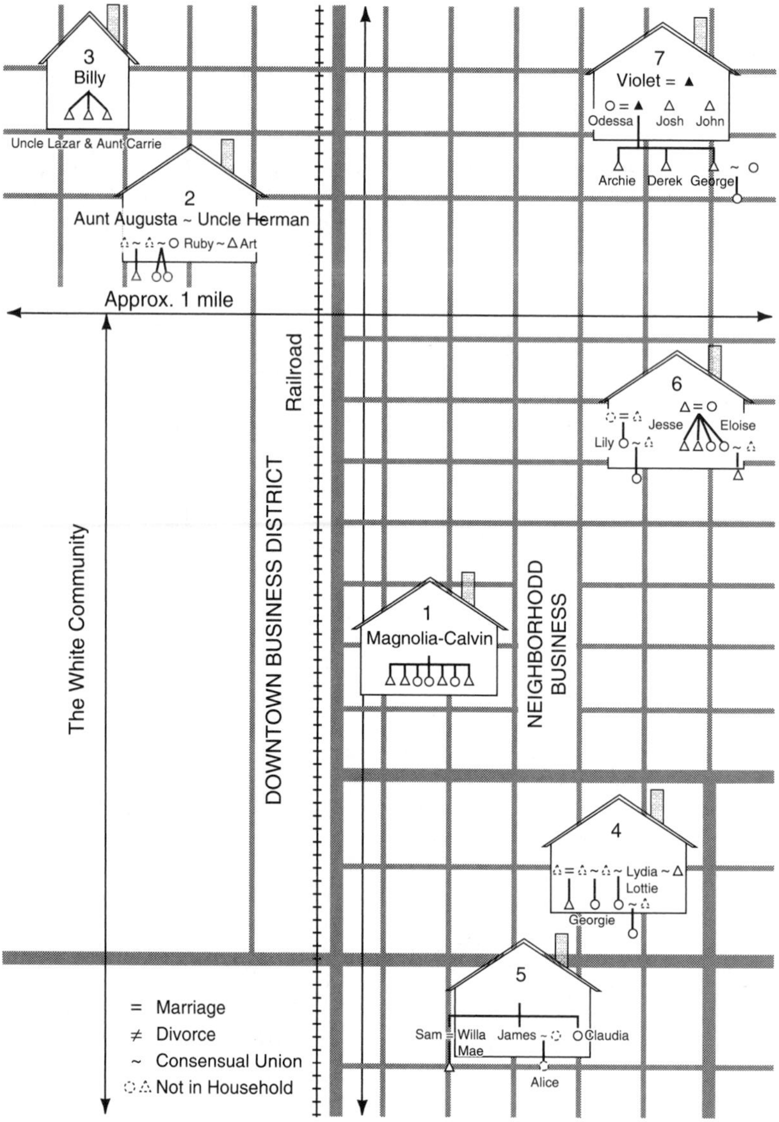

CHART 1 Spatial Relations in Magnolia and Leo's Domestic Network

JUNE 1969

Household Domestic Arrangement

1. Household composition unchanged.
2. Augusta and Herman moved out after quarreling with Ruby over housekeeping and cooking duties. They joined household #3. Ruby and Art remained in household #2 and began housekeeping with Ruby's children.
3. Billy and her three sons remained on the first floor and Lazar remained in the basement. Augusta and Herman rented a small, one-room apartment upstairs.

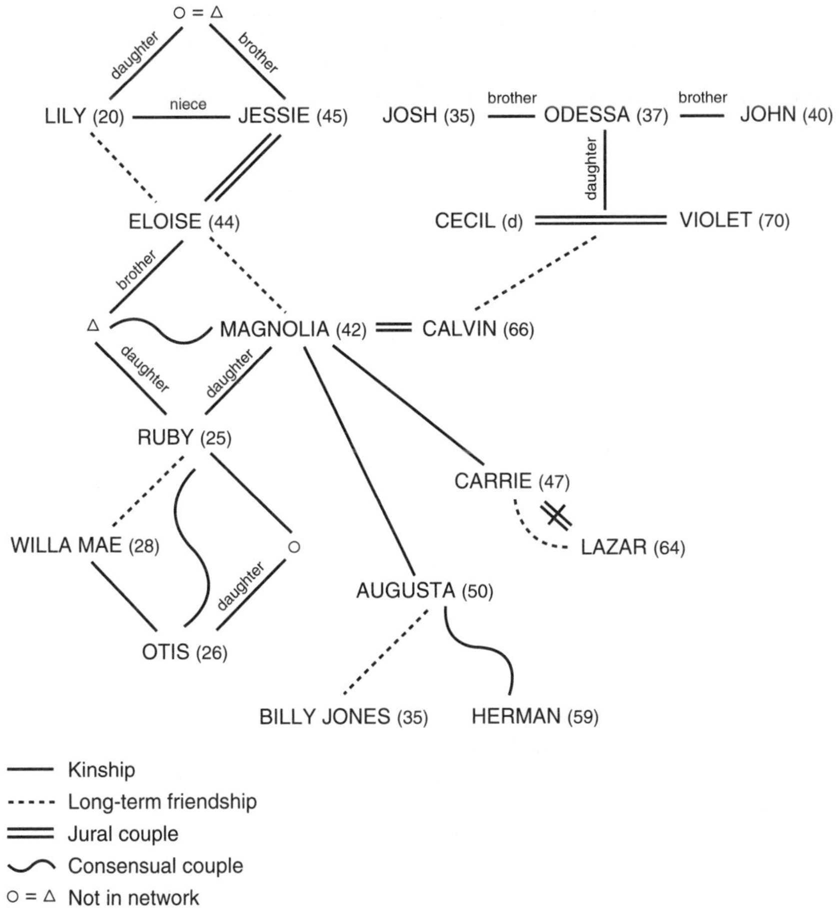

CHART 2 Kin-structured Domestic Network

4. Lottie and her daughter moved out of Lydia's house to a large apartment down the street, which they shared with Lottie's girl friend and the friend's daughter. Georgia moved into her boyfriend's apartment. Lydia and her son (17) remained in the house with Lydia's "old man."
5. James began housekeeping with a new girl friend who lived with her sister, but he kept most of his clothes at home. His brother moved into his room after returning from the service. Willa Mae, her husband, and son remained in the house.
6. Household composition unchanged.
7. Odessa's son Raymond is the father of Clover's baby. Clover and the baby joined the household which includes Violet, her two sons, her daughter, Odessa, and Odessa's three sons and one daughter and John's daughter.

Typical residential alignments in The Flats are those between adult mothers and sisters, mothers and adult sons and daughters, close adult female relatives, and friends defined as kin within the idiom of kinship. Domestic organization is diffused over these kin-based households.

Residence patterns among the poor in The Flats must be considered in the context of domestic organization. The connection between residence and domestic organization is apparent in examples of a series of domestic and child-care arrangements within Magnolia and Calvin's network a few years ago. Consider the following four kin-based residences among Magnolia and Calvin's kin in 1966.

Household Domestic Arrangement

1. Magnolia, Calvin, and seven young children.
2. Magnolia's mother, Magnolia's brother, Magnolia's sister and her sister's husband, Magnolia's oldest daughter, Ruby, and Ruby's first child.
3. Magnolia's oldest sister, Augusta, Augusta's "old man," Augusta's sister's (Carrie) son, and Magnolia's twelve-year-old son.
4. Magnolia's oldest son, his father, and the father's "old lady."

Household composition *per se* reveals little about domestic organization even when cooperation between close adult females is assumed. Three of these households (1, 2, 3) were located on one city block. Magnolia's mother rented a rear house behind Magnolia's house, and Magnolia's sister Augusta lived in an apartment down the street. As we have seen, they lived and shared each other's lives. Magnolia, Ruby, and Augusta usually pooled the food stamps they received from the welfare office. The women shopped together and everyone shared the evening meal with their men and children at Magnolia's mother's house or at Magnolia's. The children did not always have a bed of their own or a bed which they were expected to share with another child. They fell asleep and slept through the night wherever the late evening visiting patterns of the adult females took them.

The kinship links which most often are the basis of new or expanded households are those links children have with close adult females such as the child's mother, mother's mother, mother's sister, mother's brother's wife, father's mother, father's sister, and father's brother's wife.

Here are some examples of the flexibility of the Blacks' adaptation to daily, social, and economic problems (Stack 1970, p. 309).

Relational Link	*Domestic Arrangement*
Mother	Viola's brother married his first wife when he was sixteen. When she left him she kept their daughter.
Mother's mother	Viola's sister Martha was never able to care for her children because of her nerves and high blood. In between husbands, her mother kept her two oldest children, and after Martha's death, her mother kept all three of the children.
Mother's brother	A year after Martha's death, Martha's brother took Martha's oldest daughter, helping his mother out since this left her with only two children to care for.
Mother's mother	Viola's daughter (20) was living at home and gave birth to a son. The daughter and her son remained in the Jackson household until the daughter married and set up a separate household with her husband, leaving her son to be raised by her mother.
Mother's sister	Martha moved to Chicago into her sister's household. The household consisted of the two sisters and four of their children.
Father's mother	Viola's sister Ethel had four daughters and one son. When Ethel had a nervous breakdown, her husband took the three daughters and his son to live with his mother in Arkansas. After his wife's death, the husband took the oldest daughter, to join her siblings in his mother's home in Arkansas.
Father's mother	When Viola's younger sister, Christine, left her husband in order to harvest fruit in Wis-

	consin, Christine left her two daughters with her husband's mother in Arkansas.
Father's sister	When Viola's brother's wife died, he decided to raise his two sons himself. He kept the two boys and never remarried although he had several girl friends and a child with one. His residence has always been near Viola's and she fed and cared for his sons.

The basis of these cooperative units is mutual aid among siblings of both sexes, the domestic cooperation of close adult females, and the exchange of goods and services between male and female kin (Stack 1970). R.T. Smith (1970, p. 66) has referred to this pattern and observes that even when lower-class Blacks live in a nuclear family group, what is "most striking is the extent to which lower-class persons continue to be involved with other kin." Nancie Gonzalez (1970, p. 232) suggests that "the fact that individuals have simultaneous loyalties to more than one such grouping may be important in understanding the social structure as a whole."

These co-residential socializing units do indeed show the important role of the black female. But the cooperation between male and female siblings who share the same household or live near one another has been underestimated by those who have considered the female-headed household and the grandmother-headed household (especially the mother's mother) as the most significant domestic units among the urban black poor.

The close cooperation of adults arises from the residential patterns typical of young adults. Due to poverty, young females with or without children do not perceive any choice but to remain living at home with their mother or other adult female relatives. Even if young women are collecting AFDC, they say that their resources go further when they share goods and services. Likewise, jobless males, or those working at part-time or seasonal jobs, often remain living at home with their mother or, if she is dead, with their sisters and brothers. This pattern continues long after men have become fathers and have established a series of sexual partnerships with women, who are living with their own kin, friends, or alone with their children. A result of this pattern is the striking fact that households almost always have men around: male relatives, by birth or marriage, and boyfriends. These men are often intermittent members of the households, boarders, or friends who come and go; men who usually eat, and sometimes sleep, in the households. Children have constant and close contact with these men, and especially in the case of male relatives, these relationships last over the years.

The most predictable residential pattern in The Flats is that men and women reside in one of the households of their natal kin, or in the households of those who raised them, long into their adult years. Even when persons temporarily move out of the household of their mother or of a close relative, they have the option to return to the residences of their kin if they have to.

GENEROSITY AND POVERTY

The combination of arbitrary and repressive economic forces and social behavior, modified by successive generations of poverty, make it almost impossible for people to break out of poverty. There is no way for those families poor enough to receive welfare to acquire any surplus cash which can be saved for emergencies or for acquiring adequate appliances or a home or a car. In contrast to the middle class, who are pressured to spend and save, the poor are not even permitted to establish an equity.

The following examples from Magnolia and Calvin Waters' life illustrates the ways in which the poor are prohibited from acquiring any surplus which might enable them to change their economic condition or life style.

In 1971 Magnolia's uncle died in Mississippi and left an unexpected inheritance of $1,500 to Magnolia and Calvin Waters. The cash came from a small run-down farm which

Magnolia's uncle sold shortly before he died. It was the first time in their lives that Magnolia or Calvin ever had a cash reserve. Their first hope was to buy a home and use the money as a down payment.

Calvin had retired from his job as a seasonal laborer the year before and the family was on welfare. AFDC allotted the family $100 per month for rent. The housing that the family had been able to obtain over the years for their nine children at $100 or less was always small, roach infested, with poor plumbing and heating. The family was frequently evicted. Landlords complained about the noise and often observed an average of ten to fifteen children playing in the household. Magnolia and Calvin never even anticipated that they would be able to buy a home.

Three days after they received the check, news of its arrival spread throughout their domestic network. One niece borrowed $25 from Magnolia so that her phone would not be turned off. Within a week the welfare office knew about the money. Magnolia's children were immediately cut off welfare, including medical coverage and food stamps. Magnolia was told that she would not receive a welfare grant for her children until the money was used up, and she was given a minimum of four months in which to spend the money. The first surplus the family ever acquired was effectively taken from them.

During the weeks following the arrival of the money, Magnolia and Calvin's obligations to the needs of kin remained the same, but their ability to meet these needs had temporarily increased. When another uncle became very ill in the South, Magnolia and her older sister, Augusta, were called to sit by his side. Magnolia bought round-trip train tickets for both of them and for her three youngest children. When the uncle died, Magnolia bought round-trip train tickets so that she and Augusta could attend the funeral. Soon after his death, Augusta's first "old man" died in The Flats and he had no kin to pay for the burial. Augusta asked Magnolia to help pay for digging the grave. Magnolia was unable to refuse. Another sister's rent was two months overdue and Magnolia feared that she would get evicted. This sister was seriously ill and had no source of income. Magnolia paid her rent.

Winter was cold and Magnolia's children and grandchildren began staying home from school because they did not have warm winter coats and adequate shoes or boots. Magnolia and Calvin decided to buy coats, hats, and shoes for all of the children (at least fifteen). Magnolia also bought a winter coat for herself and Calvin bought himself a pair of sturdy shoes.

Within a month and a half, all of the money was gone. The money was channeled into the hands of the same individuals who ordinarily participate in daily domestic exchanges, but the premiums were temporarily higher. All of the money was quickly spent for necessary, compelling reasons.

Thus random fluctuations in the meager flow of available cash and goods tend to be of considerable importance to the poor. A late welfare check, sudden sickness, robbery, and other unexpected losses cannot be overcome with a cash reserve like more well-to-do families hold for emergencies. Increases in cash are either taken quickly from the poor by the welfare agencies or dissipated through the kin network.

Those living in poverty have little or no chance to escape from the economic situation into which they were born. Nor do they have the power to control the expansion or contraction of welfare benefits (Piven and Cloward 1971) or of employment opportunities, both of which have a momentous effect on their daily lives. In times of need, the only predictable resources that can be drawn upon are their own children and parents, and the fund of kin and friends obligated to them.

REFERENCES

Fortes, Meyer. 1962. "Marriage in Tribal Societies." *Cambridge Papers in Social Anthropology,* No. 3. Cambridge: Cambridge University Press.

Gonzalez, Nancie. 1970. "Toward a Definition of Matrifocality." In *Afro-American Anthropology:*

Contemporary Perspectives, eds. N. E. Whitten and John F. Szwed. New York: The Free Press.

Goodenough, Ward H. 1962. "Kindred and Hamlet in Lakalai, New Britain." *Ethnology* 1:5–12.

———. 1970. *Description and Comparison in Cultural Anthropology.* Chicago: Aldine Publishing Company.

Helm, June. 1965. "Bilaterality in the Socio-Territorial Organization of the Arctic Drain Age Dene." *Ethnology,* 4:361–385.

Piven, Frances Fox and Richard A. Cloward. 1971. *Regulating the Poor: The Functions of Public Welfare.* New York: Vintage Books.

Smith, Raymond T. 1970. "The Nuclear Family in Afro-American Kinship." *Journal of Comparative Family Studies* 1(1):55–70.

Stack, Carol B. 1970. "The Kindred of Viola Jackson: Residence and Family Organization of an Urban Black American Family." In *Afro-American Anthropology: Contemporary Perspectives,* eds. N. E. Whitten and John F. Szwed. New York: The Free Press, pp. 303–312.

MATRIFOCALITY, POWER, AND GENDER RELATIONS IN JAMAICA

Marsha Prior

Anthropologists have long recognized kinship units in which women maintain considerable control over the household earnings and decision making. While numerous studies have provided pertinent data and have contributed to the theory of social organization, the subject of female-focused kinship units has always been controversial, subject to bias, and confusing. The variations in terminology and a preoccupation with the origin of these units is responsible for much of the confusion. In addition, two biases, prevalent throughout the twentieth century, have influenced our understanding and acceptance of female-focused units. One bias has been the predominant view that nuclear families are "normal"; the other bias is the failure to recognize the full extent of female roles in society. The unfortunate result of this is that very little is known about the dynamics within and between female-focused kinship units.

The term *matrifocal,* which is most commonly used to refer to households composed of a key female decision maker, was coined by R.T. Smith in 1956. Recognition of such households precedes the usage of this term, however. As early as the 1930s scholars noted that African-American and African-Caribbean households were not composed of nuclear families as were the majority of middle-class households in the United States and Great Britain. Observers were struck by the authoritative role of women in these households and the limited role of the father in the family. Mothers controlled the earnings brought into the household and made key decisions. Fathers were either absent or did not appear to play a major role in economic contributions and in household decision making. However, attempts to address this situation reveal more the attitudes and biases prevalent at that time—many of which remain with us today—than any real insight as to the nature of such units. These *maternal families,* as they were often called during this early period, were viewed by scholars as deviant structures (Mohammed 1988). The high rate of illegitimacy and instability among mating partners was cited as proof that these families were disorganized and detrimental to the well-being of their members (Henriques 1953; Simey 1946; see also Moynihan 1965).

The bias toward nuclear family organization that dominated early studies stems from nineteenth century evolutionists who viewed the nuclear family as a superior system of kin-

Original material prepared for this text.

ship organization and from Malinowski who argued that nuclear families are universal (Collier, Rosaldo, and Yanigisako 1982). Thus, societies that exhibited large numbers of non-nuclear households were considered abnormal, and it was essential that their development be explained.

Scholars naturally turned to the common characteristics of these female-focused societies, noting that they were former slave societies from Africa. One explanation, suggested by Frazier (1939), held that maternal families were an adaptive strategy to the slave system that defined slaves as individual property who could be traded to another plantation at any time. Nuclear families would have been torn apart with frequent trading of adult slaves. Plantation owners were less likely, though, to tear apart mother-child dyads, at least until the child reached adolescence. Thus, the stable unit in a slave system was a household consisting of mothers and their children. The other explanation common during this time period, argued that the maternal family stemmed from the traditional African system that survived in spite of the Africans' forced migration and subsequent integration into the slave system (Herskovits 1941). These two theories enjoyed a lively debate until the mid-1950s when scholars moved away from historical explanations and emphasized the role of present social or economic conditions.

M.G. Smith (1962) argued that family structure in the West Indies was determined by the already existing mating systems that vary somewhat throughout the region. Clarke (1957), R.T. Smith (1956), and Gonzalez (1960) focused more on the effect that the current economic system had on household organization. The prevalent household structure found among African descendants in the United States and the Caribbean was viewed as an adaptive strategy to poverty, unemployment, or male migration. Nuclear families with only two working adults per household are believed by some to be at risk in socioeconomic environments in which poverty conditions exist, unemployment is high, and adult men must migrate to find work (see Durant-Gonzalez 1982; Gonzalez 1970:242). Thus, in such societies we are more likely to see households composed of a mother, a grandparent, and children; a mother and children; adult siblings and their children; or adult siblings, their children, and a grandparent.

The emphasis placed on the socioeconomic environment marked a new trend in matrifocal studies whereby the relationship between men and women took a more prominent position. However, the studies placed more emphasis on the "marginal" or absent man than on the ever-present woman and were criticized for ignoring the wide range of roles and tasks performed by women. Furthermore, Smith noted (1962:6) specific ethnographic data were used to generalize about matrifocal societies throughout the Caribbean. This proved to be problematic in understanding matrifocal societies theoretically, and it generated confusion as scholars used different terms to refer to similar types of kinship and household organizations.

R.T. Smith used the term *matrifocal* to refer to the type of structure he originally witnessed among lower class British Guianese (1956). Taking a developmental approach, Smith noted that matrifocal households arise with time after a man and woman begin to cohabitate. Early in the cycle the woman is economically dependent on the male partner. Her primary role is to provide care for the children, but as the children grow older and earn money for small tasks and labor it is the mother who controls their earnings. The father, meanwhile, has been unable to make significant contributions to the household economy due to his overall low status within a society that maintains prejudicial hiring policies. Smith's concept of matrifocality focuses on two criteria—the salience of women in their role as mothers and the marginality of men (i.e., their inability to contribute economically to the household) (1956; 1973; 1988).

The study of household structure conducted by Gonzalez on the Garifuna (Black

Carib) of Guatemala was not intended, nor originally identified, as a study on matrifocality per se, but Gonzalez did note the effect that male emigration had on household structure (1960). Gonzalez observed that households were comprised of members who were related to each other consanguineally (through blood); no two members of the household were bound by marriage. These consanguineal households developed in response to a socioeconomic environment that encouraged men to migrate as they sought employment (see also Gonzalez 1984 for comments regarding the applicability of dividing households into consanguineal and affinal types).

The terms and definitions for the household structures observed by R.T. Smith and Gonzalez were created to fit specific ethnographic data. They were later applied by various scholars to other societies that exhibited similar structures, which created confusion (see Kunstadter 1963; Randolph 1964; M.G. Smith 1962:6; and R.T. Smith 1973:126) and was exacerbated by the use of other terms to rectify the problem (e.g., the use of matricentric or female headed). Thus, in the literature we see these terms used interchangeably to refer to structures in which women control household earnings and decision making and men are viewed as marginal, though the impetus behind such household formation may differ from one society to the next. The whole concept became so clouded with terms and biases that Gonzalez astutely noted that depending on which scholar one is reading, matrifocality can suggest (1) that women are more important than the observer had expected, (2) that women maintain a good deal of control over money in the household, (3) that women are the primary source of income, or (4) that there is no resident male (1970:231–232).

Recent authors have criticized the emphasis on men's marginality and the focus on women's domestic tasks that arose in the study of matrifocality (Barrow 1988; Mohammed 1988; Tanner 1974). Concentration on women's *domestic* tasks ignores the full extent of women's networks, their access to resources, control over resources, relations with men, and relationship between household and society, all of which are important considerations when discussing matrifocality. Male marginality is problematic in part because the term is difficult to define. Does it mean that the father does not live in the household? Has he migrated out of the community? Does he contribute sporadically, or not at all, to the household economy? Is he not around to make household decisions?

As Tanner has remarked matrifocality should not be defined in "negative terms" (i.e., by the absence of the father). Instead, we should focus on the role of women as mothers, and note that in matrifocal systems mothers have at least some control over economic resources and are involved in decision making. According to Tanner, however, matrifocality goes beyond these two criteria. To be matrifocal a society must culturally value the role of mother—though not necessarily at the expense of fathers. In matrifocal societies the woman's role as mother is central to the kinship structure, but Tanner does not limit this role to domestic tasks. As mothers women may participate in cultivation, petty marketing, wage labor, in rituals, and so forth (1974). This broader definition allows us to recognize matrifocal units within a variety of kinship systems. Matrifocal units can exist in matrilineal or patrilineal societies, within nuclear families, and in bilateral systems. In any society with an emphasis on the mother-child dyad where this unit is culturally valued and where the mother plays an effective role in the economy and decision making of the unit, that unit can be defined as matrifocal (Tanner 1974:131–132).

Tanner's definition finally allows us to avoid some of the problems that previous studies encountered and permits us to further address issues pertinent to matrifocal units. We can examine gender relations within the context of gender hierarchies and the broader socioeconomic environment of which matrifocal households are a part. One area that has received little attention is the relationship between physical violence against women and matrifocality. Violence against women and matrifocality seem to contradict each other due to the assumptions regarding power and the authoritative role of women in matrifocal households.

Women, having access to and control over resources and authority to make household decisions, are viewed as powerful. This view has been particularly evident in studies of women in the Caribbean where a large number of matrifocal households exist (Massiah 1982). Caribbean women are frequently portrayed as powerful, autonomous individuals (Ellis 1986; Powell 1982, 1986; Safa 1986). Although Caribbean women's control and power over resources and decisions is not to be discounted, fieldwork in a low-income community in Jamaica suggests that matrifocality and physical violence against women are not mutually exclusive. To understand the relationship between these two phenomena requires knowledge of sociocultural elements that affect both gender relations and matrifocal household organization.

The community of study is a low-income urban neighborhood approximately 0.05 square miles located in the parish of St. Andrew, Jamaica. During the time at which data were collected, 1987 to 1988, there were an estimated 210 households with a population of 1,300. The majority of the households were of wooden construction, many without electricity, and very few with running water. Some of the wealthier residents maintained houses constructed of concrete. No telephones were present in any household because telephone lines were not available.

Within the community a variety of household organizational units were observed. Nuclear families based on common-law marriage, legal marriage, or coresidency existed. There were also single female-headed households, single male-headed households, and a variety of extended and collateral arrangements. Finally, there were households whose membership included kin and nonkin (i.e., a friend or acquaintance may reside in the household). This range in domestic organization demonstrates that household membership may vary in response to economic and social conditions.

What makes these arrangements more interesting is that the households are subject to change. During the course of the fieldwork households altered their membership; thus, a nuclear arrangement would shift to single female-headed with children as the father moved out, and it might have shifted again if a grandmother or sister moved in. Regardless of the various household arrangements, matrifocality was observed. Women certainly maintained control over the economic resources and were responsible for many household decisions. Women as mothers were structurally central to the kinship units, and mothers were culturally valued as indicated by both male and female informants.

Although Caribbean women are portrayed as powerful and autonomous, male-female relations, as anywhere in the world, are based on some form of interdependence. Within this community social and economic status are intricately tied to gender relations. Both genders support the basic notion that women are to provide sexual services and domestic labor for men, and men are to provide women with money and gifts. However, the relationships are not a simple equation whereby women provide sexual services and domestic labor in exchange for money. Women often spoke of sexual activity as something that they desired and enjoyed, and men felt free to request money from women with whom they have had relations (especially if she is the mother to any of his children). Nevertheless, there is an understanding that if a woman will not provide sexual services or domestic labor or if the man does not provide cash or gifts from time to time, the relationship will end. These expectations played key roles in understanding gender relations and the behavior of men and women.

In addition to these expectations, adult status is primarily attained by the birth of a child. At this socioeconomic level higher educational degrees, prestigious employment, and ownership of cars and houses are out of most community members' reach. Both men and women view the birth of a child as an opportunity to announce their own adult status. Thus, children are normally desired and are a source of pride for both the mother and father.

The instability that marks male-female relationships is recognized by community members and can be related to cultural values as well as to the socioeconomic environment that encourages men and women to seek more resourceful partners. Male and female informants readily acknowledged the shifting allegiances between men and women. Men were known to keep several girlfriends at one time, and marriage, common-law or legal, was no guarantee that monogamy will follow. Women also admitted to keeping an eye out for a better partner and said they would initiate a change if they so desired. Couples tended to set up visiting relationships whereby the couple did not coreside. Children, of course, may be born from these unions. If a Jamaican woman of this socioeconomic class married at all, it was more likely to occur after the age of thirty (see Brody 1981:253–255).

As households were observed and data collected through the course of fieldwork, it became apparent that fathers and male partners were not marginal to the households. Whether or not they resided in the same household as the woman, they could potentially be very influential. It also became clear that in certain situations female control over household issues could be jeopardized. A brief look at some of the households and the gender relations among men and women will demonstrate these points.

MARY'S HOUSEHOLD

Mary is a twenty-seven-year-old mother occupying a one-room wooden house—no electricity or running water—with four children. The two oldest children were fathered by one man; the youngest two were fathered by another. Sexual relations with the first father had ceased several years ago; however, Mary does maintain sexual relations with the younger children's father, though he keeps other girlfriends.

Mary's primary source of income stems from sporadic petty marketing. When Mary has the capital to invest in goods, she sells clothing and shoes in a downtown Kingston stall that is rented by her mother. Mary is very much involved in politics; she attends meetings, distributes literature, and talks to anyone about her party's political candidates and officials. She was able to work for a few months as an enumerator during a national campaign to register voters. Mary depends on contributions from the two fathers of her children. The first father rarely comes to visit, but he is in the National Guard, draws a steady paycheck, and consistently sends money for the children.

The father of her two youngest children, who works as a cook and a driver, is usually good about bringing money but has, on occasion, lapsed. Such lapses can be a severe stress on Mary's limited household budget and was the source of domestic violence on one occasion. Earl, the father of Mary's youngest children, had promised to bring some money. When he showed up at her doorstep she asked for the money, and he told her that he didn't have any. This made her angry so she began yelling at him, and a fight ensued. They began hitting each other with their fists, but the fight escalated when Earl picked up a shovel and hit Mary on the wrist. Mary fought back by taking a cutlass and striking him on the shoulder. Earl then left the premises, and Mary sought medical treatment for the pain in her wrist.

This was the first and only act of violence between the two in a seven-year period. Mary stated that they rarely even quarrel. Though not typical, the violence demonstrates the economic dependence of Mary on the contributions of the fathers and the stress that can surface when she is threatened by the lack of such contributions. Mary admitted that she was extremely angry when he told her that he had no money to give her because he had promised earlier that he would bring her some. She was convinced that he had the money to give but was holding out on her.

DORA'S HOUSEHOLD

Dora, twenty-eight years old, lives under similar circumstances as Mary and has had comparable experience regarding fathers and money. Dora is the mother of three children. Two live with her; one stays with relatives in the country. Dora's one-room house has neither electricity nor running water.

The father of Dora's first two children provides some money to the household. Dora is almost totally dependent on these contributions because she is confined to the house and cannot work due to a crippling disease. Ned, the father of her youngest child, provides nothing to the household, which is a continuous source of grief to Dora. Dora is quiet and normally avoids conflict. Her one attempt to address Ned's negligence resulted in violence, as had Mary's. Dora had decided that because Ned did not provide clothes or money for their son, Michael, he did not deserve to see the child. She packed up Michael's belongings and sent him over to Ned's sister's house for a short while, believing that the sister would feed Michael and buy him some clothes. When Ned arrived to take Michael for a visit to his own house, he questioned the child's whereabouts and became angry when Dora told him that he had been sent to Ned's sister's house. Ned began hitting Dora. She struck back once but relented when Ned punched her in the side and ran off. She did not see him again for several days. This incident occurred six months prior to our interview, and Dora has not asked Ned for anything since and vows that she never will.

RITA'S HOUSEHOLD

Rita lives in a household consisting of six members, including herself. Two of her four children, a granddaughter, a friend of her daughter, and Rita's boyfriend occupy a three-room apartment without electricity or running water. Rita is thirty-nine years old. Her boyfriend, Tom, is 40 and has lived with her for four years. They have no common children.

Rita runs a successful neighborhood bar, giving her control over the major portion of the household budget. She receives some financial contribution from the father of one daughter. Rita and Tom have established a reciprocal relationship regarding money. She does expect him to contribute from his earnings as a taxi driver when he is able, but she may be just as likely to provide Tom with money when he is in need. Rita is aware of Tom's other girlfriends and realizes that a good deal of his earnings go to entertaining these women. With her own successful business Rita is less financially dependent on her male partner than other women. She does look to Tom, however, for companionship and emotional support. The time he spends with other women is reluctantly accepted, though on one occasion his infidelities did result in conflict. One night, as he came home late, Rita began cursing Tom and made derogatory remarks about Tom's other girlfriend. Tom responded by punching Rita. She fought back for a few minutes then they both simply let it go. In the past year Rita has avoided comment on Tom's affairs and is determined to put up with it, for now at least, because she is not ready to end the relationship. Rita's attitude is that most men do this, so there is little point in severing this relationship to find another boyfriend who will do the same.

HANNAH'S HOUSEHOLD

Thirty-six-year-old Hannah is an articulate and ambitious woman. She lives in a two-room house with seven other people (five of her six children live with her along with a friend her age and a friend of one of her daughters). Hannah worked as a domestic but lost her job during my stay in the community. She did have a job lined up, cleaning the office of a dentist.

Hannah's first three children were fathered by one man; her fourth child was fathered by another man; and her last two children were fathered by a third man. The first man to father her children is now sick and unable to work. He does not provide any financial support to Hannah's household. The other two fathers help out every now and then, but the support is not enough for her to rely on. She rarely sees any of her children's fathers now, but Hannah did relate an incident involving the last father, Gerald, that occurred nearly five years prior to our interview. At the time of the incident Hannah and Gerald were still intimately involved but did not coreside. Hannah had grown dissatisfied with the relationship because Gerald provided no support for herself or his children. Thus, she had decided to break off the relationship. When Gerald learned of her decision he became angry and abusive. One night after everyone had gone to bed, he came to her house, began yelling at her, and proceeded to destroy some of her belongings: He broke a lamp and smashed a small table. Another night he came to her window, tore off the screen, and began yelling at her again. He threw a bucket of water on her and the children and threw stones. Hannah, not wanting the children to get hurt, went outside to confront him, and he began physically assaulting her. Hannah managed to grab a broken bottle and cut him with it. Gerald then left the premises, never bothering her much afterwards.

SUMMARY

Although women in matrifocal households often maintain control over resources and decision making within the household, the previous data indicate that the power associated with such control and authority can be compromised. Power, as defined by Adams, is the control over one's environment and the ability to control the environment of others based on access and control of resources that are of value to the other (1975:12). In the cases cited above the interdependence between men and women and the access that men have to certain resources must be addressed to understand female power and domestic violence.

As indicated previously, both genders view women as exercising control over sexual services and domestic labor, and men have access to some (though not all) of the economic resources that women need. At this socioeconomic level men may not be able to contribute significantly to the household economy. Nevertheless, women view men as a source of monetary and material needs and feel they have the right to demand these resources. Though women are constantly seeking ways to earn money and often don't want to rely on contributions from male partners, many, again due to the socioeconomic environment, are dependent on male contributions, no matter how small. The data suggest that while men are dependent on women, they can more easily circumvent the control that female partners have over desired resources than women can circumvent the resources that men control. In this culture it is acceptable for men to have more than one female partner. While women complain of this it is expected and negates the control that individual women can exert. Women, on the other hand, may try to circumvent male control over economic resources, but they are also subjected to an economic system that exploits the lower class for their cheap labor and that offers high unemployment. In addition to this interdependence these women are members of a culture that may value women *as mothers*, but women in general do not necessarily enjoy a high status. In other words the *mother* role is valued, but women are overall subordinate to men (Henry and Wilson 1975). Male informants felt it was their right to physically coerce or punish women as they saw fit, but a man would almost never physically abuse his own mother.

In relating the cases cited previously the intent is not to suggest that the women were weak, powerless, and always dominated by men. Women often fought back and worked to become as independent as possible. These cases are also not intended to promote negative images of men. I recount incidences of abuse to demonstrate the extreme to which men can affect matrifocal households, but I must emphasize that male influence can also be positive and rewarding for members of the household. Fathers were observed visiting their children, taking them to the health clinic, and providing money, food, and clothing.

The data collected from this study remind us that, in spite of a long interest in matrifocality, we still have much to learn. We must rid ourselves of biases that narrow our focus. Just as it was wrong to assume that men are marginal, that women perform only domestic tasks, and that the nuclear family is "normal," we must not assume that women in matrifocal societies are *always* powerful or that they consistently enjoy a high status within that society. The power that women exert must be documented and integrated into the overall cultural context that would also note gender relations, the socioeconomic environment, the political environment, and cultural values. Only then can studies on matrifocality provide us with a better understanding of human behavior.

REFERENCES

Adams, Richard N. 1975. *Energy and Structure: A Theory of Social Power.* Austin: University of Texas Press.

Barrow, Christine. 1988. Anthropology, the Family and Women in the Caribbean. In Patricia Mohammed and Catherine Shepherd (eds.). *Gender in Caribbean Development,* pp. 156–169. Mona, Jamaica: University of West Indies.

Brody, Eugene B. 1981. *Sex, Contraception, and Motherhood in Jamaica.* Cambridge, MA: Harvard University Press.

Clarke, Edith. 1957. *My Mother Who Fathered Me.* London: George Allen & Unwin.

Collier, Jane, Michelle Rosaldo, and Sylvia Yanagisako. 1982. Is There a Family? New Anthropological Views. In Barrie Thorne (ed.). *Rethinking the Family: Some Feminist Questions,* pp. 25–39. New York: Longman.

Durant-Gonzalez, Victoria. 1982. The Realm of Female Familial Responsibility. In Joycelin Massiah (ed). *Women and the Family,* pp. 1–27. Cave Hill, Barbados: University of the West Indies, Institute of Social and Economic Research.

Ellis, Pat. 1986. "Introduction: An Overview of Women in Caribbean Society." In Pat Ellis (ed.). *Women of the Caribbean,* pp. 1–24. Kingston: Kingston Publishers.

Frazier, E. Franklin. 1939. *The Negro Family in the United States.* Chicago: Chicago University Press.

Gonzalez, Nancie L. 1960. Household and Family in the Caribbean. *Social and Economic Studies* 9: 101–106.

———. 1970. Toward a Definition of Matrifocality. In Norman E. Whitten, Jr. and John F. Szwed (eds.). *Afro-American Anthropology,* pp. 231–244. New York: The Free Press.

———. 1984. Rethinking the Consanguineal Household and Matrifocality. *Ethnology* 23(1): 1–12.

Henriques, Fernando M. 1953. Family and Colour in Jamaica. London: Eyre and Spottiswoode.

Henry, Frances and Pamela Wilson. 1975. The Status of Women in Caribbean Societies: An Overview of Their Social, Economic and Sexual Roles. *Social and Economic Studies* 24(2): 165–198.

Herskovits, Melville J. 1941. *The Myth of the Negro Past.* New York: Harper & Brothers.

Kunstadter, Peter. 1963. A Survey of the Consanguine or Matrifocal Family. *American Anthropologist* 65: 56–66.

Massiah, Joycelin. 1982. Women Who Head Households. In Joycelin Massiah (ed.). *Women and the Family,* pp. 62–130. Cave Hill, Barbados: University of West Indies, Institute of Social and Economic Research.

Mohammed, Patricia. 1988. The Caribbean Family Revisited. In Patricia Mohammed and Catherine Shepherd (eds.). *Gender in Caribbean Development,* pp. 170–182. Mona, Jamaica: University of West Indies.

Moynihan, Daniel P. 1965. The Negro Family: The Case for National Action. U.S. Department of Labor, Washington, D.C.

Powell, Dorian. 1982. Network Analysis: A Suggested Model for the Study of Women and the Family in the Caribbean. In Joycelin Massiah (ed.). *Women and The Family,* pp. 131–162. Cave Hill, Barbados: University of the West Indies, Institute of Social and Economic Research.

———. 1986. Caribbean Women and Their Response to Familial Experiences. *Social and Economic Studies* 35(2): 83–130.

Randolph, Richard R. 1964. The `Matrifocal Family' as a Comparative Category. *American Anthropologist* 66: 628–31.
Safa, Helen. 1986. Economic Autonomy and Sexual Equality in Caribbean Society. *Social and Economic Studies* 35(3): 1–21.
Simey, Thomas. 1946. *Welfare Planning in the West Indies.* Oxford: Clarendon Press.
Smith, M.G. 1962. *West Indian Family Structure.* Seattle: University of Washington Press.
Smith, Raymond T. 1956. *The Negro Family in British Guiana: Family Structure and Social Status in the Villages.* London: Routledge and Kegan Paul.
———. 1973. The Matrifocal Family. In Jack Goody (ed.). *The Character of Kinship,* pp. 121–144. London: Cambridge University Press.
———. 1988. *Kinship and Class in the West Indies: A Genealogical Study of Jamaica and Guyana.* New York: Cambridge University Press.
Staples, Robert. 1972. The Matricentric Family System: A Cross-Cultural Examination. *Journal of Marriage and The Family* 34(1): 156–165.
Tanner, Nancy. 1974. Matrifocality in Indonesia and Africa and Among Black Americans. In Michelle Zimbalist Rosaldo and Louise Lamphere (eds.). *Woman, Culture, and Society,* pp. 129–156. Stanford: Stanford University Press.

MARIA, A PORTUGUESE FISHERWOMAN

Sally Cole

Maria lives in the small town of Vila Chã on the north coast of Portugal. She is a retired *pescadeira* (fisherwoman) who still goes to the beach each day to help bait traps or unload fish or just to talk with other fishermen and women. The illegitimate daughter of a poor, landless woman, Maria began fishing when she was only ten years old. And throughout her life she worked both at sea and on land. She fished by net and hand line in one of the small, gaily painted, open wooden boats that, until the 1960s, were powered by oar and sail and were typical in the inshore fishery; on land she, like the other women, harvested and dried seaweed and sold it to local peasant farmers for fertilizer. By the age of thirty-five she was a licensed boat skipper, had bought her own boat and gear, and was fishing daily with crew she hired to work for her. Maria says this was simply the only way she knew how to make a living. She fishes, she tells us, because she was forced to, because her husband emigrated to Brazil abandoning her with three daughters. Nonetheless, she likes her profession and knows she is good at it—as good as any man. Fisherwomen like Maria say they fished "like men," and they mean that not only did women have the skill of fishermen, but at sea they became social men. They stress that women's sexuality was never targeted when they were working with men. "There was more respect (*respeito*) on the sea than there was on the land," some say.

Maria is a large-boned woman who dresses in the characteristic manner of rural Portuguese women who were born, raised, and married during the Salazar regime before 1960. She wears her hair pulled into a bun at the back of her head and covered with a head scarf; she wears a dark wool shawl, skirt, socks, and *chinelas* (the mass-produced open-backed flat shoes that have replaced the home-made traditional clogs). Underneath her skirt she wears trousers—unheard of among women of her generation, and she walks with a masculine, lumbering gait and speaks in a deep, quiet authoritative voice.

On one hand Maria found my interest in her life surprising: "There is nothing remarkable about my life," she said. On the other hand, like other women in Vila Chã, Maria tells stories from her every day life in conversations with daughters, neighbors, relatives, and even clients for her fish. Women's daily

Original material prepared for this text. The ideas in this article are further developed in Sally Cole, *Women of the Praia* (Princeton, NJ: Princeton University Press, 1991).

activities on the beach, on the street, and at the fish auction, provide them with continual opportunities to constitute the female subject and to constitute the self. With this strong sense of self, Maria and other Vila Chã fisherwomen comfortably and skillfully constructed their life stories.

In the following narrative Maria assures us that she only did what she had to do. But we see, in her refusal of her estranged husband's request to take him back and care for him in his old age, how through her life of hard work and economic independence, she has constituted herself as an autonomous person and finds it impossible to do what her husband asks and what he considers to be a wife's duty.

> There is nothing remarkable about my life. I am a poor woman. I did what I had to do. I worked hard—all the women here did. I have worked very hard all my life.
>
> I was born in 1926, the third of four children. We had no father. I was raised in Vila Chã by my mother who worked as a *jornaleira* (an agricultural day laborer), harvested seaweed, and sold fish in order to feed us. But often there was no food, and we had to beg from our neighbors.
>
> In my childhood girls used to collect seaweed both from the beach in a hand net and from boats using a type of rake. It was also common for them to accompany relatives fishing. When only ten years old I began to accompany neighbors when they went fishing. When I was fourteen I took out my license, and I continued to fish as a crew member on boats owned by neighbors. These men are all dead now but it was they who taught me this work.
>
> I married when I was only twenty years old, and I think this is too young. My husband was a *pescador* (fisherman) from a neighboring parish. He came to live with me and my mother and my grandmother and took up fishing in Vila Chã. I continued fishing whenever I could, and after my daughters were born I left them in my mother's care so that I could go out on the sea. I also worked on the seaweed harvest often going out alone in the boat to collect seaweed.
>
> From the beginning my husband was selfish. He never helped me with my work but would instead go off to attend to his own affairs (*a vida dele*). I married too young. We had two daughters, and when I was pregnant with the third my husband emigrated to Brazil. He was gone for almost four years, during which time I heard nothing from him, and he sent no money. I decided to go to Brazil to find him. In 1955 I went by ship with my sister-in-law who was going to join her husband, my brother, in Brazil. I found my husband involved in a life of women and drink, and after a few months I returned home alone. I wanted to make my life in Vila Chã, and I missed my daughters. I took up fishing fulltime and harvested seaweed when I wasn't fishing, and in this way I supported my mother and my children. In 1961 I bought a boat of my own and took out my skipper's license.
>
> I like my profession, but I fished because I was forced to. My marriage became difficult. My husband went away to Brazil, leaving me in the street with three children, and I had to face life on my own. Fishing was not as productive then as it is now, and the life of a fisherwoman was a hard one. But I had to turn to what I knew. First I fished in a boat belonging to another pescador and then for eighteen years I owned and fished in my own boat "Três Marias." About fourteen years ago I managed to buy this small house, which, little by little, I have fixed up, and this is where I live now.
>
> Although in recent years I have been the only woman skipper, there have been no difficulties for me at all because I know my profession very well—as well as any of my comrades. Men used to like to fish with me because they knew I was strong. C., a member of my crew, used to say that I was stronger than he. Fishing holds no secrets for me, and besides I think that women have the right to face life beside men. What suits men suits women. I am respected by everyone, men and women. I have many friends, and when the weather prohibits fishing we all stay here on the beach working on the nets and enjoying conversation. I have always enjoyed my work on the sea. I was never one who liked to stay at home.
>
> When my daughters were small I used to be at sea day and night—whenever there was fish. They stayed at home with my mother. Later, when they were older and I was fishing, my daughters assisted my mother harvesting seaweed, and in this way they contributed to the maintenance of the household. As soon as I returned from fishing I would start the housework. You see, I was at the same time housewife and fisherman (*Olhe, eu era ao mesmo tempo dona de casa e pescador*).

I retired in 1979. I sold my boat, and I gave my fishing gear to my son-in-law. I sold my boat to a fisherman in Matosinhos because I could not bear to see it anymore here on the beach. In 1982 I bought a piece of land, and two of my daughters are building a duplex on it now. My youngest daughter lives with me in my house along with her husband and three children. I have helped all of my daughters to establish their households. I have been very good to them. And, now that I am old and my heart is not good, they are looking after me. When I returned from Brazil leaving my husband there, I could have found another man to live with. I could have lived with another man. But I never wanted to do that because, if things didn't work out with us, I worried that he would take it out on my daughters because they were nothing to him. I preferred to have my daughters.

Recently, my husband has begun writing to me from Brazil. He wants to return to Portugal, and he wants me to take him back. He needs someone to care for him now in his old age. But I won't take him back. It's not right at all. I liked him once, but that's all over now. The best part of the life of a couple is passed. I'm not interested in his returning. I'm not an object to be put away and then picked up, dusted off, and used again. I am not an object. I am a person. I am human. I have the right to be treated like a person, don't you think? I managed to make a good life for myself and my children here, but he arranged nothing for himself there—nothing. He's got nothing there, but he's also got nothing here. He has never done anything for me or my daughters, and now he wants to come back. Who does he think he is? I'm not crazy. He has no right whatsoever.

Maria describes her life of work in the inshore fishery as it existed in Vila Chã until the 1970s, by which time most households in the community had come to depend primarily on the wages earned by women in factories and men in construction work. This household-based maritime economy had depended on an annual round of diverse activities and on the seasonal availability of natural resources like fish and seaweed. On one hand the unpredictability of resources and weather ensured their poverty; on the other hand maritime production required the participation of all household members (including women and children) and thus created the conditions for the social and economic autonomy of women. The sale of fresh fish and seaweed fertilizer—both commodities that women controlled—enabled women like Maria to support themselves and their children without the assistance of men. Because Vila Chã, like other rural communities in northwestern Portugal, has sustained high rates of male emigration since at least the nineteenth century, the autonomy of women was also strategic.

Maria describes how she invested in property—a house, a boat and gear, and land for her daughters. Perhaps because men were often absent due to either temporary or permanent emigration, property in Vila Chã became identified primarily with women. It was a woman's responsibility to look after the house and garden plot and to look after the boat and gear—either by fishing herself or by hiring others to fish for her. Daughters were favored over sons to inherit property, and younger daughters (or the last to marry) were favored over older daughters. Daughters were favored not only because sons might emigrate but also because parents wanted a daughter to stay on in the house to care for them in old age and to tend their graves after death.

The relationship between women and property also determined residence patterns after marriage. As Maria describes after their marriage her husband came to live with her and her mother and her mother's mother. Maria was the third of four children and the youngest daughter. Maria lived with her mother all her life. Now, her own youngest daughter and her husband and children live with Maria and are caring for her in her old age.

The relations between these four generations of mothers and daughters are typical of relations among blood-related women in Vila Chã. Women's strong ties with their children, especially daughters, may be interpreted as having been among women's multiple strategies to provide for themselves and for their households in the absence of men. Thus, not only did women maximize their economic autonomy through their control of the sale of fresh fish and seaweed fertilizer and by assuming responsibility for the household property, but they also conceived of their children as a resource. Having children gave a woman adult status and the prerogatives (and responsibilities) of managing a household; having children also ensured that a woman—especially an unmarried woman or a deserted wife like Maria—would have someone to care for her in the frailty of her later years.

The importance women placed on having children may be seen in the high rates of illegitimacy that were common in Vila Chã until the 1960s and that are correlated with landlessness and male emigration. Poor, landless women were already limited to finding marriage partners who were of the same low economic position. Male emigration further created a demographic asymmetry, so there were not enough marriageable men to go around. Under these conditions poor women often were less concerned about getting married than they were desirous of having children. Maria's mother and her mother's mother are both women who never married but who had children and managed households. Although Maria herself did marry she tells us directly that her daughters were more important to her than any man could ever be, and for this reason, she says, she chose to live without a male partner when, still a young woman, she was abandoned by her husband. "I preferred to have my daughters," she said.

Finally, Maria describes how gender is negotiated through the relations of daily life and especially through work. Maria negotiated a dual or androgynous gender identity. She spent her entire life working with men in a profession that was locally defined as a masculine pursuit despite the fact that women also fished. This work enabled her to assume masculine roles and prerogatives in other spheres of life and to live without the support of a male companion. At the same time Maria fulfilled a woman's role: she was the mother of three children and the manager of a household. When Maria tells us that she was both "housewife and fisherman" she is telling us that to her children she was both nurturer and economic provider, both mother and father, and in the community she was both woman and man. Now, nearing the end of life, Maria and her husband have reversed positions: Maria once traveled to Brazil to entreat her husband to return and was refused; now her husband is begging her to take him back into her home and she is refusing. Maria, with her life of hard work behind her, cannot even entertain the contradiction. "I am not crazy," she said. "I am not an object. I am a person."

THE FEMALE WORLD OF CARDS AND HOLIDAYS: WOMEN, FAMILIES, AND THE WORK OF KINSHIP[1]

Micaela di Leonardo

Why is it that the married women of America are supposed to write all the letters and send all the cards to their husbands' families? My old man is a much better writer than I am, yet he expects me to correspond with his whole family. If I asked him to correspond with mine, he would blow a gasket.

Letter to Ann Landers

Women's place in man's life cycle has been that of nurturer, caretaker, and helpmate, the weaver of those networks of relationships on which she in turn relies.

Carol Gilligan, *In a Different Voice*[2]

Reprinted with permission of The University of Chicago Press from *Signs* 12(3): 440–453, 1987.

Feminist scholars in the past fifteen years have made great strides in formulating new understandings of the relations among gender, kinship, and the larger economy. As a result of this pioneering research, women are newly visible and audible, no longer submerged within their families. We see households as loci of political struggle, inseparable parts of the larger society and economy, rather than as havens from the heartless world of industrial capitalism.[3] And historical and cultural variations in kinship and family forms have become clearer with the maturation of feminist historical and social-scientific scholarship.

Two theoretical trends have been key to this reinterpretation of women's work and family domain. The first is the elevation to visibility of women's nonmarket activities—housework, child care, the servicing of men, and the care of the elderly—and the definition of all these activities as *labor,* to be enumerated alongside and counted as part of overall social reproduction. The second theoretical trend is the nonpejorative focus on women's domestic or kin-centered networks. We now see them as the products of conscious strategy, as crucial to the functioning of kinship systems, as sources of women's autonomous power and possible primary sites of emotional fulfillment, and, at times, as the vehicles for actual survival and/or political resistance.[4]

Recently, however, a division has developed between feminist interpreters of the "labor" and the "network" perspectives on women's lives. Those who focus on women's work tend to envision women as sentient, goal-oriented actors, while those who concern themselves with women's ties to others tend to perceive women primarily in terms of nurturance, other-orientation—altruism. The most celebrated recent example of this division is the opposing testimony of historians Alice Kessler-Harris and Rosalind Rosenberg in the Equal Employment Opportunity Commission's sex discrimination case against Sears Roebuck and Company. Kessler-Harris argued that American women historically have actively sought higher-paying jobs and have been prevented from gaining them because of sex discrimination by employers. Rosenberg argued that American women in the nineteenth century created among themselves, through their domestic networks, a "women's culture" that emphasized the nurturance of children and others and the maintenance of family life and that discouraged women from competition over or heavy emotional investment in demanding, high-paid employment.[5]

I shall not here address this specific debate but, instead, shall consider its theoretical background and implications. I shall argue that we need to fuse, rather than to oppose, the domestic network and labor perspectives. In what follows, I introduce a new concept, the work of kinship, both to aid empirical feminist research on women, work, and family and to help advance feminist theory in this arena. I believe that the boundary-crossing nature of the concept helps to confound the self-interest/altruism dichotomy, forcing us from an either-or stance to a position that includes both perspectives. I hope in this way to contribute to a more critical feminist vision of women's lives and the meaning of family in the industrial West.

In my recent field research among Italian-Americans in Northern California, I found myself considering the relations between women's kinship and economic lives. As an anthropologist, I was concerned with people's kin lives beyond conventional American nuclear family or household boundaries. To this end, I collected individual and family life histories, asking about all kin and close friends and their activities. I was also very interested in women's labor. As I sat with women and listened to their accounts of their past and present lives, I began to realize that they were involved in three types of work: housework and child care, work in the labor market, and the work of kinship.[6]

By kin work I refer to the conception, maintenance, and ritual celebration of cross-household kin ties, including visits, letters, telephone calls, presents, and cards to kin; the organization of holiday gatherings; the creation and maintenance of quasi-kin relations; decisions to neglect or to intensify particular ties; the mental work of reflection about all these activities; and the creation and communication of altering images of family and kin vis-à-vis the images of others, both folk and mass media. Kin work is a key element that has been missing in the synthesis of the "household labor" and "domestic network" perspectives. In our emphasis on individual women's responsibilities within households and on the job, we reflect the common picture of households as nuclear units, tied perhaps to the larger social and economic system, but not to *each other.* We miss the point of telephone and soft drink advertising, of women's magazines' holiday issues, of commentators' confused nostalgia for the mythical American extended family: it is kinship contact *across households,* as much as women's work within them, that fulfills our cultural expectation of satisfying family life.

Maintaining these contacts, this sense of family, takes time, intention, and skill. We tend to think of human social and kin networks as the epiphenomena of production and reproduction: the social traces created by our material lives. Or, in the neoclassical tradition, we see them as part of leisure activities, outside an economic purview except insofar as they involve consumption behavior. But the creation and maintenance of kin and quasi-kin networks in advanced industrial societies is *work;* and, moreover, it is largely women's work.

The kin-work lens brought into focus new perspectives on my informants' family lives. First, life histories revealed that often the very existence of kin contact and holiday celebration depended on the presence of an adult woman in the household. When couples divorced or mothers died, the work of kinship was left undone; when women entered into sanctioned sexual or marital relationships with men in these situations, they reconstituted the men's kinship networks and organized gatherings and holiday celebrations. Middle-aged businessman Al Bertini, for example, recalled the death of his mother in his early adolescence: "I think that's probably one of the biggest losses in losing a family—yeah, I remember as a child when my Mom was alive . . . the holidays were treated with enthusiasm and love . . . after she died the attempt was there but it just didn't materialize." Later in life, when Al Bertini and his wife separated, his own and his son Jim's participation in extended-family contact decreased rapidly. But when Jim began a relationship with Jane Batemen, she and he moved in with Al, and Jim and Jane began to invite his kin over for holidays. Jane single-handedly planned and cooked the holiday feasts.

Kin work, then, is like housework and child care: men in the aggregate do not do it. It differs from these forms of labor in that it is harder for men to substitute hired labor to accomplish these tasks in the absence of kinswomen. Second, I found that women, as the workers in this arena, generally had much greater kin knowledge than did their husbands, often including more accurate and extensive knowledge of their husbands' families. This was true both of middle-aged and younger couples and surfaced as a phenomenon in my interviews in the form of humorous arguments and in wives' detailed additions to husbands' narratives. Nick Meraviglia, a middle-aged professional, discussed his Italian antecedents in the presence of his wife, Pina:

NICK: My grandfather was a very outspoken man, and it was reported he took off for the hills when he found out that Mussolini was in power.

PINA: And he was a very tall man; he used to have to bow his head to get inside doors.

NICK: No, that was my uncle.

PINA: Your grandfather too, I've heard your mother say.

NICK: My mother has a sister and a brother.

PINA: *Two* sisters!

NICK: You're right!

PINA: Maria and Angelina.

Women were also much more willing to discuss family feuds and crises and their own roles in them; men tended to repeat formulaic statements asserting family unity and respectability. (This was much less true for younger men.) Joe and Cetta Longhinotti's statements illustrate these tendencies. Joe responded to my question about kin relations: "We all get along. As a rule, relatives, you got nothing but trouble." Cetta, instead, discussed her relations with each of her grown children, their wives, her in-laws, and her own blood kin in detail. She did not hide the fact that relations were strained in several cases; she was eager to discuss the evolution of problems and to seek my opinions of her actions. Similarly, Pina Meraviglia told the following story of her fight with one of her brothers with hysterical laughter: "There was some biting and hair pulling and choking . . . it was terrible! I shouldn't even tell you. . . ." Nick, meanwhile, was concerned about maintaining an image of family unity and respectability.

Also, men waxed fluent while women were quite inarticulate in discussing their past and present occupations. When asked about their work lives, Joe Longhinotti and Nick Meraviglia, union baker and professional, respectively, gave detailed narratives of their work careers. Cetta Longhinotti and Pina Meraviglia, clerical and former clerical, respectively, offered only short descriptions focusing on factors of ambience, such as the "lovely things" sold by Cetta's firm.

These patterns are not repeated in the younger generation, especially among younger women, such as Jane Batemen, who have managed to acquire training and jobs with some prospect of mobility. These younger women, though, have *added* a professional and detailed interest in their jobs to a felt responsibility for the work of kinship.[7]

Although men rarely took on any kin-work tasks, family histories and accounts of contemporary life revealed that kinswomen often negotiated among themselves, alternating hosting, food-preparation, and gift-buying responsibilities—or sometimes ceding entire task clusters to one woman. Taking on or ceding tasks was clearly related to acquiring or divesting oneself of power within kin networks, but women varied in their interpretation of the meaning of this power. Cetta Longhinotti, for example, relied on the "family Christmas dinner" as a symbol of her central kinship role and was involved in painful negotiations with her daughter-in-law over the issue: "Last year she insisted—this is touchy. She doesn't want to spend the holiday dinner together. So last year we went there. But I still had my dinner the next day . . . I made a big dinner on Christmas Day, regardless of who's coming—candles on the table, the whole routine. I decorate the house myself too . . . well, I just feel that the time will come when maybe I won't feel like cooking a big dinner—she should take advantage of the fact that I feel like doing it now." Pina Meraviglia, in contrast, was saddened by the centripetal force of the developmental cycle but was unworried about the power dynamics involved in her negotiations with daughters- and mother-in-law over holiday celebrations.

Kin work is not just a matter of power among women but also of the mediation of power represented by household units.[8] Women often choose to minimize status claims in their kin work and to include numbers of households under the rubric of family. Cetta Longhinotti's sister Anna, for example, is married to a professional man whose parents have considerable economic resources, while Joe and Cetta have low incomes and no other well-off kin. Cetta and Anna remain close, talk on the phone several times a week, and assist their adult children, divided by distance and economic status, in remaining united as cousins.

Finally, women perceived housework, child care, market labor, the care of the elderly, and the work of kinship as competing responsibilities. Kin work was a unique category, however, because it was unlabeled and because women felt they could either cede some tasks to kinswomen and/or could cut them back severely. Women variously cited the pressures of market labor, the needs of the elderly, and their own desires for freedom and job enrichment as reasons for cutting back Christmas card lists, organized holiday gatherings, multifamily dinners, letters, visits, and phone calls. They expressed guilt and defensiveness about this cutback process and, particularly, about their failures to keep families close through constant contact and about their failures to create perfect holiday celebrations. Cetta Longhinotti, during the period when she was visiting her elderly mother every weekend in addition to working a full-time job, said of her grown children, "I'd have the whole gang here once a month, but I've been so busy that I haven't done that for about six months." And Pina Meraviglia lamented her insufficient work on family Christmases, "I wish I had really made it traditional . . . like my sister-in-law has special stories."

Kin work, then, takes place in an arena characterized simultaneously by cooperation and competition, by guilt and gratification. Like housework and child care, it is women's work, with the same lack of clear-cut agreement concerning its proper components: How often should sheets be changed? When should children be toilet trained? Should an aunt send a niece a birthday present? Unlike housework and child care, however, kin work, taking place across the boundaries of normative households, is as yet unlabeled and has no retinue of experts prescribing its correct forms. Neither home economists nor child psychologists have much to say about nieces' birthday presents. Kin work is thus more easily cut back without social interference. On the other hand, the results of kin work—frequent kin contact and feelings of intimacy—are the subject of considerable cultural manipulation as indicators of family happiness. Thus, women in general are subject to the guilt my informants expressed over cutting back kin-work activities.

Although many of my informants referred to the results of women's kin work—cross-household kin contacts and attendant ritual gatherings—as particularly Italian-American, I suggest that in fact this phenomenon is broadly characteristic of American kinship. We think of kin-work tasks such as the preparation of ritual feasts, responsibility for holiday card lists, and gift buying as extensions of women's domestic responsibilities for cooking, consumption, and nurturance. American men in general do not take on these tasks any more than they do housework and child care—and probably less, as these tasks have not yet been the subject of intense public debate. And my informants' gender breakdown in relative articulateness on kinship and workplace themes reflects the still prevalent occupational segregation—most women cannot find jobs that provide enough pay, status, or promotion possibilities to make them worth focusing on—as well as women's perceived power within kinship networks. The common recognition of that power is reflected in Selma Greenberg's book on nonsexist child rearing. Greenberg calls mothers "press agents" who sponsor relations between their own children and other relatives; she advises a mother whose relatives treat her disrespectfully to deny those kin access to her children.[9]

Kin work is a salient concept in other parts of the developed world as well. Larissa Adler Lomnitz and Marisol Pérez Lizaur have found that "centralizing women" are responsible for these tasks and for communicating "family ideology" among upper-class families in Mexico City. Matthews Hamabata, in his study of upper-class families in Japan, has found that women's kin work involves key financial transactions. Sylvia Junko Yanagisako discovered that, among rural Japanese migrants to the United States, the maintenance of kin networks was assigned to women as the migrants adopted the American ideology of the independent nuclear family household. Maila Stivens notes that urban Australian housewives' kin ties and kin ideology "transcend women's isolation in domestic units."[10]

This is not to say that cultural conceptions of appropriate kin work do not vary, even within the United States. Carol B. Stack documents institutionalized fictive kinship and concomitant reciprocity networks among impoverished black American women. Women in populations characterized by intense feelings of ethnic identity may feel bound to emphasize particular occasions—Saint Patrick's or Columbus Day—with organized family feasts. These constructs may be mediated by religious affiliation, as in the differing emphases on Friday or Sunday family dinners among Jews and Christians. Thus the personnel involved and the amount and kind of labor considered necessary for the satisfactory performance of particular kin-work tasks are likely to be culturally constructed.[11] But while the kin and quasi-kin universes and the ritual calendar may vary among women according to race or ethnicity, their general responsibility for maintaining kin links and ritual observances does not.

As kin work is not an ethnic or racial phenomenon, neither is it linked only to one social class. Some commentators on American family life still reflect the influence of work done in England in the 1950s and 1960s (by Elizabeth Bott and by Peter Willmott and Michael Young) in their assumption that working-class families are close and extended, while the middle class substitutes friends (or anomie) for family. Others reflect the prevalent family pessimism in their presumption that neither working- nor middle-class families have extended kin contact.[12] Insofar as kin contact depends on residential proximity, the larger economy's shifts will influence particular groups' experiences. Factory workers, close to kin or not, are likely to disperse when plants shut down or relocate. Small businesspeople or independent professionals may, however, remain resident in particular areas—and thus maintain proximity to kin—for generations, while professional employees of large firms relocate at their firms' behest. This pattern obtained among my informants.

In any event, cross-household kin contact can be and is effected at long distance through letters, cards, phone calls, and holiday and vacation visits. The form and functions of contact, however, vary according to economic resources. Stack and Brett Williams offer rich accounts of kin networks among poor blacks and migrant Chicano farmworkers functioning to provide emotional support, labor, commodity, and cash exchange—a funeral visit, help with laundry, the gift of a dress or piece of furniture.[13] Far different in degree are exchanges such as the loan of a vacation home, a multifamily boating trip, or the provision of free professional services—examples from the kin networks of my wealthier informants. The point is that households, as labor- and income-pooling units, whatever their relative wealth, are somewhat porous in relation to others with whose members they share kin or quasi-kin ties. We do not really know how class differences operate in this realm; it is possible that they do so largely in terms of ideology. It may be, as David Schneider and Raymond T. Smith suggest, that the affluent and the very poor are more open in recognizing necessary economic ties to kin than are those who identify themselves as middle class.[14]

Recognizing that kin work is gender rather than class based allows us to see women's kin networks among all groups, not just among working-class and impoverished women in industrialized societies. This recognition in turn clarifies our understanding of the privileges and limits of women's varying access to economic resources. Affluent women can "buy out" of housework, child care—and even some kin-work responsibilities. But they, like all women, are ultimately responsible, and subject to both guilt and blame, as the administrators of home, children, and kin network. Even the wealthiest women must negotiate the timing and venue of holidays and other family rituals with their kinswomen. It may be that kin work is the core women's work category in which all women cooperate, while women's perceptions of the appropriateness of cooperation for housework, child care, and the care of the elderly varies by race, class, region, and generation.

But kin work is not necessarily an appropriate category of labor, much less gendered labor, in all societies. In many small-scale societies, kinship is the major organizing principle of all social life, and all contacts are by definition kin contacts.[15] One cannot, therefore, speak of labor that does not involve kin. In the United States, kin work as a separable category of gendered labor perhaps arose historically in concert with the ideological and material constructs of the moral mother/cult of domesticity and the privatized family during the course of industrialization in the eighteenth and nineteenth centuries. These phenomena are connected to the increase in the ubiquity of productive occupations *for men* that are not organized through kinship. This includes the demise of the family farm with the capitalization of agriculture and rural-urban migration; the decline of family recruitment in factories as firms grew, ended child labor, and began to assert bureaucratized forms of control; the decline of artisanal labor and of small entrepreneurial enterprises as large firms took greater and greater shares of the commodity market; the decline of the family firm as corporations—and their managerial work forces—grew beyond the capacities of individual families to provision them; and, finally, the rise of civil service bureaucracies and public pressure against nepotism.[16]

As men increasingly worked alongside of non-kin, and as the ideology of separate spheres was increasingly accepted, perhaps the responsibility for kin maintenance, like that for child rearing, became gender-focused. Ryan points out that "built into the updated family economy . . . was a new measure of voluntarism." This voluntarism, though, "perceived as the shift from patriarchal authority to domestic affection," also signaled the rise of women's moral responsibility for family life. Just as the "idea of fatherhood itself seemed almost to wither away" so did male involvement in the responsibility for kindred lapse.[17]

With postbellum economic growth and geographic movement, women's new kin burden involved increasing amounts of time and labor. The ubiquity of lengthy visits and of frequent letter-writing among nineteenth-century women attests to this. And for visitors and for those who were residentially proximate, the continuing commonalities of women's domestic labor allowed for kinds of work sharing—nursing, childkeeping, cooking, cleaning—that men, with their increasingly differentiated and controlled activities, probably could not maintain. This is not to say that some kin-related male productive work did not continue; my own data, for instance, show kin involvement among small businessmen in the present. It is, instead, to suggest a general trend in material life and a cultural shift that influenced even those whose productive and kin lives remained commingled. Yanagisako has distinguished between the realms of domestic and public kinship in order to draw attention to anthropology's relatively "thin descriptions" of the domestic (female) domain. Using her typology, we might say that kin work as gendered labor comes into existence within the domestic domain with the relative erasure of the domain of public, male kinship.[18]

Whether or not this proposed historical model bears up under further research, the question remains, Why do women do kin work? However material factors may shape activities, they do not determine how individuals may perceive them. And in considering issues of motivation, of intention, of the cultural construction of kin work, we return to the altruism versus self-interest dichotomy in recent feminist theory. Consider the epigraphs to this article. Are women kin workers the nurturant weavers of the Gilligan quotation, or victims, like the fed-up woman who writes to complain to Ann Landers? That is, are we to see kin work as yet another example of "women's culture" that takes the care of others as its primary desideratum? Or are we to see kin work as another way in which men, the economy, and the state extract labor from women without a fair return? And how do women themselves see their kin work and its place in their lives?

As I have indicated above, I believe that it is the creation of the self-interest/altruism dichotomy that is itself the problem here. My women informants, like most American women, accepted their primary responsibility for housework and the care of dependent children. Despite two major waves of feminist activism in this century, the gendering of certain categories of unpaid labor is still largely unaltered. These work responsibilities clearly interfere with some women's labor force commitments at certain life-cycle stages; but, more important, women are simply discriminated against in the labor market and rarely are able to achieve wage and status parity with men of the same age, race, class, and educational background.[19]

Thus for my women informants, as for most American women, the domestic domain is not only an arena in which much unpaid labor must be undertaken but also a realm in which one may attempt to gain human satisfactions—and power—not available in the labor market. Anthropologists Jane Collier and Louise Lamphere have written compellingly on the ways in which varying kinship and economic structures may shape women's competition or cooperation with one another in domestic domains.[20] Feminists considering Western women and families have looked at the issue of power primarily in terms of husband-wife relations or psychological relations between parents and children. If we adopt Collier and Lamphere's broader canvas, though, we see that kin work is not only women's labor from which men and children benefit but also labor that women undertake in order to create obligations in men and children and to gain power over one another. Thus Cetta Longhinotti's struggle with her daughter-in-law over the venue of Christmas dinner is not just about a competition over altruism, it is also about the creation of future obligations. And thus Cetta's and Anna's sponsorship of their children's friendship with each other is both an act of nurturance and a cooperative means of gaining power over those children.

Although this was not a clear-cut distinction, those of my informants who were more explicitly antifeminist tended to be most invested in kin work. Given the overwhelming historical shift toward greater autonomy for younger generations and the withering of children's financial and labor obligations to their parents, this investment was in most cases tragically doomed. Cetta Longhinotti, for example, had repaid her own mother's devotion with extensive home nursing during the mother's last years. Given Cetta's general failure to direct her adult children in work, marital choice, religious worship, or even frequency of visits, she is unlikely to receive such care from them when she is older.

The kin-work lens thus reveals the close relations between altruism and self-interest in women's actions. As economists Nancy Folbre and Heidi Hartmann point out, we have inherited a Western intellectual tradition that both dichotomizes the domestic and public domains and associates them on exclusive axes such that we find it difficult to see self-interest in the home and altruism in the workplace.[21] But why, in fact, have women fought for better jobs if not, in part, to support their children? These dichotomies are Procrustean beds that warp our understanding of women's lives both at home and at work. "Altruism" and "self-interest" are cultural constructions that are not necessarily mutually exclusive, and we forget this to our peril.

The concept of kin work helps to bring into focus a heretofore unacknowledged array of tasks that is culturally assigned to women in industrialized societies. At the same time, this concept, embodying notions of both love and work and crossing the boundaries of households, helps us to reflect on current feminist debates on women's work, family, and community. We newly see both the interrelations of these phenomena and women's roles in creating and maintaining those interrelations. Revealing the actual labor embodied in what we culturally conceive as love and considering the political uses of this labor helps to deconstruct the self-interest/altruism dichotomy and to connect more closely women's domestic and labor-force lives.

The true value of the concept, however, remains to be tested through further historical and contemporary research on gender, kinship, and labor. We need to assess the suggestion that gendered kin work emerges in concert with the capitalist development process; to probe the historical record for women's and men's varying and changing conceptions of it; and to research the current range of its cultural constructions and material realities. We know that household boundaries are more porous than we had thought—but they are undoubtedly differentially porous, and this is what we need to specify. We need, in particular, to assess the relations of changing labor processes, residential patterns, and the use of technology to changing kin work.

Altering the values attached to this particular set of women's tasks will be as difficult as are the housework, child-care, and occupational-segregation struggles. But just as feminist research in these latter areas is complementary and cumulative, so researching kin work should help us to piece together the home, work, and public-life landscape—to see the female world of cards and holidays as it is constructed and lived within the changing political economy. How female that world is to remain, and what it would look like if it were not sex-segregated, are questions we cannot yet answer.

NOTES

Many thanks to Cynthia Costello, Rayna Rapp, Roberta Spalter-Roth, John Willoughby, and Barbara Gelpi, Susan Johnson, and Sylvia Yanagisako of *Signs* for their help with this article. I wish in particular to acknowledge the influence of Rayna Rapp's work on my ideas.

1. Acknowledgment and gratitude to Carroll Smith-Rosenberg for my paraphrase of her title, "The Female World of Love and Ritual: Relations between Women in Nineteenth-Century America," *Signs: Journal of Women in Culture and Society* 1, no. 1 (Autumn 1975): 1–29.
2. Ann Landers letter printed in *Washington Post* (April 15, 1983); Carol Gilligan, *In a Different Voice* (Cambridge, Mass.: Harvard University Press, 1982), 17.
3. Heidi I. Hartmann, "The Family as the Locus of Gender, Class, and Political Struggle: The Example of Housework," *Signs* 6, no. 3 (Spring 1981): 366–94; and Christopher Lasch, *Haven in a Heartless World: The Family Besieged* (New York: Basic Books, 1977).
4. Representative examples of the first trend include Joann Vanek, "Time Spent on Housework," *Scientific American* 231 (November 1974): 116–20; Ruth Schwartz Cowan, "A Case Study of Technological and Social Change: The Washing Machine and the Working Wife," in *Clio's Consciousness Raised,* ed. Mary Hartmann and Lois Banner (New York: Harper & Row, 1974), 245–53; Ann Oakley, *Women's Work: The Housewife, Past and Present* (New York: Vintage, 1974); Hartmann; and Susan Strasser, *Never Done: A History of American Housework* (New York: Pantheon Books, 1982). Key contributions to the second trend include Louise Lamphere, "Strategies, Cooperation and Conflict among Women in Domestic Groups," in *Woman, Culture and Society,* ed. Michelle Zimbalist Rosaldo and Louise Lamphere (Stanford, Calif.: Stanford University Press, 1974), 97–112; Mina Davis Caulfield, "Imperialism, the Family and the Cultures of Resistance," *Socialist Revolution* 20 (October 1974): 67–85; Smith-Rosenberg; Sylvia Junko Yanagisako, "Women-centered Kin Networks and Urban Bilateral Kinship," *American Ethnologist* 4, no. 2 (1977): 207–26; Jane Humphries, "The Working Class Family, Women's Liberation and Class Struggle: The Case of Nineteenth Century British History," *Review of Radical Political Economics* 9 (Fall 1977): 25–41; Blanche Weisen Cook, "Female Support Networks and Political Activism: Lillian Wald, Crystal Eastman, Emma Goldman," in *A Heritage of Her Own,* ed. Nancy F. Cott and Elizabeth H. Pleck (New York: Simon & Schuster, 1979); Temma Kaplan, "Female Consciousness and Collective Action: The Case of Barcelona, 1910–1918," *Signs* 7, no. 3 (Spring 1982): 545–66.
5. On this debate, see Jon Weiner, "Women's History on Trial," *Nation* 241, no. 6 (September 7, 1985): 161, 176, 178–80; Karen J. Winkler, "Two Scholars' Conflict in Sears Sex-Bias Case Sets Off War in Women's History," *Chronicle of Higher Education* (February 5, 1986), 1, 8; Rosalind Rosenberg, "What Harms Women in the Workplace," *New York Times* (February 27, 1986); Alice Kessler-Har-

ris, "Equal Employment Opportunity Commission vs. Sears Roebuck and Company: A Personal Account," *Radical History Review* 35 (April 1986): 57–79.

6. Portions of the following analysis are reported in Micaela di Leonardo, *The Varieties of Ethnic Experience: Kinship, Class and Gender among California Italian-Americans* (Ithaca, N.Y.: Cornell University Press, 1984), chap. 6.
7. Clearly, many women do, in fact, discuss their paid labor with willingness and clarity. The point here is that there are opposing gender tendencies in an identical interview situation, tendencies that are explicable in terms of both the material realities and current cultural constructions of gender.
8. Papanek has rightly focused on women's unacknowledged family status production, but what is conceived of as "family" shifts and varies (Hanna Papanek, "Family Status Production: The 'Work' and 'Non-Work' of Women," *Signs* 4, no. 4 [Summer 1979]: 775–81).
9. Selma Greenberg, *Right from the Start: A Guide to Nonsexist Child Rearing* (Boston: Houghton Mifflin Co., 1978), 147. Another example of indirect support for kin work's gendered existence is a recent study of university math students, which found that a major reason for women's failure to pursue careers in mathematics was the pressure of family involvement. Compare David Maines et al., *Social Processes of Sex Differentiation in Mathematics* (Washington, D.C.: National Institute of Education, 1981).
10. Larissa Adler Lomnitz and Marisol Pérez Lizaur, "The History of a Mexican Urban Family," *Journal of Family History* 3, no. 4 (1978): 392–409, esp. 398; Matthews Hamàbata, Crested Kimono Power and Love in the Japanese Business Family (Ithaca, N.Y.: Cornell University Press, 1990); Sylvia Junko Yanagisako, "Two Processes of Change in Japanese-American Kinship," *Journal of Anthropological Research* 31 (1975): 196–224; Maila Stivens, "Women and Their Kin: Kin, Class and Solidarity in a Middle-Class Suburb of Sydney, Australia," in *Women United, Women Divided,* ed. Patricia Caplan and Janet M. Bujra (Bloomington: Indiana University Press, 1979), 157–84.
11. Carol B. Stack, *All Our Kin: Strategies for Survival in a Black Community* (New York: Harper & Row, 1974). These cultural constructions may, however, vary within ethnic/racial populations as well.
12. Elizabeth Bott, *Family and Social Network,* 2d ed. (New York: Free Press, 1971): Michael Young and Peter Willmott, *Family and Kinship in East London* (London: Routledge & Kegan Paul, 1957), and *Family and Class in a London Suburb* (London: Routledge & Kegan Paul, 1960). Classic studies that presume this class difference are Herbert Gans, *The Urban Villagers: Group and Class in the Life of Italian-Americans* (New York: Free Press, 1962); and Mirra Komarovsky, *Blue-Collar Marriage* (New York: Random House, 1962). A recent example is Ilene Philipson, "Heterosexual Antagonisms and the Politics of Mothering," *Socialist Review* 12, no. 6 (November–December 1982): 55–77. Edward Shorter, *The Making of the Modern Family* (New York: Basic Books, 1975), epitomizes the pessimism of the "family sentiments" school. See also Mary Lyndon Shanley. "The History of the Family in Modern England: Review Essay," *Signs* 4, no. 4 (Summer 1979): 740–50.
13. Stack; and Brett Williams, "The Trip Takes Us: Chicano Migrants to the Prairie" (Ph.D. diss., University of Illinois at Urbana-Champaign, 1975).
14. David Schneider and Raymond T. Smith, *Class Differences and Sex Roles in American Kinship and Family Structure* (Englewood Cliffs, N.J.: Prentice-Hall, Inc., 1973), esp. 27.
15. See Nelson Graburn, ed., *Readings in Kinship and Social Structure* (New York: Harper & Row, 1971), esp. 3–4.
16. The moral mother/cult of domesticity is analyzed in Barbara Welter, "The Cult of True Womanhood, 1820–1860," *American Quarterly* 18, no. 2 (Summer 1966): 151–74; Nancy Cott, *The Bonds of Womanhood: "Women's Sphere" in New England,* 1780–1835 (New Haven, Conn.: Yale University Press, 1977); and Ruth Bloch, "American Feminine Ideals in Transition: The Rise of the Moral Mother, 1785–1815," *Feminist Studies* 4, no. 2 (June 1978): 101–26. The description of the general political-economic shift in the United States is based on Harry Braverman, *Labor and Monopoly Capital: The Degradation of Work in the Twentieth Century* (New York: Monthly Review Press, 1974); Peter Dobkin Hall, "Family Structure and Economic Organization: Massachusetts Merchants, 1700–1850," in *Family and Kin in Urban Communities, 1700–1950,* ed. Tamara K. Hareven (New York: New Viewpoints, 1977), 38–61; Michael Anderson, "Family, House-

hold and the Industrial Revolution," in *The American Family in Social-Historical Perspective,* ed. Michael Gordon (New York: St. Martin's Press, 1978), 38–50; Tamara K. Hareven, *Amoskeag: Life and Work in an American Factory City* (New York: Pantheon Books, 1978); Richard Edwards, *Contested Terrain: The Transformation of the Workplace in the Twentieth Century* (New York: Basic Books, 1979); Mary Ryan, *The Cradle of the Middle Class: The Family in Oneida County, New York, 1790–1865* (Cambridge: Cambridge University Press, 1981); Alice Kessler-Harris, *Out to Work: A History of Wage-earning Women in the United States* (New York: Oxford University Press, 1982).

17. Ryan, 231–32.
18. Sylvia Junko Yanagisako, "Family and Household: The Analysis of Domestic Groups," *Annual Review of Anthropology* 8 (1979): 161–205.
19. See Donald J. Treiman and Heidi I. Hartmann, eds., *Women, Work and Wages: Equal Pay for Jobs of Equal Value* (Washington, D.C.: National Academy Press, 1981).
20. Lamphere (n. 4 above); Jane Fishburne Collier, "Women in Politics," in Rosaldo and Lamphere, eds. (n. 4 above), 89–96.
21. Nancy Folbre and Heidi I. Hartmann, "The Rhetoric of Self-Interest: Selfishness, Altruism, and Gender in Economic Theory," in *The Consequences of Economic Rhetoric,* ed. Arjo Klamer and Donald McCloskey (New York: Cambridge University Press, 1988).

IX

GENDER, RITUAL, AND RELIGION

In many non-western societies women's ritual roles are central and indispensable to community cohesion and well-being. In contrast, in Anglo-European cultures women's religious activities tend to be secondary and marginal because of the preeminence of men in both organizational hierarchies and doctrine. Anthropological research has long recognized that religious systems reflect, support, and carry forward patterns of social organization and central values of a society. What has not been sufficiently recognized is the interrelationships of men and women in the perpetuation of social life through religious activities.

The study of the ritual activities of women has often been embedded in analyses of life cycle events, such as the Nkang'a girl's puberty ritual among the Ndembu of Central Africa (Turner 1968: 198) or pregnancy and childbirth rituals in Asia (Jacobson 1989; Laderman 1983). With the exception of this area of research, the study of women and religion has often been neglected, despite the fact that women are prominent in religious activities. As a result of a renewed interest in gender in various cultures, scholars have begun to explore how the religious experience of women is different from that of men; whether and how women become ritual specialists; what religious functions they perform and the degree to which these are private or public; and, finally, what implications these ritual activities have for female prestige and status.

This has led, in some cultural contexts, to an attempt to formulate a more complete ethnographic picture. For example, in the literature on Australian aborigines, where there is a good deal of debate about gender roles, a number of ethnologists have asserted that the dominance of senior men is sustained by their control of sacred knowledge and that their position is recognized by both men and women in the culture (Warner 1937; White 1975; Bern 1979). This viewpoint has been challenged by Diane Bell (1981, 1983), who notes that male anthropologists have underestimated and under-reported the religious life of Australian aboriginal women. She argues that "Both men and women have rituals that are closed to the other, both men and women allow the other limited attendance at certain of their rituals, and, finally, there are ceremonies in which both men and women exchange knowledge and together celebrate their membership in one society and their duty to maintain the law of their ancestors" (1981: 319).

Bell focuses in particular on the love rituals of women, rituals that originally were viewed by ethnologists as magic and therefore deviant, unimportant, and marginal to the central decision-making realm of men. In contrast, Bell suggests that in the celebration of these rituals, used by women to establish and maintain marriages of their own choosing, "Women clearly perceived themselves as independent operators in a domain where they exercised power and autonomy based on their dreaming affiliations with certain tracts of lands. These rights are recognized and respected by the whole society" (1981: 322). The love rituals of Australian aboriginal women are, in short, by no means peripheral to the society. They are underwritten by Dreamtime Law and feared by men who are often unaware that they are being performed and unable to negate their power. Through their rituals some Australian aboriginal women have, as Hamilton (1981) suggests, a mechanism with which to challenge the ideology of male superiority that is expressed in male ritual.

Mathews (1985) provides us with another example of an important arena of religious activity—the civil-religious hierarchy or cargo system in Mesoamerica—that has long been considered a public and exclusively male arena. If women were mentioned at all in studies of the cargo system, it was for their peripheral roles in food preparation. Based on her research in the state of Oaxaca in Mexico, Mathews begins by pointing out that an application of the domestic-public model (see Section III) to an understanding of these religious ceremonies obscures the significant ritual roles of women because it places the cargo system in the public sphere of activity and fails to acknowledge the importance of the household unit. Rather than oppose men and women within a rigid domestic-public model, Mathews emphasizes the parallel and interdependent roles of men and women in the execution of cargo. Male cargo holders (*mayordomos*) organize and coordinate the activities of men, and female cargo holders (*mayordomas*) organize and coordinate the activities of women. At the end of their year of responsibility, both share in the prestige gained from service.

If Oaxacan women have an important and prestige-conferring role within the religious sphere of cargo activity, similar opportunities are denied them within the civil sphere. Thus Mathews explores the impact of the penetration of the state (see Section VII) on the lives of women. A sexual divide-and-rule state policy, she argues, makes men into social adults and women into domestic wards whose dealings with the public sphere become restricted. Prestige in local institutions is undermined by its absence in extracommunity institutions, and as civil offices assume increasing importance at the expense of cargo offices, the position of women is eroded.

In contrast to the underestimation of women's religious roles in the literature on Australian aborigines and the Mesoamerican cargo system, studies of sub-Saharan Africa have long recognized that the ritual life of women is both significant and highly elaborated. In this region, women are involved in complex ceremonies of initiation; they are engaged in witchcraft and divination (Mendonsa 1979; Ngubane 1977); they act as spirit mediums and healers (Green 1989; Sargent 1989); they lead and participate in possession cults (Berger 1976); and they form their own secret societies (MacCormack 1979).

In Africa, and elsewhere around the world, female religious practitioners are often conceived of as women apart. They frequently transcend local cultural definitions of womanhood and are recognized as having extraordinary characteristics. Kendall (in this book) notes that Korean women who become shamans (*mansin*) stand above the social and economic constraints generally imposed on a proper Korean wife and mother. The *mansin* occupies an ambiguous status similar to that of other "glamorous but morally dubious female marginals, the actress, the female entertainer, and the prostitute." Though not always accorded respect, the *mansin* wears the costumes and speaks with the authority of the gods. *Mansin* and their rituals are, in Kendall's view, "integral components of Korean family and village religion. Within this religious system, women and shamans perform essential ritual tasks that complement men's ritual tasks" (1985: 25).

Women in other cultural contexts use spirit possession and trance as an outlet for the stress that results from their social and material deprivation and subordination (Broch 1985; Hamer and Hamer 1966; Lewis 1966, 1969; Morsy 1979; Pressel 1973). As Danforth (1989: 99) argues with regard to Firewalking (*Anastenaria*) in northern Greece, "Through these rituals women seek to address the discrepancies that characterize the relationship between an official ideology of male dominance and a social reality in which women actually exercise a significant degree of power. Spirit possession . . . provides a context for the resolution of conflict often associated with gender roles and gender identity." However, in Korea, rather than serving as an outlet for stress, possession is the vehicle whereby a *mansin,* as a recognized ritual practitioner, ministers to the needs of other women who are in turn the ritual representatives of their families.

Korean housewives come to the *mansin* for therapeutic answers to a range of personal and household problems; for divinations about the future and prospects for the coming year; and for female solidarity and a "venting of the spleen" (Kendall 1985: 25). Women's rituals in Korea, like those in some other parts of the world, are both practical and expressive. As Mernissi (1978) suggests, based on her research in Morocco, female devotional societies provide a tightly knit community of supporters and advisers. The Christian Science movement founded in America by Mary Baker Eddy in the late nineteenth century was a healing religion that also offered middle-class women a "socially acceptable alternative to the stifling Victorian stereotypes then current" (Fox 1989: 98).

In Nahua-speaking communities in Mexico women also have narrowly defined social roles (Huber, in this book). They are expected to engage in domestic responsibilities, remain subservient to their mothers-in-law, and they have fewer outlets for reducing stress than do men. Women are believed to be prone to soul loss in response to the many stresses they experience. Since soul loss is considered a likely indicator of a mandate to cure, more young women than men become healers. In addition, the healing role may appear to be a continuation of the nurturing role women ideally play in local society. Indeed, women curers tend to serve patients in the privacy of their own homes while male curers are more likely to engage in prestigious public rituals that provide greater economic benefits than do the restricted curing roles of women.

Mama Lola, the Vodou priestess (*manbo*) described by Brown (in this book) is a ritual specialist, diviner, and healer working in New York who, when she is possessed, "acts out the social and psychological forces that define and often contain the lives of contemporary Haitian woman." Through ritual, Mama Lola empowers her clients. This phenomenon of psychological empowerment is characteristic of other religious systems; it is described by Danforth (1989) in his discussion of the New Age Firewalking cult in the United States and by Wadley (1989) in her analysis of the active control over their lives that north Indian village women gain through their ritual activities.

Mama Lola maintains a very personal relationship with two female spirits. To one she stands in the role of child to a spiritual mother, thereby metaphorically expressing an important bond within Haitian culture and society that is manifested in her own relationship with her daughter Maggie. This ritually embedded mother-child metaphor can be found in other parts of the world where women healers meet the physical and emotional needs of their patients just as mothers meet the needs of their children (Wedenoja 1989; Kerewsky-Halpern 1989). If one of Mama Lola's female spirits represents the nurturing side of women in relation to their children, the other represents the romantic side in relation to men.

In Haitian Vodou the diverse roles of women are projected into the religious sphere. This is equally true of other religious traditions. In Catholic cultures values about ideal womanhood are sanctified by the image of the Virgin Mary, who represents submission, humility, serenity, and long suffering (Stevens 1973). In Mexico, for example, Eve and the Virgin Mary are contrasting images that "encode the cycle of reproduction within the domestic group. When a woman is nursing and sexually continent she resembles the Virgin. When she submits to sex, she is more like Eve" (Ingham 1986: 76). Hindu goddesses are also multifaceted; they are mothers, mediators, and protectresses. According to Preston (1985: 13), there is a connection "between the role of women in Indian life and the special position of female deities in the Hindu pantheon. Though Indian women are supposed to be absolutely devoted to their husbands who are respected as embodiments of the deity, women may also reign supreme in their own domains as mothers of their children." In Dinaan Hinduism the Great Goddess takes several forms, some good and some evil. Babb (1975: 226) suggests that these two aspects reflect an opposition in male and female principles: "When female dominates male, the pair is sinister; when male dominates female the pair is benign."

Of importance, then, to some students of the relationship between gender and religion is the question of how women are portrayed in religious symbolism and doctrine. One of the most intriguing representations of women in religious thought is the Shaker conception of a female God. The Shakers were a millenarian Christian group who arrived on the shores of America in the late eighteenth century. As Procter-Smith (in this book) points out, long before recent feminists began to refer to God as "she," the Shakers believed in God the mother to complement God the father and conceived of their leader, Ann Lee, as a manifestation of the second coming of Christ in female form.

This millenial thinking empowered women and permitted the eradication of women's subordination. Shaker men and women shared spiritual authority and the leadership roles that were specified by this authority. Long before Engels (see Section VII), the Shakers appear to have recognized that property, marriage, and sexuality may undermine the status of women, and they therefore worked to eliminate these phenomena both ideologically and practically from their way of life. They upheld celibacy and the communal ownership of property. Procter-Smith observes, however, that the Shakers were not fully successful in their efforts. A patriarchal and hierarchical model persisted, as did a division of labor that followed broader societal patterns for what men and women do. To this Setta (1989: 231) has added the observation that Shaker theology was dominated by men while women were the spirit mediums, a distinction in her view that parallels a frequent human division "between men as scholars and thinkers and women as vehicles for religious experience."

Shakerism in its original form had much in common with some of the female-oriented religious cults described by anthropologists working in other parts of the world. It too was based in spirit possession and other forms of ecstatic behavior. It too was organized around the metaphor of mother who gives birth to, nurtures, and protects her child believers. It too provided an outlet for women who were otherwise constrained by the social institutions of nineteenth-century American society.

In this book, we have taken the approach that what it means to be male and female (i.e., gender) is learned and shaped within a cultural context. Religious symbols are a powerful mechanism by which culturally appropriate gender messages are transmitted. As Bynum observes, "It is no longer possible to study religious practice or religious symbols without taking gender—that is, the cultural experience of being male or female—into account" (1986: 1–2). In addition, through participation and leadership in ritual, women may enhance their social position. Involvement in religious activities may also generate a sense of female or community solidarity through membership in a congregation or participation in ritual functions.

REFERENCES

Babb, Lawrence. 1975. *The Divine Hierarchy.* New York: Columbia University Press.

Bell, Diane. 1981. "Women's Business Is Hard Work: Central Australian Aboriginal Women's Love Rituals." *Signs* 7: 314–337.

———. 1983. *Daughters of the Dreaming.* London: George Allen and Unwin.

Berger, Iris. 1976. "Rebels or Status-Seekers? Women as Spirit Mediums in East Africa." In Nancy J. Hafkin and Edna G. Bay (eds.). *Women in Africa,* pp. 157–182. Stanford: Stanford University Press.

Bern, J. 1979. "Ideology and Domination: Toward a Reconstruction of Australian Aboriginal Social Formation." *Oceania* 50: 118–132.

Broch, Harald Meyer. 1985. "'Crazy Women Are Performing in Sombali': A Possession-Trance Ritual on Bonerate, Indonesia." *Ethos* 13: 262–282.

Bynum, Caroline Walker. 1986. "Introduction: The Complexity of Symbols." In Caroline Walker Bynum, Steven Harrell, and Paula Richman (eds.). *Gender and Religion: On the Complexity of Symbols,* pp. 1–20. Boston: Beacon.

Danforth, Loring M. 1989. *Firewalking and Religious Healing: The Anastenaria of Greece and the American Firewalking Movement.* Princeton: Princeton University Press.

Fox, Margery. 1989. "The Socioreligious Role of the Christian Science Practitioner." In Carole Shepherd McClain (ed.). *Women as Healers: Cross-Cultural Perspectives,* pp. 98–114. New Brunswick, NJ: Rutgers University Press.

Green, Edward C. 1989. "Mystical Black Power: The Calling to Diviner-Mediumship in Southern Africa." In Carole Shepherd McClain (ed.). *Women as Healers: Cross-Cultural Perspectives,* pp. 186–200. New Brunswick, NJ: Rutgers University Press.

Hamer, J. and I. Hamer. 1966. "Spirit Possession and its Socio-psychological Implications among the Sidamo of Southwest Ethiopia." *Ethnology* 5: 392–408.

Hamilton, Annette. 1981. "A Complex Strategical Situation: Gender and Power in Aboriginal Australia." In N. Grieve and P. Grimshaw (eds.). *Australian Women: Feminist Perspectives,* pp. 69–85. Melbourne: Oxford University Press.

Ingham, John. 1986. *Mary, Michael and Lucifer.* Austin: University of Texas Press.

Jacobson, Doranne. 1989. "Golden Handprints and Red-painted Feet: Hindu Childbirth Rituals in Central India." In Nancy Auer Falk and Rita M. Gross (eds.). *Unspoken Worlds: Women's Religious Lives,* pp. 59–71. Belmont, CA: Wadsworth Publishing Co.

Kendall, Laurel. 1985. *Shamans, Housewives, and Other Restless Spirits: Women in Korean Ritual Life.* Honolulu: University of Hawaii Press.

Kerewsky-Halpern, Barbara. 1989. "Healing with Mother Metaphors: Serbian Conjurers' Word Magic." In Carole Shepherd McClain (eds.). *Women as Healers: Cross-Cultural Perspectives,* pp. 115–135. New Brunswick, NJ: Rutgers University Press.

Laderman, Carol. 1983. *Wives and Midwives: Childbirth and Nutrition in Rural Malaysia.* Berkeley: University of California Press.

Lewis, L. M. 1966. "Spirit Possession and Deprivation Cults." *Man* 1: 307–329.

———. 1969. *Religion in Context: Cults and Charisma.* Cambridge: Cambridge University Press.

MacCormack, Carol P. 1979. "Sande: The Public Face of a Secret Society." In Bennetta Jules-Rosette (ed.). *New Religions of Africa,* pp. 27–39. Norwood, NJ: Ablex.

Mathews, Holly F. 1985. "'We are Mayordomo': A Reinterpretation of Women's Roles in the Mexican Cargo System." *American Ethnologist* 12 (2): 285–301.

Mendonsa, Eugene L. 1979. "The Position of Women in the Sisala Divination Cult." In Bennetta Jules-Rosette (ed.). *The New Religions of Africa,* pp. 57–67. Norwood, NJ: Ablex.

Mernissi, Fatima. 1978. "Women, Saints and Sanctuaries." *Signs* 3: 101–12.

Morsy, Soheir. 1979. "Sex Roles, Power, and Illness." *American Ethnologist* 5: 137–150.

Ngubane, H. 1977. *Body and Mind in Zulu Medicine: An Ethnography of Health and Disease In*

Nyuswa-Zulu Thought and Practice. New York: Academic Press.

Pressel, Ester. 1973. "Umbanda in Sao Paulo: Religious Innovations in a Developing Society." In Erika Bourguignon (ed.). *Religion, Altered States of Consciousness and Social Change,* pp. 264–318. Columbus: Ohio State University Press.

Preston, James J. 1985. *Cult of the Goddess: Social and Religious Change in a Hindu Temple.* Prospect Heights, IL: Waveland. (Orig pub. 1980.)

Sanday, Peggy. 1974. "Female Status in the Public Domain." In Michelle Z. Rosaldo and Louise Lamphere (eds.). *Woman, Culture, and Society,* pp. 189–206. Stanford: Stanford University Press.

Sargent, Carolyn. 1989. "Women's Roles and Women Healers in Contemporary Rural and Urban Benin." In Carole Shepherd McClain (ed.). *Women as Healers: Cross-Cultural Perspectives,* pp. 204–218. New Brunswick, NJ: Rutgers University Press.

Setta, Susan M. 1989. "When Christ Is a Woman: Theology and Practice in the Shaker Tradition." In Nancy Auer Falk and Rita M. Gross (eds.). *Unspoken Worlds: Women's Religious Lives,* pp. 221–234. Belmont, CA: Wadsworth.

Stevens, Evelyn. 1973. "Marianismo: The Other Face of Machismo in Latin America." In Ann Pescatello (ed.). *Female and Male in Latin America,* pp. 89–101. Pittsburgh: University of Pittsburgh Press.

Turner, Victor. 1968. *Drums of Affliction.* Oxford: Clarendon Press.

Wadley, Susan S. 1989. "Hindu Women's Family and Household Rites in a North Indian Village." In Nancy Auer Falk and Rita M. Gross (eds.). *Unspoken Worlds: Women's Religious Lives,* pp. 72–81. Belmont, CA: Wadsworth.

Warner, William Lloyd. 1937. *A Black Civilization: A Study of an Australian Tribe.* New York: Harper & Row.

Wedenoja, William. 1989. "Mothering and the Practice of 'Balm' in Jamaica." In Carole Shepherd McClain (ed.). *Women as Healers: Cross-Cultural Perspectives,* pp. 76–97. New Brunswick, NJ: Rutgers University Press.

White, I. 1975. "Sexual Conquest and Submission in the Myths of Central Australia." In L. Hiatt (ed.). *Australian Aboriginal Mythology,* pp. 123–142. Canberra: Australian Institute of Aboriginal Studies.

DIVINE CONNECTIONS: THE *MANSIN* AND HER CLIENTS

Laurel Kendall

> This order is recruited from among hysterical and silly girls as well as from women who go into it for a livelihood or for baser reasons.
>
> —H. N. Allen, *Some Korean Customs*

> The magistrate said, "Alas! I thought *mutangs* were a brood of liars, but now I know that there are true *mutangs* as well as false." He gave her rich rewards, sent her away in safety, recalled his order against witches, and refrained from any matters pertaining to them for ever after.
>
> —Im Bang, from "The Honest Witch"

Excerpted with permission from Laurel Kendall, *Shamans, Housewives, and Other Restless Spirits: Women in Korean Ritual Life* (Honolulu: University of Hawaii Press, 1985), pp. 54–85.

The *mansin's* house is much like any other country residence. She hangs no sign outside. Women seek out the *mansin's* house by word of mouth or on the recommendation of kinswomen or neighbors. Once inside, a client makes herself comfortable, sitting on the heated floor. She should feel at home in the *mansin's* inner room, for the place resembles her own. The room where Yongsu's Mother divines could be the main room of any prosperous village home, crammed with the stuff of everyday life. Here are cabinets full of clothes and dishes, a dressing table with a neatly arranged collection of bottled cosmetics, an electric rice warmer, and a television set decorated with an assortment of rubber dolls and pink furry puppies.

THE GODS AND THEIR SHRINE

Yongsu's Mother's shrine, tucked away behind the sliding doors of the one spare room, resembles a rural temple. Gilt-plaster Buddha statues sit on the front altar. Bright printed portraits of Yongsu's Mother's gods hang on the walls. Incense burners, brass candleholders, aluminum fruit plates, water bowls, and stemmed offering vessels clutter the main and side altars. Each utensil and the three brass bells above the altar all bear the engraved phrase "Grant the wish of," followed by the name of the client. These are clients' gifts. The *mansin* advises a client to secure a particular god's good offices with appropriate tribute. One incense burner and water bowl bear my name. Yongsu's Mother told me, with some embarrassment, that the Buddhist Sage and the Mountain God requested gifts since I was doing my research through their will. She told a soldier's wife worried about her husband's fidelity and a young wife worried about her husband's job prospects to dedicate brass bells. She told another young wife to dedicate a water bowl because the Mountain God has helped her husband. Other clients gave the *mansin* her drum and battle trident, her cymbals and knives, her robes and hats, all the equipment she uses to perform *kut* [the most elaborate Shaman ritual]. She stores this equipment out of sight under the altar. Like the shrine fittings, each of these accoutrements bears a client's name. A shrine littered with bells, water vessels, and incense pots advertises a successful *mansin.* In the early morning the *mansin* burns incense, lights candles, and offers cold water inside the shrine. Clients leave incense and candles, and the *mansin* echoes their requests in her own prayers.

A *mansin's* shrine is called a god hall (*sindang*) or hall of the law (*pŏptang*), a Buddhist term. In casual conversation Yongsu's Mother calls her shrine the grandfather's room (*harabŏjiŭi pang*). When I first visited her, I mistook the unmarked plural and thought she was renting a spare room to an older man. "Grandmother" and "grandfather" are honorific, but not excessively formal, terms. In Korea all old men and all old women, by virtue of the status white hair confers, are politely addressed as grandfather and grandmother. Gods also carry a faint connotation of kinship. Although both power and position set gods (*sillyŏng*) above ancestors (*chosang*), some gods, like the Chŏns' Great Spirit Grandmother, are also known ancestors. They are grandfathers and grandmothers writ large. Whether venerable distant kin or generalized venerable elders, Yongsu's Mother owes her gods respect and good treatment. Her gods are not distant, awesome beings; with a common term of address, she brings them close. She dreads their anger and anticipates their will, but she also expects them to help her, as a Korean child looks to a grandparent for small indulgences.

Standing before the gods in her shrine, Yongsu's Mother assumes the self-consciously comic pose of a young child, head slightly bowed, eyes wide with pleading. Speaking in a high, soft voice, she says, "Grandfather, please give me some money. I'm going to the market." She takes a bill from the altar and stuffs it into her coin purse. "I'll be right back," and she brings her hands together and nods her head in a quick bow.

Yongsu's Mother originally kept her gods in a narrow storage alcove off the porch and rented her spare room. She began to suspect that the gods disliked the alcove when she, her son, and her roomers' child were all sick at the same time in the middle of winter. One night her dead husband appeared in a dream. He boldly marched into the spare room while its occupants were in Seoul. Yongsu's Mother yelled at him, "You can't go in there when people are away. They'll think you're going to take something." Her husband answered, "This is my room. I'll give you the rent money." Yongsu's Mother continued to quarrel with her husband until she woke up.

The very next day, her roomers announced that they were moving to Seoul. Someone else wanted to rent the room immediately, but Yongsu's Mother said that she would have to think about it. That night she dreamed that all of the grandmothers and grandfathers in her shrine left the alcove and followed Yongsu's Father into the spare room, calling as they passed, "We'll give you the rent money, we'll give you the rent money."

She told her dream to the Chatterbox Mansin who agreed that Yongsu's Mother must make the spare room into a shrine. Thereafter, she prospered as a *mansin*. Her grandmothers and grandfathers gave her the rent money.

This incident is typical of Yongsu's Mother's ongoing tug-of-war with her grandmothers and grandfathers. Her gods do well by her, but they are even more demanding than her clients' gods. She intended to give a *kut* every three years for their pleasure, but after a prosperous early spring, they made her ill to let her know that they wanted an annual *kut*. The next year, in the fall, she gave the grandmothers and grandfathers special feast food (*yŏt'am*) before her stepdaughter's wedding. The gods were angry because she hit the hourglass drum and roused them but did not give them a *kut*. Her luck was bad for several months. She purchased fabric to make new robes for the General and the Warrior, and gave another *kut* the following spring.

Like many children from Enduring Pine Village, her son Yongsu goes to the private Christian middle school in Righteous Town. The fees at the school are minimal and admissions relatively open, but pressure to convert is high. The gods in the shrine do not like Yongsu's daily brush with Christianity. They make his thoughts wander in school. He says he feels an urge to rush home. Yongsu's Mother told the principal that Yongsu's family had "honored Buddha from long ago," and asked him to understand that Yongsu cannot become a Christian. Then she went to her shrine, hit the cymbals, and implored her grandmothers and grandfathers: "Please understand, please forgive. Yongsu has to get an education. Let him go to that place until he's gotten his education."

THE DESCENT OF THE GODS

A *mansin* engages in a battle of wills with the gods from the very beginning of her career. A woman is expected to resist her calling and struggle against the inevitable, but village women say that those who resist the will of the gods to the very end die raving lunatics. Strange, wild behavior marks a destined *mansin*. Yongsu's Mother describes the struggle:

> They don't know what they're doing. They yell, "Let's go, let's go!" and go running out somewhere. They snatch food from the kitchen and run out into the road with it. God-descended people swipe things and run away. They strike at people and shout insults.
>
> If I were a god-descended person and my husband were hitting me and calling me crazy woman, I'd shout back at him, "You bastard! Don't you know who I am, you bastard?" That's what the Clear Spring Mansin did. Then she sat beside the road talking to the chickens. So funny!

The destined *mansin*, or god-descended person (*naerin saram*), can experience a variety of symptoms. According to Yongsu's Mother,

> It's very difficult for them. They're sick and they stay sick, even though they take medicine. And there are people who get better even without taking medicine. There are some who can't eat the least bit of food; they just go hungry. There are some who sleep with their eyes open, and some who can't sleep at all. They're very weak but they get well as soon as the gods descend in the initiation *Kut*. For some people the gods descend gently, but for others the gods don't descend gently at all. So they run around like crazy women.

Although the destined *mansin* acts like a "crazy woman," Yongsu's Mother makes a distinction between the god-descended person (*naerin saram*) and someone struck temporarily insane (*mich'ida*) by angry household gods or ancestors. "You just have to see them to tell the difference. Insane people look like they're in pain somewhere. The god-descended person wanders here and there singing out, 'I'm this god, I'm that god.'" The *mansin* exorcise insane people as swiftly as possible in a healing *kut* for fear that the possessing spirits will torment their victims to death. The *mansin* flourish knives and flaming torches, threatening, cajoling, and pleading with the offending spirits, urging them to depart (Kendall 1977a). In the initiation *kut* for a god-descended person (*naerim kut*), the initiating *mansin* invites the gods to complete their descent and allow their chosen one to dance and sing as a *mansin*.

A woman often endures considerable anguish before her initiation. The Chatterbox Mansin's story is typical. She was a young matron when the gods descended, a first son's wife living with her mother-in-law. She had already produced two healthy sons. Her husband was away in the air force when she began to exhibit bizarre behavior. She would wander about, talking in a distracted fashion. Worried, her mother-in-law sent for Chatterbox's sister, but when the sister arrived, Chatterbox was sitting in the main room, calmly sewing. She said that every night an old woman—a grandmother—came and asked her to go wandering about with her.

Her sister thought that if Chatterbox was normal enough in the daytime and only behaved strangely at night, she would be all right soon enough. But a few days later, Chatterbox came back to her natal home, clapping her hands together and shrieking like a lunatic. She looked like a beggar woman in torn clothes. Her hair was a tangled mass down her back and her face was filthy. When her mother-in-law came to take her back home, she just sat on the porch and screamed. They tried to pull her up, but her legs stuck fast to the wooden boards of the porch. She asked for some water and poured it all over her body. That night she wandered away. She went into a house and stole a Buddha statue. When her family asked her why she did this, she said, "I was told to do it." For two weeks she went about clapping her hands and pilfering small objects. Then she disappeared completely.

Her family thought she was dead. Much later they heard that she had become the apprentice spirit daughter of the Boil-face Mansin, a great shaman (*k'ŭn mudang*) in the next county. The Boil-face Mansin had taken her in, initiated her, and was training her to perform *kut*. Over the years she learned chants, dances, and ritual lore.

During Chatterbox's distracted wanderings her mother-in-law began divorce proceedings. The woman never lived with her husband again and was forbidden to see her children. But when sorrow overwhelmed her, she would go to the school and, from a safe distance, watch her sons playing in the school yard. A quarrel with his stepmother prompted the oldest son to search out Chatterbox in the countryside. After the boy's flight her sons visited her every summer.

Chatterbox prospered as a *mansin* and built up her own clientele. She broke with her spirit mother after a bitter fight, claiming the shaman overworked and underpaid her. Today, some twenty years after the gods' initial descent, no trace of the haunted young matron remains. Well dressed in Western-style clothing, Chatterbox walks through the streets of the county seat where she has just purchased a new house. Today people in the area consider her a "great shaman" and her own spirit daughter accuses her of stinginess.

By her own admission, Yongsu's Mother had an easy experience as a god-descended person. Widowed after only two years of marriage, she was left with two stepchildren and her own small son. She worked as a peddler, one of a limited number of occupations open to a woman who must support a family. At the end of the mourning period, she went to a *kut* at Chatterbox's shrine.

During an interlude in the *kut*, women danced the *mugam* in the Chatterbox Mansin's costumes to amuse their personal guardian gods and bring luck to their families. The Chatterbox Mansin told Yongsu's Mother to use the *mugam* and dance for success in her precarious business ventures. As Yongsu's Mother remembers it,

> I said, "What do you mean 'use the *mugam?*' It's shameful for me to dance like that." But the Chatterbox Mansin kept saying, "It'll give you luck. You'll be lucky if you dance." So I put on the clothes and right away began to dance wildly. I ran into the shrine, still dancing, and grabbed the Spirit Warrior's flags. I started shouting, "I'm the Spirit Warrior of the Five Directions," and demanded money. All of the women gave me money. I ran all the way home. My heart was thumping wildly. I just wanted to die like a crazy woman. We talked about it this way and that way and decided there was no way out. So the next year I was initiated as a *mansin.*

Although Yongsu's Mother's possession was sudden and unique in its relative painlessness, there had been suggestions throughout her life that she would become a *mansin.*[1] In her early teens during the Korean War, she was fingered as a member of a right-wing youth organization and arrested by North Korean soldiers just before their retreat. Taken on the march north, she made a bold escape on the same night that the Mountain God appeared to her in a dream and said, "It's already getting late."

In late adolescence she had frightening hallucinations. The little Buddha statue a friend brought her from Japan burst into flames in the middle of the room. She watched her mother's face turn into a tiger's face. She wandered about at night, drawn to the stone Buddha near a neighborhood temple. Her mother held a healing *kut.* During the *kut* the girl fell asleep. A white-haired couple appeared and gave her a bowl of medicinal water to drink. When she woke up, she told her dream to the *mansin,* who was pleased. The *mansin* asked her to become her spirit daughter and be initiated as a *mansin,* but she and her mother refused.

Years later, on her wedding night, her sister-in-law dreamed that the new bride was sitting in the inner room hitting a drum. Overhead, on a rope line, hung all of the gods' clothes, as if a *kut* were in progress. Later, when her husband was fatally ill, Yongsu's Mother went to a *mansin's* shrine for an exorcism. She set out her offerings and the *mansin* began to chant, but when Yongsu's Mother went to raise her arms over her head and bow to ground, her arms stuck to her sides as if someone were holding them down. She could not budge them. It was destined that her husband would die and she would become a *mansin.* There was nothing she could do about it.

Yongsu's Mother was a young widow awash in economic difficulties when the gods descended. The Chatterbox Mansin was separated from her husband but living with her mother-in-law, the woman who would later insist on divorce. I am reluctant to speculate on the two initiates' subconscious motivations, but Harvey (1979, 1980) suggests that severe role stress propels women like the Chatterbox Mansin and Yongsu's Mother into god-descended behavior. It is true that, as *mansin,* such women stand above the social and economic constraints imposed on a proper Korean wife, and as *mansin,* they wear the gods' costumes and speak with the gods' authority. But whatever personal and economic gratification she enjoys, the *mansin* and her family pay a price. Shamans were listed, under the occupational classification system of the Yi dynasty, among the despised "mean people" (*ch'ŏnmin*) along with butchers, fortune-tellers, roving players, monks, and female entertainers. According to one early missionary, "Sometimes the daughter of a genteel family may become a Mootang, though this is rare, as her people would rather kill her than have her madness take this form" (Allen 1896, 164).

Like the female entertainer, the *kisaeng,* the shaman engages in public display, singing and dancing. An element of ambiguous sexuality wafts about the *mansin's* performance. In folklore and literature *mudang* are portrayed as "lewd women," and so they are often perceived (Wilson 1983). The *mansin* Cho Yŏng-ja told Ch'oe and Chang that the county chief had come to her home on the pretext of having his fortune told and had then insisted on sleeping with her. Disgusted, she contrived an escape. Thereafter all was coldness between the *mansin* and the county chief (Ch'oe and Chang 1967, 32–33).

The *mansin* play to their female audience, but when the supernatural Official sells "lucky wine," the costumed *mansin* roams through the house seeking male customers. The men have been drinking by themselves in a corner of the house, as far removed from the *kut* as possible. Now they emerge, red faced, and the bolder of their company dance a few steps on the porch. Men buy the Official's wine and tease the *mansin,* flourishing their bills in front of her face before securing the money in her chestband. An audacious man may try to tweak the *mansin's* breast as he secures his bill.

The *mansin* is caught at cross purposes. By her coy, flirtatious performance, she encourages the men to spend more money on wine. But as a woman alone, she must defend herself from harassment and protect her reputation. Yongsu's Mother was resourceful.

> It doesn't happen so much anymore, but when I first started going to *kut,* men would bother me. We were doing a *kut* at a house way out in the country, and I was going around selling the Official's wine. Some son-of-a-bitch grabbed my breast. I put out my hand so the drummer would go faster, then brought my arms up quick to start dancing. I knocked that guy against the wall. Afterwards, he asked me, "What did you mean by that?" I said, "Oh, that wasn't me, it was the honorable Official who did that." Other times, I'd be drumming and some guy would say, "Auntie, where is Uncle? What is Uncle doing now?" and go on like that. I'd reach out to beat the drum faster and slap the guy with the drumstick.

At the *kut* for the dead, performed outside the house gate, men gather off to the side. They gaze at the *mansin* garbed like a princess who sings the long ballad tale of Princess Pari, rapping the drum with elegant flicks of her wrist. My landlady told me of a famous *mansin,* now aged, who was once a beauty. "When she did the *kut* for the dead, it would take forever. This one would carry her off on his back, and that one would embrace her."

To the exemplar of Confucian virtue, the *mansin* offends simply because she dances in public. When an officer from the district police station tried to stop a *kut* in Enduring Pine Village, he threatened to arrest the *mansin* because "they were dancing to drum music and students were watching." The moral education of the young was thereby imperiled. An envelope of "cigarette money" finally silenced this paragon.

It would be a distortion to paint the *mansin* I knew in northern Kyŏnggi Province as social pariahs. Since she has no husband, Yongsu's Mother's house is a favorite gathering place for village women. In their leisure moments they drop by to chat about the latest school fee, the inept village watch system, the new neighborhood loan association, or simply to gossip. Even the wife of the progressive village chief, though she disdains "superstition," seeks out the company of the articulate, loquacious *mansin.* Yongsu's Mother is a favorite guest at birthday parties. She gets the singing started and makes people laugh. She can sometimes be persuaded to bring her drum so the women can dance.

But Yongsu's Mother lives under the shadow of potential insult. Village people say, "Not so many years ago, even a child could use blunt speech [*panmal*] to a shaman."[2] Although this is no longer true, when tempers flare Yongsu's Mother's occupation is still flung in her face. Yongsu's Mother and the widowed Mr. Yun were great friends. Village gossips expected them to marry. Mr. Yun's daughter-in-law rankled at the possibility. She finally exploded in a fit of rage, shrieking at Yongsu's Mother, "Don't come into my house! I don't want a shaman to come into my house! It's bad luck if a shaman comes into your house." Pride wounded to the quick, Yongsu's Mother avoided the Yun family and there was no more talk of marriage.

After her stepdaughter's marriage Yongsu's Mother was anxious lest the groom discover her occupation. She did only one hasty New Year Rite for a client on the second day of the New Year since she expected a visit from the newlyweds on that day. She dreaded the thought of them walking in and catching her banging her cymbals in the shrine.

The Chatterbox Mansin's sister-in-law found her own children dancing in time to the drum rhythm during a *kut.* She slapped them soundly, then howled at her miserable fortune to have married into a shaman's house. Since this was all in the family, and the Chatterbox mansin is never at a loss for words, whatever the circumstance, she snapped back, "Well then, you knew this was a shaman's house. You didn't have to marry my brother and come to live here."

The *mansin* shares in the ambiguous status of other glamorous but morally dubious female marginals, the actress, the female entertainer, and the prostitute. Like the others, she makes a living, often a comfortable living, by public performance in a society where so-called good women stay home. But the *mansin* is neither an actress nor a courtesan. She is the ritual specialist of housewives. The good women who stay home need her. She came from their midst, lives like them, and speaks to their anxieties and hopes.

The gods who have claimed a woman as a *mansin* leave her one lingering shred of respectability. It is well known that only by virtue of divine calling is she a shaman, and that is a compulsion fatal to resist.[3] Her neighbors assume that she did not want to become a *mansin.* She tells her story to clients, describes how she resisted the call with the last ounce of her strength and succumbed only after considerable suffering and in fear for her very life. . . .

WOMEN WHO COME TO THE *MANSIN*'S HOUSE

A shaman's divination (*mugŏri*) is the first step in any ritual therapy. Women like Grandmother Chŏn come to the *mansin's* house when they suspect that malevolent forces lurk behind a sudden or persistent illness or domestic strife. In Yongsu's Mother's shrine I heard reports of inflamed lungs, an infected leg, fits of possession "craziness," alcoholism, and dreamy, wandering states of mind. One woman, afflicted with this last complaint, feared that she was god-descended, but Yongsu's Mother laughed off her worries and divined more commonplace godly displeasure as the source of her problems. Other women who came to the shrine worried about their husbands' or sons' career prospects, or about sudden financial reverses. Should the husband switch jobs? Would the son receive his security clearance to work in Saudi Arabia? Thieves had broken into the family rice shop, what did that presage? Other women were anxious that adulterous husbands might abandon them. Some had only the vaguest suspicion that their spouses had "smoked the wind," but one young woman was certain that her husband took the grain his mother sent up from the country and shared it with his mistress. One woman, caught in a compromising position by her enraged spouse, had fled to the *mansin* in fear of life and limb. And still other women asked about wayward children, stepchildren, or grandchildren whose transgressions ranged from mild rebelliousness to Christian zealotry, petty theft, and delinquency. A mother-in-law asked how she should deal with a runaway daughter-in-law. A daughter-in-law who had fled home asked if she should divorce her husband. An older woman wondered if she should join a married son's household. . . .

The *mansin* chats with the women before fetching the divination tray. Sometimes the women begin to discuss their anxieties before the actual divination, but these are usually long-standing clients. Clients who come to the *mansin* for the first time tend to hold back and see how much the *mansin* can uncover in the divination.

The *mansin* brings in the divination tray, an ordinary low tray of the sort used for meals in any Korean home. The tray bears a mound or rice grains, a handful of brass coins (imitations of old Chinese money), and the brass bell rattle a *mansin* uses to summon up her visions.

"Well now, let's see," says the *mansin,* settling down to a kneeling posture behind her tray. The client places a bill under the pile of grain on the tray. At Yongsu's Mother's shrine in 1977 and 1978, this fee was usually five-hundred or a thousand won. Now the *mansin* shakes the brass bells beside her own ear and chants, asking the gods to send "the correct message." She receives a message for each member of the client's family, beginning with the client's husband if he is alive. She announces each subject's name and age to the gods, tosses her coins on the tray, and spills handfuls of rice grains until the Great Spirit Grandmother speaks and sends visions.

Coin and rice configurations hint at the client's concerns. A broad spread of coins bespeaks quarrels between husband and wife or parent and child, or betrays financial loss. A long line of coins broken by one or two solitary coins at the end tells of someone leaving home, a change of employment, a death, or the inauspicious influence of an ancestor who died far from home. A few grains spilled on the floor caution financial prudence; the client should postpone switching jobs or buying a house.

The *mansin* describes a situation and asks for confirmation. "Your husband has a cold or something, is that it?" "Your thirteen-year-old daughter doesn't get along with her father, is that right?" The *mansin* develops the theme, weaving her visions together with her client's information. With more tosses of coins and grain, the Great Spirit Grandmother sends more specific visions. "I see a steep embankment. Is there something like that near your house?" The woman and her neighbor nod affirmation. "Be careful of that place." To another woman, "Your daughter has two suitors. One is quite handsome. The other is extremely clever but also very meticulous. Since your daughter isn't especially clever herself, she'll have a better life if she marries the second suitor, but she must watch her step and scrupulously manage her house."

Sometimes she sights the discontented gods and ancestors of her clients' households. "Is there a distant grandfather in your family who carried a sword and served inside the palace?" "Did someone in your family die far from home and dripping blood?" She circles in on the supernatural source of her client's problems and suggests an appropriate ritual to mollify a greedy god's demands or send a miserable and consequently dangerous soul "away to a good place."

For a housewife to evaluate the skill of an individual *mansin* and trust her diagnosis, she must know the supernatural history of her husband's family and of her own kin. And if the *mansin* is convinced that there was "a grandmother who worshiped Buddha," or "a bride who died in childbirth," she tells her client, "Go home and ask the old people, they know about these things. . . ."

SEEING THE YEAR'S LUCK

During the first two weeks of the lunar year, women crowd the *mansin's* house to "see the year's luck" (*illyŏn sinsurŭl poda*). The New Year marks a fresh, auspicious start for each household. A woman therefore gets a prognosis on each member of her family. If noxious influences threaten someone in her charge, she can "make them clean" by performing simple rituals under the first full moon.

This is the peasants' winter slack season and the women are in a holiday mood when they come to the *mansin's* house. Most arrive in groups. Waiting their turn, they bunch together in the hot-floor inner room. If the wait is long, they play cards, doze, or listen to other divinations. They sigh sympathetically for the woman whose divination reveals an adulterous husband, unruly child, or pitiable ghost. They coach the young matron who does not yet know the vocabulary of women's rituals. Not for them, the confidential atmosphere of the Western doctor's or analyst's office. The confessional's anonymity is missing here. The women enjoy each other's stories and accept each other's sympathy.

A woman, as a matter of course, receives divinations for her husband, herself, living parents-in-law, sons, unmarried daughters, sons' wives, and sons' children. Many women, however, pay an extra hundred or two hundred won for the fortunes of those whose ties stretch outside the woman's "family," the family she enters at marriage and represents in the *mansin's* shrine. Some women ask about a married daughter, her husband, and their children, or about other natal kin. During New Year divinations in 1978, one woman asked about her own mother, brother, and brother's wife, another about her own elder sister. Yongsu's Mother teased, "What do you want to know about them for?" but provided the divinations. Women acknowledge their concern for mothers, married daughters, and siblings, but it costs more, an extra coin or two.

In the New Year divination the *mansin* predicts dangerous and advantageous months, warns against potentially dangerous activities, and suggests preventive ritual action. The following condensation of Yongsu's Mothers New Year divination for a seventy-year-old widow is an example.

> My seventy-year-old lady, you shouldn't go on long trips; you must be careful now. Your children will receive succor; someone will come with aid in the seventh or eighth month. You will have some good news in the third or fourth month.
>
> Your thirty-nine-year-old son should not visit anyone who is sick [since in this horoscope year, he is vulnerable to noxious influences]. His thirty-five-year-old wife should be heedful of things other people say about her. Their twelve-year-old son should be exorcised with five-grain rice left at the crossroads and by casting out a scarecrow stuffed with his name [because he has acquired an accretion of noxious influences and his year fate is bad]. The eight-year-old daughter will be lucky but you should burn a string of pine nuts, one for each year of her life, and address the moon on the night of the first full moon.
>
> Your thirty-five-year-old son is troubled with sorrow and regret, but his luck is changing. There is no trouble between husband and wife, nothing to worry about there. Their seven-year-old child has a cold or something. This is a dangerous time for him so they must guard him carefully. Your unmarried thirty-year-old son doesn't even have a girl friend, but next year his prospects will improve. He should marry when he's thirty-two. He'll succeed in life when he's thirty-five or thirty-seven.

The scarecrow, five-grain rice left at the crossroads, and pine nuts burned under the moon are minor rituals performed on the fifteenth day of the lunar year. The first full moon marks the end of the New Year holidays, a time when women immunize a threatened family member, usually a child, against noxious influences lurking in the year's fortune. When the *mansin's* visions reveal a swarm of noxious influences on the road, a growing splotch of red, she tells the child's mother or grandmother to leave five-grain rice at a crossroads, then wave it over the child's head and cast it out. A mother must warn her child to be especially mindful of traffic. When the *mansin* sees swimming fish, she tells the woman to write the child's name, age, and birthdate on a slip of paper and wrap the paper around a lump of breakfast rice on the morning of the fifteenth. The woman throws the packet into a well or stream saying, "Take it, fish!" She substitutes the rice for a child with a drowning fate.

The *mansin* also cautions that children should not swim, go fishing, or climb mountains in certain months. Here the women sigh, "How can I do that?" The *mansin* tells the housewife which family members, according to the particular vulnerability of their year horoscope, must disdain funerals, feasts, or visits to sick friends. She advises switching a sixty-first birthday celebration to a more auspicious month. She predicts the compatibility of a son's or daughter's lover or a matchmaker's candidate. She determines when "the ancestors are hungry and the gods want to play," and advises these families to hold *kut* early in the new year. The early spring is a busy season for the *mansin*. . . .

A woman goes to the *mansin* with some ambivalence. She assumes the *mansin* will discern a supernatural problem and suggest ritual action. Rituals, be it an inexpensive exorcism or an elaborate *kut,* require cash. Hangil's Mother told me, "I don't go to the *mansin's* house anymore. They always tell you to do things that cost money, and I can't afford to do that. I'm just like a Christian now, only I don't believe in Jesus." Though some women are cynical, Hangil's Mother is not. She advised me on the rituals I should perform for my own spirits and was almost invariably among the women watching a *kut* in Yongsu's Mother's shrine. A divination is the essential first step in a *mansin's* treatment, but the whole process may stop here. Whenever Yongsu's Mother counseled a woman to dedicate a brass bell or sponsor a ritual, the client would almost always say, "I'll have to talk it over with my husband," or "I'll have to see what the old people say." At home she weighs the potential benefits against the household budget. A woman told me, "They say we ought to do a *kut* because a grandmother of this house was a great shaman, but it takes too much money." Some women decide to wait and see if their problems will improve over time. There was, for example, the woman who said,

> Years ago, I went to a *mansin* in Righteous Town. Someone told me she was good, so I went to her by myself. My husband was losing money and I felt uneasy. The *mansin* said, "Do a *kut*," but I didn't.

Others are satisfied with the *mansin's* actions on their behalf:

> I was sick last year. I felt exhausted and my whole body ached. I went to the hospital for treatment and that took a lot of money. . . . After the exorcism I got better.

or:

> We did a *kut* two years ago for my eldest son. He drank too much and had pains in his chest. He took Western medicine, but that didn't work. The Brass Mirror Mansin did a *kut* and he got better, so he didn't have to go to the hospital.

Some of the women were reluctant to attribute a successful cure directly and exclusively to the *mansin's* efforts. "The *mansin* did an exorcism and my daughter took medicine; she recovered." There are also clients who claim total dissatisfaction with the *mansin's* cure. Everyone in the Song family's immediate neighborhood knew that the entire household of the minor line became Christian when their healing *kut* did not cure the son's acute headaches. He recovered slowly over the next few months. Another woman said that she stopped believing when she learned that she had cancer of the womb. On the other side of the ledger was a young woman who, years ago, had prayed to the Christian god to spare her ailing parents. They died and she stopped believing. Now she was sponsoring a *kut*. Other women wonder if the *kut* the *mansin* advised might have saved an afflicted family member:

> Three years ago, I went to a *mansin* I'd heard was good. I went for my husband who was paralyzed. The *mansin* did an exorcism and told us to do a *kut*. We didn't do the *kut*, and my husband died.

or:

> My son died when he was sixteen years old. We should have gone to a *mansin*, but we didn't. There was something wrong with his thigh. It seemed fine from the outside. We couldn't see anything wrong and neither did the hospital. We went to the Western hospital and the hospital for Chinese medicine. . . .

HOUSEHOLD TRADITIONS AND WOMEN'S WORK

Women go to *mansin's* shrines and to Buddhist temples as the ritual representatives of their families and households. They sponsor *kut* in the shrine and in their own homes, but never in other houses. Other houses have their own house gods. A bond like an electrical connection links the *mansin's* house to the housewife's own dwelling. When clients leave after making offerings in the shrine or sponsoring a *kut* there, they give no farewell salutation. The *mansin* carefully reminds new clients of this necessary breach of etiquette, and tells the women to go straight home. A woman brings blessings from the shrine directly to her own house lest they be lost along the way. The woman leaves the shrine without a farewell and enters her own home without a greeting. Salutations mark boundaries and transitions; they are inappropriate here.

Any woman, old or young, married or single, can visit the *mansin's* house and receive a divination, but the *tan'gol* [regular customer] who make seasonal offerings in the shrine and sponsor *kut* are female househeads, the senior women in their households. Commensurate with their temporal responsibilities, they come to the shrine on behalf of husbands, children, and retired parents-in-law. Some *tan'gol* are young matrons, but others are grandmothers whose concerns stretch beyond their own households to their married sons' households. They pray on behalf of sons, daughters-in-law, and grandchildren. Sometimes a worried mother brings her own daughter to the *mansin.* Occasionally mothers press their married daughters to hold a *kut* or perform a clandestine conception ritual, and mothers often pay an extra fee to include a married daughter's household in their divinations. A mother's concern for her own daughter might suggest pity for the suffering shared by all women, but it also suggests a mother's assumed ability to aid all of her children, even those who have left the ritual family she represents in the shrine. . . .

In the ideal flow of tradition, a daughter-in-law continues her mother-in-law's relationship with a particular *mansin.* The *mansin's* spirit daughter inherits the shrine and the old *mansin's* clients or her clients' daughters-in-law. In practice, the relationship is far more flexible. The daughter-in-law sometimes favors a *mansin* close to her own age over the white-haired *mansin* her mother-in-law patronized. A spirit daughter may not enjoy the rapport her spirit mother had with clients. Some women switch *mansin* when they are dissatisfied with a diagnosis and cure. Other clients, like the Songs who converted to Christianity, stop visiting *mansin* altogether out of disappointment or because of diminishing returns. Other women said they stopped going to the *mansin's* shrine because their present lives were "free of anxiety" (*uhwani ŏptta*). Yongsu's Mother said, "When things are fine, people don't do anything. When someone is sick, when they lose money, or when there's trouble with the police, then they do things like exorcisms and *kut.*"

Yongsu's Mother acknowledges her role as a specialist. The women who seek her services share with her a rich lore of belief and practice aimed at securing the health, harmony, and prosperity of households. At the new year or in time of crisis, she helps them order their world. Across her divination table, ordinary women's concerns and stories mingle with the painful tales of a shaman's destiny.

NOTES

1. Pyongyang-mansin, one of Harvey's informants, reports a similar experience (Harvey 1979:109).
2. Like the Japanese language, spoken Korean sentence endings are shorter or longer depending on the relative status of the speaker and the addressee. Adults use blunt endings, *panmal,* when addressing children, and children use them when addressing dogs.
3. There are hereditary *mundang* families in the southernmost provinces. Whether by birth or divine will, the point is the same: The female religious practitioner does not voluntarily assume her role.

REFERENCES

Allen, H. N. 1896. Some Korean Customs: The Mootang. *Korean Repository* 3: 163–168.

Ch'oe, Kil-sŏng, and Chang Chu-gŭn. 1967. *Kyŏnggido Chiyŏk Musok (Shaman Practices of Kyŏnggi Province).* Seoul: Ministry of Culture.

Harvey, Youngsook Kim. 1979. *Six Korean Women: The Socialization of Shamans.* St. Paul: West Publishing Company.

———. 1980. Possession Sickness and Women Shamans in Korea. In N. Falk and R. Gross (eds.). *Unspoken Worlds: Women's Religious Lives in Non-Western Cultures,* pp. 41–52. New York: Harper and Row.

Kendall, Laurel. 1977. Caught Between Ancestors and Spirits: A Korean Mansin's Healing Kut. *Korea Journal* 17(8): 8–23.

Wilson, Brian. 1983. The Korean Shaman: Image and Reality. In L. Kendall and M. Peterson (eds.). *Korean Women: View from the Inner Room,* pp. 113–128. New Haven: East Rock Press.

THE RECRUITMENT OF NAHUA CURERS: ROLE CONFLICT AND GENDER[1]

Brad R. Huber

Josefa,[2] age 43, explains the role illness plays as a sign of an individual's destiny to cure in Nahua-speaking communities in Mexico:

> Lightning struck me when I was feeding the pigs. A pig fell down because it was also hit. It got back up, but as soon as it got up it fell over dead. To one side we had a jar of holy water so that the bats wouldn't come to suck the blood of the pigs. When the lightning-bolt killed the pig, it then struck me and finally it broke the jar of holy water. My illnesses began when the lightning-bolt frightened me and when the pig died next to me. [I began to suffer soul loss.] It must always be like that . . . Afterwards one cures.

This paper has three primary goals. The first is to make an ethnographic contribution to the study of Nahua curers. Though curers are one of the most important types of medical specialists serving Nahua-speaking communities, no scholar has described their mode of recruitment, the various roles they play, or their relationship to other types of religious personnel in any detail. Research in Hueyapan resulted in the collection of a significant amount of new information that is of interest to ethnohistorians, linguists, and ethnographers working in Mesoamerica.

The second goal of this paper is to make an analytical contribution to the study of shamanism and its relationship to gender. This area of research is currently receiving considerable attention (McClain 1989; Lewis 1989; Welch 1982). The author's fieldwork with Nahua curers isolated several factors associated with the recruitment of either male or female practitioners. They include: (1) an individual's social, economic, and genealogical status, (2) role stress, continuity, and compatibility, and (3) the scope of the curing role.

The final goal is to critically appraise Lewis's (1989) cross-cultural study of shamanism. Several modifications to his theoretical framework are suggested here. When modified, Lewis's framework provides a new way to look at medical and religious specialists in Nahua communities.

RESEARCH SITE AND METHODS

The author conducted fieldwork in the municipality of Hueyapan[3] for a total of eighteen months between August 1983 and August 1987. Hueyapan is located in the Sierra Norte de Puebla, Mexico. It is divided into ten administrative sections with slightly more than one-third of its 6,000 residents living in the municipal seat. Members of nearly every household raise domesticated animals and cultivate subsistence and cash crops. In addition, the majority of women produce woven garments for domestic use and sale, and most men migrate as wage laborers. With very few exceptions, residents speak both Nahuat and Spanish, though they vary considerably in their proficiency in the latter language.

Eighteen curers (thirteen women and five men) reside in Hueyapan, an average of one practitioner per 335 residents. Structured interviews were administered in Nahuat by the investigator and a trained field assistant to eight curers (seven women and one man). These eight curers range in age from 43 to more than 80 years, with a mean age of approximately 54. Table 1 summarizes this information.

Some curers were interviewed on two or more occasions. The interviews lasted approximately 90 minutes and were tape recorded.

Reprinted with permission of Brad Huber and from *Ethnology* 29 (2): 159–176.

Table 1 Hueyapan's Curers

Name	*Primary Specialty*	*Secondary Specialty*	*Sex*	*Age**
Andrés	Curer	Bonesetter	Male	55 (—)
Antonia	Curer	———	Female	58 (22)
Concepciona	Curer	———	Female	43 (—)
Feliciana	Curer	———	Female	50 (30)
Francisca	Curer	———	Female	80 (13)
Josefa	Curer	———	Female	43 (35)
Juana	Curer	Midwife	Female	50 (34)
Maria	Curer	———	Female	46 (20)

*All ages are based upon self-reports. The numbers in parentheses indicate the ages when curers began treating patients on a more or less regular basis.

Structured interviews were supplemented with information collected informally from three additional curers (two men and one woman). The research reported here is part of a larger project which also includes work with Nahua midwives and bonesetters.

THE DIVISION OF MEDICAL LABOR

In Hueyapan, the division of medical labor is fairly rigid (Huber 1990). In general, one type of medical specialist will not attend illnesses treated by another.[4] A bonesetter treats broken bones, dislocations, sprains, and bruises. A midwife assists women prior to, during, and after parturition. A curer (*tepahtihqui,*[5] *tepahtiani*) attends almost all other medical problems, including those thought to have supernatural causes. He or she serves in the capacity of pharmacist, diagnostician, diviner, doctor, and ritual specialist.

In other Nahua communities, the division of medical labor is somewhat different. For example, medical roles may overlap more. In the southern Huasteca, midwives (or even bonesetters) may perform a curer-like role during certain rituals and at certain times of the year (Alan Sandstrom, personal communication). In some communities of the states of Mexico, Morelos, Puebla, Tlaxcala, and Veracruz, the curer's role is more broadly defined than it is in Hueyapan. Individuals who cure illness may also officiate at public-communal rites concerning animal and crop fertility, the control of the weather, the installation of public officials, and events associated with the church calendar (Barrios 1949:64–66; Bonfil Batalla 1968:113–114, 121–122; Cook de Leonard 1966:295; Medellín Zenil 1979:114–118; Nutini and Isaac 1974:364; Sandstrom and Sandstrom 1986:106–107). Finally, the curer's role may be more narrowly defined than it is in Hueyapan. Nahua curers of San Bernardino Contla (Tlaxcala) and Tepoztlán (Morelos) serve only as herbalists, diagnosticians, and doctors, and claim little or no contact with supernatural entities (Nutini and Isaac 1974: 48–49; Redfield 1930:152).

THE NAHUA CURER'S ROLE

As pharmacists, Hueyapan's curers possess considerable knowledge of the preparation, qualities, uses, and effects of herbs, plants, fruits, animal parts and patent medicines. Medicines are prescribed according to the principle of opposites ("hot" medicines for "cold" illnesses and vice versa), their sympathetic qualities, or because they have been observed to alleviate the symptoms of an illness in the past (Foster 1988).

Illness is diagnosed by verbally, visually, and physically examining a patient. However, Hueyapan's curers claim that "pulsing" is the most reliable method of diagnosis. Pulsing is a widely distributed form of divination used in Mesoamerica (Tedlock 1982:133–138). In Hueyapan, curers pulse patients at their wrists, neck, temples, waist, and chest. The type of pulse (weak or strong, fast or slow) is used to determine the kind of illness a person has, the appropriate medicinal and ritual therapy, the location of a patient's lost soul, and whether a person is destined to cure. In cases of illness caused by sorcery, curers state that the blood of patients accuses the guilty person.

Hueyapan's curers also use two other types of divination. Corn kernel divination is used to discover the identities of saints who will assist in the recovery of an extremely-ill patient. Curers drop seven corn kernels one-by-one into a bowl of water while simultaneously naming a saint. A kernel which "stands on end" at the bottom of the bowl indicates that the saint who was named should be petitioned for assistance.

Water vapor divination is used to determine an ill patient's godparent. Dried flowers from Hueyapan's main church are boiled in water. Curers then sprinkle the cooling water on specific points of the patient's head and neck. The identity of the patient's godparent is revealed by observing the point where water vapor rises. This individual later accompanies his or her ill godchild on a pilgrimage to a saint's image, and sponsors a fiesta after the godchild's recovery.

Variations of the above methods as well as egg, copal incense, quartz crystal, and obsidian divination are reported in several other Nahua communities. In addition, dream revelation, and entering trance-like states after becoming intoxicated with rum, marijuana, and hallucinogenic substances are used by some Nahua curers to diagnose illness (Barrios 1949:65–70; Bonfil Batalla 1968:105, 113–114; Cook de Leonard 1966:291–293; García de León 1968:284, 289; Lewis 1963:282; C. Madsen 1965:104; W. Madsen 1955:51–52; Montoya Briones 1964:156; Münch Galindo 1983:201; Sandstrom 1975:263–265; Signorini 1982:316).

Hueyapan's curers perform a wide variety of rituals (e.g., ritual cleansings, soul callings) to alleviate suffering caused by sorcery, object and spirit intrusion, soul loss, etc. Since detailed accounts of these healing rituals can be found elsewhere (Barrios 1949:70–72; Huber 1985:12–127, 174–178; Montoya Briones 1964: 156–165; Münch Galindo 1983:194–205, 234–240; Reyes García 1976:92–95; Robinson 1961: 348–353; Sandstrom 1975:135–301; and Sandstrom and Sandstrom 1986:35–51, 100–108), they are not discussed here. It is worthwhile noting, however, that a few of Hueyapan's curers claim making face-to-face contact with supernatural beings, the lost souls of their patients, and spirits of deceased people. The following is an account of Juana's experience with a *tamatini* (one who customarily knows things; plural, *tamatinime*). In this case, a *tamatini* appeared to Juana in the form of a female lightning-bolt spirit. It was holding her male patient's soul captive in a cave, and Juana went to recover it. She recalls:

> At one side of the waterfall was a cave and I entered it to call the [man's soul]. Then a woman appeared and I saw her dancing. I went to the entrance to wait for that lightning-bolt and she said, "What do you want?" and I said, "Please . . . give me the man." She said "I'll give him to you right now, [but] you're going to pay me." I told her I would and asked her how much.
>
> She said she wanted 7000 pesos but that wasn't really true. She wanted seven centavos.[6] I put down seven centavos, a cross, and flowers. After I had called the man, I saw the man leaving but it wasn't really him . . . , it was his soul. The man passed by me. I went with him and said good-bye [to the tamatini]. The man was in front of me and we went over a bridge and saw three dead men. I asked [my patient] to help me because I thought perhaps my soul would remain there. But that didn't happen.

Madsen (1955:50–51, 1957:164, 1983:114–116) and Knab (1983:383–466) indicate that Nahua curers in the Milpa Alta area and the Sierra Norte de Puebla, respectively, claim making direct contact with similar kinds of supernatural beings.

Hueyapan's curers do not charge a fixed sum of money for their services. Instead, fees are negotiated. The amount of cash, food, liquor, and cigarettes curers receive depends upon the severity of the illness, the economic circumstances of the patient, the curer's reputation, etc. In July 1987, a curer received approximately 1000 pesos ($0.65 U.S.) in cash or kind for curing soul loss, a particularly serious illness. For other illnesses, curers receive considerably less. The compensation Hueyapan's curers receive is neither exceptionally low nor high when compared to that of curers in other Nahua communities.

THE RECRUITMENT OF NAHUA CURERS

The process by which Nahua curers are recruited shares many characteristics with a rite of initiation, including a quasi-liminal period (Eliade 1958, 1960, 1964; Paul 1975:464; Turner 1979). When individuals enter this liminal period, they are forced to decide either for or against becoming a curer, a decision that is both traumatic and disorienting. This decision-making period is charged with ambiguity, psychological stress, themes of life and death, and encounters with supernatural beings. Analogous to a liminal period in a rite of initiation, it startles "neophytes into thinking about objects, persons, relationships, and features of the environment they have hither taken for granted" (Turner 1979:240).

Hueyapan's curers claim that *tamatinime* played an important role during the liminal phase of their recruitment. *Tamatinime* are thought to be wise and powerful spirits who live in caves, and frequent streams, waterfalls, forests, mountainous areas, and the ocean. They are referred to by several additional names depending upon the form they take and the function they perform (cf., Taggart 1983:60–61, 73–74, 138–148). As *rayos* (lightning-bolts), they punish people with illness who show disrespect for nature or for other people. As *achihualime* (rainmakers), they appear as small naked children with light curly hair. San Miguel Arcangel and the Virgen del Rayo (also known as the Virgen del Carmen) command seven male and thirteen female rainmakers, respectively. *Tamatinime* may also appear as snakes, men, and women, and are sometimes thought to be actual individuals with lightning-bolt companion spirits.

Supernatural beings which are similar to Hueyapan's *tamatinime* and who are said to play an important role in the recruitment of curers in other Nahua communities include: *enanitos* (literally, dwarfs), *rayos* (lightning bolts), *aires* (literally airs), *ahuahque* (water-possessors), and *chaneques* (residents) (Bonfil Batalla 1968: 102; Madsen 1965:102–104; Madsen 1955:50, 1957:164–165, 1983:114; Montoya Briones 1964:155, 173, 1981:12–15; Münch Galindo 1983:173–175). Adams and Rubel (1967:337–339) and Mendelson 1967: 406–409) suggest that a belief in such beings is widespread in Mesoamerica. For an excellent description of the residences of these beings see Grigsby (1986).

According to Hueyapan's curers, *tamatinime* forced them to assure their medical role after they appeared to them in dreams,[7] or attacked them in snake, human, or lightning-bolt form. *Tamatinime* appeared to most of Hueyapan's curers prior to or during adolescence. At age fifteen, Antonia recalls:

> I use to dream a lot. I dreamt, for example, that snakes attacked me and that men grabbed me. This is said to show you [that you're destined to be a curer]. Also, I dreamt of many bundles of flowers, that I parted them and some angry people [i.e., tamatinime] shot at me [with guns]. Also, I dreamt of mountains and the ocean. They came and pushed me in [the ocean] but I had the strength to get myself out. I was frightened but I knew then the kind of work they were going to give me.

Though premonitory dreams are the most frequent means by which Hueyapan's curers are divinely called, Francisca encountered three *tamatinime* in snake form as a young girl of thirteen. She remembers:

> Before I started to cure I encountered some enormous snakes in [a remote hamlet of Hueyapan]. I was walking with my mother when some snakes wrapped themselves around my body. There were three, and they scared me. It was their nature to do this or rather it was predestined that they frighten me. And well . . . that's the way it had to be.

Some of Hueyapan's curers also report being instructed to cure during their encounters with *tamatinime*. Josefa states:

> I used to dream a lot about mountains and snakes. [Once] when I was dreaming, I saw some snakes who threw me down a ravine . . . They told me, "Please don't be bad [i.e., a sorcerer]," and I paid attention to them. I went with them [to see their sick son]. I dreamt that I remained with the tamatinime for three days without food or water. [Then], they threw an herb at me . . . , and also some [medicinal] roots . . . I prepared their son's medicine and cleansed him. After curing him, I left them. I don't really remember if they took me out or if I left on my own.

García de León (1969:282), Kaufman (1988), and Signorini (1982:322) also report that Nahua curers experience premonitory dreams. Scholars working in other Nahua communities report individuals are alerted to their calling after being struck unconscious by lightning, attacked by a mal aire, or having taken hallucinogenic drugs (Barrios 1949: 65–67; Bonfil Batalla 1968:102–106; Cook de Leonard 1966:293; Madsen 1965:102–104; Madsen 1955:50–51, 1957:164–65, 1983:114; Montoya Briones 1964:155; Münch Galindo 1983:210). Nutini and Nutini (1987:335) report that some individuals first realize they will become curers in Tlaxcala after they discover they have extraordinary visual and auditory abilities.

As can be seen, many Nahua curers report first becoming aware of their calling when their bodies have been "de-possessed" of their souls. It is during this time that their detached souls encounter spirits that oblige them to assume the medical role for which they are destined to undertake. No scholar makes mention of Nahua curers being recruited by means of spirit possession, the other major mystical theory of divine election (Lewis 1989).

In Hueyapan, encounters with *tamatinime* are followed by a patterned series of events. Subsequent events include: severe and recurrent illnesses, an experienced curer's revelation that the afflicted individual must either begin curing or die, a display of reluctance to assume the healing role, a short apprenticeship (optional), the novice's successful healing of his or her first few patients, and a corresponding increase in prestige and clientele. Antonia describes the role illness and an experienced curer's revelation played in her recruitment (Madsen 1965:102):

> It was my mother who took care of me when I was sick for nine complete months. I couldn't even turn myself over in bed. I changed curers many times . . . [Finally] I went to a curer in [a hamlet in section seven]. He told my parents to ask God to help me. After visiting seven churches, my curer told me that I too would start to cure people and that I should not deny [sick people my help]. My curer told me that if I didn't cure them I would get sick like before.

Francisca reports that after her encounter with *tamatinime* in the guise of three enormous snakes, she became ill with soul loss. Shortly thereafter:

> I went to see my curer and she told me that I had to take an [herbal medicine] for twenty days. And if in those twenty days of eating this herb I survived, I would then get better. And I survived! My curer told me that the snakes attacked me in order to see if I would survive or not. [She also told me that] it was my fate [to cure] and that I shouldn't deny that when sick people come to me even if they come at midnight because this is my obligation.

Though it was clear to Hueyapan's initiates that the consequences of not curing are sickness and death, many report having been reluctant to assume the curing role. Before Josefa started to cure, she remembers, "I was afraid and at the same time I was ashamed. For example, I thought, 'What if I don't cure' [my patients]?' Similarly, Feliciana recalls after helping her mentor to cure a young infant, "I started to doubt myself again and I asked my curer, 'Do you believe that I'm going to cure?' And he answered me, 'Of course [you will], and [you will] always [cure]. You must have faith in what you are doing'."

Hueyapan's curers resist assuming the healing role for a number of years. Most do not begin treating patients on a regular basis until early adulthood (see Table 1). However, the continuation of dreams and illness, and the threat of death eventually encourage them to overcome their reluctance, self-doubt, and ambivalence. Similar accounts of the psychological conflicts experienced by Nahua curers during their recruitment can be found in Madsen (1965:103–104), Madsen (1955:50, 1957:164, 1983:114), and Montoya Briones (1964:155). Reluctance to become a curer is probably more common than published reports indicate. Initially resisting commands or offers (e.g., a proposal of marriage, ritual kinship, a religious office) is a norm found in many parts of Mesoamerica (Paul and Paul 1975:139).

Five of Hueyapan's curers also report a short period of apprenticeship, and that this training had a decisive impact on overcoming their reluctance to become active practitioners. Feliciana's description of her relationship to her mentor is the most explicit:

> When I turned fourteen, they took me to the house of Miguel Romero, [a curer in a nearby town]. He told me, "Right now we have an eight-month-old who is gravely ill, and you are going to help him." I told him, "But I don't know how." Then the curer said to me, "You must do it like this and like that, and if you don't [try to heal him], you're going to get sick and you're going to die. And if you die it's not my fault; it will be your problem."
>
> [I was reluctant to attend this infant], but don Miguel insisted. Thus, we got down on our knees before the altar where there [were images] of the Virgin of Carmen, the Virgin Guadalupe, the [Sacred] Heart of Jesus, the [Sacred] Heart of Mary, Saint Peter, and Saint Joseph. [We kneeled] there where we had been when I arose from my illness.
>
> And at this time, he advised me to work and not to be ashamed. Well, I started to work and [afterwards] don Miguel took me with him. And when we arrived [at a patient's home] to cure, he sat down and allowed me to begin curing. Of course, he only watched me. And [so], I rather weakly started the struggle to cure.

Nahua curers who deny serving an apprenticeship, or deny even the possibility of learning to cure from other individuals are reported by Barrios (1949:66), Bonfil Batalla (1968:104), Madsen (1965:102), and Madsen (1955:54). Curers from Pajapan (Veracruz), Atla (Puebla), and Tlaxcalan communities surrounding Malintzi volcano report receiving formal training (García de León 1968: 282, Montoya Briones 1964:155; Nutini and Nutini 1987:336). Curers in these communities appear to hold an opinion similar to that of Hueyapan's curers: training is of little use to individuals unless they first show signs of having been divinely elected. Finally, Sandstrom and Sandstrom (1986:72) indicate that any adult may become a curer in Ixhuatlán de Madero, Veracruz. Novices serve a one to six-year apprenticeship under a master. This relatively long period of apprenticeship may reflect the complexity and range of rituals curers will be asked to conduct in this region (Alan Sandstrom, personal communication).

In Hueyapan, the first few patients a novice curer attends play an important role in his or her recruitment. Six of the eight curers who were interviewed report that their first patients were relatives or neighbors who had been unsuccessfully treated by doctors and other curers with an established practice. Despite the odds, these curers report success in treating these difficult cases. According to Juana:

> First my aunt came to me and she told me, "I have pain [in my back]. I went to a doctor, paid him a lot of money and he didn't help me." I told her to take a pill, bathe with soap, and not to [work]. Also, I rubbed her with an ointment, after which she sweated. I covered her up well and with this she was cured.
>
> My aunt told another person [about her being healed], a man who had been to a doctor who said he was going to die. I told my aunt, "This man isn't going to die." I told this man he had soul loss. All I did was take his pulse.

After recounting the difficulty she experienced in retrieving his lost soul, Juana goes on to say, "The next day he ate a tortilla. The man lived another four years and then he died, but of old age [not soul loss]."

After these early successes, word of the novice's healing ability is spread in Hueyapan, often by family members, grateful patients or by the curer to whom he or she was apprenticed. Soon the curer's reputation and clientele grow. The same events may be important in the recruitment histories of curers in other Nahua communities, though only one scholar makes brief mention of them (Madsen 1983:114).

CURING AND ROLE CONFLICT

After individuals become active practitioners, they find that their relationships with family, friends, and neighbors have been radically altered. Both men and women report that the responsibilities associated with curing conflict with those of their other roles. For Feliciana, this conflict was especially intense:

> [My husband] wouldn't let me leave [the house] to go to work [i.e., attend patients]. He would say, "Why are you leaving? You're only leaving [in order] to put your arms around men . . ." [My husband also used to] hit me a lot. My nose would bleed and I would wipe it with my shawl. I used to squeeze [my shawl] until only blood dripped out. [Finally] my mother-in-law helped me. When he started to beat me all the time, my mother-in-law took me to my [parent's] home and that's where I stayed [for awhile].

After staying with her parents for a short period time, Feliciana returned to live with her husband because he became extremely ill. She claims his illness was God's punishment for not allowing her to cure. He died four years later in excruciating pain:

> [My husband used] to cry a lot because of what was happening to him. He wasn't even able to talk. His mouth was twisted and his head was bent to one side. During this time he yelled [at me and said] it was I who bewitched him. And [he would ask] why did I have to be a woman of the street.

Feliciana also reports that her sons and some of the community's residents criticize her when she visits patients:

> This makes me angry because when I go to cure someone, they say, "Here comes that starving person. Here comes that woman who doesn't know how to work and who only deceives people in order to eat. She's just lazy." Even one of my sons said to me, "Look . . . it's better to stop doing this work." But, I told him, "It would be a shame if you became sick after I stop." Another son, the oldest, said to me, "It's better if you don't walk around [visiting patients]. All you get is criticism."

Other curers in Hueyapan report that they have been accused of being lazy, interested only in money, sexually promiscuous, and of practicing sorcery. However, some have reduced this conflict somewhat by making adjustments in their relationships with spouses and patients. Josefa indicates that:

> [My husband] tells me not to go [visit patients] because I [won't be able to] feed him or wash clothes. Now if I had a daughter, well . . . at least she would be here [in the home] making meals. But when I see that he always gets angry [when I leave to cure], it's better that I don't go anywhere. We'll just get disgusted with each other. Now instead of going [to see patients] I tell them to come see me. And I really am afraid of my husband's anger. Because . . . truly I am afraid.

Antonia seems to have worked out the most satisfying arrangement to reduce marital conflict. Her husband used to get angry when she left at night to cure people, but now that he assists her in curing,[8] she says he is content. "Yes [he's happier] now. There are times that I [have to go out] at night and now he goes with me." According to Antonia, her husband has even been instrumental in increasing her (and his) clientele:

> A little while ago, my husband went to buy things at the store and met a man from [an adjacent municipality] whose son was sick. My husband told him I cured. So the man brought

> me cigarettes and beer, and requested that I come with him to see his son. We went there and waited for [them to bring back] the medicines. The next day, they came to advise us that [their son] was now cured.

In previously published reports, Nahua scholars have noted that curers are respected for the good work they perform and feared because of the harm they might do as sorcerers. Curers suspected of performing sorcery may even be murdered by outraged family members of people they have victimized (Lewis 1963:106; Madsen 1965:102–104; Madsen 1955:49–50; Montoya Briones 1964:154–155, 158; Nutini and Nutini 1987:338; Sandstrom and Sandstrom 1986:73; Soustelle 1958:151; cf., Adams and Rubel 1967:340). However, materials collected in Hueyapan suggested that the role of Nahua curers is considerably more complex. Curers enter this role with self-doubt, fear, embarrassment and ambivalence. Active practitioners encounter strong resistance from their spouses and family, as well as accusations of sexual promiscuity, laziness, and of being interested only in financial gain. Though the curing role provides practitioners with additional income and some measure of respect and prestige, the psychological and social costs are considerable.

GENDER AND HEALING

A number of factors leading to the recruitment of men and women to the curing role are examined in this section. They include the social, economic, and genealogical status of individuals prior to their recruitment, role stress, continuity and compatibility, and the scope of the curing role. The discussion begins with a consideration of the family backgrounds of Hueyapan's curers.

Hueyapan's curers had a similar status prior to their recruitment. Four of the curers who were interviewed report that one or both of their parents died when they were young children; six curers indicate their natal families were extremely poor by local standards. As a consequence, some of Hueyapan's future curers were forced to live with relatives, godparents, or neighbors. They describe this time in their lives as one of hardship and loneliness. Presumably, socially disadvantaged individuals such as these would be inclined to assume a role that promises some measure of positive recognition and additional income.

Appropriate role models were also present prior to the recruitment of Hueyapan's curers. Though none of the curers' parents were healers, five curers report they had relatives who were bonesetters, midwives, or curers. Three report having observed their relatives heal prior to their recruitment. Surprisingly, there is apparently no one type of relative who served as a role model for Hueyapan's curers. Role models include maternal and paternal grandparents, aunts, uncles, and sisters.

These factors explain why individuals of both sexes might be inclined to become curers in Hueyapan. However, they do not account for the disproportionate number of female curers (thirteen of eighteen) in this community. In order to understand why female curers predominate in Hueyapan, differences in the roles men and women generally play must be taken into account.

Role Stress, Soul Loss, and Female Curers

O'Nell defines role stress as "stress generated in an individual as a result of his or her self-perceived failure to respond adequately to the essential expectations accruing to a given role, which the person legitimately fills by virtue of membership in his cultural group" (1975:43). O'Nell and Selby claim that Zapotec women experience role stress more frequently than men because the woman's role: (1) is more narrowly defined and (2) provides fewer outlets to escape stress. Susto (one of several terms used to refer to soul loss) and the asustado role provide a temporary "channel of escape for the relief of psychological stress" (O'Nell and Selby 1968:97). As a consequence, more Zapotec women than men experience this folk illness (cf., Rubel 1964:280; Rubel, O'Nell, and Collado-Ardón 1984:122; Uzzell 1974).

A very narrowly defined role is also ascribed to women in Hueyapan. A young girl is often more severely disciplined than a boy for laziness. As an adult, a woman is expected to be faithful to her husband, assume few responsibilities outside the domestic sphere, and respect the demands of her mother-in-law with whom she often lives. In addition, few outlets are open to women to reduce stress. Traveling outside of Hueyapan, visiting, and drinking alcoholic beverages are not encouraged (cf., Brown 1982:144–145; Paul and Paul 1975:139; Vexler 1981:167–169).

Of special interest is the fact that the majority of Hueyapan's curers report first suffering soul loss as adolescents. Adolescence would appear to be an especially stressful period for Nahua women (Taggart 1983:24). They are often expected to marry at this time, leave familiar surroundings, and join their husband's household in another part of Hueyapan. Feliciana seems to have been especially unprepared for this transition:

> I didn't live long with [my parents] because I married [young]. I didn't even know they had arranged my marriage. [My future husband's family] came to get me with a godfather at the age of thirteen. This meant that I was married ... [Later] my brothers really got angry because I married and returned home.

The following relationship between role stress, soul loss, and the election of adolescent females to the curing role is suggested: In Hueyapan, more women than men experience soul loss because the woman's role is very narrowly defined and provides few outlets to reduce stress. Soul loss is often first experienced during adolescence, a particularly stressful period for females. Since experienced curers interpret frequent and severe cases of soul loss as signs of their patient's destiny to cure, more young women than men are encouraged to become healers.

Role Continuity and Compatibility

As was previously mentioned, individuals seriously entertaining the idea of becoming a curer express great reluctance to begin healing. Among other considerations, potential recruits face the prospect of encountering life-threatening accusations of sorcery and strong resistance from their spouses, family members, and residents. This section explores why women would be more likely than men to overcome their reluctance to become active practitioners.

First, the curing role offers women some measure of role continuity. In Hueyapan, women are expected to be supportive, concerned about the health of household members, provide their family with a proper balance of "hot" and "cold" foods, and treat minor illnesses. The curing role can be viewed as an extension and amplification of the role women ideally play in Hueyapan (Hock-Smith and Spring 1977:2, 15; Marcos 1987:25).

Second, curing is compatible with the economic role women undertake in Hueyapan. As in other indigenous Mesoamerican communities, the economic relationship between men and women in Hueyapan tends to be "a partnership based upon mutual dependency, where the work of both sexes is valued and respected" (Bossen 1983:40; Taggart 1983:21). In general, Hueyapan's men perform most of the agricultural work and periodically migrate as wage laborers. Women prepare meals, wash clothing, care for small children, and earn a cash income through weaving and sewing.

Though their work is complementary, there are some important differences in the scheduling of men's and women's work. The timing of hoeing, planting, weeding, and harvesting is somewhat unpredictable since these activities depend upon variable climatic factors. However, once these tasks are begun, they take precedence over all other activities engaged in by men. It is only during periods of little or no agricultural activity that men are able to work outside of Hueyapan.

The demands made of curers are often incompatible with the scheduling of men's work. The curing role is occasionally very time consuming and almost always unpredictable. Reliable curers must be easily accessible to their patients and available day and night throughout the year. Since men frequently migrate and are reluctant to reschedule their agricultural duties, it is not surprising so few men in Hueyapan find a way to incorporate the unpredictable duties of curing with their other responsibilities.

In contrast, very few women leave Hueyapan in search of work. Moreover, tasks such as washing and weaving can be delayed during busy periods of attending patients with fewer of the long-term consequences associated with postponing agricultural work. The fit between the work generally undertaken by women and the responsibilities of curing is better.

The Scope of the Curer's Role

The exact number of male and female curers serving a specific community is not always reported. Nevertheless, in addition to Hueyapan, curers tend to be women in the Nahua communities of Atla and Huauchinango, Puebla (Montoya Briones 1964:155; Nutini and Isaac 1974:223), Mecayapan, Veracruz (Münch Galindo 1983:201), and Tepoztlán, Morelos (Lewis 1963:101–102; Redfield 1930:152). Male curers predominate in Ixhuatlán de Madero, Veracruz (Sandstrom 1975:93; Sandstrom and Sandstrom 1986:72), in Tlaxcalan communities surrounding La Malintzi volcano (Nutini and Nutini 1987:335), and communities of the Sierra Nevada (Bonfil Batalla 1968:117).

After reviewing the responsibilities of curers in these areas, a relationship was discovered between the scope of the curing role and sex of the practitioner. In communities where male curers predominate, curers may also officiate at public-communal rites concerning animal and crop fertility, the control of the weather, the installation of public officials, and events associated with the Catholic church calendar. Their broadly defined role can be characterized as that of a shaman-priest (Tedlock 1982:47–53). In communities where female curers predominate, there is no report of their participation in public-communal rituals of this kind.[9] Their role is restricted to healing illnesses. They serve residents of their community on an individual basis and in the privacy of their own homes.

There is no evidence that indicates women are less willing than men to undertake the role of shaman-priest. Thus, the possibility that women are being excluded from this role should be seriously considered. In a cross-cultural study, Welch (1982) reviews a wide variety of explanations that have been used to account for the exclusion of women from priestly roles. These explanations can be subsumed under three broad types: (1) men fear women holding positions of power, (2) women have difficulty marshalling the economic and social support necessary to secure access to privileged positions, and (3) community norms limit female participation in the public sector. It seems quite reasonable to employ one or more of these explanations to account for the relative absence of female shaman-priests in Nahua communities. Nevertheless, Welch concluded that none of the above explanations adequately accounted for the exclusion of females from priestly roles in his sample of 93 societies.[10]

Though it is not clear why so few women become shaman-priests, several factors have been identified that would encourage men in Nahua communities to undertake this religious specialty. First, men may view the role of shaman-priest as similar to that of sponsoring a saint's feast day, i.e, a religious steward. Both roles provide men with the opportunity to perform valued public-communal services, and both are means by which they can acquire status and prestige. In some Nahua communities, shaman-priests are even ranked in a formal hierarchy similar to that of religious stewards (Bonfil Batalla 1968:103).

Second, men in Nahua communities would also find the shaman-priest role attractive for economic reasons. Because Nahua shaman-priests engage in a wide variety of paid ritual activities, the income derived from the shaman-priest role is potentially greater than that of the more narrowly defined curing role. The economic benefits of this role may more than offset the costs of curtailing agricultural activities and forgoing wage labor opportunities outside the community. Furthermore, male shaman-priests would be engaged in activities designed to enhance animal and crop fertility, activities that promote their primary economic interests. In sum, men in Nahua communities may view the shaman-priest role as a viable alternative to wage labor, compatible with their economic role, and similar to other status-enhancing roles they are expected to play. They generally find the more narrowly defined curing role unattractive because it conflicts with their work schedule, confers little prestige, and provides relatively few economic benefits.

CONCLUSIONS

Lewis (1989: 26–27, 63, 152–59) identifies three basic religious patterns. They are: (1) the central non-ecstatic cult headed by male priests whose claim to authority is validated by their knowledge of ritual and religious doctrine, (2) the central ecstatic cult typically led by men who are divinely elected, and (3) the peripheral ecstatic cult composed primarily of female shamans.

Male priests and shamans of central cults are recruited from relatively advantaged social strata. They, in conjunction with other elite members of society, directly regulate basic social, economic, and political relationships. Because leaders of central cults regulate human relationships, they are said to have a moral focus.

In contrast, female shamans of peripheral cults are recruited from the most disadvantaged ranks of society. Though the peripheral healing role does not provide women with a direct means to influence public affairs, it does provide women with "the opportunity to gain ends (material and nonmaterial) which they cannot readily secure more directly" (Lewis 1989:77). Peripheral cults are said to be amoral because their leaders attempt to regulate spirit-human relationships, rather than relationships among people.

It should now be clear how Lewis's theoretical framework can be employed to analyze the relationship between type of medico-religious avocation and gender in Nahua communities. The central cults of Nahua communities include those dedicated to Catholic saints, and other locally important deities associated with meteorological phenomenon, and animal and crop fertility. Leaders of these cults are almost always men and include Catholic priests, religious stewards, and shaman-priests. As is well known, the leaders of these cults often attempt to regulate economic and political relationships that are central to their community's social organization.

Peripheral cults in Nahua communities are led by individuals who occupy the more narrowly defined curing role. Individuals undertaking this role are predominately women who are socially and economically disadvantaged, and who fail to meet social role expectations. From Lewis's perspective, recruits to this healing role are given an opportunity to moderately increase their status and economic standing. As such they are engaging in an indirect type of social protest. In response to the moderate success of these indirect protests, spouses, family members, and residents attempt to regulate the curers' gains either directly through verbal criticism and physical abuse or indirectly through the use of sorcery accusations (Lewis 1989: 195–113).

Three observations about Lewis's analysis of the relationship of gender to religious avocation can now be made. First, Lewis's theoretical framework is based upon his cross-cultural study of religious specialists whose mode of recruitment is spirit possession. Until now, it was not known whether his generalizations could be applied to specialists who claim to have been divinely elected after having suffered soul loss. The materials presented in this paper clearly suggest his framework can be extended to societies in which the recruitment of medical and religious personnel is based upon this alternate mystical theory of divine election.

Second, the materials presented is this paper indicate that social deprivation is a necessary, but not a sufficient cause of the recruitment of individuals to peripheral healing roles. Additional factors include an individual's genealogical status, role stress, continuity and compatibility, the material (and nonmaterial) costs and benefits of the role, etc. One of the positive features of Lewis's theoretical framework is that these additional variables can quite easily be incorporated within it.

Third, the materials presented on Nahua curers call into question Lewis's claim that spirits of peripheral cults are "amoral" (cf., Bourguignon 1976:34–36; Green 1989:198; Kendall 1989:155). In addition to recruiting curers, *tamatinime* are thought to punish individuals with illness who think badly of other people or who desire to harm them. When patients consult curers, they point out to them the danger of entertaining immoral thoughts and breaking social norms. The underlying message curers convey is that socially approved behavior is therapeutic.

It is difficult to predict how the sexual division of medical labor in Nahua communities will change in the future. Bossen makes the important observation that "the modern cash economy and occupational structure [of Mesoamerica] offer men wider and better opportunities" (1983:42). If this trend continues, then it is predicted that (1) curing will attract fewer and fewer men in Nahua communities as more and better economic opportunities become available to them, and (2) more women will become curers as they become more socially, economically, and politically disadvantaged.

NOTES

1. An abbreviated version of this article was presented at the annual meeting of the American Anthropological Association, Washington D.C., on November 25, 1989. The research reported here was supported in part by two Tinker Summer Research grants. I thank Laurel Bossen, Linda Brown, Lynn Mayo, Sharon Gormley, Thomas L. Grigsby, Carol McClain, Hugo G. Nutini, and Alan R. Sandstrom for their valued criticism and assistance with earlier drafts.
2. The names of Hueyapan's curers are pseudonyms.
3. For a general ethnographic description of Hueyapan and some of the changes it has recently undergone see Huber (1985, 1987).
4. One female curer (Juana) is also a midwife, and one male curer (Andrés) is a bonesetter. In addition, several of Hueyapan's midwives and one bonesetter report using techniques typically employed by curers.
5. Nahua curers are referred to by a variety of names. This variation is due, in part, to regional dialectical differences, the various roles curers may play, and the use of different orthographic systems by ethnographers. In Spanish, the names reported include: *adivino* (diviner), *brujo* (witch), *curandero* (curer), *hechicero* (sorcerer), and *yerbatero* (herbalist). Some of the more common Nahua names include: *huehuetlacatl* (literally, a big or old person), *pachiquetl* (a variant of *pachiuhqui,* medicine maker), *tapahtiani, tepahe* and *tepaxtial* (variants of *tepahtiani,* one who customarily treats people with medicine), and *tlamatiquetl* and *tlamatki* (variants of either *tlamatqui,* wise person or *tlahmatqui,* one who practices deception) Barrios 1949:66; García de León 1968:283; Madsen 1965:102; Medellín Zenil 1979:114; Montoya Briones 1964: 154; Nutini and Isaac 1974:196, 230, 364; Nutini and Nutini 1987:334; Sandstrom and Sandstrom 1986:72; Soustelle 1958: 147).
6. Tamatinime evidently count one centavo as one thousand pesos (Dow 1986:52).
7. In Hueyapan, dreams represent real experiences of the spirit (Madsen 1983:114; Paul 1975:458; Tedlock 1981:315).
8. Antonia's husband as well as Concepcion's are curers. Both husbands serve primarily as their wive's assistants.
9. Montoya Briones (1964:153) reports that Atla's curers petitioned rain in the past. At the present time, most curers are women. Barrios (1949:64) and Cook de Leonard (1966:295) make mention of women in the states of Morelos and Mexico, respectively, who both cure and petition rain. Neither indicates whether most curers in these areas petition rain nor whether curers tend to be female.
10. Welch's "counter-intuitive" finding that low control of property is conducive to women becoming shamans is consistent with the fact that many of Hueyapan's female curers came from impoverished natal households.

REFERENCES

Adams, R. N., and A. J. Rubel. 1967. "Sickness and Social Relations." *Handbook of Middle American Indians,* ed. R. Wauchope, Vol. 6, pp. 333–356. Austin.

Barrios E., M. 1949. "Textos de Hueyapan, Morelos." *Tlalocan* 3:53–75.

Bonfil Batalla, G. 1968. "Los que trabajan con el tiempo: Notas etnográficas sobre los graniceros de la Sierra Nevada, México." *Anales de Antropología* 5:99–128.

Bossen, L. 1983. "Sexual Stratification in Mesoamerica." *Heritage of Conquest: Thirty Years Later,* eds. C. Kendall, J. Hawkins, and L. Bossen, pp. 35–71. Albuquerque.

Bourguignon, E. 1976. *Possession.* San Francisco.

Brown, J. K. 1982. "Cross-Cultural Perspectives on Middle-Age Women." *Current Anthropology* 23: 143–156.

Cook de Leonard, C. 1966. "Roberto Weitlaner y los graniceros." *Summa Anthropologica en homenaje a Roberto J. Weitlaner,* pp. 291–298. Mexico.

Dow, J. 1986. *The Shaman's Touch: Otomí Indian Symbolic Healing.* Salt Lake City.

Eliade, M. 1958. *Rites and Symbols of Initiation: The Mysteries of Birth and Rebirth,* trans. W. R. Trask. New York.

———. 1960. *Myths, Dreams and Mysteries: The Encounter between Contemporary Faiths and Archaic Realities,* trans. P. Mairet. London.

———. 1964. *Shamanism: Archaic Techniques of Ecstasy,* trans. W. R. Trask. New York.

Foster, G. M. 1988. "The Validating Role of Humoral Theory in Traditional Spanish-American Therapeutics." *American Ethnologist* 15:120–135.

García de León, A. 1968. "El universo de lo sobrenatural entre los Nahua de Pajapan, Veracruz." *Estudios de Cultura Nahuatl* 8: 279–311.

Green, E. C. 1989. "Mystical Black Power: The Calling to Diviner-Mediumship in Southern Africa." In *Women as Healers: Cross-Cultural Perspectives,* ed. C. S. McClain, pp. 186–200. New Brunswick.

Grigsby, T. 1986. "In the Stone Warehouse: The Survival of a Cave Cult in Central Mexico." *Journal of Latin American Lore* 12:161–179.

Hoch-Smith, J., and A. Spring. 1977. *Women in Ritual and Symbolic Roles.* New York.

Huber, B. R. 1985. "Category Prototypes and the Reinterpretation of Household Fiestas in a Nahuat-Speaking Community of Mexico." Ph.D. dissertation, University of Pittsburgh.

———. 1987. "The Reinterpretation and Elaboration of Fiestas in the Sierra Norte de Puebla, Mexico." *Ethnology* 26 : 281–296.

———. 1990. "Curers, Illness, and Healing in San Andrés Hueyapan, a Nahuat-Speaking Community of the Sierra Norte de Puebla, Mexico." *Notas Mesoamericanas* 12 (forthcoming).

Kaufman, T. 1988. "Ethnomedical Research in Huastec Country: Commentary on Work in Progress" (unpublished manuscript).

Kendall, L. 1989. "Old Ghosts and Ungrateful Children: A Korean Shaman's Story." In *Women as Healers: Cross-Cultural Perspectives,* ed. C. S. McClain, pp. 138–156. New Brunswick.

Knab, T. J. 1983. "Words Great and Small: Sierra Nahuat Narrative Discourse in Everyday Life." Ph.D. dissertation, State University of New York-Albany.

Lewis, I. M. 1989. *Ecstatic Religion: A Study of Shamanism and Spirit Possession,* 2nd edition. New York.

Lewis, O. 1963. *Life in a Mexican Village: Tepoztlán Restudied.* Urbana.

McClain, C. S. (ed.). 1989. *Women as Healers: Cross-Cultural Perspectives.* New Brunswick.

Madsen, C. 1965. "A Study of Change in Mexican Folk Medicine." *Middle American Research Institute,* Publication 25. New Orleans.

Madsen, W. 1955. "Shamanism in Mexico." *Southwestern Journal of Anthropology* 11:48–57.

———. 1957. "Christo-Paganism: A Study of Mexican Religious Syncretism." *Middle American Research Institute,* Publication 19. New Orleans.

———. 1983. "Death of a Curandero." *Notas Mesoamericanas* 9:112–116.

Marcos, S. 1987. "Curing and Cosmology: The Challenge of Popular Medicines." In *Development: Seeds of Change* 1:20–25.

Medellín Zenil, A. 1976. "Muestrario ceremonial de la región de Chicontepec, Veracruz." *Actes du XLIIe Congres International des Americanistes* (Paris) 9B:113–120.

Mendelson, E. M. 1967. "Ritual and Mythology." In *Handbook of Middle American Indians,* ed. R. Wauchope, Vol. 6, pp. 392–415. Austin.

Montoya Briones, J. de J. 1964. *Etnografía de un pueblo Nahuatl.* Mexico.

———. 1981. "Significado de los aires en la cultura indégena." *Cuadernos del Museo Nacional de Antropología.* Mexico.

Montoya Briones, J. de J., and G. Moedano Navarro. 1969. "Esbozo analítico de la estructura socioeconómica y el folklore de Xochitlán, Sierra Norte de Puebla." *Anales del Instituto Nacional de Antropología e Historia* 2:257–299.

Morsy, S. 1978. "Sex Roles, Power, and Illness." *American Ethnologist* 5:137–150.

Münch Galindo, G. 1983. *Etnología del Istmo Veracruszano.* Mexico.
Nutini, H. G. 1968. *San Bernardino Contla: Marriage and Family Structure in a Tlaxcalan Municipio.* Pittsburgh.
Nutini, H. G., and J. Forbes de Nutini. 1987. "Nahualismo, control de los elementos y hechiceria en Tlaxcala rural." *La heterodoxia recuperada en torno a Angel Palerm,* ed. S. Glantz, pp. 321–346. Mexico.
Nutini, H. G., and B. L. Isaac. 1974. *Los pueblos de habla Nahuatl de la region de Tlaxcala y Puebla.* Mexico.
O'Nell, C. W. 1975. "An Investigation of Reported 'Fright' as a Factor in the Etiology of Susto, 'Magical Fright'" *Ethos* 3: 41–76.
O'Nell, C. W., and H. A. Selby. 1968. "Sex Differences in the Incidence of Susto in Two Zapotec Pueblos: An Analysis of the Relationships between Sex Role Expectations and a Folk Illness." *Ethnology* 7:96–105.
Paul. L. 1975. "Recruitment to a Ritual Role: The Midwife in a Maya Community." *Ethos* 3: 449–467.
Paul, L., and B. D. Paul. 1975. "The Maya Midwife as Sacred Specialist: A Guatemalan Case." *American Ethnologist* 2:131–148.
Redfield, R. 1930. *Tepoztlán, A Mexican Village: A Study of Folk Life.* Chicago.
Reyes García, L. 1976. *Der Ring Aus Tlalocan: Mythen und Gebete, Lieder und Erzählungen der heutigen Nahua in Veracruz and Puebla, Mexiko.* Berlin.
Robinson, D. F. 1961. "Textos de medicina Nahuat." *America Indígena* 21: 345–353.
Rubel, A. J. 1964. "The Epidemiology of a Folk Illness: Susto in Hispanic America." *Ethnology* 3:268–283.
Rubel, A. J., C. W. O'Nell, and R. Collado-Ardón. 1984. *Susto, A Folk Illness.* Berkeley.
Sandstrom, A. R. 1975. "Ecology, Economy, and the Realm of the Sacred: An Interpretation of Ritual in a Nahua Community of the Southern Huasteca, Mexico." Ph.D. dissertation, Indiana University, Bloomington.
Sandstrom, A. R., and P. E. Sandstrom. 1986. *Traditional Papermaking and Paper Cult Figures of Mexico.* Norman.
Signorini, I. 1982. "Patterns of Fright: Multiple Concepts of Susto in a Nahua-Ladino Community of the Sierra de Puebla (Mexico)." *Ethnology* 21:313–323.
Soustelle, G. 1958. *Tequila: Un Village Nahuatl du Mexique Oriental.* Paris.
Taggart, J. M. 1983. *Nahuat Myth and Social Structure.* Austin.
Tedlock, B. 1982. *Time and the Highland Maya.* Albuquerque.

MAMA LOLA AND THE EZILIS: THEMES OF MOTHERING AND LOVING IN HAITIAN VODOU

Karen McCarthy Brown

Mama Lola is a Haitian woman in her mid-fifties who lives in Brooklyn, where she works as a Vodou priestess. This essay concerns her relationship with two female *lwa,* Vodou spirits whom she "serves." By means of trance states, these spirits periodically speak and act through her during community ceremonies and private healing sessions. Mama Lola's story will serve as a case study of how the Vodou spirits closely reflect the lives of those who honor them. While women and men routinely and meaningfully serve both male and female spirits in Vodou, I will focus here on only one strand of the complex web of relations between the "living" and the Vodou spirits, the strand that connects women and female spirits. Specifically I will demonstrate how female spirits, in their iconography and

Reprinted with permission from Nancy Falk and Rita Gross (eds.), *Unspoken Worlds: Women's Religious Lives* (Belmont, Calif.: Wadsworth Publishing Co.), pp. 235–245. The main ideas in this article are developed further in a chapter of *Mama Lola: Vodou Priestess in Brooklyn* (Berkeley: University of California Press, 1991).

possession-performance, mirror the lives of contemporary Haitian women with remarkable specificity. Some general discussion of Haiti and of Vodou is necessary before moving to the specifics of Mama Lola's story.

Vodou is the religion of 80% of the population of Haiti. It arose during the eighteenth century on the giant sugar plantations of the French colony of Saint Domingue, then known as the Pearl of the Antilles. The latter name was earned through the colony's veneer of French culture, the reknowned beauty of its Creole women, and most of all, the productivity of its huge slave plantations. Haiti is now a different place (it is the poorest country in the Western hemisphere) and Vodou, undoubtedly, a different religion from the one or ones practiced by the predominantly Dahomean, Yoruba, and Kongo slaves originally brought there. The only shared language among these different groups of slaves was French Creole, yet they managed before the end of the eighteenth century to band together (most likely through religious means) to launch the only successful slave revolution during this immoral epoch. As contemporary Haitian history has made amply clear, a successful revolution did not lead to a free and humane life for the Haitian people. Slave masters were quickly replaced by a succession of dictators from both the mulatto and black populations.

Haitians started coming to the United States in large numbers after François Duvalier took control of the country in the late 1950s. The first wave of immigrants was made up of educated, professional people. These were followed by the urban poor and, most recently, the rural poor. All were fleeing dead-end lives in a society drenched in corruption, violence, poverty, and disease. There are now well over one-half million Haitians living in the U.S.

Alourdes, the name by which I usually address Mama Lola, came to New York in 1963 from Port-au-Prince, the capital of Haiti and a city of squalor and hopelessness where she had at times resorted to prostitution to feed three small children. Today, twenty-five years later, Alourdes owns her own home, a three-story rowhouse in the Fort Greene section of Brooklyn. There she and her daughter Maggie run a complex and lively household that varies in size from six people (the core family, consisting of Alourdes, Maggie, and both their children) to as many as a dozen. The final tally depends on how many others are living with them at any given time. These may be recent arrivals from Haiti, down-on-their-luck friends and members of the extended family, or clients and members of the extended family, or clients of Alourdes's Vodou healing practice.

Maggie, now in her thirties, has been in the United States since early adolescence and consequently is much more Americanized than her mother. She is the adult in the family who deals with the outside world. Maggie does the paperwork which life in New York requires and negotiates with teachers, plumbers, electricians, and an array of creditors. She has a degree from a community college and currently works as a nurse's aide at a New York hospital.

Most of the time Alourdes stays at home where she cares for the small children and carries on her practice as a *manbo,* a Vodou priestess. Many Haitians and a few others such as Trinidadians, Jamaicans, and Dominicans come to her with work, health, family, and love problems. For diagnostic purposes, Alourdes first "reads the cards." Then she carries out healing "work" appropriate to the nature and severity of the problem. This may include: counseling the client, a process in which she calls on her own life experience and the shared values of the Haitian community as well as intuitive skills bordering on extrasensory perception; administering baths and other herbal treatments; manufacturing talismans; and summoning the Vodou spirits to "ride" her through trance-possession in order that spiritual insight and wisdom may be brought to bear on the problem.

Vodou spirits (Haitians never call them gods or goddesses) are quite different from deities, or even saints, in the way that we in North America usually use those terms. They are not moral exemplars, nor are their stories characterized by deeds of cosmic or even heroic proportion. Their scale (what makes them larger than life though not other than it) comes, on the one hand, from the key existential paradoxes they contain and, on the other, from the caricature-like clarity with which they portray those pressure points in life. The *lwa* are full-blown personalities who preside over some particular social arena, and the roles they exemplify contain, as they do for the living who must fill them, both positive and negative possibilities.

Trance-possession within Vodou is somewhat like improvisational theater.[1] It is a delicate balancing act between traditional words and gestures which make the spirits recognizable and innovations which make them relevant. In other words, while the character types of the *lwa* are ancient and familiar, the specific things they say or do in a Vodou ritual unfold in response to the people who call them. Because the Vodou spirits are so flexible and responsive, the same spirit will manifest in different ways in the north and in the south of Haiti, in the countryside and in the cities, in Haiti and among the immigrants in New York. There are even significant differences from family to family. Here we are considering two female spirits as they manifest through a heterosexual Haitian woman who has lived in an urban context all her life and who has resided outside of Haiti for a quarter of a century. While most of what is said about these spirits would apply wherever Vodou is practiced, some of the emphases and details are peculiar to this woman and her location.

Vodou is a combination of several distinct African religious traditions. Also, from the beginning, the slaves included Catholicism in the religious blend they used to cope with their difficult lives. Among the most obvious borrowings were the identifications of African spirits with Catholic saints. The reasons why African slaves took on Catholicism are complex. On one level it was a matter of habit. The African cultures from which the slaves were drawn had traditionally been open to the religious systems they encountered through trade and war and had routinely borrowed from them. On another level it was a matter of strategy. A Catholic veneer placed over their own religious practices was a convenient cover for the perpetuation of these frequently outlawed rites. Yet this often cited and too often politicized explanation points to only one level of the strategic value of Catholicism. There was something deep in the slaves' religious traditions that very likely shaped their response to Catholicism. The Africans in Haiti took on the religion of the slave master, brought it into their holy places, incorporated its rites into theirs, adopted the images of Catholic saints as pictures of their own traditional spirits and the Catholic calendar as descriptive of the year's holy rhythms, and in general practiced a kind of cultural judo with Catholicism. They did this because, in the African ethos, imitation is not the sincerest form of flattery but the most efficient and direct way to gain understanding and leverage.

This epistemological style, exercised also on secular colonial culture, was clearly illustrated when I attended Vodou secret society[2] ceremonies in the interior of Haiti during the 1983 Christmas season. A long night of thoroughly African drumming and dancing included a surprising episode in which the drums went silent, home-made fiddles and brass instruments emerged, and a male and female dancer in eighteenth-century costume performed a slow and fastidious *contradans.* So eighteenth-century slaves in well-hidden places on the vast sugar plantations must have incorporated mimicry of their masters into their traditional worship as a way of appropriating the masters' power.

I want to suggest that this impulse toward imitation lies behind the adoption of Catholicism by African slaves. Yet I do not want to reduce sacred imitation to a political maneuver. On a broader canvas this way of getting to know the powers that be by imitating them is a pervasive and general characteristic of all the African-based religions in the New World. Grasping this important aspect of the way Vodou relates to the world will provide a key for understanding the nature of the relationship between Alourdes and her female spirits. When possessed by her woman spirits, Alourdes acts out the social and psychological forces that define, and often confine, the lives of contemporary Haitian women. She appropriates these forces through imitation. In the drama of possession-performance, she clarifies the lives of women and thereby empowers them to make the best of the choices and roles available to them.

Sacred imitation is a technique drawn from the African homeland, but the kinds of powers subject to imitation shifted as a result of the experience of slavery. The African religions that fed into Haitian Vodou addressed a full array of cosmic, natural, and social forces. Among the African spirits were those primarily defined by association with natural phenomena such as wind, lightning, and thunder. As a result of the shock of slavery, the lens of African religious wisdom narrowed to focus in exquisite detail on the crucial arena of social interaction. Thunder and lightning, drought and pestilence became pale, second-order threats compared with those posed by human beings. During the nearly 200 years since their liberation from slavery, circumstances in Haiti have forced Haitians to stay focused on the social arena. As a result, the Vodou spirits have also retained the strong social emphasis gained during the colonial period. Keeping these points in view, I now turn to Alourdes and two female Vodou spirits she serves. They both go by the name Ezili.

The Haitian Ezili's African roots are multiple.[3] Among them is Mammy Water, a powerful mother of the waters whose shrines are found throughout West Africa. Like moving water, Ezili can be sudden, fickle, and violent, but she is also deep, beautiful, moving, creative, nurturing, and powerful. In Haiti Ezili was recognized in images of the Virgin Mary and subsequently conflated with her. The various manifestations of the Virgin pictured in the inexpensive and colorful lithographs available throughout the Catholic world eventually provided receptacles for several different Ezilis as the spirit subdivided in the New World in order to articulate the different directions in which women's power flowed.

Alourdes, like all Vodou priests or priestesses, has a small number of spirits who manifest routinely through her. This spiritual coterie, which differs from person to person, both defines the character of the healer and sets the tone of his or her "temple." Ezili Dantor is Alourdes's major female spirit, and she is conflated with Mater Salvatoris, a black Virgin pictured holding the Christ child. The child that Dantor holds (Haitians usually identify it as a daughter!) is her most important iconographic detail, for Ezili Dantor is above all else the woman who bears children, the mother par excellence.

Haitians say that Ezili Dantor fought fiercely beside her "children" in the slave revolution. She was wounded, they say, and they point to the parallel scars that appear on the right cheek of the Mater Salvatoris image as evidence for this. Details of Ezili Dantor's possession-performance extend the story. Ezili Dantor also lost her tongue during the revolution. Thus Dantor does not speak when she possesses someone. The only sound the spirit can utter is a uniform "de-de-de." In a Vodou ceremony, Dantor's mute "de-de-de" becomes articulate only through her body language and the interpretive efforts of the gathered community. Her appearances are thus reminiscent of a somber game of charades. Ezili Dantor's fighting spirit is reinforced by her identification as a member of the Petro pantheon of Vodou spirits, and as such she is associated with what is hot, fiery, and strong. As a Petro spirit Dantor is handled with care. Fear and caution are always somewhere in the mix of attitudes that people hold toward the various Petro spirits.

Those, such as Alourdes, who serve Ezili Dantor become her children and, like children in the traditional Haitian family, they owe their mother high respect and unfailing loyalty. In return, this spiritual mother, like the ideal human mother, will exhaust her strength and resources to care for her children. It is important to note here that the sacrifice of a mother for her children will never be seen by Haitians in purely sentimental or altruistic terms. For Haitian women, even for those now living in New York, children represent the main hope for an economically viable household and the closest thing there is to a guarantee of care in old age. The mother-child relationship among Haitians is thus strong, essential, and in a not unrelated way, potentially volatile. In the countryside, children's labor is necessary for family survival. Children begin to work at an early age, and physical punishment is often swift and severe if they are irresponsible or disrespectful. Although in the cities children stay in school longer and begin to contribute to the welfare of the family at a later age, similar attitudes toward childrearing prevail.

In woman-headed households, the bond between mother and daughter is the most charged and the most enduring. Women and their children form three- and sometimes four-generation networks in which gifts and services circulate according to the needs and abilities of each. These tight family relationships create a safety net in a society where hunger is a common experience for the majority of people. The strength of the mother-daughter bond explains why Haitians identify the child in Ezili Dantor's arms as a daughter. And the importance and precariousness of that bond explain Dantor's fighting spirit and fiery temper.

In possession-performance, Ezili Dantor explores the full range of possibilities inherent in the mother-child bond. Should Dantor's "children" betray her or trifle with her dignity, the spirit's anger can be sudden, fierce, and uncompromising. In such situations her characteristic "de-de-de" becomes a powerful rendering of women's mute but devastating rage. A gentle rainfall during the festivities at Saut d'Eau, a mountainous pilgrimage site for Dantor, is readily interpreted as a sign of her presence but so is a sudden deluge resulting in mudslides and traffic accidents. Ezili's African water roots thus flow into the most essential of social bonds, that between mother and child, where they carve out a web of channels through which can flow a mother's rage as well as her love.

Alourdes, like Ezili Dantor, is a proud and hard-working woman who will not tolerate disrespect or indolence in her children. While her anger is never directed at Maggie, who is now an adult and Alourdes' partner in running the household, it can sometimes sweep the smaller children off their feet. I have never seen Alourdes strike a child, but her wrath can be sudden and the punishments meted out severe. Although the suffering is different in kind, there is a good measure of it in both Haiti and New York, and the lessons have carried from one to the other. Once, after Alourdes disciplined her ten-year-old, she turned to me and said: "The world is evil. . . . You got to make them tough!"

Ezili Dantor is not only Alourdes's main female spirit, she is also the spirit who first called Alourdes to her role as priestess. One of the central functions of Vodou in Haiti, and among Haitian emigrants, is that of reinforcing social bonds. Because obligations to the Vodou spirits are inherited within families, Alourdes's decision to take on the heavy responsibility of serving the spirits was also a decision to opt for her extended family (and her Haitian identity) as her main survival strategy.

It was not always clear that this was the decision she would make. Before Alourdes came to the United States, she had shown little interest in her mother's religious practice, even though an appearance by Ezili Dantor at a family ceremony had marked her for the priesthood when she was only five or six years old. By the time Alourdes left Haiti she was in her late twenties and the memory of that message from Dantor had either disappeared or ceased to feel relevant. When Alourdes left Haiti, she felt she was leaving the spirits behind along with a life marked by struggle and suffering. But the spirits sought her out in New York. Messages from Ezili and other spirits came in the form of a debilitating illness that prevented her from working. It was only after she returned to Haiti for initiation into the priesthood and thus acknowledged the spirits' claim on her that Alourdes's life in the U.S. began to run smoothly.

Over the ten years I have known this family, I have watched a similar process at work with her daughter Maggie. Choosing the life of a Vodou priestess in New York is much more difficult for Maggie than it was for her mother. To this day, I have yet to see Maggie move all the way into a trance state. Possession threatens and Maggie struggles mightily; her body falls to the floor as if paralyzed, but she fights off the descending darkness that marks the onset of trance. Afterwards, she is angry and afraid. Yet these feelings finally did not prohibit Maggie from making a commitment to the *manbo's* role. She was initiated to the priesthood in the summer of 1982 in a small temple on the outskirts of Port-au-Prince. Alourdes presided at these rituals. Maggie's commitment to Vodou came after disturbing dreams and a mysterious illness not unlike the one that plagued Alourdes shortly after she came to the United States. The accelerated harassment of the spirits also started around the time when a love affair brought Maggie face to face with the choice of living with someone other than her mother. Within a short period of time, the love affair ended, the illness arrived, and Maggie had a portentous dream in which the spirits threatened to block her life path until she promised to undergo initiation. Now it is widely acknowledged that Maggie is the heir to Alourdes's successful healing practice.

Yet this spiritual bond between Alourdes and Maggie cannot be separated from the social, economic, and emotional forces that hold them together. It is clear that Alourdes and Maggie depend on one another in myriad ways. Without the child care Alourdes provides, Maggie could not work. Without the check Maggie brings in every week, Alourdes would have only the modest and erratic income she brings in from her healing work. These practical issues were also at stake in Maggie's decision about the Vodou priesthood, for a decision to become a *manbo* was also a decision to cast her lot with her mother. This should not be interpreted to mean that Alourdes uses religion to hold Maggie against her will. The affection between them is genuine and strong. Alourdes and Maggie are each other's best friend and most trusted ally. In Maggie's own words: "We have a beautiful relationship . . . it's more than a twin, it's like a Siamese twin. . . . She is my soul." And in Alourdes's: "If she not near me, I feel something inside me disconnected."

Maggie reports that when she has problems, Ezili Dantor often appears to her in dreams. Once, shortly after her arrival in the United States, Maggie had a waking vision of Dantor. The spirit, clearly recognizable in her gold-edged blue veil, drifted into her bedroom window. Her new classmates were cruelly teasing her, and the twelve-year-old Maggie was in despair. Dantor gave her a maternal backrub and drifted out the window, where the spirit's glow was soon lost in that of a corner streetlamp. These days, when she is in trouble and Dantor does not appear of her own accord, Maggie goes seeking the spirit. "She don't have to talk to me in my dream. Sometime I go inside the altar, just look at her statue . . . she says a few things to me." The image with which Maggie converses is, of course, Mater Salvatoris, the black virgin, holding in her arms her favored girl child, Anaise.

It is not only in her relationship with her daughter that Alourdes finds her life mirrored in the image of Ezili Dantor. Ezili Dantor is also the mother raising children on her own, the woman who will take lovers but will not marry. In many ways, it is this aspect of Dantor's story that most clearly mirrors and maps the lives of Haitian women.

In former days (and still in some rural areas) the patriarchal, multigenerational extended family held sway in Haiti. In these families men could form unions with more than one woman. Each woman had her own household in which she bore and raised the children from that union. The men moved from household to household, often continuing to rely on their mothers as well as their women to feed and lodge them. When the big extended families began to break up under the combined pressures of depleted soil, overpopulation, and corrupt politics, large numbers of rural people moved to the cities.

Generally speaking, Haitian women fared better than men in the shift from rural to urban life. In the cities the family shrank to the size of the individual household unit, an arena in which women had traditionally been in charge. Furthermore, their skill at small-scale commerce, an aptitude passed on through generations of rural market women, allowed them to adapt to life in urban Haiti, where the income of a household must often be patched together from several small and sporadic sources. Urban women sell bread, candy, and herbal teas which they make themselves. They also buy and re-sell food, clothing, and household goods. Often their entire inventory is balanced on their heads or spread on outstretched arms as they roam through the streets seeking customers. When desperate enough, women also sell sex. They jokingly refer to their genitals as their "land." The employment situation in urban Haiti, meager though it is, also favors women. Foreign companies tend to prefer them for the piecework that accounts for a large percentage of the jobs available to the poor urban majority.

By contrast, unemployment among young urban males may well be as high as 80%. Many men in the city circulate among the households of their girlfriends and mothers. In this way they are usually fed, enjoy some intimacy, and get their laundry done. But life is hard and resources scarce. With the land gone, it is no longer so clear that men are essential to the survival of women and children. As a result, relationships between urban men and women have become brittle and often violent. And this is so in spite of a romantic ideology not found in the countryside. Men are caught in a double bind. They are still reared to expect to have power and to exercise authority, and yet they have few resources to do so. Consequently, when their expectations run up against a wall of social impossibility, they often veer off in unproductive directions. The least harmful of these is manifest in a national preoccupation with soccer; the most damaging is the military, the domestic police force of Haiti, which provides the one open road toward upward social mobility for poor young men. Somewhere in the middle of this spectrum lie the drinking and gambling engaged in by large numbers of poor men.

Ezili Dantor's lover is Ogou, a soldier spirit sometimes pictured as a hero, a breathtakingly handsome and dedicated soldier. But just as often Ogou is portrayed as vain and swaggering, untrustworthy and self-destructive. In one of his manifestations Ogou is a drunk. This is the man Ezili Dantor will take into her bed but would never depend on. Their relationship thus takes up and comments on much of the actual life experience of poor urban women.

Ezili Dantor also mirrors many of the specifics of Alourdes's own life. Gran Philo, Alourdes's mother, was the first of her family to live in the city. She worked there as a *manbo.* Although she bore four children, she never formed a long-term union with a man. She lived in Santo Domingo, in the Dominican Republic, for the first years of her adult life. There she had her first two babies. But her lover proved irrational, jealous, and possessive. Since she was working as hard or harder than he, Philo soon decided to leave him. Back in Port-au-Prince, she had two more children, but in neither case did the father participate in the rearing of the children. Alourdes, who is the youngest, did not know who her father was until she was grown. And when she found out, it still took time for him to acknowledge paternity.

In her late teens, Alourdes's fine singing voice won her a coveted position with the Troupe Folklorique, a song and dance group that drew much of its repertoire from Vodou. During that period Alourdes attracted the attention of an older man who had a secure job with the Bureau of Taxation. During their brief marriage Alourdes lived a life that was the dream of most poor Haitian women. She had a house and two servants. She did not have to work. But this husband, like the first man in Philo's life, needed to control her every move. His jealousy was so great that Alourdes was not even allowed to visit her mother without supervision. (The man should have known better than to threaten that vital bond!) Alourdes and her husband fought often and, after less than two years, she left. In the years that followed, there were times when Alourdes had no food and times when she could not pay her modest rent but, with pride like Ezili Dantor's, Alourdes never returned to her husband and never asked him for money. During one especially difficult period Alourdes began to operate as a Marie-Jacques, a prostitute, although not the kind who hawk their wares on the street. Each day she would dress up and go from business to business in downtown Port-au-Prince looking for someone who would ask her for a "date." When the date was over she would take what these men offered (everyone knew the rules), but she never asked for money. Alourdes had three children in Haiti, by three different men. She fed them and provided shelter by juggling several income sources. Her mother helped when she could. So did friends when they heard she was in need. For a while, Alourdes held a job as a tobacco inspector for the government. And she also dressed up and went out looking for dates.

Maggie, like Alourdes, was married once. Her husband drank too much and one evening, he hit her. Once was enough. Maggie packed up her infant son and returned to her mother's house. She never looked back. When Maggie talks about this marriage, now over for nearly a decade, she says he was a good man but alcohol changed him. "When he drink, forget it!" She would not take the chance that he might hit her again or, worse, take his anger and frustration out on their son.

Ezili Dantor is the mother—fierce, proud, hard-working, and independent. As a religious figure, Dantor's honest portrayal of the ambivalent emotions a woman can feel toward her lovers and a mother can feel toward her children stands in striking contrast to the idealized attitude of calm, nurture, and acceptance represented by more standard interpretations of the Holy Mother Mary, a woman for whom rage would be unthinkable. Through her iconography and possession-performances, Ezili Dantor works in subtle ways with the concrete life circumstances of Haitian women such as Alourdes and Maggie. She takes up their lives, clarifies the issues at stake in them, and gives them permission to follow the sanest and most humane paths. Both Alourdes and Maggie refer to Ezili Dantor as "my mother."

Vodou is a religion born of slavery, of wrenching change and deep pain. Its genius can be traced to long experience in using the first (change) to deal with the second (pain). Vodou is a religion in motion, one without canon, creed, or pope. In Vodou the ancient African wisdom is preserved by undergoing constant transformation in response to specific life circumstances. One of the things which keeps Vodou agile is its plethora of spirits. Each person who serves the spirits has his or her own coterie of favorites. And no single spirit within that group can take over and lay down the law for the one who serves. There are always other spirits to consult, other spirit energies to take into account. Along with Ezili Dantor, Alourdes also serves her sister, Ezili Freda.

Ezili Freda is a white spirit from the Rada pantheon, a group characterized by sweetness and even tempers. Where Dantor acts out women's sexuality in its childbearing mode, Freda, the flirt, concerns herself with love and romance. Like the famous Creole mistresses who lent charm and glamour to colonial Haiti, Ezili Freda takes her identity and worth from her relationship with men. Like the mulatto elite in contemporary Haiti who are the heirs of those Creole women, Freda loves fine clothes and jewelry. In her possession-performances, Freda is decked out in satin and lace. She is given powder and perfume, sweet smelling soaps and rich creams. The one possessed by her moves through the gathered community, embracing one and then another and then another. Something in her searches and is never satisfied. Her visits often end in tears and frustration.[4]

Different stories are told about Freda and children. Some say she is barren. Others say she has a child but wishes to hide that fact in order to appear fresher, younger, and more desirable to men. Those who hold the latter view are fond of pointing out the portrait of a young boy that is tucked behind the left elbow of the crowned Virgin in the image of Maria Dolorosa with whom Freda is conflated. In this intimate biographical detail, Freda picks up a fragment from Alourdes's life that hints at larger connections between the two. When Alourdes was married she already had two children by two different men. She wanted a church wedding and a respectable life, so she hid the children from her prospective in-laws. It was only at the wedding itself, when they asked about the little boy and girl seated in the front row, that they found out the woman standing before the altar with their son already had children.

Alourdes does not have her life all sewn up in neat packages. She does not have all the questions answered and all the tensions resolved. Most of the time when she tells the story of her marriage, Alourdes says flatly: "He too jealous. That man crazy!" But on at least one occasion she said: "I was too young. If I was with Antoine now, I never going to leave him!" When Alourdes married Antoine Lovinsky she was a poor teenager living in Port-au-Prince, a city where less than 10% of the people are not alarmingly poor. Women of the elite class nevertheless structure the dreams of poor young women. These are the light-skinned women, who marry in white dresses in big Catholic churches and return to homes that have bedroom sets and dining room furniture and servants. These are the women who never have to work. They spend their days resting and visiting with friends and emerge at night on the arms of their men dressed like elegant peacocks and affecting an air of haughty boredom. Although Alourdes's tax collector could not be said to be a member of the elite, he provided her with a facsimile of the dream. It stifled her and confined her, but she has still not entirely let go of the fantasy. She still loves jewelry and clothes and, in her home, manages to create the impression, if not the fact, of wealth by piling together satin furniture, velvet paintings, and endless bric-a-brac.

Alourdes also has times when she is very lonely and she longs for male companionship. She gets tired of living at the edge of poverty and being the one in charge of such a big and ungainly household. She feels the pull of the images of domesticity and nuclear family life that she sees everyday on the television in New York. Twice since I have known her, Alourdes has fallen in love. She is a deeply sensual woman and this comes strongly to the fore during these times. She dresses up, becomes coquettish, and caters to her man. Yet when describing his lovable traits, she always says first: "He help me so much. Every month, he pay the electric bill," and so forth. Once again the practical and the emotional issues cannot be separated. In a way, this is just another version of the poor woman selling her "land." And in another way it is not, for here the finances of love are wound round and round with longing and dreams.

Poor Haitian women, Alourdes included, are a delight to listen to when their ironic wit turns on what we would label as the racism, sexism, and colonial pretense of the upper-class women Freda mirrors. Yet these are the values with power behind them both in Haiti and in New York, and poor women are not immune to the attraction of such a vision. Ezili Freda is thus an image poor Haitian women live toward. She picks up their dreams and gives them shape, but these women are mostly too experienced to think they can live on or in dreams. Alourdes is not atypical. She serves Freda but much less frequently than Dantor. Ezili Dantor is the one for whom she lights a candle every day; she is the one Alourdes turns to when there is real trouble. She is, in Alourdes' words, "my mother." Yet I think it is fair to say that it is the tension between Dantor and Freda that keeps both relevant to the lives of Haitian women.

There is a story about conflict between the two Ezilis. Most people, most of the time, will say that the scars on Ezili Dantor's cheek come from war wounds, but there is an alternative explanation. Sometimes it is said that because Dantor was sleeping with her man, Maria Dolorosa took the sword from her heart and slashed the cheek of her rival.

A flesh and blood woman, living in the real world, cannot make a final choice between Ezili Dantor and Ezili Freda. It is only when reality is spiced with dreams, when survival skills are larded with sensuality and play, that life moves forward. Dreams and play alone lead to endless and fruitless searching. And a whole life geared toward survival becomes brittle and threatened by inner rage. Alourdes lives at the nexus of several spirit energies. Freda and Dantor are only two of them, the two who help her most to see herself clearly as a woman.

To summarize the above discussion: The Vodou spirits are not idealized beings removed from the complexity and particularity of life. On the contrary, the responsive and flexible nature of Vodou allows the spirits to change over space and time in order to mirror people's life circumstances in considerable detail. Vodou spirits are transparent to their African origins and yet they are other than African spirits. Ancient nature connections have been buried deep in their iconographies while social domains have risen to the top, where they have developed in direct response to the history and social circumstances of the Haitian people. The Vodou spirits make sense of the powers that shape and control life by imitating them. They act out both the dangers and the possibilities inherent in problematic life situations. Thus, the moral pull of Vodou comes from clarification. The Vodou spirits do not tell the people what should be; they illustrate what is.

Perhaps Vodou has these qualities because it is a religion of an oppressed people. Whether or not that is true, it seems to be a type of spirituality with some advantages for women. The openness and flexibility of the religion, the multiplicity of its spirits, and the detail in which those spirits mirror the lives of the faithful makes women's lives visible in ways they are not in the so-called great religious traditions. This visibility can give women a way of working realistically and creatively with the forces that define and confine them.

NOTES

1. I use terms such as possession-performance and theater analogies in order to point to certain aspects of the spirits' self-presentation and interaction with devotees. The terms should not be taken as indicating that priestesses and priests simply pretend to be spirits during Vodou ceremonies. The trance states they enter are genuine, and they themselves will condemn the occasional imposter among them.
2. In an otherwise flawed book, E. Wade Davis does a very good job of uncovering and describing the nature and function of the Vodou secret societies. See *The Serpent and the Rainbow* (New York: Simon and Schuster, 1985).
3. Robert Farris Thompson traces Ezili to a Dahomean "goddess of lovers." *Flash of the Spirit: African and Afro-American Art and Philosophy* (New York: Random House, 1983), p. 191.
4. Maya Deren has drawn a powerful portrait of this aspect of Ezili Freda in *The Divine Horsemen: The Living Gods of Haiti* (New Paltz, N.Y.: Documentext, McPherson and Co., 1983), pp. 137–45.

FURTHER READINGS

Brown, Karen McCarthy. "The Center and the Edges: God and Person in Haitian Vodou." *The Journal of the Interdenominational Theological Center* 7, no. 1 (Fall 1979).

———. "Olina and Erzulie: A Woman and a Goddess in Haitian Vodou." *Anima,* Spring 1979.

———. "Systematic Forgetting, Systematic Remembering: Ogou in Haiti." In *Africa's Ogun: Old World and New.* ed. by Sandra T. Barnes. Bloomington, Ind.: University of Indiana Press, 1988.

———. "Alourdes: A Case Study of Moral Leadership in Haitian Vodou." In *Saints and Virtues,* ed. by John S. Hawley. Berkeley, Calif.: University of California Press, 1987.

———. "Afro-Caribbean Spirituality." In *Caring and Curing: Health and Medicine in the Western Religious Traditions,* ed. by Lawrence Eugene Sullivan. New York: Macmillan Press, 1988.

———. "The Power to Heal: Reflections on Women, Religion and Medicine." In *Shaping*

New Vision: Gender and Values in American Culture. Ann Arbor, Mich.: UMI Press, 1987.

Deren, Maya. *Divine Horsemen: The Living Gods of Haiti.* New Paltz, N.Y.: Documentext, McPherson and Co., 1983.

Metraux, Alfred. *Voodoo in Haiti.* New York: Schocken Books, 1972.

Thompson, Robert Farris. *Flash of the Spirit: African and Afro-American Art and Philosophy.* New York: Random House, 1983.

BLESSED MOTHER ANN, HOLY MOTHER WISDOM: GENDER AND DIVINITY IN SHAKER LIFE AND BELIEF

Marjorie Procter-Smith

Can Christians speak of God the Creator and God the Savior in any terms but male? "I believe in God, the Father Almighty, maker of heaven and earth; and in Jesus Christ his only Son, our Lord." "Glory be to the Father and to the Son and to the Holy Ghost." These phrases, recited or sung by generations of Christians, make it clear that the traditional Christian emphasis rests on a male God and his divine male son. Centuries of Christian doctrine, ritual, prayer, and song have repeated and developed the Father-Son imagery so thoroughly that it is difficult for many to imagine Christianity using any other language. When some contemporary feminists propose calling God Mother or imagining a woman Christ, they are often ridiculed or accused of abandoning the Christian tradition.

But in fact 200 years ago a Christian sect known as the Shakers spoke of God as Mother and believed that their founder, Ann Lee, was the second coming of Christ in female form. This essay discusses who the Shakers were, why they used female language for God, and how that language related to the roles and lives of women in the community.

Original material prepared for this text.

WHO ARE THE SHAKERS?

In 1774, nine English passengers disembarked at New York harbor after a seventy-nine-day voyage from Liverpool. The passengers were Ann Lee, a prophetess and religious leader from Manchester in England, and her eight followers (six men and two women). These voyagers had been members of a group known in England as "Shaking Quakers." One of many small sects who prophesied the imminent end of the world and return of Christ to earth, the Shaking Quakers were chiefly known in England for disrupting church services with their ecstatic speech, singing, and prophesying.

When Ann Lee joined the group, they were guided by a charismatic woman, Jane Wardley. However, sometime around 1770, Ann Lee had an extraordinary religious experience, which propelled her into prominence among them. She later described this experience in language borrowed from her own experience of childbirth:

> Thus I labored, in strong cries and groans to God, day and night, till my flesh wasted away, and I became like a skeleton, and a kind of down came upon my skin, until my soul broke forth to God; which I felt as sensibly as ever a woman did a child, when she was delivered of it.[1]

As a result of this experience of new birth, Lee was favored with ecstatic visions of God and Jesus, Heaven and Hell. In the course of these visions, it was revealed to Lee by Jesus Christ that the "sin which is the root of all evil" is sexual intercourse, even within lawful marriage. Ann Lee's witness against "the doleful works of the flesh," an insistence on absolute celibacy, became one of the central tenets of Shaker faith and a foundation for the development of Shaker community life.

Armed with these powerful heavenly visions, Lee claimed authority as leader of the group and convinced her followers of the necessity of resettling in America, where new missionary fields lay open to them. Once in America, Ann Lee and her small group settled in the wilderness of New York state in a village called Niskeyuna (now Watervliet, New York, near Albany) and began to gather new believers in Lee's message.

Lee taught that perfection was possible in this life, provided one "took up a full cross," which meant, practically speaking, willingness to confess all known sins to a Shaker leader (either Mother Ann or someone designated by her); to accept a celibate life, regardless of marital status; and to live a sinless life after the manner of Christ.

The term "Shaker" was a derisive one, given by non-Shakers who observed the ecstatic religious behavior of Ann Lee and her followers. Typical Shaker worship included shouting, leaping, dancing, whirling about, singing in unknown tongues, and falling into trances. Prophetic announcements and gestures were common, and Shaker worshippers thereby gained access to the spiritual world.

Lee's visions, however, were exceptional. To the observer, she appeared strange, otherworldly, and perhaps a bit frightening. One early follower remembered seeing Lee

> sit in her chair, from early in the morning, until afternoon, under great operations and power of God. She sung in unknown tongues, the whole of the time; and seemed to be wholly divested of any attraction to material things. All her sensations appeared to be engaged in the spiritual world.[2]

Lee reported that her visions during such periods included face-to-face conversations with God and with Jesus, visions of Heaven and the saints, and harrowing views of the suffering of the damned in Hell. In particular she described her relationship with Jesus as especially intimate:

> I have been walking in fine valleys with Christ, as with a lover. . . . Christ is ever with me, both in sitting down and rising up; in going out and coming in. If I walk in groves and valleys, there he is, with me; and I converse with him as one friend converses with another, face to face.[3]

She also referred to Christ as her husband, her "Lord and Head," who preempts the authority of any human man. Lee's earthly husband, who had accompanied her to America, had not found Shaker doctrine and life satisfactory and apparently left the group early on.

At first Lee and the other leaders of the group advised new converts to return to their families and live in peace and holiness with them, an evangelical strategy that often seemed to work, because many of the first converts to Shakerism in America were members of a few large New England families. However, by 1782 or so necessity was conspiring with religious disposition to encourage the development of communal living, at least in a rather informal way. Clusters of Believers (as Shakers preferred to call themselves) began pooling their financial resources to provide support for poorer families and to provide food and lodging for traveling Shaker missionaries and visitors who gathered to hear the Shaker message.

When Ann Lee died in 1784 the remaining leaders recognized that for their movement to survive they needed to establish a more formal order and structure for living the Shaker life. Lee's successor, James Whittaker, began the process of organizing Believers into communities on the basis of common ownership of property and goods, or "joint interest." This process of "gathering into order" was continued by Whittaker's successor, Joseph Meacham, and his associate and successor, Lucy Wright.

Shaker communities, organized into units called "families," were constructed in part to replace the natural families that celibate Shakers were required to give up. All members were called "brother" or "sister," with those in leadership designated as "elders" and "eldresses." Each family had two elders and two eldresses who held spiritual authority over the brothers and sisters; two deacons and two deaconesses who were responsible for the material well-being of the family (providing for food, clothing, upkeep of buildings and grounds, and so forth); and several trustees, who handled all business dealings with the "World," as non-Shakers were called.[4]

Overall, there have been eighteen major Shaker communities and several smaller and short-lived ones. During the middle of the nineteenth century the Shakers reached their peak membership of perhaps as many as 6,000.[5] Membership began to decline soon after this, however, and now only a very few individuals remain.[6]

SHAKER RELIGIOUS LANGUAGE

Shakerism grew in a religious environment in which many Christians believed in the imminent return of Jesus Christ to earth. This millennialism, as it is called, predisposed people to expect miraculous signs of various kinds. For example, on May 19, 1780, settlers clearing land in New England burned off brush and trees, and the resulting smoke hid the sun, making the day as dark as night. Terrified New Englanders, seeing birds and farm animals go to sleep as if it were night and remembering apocalyptic Biblical prophecy about the sun becoming "black as sackcloth," cried, "The day of judgment is come!" During Ann Lee's missionary journey through New England between 1781 and 1783 she and some of her followers saw a particularly spectacular display of the Northern Lights. One commented that the lights were "a sign of the coming of the Son of Man in the clouds of heaven." Although Ann Lee rejected this interpretation, clearly Shakers shared the general disposition of people to look for "signs and portents."

Likewise, millennialist expectations predisposed people to look for prophets and visionists. In such a milieu, then, Ann Lee's extraordinary visions and prophecies, her singing in unknown tongues, and astonishing messages about sin and perfection aroused intense interest. The extravagant singing and dancing in Shaker gatherings and the charismatic presence of Ann Lee combined to convince many New Englanders that the Second Coming was upon them.

In this religious context, believers concluded that Ann Lee had been the instrument of initiating the millennial church and had opened to the world the possibility of a life of Gospel perfection. The official name of the Shakers was the United Society of Believers in Christ's Second Appearing, also sometimes called the Millennial Church.

Some of the earliest Shaker theological works are explicit that Ann Lee herself is the one "in whom Christ did visibly make his second appearance."[7] Ann Lee and Jesus Christ are described in parallel terms as embodiments of the Christ-Spirit:

> The man who was called Jesus and the woman who was called Ann, are verily the two foundation pillars of the Church of Christ.[8]

Fundamental to this interpretation of Ann Lee as parallel to Jesus is Lee's own claim to have been married to Christ.

Another important element in the development of Shaker religious language is the title by which most Believers addressed Ann Lee during her life and remembered her after her death: "Mother" Ann. Perhaps because Lee was older than many of her American converts and because of the emotional attachment Believers felt for Ann Lee, the title of "Mother" became synonymous with Ann Lee, and Shaker documents routinely assume that the reader will know that any reference to "Mother" is a reference to Ann Lee.

Although Lee is often remembered as a rather stern mother who chastised her errant children and spoke sharply to them, she is represented predominantly as a loving mother who gave birth to her children in the faith, who labored over them and for them, and who guided them in the faith. A Shaker hymn expresses this idea:

> Born by our Mother, we were led,
> By her our infant souls were fed;
> And by her suff'rings and her toils
> She brought salvation to our souls.[9]

Thus, Jesus and Mother Ann were Believers' "Gospel Parents," as described in this hymn:

> Our Father and our Mother
> Have borne us in the birth,
> Their union is together,
> Redeemed from the earth:
> We children born, are not forlorn,
> But like our Parents dear,
> We've overcome the wicked one,
> And reign in Zion here.[10]

Having worked out the theological significance of Ann Lee as Mother and as Second appearing of Christ, Shakers turned their thoughts to the question of God. Unlike the theological development of an understanding of Ann Lee, which was based on personal experience of her as their spiritual mother, the Shaker doctrine of God was largely based on intellectual conviction.

The reasoning went something like this: If Ann Lee is our Mother and she is the female embodiment of the Christ-Spirit, then she holds a parallel position to Jesus as the first and male embodiment of the Christ-Spirit. If Jesus as the Christ reveals God the Father to humankind, then Mother Ann must also reveal God, and the God she reveals must necessarily be God the Mother. A major Shaker theological work puts it this way:

> The first appearing of Christ, in the simplest terms of language, is the Revelation of the Father, and the second appearing of Christ is the Revelation of the Mother; but for the subject under consideration we have preferred the title, "The Revelation of the Holy Ghost," as the most forcible and striking of all other scripture terms.[11]

This Mother-Holy Ghost God whom Ann Lee was said to reveal was later called Holy Mother Wisdom, who was said to reign with God the Father in heaven, as described in this hymn:

> Long ere this fleeting world began
> Or dust was fashioned into man,
> There *Power* and *Wisdom* we can view,
> Names of the *Everlasting Two*.
>
> The Father's high eternal throne
> Was never fill'd by one alone:
> There Wisdom holds the Mother's seat
> And is the Father's helper-meet.[12]

Shaker theologians regarded their dual Father-Mother God as logically superior to the trinitarian God of more traditional Christian theology. "As every individual on the world sprang from a father and a mother, the conclusion is self-evident, that the whole sprang from one joint parentage," argued Shaker theologian Benjamin Seth Youngs in 1808. It makes more sense, he reasoned, to talk about a God who is male and female than a God who is all male. Ridiculing "defective" trinitarian doctrine, Youngs wrote:

> First the Father, second the Son, and third the Holy Ghost; He proceeding from Father and Son . . . without the attribute of either Mother or Daughter . . . and [they] finally look for the mystery of God to be finished in the odd number of three males. . . . Where then is the correspondent cause of the woman's existence?[13]

The cause of woman's existence, Shakers believed, had been revealed by Mother Ann, a Mother God, who shared God the Father's throne and represented "wisdom" to God the Father's "power."

Beginning in the 1830s a period of intense internal revival affected all the Shaker communities and brought the image of God the Mother into prominence in Shaker experience. Beginning with trance-like experiences similar to the ecstatic worship of the earliest days of Shakerism, the revival swept through all of the communities and lasted for more than ten years. Believers once again sang heavenly songs in unknown tongues, leaped and whirled about uncontrollably, and fell into trances in which they saw and spoke to long-dead Shaker leaders, including Mother Ann, Father William Lee (Ann Lee's brother), Father Joseph (Meacham), and others. This period became known as "Mother Ann's Work," because it was believed that Mother Ann, seeing the loss of vitality in the faith of her children, had sent them this revival.

Most notably, certain Believers claimed to have been chosen as "instruments" of various heavenly beings, usually angels, who delivered messages from Mother Ann and other heavenly denizens to Believers. For the most part these claims were accepted by the leadership and by the members, and their messages were received with great respect and awe.[14] A disproportionate number of these instruments were women.

During the height of the revival, between 1840 and 1843, Holy Mother Wisdom made a series of visits to the communities in the person of a female instrument. Sometimes the visits lasted several days and included individual interviews by Holy Mother Wisdom of each member of the community. These visits were carefully prepared for by periods of fasting, prayer, confessions of sin, and intensive cleaning of the grounds and buildings. The visit normally concluded with Holy Mother Wisdom bestowing her "mark" on the forehead of each Believer or granting them some similar spiritual blessing. One contemporary observer remembered Holy Mother Wisdom concluding the visit with these words: "Around thy head I place a golden band. On it is written the name of me, Holy Mother Wisdom! the Great Jehovah! the Eternal God! Touch not mine anointed!"[15]

SHAKER WOMEN

Shaker women had before them the example of Ann Lee. On the one hand, she was extraordinarily gifted: prophetess, visionary, bride, and companion of Christ; teacher; judge; and loving but strict spiritual mother. On the other hand she shared the experiences of many of the women who were drawn to Shakerism: She was poor and illiterate; she had been married to a man she described as "very kind, according to nature," and had given birth to four children and had seen them all die in infancy; she had suffered persecution for her religious beliefs; and she had struggled to make a living and survive in a new land. Lee's exceptional ability to infuse with religious meaning her own struggles and sufferings as a woman provided a rich resource to her female followers who shared many of her experiences.

Later theological speculation interpreted Ann Lee as the Second Christ, an object not only of loving memory but also a figure of cosmic significance: one of the two "foundation pillars" of the Church, the Daughter of God, the Mother of All Living, the Revelation of God the Mother. Shaker women had not only the memory of a spiritually powerful woman who was like them in many ways, but they also had access to a positive, powerful female Christ and a loving Mother God.

The loving Mother God came to be known as Holy Mother Wisdom and was presented to them materially in the form of a woman visionist. During the visitations of Holy Mother Wisdom each woman and man in the community received at the hands of a woman a gift directly from God, the mark of Holy Mother Wisdom, and heard from the mouth of a woman words of judgment or blessing. Although female instruments did not always speak only in the name of Holy Mother Wisdom or Mother Ann, the strength of the communities' belief in these figures legitimated women's exercise of their prophetic gifts in general.

Shaker women's more temporal gifts were also legitimated by Shaker community structures. The development of a centralized and tightly structured leadership after the "gathering into order" might have excluded women, after the pattern of many other religious movements founded by women. Indeed leadership did not automatically pass to other women on Ann Lee's death. On the contrary Lee was succeeded by two men before a pattern of female leadership was established with the appointment by Joseph Meacham of

Lucy Wright as "Mother" of the entire sect alongside himself as "Father."

At first there was considerable resistance to Mother Lucy's leadership from male Shakers who were offended by the idea of a woman in a position of religious authority over them, and many people left the community in protest. However, the pattern of dual male and female leadership was established and remained the norm for all Shaker communities. This requirement gave Shaker women greater access to positions of religious leadership than women in most other Christian groups. Appointment to eldress of a community meant the opportunity to exercise temporal and spiritual leadership, greater responsibility, and chances to travel to other communities.

At the same time along with the advantages of the Shaker theological and communal system for woman came some disadvantages. The theological interpretation of Holy Mother Wisdom, for example, depended a great deal on popular nineteenth-century views of "women's sphere" and the "cult of True Womanhood."[16] Holy Mother Wisdom was described by one Shaker writer as "endless love, truth, meekness, long forbearance, and loving kindness . . . the Mother of all Godliness, meekness, purity, peace, sincerity, virtue, and chastity."[17] Although in theory such virtues were to apply to all Shakers, in fact they were associated with women primarily, even divine women.

The Shaker communal system provided opportunities for leadership for women, but it did so in the context of a strictly hierarchical system in which leaders were not elected but appointed by their superiors, and virtually absolute obedience to the leaders was expected. Work in the communities was rigidly divided, with women largely confined to traditional "women's work": food preparation, clothing manufacture and maintenance, and household maintenance. This pragmatic division of labor was interpreted as being of divine origin, and Shaker women were advised that true freedom for them lay in remaining within "woman's sphere."

CONCLUSIONS

It is striking how many contemporary feminist religious issues are found in the history of Shakerism. Contemporary feminists have challenged mainstream religious groups to expand women's opportunities for religious leadership, to reconsider the use of exclusively male language about God and Christ, and to develop religious language that draws on women's experience. From an examination of Shaker history we may see a Christian group that struggled to preserve women's religious leadership, that worshipped God as Mother as well as Father, and that drew some of its central religious terms from women's traditional childbearing and household work.

Most radical of the Shakers' ideas about women and religion, and most startlingly contemporary, is their grasp of the connection between an exclusively male representation of God and a male-dominated society. Antoinette Doolittle, editor of the Shaker journal *Shaker and Shakeress* from 1873 to 1875, observed, "As long as we have all male Gods in the heavens we shall have all male rulers on the earth."[18] They also insisted that the recognition of the female in deity was essential to women's social and religious emancipation, and they were unflinching in their criticism of male-centered theology and church.

However, their answer to their critique of male-centered religion was a highly dualistic system based on the fundamental difference between men and women. In this oppositional system women's "sphere" was diametrically opposed to that of men, and it left women in the same place reserved for them by conventional wisdom. Although redeemed Shaker women were spiritually superior to all unredeemed women and men, women by nature were understood to be more sinful than men. Indeed, this greater sinfulness of women necessitated, in part, the Second Coming of Christ in female form. A Shaker hymn says,

> As disobedience first began
> In Eve, the second part of man
> The second trumpet could not sound
> Til second Eve her Lord had found.[19]

"Second Eve" here refers to Ann Lee, whose Lord is Christ.

The questions these limitations of the Shaker system raise are several and are now being dealt with in contemporary feminist critiques of religion. First, there is the question of valorizing women's traditional experience. Such valorization recognizes that the work women have done for eons—care of children, care of households, concern for maintenance of human relationships—is the work of world-construction and world-maintenance, and as such it is religious work. The risk of such valorization, as the Shaker history shows, is that it reinforces the cultural notion that such work is women's sole work and that it is solely women's work. Such a view restricts women's access to other kinds of work and suggests that men need not concern themselves with such work, a bifurcation that feminism has taken some pains to correct.

Second, the Shaker story raises questions about essentialism. Is there some essential female character or virtue? Some Shaker theologians assumed that there was such a thing and that they knew what it was. Both arguments that female character is essentially flawed or sinful and that female character is essentially nurturant, loving, and caring claim such knowledge, and both views can be found not only in Shakerism but in other religions as well. Some contemporary feminists have challenged such claims about women, insisting instead that while women share some oppressions in common as women, women's experiences are diverse and complex and cannot be simplified into claims of innate evil or innate goodness.

Third, the Shakers demonstrate both the difficulties of preserving and perpetuating strong female leadership and the value of having the example of a female founder as a living memory in the community's life. The Shaker's most effective method of ensuring the continuation of female leadership, however, was their ideological system, which demanded equal leadership by men and women and recruited and developed strong women for leadership positions. Without such structural demands even the memory of Ann Lee would not have sufficed to preserve women's religious leadership.

NOTES

1. *Testimonies of the Life, Character, Revelations and Doctrines of our Ever Blessed Mother Ann Lee, and the Elders With Her* (Hancock, MA: J. Talcott and J. Deming, Junrs., 1816), p. 47.
2. Ibid., p. 200.
3. Ibid., p. 211.
4. For further information on the Shakers' business dealings, see Edward Deming Andrews, *The Community Industries of the Shakers* (University of the State of New York, 1933; New York State Museum Handbook No. 15).
5. The actual peak population of Shaker communities is disputed. Compare Edward Deming Andrews, *The People Called Shakers* (New York: Dover Publications, 1953), p. 224; Priscilla J. Brewer, *Shaker Communities, Shaker Lives* (Hanover, NH: University Press of New England, 1986), p. 156; and William Sims Bainbridge, "Shaker Demographics 1840–1900: An Example of the Use of U.S. Census Enumeration Schedule," *Journal For the Scientific Study of Religion* 21 (1982), p. 355.
6. At present the Shaker communities of Sabbathday Lake, Maine, and Canterbury, New Hampshire, are the only occupied communities.
7. *Testimonies* (1816), p. 2.
8. Benjamin Seth Youngs, *The Testimony of Christ's Second Appearing* (Albany: The United Society, 1810, Second Edition), p. 440.
9. Seth Y. Wells, compiler, *Millennial Praises* (Hancock, MA: Josiah Talcott, 1813), p. 105.
10. Ibid., p. 35.
11. Youngs, p. 537.
12. Wells, p. 1.
13. Youngs, p. 454.
14. Shaker manuscript collections such as those found at the Western Reserve Historical Society, the Shaker Museum at Old Chatham, New York, and the Archives and Manuscript Division of the New York Public Library have large numbers of recorded gift drawings and messages from this period, most of them by women.
15. David R. Lamson, *Two Years' Experience Among the Shakers* (West Boylston, MA: Published by the Author, 1848), p. 95.
16. See Barbara Welter, "The Cult of True Wom-

anhood," *American Quarterly* 18 (1966), pp. 151–174.

17. Paulina Bates, *The Divine Book of Holy Wisdom* (Canterbury, NH: n.p., 1849), p. 661.
18. "Address of Antoinette Doolittle, Troy, NY, March 24, 1872," *The Shaker* 2.6 (June 1872), p. 43.
19. Wells, p. 250.

REFERENCES

Andrews, Edward Deming. 1953. *The People Called Shakers*. New York: Dover Publications.

Foster, Lawrence. 1984. *Religion and Sexuality: The Shakers, the Mormons, and the Oneida Community*. Urbana: University of Illinois Press.

Garrett, Clarke. 1989. *Spirit Possession and Popular Religion: From the Camisards to the Shakers*. Baltimore: Johns Hopkins.

Humez, Jean. 1981. *Gifts of Power: The Writings of Rebecca Jackson, Black visionary, Shaker Eldress*. Amherst: University of Massachusetts Press.

Mercadante, Linda. 1990. *Gender, Doctrine, and God: The Shakers and Contemporary Theology*. Nashville: Abingdon Press.

Patterson, Daniel W. 1979. *The Shaker Spiritual*. Princeton: Princeton University Press.

Procter-Smith, Marjorie. 1985. *Women in Shaker Community and Worship*. Lewiston, NY: Edwin Mellen Press.

Sasson, Diane. 1983. *The Shaker Spiritual Narrative*. Knoxville: University of Tennessee.

X

GENDER, POLITICS, AND REPRODUCTION

All human reproductive behavior is culturally patterned. This cultural patterning includes menstrual beliefs and practices; restrictions on the circumstances in which sexual activity may occur; beliefs and practices surrounding pregnancy, labor, and the postpartum period; understanding and treatment of infertility; and the significance of menopause. While research on human biological reproduction has been dominated by medical concerns such as normal and abnormal physiological functioning, an increasing anthropological literature emphasizes the centrality of reproduction to global social, political, and economic processes (Ginsburg and Rapp 1995; Sargent and Brettell 1996). Biological reproduction refers to the production of human beings, but this process is always a social activity, leading to the perpetuation of social systems and social relations. The ways in which societies structure human reproductive behavior reflect core social values and principles, informed by changing political and economic conditions (Browner and Sargent 1990: 215).

Much of the available anthropological data on reproduction prior to 1970 is to be found within ethnographies devoted to other subjects. For example, Montagu (1949) analyzed concepts of conception and fetal development among Australian aborigines, and Malinowski (1932) wrote about reproductive concepts and practices among the Trobriand Islanders. Several surveys of ethnographic data on reproduction were compiled, such as Ford's (1964) study of customs surrounding the reproductive cycle or Spencer's (1949–1950) list of reproductive practices around the world.

In the past 20 years anthropologists have sought to use cross-cultural data from preindustrial societies to help resolve women's health problems in the industrialized world (Oakley 1977; Jordan 1978). For example, comparative research on birth practices has raised questions regarding the medicalization of childbirth in the United States. Anthropologists have also involved themselves in international public health efforts to improve maternal and child health around the world. In addition, anthropological research has helped clarify the relationship between population growth and poverty. While some analysts have held the view that overpopulation is a determinant of poverty and the poor must control their fertility to overcome impoverishment, others argue the reverse: People have many children *because* they are poor (Rubinstein and Lane 1991: 386).

Concern with population growth has often focused on women as the potential users of contraceptives, although women's personal desires to limit fertility may not be translated into action because of opposition from husbands, female relations, or others with influence or decision-making power. In this area of research anthropologists have an important contribution to make in examining such factors as cultural concepts regarding fertility and family size, the value of children, dynamics of decision making within the family and community, and the relationship between women's reproductive and productive roles.

Since the 1970s anthropological interest has turned to the linkages between cultural constructions of gender, the cultural shaping of motherhood, and reproductive beliefs and practices. In many societies throughout the world the relationship between women's status and maternity is clear: A woman attains adult status by childbearing, and her prestige may be greatly enhanced by bearing numerous male children (Browner and Sargent 1990: 218). Thus, in the Middle East a woman is "raised for marriage and procreation [and] acquires her own social status only by fecundity" (Vieille 1978: 456), while in parts of Africa pressures to be prolific weigh heavily on women (Sargent 1982).

In much of the world infertility is dreaded by men and women alike but is a particular burden to women (Browner and Sargent 1990: 219). Such pressure to reproduce is especially intense in agrarian societies, which have a high demand for labor. However, in many hunter-gatherer and horticultural societies, motherhood and reproduction are less emphasized. As Collier and Rosaldo observe, "Contrary to our expectation that motherhood provides women everywhere with a natural source of emotional satisfaction and cultural value, we found that neither women nor men in very simple societies celebrate women as nurturers or women's unique capacity to give life" (1981: 275).

Just as beliefs and practices regarding fertility are culturally patterned, birth itself is a cultural production (Jordan 1978). As Romalis notes, "The act of giving birth to a child is never simply a physiological act but rather a performance defined by and enacted within a cultural context" (1981: 6). Even in advanced industrial societies such as the United States, childbirth experiences are molded by cultural, political, and economic processes (Oakley 1980; Martin 1987; Michaelson et al. 1988). Studying the cultural patterning of birth practices can illuminate the nature of domestic power relations and the roles of women as reproductive health specialists, and it can increase our understanding of the relations between men and women cross-culturally.

Davis-Floyd (in this book) illustrates how gender ideology is revealed in the management of American pregnancy and birth. Childbirth in the United States is standardized, and it is usually highly technological. Davis-Floyd argues that core beliefs in American society about science, technology, and patriarchy shape American birth. Through the routinizing of high-tech childbirth, a message is conveyed to American women that their bodies are defective machines and that they must therefore rely on more efficient machines to give birth. Drawing on centuries-old Western European notions of nature, culture, and society, today's dominant medical model regards the male body as the ideal body-machine, while the female body is considered abnormal and inherently inadequate. Hospital birth "rituals" work to transform the birthing woman into an "American mother," who has been socialized through the birth experience to accept core values of the society. Thus birth is a cultural *rite of passage,* in which the patriarchal status quo is reproduced and reaffirmed.

While reproduction is culturally patterned, not all individuals in a society share reproductive goals. As Browner (in this book) points out, reproductive behavior is influenced by the interests of a woman's kin, neighbors, and other members of the community, and these interests may conflict. Government policies regarding the size and distribution of population may differ from the interests of reproducing women. Women's goals in turn may not be shared by their partners or other individuals and groups in the society. Browner examines the ways in which access to power in a society determines how conflicts concerning reproduction are carried out and dealt with by analyzing population practices in a Chinantec-Spanish-speaking township in Oaxaca, Mexico.

In this community the government's policy to encourage fertility reduction was imposed on a pre-existing conflict between the local community as a whole, which encouraged increased fertility, and women of the community, who sought to limit family size. Women and men manifested very different attitudes concerning fertility desires: Women sought much smaller families than men. As children increasingly attend school their economic benefits appeared slight to their mothers. Further, women viewed pregnancy as stressful and debilitating. Yet despite these negative views, women felt they could not ignore pressures to reproduce.

Such pressure came from community men, who valued a large population for the defense and well-being of the collectivity, and from women, who, while not desiring more children themselves, wanted other women to bear children in the interests of the group. In spite of the ease of obtaining government contraceptives, women rejected their use. Some felt that state policy promoting family planning was in fact cultural genocide, designed to eliminate indigenous Indian populations. In this cultural, political, and economic context, local women experienced conflict between personal desires to have few children and local pressures to be prolific.

Ginsburg (in this book) also discusses reproduction as a contested domain, using the example of abortion in American culture. She suggests that the focus of this conflict of interests is the relationship between reproduction, nurturance, sex, and gender. Using life histories of pro-life and pro-choice activists in Fargo, North Dakota, she reveals how different historical conditions affect reproductive decisions. The activist protesters in Fargo vie for the power to define womanhood in light of a basic American cultural script in which, in the context of marriage, pregnancy results in childbirth and motherhood. Ginsburg argues that the struggle over abortion rights is a contest for control over the meanings attached to reproduction in America and suggests that "female social activism in the American context operates to mediate the construction of self and gender with larger social, political, and cultural processes."

Similarly, Whitbeck argues that controversy over abortion rights in the United States must be understood in relation to a cultural context that neglects women's experiences and the status of women as "moral individuals." Rather, American culture regards women and women's bodies as "property to be bartered, bestowed, and used by men" (Whitbeck 1983: 259). Concern with restricting access to abortions derives from the interest of the state or others in power to control women's bodies and their reproductive capacity (Whitbeck 1983: 260).

Ginsburg's research shows that pro-choice activists in Fargo cluster in a group born in the 1940s and influenced by the social movements of the 1960s and 1970s. These movements offered a new vision of a world defined not only by reproduction and motherhood, but filled with broader possibilities. Right-to-life women comprised one cohort born in the 1920s and a second cohort born in the 1950s. Many of these women experienced their commitment to the right-to-life movement as a sort of conversion, occurring at the time they moved out of the paid work force to stay home with children. Women's life histories indicate that embracing a pro-life or pro-choice position "emerges specifically out of a confluence of reproductive and generational experiences." Reproduction, often defined in American culture as a biological domain, takes on meaning within a historically specific set of cultural conditions.

While Ginsburg discusses how abortion activists seek to define American womanhood in relation to cultural ideals of motherhood and nurturance, Gruenbaum (in this book) shows that cultural expectations of marriage and motherhood in Sudan form the context for the deeply embedded practice of female circumcision. Female circumcision is reported to exist in at least 26 countries, and estimates of the number of women of all ages who have been circumcised in Africa reach 80 million; other estimates suggest that as many as 5 million children are operated on each year (Kouba and Muasher 1985; Sargent 1991). The various forms of female circumcision present serious risks, such as infection and hemorrhage at the time of the procedure and future risks to childbearing; therefore, social scientists, feminists, and public health organizations have opposed the practices. However, as Gruenbaum observes, female circumcision "forms part of a complex sociocultural arrangement of female subjugation in a strongly patrilineal, patriarchal society" and continues to be most strongly defended by women, who carry out the practice.

Women in Sudan derive status and security as wives and mothers. Virginity is a prerequisite for marriage, and in this context clitoridectomy and infibulation, the major forms of circumcision, are perceived as protecting morality. Thus, these practices persist because they are linked to the important goal of maintaining the reputation and marriageability of daughters. Forty years of policy formulated by the Sudanese government and by international health organizations emphasizing the physically dangerous dimensions of female circumcision and prohibiting the most extensive forms of the practice have not resulted in its elimination.

As Gruenbaum notes, clitoridectomy and infibulation are considered by Sudanese men and women to enhance a woman's ability to please her husband sexually, while attenuating inappropriate sexual desire outside marriage. Insofar as women are dependent on husbands for social and economic support and have few opportunities for educational advancement or viable employment, female circumcision is unlikely to be eradicated on medical grounds.

Miller's discussion of female infanticide and child neglect in North India (in this book) is also set in a strongly patrilineal, patriarchal society and dramatically illustrates the links between gender ideology, reproduction, and health. In North India family survival depends on the reproduction of sons for the rural labor force, and preference for male children is evident in substantial ethnographic data documenting discrimination against girls. In this region preferences for male children result in celebrations at the birth of a boy, while a girl's birth goes unremarked. Sex-selective child care and female infanticide also indicate cultural favoring of male children.

Reports of female infanticide in India have occurred since the eighteenth century. There is evidence that a few villages in North India have never raised one daughter. In spite of legislation prohibiting female infanticide, the practice has not totally disappeared, although Miller argues that direct female infanticide has been replaced by indirect infanticide or neglect of female children. Indirect female infanticide is accomplished by nutritional and health care deprivation of female children, a phenomenon also discussed by Charlton (1984). Miller argues that the strong preference for sons in rural North India is related to their economic and social functions.

The preference for male children has important repercussions in the increasing demand for abortion of female fetuses following amniocentesis. For example, in one clinic in North India 95 percent of female fetuses were aborted following prenatal sex determination. Thus, new reproductive technologies such as amniocentesis are seen to be manipulated by patriarchal interests. Miller suggests that, ultimately, understanding the patriarchal culture of north India may help promote more effective health care and enhanced survival chances for female children.

The readings in this section illustrate the ways in which human reproductive behavior is socially constructed and influenced by economic and political processes (Ginsburg and Rapp 1991). Rather than perceiving reproductive health in a narrow biological or purely personal framework, cross-cultural research suggests that women's health needs should be addressed in the context of their multifaceted productive, reproductive, and social roles. Consequently, decisions about such reproductive health issues as family size and composition are never left to the individual woman, but are influenced by kin, community, and state interests. These interests are often contested with the introduction of new reproductive technologies enabling sophisticated prenatal testing, treatment for infertility, and surrogate mothering. As these technologies increasingly spread throughout the world, their availability will raise important questions regarding cultural definitions of parenting, concepts of personhood, and gender roles and relations.

REFERENCES

Browner, Carole and Carolyn Sargent. 1990. "Anthropology and Studies of Human Reproduction." In Thomas M. Johnson and Carolyn Sargent (eds.). *Medical Anthropology: Contemporary Theory and Method,* pp. 215–229. New York: Praeger Publishers.

Charlton, Sue Ellen M. 1984. *Women in Third World Development.* Boulder: Westview Press.

Collier, Jane F. and Michelle Z. Rosaldo. 1981. "Politics and Gender in Simple Societies." In Sherry B. Ortner and Harriet Whitehead (eds.). *Sexual Meanings: The Cultural Construction of Gender and Sexuality.* Cambridge: Cambridge University Press.

Ford, Clellan Stearns. 1964. "A Comparative Study of Human Reproduction." *Yale University Publications in Anthropology* No. 32: Human Relations Area Files Press.

Ginsburg, Faye and Rayna Rapp. 1991. "The Politics of Reproduction." *Annual Review of Anthropology* 20: 311–43.

Ginsburg, Faye and Rayna Rapp (eds.). 1995. *Conceiving the New World Order: The Global Politics of Reproduction.* Berkeley: University of California Press.

Jordan, Brigitte. 1978. *Birth in Four Cultures.* Montreal: Eden Press Women's Publications.

Kouba, Leonard J. and Judith Muasher. 1985. "Female Circumcision in Africa: An Overview." *African Studies Review* 28 (1): 95–110.

Malinowski, Bronislaw. 1932. *The Sexual Life of Savages in Northwestern Melanesia.* London: Routledge and Kegan Paul.

Martin, Emily. 1987. *The Woman in the Body: A Cultural Analysis of Reproduction.* Boston: Beacon Press.

Michaelson, Karen, et al. 1988. *Childbirth in America: Anthropological Perspectives.* South Hadley, MA: Bergin and Garvey.

Montagu, M. F. Ashley. 1949. "Embryology from Antiquity to the End of the 18th Century." Ciba Foundation Symposium 10 (4): 994–1008.

Oakley, Ann. 1977. "Cross-cultural Practices." In Tim Chard and Martin Richards (eds.). *Benefits and Hazards of the New Obstetrics.* London: William Heinemann Medical Books.

———. 1980. *Women Confined: Towards a Sociology of Childbirth.* New York: Schocken Books.

Romalis, Shelly (ed.). 1981. *Childbirth: Alternatives to Medical Control.* Austin: University of Texas Press.

Rubinstein, Robert A. and Sandra D. Lane. 1991. "International Health and Development." In Thomas M. Johnson and Carolyn Sargent (eds.). *Medical Anthropology: Contemporary Theory and Method,* pp. 367–391. New York: Praeger Publishers.

Sargent, Carolyn. 1982. *The Cultural Context of Therapeutic Choice.* Dordrecht, Holland: D. Reidel Publishing Company.

———. 1991. "Confronting Patriarchy: The Potential for Advocacy in Medical Anthropology." *Medical Anthropology Quarterly* 5 (1): 24–25.

Sargent, Carolyn F. and Caroline B. Brettell (eds.).

1996. *Gender and Health: An International Perspective.* Upper Saddle River, NJ: Prentice Hall, Inc.
Spencer, Robert. 1949–1950. "Introduction to Primitive Obstetrics." Ciba Foundation Symposium 11 (3): 1158–88.
Vieille, Paul. 1978. "Iranian Women in Family Alliance and Sexual Politics." In Lois Beck and Nikki Keddie (eds.). *Women in the Muslim World,* pp. 451–472. Cambridge: Harvard University Press.
Whitbeck, Caroline. 1983. "The Moral Implications of Regarding Women as People: New Perspectives on Pregnancy and Personhood." In William B. Bondeson et al. (eds.). *Abortion and the Status of the Fetus,* pp. 247–272. Dordrecht, Holland: D. Reidel Publishing.

GENDER AND RITUAL: GIVING BIRTH THE AMERICAN WAY

Robbie E. Davis-Floyd

Although the array of new technologies that radically alter the nature of human reproduction is exponentially increasing, childbirth is still an entirely gendered phenomenon. Because only women have babies, the way a society treats pregnancy and childbirth reveals a great deal about the way that society treats women. The experience of childbirth is unique for every woman, and yet in the U.S. childbirth is treated in a highly standardized way. No matter how long or short, how easy or hard their labors, the vast majority of American women are hooked up to an electronic fetal monitor and an IV (intravenously administered fluids and/or medication), are encouraged to use pain-relieving drugs, receive an episiotomy (a surgical incision in the vagina to widen the birth outlet in order to prevent tearing) at the moment of birth, and are separated from their babies shortly after birth. Most women also receive doses of the synthetic hormone pitocin to speed their labors, and they give birth flat on their backs. Nearly one quarter of babies are delivered by Cesarean section.

Many Americans, including most of the doctors and nurses who attend birth, view these procedures as medical necessities. Yet anthropologists regularly describe other, less technological ways to give birth. For example, the Mayan Indians of Highland Chiapas hold onto a rope while squatting for birth, a position that is far more beneficial than the flat-on-your-back-with-your-feet-in-stirrups (lithotomy) position. Mothers in many low-technology cultures give birth sitting, squatting, semi-reclining in their hammocks, or on their hands and knees, and are nurtured through the pain of labor by experienced midwives and supportive female relatives. What then might explain the standardization and technical elaboration of the American birthing process?

One answer emerges from the field of symbolic anthropology. Early in this century, Arnold van Gennep noticed that in many societies around the world, major life transitions are ritualized. These cultural *rites of passage* make it appear that society itself effects the transformation of the individual. Could this explain the standardization of American birth? I believe the answer is yes.

I came to this conclusion as a result of a study I conducted of American birth between 1983 and 1991. I interviewed over 100 mothers, as well as many of the obstetricians, nurses, childbirth educators, and midwives who attended them.[1] While poring over my interviews, I began to understand that the forces shaping American hospital birth are invisible to us because they stem from the conceptual foundations of our society. I realized that American society's deepest beliefs center around science, technology, patriarchy, and the institutions that control and disseminate them, and that there could be no better transmitter of these core values and beliefs than the hospital procedures so salient in American birth. Through these procedures, American women are repeatedly told, in dozens of visible and invisible ways, that their bodies are defective machines incapable of giving birth without the assistance of these other, male-created, more perfect machines.

RITES OF PASSAGE

A *ritual* is a patterned, repetitive, and symbolic enactment of a cultural belief or value; its primary purpose is alignment of the belief system of the individual with that of society. A *rite of passage* is a series of rituals that move individuals from one social state or status to another as, for example, from girlhood to womanhood, boyhood to manhood, or from the womb to the world of culture. Rites of passage transform both society's perception of individuals and individuals' perceptions of themselves.

Rites of passage generally consist of three stages, originally outlined by van Gennep: (1) *separation* of the individuals from their preceding social state; (2) a period of *transition* in which they are neither one thing nor the other; and (3) an *integration* phase, in which, through various rites of incorporation, they are absorbed into their new social state. In the year-long pregnancy/childbirth rite of passage in American society, the separation phase begins with the woman's first awareness of pregnancy; the transition stage lasts until several days after the birth; and the integration phase ends gradually in the newborn's first few months of life, when the new mother begins to feel that, as one woman put it, she is "mainstreaming it again."

Victor Turner, an anthropologist famous for his writings on ritual, pointed out that the most important feature of all rites of passage is that they place their participants in a transitional realm that has few of the attributes of the past or coming state. Existing in such a non-ordinary realm, he argues, facilitates the gradual psychological opening of the initiates to profound interior change. In many initiation rites involving major transitions into new social roles (such as military basic training), ritualized physical and mental hardships serve to break down initiates' belief systems, leaving them open to new learning and the construction of new cognitive categories.

Birth is an ideal candidate for ritualization of this sort, and is, in fact, used in many societies as a model for structuring other rites of passage. By making the naturally transformative process of birth into a cultural rite of passage, a society can ensure that its basic values will be transmitted to the three new members born out of the birth process: the new baby, the woman reborn into the new social role of mother, and the man reborn as father. The new mother especially must be very clear about these values, as she is generally the one primarily responsible for teaching them to her children, who will be society's new members and the guarantors of its future.

THE CHARACTERISTICS OF RITUAL

Some primary characteristics of ritual are particularly relevant to understanding how the initiatory process of cognitive restructuring is accomplished in hospital birth. We will examine each of these characteristics in order to understand (1) how ritual works; (2) how the natural process of childbirth is transformed in the United States into a cultural rite of passage; and (3) how that transformation works to cement the patriarchal status quo.

Symbolism

Above all else, ritual is symbolic. Ritual works by sending messages in the form of symbols to those who perform and those who observe it. A *symbol* is an object, idea, or action that is loaded with cultural meaning. The left hemisphere of the human brain decodes and analyzes straightforward verbal messages, enabling the recipient to either accept or reject their content. Complex ritual symbols, on the other hand, are received by the right hemisphere of the brain, where they are interpreted holistically. Instead of being analyzed intellectually, a symbol's message will be *felt* through the body and the emotions. Thus, even though recipients may be unaware of incorporating the symbol's message, its ultimate effect may be extremely powerful.

Routine obstetric procedures are highly symbolic. For example, to be seated in a wheelchair upon entering the hospital, as many laboring women are, is to receive through their bodies the symbolic message that they are disabled; to then be put to bed is to receive the symbolic message that they are sick. Although no one pronounces, "You are disabled; you are sick," such graphic demonstrations of disability and illness can be far more powerful than words. Suzanne Sampson told me:

> I can remember just almost being in tears by the way they would wheel you in. I would come into the hospital, on top of this, breathing, you know, all in control. And they slap you in a wheelchair! It made me suddenly feel like maybe I wasn't in control any more.

The intravenous drips commonly attached to the hands or arms of birthing women make a powerful symbolic statement: They are umbilical cords to the hospital. The cord connecting her body to the fluid-filled bottle places the woman in the same relation to the hospital as the baby in her womb is to her. By making her dependent on the institution for her life, the IV conveys to her one of the most profound messages of her initiation experience: In American society, we are all dependent on institutions for our lives. The message is even more compelling in her case, for *she* is the real giver of life. Society and its institutions cannot exist unless women give birth, yet the birthing woman in the hospital is shown, not that *she* gives life, but rather that the *institution* does.

A Cognitive Matrix

A *matrix* (from the Latin *mater,* mother), like a womb, is something from within which something else comes. Rituals are not arbitrary; they come from within the belief system of a group. Their primary purpose is to enact, and thereby, to transmit that belief system into the emotions, minds, and bodies of their participants. Thus, analysis of a culture's rituals can lead to a profound understanding of its belief system.

Analysis of the rituals of hospital birth reveals their cognitive matrix to be the *technocratic model* of reality which forms the philosophical basis of both Western biomedicine and American society. All cultures develop technologies. But most do not supervalue their technologies in the particular way that we do. This point is argued clearly by Peter C. Reynolds (1991) in his book *Stealing Fire: The Mythology of the Technocracy* (a *technocracy* is a hierarchical, bureaucratic society driven by an ideology of technological progress). There he discusses how we "improve upon" nature by controlling it through technology. The technocratic model is the paradigm that charters such behavior. Its early forms were originally developed in the 1600s by Descartes, Bacon, and Hobbes, among others. This model assumes that the universe is mechanistic, following predictable laws that the enlightened can discover through science and manipulate through technology, in order to decrease their dependence on nature. In this model, the human body is viewed as a machine that can be taken apart and put back together to ensure proper functioning. In the seventeenth century, the practical utility of this body-as-machine metaphor lay in its separation of body, mind, and soul. The soul could be left to religion, the mind to the philosophers, and the body could be opened up to scientific investigation.

The dominant religious belief systems of Western Europe at that time held that women were inferior to men—closer to nature and feebler both in body and intellect. Consequently, the men who developed the idea of the body-as-machine also firmly established the male body as the prototype of this machine. Insofar as it deviated from the male standard, the female body was regarded as abnormal, inherently defective, and dangerously under the influence of nature.

The metaphor of the body-as-machine and the related image of the female body as a defective machine eventually formed the philosophical foundations of modern obstetrics. Wide cultural acceptance of these metaphors accompanied the demise of the midwife and the rise of the male-attended, mechanically manipulated birth. Obstetrics was thus enjoined by its own conceptual origins to develop tools and technologies for the manipulation and improvement of the inherently defective, and therefore anomalous and dangerous, process of birth.

The rising science of obstetrics ultimately accomplished this goal by adopting the model of the assembly-line production of goods as its template for hospital birth. Accordingly, a woman's reproductive tract came to be treated like a birthing machine by skilled technicians working under semiflexible timetables to meet production and quality control demands. As one fourth-year resident observed:

> We shave 'em, we prep 'em, we hook 'em up to the IV and administer sedation. We deliver the baby, it goes to the nursery, and the mother goes to her room. There's no room for niceties around here. We just move 'em right on through. It's hard not to see it like an assembly line.

The hospital itself is a highly sophisticated technocratic factory; the more technology the hospital has to offer, the better it is considered to be. Because it is an institution, the hospital constitutes a more significant social unit than an individual or a family. Therefore it can require that the birth process conform more to institutional than personal needs. As one resident explained,

> There is a set, established routine for doing things, usually for the convenience of the doctors and the nurses, and the laboring woman is someone you work around, rather than with.

The most desirable end-product of the birth process is the new social member, the baby; the new mother is a secondary by-product. One obstetrician commented, "It was what we were all trained to always go after—the perfect body. That's what we were trained to produce. The quality of the mother's experience—we rarely thought about that."

Repetition and Redundancy

Ritual is marked by repetition and redundancy. For maximum effectiveness, a ritual concentrates on sending one basic set of messages, repeating it over and over again in different forms. Hospital birth takes place in a series of ritual procedures, many of which convey the same message in different forms. The open and exposing hospital gown, the ID bracelet, the intravenous fluid, the bed in which she is placed—all these convey to the laboring woman that she is dependent on the institution.

She is also reminded in myriad ways of the potential defectiveness of her birthing machine. These include periodic and sometimes continuous electronic monitoring of that machine, frequent manual examinations of her cervix to make sure that it is dilating on schedule, and, if it isn't, administration of the synthetic hormone pitocin to speed up labor so that birth can take place within the required 26 hours.[2] All three of these procedures convey the same messages over and over: *Time is important, you must produce on time, and you cannot do that without technological assistance because your machine is defective.* In the technocracy, we supervalue time. It is only fitting that messages about time's importance should be repeatedly conveyed during the births of new social members.

Cognitive Reduction

In any culture, the intellectual abilities of ritual participants are likely to differ, often markedly. It is not practical for society to design different rituals for persons of different levels of intellectual ability. So ritual utilizes specific techniques, such as rhythmic repetition, to reduce all participants to the same narrower level of cognitive functioning. This low level involves thinking in either/or patterns that do not allow for consideration of options or alternative views.

Four techniques are often employed by ritual to accomplish this end. One is the *repetition* already discussed above. A second is *hazing*, which is familiar to undergraduates who undergo fraternity initiation rites but is also part of rites of passage all over the world. A third is *strange-making*—making the commonplace appear strange by juxtaposing it with the unfamiliar. Fourth is *symbolic inversion*—metaphorically turning things upside-down and inside-out to generate, in a phrase coined by Roger Abrahams (1973), "The power attendant upon confusion."

For example, in the rite of passage of military basic training, the initiate's normal patterns of action and thought are turned topsy-turvy. He is made strange to himself: His head is shaved, so that he does not even recognize himself in the mirror. He must give up his clothes, those expressions of his past individual identity and personality, and put on a uniform identical to that of the other initiates. Constant and apparently meaningless hazing, such as orders to dig six ditches and then fill them in, further breaks down his cognitive structure. Then through repetitive and highly symbolic rituals, such as sleeping with his rifle, the basic values, beliefs, and practices of the Marines are incorporated into his body and his mind.

In medical school and again in residency, the same ritual techniques that transform a youth into a Marine are employed to transform college students into physicians. Reduced from the high status of graduate to the lowly status of first-year medical student, initiates are subjected to hazing techniques of rote memorization of endless facts and formulas, absurdly long hours of work, and intellectual and sensory overload. As one physician explained:

> You go through, in a six-week course, a thousand-page book. You have pop quizzes in two or three courses every day the first year. We'd get up around 6, attend classes till 5, go home and eat, then head back to school and be in anatomy lab working with a cadaver, or something, until 1 or 2 in the morning, and then go home and get a couple of hours sleep, and then go out again.

Subjected to such a process, medical students often gradually lose any broadminded goals of "helping humanity" they had upon entering medical school. A successful rite of passage produces new professional values structured in accordance with the technocratic and scientific values of the dominant medical system. The emotional impact of this cognitive narrowing is aptly summarized by a former resident:

> Most of us went into medical school with pretty humanitarian ideals. I know I did. But the whole process of medical education makes you inhuman. . . . you forget about the rest of life. By the time you get to residency, you end up not caring about anything beyond the latest techniques and most sophisticated tests.

Likewise, the birthing woman is socialized by ritual techniques of cognitive reduction. She is made strange to herself by being dressed in a hospital gown, tagged with an ID bracelet, and by the shaving or clipping of her pubic hair, which symbolically de-sexualizes the lower portion of her body, returning it to a conceptual state of childishness. (In many cultures, sexuality and hair are symbolically linked.) Labor itself is painful, and is often rendered more so by the hazing technique of frequent and very painful insertion of someone's fingers into her vagina to see how far her cervix has dilated. This technique also functions as a strange-making device. Since almost any nurse or resident in need of practice may check her cervix, the birthing woman's most private parts are symbolically inverted into institutional property. One respondent's obstetrician observed, "It's a wonder you didn't get an infection, with so many people sticking their hands inside of you."

Cognitive Stabilization

When humans are subjected to extremes of stress and pain, they may become unreasonable and out of touch with reality. Ritual assuages this condition by giving people a conceptual handle-hold to keep them from "falling apart" or "losing it." When the airplane starts to falter, even passengers who don't go to church are likely to pray! Ritual mediates between cognition and chaos by making reality appear to conform to accepted cognitive categories. In other words, to perform a ritual in the face of chaos is to restore order to the world.

Labor subjects most women to extremes of pain, which are often intensified by the alien and often unsupportive hospital environment. They look to hospital rituals to relieve the distress resulting from their pain and fear. They utilize breathing rituals taught in hospital-sponsored childbirth education classes for cognitive stabilization. They turn to drugs for pain relief, and to the reassuring presence of medical technology for relief from fear. LeAnn Kellog expressed it this way:

> I was terrified when my daughter was born. I just knew I was going to split open and bleed to death right there on the table, but she was coming so fast, they didn't have any time to do anything to me. . . . I like Cesarean sections, because you don't have to be afraid.

When you come from within a belief system, its rituals will comfort and calm you. Accordingly, those women in my study who were in basic agreement with the technocratic model of birth before going into the hospital (70%) expressed general satisfaction with their hospital births.

Order, Formality, and a Sense of Inevitability

Its exaggerated and precise order and formality set ritual apart from other modes of social interaction, enabling it to establish an atmosphere that feels both inevitable and inviolate. To perform a series of rituals is to feel oneself locking onto a set of "cosmic gears" that will safely crank the individual through danger to safety. For example, Trobriand sea fishermen described by anthropologist Bronislaw Malinowski (1954) regularly performed an elaborate series of rituals on the beach before embarking. The fishermen believed that these rituals, when carried out with precision, would obligate the gods of the sea to do their part to bring the fishermen safely home. Likewise, obstetricians, and many birthing women, feel that correct performance of standardized procedures ought to result in a healthy baby. Such rituals generate in humans a sense of confidence that makes it easier to face the challenge and caprice of nature.

When women who have placed their faith in the technocratic model are denied its rituals, they often react with fear and a feeling of being neglected:

> My husband and I got to the hospital, and we thought they would take care of everything. I kept sending my husband out to ask them to give me something for the pain, to check me, but they were short-staffed and they just ignored me until the shift changed in the morning.

Hospital rituals such as electronic monitoring work to give the laboring woman a sense that society is using the best it has to offer—the full force of its technology—to inevitably ensure that she will have a safe birth.

However, once those "cosmic gears" have been set into motion, there is often no stopping them. The very inevitability of hospital procedures makes them almost antithetical to the possibility of normal, natural birth. A "cascade of intervention" occurs when one obstetric procedure alters the natural birthing process, causing complications, and so inexorably "necessitates" the next procedure, and the next. Many of the women in my study experienced such a "cascade" when they received some form of pain relief, such as an epidural, which slowed their labor. Then pitocin was administered through the IV to speed up the labor, but pitocin very suddenly induced longer and stronger contractions. Unprepared for the additional pain, the women asked for more pain relief, which ultimately necessitated more pitocin. Pitocin-induced contractions, together with the fact that the mother must lie flat on her back because of the electronic monitor belts strapped around her stomach, can cause the supply of blood and oxygen to the fetus to drop, affecting the fetal heart rate. In response to the "distress" registered on the fetal monitor, an emergency Cesarean is performed.

Acting, Stylization, Staging

Ritual's set-apartness is enhanced by the fact that it is usually highly stylized and self-consciously acted, like a part in a play. Most of us can easily accept this view of the careful performances of TV evangelists, but it may come as a surprise that those who perform the rituals of hospital birth are often aware of their dramatic elements. The physician becomes the protagonist. The woman's body is the stage upon which he performs, often for an appreciative audience of medical students, residents, and nurses. Here is how one obstetrician played to a student audience observing the delivery he was performing:

> "In honest-to-God natural conditions babies were *sometimes* born without tearing the perineum and without an episiotomy, but without artificial things like anesthesia and episiotomy, the muscle is torn apart and if it is not cut, it is usually not repaired. Even today, if there is no episiotomy and repair, those women quite often develop a rectocoele and a relaxed vaginal floor. This is what I call the saggy, baggy bottom." (Laughter by the students. A student nurse asks if exercise doesn't help strengthen the perineum.) "No, exercises may be for the birds, but they're not for bottoms. . . . When the woman is bearing down, the leveator muscles of the perineum contract too. This means the baby is caught between the diaphragm and the perineum. Consequently, anesthesia and episiotomy will reduce the pressure on the head, and hopefully, produce more Republicans." (More laughter from the students) (Shaw 1974: 90).

Cognitive Transformation

The goal of most initiatory rites of passage is cognitive transformation. It occurs when the symbolic messages of ritual fuse with individual emotion and belief, and the individual's entire cognitive structure, reorganize around the newly internalized symbolic complex. The following quote from a practicing obstetrician presents the outcome for him of such transformative learning:

> I think my training was valuable. The philosophy was one of teaching one way to do it, and that was the right way. . . . I like the set hard way. I like the riverbanks that confine you in a direction. . . . You learn one thing real well, and that's *the* way.

For both nascent physicians and nascent mothers, cognitive transformation of the initiate occurs when reality as presented by the technocratic model, and reality as the initiate perceives it, become one and the same. This process is gradual. Routine obstetric procedures cumulatively map the technocratic model of birth onto the birthing woman's perceptions of her labor experience. They align her belief system with that of society.

Take the way many mothers come to think about the electronic fetal monitor, for example. The monitor is a machine that uses ultrasound to measure the strength of the mother's contractions and the rate of the baby's heartbeat through electrodes belted onto the mother's abdomen. This machine has become *the* symbol of high technology hospital birth. Observers and participants alike report that the monitor, once attached, becomes the focal point of the labor.[3] Nurses, physicians, husbands, and even the mother herself become visually and conceptually glued to the machine, which then shapes their perceptions and interpretations of the birth process. Diana Crosse described her experience this way:

> As soon as I got hooked up to the monitor, all everyone did was stare at it. The nurses didn't even look at me anymore when they came into the room—they went straight to the monitor. I got the weirdest feeling that *it* was having the baby, not me.

This statement illustrates the successful conceptual fusion between the woman's perceptions of her birth experience and the technocratic model. So thoroughly was this model mapped on to her psyche that she began to *feel* that the machine was having the baby, that she was a mere onlooker. Soon after the monitor was in place, she requested a Cesarean section, declaring that there was "no more point in trying."

Consider the visual and kinesthetic images that the laboring woman experiences—herself in bed, in a hospital gown, staring up at an IV pole, bag, and cord, and down at a steel bed and a huge belt encircling her waist. Her entire sensory field conveys one overwhelming message about our culture's deepest values and beliefs: Technology is supreme, and the individual is utterly dependent upon it.

Internalizing the technocratic model, women come to accept the notion that the female body is inherently defective. This notion then shapes their perceptions of the labor experience, as exemplified by Merry Simpson's story:

> It seemed as though my uterus had suddenly tired! When the nurses in attendance noted a contraction building on the recorder, they instructed me to begin pushing, not waiting for the *urge* to push, so that by the time the urge pervaded, I invariably had no strength remaining but was left gasping and dizzy. . . . I felt suddenly depressed by the fact that labor, which had progressed so uneventfully up to this point, had now become unproductive.

Note that she does not say "The nurses had me pushing too soon," but "My uterus had tired," and labor had "become unproductive." These responses reflect her internalization of the technocratic tenet that when something goes wrong, it is her body's fault.

Affectivity and Intensification

Rituals tend to intensify toward a climax. Behavioral psychologists have long understood that people are far more likely to remember, and to absorb lessons from, those events that carry an emotional charge. The order and stylization of ritual, combined with its rhythmic repetitiveness and the intensification of its messages, methodically create just the sort of highly charged emotional atmosphere that works to ensure long-term learning.

As the moment of birth approaches, the number of ritual procedures performed upon the woman will intensify toward the climax of birth, whether or not her condition warrants such intervention. For example, once the woman's cervix reaches full dilation (10 cm), the nursing staff immediately begins to exhort the woman to push with each contraction, whether or not she actually feels the urge to push. When delivery is imminent, the woman must be transported, often with a great deal of drama and haste, down the hall to the delivery room. Lest the baby be born *en route,* the laboring woman is then exhorted, with equal vigor, *not* to push. Such commands constitute a complete denial of the natural rhythms of the woman's body. They signal that her labor is a mechanical event and that she is subordinate to the institution's expectations and schedule. Similar high drama will pervade the rest of her birthing experience.

Preservation of the Status Quo

A major function of ritual is cultural preservation. Through explicit enactment of a culture's belief system, ritual works both to preserve and to transmit the culture. Preserving the culture includes perpetuating its power structure, so it is usually the case that those in positions of power will have unique control over ritual performance. They will utilize the effectiveness of ritual to reinforce both their own importance and the importance of the belief and value system that legitimizes their positions.

In spite of tremendous advances in equality for women, the United States is still a patriarchy. It is no cultural accident that 99 percent of American women give birth in hospitals, where only physicians, most of whom are male, have final authority over the performance of birth rituals—an authority that reinforces the cultural privileging of patriarchy for both mothers and their medical attendants.

Nowhere is this reality more visible than in the lithotomy position. Despite years of effort on the part of childbirth activists, including many obstetricians, the majority of American women still give birth lying flat on their backs. This position is physiologically dysfunctional. It compresses major blood vessels, lowering the mother's circulation and thus the baby's oxygen supply. It increases the need for forceps because it both narrows the pelvic outlet and ensures that the baby, who must follow the curve of the birth canal, quite literally will be born heading upward, against gravity. This lithotomy position completes the process of symbolic inversion that has been in motion ever since the woman was put into that "upside-down" hospital gown. Her normal bodily patterns are turned, quite literally, upside-down—her legs are in the air, her vagina totally exposed. As the ultimate symbolic inversion, it is ritually appropriate that this position be reserved for the peak tranformational moments of the initiation experience—the birth itself. The doctor—society's official representative—stands in control not at the mother's head nor at her side, but at her bottom, where the baby's head is beginning to emerge.

Structurally speaking, this puts the woman's vagina where her head should be. Such total inversion is perfectly appropriate from a social perspective, as the technocratic model promises us that eventually we will be able to grow babies in machines—that is, have them with our cultural heads instead of our natural bottoms. In our culture, "up" is good and "down" is bad, so the babies born of science and technology must be delivered "up" toward the positively valued cultural world, instead of down toward the negatively valued natural world. Interactionally, the obstetrician is "up" and the birthing woman is "down," an inversion that speaks eloquently to her of her powerlessness and of the power of society at the supreme moment of her own individual transformation.

The episiotomy performed by the obstetrician just before birth also powerfully enacts the status quo in American society. This procedure, performed on over 90 percent of first-time mothers as they give birth, expresses the value and importance of one of our technocratic society's most fundamental markers—the straight line. Through episiotomies, physicians can deconstruct the vagina (stretchy, flexible, part-circular and part-formless, feminine, creative, sexual, non-linear), then reconstruct it in accordance with our cultural belief and value system. Doctors are taught (incorrectly) that straight cuts heal faster than the small jagged tears that sometimes occur during birth. They learn that straight cuts will prevent such tears, but in fact, episiotomies often cause severe tearing that would not otherwise occur (Klein 1992; Shiono et al. 1990; Thorp and Bowes 1989; Wilcox et al. 1989[4]). These teachings dramatize our Western belief in the superiority of culture over nature. Because it virtually does not exist in nature, the line is most useful in aiding us in our constant conceptual efforts to separate ourselves from nature.

Moreover, since surgery constitutes the ultimate form of manipulation of the human body-machine, it is the most highly valued form of medicine. Routinizing the episiotomy, and increasingly, the Cesarean section, has served both to legitimize and to raise the status of obstetrics as a profession, by ensuring that childbirth will be not a natural but a surgical procedure.

Effecting Social Change

Paradoxically, ritual, with all of its insistence on continuity and order, can be an important factor not only in individual transformation but also in social change. New belief and value systems are most effectively spread through new rituals designed to enact and transmit them; entrenched belief and value systems are most effectively altered through alterations in the rituals that enact them.

Nine percent of my interviewees entered the hospital determined to avoid technocratic rituals in order to have "completely natural childbirth," yet ended up with highly technocratic births. These nine women experienced extreme cognitive dissonance between their previously held self-images and those internalized in the hospital. Most of them suffered severe emotional wounding and short-term post-partum depression as a result. But 15 percent did achieve their goal of natural childbirth, thereby avoiding conceptual fusion with the technocratic model. These women were personally empowered by their birth experiences. They tended to view technology as a resource that they could choose to utilize or ignore, and often consciously subverted their socialization process by replacing technocratic symbols with self-empowering alternatives. For example, they wore their own clothes and ate their own food, rejecting the hospital gown and the IV. They walked the halls instead of going to bed. They chose perineal massage instead of episiotomy, and gave birth like "primitives," sitting up, squatting, or on their hands and knees. One of them, confronted with the wheelchair, said "I don't need this," and used it as a luggage cart. This rejection of customary ritual elements is an exceptionally powerful way to induce change, as it takes advantage of an already charged and dramatic situation.

During the 1970s and early 1980s, the conceptual hegemony of the technocratic model in the hospital was severely challenged by the natural childbirth movement which these 24 women represent. Birth activists succeeded in getting hospitals to allow fathers into labor and delivery rooms, mothers to birth consciously (without being put to sleep), and mothers and babies to room together after birth. They fought for women to have the right to birth without drugs or interventions, to walk around or even be in water during labor (in some hospitals, Jacuzzis were installed). Prospects for change away from the technocratic model of birth by the 1990s seemed bright.

Changing a society's belief and value system by changing the rituals that enact it is possible, but not easy. To counter attempts at change, individuals in positions of authority often intensify the rituals that support the status quo. Thus a response to the threat posed by the natural childbirth movement was to intensify the use of high technology in hospital birth. During the 1980s, periodic electronic monitoring of nearly all women became standard procedure, the epidural rate shot up to 80 percent, and the Cesarean rate rose to nearly 25 percent. Part of the impetus for this technocratic intensification is the increase in malpractice suits against physicians. The threat of lawsuit forces doctors to practice conservatively—that is, in strict accordance with technocratic standards. As one of them explained.

> Certainly I've changed the way I practice since malpractice became an issue. I do more C-sections . . . and more and more tests to cover myself. More expensive stuff. We don't do risky things that women ask for—we're very conservative in our approach to everything. . . . In 1970 before all this came up, my C-section rate was around 4 percent. It has gradually climbed every year since then. In 1985 it was 16 percent, then in 1986 it was 23 percent.

The money goes where the values lie. From this macro-cultural perspective, the increase in malpractice suits emerges as society's effort to make sure that its representatives, the obstetricians, perpetuate our technocratic core value system by continuing through birth rituals to transmit that system. Its perpetuation seems imperative, for in our technology we see the promise of our eventual transcendence of bodily and earthly limitations—already we replace body parts with computerized devices, grow babies in test tubes, build space stations, and continue to pollute the environment in the expectation that someone will develop the technologies to clean it up!

We are all complicitors in our technocratic system, as we have so very much invested in it. Just as that system has given us increasing control over the natural environment, so it has also given not only doctors but also women increasing control over biology and birth. Contemporary middle-class women *do* have much greater say over what will be done to them during birth than their mothers, most of whom gave birth during the 1950s and 1960s under general anesthesia. When what they demand is in accord with technocratic values, they have a much greater chance of getting it than their sisters have of achieving natural childbirth. Even as hospital birth still perpetuates partriarchy by treating women's bodies as defective machines, it now also reflects women's greater autonomy by allowing them conceptual separation from those defective machines.

Epidural anesthesia is administered in about 80 percent of American hospital births. So common is its use that many childbirth educators are calling the 1990s the age of the "epidural epidemic." As the epidural numbs the birthing woman, eliminating the pain of childbirth, it also graphically demonstrates to her through lived experience the truth of the Cartesian maxim that mind and body are separate, that the biological realm can be completely cut off from the realm of the intellect and the emotions. The epidural is thus the perfect technocratic tool, serving the interests of the technocratic model by transmitting it, and of women choosing to give birth under that model, by enabling them to use it to divorce themselves from their biology:

> Ultimately the decision to have the epidural and the Cesarean while I was in labor was mine. I told my doctor I'd had enough of this labor business and I'd like to . . . get it over with. So he whisked me off to the delivery room and we did it. (Elaine)

For many women, the epidural provides a means by which they can actively witness birth while avoiding "dropping into biology." Explained Joanne, "I'm not real fond of things that remind me I'm a biological creature—I prefer to think and be an intellectual emotional person." Such women tended to define their bodies as tools, vehicles for their minds. They did not enjoy "giving in to biology" to be pregnant, and were happy to be liberated from biology during birth. And they welcomed advances in birth technologies as extensions of their own ability to control nature.

In dramatic contrast, six of my interviewees (6%), insisting that "I am my body," rejected the technocratic model altogether. They chose to give birth at home under an alternative paradigm, the *holistic model*. This model stresses the organicity and trustworthiness of the female body, the natural rhythmicity of labor, the integrity of the family, and self-responsibility. These homebirthers see the safety of the baby and the emotional needs of the mother as one. The safest birth for the baby will be the one that provides the most nurturing environment for the mother.[5] Said Ryla,

> I got criticized for choosing a home birth, for not considering the safety of the baby. But that's exactly what I was considering! How could it possibly serve my baby for me to give birth in a place that causes my whole body to tense up in anxiety as soon as I walk in the door?

Although homebirthers constitute only about 2 percent of the American birthing population, their conceptual importance is tremendous, as through the alternative rituals of giving birth at home, they enact—and thus guarantee the existence of—a paradigm of pregnancy and birth based on the value of connection, just as the technocratic model is based on the principle of separation.

The technocratic and holistic models represent opposite ends of a spectrum of beliefs about birth and about cultural life. Their differences are mirrored on a wider scale by the ideological conflicts between biomedicine and holistic healing, and between industrialists and ecological activists. These groups are engaged in a core value struggle over the future—a struggle clearly visible in the profound differences in the rituals they daily enact.

CONCLUSION

Every society in the world has felt the need to thoroughly socialize its citizens into conformity with its norms, and citizens derive many benefits from such socialization. If a culture had to rely on policemen and make sure that everyone would obey its laws, it would disintegrate into chaos, as there would not be enough policemen to go around. It is much more practical for cultures to find ways to socialize their members from the *inside,* by making them *want* to conform to society's norms. Ritual is one major way through which such socialization can be achieved.

American obstetrical procedures can be understood as rituals that facilitate the internalization of cultural values. These procedures are patterned, repetitive, and profoundly symbolic, communicating messages concerning our culture's deepest beliefs about the necessity for cultural control of natural processes. They provide an ordered structure to the chaotic flow of the natural birth process. In so doing, they both enhance the natural affectivity of that process and create a sense of inevitability about their performance. Obstetric interventions are also transformative in intent. They attempt to contain and control the process of birth, and to transform the birthing woman into an American mother who has internalized the core values of this society. Such a mother believes in science, relies on technology, recognizes her biological inferiority (either consciously or unconsciously), and so at some level accepts the principles of patriarchy. She will tend to conform to society's dictates and meet the demands of its institutions, and will teach her children to do the same.

Yet it is important to note that human beings are not automatons. Human behavior varies widely even within the restraints imposed by particular cultures, including their rituals. As July Sanders sums it up:

> It's almost like programming you. You get to the hospital. They put you in this wheelchair. They whisk you off from your husband, and I mean just start in on you. Then they put you in another wheelchair, and send you home. And then they say, well, we need to give you something for the depression. [Laughs] Get away from me! That will help my depression!

Through hospital ritual procedures, obstetrics deconstructs birth, then inverts and reconstructs it as a technocratic process. But unlike most transformations effected by ritual, birth does *not* depend upon the performance of ritual to make it happen. The physiological process of labor itself transports the birthing woman into a naturally transitional situation that carries its own affectivity. Hospital procedures take advantage of that affectivity to transmit the core values of American society to birthing women. From society's perspective, the birth process will not be successful unless the woman and child are properly socialized during the experience, transformed as much by the rituals as by the physiology of birth. In the latter half of this century, women have made great strides in attaining equality with men on many cultural fronts. Yet, as I noted at the beginning, the cultural treatment of birth is one of the most revealing indicators about the status of women in a given society. In the United States, through their ritual transformation during birth, women learn profound lessons about the weakness and defectiveness of their bodies and the power of technology. In this way, every day in hospitals all over the country, women's status as subordinate is subtly reinforced, as is the patriarchal nature of the technocracy.

NOTES

1. The full results of this study appear in Davis-Floyd 1992.
2. In Holland, by way of contrast, most births are

attended by midwives who recognize that individual labors have individual rhythms. They can stop and start; can take a few hours or several days. If labor slows, the midwives encourage the woman to eat to keep up her strength, and then to sleep until contractions pick up again (Beatriz Smulders, Personal Communication, 1994; Jordan 1993).

3. As is true for most of the procedures interpreted here as rituals, there is no scientific justification for the routine use of the electronic fetal monitor: Numerous large-scale studies have shown no improvement in outcome (Leveno et al. 1986; Prentice and Lind 1987; Sandmire 1990; Shy et al. 1990). What these studies do show is that a dramatic increase in the rate of Cesarean section accompanies routine electronic monitoring. Most commonly, this increase is due both to the occasional malfunctioning of the machine, which sometimes registers fetal distress when there is none, and to the tendency of hospital staff to overreact to fluctuations on the monitor strip.
4. See Goer 1995: 274–284 for summaries and interpretations of these studies and others concerning electronic fetal monitoring.
5. For summaries of studies that demonstrate the safety of planned, midwife-attended home birth relative to hospital birth, see Davis-Floyd 1992, Chapter 4, and Goer 1995.

REFERENCES

Abrahams, Roger D. 1973. "Ritual for Fun and Profit (or The Ends and Outs of Celebration)." Paper delivered at the Burg Wartenstein Symposium No. 59, on "Ritual: Reconciliation in Change." New York: Wenner-Gren Foundation for Anthropological Research.

Davis-Floyd, Robbie E. 1992. *Birth as an American Rite of Passage.* Berkeley: University of California Press.

Goer, Henci. 1995. *Obstetric Myths Versus Research Realities: A Guide to the Medical Literature.* Westport, CT: Bergin and Garvey.

Jordan, Brigitte. 1993. *Birth in Four Cultures: A Cross-Cultural Investigation of Birth in Yucatan, Holland, Sweden and the United States* (4th edition revised). Prospect Heights: Waveland Press.

Klein, Michael et al. 1992. "Does Episiotomy Prevent Perineal Trauma and Pelvic Floor Relaxation?" *Online Journal of Current Clinical Trials* 1 (Document 10).

Leveno K. J., F. G. Cunningham, S. Nelson, M. Roark, M. L. Williams, D. Guzick, S. Dowling, C. R. Rosenfeld, A. Buckley. 1986. "A Prospective Comparison of Selective and Universal Electronic Fetal Monitoring in 34,995 Pregnancies." *New England Journal of Medicine* 315 (10): 615–619.

Malinowski, Bronislaw. 1954. (orig. pub. 1925). "Magic, Science, and Religion." In *Magic, Science and Religion and Other Essays,* pp. 17–87. New York: Doubleday/Anchor.

Prentice, A. and T. Lind. 1987. "Fetal Heart Rate Monitoring During Labor—Too Frequent Intervention, Too Little Benefit." *Lancet* 2: 1375–1877.

Reynolds, Peter C. 1991. *Stealing Fire: The Mythology of the Technocracy.* Palo Alto, CA: Iconic Anthropology Press.

Sandmire, H. F. 1990. "Whither Electronic Fetal Monitoring?" *Obstetrics and Gynecology* 76 (6): 1130–1134.

Shaw, Nancy Stoller. 1974. *Forced Labor: Maternity Care in the United States.* New York: Pergamon Press.

Shiono, P., M. A. Klebanoff, and J. C. Carey. 1990. "Midline Episiotomies: More Harm Than Good?" *American Journal of Obstetrics and Gynecology* 75 (5): 765–770.

Shy, Kirkwood, David A. Luthy, Forrest C. Bennett, Michael Whitfield, Eric B. Larson, Gerald van Belle, James P. Hughes, Judith A. Wilson, Martin A. Stenchever. 1990. "Effects of Electronic Fetal Heart Rate Monitoring, as Compared with Periodic Auscultation, on the Neurologic Development of Premature Infants." *New England Journal of Medicine* 322 (9): 588–593.

Thorp J. M. and W. A. Bowes. 1989. "Episiotomy: Can Its Routine Use Be Defended?" *American Journal of Obstetrics and Gynecology* 160 (5Pt1): 1027–1030.

Turner, Victor. 1979. (orig. pub. 1964). "Betwixt and Between: The Liminal Period in Rites de Passage." In W. Lessa and E. Z. Vogt (eds.). *Reader in Comparative Religion,* pp. 234–243. 4th edition. New York: Harper and Row.

Van Gennep, Arnold. 1966 (orig. pub. 1908). *The Rites of Passage.* Chicago: University of Chicago Press.

Wilcox, L. S. et al. 1989. "Episiotomy and Its Role in the Incidence of Perineal Lacerations in a Maternity Center and a Tertiary Hospital Obstetric Service." *American Journal of Obstetrics and Gynecology* 160 (5Pt1): 1047–1052.

THE POLITICS OF REPRODUCTION IN A MEXICAN VILLAGE

Carole H. Browner

Although women in all societies bear children in private, or with only a select few present, human reproduction is never entirely a personal affair. Kin, neighbors, and other members of the larger collectives of which women are a part seek to influence reproductive behavior in their groups. Their concerns, however, about who reproduces, how often, and when frequently conflict quite sharply with the desires of the reproducers themselves.[1] At the state level, governments develop policies with which they try to shape the size, composition, and distribution of their populations. These policies inevitably seek to influence the reproductive activities of individuals. They may be directed toward the fertility of the whole society or selectively imposed on particular classes, subcultures, or other internal groups,[2] but they are usually promoted without much consideration for the individual women who bear and raise the children, and, as a result, they may not be embraced by their target groups. Further, state-initiated population policies are sometimes challenged by internal groups whose objectives differ from those of the state.[3]

It is surprising that conflicts between the reproductive desires of a society's fecund women and the demographic interests of other individuals, groups, and political entities are rarely explored. After a comprehensive review of research in demography, population studies, and the anthropology and sociology of reproduction, Rosalind Pollack Petchesky reports, "Utterly lacking [in these fields] is any sense that the methods and goals of reproduction, and control over them, may themselves be a contested area within [a] culture."[4] Also absent from this research is the recognition that differential access to a society's sources of power determines how conflicts over reproduction are conducted and resolved, and even whether resolution ever occurs.

The following account analyzes the relationship between the population practices in one indigenous community in Mexico and the Mexican government's recent effort to reduce population growth. It shows that the government's fertility-reducing policy was superimposed on a long-standing local conflict between this community's women, who wished to limit the size of their own families, and the community as a whole, which wanted all of its female members to reproduce abundantly. Despite their apparent concordance with the goals of the state, the women refused the government's contraceptive services. They continued to have many children instead. The discussion will consider both why these indigenous rural women did not act on the fertility desires they expressed and why the demographic policies of Mexico have met uncertain success; for the two are outcomes of the same phenomenon: an overriding cultural prohibition in that community against any kind of fertility control.

BACKGROUND

The data presented here were collected in 1980–81 in a community I will call San Francisco, a Chinantec-Spanish-speaking *municipio* (township) located five hours by bus from the capital of the state of Oaxaca. The *municipio* was made up of a *cabecera* (head town) and a number of *ranchos* (hamlets) spread over a fifty-kilometer range. A year's participant observation was combined with interviews from a sample selected from the 336

Reprinted with permission of The University of Chicago Press from *Signs* 11(4):710–724, 1986 adult women who lived in San Francisco. This sample consisted of 180 women selected to represent the age, residence, and linguistic background of the women. The husbands of the married women were also interviewed, a total of 126 men.

Historically, an important element in women's attempts to control their fertility was the use of medicinal plants. In addition to learning the respondents' reproductive desires and attitudes toward childbearing and child rearing, one aim of the interviews was to determine how the knowledge and use of such plants for management of reproduction and the maintenance of reproductive health were distributed and what might be the social implications of this distribution of knowledge before and after the Mexican government's introduction of modern birth control techniques. Demographic, economic, and health data were also obtained.

The *municipio* consisted of just over three hundred families of subsistence farmers who lived dispersed over its 18,300 hectares. Nearly two-thirds of the households (65 percent) cultivated the community's abundant communal landholdings in the tropical lowlands thirty miles east of the *cabecera,* or three hours from there by bus. The remainder used private plots located either in the *cabecera* or in the highland territory that individual Franciscanos purchased in 1930 from a neighboring *municipio,* or they farmed in both places. About a third of the families (32 percent) lived permanently on lowland ranches while most of the rest divided their time between the town center and the lowlands. Although only 5 percent of the households worked solely for wages, another 80 percent reported cash income from at least occasional wage labor.

Most full-time *rancho* residents had regular contact with the *cabecera.* Men made the trip several times each year to attend mandatory town assemblies. Men were also required to reside in the head town during their terms of civil and/or religious community service (*cargos*), which required several years of full-time commitment over the course of their lifetimes. Women had no formal reason for regular visits to the *cabecera,* but they sometimes went during holidays. In addition, they were expected to help their husbands carry out *cargo* responsibilities and often moved with them to the *cabecera* during their husbands' terms of office.

Until about 1965, the *municipio* fit the model of a closed corporate peasant community,[5] maintaining only sporadic contact with the world outside. Since that time, San Francisco's isolation had been sharply reduced by mandatory primary education, the construction of the Oaxaca-Tuxtepec highway and a feeder road connecting the *cabecera* in it, and a growing stream of migrants leaving the area for Oaxaca City, Mexico City, and the United States. Nevertheless, for many residents, daily life was much as it had always been: 42 percent of the women interviewed and 16 percent of the men had never been more than a few miles outside the community.

WOMEN'S ATTITUDES TOWARD PREGNANCY AND CHILDREN

Women in San Francisco expressed sharply negative attitudes about childbearing and child rearing, an unexpected finding that is contrary to the results of most other studies of peasants' attitudes toward fertility in Latin America.[6] While most research has suggested that peasant women want fewer children than they actually have, it has also suggested that, among these women, three to five children is considered the ideal family size and childlessness is considered a great misfortune. In San Francisco, a very different picture emerged. Among my study population, it was not unusual for women to volunteer that they would have preferred to remain childless or to have far smaller families than they did have. (Sixty of the 180 women interviewed had five or more children.) Sixty-three percent believed that there were women in their community who would choose childlessness if they could. As one informant explained, "The women without children, they're the smart ones"; and yet, as we shall see, choosing childlessness was socially very problematic.[7]

The differences in fertility desires between women and men in San Francisco underscored the women's negative attitudes. Respondents were asked whether they wanted to have more children. The majority of both sexes who still considered themselves of childbearing age said they wanted no more (see Table 1), but women were satisfied with far smaller families than were men. The overwhelming majority of the women (80 percent) who had at least one living child said they were content with their present family size. Moreover, of the small number of childless women ($N = 9$), one-third indicated that they were satisfied to remain so. However, most of the men who were satisfied with family size had at least four children (60 percent), and of the childless men ($N = 6$), none indicated that he was satisfied.

Women with large families said they resented the demands of child care and the limitations it placed on them. Many saw children as a burden. They considered them too much work, too hard to raise, a source of problems, "war," and domestic strife. They viewed children as pesky disturbances who kept them tied to the house. One woman told me, "[The people of the community] want us to have many children. That's fine for them to say. They don't have to take care of them and keep them clean. My husband sleeps peacefully through the night, but I have to get up when the children need something. I'm the one the baby urinates on; sometimes I have to get out of bed in the cold and change both our clothes. They wake me when they're sick or thirsty, my husband sleeps through it all."

This resentment was balanced to some extent by the women's perception of advantages associated with children. They particularly valued the physical and emotional companionship of their children, in part because the women were extremely reluctant to be at home alone, especially at night. They feared ghosts, phantoms, and spirits and worried about drunks reputed to harass solitary women. Women also tried to avoid going alone on errands out of town, for they feared wild animals and unknown men. They always sought out a child—their own or someone else's—if no other companion could be found.

Overall, however, most Franciscanas did not perceive much practical advantage in rearing large families. There was little economic benefit seen, for the women considered their offspring lazy or too busy with other activities to be of much help. Since mandatory school attendance was strictly enforced in San Francisco, and children were encouraged by school authorities to attend

TABLE 1 Fertility Goals of Adults in a Mexican Municipio, 1980

Living Children (N)	*Women*				*Men*			
	No	*Yes*	*Total*	*Yes (%)*	*No*	*Yes*	*Total*	*Yes (%)*
0	3	6	9	67	0	6	6	100
1	7	4	11	36	3	3	6	50
2	9	4	13	31	5	5	10	50
3	16	7	23	30	10	13	23	57
4	11	3	14	21	13	2	15	13
5	11	3	14	21	6	4	10	40
6+	31	1	32	3	23	1	24	4
Totals	88	28	116	24	60	34	94	36

Note—Number of responses to the question. "Do you want more children?" by number of living children. The remaining responses among women and men are: Women ($N = 180$): too old, 47; no husband, 8; ambiguous, 3; missing data, 6. Men ($N = 126$): too old, 25; ambiguous, 3; missing data, 4. (The response "no wife" was not possible since all men in the sample were the husbands of women interviewed.)

frequent after-school activities, mothers often felt saddled with chores that their children should have done. Although women hoped their offspring would care for them in their old age, the expectation that they would actually do so was changing as children left the village to find employment elsewhere. Interestingly, mothers expressed greater support for their children's migration than did fathers.[8] Nevertheless, the women felt disappointed when they realized that they had been forgotten at home.

In addition to resenting the hard work of raising children and the frustrations of its uncertain rewards, the women in this sample saw frequent pregnancies as physically stressful and even debilitating. In their view, much of a woman's blood supply during pregnancy was devoted to nourishing the developing fetus. This left their own bodies unbalanced and susceptible to the large number of disorders that could be caused by penetration of cold and *aire* (air, winds). They also saw parturition as a threat to their health, believing that, during childbirth, the womb—and the rest of the body—must "open" to expel the newborn and that this process increased the body's already heightened vulnerability to *aire*.

Postpartum complications were common among Franciscanas. Of the 180 interviewed, two-thirds reported at least one. They ranged from conditions the women considered relatively minor, such as facial swelling and backaches, to such serious conditions as uterine prolapsis and uncontrolled bleeding. Emotional complications were sometimes mentioned as well. For instance, one woman reported that, after the birth of her second child, she was unable to tolerate criticism from her husband's relatives, with whom she and her family then lived. "I wanted to get up and run and run, I had no idea to where," she told me. In addition to the complications of pregnancy per se, women also feared that frequent childbirth and short birth intervals caused menstrual hemorrhaging, exhaustion, and early death. There are no reliable data on postpartum mortality for this particular population, but examples existed in the memories of all women interviewed.

The women's illness experiences that were not related to pregnancy reinforced their understanding that frequent pregnancies harmed their general health. Those who had had four or more pregnancies were significantly more likely than the rest to report at least one serious illness ($\chi^2 = 7.06$, $P < .001$). Even when age was controlled for, this pattern occurred. Women with four or more pregnancies were also significantly more likely to report a greater number of minor health problems overall, including headaches, backaches, breast problems, and *coraje* (anger sickness; $\chi^2 = 6.38$, $P < .025$). Again with age controlled for, women who had had four or more pregnancies were less healthy overall than women who had had fewer pregnancies.

THE CASE FOR LARGE FAMILIES

Despite the desires of many Franciscanas to have few (or no) children, they did not think that they could actually do so. The pressures on them to reproduce were simply too great to ignore. These pressures came most often and overtly from the community's men, who argued that a populous community was vital to the defense of the collectivity and its interests. Women were another source of pressure. Although most wanted few children themselves, they felt that other women were obligated by the needs of the collectivity to bear many children.

Maintaining a sufficient population base was a constant source of concern. San Francisco was surrounded by communities that coveted its comparatively large landholdings. It needed a sizable male population to defend its borders in case of armed attack by neighboring enemy communities who still threatened the *municipio*. One particularly bloody battle in the 1950s claimed the lives of thirteen Franciscanos. Residents also felt threatened by indications that the federal government might resettle members of other communities or ethnic groups onto San Francisco's lands or allocate territory to other *mu-*

nicipios that were litigating for it because, unlike many rural *municipios*, San Francisco had more land than its population required. Residents were also concerned about the regional government's proposals to consolidate San Francisco with neighboring *municipios* because it was considered far too small to remain independent. The most likely of these plans would combine San Francisco with its most hated and feared enemy.

A number of endogenous factors also threatened the community's population base. Despite the presence in the *cabecera* of two government health centers, disease continued to take a significant toll. The rate of infant mortality in the state was one of Mexico's highest. On average, deaths from all causes in San Francisco had not declined during the past fifteen years.[9] Migration from the community to the state and national capitals and to the United States was also taking increasing numbers of the most able-bodied women and men. In the past two decades, the state of Oaxaca had experienced Mexico's highest rate of out-migration, suffering a net population loss of 290,000 between 1960 and 1970 alone. Because this trend had continued, Oaxaca's population had grown more slowly than that of any other Mexican state.[10] San Francisco had been acutely affected by these broader demographic trends. Of the women interviewed whose children were grown, nearly two-thirds reported having at least one child who resided outside the *municipio*, and more than one-fourth reported that all their grown children lived elsewhere.

Half of San Francisco's adult population was now over forty years old. As a result of this aging trend, an increasing proportion of the population were experiencing declining physical strength and productivity, which residents felt boded ill for the community's future. One concrete and very important manifestation of these difficulties was the inability of the *municipio* to find enough men to fill the annual eighteen-man quota for civil and religious *cargo* positions. Moreover, there had been increasing pressure for independence from San Francisco on the part of some of the lowland *rancho* subcommunities (*agencias*); two had already won semiautonomous status from the regional government, and at least one of these was continuing to press for even greater independence.[11] All of these trends led residents of San Francisco to worry about the collectivity's future and to seek ways to diminish the impact of depopulation.

THE BIRTH CONTROL TREE

Although some of the reasons for the depopulation of San Francisco were new, concern about the size and strength of the collectivity was not. The conflict between the collective desire for a large and populous community and individual women's wishes to have few children had had a long, dramatic history in the *municipio*.

On many occasions during my fieldwork, men told me how, some twenty years before, they had cut down a tree whose bark was used by women as a contraceptive. They needed to eliminate the tree, they said, because so many women were refusing to bear children. This is the story the men told: Not far from the town center and just off a popular path to the lowland hamlets was a tree without a name. Its bark turned red when stripped from its trunk and was said to prevent conception. The large old tree was the only one of its kind known to the people of San Francisco. "Who knows where the seed came from," said one elderly resident; "strange it was the only one." Women who wished to avoid pregnancy brewed tea from the bark and drank it prior to intercourse. This would "burn" their wombs and render them temporarily sterile. This tea was dangerous and powerful, "like poison," some said. It could kill an incautious user. Women who drank the tea several times grew emaciated and weak. Even if they subsequently wished to bear children, as many as eight years might pass before a pregnancy.

Some said the users went secretly at night to get bark from the tree. Others thought that itinerant peddler women from an enemy town secretly sold Franciscanas strips of the dried bark along with other wares. Said one man, "It was they who deceived our women into not wanting children because they didn't want our town to grow."

A group of San Francisco's men were at work one day cutting back brush from the path that passed near the tree. They could see it from where they worked, almost stripped of its bark from frequent use. "Let's get rid of it," one of them said quietly; "we must have more children in this town." The others quickly agreed. "So," explained one who had been there, "we cut down the tree and tore its roots right out." They used the trunk to restore a nearby bridge in disrepair and returned home tired but satisfied with their work. (In an alternate version of the story, the men saw the tree, were angered, and stripped it entirely of its bark, causing it to die.)

I asked some of the men who said they were responsible for the act why they had killed the tree. "We were angry," one told me. "The women weren't having babies. They were lazy and didn't want to produce children." Another said that the women "had stopped making children. We were working hard with our men's work, but they weren't doing any of their women's work." One who said he remembered the incident explained that "the town was small and we wanted it to grow. We wanted a big town and we needed more people. But the women wouldn't cooperate." A woman I interviewed saw the men's motives differently. "The men depended on the women," she said. "They couldn't have their children by themselves. But the women were walking free. The men pulled out the tree to control the women so they'd have children for them."

My research in San Francisco led me to ask often about the birth control tree. Every man I asked had heard of it although none could tell me its name or show me one like it. These days, they explained, people seldom passed the spot where it had grown because a better road to the lowlands had been built. After weeks of asking, I nearly concluded that the tree was only a myth. Persistence finally led me to a woman who said her husband could show me the tree. He was more than reluctant to comply. "What if people found out that it has grown back?" he said. "What if they began to use it again? Then what would happen to the town?"

I continued to press him. Finally, he said he would not show me the tree but would take my field assistant's nine-year-old son to see it. The boy could later lead me to the spot. During the same period, one of the men who said he had participated in the destruction of the tree agreed to see if it had possibly regenerated. During different weeks, each of the two informants independently led me to the same clump of *Styrax argenteus*. As the second man showed me the abundant young growth, he expressed surprise that several had grown where only one had been.

The women I asked about the tree were consistently less informative than the men. While all the men knew of the birth control tree, the majority of women said they had never even heard of it, let alone used it to avoid pregnancy. The men did not believe the women were as ignorant as they claimed. I asked one man how the men had learned of the tree if the women had used it only in secret. He replied, "Of course the women think they have their secrets. But we men were able to find out. They have no secrets from us."

THE WOMEN'S RESPONSES TO PRESSURES TO REPRODUCE

There are several morals to this story, but the inevitability of negative reactions to behaviors that place individual interests above those of the collectivity is a very important one. In San Francisco, married women with few or no children were seen as selfish and socially negligent regardless of whether their low fertility was natural or willfully induced. Such women were particularly vulnerable to gossip, much of which centered on their fertility behavior. They were sharply and repeatedly criticized for causing miscarriages and using contraceptives. Some were even accused of infanticide. All of their acts were carefully monitored by relatives and other interested parties to detect any efforts to avoid pregnancy. For example, lemon juice was widely regarded as a contraceptive and an abortifacient.[12] After failing to conceive during her first year of marriage, one woman fell subject to her mother-in-law's constant gossip and criticism for avoiding her reproductive responsibilities by eating too much of the fruit. Another woman determinedly broke her young daughter of the habit of enjoying lemons, for she feared that they would damage her daughter's fertility.

Women with small families were susceptible to gossip about marital infidelity, which diminished the social status of their husbands as well. As a middle-aged mother of six explained, "The women who are most likely to go with other men are the ones who don't have much work to do. They have time for sex. But if you have a lot of kids like I do, you have to work very hard all the time. The tiredness takes over at the end of the day and you don't have time to think about the husbands of other women. You don't have time to go out looking for men." The targets of such gossip attributed it to envy of the relative wealth and freedom they enjoyed as a result of having small families—and they adamantly denied that their low fertility was due to contraceptives.

Contraceptives were, however, readily available at the town's two government-run health centers; one even provided the services free of charge. The Mexican government's interest in lowering its national birth rate had led it since 1972 to promote family planning aggressively.[13] The walls of both clinics were decorated almost exclusively with posters demonstrating the benefits of small families and *paternidad responsable* (responsible parenthood).[14] They were written in simple language with humorous illustrations. The text of a typical one read: "What will happen when we are more? We will have less money . . . less food . . . less education . . . less space . . . less clothing . . . less peace. You can avoid these problems if you plan your family. Now planning is easier! Consult the family doctor at the Social Security Clinic although you may not be insured. *The consultation is free.*"[15] Each clinic assigned its staff monthly inscription quotas for new contraceptive users. Health center personnel were expected to undertake house-to-house campaigns to introduce fecund women to modern birth control techniques.

Overwhelmingly, Franciscanas rejected these government services. For the period between January 1980 and February 1981, records from the two clinics indicated that thirteen Franciscanas initiated contraceptive use—only 7 percent of women between the ages of eighteen and forty-five. These women used contraceptives for an average of just 3.5 months before stopping, and only one continued using contraceptives for longer than six months.

When I asked several who said they wanted no more children why they did not seek the means to avoid pregnancy, they revealed an extreme reluctance to engage in socially disapproved behavior. Some indicated they would never consider obtaining birth control from government clinics because they would be ashamed to be publicly "registered" as a user of contraceptives. This same fear of community censure led women to avoid other means of fertility control and even the kinds of behavior that could be construed as attempts at fertility limitation. When I naively asked one of the town midwives if she had ever been asked to perform an abortion, she looked at me and said, "They wouldn't dare." Similarly, a Franciscana suffering from menstrual delay was afraid to inquire locally for a remedy. Even though she was convinced that she was not pregnant, she was sure she would be accused of abortion if she took a remedy to induce menstrual bleeding.

The women responded to these pressures to reproduce not simply by refusing to use contraceptives but also by denying they knew anything whatsoever about ways to limit fertility. It seemed they felt that merely possessing information would be interpreted as evidence of their malevolent intentions. When I asked women the direct question, "Do you know of any herbs or other remedies that can be used to avoid pregnancy?" only 11 percent mentioned specific techniques such as the infamous birth control tree. Another 6 percent said they believed that ways existed but knew of none themselves. The remaining 83 percent said they believed there were no traditional ways to avoid getting pregnant. An even larger proportion (86 percent) said they knew no ways to induce an abortion. Even Franciscanas who considered themselves authorities on a great many subjects pleaded ignorance when it came to birth limitation.

Denial, however, did not necessarily imply ignorance. Probes revealed that 60 percent who had initially said they knew no ways to limit births had at least heard of the existence of techniques for fertility limitation. The vast majority of these respondents named modern rather than traditional methods and the responses were often quite oblique. For example, to the questions, "Is there *anything* that can be done to not have children if one doesn't want to have them? If so, what things?" typical responses were: "Yes, in the health center"; "I know the doctor has some"; "They say there are pills, medicines." Other replies explicitly identified the government as the source of contraceptives, shifting the question away from indigenous techniques for birth limitation to methods made available from outside the community. For example, "These days the government doesn't allow people to have so many children. It gives them medicines so they won't"; and "There used to be lots of herbs. Now, the government sends us doctors."

Yet none of the affirmative responses to the questions about knowledge of birth control could be interpreted as endorsements of contraceptive use. No respondent seemed to regard the available fertility-limiting techniques as liberating or as helping them to achieve their expressed goals of having small families. In fact, when responding affirmatively to the probe concerning their knowledge of contraceptives, the women would frequently volunteer a disclaimer in an apparent effort to dissociate themselves even further from the information, even though the probe did not concern their own experiences with contraceptives. For instance; "Well, yes, I have heard that there are medicines available, but I haven't tried them"; "Yes, there are remedies in the health center, but I haven't looked into it"; and, "They say there are medicines in the health center, but I myself haven't used any." Even most of those few in my study population (four out of six women) whose health center records revealed a history of contraceptive use strenuously denied use when directly asked during interviews.

Others told me with extreme caution what they knew about contraception. Some who during interviews had denied all knowledge of contraceptive methods subsequently came to my house to tell me about plants or other techniques that had previously "escaped" their memories. Even knowledge that seemed to me benign was very reluctantly conveyed if it pertained to birth limitation. For example, after initially denying she knew any remedies to induce an abortion, one woman reconsidered and whispered, "I don't know if this would really work, but some say that it can: carrying heavy loads, carrying heavy tumplines of firewood every day, doing a lot of laundry. It's said this can make one abort." Although this idea might be inferred from the circumstances under which miscarriages were observed to have occurred, women carefully guarded even this much knowledge, for they feared it would be incriminating.

IMPLICATIONS OF THE RESEARCH

These data shed light on the context in which a national population planning program was experienced in a rural indigenous community. The context was political, economic, civic, and cultural. On the part of the Mexican government, the decision to promote family planning among indigenous populations was politically delicate, for many Mexican nationalists regard the preservation of their Indian cultural heritage as fundamental to their cultural identity as Mexicans, and aggressive programs to limit the growth of indigenous groups may be perceived as cultural genocide.[16] However, because economic development could not keep pace, the need to check population growth proved more pressing than the state's concerns with the politics of ethnic preservation. Terry L. McCoy has shown, moreover, that the recognition that the government could be destabilized by unchecked growth among less than fully loyal social classes and cultural groups provided significant impetus for the Mexican population policy.[17] In Mexico, as in other developing countries, such policies are used to further state consolidation.

A reduction in San Francisco's rate of population growth was, as we have seen, the last thing the male guardians of the collectivity wanted. While appreciating the value of birth control for the nation in the abstract, and in some cases even wishing for relatively small families themselves, the men unambivalently rejected family planning for the people of San Francisco. In contrast, the women were caught between their desires to have very few children and inexorable local social pressures to be prolific. Because of this pressure, government family planning services could not help the women achieve their own fertility goals. In fact, the existence of these services may have made it even more difficult for the women to practice covert fertility limitation: with the availability of modern contraceptives in the community, women fell under even more suspicion than before.

It has all too often been assumed that women's reproductive goals could be understood by analyzing those of the larger collectivities of which they are a part. However, when collectivities have specific fertility goals, it is reasonable to expect that these goals will conflict with the reproductive desires of at least some of the female members of the group. The extent to which women successfully implement their individual fertility goals depends on a number of factors that vary according to the characteristics of the particular society in which they live. These include the nature of the gender-based power relations and the extent to which women feel they can support one another in controversy. In stratified societies, issues related to social class and ethnicity also play a part, and women may be torn by conflicting sets of interests.[18] Studies that fail to consider *both* these broad sociopolitical conditions and the interests and desires of individual women will understate the complexity, misrepresent the realities, and yield questionable conclusions about reproductive policy and reproductive behavior.

NOTES

Support for this research was generously provided by grants from the National Science Foundation (BNS-8016431), National Institute for Child Health Development (HD-04612), and the Wenner-Gren Foundation for Anthropological Research (3387). Arthur J. Rubel provided truly valuable assistance during all phases of this research, including the production of this report. Judith Friedlander's suggestions also contributed importantly to the manuscript.

1. Burton Benedict, "Social Regulation of Fertility," in *The Structure of Human Populations,* ed. G. A. Harrison and A. J. Boyce (Oxford: Clarendon Press, 1972), 73–89; Carole Browner, "Abortion Decision Making: Some Findings from Colombia," *Studies in Family Planning* 10, no. 3 (1979): 96–106; Thomas K. Burch and Murray Gendall, "Extended Family Structure and Fertility: Some Conceptual and Methodological Issues," in *Culture and Population: A Collection of Current Studies,* ed. Steven Polgar (Cambridge, Mass.: Schenkman Publishing Co.; Chapel Hill, N.C.: Carolina Population Center, 1971), 87–104; Ronald Freedman, "The Sociology of Human Fertility: A Trend Report and Bibliography," *Current Sociology* 10/11, no. 2 (1961–62): 35–121; Frank Lorimer, *Culture and Human Fertility: A Study of the Relation of Cultural Conditions to Fertility in Nonindustrial and Transitional Societies* (Paris: Unesco, 1958); John F. Marshall, Susan Morris, and Steven Polgar, "Culture and Natality: A Preliminary Classified Bibliography," *Current Anthropology* 13, no. 2 (April 1972): 268–78; Moni Nag, *Factors Affecting Human Fertility in Nonindustrial Societies: A Cross-cultural Study* (New Haven, Conn.: Human Relations Area Files Press, 1976); Steven Polgar, "Population History and Population Policies from an Anthropological Perspective." *Current Anthropology* 13, no. 2 (April 1972): 203–11.

2. Bernard Berelson, *Population Policy in Developed Countries* (New York: McGraw-Hill Book Co., 1974); J. C. Caldwell, "Population Policy: A Survey of Commonwealth Africa," in *The Population of Tropical Africa,* ed. John C. Caldwell and Chukuka Okonjo (New York: Columbia University Press, 1968), 368–75; Leslie Corsa and Deborah Oakley, *Population Planning* (Ann Arbor: University of Michigan Press, 1979), chap. 5, 155–94; William L. Langer, "Checks on Population Growth, 1750–1850," *Scientific American* 226, no. 2 (1972): 92–99; Benjamin White, "Demand for Labor and Population Growth in Colonial Java," *Human Ecology* 1, no. 3 (1973): 217–39.
3. Ad Hoc Women's Studies Committee against Sterilization Abuse, *Workbook on Sterilization and Sterilization Abuse* (Bronxville, N.Y.: Sarah Lawrence College, 1978); Toni Cade, "The Pill: Genocide or Liberation?" in *The Black Woman,* ed. Toni Cade (New York: New American Library, 1970), 162–69; Lucinda Cisler, "Unfinished Business: Birth Control and Women's Liberation," in *Sisterhood Is Powerful: An Anthology of Writings from the Women's Liberation Movement,* ed. Robin Morgan (New York: Vintage Books, 1970), 245–89; Sally Covington, "Is 'Broader' Better? Reproductive Rights and Elections '84," *Taking Control: The Magazine of the Reproductive Rights National Network* 1, no. 1 (1984): 6–8; Boston Women's Health Book Collective, *Our Bodies, Ourselves: A Book by and for Women* (New York: Simon & Schuster, 1971); Reproductive Rights National Network, "Caught in the Crossfire: Third World Women and Reproductive Rights," *Reproductive Rights Newsletter* 5, no. 3 (Autumn 1983): 1–13; Helen Rodriguez-Trias, *Sterilization Abuse* (New York: Barnard College, Women's Center, 1978).
4. Rosalind Pollack Petchesky, *Abortion and Woman's Choice: The State, Sexuality, and Reproduction Freedom* (New York and London: Longman, Inc., 1984), esp. 10.
5. Eric R. Wolf, "Types of Latin American Peasantry: A Preliminary Discussion," *American Anthropologist* 57 (1955): 452–71, and "Closed Corporate Peasant Communities in Mesoamerica and Central Java," *Southwestern Journal of Anthropology* 13 (1957): 1–18.
6. Clifford R. Barnett, Jean Jackson, and Howard M. Cann, "Childspacing in a Highland Guatemala Community," in Polgar, ed. (n. 1 above), 139–48; Paula H. Hass, "Contraceptive Choices for Latin American Women," *Populi* 3 (1976): 14–24; Jenifer Oberg, "Natality in a Rural Village in Northern Chile," in Polgar, ed., 124–38; Michele Goldzieher Shedlin and Paula E. Hollerbach, "Modern and Traditional Fertility Regulation in a Mexican Community: The Process of Decision-Making," *Studies in Family Planning* 12, no. 6/7 (1981): 278–96. John Mayone Stycos, *Ideology, Faith, and Family Planning in Latin America: Studies in Public and Private Opinion on Fertility Control* (New York: McGraw-Hill Book Co., 1971).
7. It should be noted that the women's professed negative attitudes toward childbearing and child rearing generally were not apparent in their behavior toward their children.
8. C. H. Browner, "Gender Roles and Social Change: A Mexican Case," *Ethnology* 25, no. 2 (April 1986): 89–106.
9. Arthur J. Rubel, "Some Unexpected Health Consequences of Political Relations in Mexico" (paper presented at the eighty-second annual meeting of the American Anthropological Association, Chicago, 1983).
10. Consejo Nacional de Población México (CONAPO), *México Demográfico: Breviario* (Mexico City: CONAPO, 1979), 52, 78. More recent statistics on out-migration are not available.
11. Anselmo Hernandez Lopez, personal communication, Oaxaca, Mexico, 1981.
12. C. H. Browner and Bernard Ortiz de Montellano, "Herbal Emmenagogues Used by Women in Columbia and Mexico," in *Plants Used in Indigenous Medicine: A Biocultural Approach,* ed. Nina Etkin (New York: Docent Publishers, 1986), 32–47.
13. Victor Urquidi et al., *La explosión humana* (Mexico City: Litoarte, 1974); Frederick C. Turner, *Responsible Parenthood: The Politics of Mexico's New Population Policies* (Washington, D.C.: American Enterprise Institute for Public Policy Research, 1974).
14. This official slogan of the government's population control program was chosen to emphasize the concrete advantages of small families to individual couples rather than the macrodemographic benefits of a reduced national birth rate (Terry L. McCoy, "A Paradigmatic Analysis of Mexican Population Policy," in *The Dynamics of Population Policy in Latin America,* ed. Terry L. McCoy [Cambridge, Mass.: Ballinger Publishing Co., 1974], 377–408, esp. 397).

15. Mexico City: Instituto Mexicano de Seguro Social (IMSS); italics in original. In the mid-1960s, the government's Social Solidarity Program (*Solidaridad Social*) extended the social security health system to cover the health needs of some rural areas. Family planning services were part of the coverage.
16. [Gonzalo] Aquirre Beltrán, *Obra polémica* (Mexico City: Instituto Nacional de Antropología e Historia, 1976); Luis Leñero Otero, *Valores ideológicos y las políticas de población en México* (Mexico City: Editorial Edicol, 1979), 115–17.
17. McCoy, 377–408.
18. Floya Anthias and Nira Yuval-Davis, "Contextualizing Feminism: Gender, Ethnic and Class Divisions," *Feminist Review* 15 (Winter 1983): 62–75, esp. 70–71.

PROCREATION STORIES: REPRODUCTION, NURTURANCE, AND PROCREATION IN LIFE NARRATIVES OF ABORTION ACTIVISTS

Faye Ginsburg

The residents of Fargo, North Dakota—a small metropolitan center providing commercial and service industries for the surrounding rural area—pride themselves on their clean air, regular church attendance, rich topsoil, and their actual and metaphorical distance from places like New York City. The orderly pace of Fargo's daily life was disrupted in the fall of 1981 when the Fargo Woman's Health Center—the first free-standing facility in the state to publicly offer abortions—opened for business. A right-to-life[1] coalition against the clinic formed immediately. Soon after, a pro-choice group emerged to respond to the antiabortion activities. Each side asked for support by presenting itself as under attack, yet simultaneously claimed to represent the "true" interests of the community. The groups have evolved and fissioned. There are approximately 1000 potentially active supporters on each side and a hard core of 10 to 20 activists.

Broadly sketched, two positions emerged. For the pro-life movement in Fargo, the availability of abortion in their own community represented the intrusion of secularism, narcissism, materialism, and anomie, and the reshaping of women into structural men. Prochoice activists reacted to right-to-life protesters as the forces of narrow-minded intolerance who would deny women access to a choice that is seen as fundamental to women's freedom and ability to overcome sexual discrimination.

When pro-life forces failed to close the clinic through conventional political tactics,[2] they shifted their strategy. They currently are engaged in a battle for the clinic's clientele. Competition is focused increasingly on winning the minds, bodies, and power to define the women who might choose to violate a basic cultural script—the dominant American procreation story—in which pregnancy necessarily results in childbirth and motherhood, preferably within marriage.

The local controversy over the clinic opening in Fargo revealed at close range how the struggle over abortion rights has become a contested domain for control over the constellation of meanings attached to reproduction in America. In the course of fieldwork,[3] it became clear to me that this conflict does not indicate two fixed and irreconcilable positions. Rather, the social movements orga-

Reproduced by permission of the American Anthropological Association from *American Ethnologist* 14:4, November 1987. Not for further reproduction.

nized around abortion provide arenas for innovation where cultural and social definitions of gender are in the process of material and semiotic reorganization.

In each movement, then, a particular understanding of reproduction is demonstrated through abortion activism. This was especially apparent in life stories[4]—narratively shaped fragments of more comprehensive life histories—I collected with female abortion activists.[5] Such narratives, which I am calling procreation stories, reveal the way in which women use their activism to frame and interpret their experiences—both historical and biographical. The stories create provisional solutions to disruptions in a coherent cultural model for the place of reproduction and motherhood in the female life course in contemporary America. They illuminate how those dimensions of experience considered "private" in American culture intersect with particular social and historical conditions that distinguish the memberships of each group. In the ways that the rhetoric and action of abortion activism are incorporated into life stories, one can see how cultural definitions of the female life course, and the social consequences implied, are selected, rejected, reordered, and reproduced in new form.

This paper is based on my own fieldwork with local women activists engaged in the Fargo abortion controversy from 1981 to 1983. I chose subjects who were most prominent in local activity at the time and who reflected, in my estimation, the range of diversity encompassed in the active memberships of both pro-life and pro-choice groups in terms of age, socioeconomic status, religious affiliation, household and marriage arrangements, style of activism, and the like. Altogether I collected 21 life stories from right-to-life activists and 14 from pro-choice activists. While most of these people are still active, each side continues to undergo rapid permutations both locally and nationally. Thus, the benefits of in-depth participant observation research must be balanced against the debits of a small sample bound by the conditions of a particular time and setting. In addition, because of space limitations, I can present only a few cases, which are illustrative of themes that are prominent in the narratives more generally. However, my conclusions are confirmed in other qualitative studies of abortion activists (for example, Luker 1984), which also find abortion activism linked to a more general integrative process. For example, in an article discussing the role abortion seems to play in activists' lives, authors Callahan and Callahan write:

> The general debate has seen an effort, on all sides, to make abortion fit into some overall coherent scheme of values, one that can combine personal convictions and consistency with more broadly held social values. Abortion poses a supreme test in trying to achieve that coherence. It stands at the juncture of a number of value systems, which continually joust with each other for dominance, but none of which by itself can do full justice to all the values that, with varying degrees of insistence and historical rootedness, clamor for attention and respect [1984:219].

On the basis of such findings, it seems appropriate to use life stories as texts in which abortion is a key symbol around which activists are interpreting and reorienting their lives. More generally, this suggests a model for understanding how female social activism in the American context operates to mediate the construction of self and gender with larger social, political, and cultural processes.

REPRODUCTION, GENERATION, AND NURTURANCE

Surveys of representative samples of pro-life and pro-choice activists have not established any clear correlations between such activity and conventional social categories. Activists span and divide religious, ethnic, and occupational lines. The core of membership on both sides is primarily white, middle class,[6] and female[7] (Granberg 1981). Ideologically, the connections drawn between abortion activism and other social issues are diverse

(Ginsburg 1986:76–81). Of the life stories I collected from abortion activists in Fargo, in almost all cases, pro-choice and pro-life alike, women described a coming to consciousness regarding abortion in relation to some critical realignment of personal and social identity, usually related to reproduction. Initially, this recognition only seemed to confound the problem of trying to understand the differences between the women on opposite sides of the issue. From accounts of the early histories of Fargo activists, up to the age of 18 or so, it would be hard to predict whether women would end up pro-choice or pro-life in their views. Devout Catholics became ardent feminists; middle-class, college-educated, liberal Protestants became staunch pro-lifers. As I puzzled over the seeming convergences in catalyzing experiences, social backgrounds, and even sentiments—most see themselves as working toward the reform of society as a whole—I began to notice a generational distinction.

The pro-choice activists cluster in a group born in the 1940s. For the most part, they had reached adulthood—which generally meant marriage and children—in the late 1960s and early 1970s. Their life stories indicate that contact with the social movements of that period, particularly the second wave of feminism, was a central experience for nearly all of them. They describe their encounter with these movements as a kind of awakening or passage from a world defined by motherhood into one seen as filled with broader possibilities. For most of these women, feminism offered new resources with which to understand and frame their lives; it provided an analysis, a community of others, and a means for engaging in social change that legitimated their own experience.

By contrast, the right-to-life women cluster in two groups. Those born in the 1920s were most active in pro-life work in the early 1970s. A second cohort, the one currently most active, was born in the 1950s. Typically, this latter group was made up of women who had worked prior to having children and left wage labor when they became mothers. This transition occurred in the late 1970s or even more recently, a period when feminism was on the wane as an active social movement and pro-life and anti-ERA activity were on the rise. This latter group claims to have been or even be feminist in many respects (that is, on issues such as comparable worth). Many describe their commitment to the right-to-life movement as a kind of conversion; it occurs most frequently around the birth of a first or second child when many women of this group decided to move out of the paid work force to stay home and raise children.

Let me clarify that I am not arguing that all abortion activists fall neatly into one or another historical cohort. As is the case in most anthropological studies in complex societies, my study is small and local, allowing for fine-grained, long-term study that can reveal new understandings but not necessarily support broad generalizations. In this case, the appearance of a generational shift, even in this small sample, is intended less as an explanation and more as a reminder of the importance of temporal factors in the dialectics of social movements. In other words, social activists may hold different positions due not only to social and ideological differences. Differing views may also be produced by historical changes, which include their experience of the opposition at different points over the life course. On the basis of my research, I would argue that this might be particularly relevant in conflicts tied so closely to life cycle events. In the narratives, *all* the women are struggling to come to terms with problematic life-cycle transitions, but in each group, the way they experience those as problematic is associated with very particular historical situations. Abortion activism seems to mediate between these two domains, as a frame for action and interpretation of the self in relation to the world. For most of these women, their procreation stories create harmonious narrative out of the dissonance of history, both personal and generational.

In his classic essay "The Problem of Generations," Karl Mannheim underscores the importance of this nexus between the individual life cycle and rapidly changing historical conditions in understanding generational shifts in the formation of political consciousness and social movements:

> In the case of generations, the "fresh contact" with the social and cultural heritage is determined not by mere social change but by fundamental biological factors. We can accordingly differentiate between two types of "fresh contact": one based on a shift in social relations, and the other in vital factors [1952:383].
>
> The *sociological* problem of generations . . . begins at that point where the sociological relevance of these biological factors is discovered [1952:381].

To use Mannheim's suggestion, one must consider the intersection of two unfolding processes in order to understand what attracts women to opposing movements in the abortion controversy. One is the "biological factors," the trajectory of a woman's sexual and reproductive experiences over her life course and her interpretation of those events. The second is the historical moment shaping the culture when these key transitional points occur. It is this moment of "fresh contact" that creates the conditions of "a changed relationship" and a "novel approach" to the culture that ensures its continual reorganization. Such "fresh contact" is manifest in the self-definition and social actions of women engaged in the abortion controversy, some of whose life stories are analyzed below. Their narratives reveal how the embracing of a pro-life or pro-choice position emerges specifically out of a confluence of reproductive and generational experiences. In the negotiation of critical moments in the female life course with an ever-shifting social environment, the contours of their own biographies and the larger cultural and historical landscape are measured, reformulated, and given new meaning.

Such reconstructing is most marked at critical transitional points in the life course. In situations of rapid change when the normative rules for an assumed life trajectory are in question, these life-cycle shifts are experienced as crises, revealing contention over cultural definitions. In other words, when the interpretation of a particular life event—abortion or more generally the transition to motherhood, for example—becomes the object of political struggle, it indicates a larger disruption occurring in the social order as well. What emerges in the biographical narratives of these women is an apparent dissonance between cultural codes, social process, and individual transformation in the life course. Analytically, then, life stories can be seen as the effort of individuals to create continuity between subjective and social experience, the past and current action and belief.

These orientations provide a useful framework for interpreting the narratives of abortion activists in relation to the social movements that engage them. The battles they fight are loci for potential cultural and social transformation; in life stories, change is incorporated, ordered, and assigned meaning by and for the individual. This process is central to the "changed relationships" of many women to American culture that have generated struggles over conflicting views of the interpretation of gender in the last two decades. Thus, in the case of abortion, two mutually exclusive interpretations and arenas of action are formulated, which give the narrator symbolic control over problematic transitions in the female life cycle.

I am arguing that these transitions constitute life crises for women at this moment in American history because of the gap between experiences of discontinuous changes in their own biographies and the available cultural models for marking them, both cognitively and socially. As increasing numbers of women are entering the wage labor market and traditional marriage and familial arrangements seem to be in disarray, it is hardly surprising that the relationship of women to reproduction, and mothering in particular, has been thrown open to reinterpretation.

In the United States, where the culture and economy are underwritten by an ideal of individual autonomy and achievement and the separation of workplace and home, the fact of dependency over the life course has been hidden in the household. Assigned to the "private realm"—the domain of unpaid labor performed by women serving as emotional and often material providers for infants, children, the sick, the elderly—nurturance thus escapes consideration as a larger cultural concern. Rather, the general social problem of caring for dependent human beings is linked to biological reproduction and childrearing in heterosexually organized families, all of which are conflated with the category female.[8] When women vote with their bodies to eschew the imperatives of American domesticity by remaining single, childless, and/or entering wage labor in large numbers, both the conditions and native understandings of nurturance and reproduction necessarily change.

Such changes are central themes in the procreation stories of abortion activists. While their "life scripts" are cast against each other, both provide ways for managing the structural opposition in America between work and parenthood that still shapes the lives of most women and men in this culture. Because contrasting definitions of the cultural and personal meaning of reproduction are being created in a contested domain, they are shaped dialectically. Each side attempts to both incorporate and repudiate the claims to truth of their opposition, casting as unnatural, immoral, or false other possible formulations. In the abortion debate, both positions serve to "naturalize" constructions regarding women's work, sexuality, and motherhood, and the relationships among them, thus claiming a particular view of American culture and the place of men and women in it in a way that accommodates discontinuities and contradictions.

The location of and responsibility for nurturance in relationship to biological reproduction is of critical concern, the salient value and contradiction for women on both sides of the debate. Nurturance is claimed by activists as a source of moral authority for female action. Yet, it is also understood as the culturally assigned attribute that puts women at a disadvantage socially, economically, and politically, confining them to the unappreciated tasks of caring for dependent people. These two views of the "proper" place of reproduction and nurturance in the female life course are the poles around which activists' life stories are constituted.

Activists' views on abortion are linked to a very diverse range of moral, ethical, and religious questions, which I discuss in more detail elsewhere (Ginsburg 1986).[9] In this paper, however, I have confined my analysis to the issues that emerge in their life stories. My goal here is an effort to understand how abortion activism and abstract notions tied to it mediate between historical experience, construction of self, and social action. What I think is striking about the emergence of nurturance as a central theme in these narratives is that it ties female life-cycle transitions to the central philosophical questions of each side: the pro-life concern with the protection of nascent life, and the pro-choice concern with the rights and obligations of women, those to whom the care of that nascent life is culturally assigned.

THE LIFE STORIES

The Pro-Choice Narratives

The pro-choice narratives were drawn from women activists who organized to defend the Fargo abortion clinic; most were born between 1942–52. They represent a range of backgrounds in terms of their natal families, yet all were influenced as young adults by the social unrest of the late 1960s and early 1970s, and by the women's movement in particular. While their current household, conjugal, and work arrangements differ, for almost all, the strong commitment to pro-choice activism was connected to specific life-cycle events, generally having to do with experiences and choices around sexuality, pregnancy, and childbearing, including the choice not to have children.

A central figure of the current controversy in Fargo is Kay Bellevue, an abortion rights activist since 1972. Kay grew up in the Midwest, the oldest of seven children. Her father was a Baptist minister; her mother worked as a homemaker and part-time public school teacher. In her senior year of college, Kay got pregnant and married. Like almost *all* of the women activists, regardless of their position on abortion, Kay's transition to motherhood was surrounded by ambivalence.

> I enjoyed being home, but I could never stay home all the time. I have never done that in my life. After being home one year and taking care of a kid, I felt my mind was a wasteland. And [my husband and I] were so poor we could almost never go out together.

Although her *behavior* was not that different from that of many right-to-life women—that is, as a young mother she became involved in community associations—Kay's interpretation of her actions stresses the limitations of motherhood; by contrast, pro-life women faced with the same dilemma emphasize the drawbacks of the workplace. Not surprisingly, for both groups of women, voluntary work for a "cause" was an acceptable and satisfying way of managing to balance the pleasures and duties of motherhood with the structural isolation of that work as it is organized in America. La Leche League, for example, is a group where one stands an equal chance of running into a pro-life or pro-choice women. In her early 20s, Kay became active in a local chapter of that organization, an international group promoting breast-feeding and natural childbirth. She marks this as a key event.

> My first child had not been a pleasant birth experience so I went [to a La Leche meeting] and I was really intrigued. There were people talking about this childbirth experience like it was the most fantastic thing you'd ever been through. I certainly didn't feel that way. I had a very long labor. I screamed, I moaned, my husband thought I was dying. So . . . this group introduced me to a whole different conception of childbirth and my second experience was so different I couldn't believe it.
>
> And the way I came to feminism was that through all of this, I became acutely aware of how little physicians actually knew about women's bodies . . . So I became a real advocate for women to stand up for their rights, starting with breastfeeding.

Surprisingly, the concerns Kay voices are not so different from those articulated by her neighbors and fellow citizens who so vehemently oppose her work.

In 1972, Kay moved to Fargo; she remembers this transition as a time of crisis. Her parents were divorcing, one of her children was having problems, and Kay became pregnant for the fifth time.

> Then I ended up having an abortion myself. My youngest was 18 months old and I accidentally got pregnant. We had four small kids at the time and we decided if we were going to make it as a family unit, we had all the stress we could tolerate if we were going to survive.

In her more public role, as was the case in these personal decisions regarding abortion, Kay always linked her activism to a strong commitment to maintain family ties. As such, she was responding to accusations made by right-to-life opponents that abortion advocacy means an oppositional stance toward marriage, children, and community.

> I think it's easy for them to stereotype us as having values very different than theirs and that's not the case at all. Many of the people who get abortions have values very similar to the anti-abortion people. The Right-to-lifers don't know how deeply I care for my own family and how involved I am, since I have four children and spent the early years of my life working for a breast-feeding organization.

Kay particularly resents the casting of pro-choice activists by right-to-lifers as not only "antifamily" but "godless" as well. Although she stopped attending church services when she got married—something she feels could stigmatize her in a community noted for its church attendance—Kay nonetheless connects her activism to religious principles of social justice learned in her natal family.

> I have always acted on what to me are Judeo-Christian principles. The Ten Commandments, plus love thy neighbor. I was raised by my family to have a very strong sense of ethics and it's still with me. I have a strong concern about people and social issues. I've had a tough time stomaching what goes on in the churches in the name of Christianity. I've found my sense of community elsewhere. I think pro-choice people have a very strong basis in theology for their loving, caring perspective. . . . It's very distressing to me that, particularly the people opposed to abortion will attempt to say their moral beliefs are the only correct ones.

Such stereotypes, to which most of the pro-choice women in Fargo were extremely sensitive, are addressed implicitly or explicitly in the repeated connections these activists made between abortion rights and a larger claim to the cultural values of nurturance which, in their view, women represent.

These concerns are prominent, for example, in the narratives of other abortion rights advocates. Janice Sundstrom, like most of the pro-choice activists in Fargo, frames her story by emphasizing her differentiation from, rather than integration with, her childhood milieu.

> In 1945, shortly after I was born, my mom and dad moved here and brought me along and left all the other children with relations back in Illinois. I think I'm different from the rest of them because I had the experience of being the only child at a time when they had far too many children to deal with.

While the transformations Janice eventually experienced are cast, in her story, as almost predictable, they hardly seem the inevitable outcome of her youth and adolescence: 12 years in Catholic parochial school and marriage to her high-school sweetheart a year after graduation, followed immediately by two pregnancies.

> We were both 19 then and I didn't want to have another child. We were both in school and working and there we were with this kid. But I didn't have any choice. There was no option for me about birth control because I was still strongly committed to the Church's teaching. And then, three months later, I was pregnant again. After Jodie was born I started taking pills and that's what ended the Church for me.

For Janice, ambivalent encounters with reproduction—in this case the problem of birth control that made her question her church—are key events in her story. In this way, her interpretation of her experiences resembles the way that pregnancy and pro-life activism are linked in the right-to-life narratives discussed later on. It is a central pivoting moment in her life, which turned her toward alternative cultural models.

> Up to that time, I felt very strongly about abortion as my church had taught me to think and somehow between 1968 and 1971—those years were crucial to the political development of a lot of people in my generation—I came to have different feelings about abortion. My feeling toward abortion grew out of my personal experiences with friends who had abortions and a sensitivity to the place of women in this society.

What is striking in the connections Janice goes on to make to her abortion rights position is not its *difference* from that of her opponents, but its similarities. She is disturbed by cultural currents that promote, in her view, narcissistic attitudes toward sexuality and personal fulfillment in which the individual denies any responsibility to kin, community, and the larger social order. Several pro-choice women referred to this constellation of concerns as "midwestern feminism." They are described as natural attributes possessed and represented by women. In Janice's words,

> It's important that we remember our place, that we remember we are the caregivers, that we remember that nurturing is important, that we maintain the value system that has been given to us and that has resided in us and that we bring it with us into that new structure. . . . It's impor-

tant that we bring to that world the recognition that 80-hour work weeks aren't healthy for anyone—that children suffer if they miss relationships with their fathers and that fathers suffer from missing relationships with their children. This society has got to begin recognizing its responsibility for caring for its children.

Such concerns are emblematic of a broader goal of pro-choice women to improve conditions in a less than perfect world. More generally, the agenda of women on the pro-choice side is to use legal and political means to extend the boundaries of the domain of nurturance into the culture as a whole. They are attempting to reformulate the requirements of human reproduction and dependency as conditions to be met collectively. Their narratives reveal both an embracing of nurturance as a valued quality natural to women and the basis of their cultural authority, and their rejecting of it as an attribute that assigns women to childbearing, caretaking, and domesticity. These themes emerge in pro-choice stories as well as in action. In their view, nurturance is broadly defined. It includes the stated and actual preference for nonhierarchical relationships and group organization, and an insistence that their activism is not for personal gain or individual indulgence but in the interests of women and social justice. This utopian subtext of their position is rooted in their historical encounter with feminism. More directly, it is expressed as a desire to create a society more hospitable to the qualities and tasks they identify as female: the reproduction of generative, compassionate, or at least tolerant relationships between family, friends, members of the community, people in the workplace, and even the nation as a whole. In the narratives they construct, their desire to control their own reproduction is linked to a larger goal of (re)producing cultural values of nurturance on a large social scale.

The Right-to-Life Narratives

Right-to-life activists express a similar concern for the preservation of female nurturance. While it is linked directly to biological reproduction, nurturance in their narratives is not natural but achieved. In all the stories of pregnancy and birth told by right-to-life women, the ambivalence of the mother towards that condition—either through reference to the storyteller's own mother or children, or experience of motherhood herself—is invoked and then overcome through a narrative strategy that stresses continuities between generations, as the following quote illustrates. The speaker is Shirley, a 63-year-old widow, part-time nurse, mother of six, and a well-known member of Fargo's comfortable middle class.

> Our Senator, he's not pro-life, sent me a congratulations letter when [my son] John got a teacher of the year award in 1980. I wanted to take the letter back to him and say, 'It was very inconvenient to have this son. My husband was in school and I was working. We thought we needed other things besides a child. And had abortion been available to me, I might have aborted the boy who was teacher of the year.' What a loss to society that would have been. What losses are we having in society now?

The first wave of right-to-life activity in Fargo received much of its support from women of Shirley's cohort, many of whom had recently been widowed and were facing the loss of children from their immediate lives as well. At a moment in their life cycles when the household and kin context for a lifelong vocation of motherhood was diminishing, pro-life work provided an arena for extending that work beyond the boundaries of home and family.

Another woman of that cohort, Helen, also drew cross-generational connections through her right-to-life commitment. Raised in one of Fargo's elite Lutheran families, Helen fulfilled her mother's dream by attending an eastern "seven sisters' school" and going on for a master's degree in social work. After World War II, she married, returned to Fargo, and had three children. There, she has led the life appropriate for the wife of a local retail magnate. She was, until recently, a pro-choice advocate, a position of which her mother disapproved.

> Years ago, as a social worker, even though I reverenced life, I can still see some of those families and how they lived. I was pro-choice because I thought of those little children and how they lived. And I remember my mother saying 'Helena,' (she always called me Helena when it was serious) 'That's murder . . .' And I said, 'Better those children were never born, mother. They live a hell on earth . . .' and she never talked about it to me after that but I'm sure it hurt.

When the clinic opened in 1981, Helen was asked by a member of one of her prayer groups to join the pro-life coalition against the clinic, which she did. She saw her "conversion" to the right-to-life movement as a repudiation of a prior sense of self that had separated her from her mother, who recently died. She links all of these to the circumstances of her own birth.

> I had a sister killed in a car accident before I was born and . . . I don't know if I ever would have been if she hadn't died . . . My mother was so sick when she was pregnant with me because she was still grieving. They wanted to abort her and she said, 'No way.'
>
> So when she died last year and all these checks came in, I gave them to LIFE Coalition and as a thank you note to people, I told them about her story . . . It brought life to me that at her death this could go on.
>
> You know there is one scripture in Isaiah 44 that I especially pray for my family and that says "I knew you before you were formed in your mother's womb. Fear not, for you are my witness."

In this fragment, Helen establishes metaphorical continuity between her pro-life conviction and the opening story of her narrative, in which she reconstucts her own sojourn in her mother's womb, identifying herself simultaneously with her earliest moments of existence and with her mother's trauma as well. As in Shirley's story, the denial and acceptance of mother and child of each other's lives are merged, and then given larger significance as reproductive events are linked figuratively and materially to the right-to-life movement and given new meaning.

The connections of the right-to-life position with overcoming ambivalence toward pregnancy, and the merging of divergent generational identities in the act of recollection are present, though less prominent, in the procreation stories of younger pro-life women as well. Sally Nordsen is part of a cohort of women born between 1952–62 who make up the majority and most dedicated members of Fargo's antiabortion activists. Like most of the other pro-life women of this group, Sally went to college and married soon after her graduation; she worked for seven years as a social worker. In her late 20s, she got pregnant and decided to leave the work force in order to raise her children. Sally regards this decision as a positive one; nonetheless, it was marked by ambivalence.

> I had two days left of work before my resignation was official but Dick was born earlier than expected. So I left the work on my desk and never went back to it. There were so many things that were abrupt. When I went into the hospital it was raining, and when I came out it was snowing. A change of seasons, a change of work habits, a new baby in my life. It was hard. I was so anxious to get home and show this baby off. And when I walked in the door, it was like the weight of the world and I thought, 'What am I going to do with him now?' Well, these fears faded.
>
> So it was a change. When Ken would come home, I would practically meet him at the door with my coat and purse 'cause I wanted to get out of there. I couldn't stand it, you know. And that's still the case sometimes. But the joys outweigh the desire to go back to work.

For Sally and the other pro-life activists her age, the move from wage labor to motherhood occurred in the late 1970s or more recently. Feminism was identified, more often than not, with its distorted reconstruction in the popular media. Women like Sally, who have decided to leave the work force for a "reproductive phase" of their life cycle, are keenly aware that the choices they have made are at odds with the images they see in the popular media of young, single, upwardly mobile corporate women. Sally's colleague, Roberta makes the case succinctly.

> They paint the job world as so glamorous, as if women are all in executive positions. But really, what is the average woman doing? Mostly office work, secretarial stuff. When you watch TV, there aren't women being pictured working at grocery store check-outs.

For Roberta, her decision to leave the workplace represents a critique of what she considers to be the materialism of the dominant culture. For example, she sees in abortion a reevaluation of biological reproduction in the cost-benefit language and mores of the marketplace, and an extension of a more pervasive condition, the increasing commercialization of human relations, especially those involving dependents.

> You know, reasons given for most abortions is how much kids cost. How much work kids are, how much they can change your lifestyle, how they interrupt the timing of your goals. What is ten years out of a 70-year life span? . . . If you don't have your family, if you don't have your values, then what's money, you know?

In this view, legal abortion represents the loss of a locus of unconditional nurturance in the social order and the steady penetration of the forces of the market. In concrete terms, the threat is constituted in the public endorsement of sexuality disengaged from motherhood. From the right-to-life perspective, this situation serves to weaken social pressure on men to take responsibility for the reproductive consequences of intercourse. Pro-life women are fully cognizant of the fragility of traditional marriage arrangements and recognize as well the lack of other social forms that might ensure the emotional and material support of women with children or other dependents. Nonetheless, the movement's supporters continue to be stereotyped as reactionary right-wing housewives unaware of alternative possibilities. Almost all of the Fargo pro-life activists were aware of these representations and addressed them in a dialectical fashion, using them to confirm their own position. As Roberta explained,

> The image that's presented of us as having a lot of kids hanging around and that's all you do at home and you don't get anything else done, that's really untrue. In fact, when we do mailings here, my little one stands between my legs and I use her tongue as a sponge. She loves it and that's the heart of grassroots involvement. That's the bottom. That's the stuff and the substance that makes it all worth it. Kids are what it boils down to. My husband and I really prize them; they are our future and that is what we feel is the root of the whole pro-life thing.

The collective portrait that emerges from these stories, then, is much more complex than the media portrayals of right-to-life women as housewives and others passed by in the sweep of social change. It is not that they discovered an ideology that "fit" some prior sociological category (see notes 6 and 7). Their sense of identification evolves from their own changing experiences with motherhood and wage labor, and in the very process of voicing their views against abortion. In their narratives and the regular performance of their activism, they are, simultaneously, transforming themselves, projecting their vision of the culture onto their own past and future, both pragmatically and symbolically. Sally, for example, describes her former "liberated" ideas about sexuality as a repression of her true self:

> You're looking at somebody who used to think the opposite. I used to think that sex outside of marriage was fine. I think there was part of me that never fully agreed. It wasn't a complete turnaround. It was kind of like inside you know it's not right but you make yourself think it's OK.

Rather than simply defining themselves in opposition to what they understand feminist ideology and practice to be, many of the younger right-to-life women claim to have held that position and to have transcended it. For example, a popular lecture in Fargo in 1984 was entitled, "I Was A Pro-choice Feminist But Now I'm Pro-Life." Much in the same way that pro-choice women embraced feminism, right-to-life women find in *their* movement a particular symbolic frame that integrates their experiences of work, reproduction, and marriage with shifting ideas of gender and politics that they encounter around them.

In the pro-life view of the world, to subvert the fertile union of men and women, either by denying procreative sex or the differentiation of male and female character, is to destroy the bases of biological, cultural, and social reproduction. This chain of associations to reproductive, heterosexual sex is central to the organization of meaning in pro-life discourse. For most right-to-lifers, abortion is not simply the termination of an individual potential life, or even that act multiplied a million-fold. It represents an active denial of the reproductive consequences of sex and a rejection of female nurturance, and thus sets forth the possibility of women structurally becoming men. This prospect threatens the union of opposites on which the continuity of the social whole is presumed to rest. In the words of a national pro-life leader

> Abortion is of crucial importance because it negates the one irrefutable difference between men and women. It symbolically destroys the precious essence of womanliness—nurturance. . . . Pro-abortion feminists open themselves to charges of crass hypocrisy by indulging in the very same behavior for which they condemn men: the unethical use of power to usurp the rights of the less powerful.

For pro-life women, then, their work is a gesture against what they see as the final triumph of self-interest. In their image of the unborn child ripped from the womb, they have symbolized the final penetration and destruction of the last arena of women's domain thought to be exempt from the truncated relations identified with both male sexuality and commercial exchange: reproduction and motherhood. At a time when wombs can be rented and zygotes are commodities, abortion is understood by right-to-lifers as an emblematic symbol for the increasing commercialization of human dependency. Their perception of their opponents' gender identity as culturally male—sexual pleasure and individual ambition separated from procreation and nurturant social bonds—is set against their own identification of "true femininity" with the self-sacrificing traits our culture conflates with motherhood. The interpretation of gender that underpins pro-life arguments, however, is based not on a woman's possession of but in her *stance toward* her reproductive capacities. Nurturance is achieved rather than natural, as illustrated in the procreation stories in which the point of the narrative is to show that pregnancy and motherhood are accepted *despite* the ambivalent feelings they produce. In their view, a woman who endorses abortion stresses the other side of the ambivalence and thus is "like a man," regardless of the shape of her body. Conversely, pro-life men encourage and take on a nurturant stance culturally identified as female, often at the urging of their activist wives.

CONCLUSION

This paper examines how American concepts of gender are being redefined by female activists in life story narratives and collective movements. While the analysis is specific to the abortion controversy as it developed in one locale, it is part of two interrelated areas of research: the cultural and social meanings of gender, reproduction, and sexuality; and arenas of conflict in contemporary American culture.[10] The common theoretical assumption of such work (cf. Colen 1986; Harding 1981; Martin 1986; Rapp 1986; Vance 1986) is that understandings of gender and its attendant meanings in American culture are not unified but multiple, and most clearly visible in moments of social and cultural discord. Methodologically, those interested in such dialectical processes focus on contested domains in America in which the definitions and control of procreation, sexuality, family, and nurturance are in contention.

At such moments of reformulation of cultural definitions, models from other societies offer instructive (or deconstructive) counterpoints to our own arrangements. New Guinea and Australia provide notable cases in which a high valuation is placed on nurturance and reproduction, broadly defined, and the role of men as well as women in "growing up" the next generation. Writing on the Trobriand Islanders, Annette Weiner points out:

> All societies make commitments to the reproduction of their most valued resources, i.e. resources that encompass human reproduction as well as the regeneration of social, material, and cosmological phenomena. In our Western tradition, however, the cyclical process of the generation of elements is not of central concern. Even the value of biological reproduction remains a secondary order of events in terms of power and immortality achieved through male domains. Yet in other societies, reproduction, in its most inclusive form, may be a basic principle through which other major societal structures are linked [Weiner 1979].

Similarly, the abortion struggle demonstrates how reproduction, so frequently reified in American categorizations as a biological domain of activity, is always given meaning and value within a historically specific set of cultural conditions. Looked at in this way, the conflict over abortion, regardless of its particular substance, presents a paradox. The claims of opponents to each represent "the truth" about women are at odds with the fact of the controversy. The very existence of the contest that they have created draws attention to reproduction as an "open" signifier in contemporary America. Yet, both pro-life and pro-choice women are trying, in their activism and procreation stories, to "naturalize" their proposed solutions to the problems created by the differential consequences of biological reproduction for men and women in American culture.

Activists, as narrators of their life stories, create symbolic continuity between discontinuous transitions in the female life cycle, particularly between motherhood and wage work, that, for larger reasons, are particularly problematic for specific cohorts in ways that mark them as "generations." In the procreation stories, abortion not only provides a framework for organizing "disorderly" life transitions and extending a newly articulated sense of self in both space and time, it also provides narrators a means of symbolically controlling their opposition. The narratives show how these activists require the "other" in order to exist. This is what gives these stories their dialectical quality; in them the two sides are, by definition, in dialogue with each other, and thus must address the position of their opposition in constituting their own identities.

The signification attached to abortion provides each position with opposed but interrelated paradigms which reconstitute and claim a possible vision of being female. Reformulated to mesh with different historical and biographical experiences, the authority of nurturance remains prominent in both positions. As historian Linda Gordon points out:

> Contemporary feminism, like feminism a century ago, contains an ambivalence between individualism and its critique. [Right-to-lifers] fear a completely individualized society with all services based on cash nexus relationships, without the influence of nurturing women counteracting the completely egoistic principles of the economy, and without any forms in which children can learn about lasting human commitments to other people. Many feminists have the same fear [1982:50–51].

Grassroots pro-life and pro-choice women alike envision their work as a full-scale social crusade to enhance rather than diminish women's position in American culture. While their solutions differ, both sides share a critique of a society that increasingly stresses materialism and self-enhancement while denying the value of dependents and those who care for them. These conditions are faced by all parties to the debate. Nonetheless, the abortion issue persists as a contested domain in which the struggle over the place and meaning of work, reproduction, and nurturance, and their relationship to the category female, are being reorganized in oppositional terms. By casting two possible interpretations of this situation in opposition, the abortion debate masks their common roots in, and circumvents effective resistance to, problematic conditions engendered by a central contradiction for women living in a system in which motherhood and wage labor are continually placed in conflict.

The procreation stories told by women on each side—spun from the uneven threads of women's daily experience and woven into life stories—give compelling shape to the reproductive experiences of different generations, which stress one side of the contradiction. It is not surprising that the abortion contest arouses such passion. Its effects, played out on women's bodies and lives in particular, are the evidence and substance on which activists draw. Their verbal and political performances are created to fix with irreversible meaning events in the female life course that are inherently contingent, variable, and liminal. Yet, the narrative and political actions of activists are intended to close off other possible interpretations, as each side claims to speak the truth regarding contemporary as well as past and future generations of American women.

NOTES

Acknowledgments. I gratefully acknowledge research support from the following sources: American Association for University Women Dissertation Fellowship; a Newcombe Fellowship for Studies in Ethics and Values; the David Spitz Distinguished Dissertation Award, CUNY; and a Sigma Xi research grant. I would also like to thank the women in Fargo with whom I worked, who were so generous with their time and insights. They shall remain anonymous, as was agreed. This paper is a longer version of a talk delivered at the 1986 meetings of the American Ethnological Society. It has improved, I hope, from the many helpful comments I received in the discussion there as well as from the thoughtful critiques of the anonymous reviewers of the first draft of this paper. In addition, I would like to thank Susan Harding, Fred Myers, and Rayna Rapp for their invaluable intellectual support.

1. There is considerable argument in the debate over abortion regarding the proper name for each position. Those advocating abortion rights prefer to call their opposition "anti-choice" while those opposed to legal abortion refer to their opponents as "pro-abortion." Following Malinowski's axiom that the anthropologist's task is, in part, to represent the world from the native's point of view, I have used the appellation each group chooses for itself.
2. For a description and analysis of the "social drama" that took place over the clinic opening, see Faye Ginsburg (1984), "The Body Politic: The Defense of Sexual Restriction by Anti-Abortion Activists," in *Pleasure and Danger,* C. Vance, ed.; and Part III of *Reconstructing Gender in America: Self-Definition and Social Action Among Abortion Activists* (1986).
3. I carried out research in Fargo during 1981–82, as a producer for WCCD-TV Minneapolis, for a documentary on the clinic conflict, "Prairie Storm," broadcast in 1982. I am grateful to Joan Arnow, the George Gund Foundation, Michael Meyer, and the Money for Women Fund for their financial assistance; and to Jan Olsen, Greg Pratt, and Mike Sullivan with whom I worked on that project. I returned for another eight months of participant observation fieldwork in 1983.
4. In a 1984 review article on life histories in the *Annual Review of Sociology,* Daniel Bertaux and Martin Kohli use the term "life story" to distinguish such oral autobiographical fragments from more comprehensive, fully developed narrative texts that would more properly be called life histories, such as Vincent Crapanzano's *Tuhami* (Chicago: University of Chicago Press, 1980); Sidney Mintz's *Worker in the Cane* (New York: Norton, 1974); or Marjorie Shostak's *Nisa* (New York: Vintage, 1983). See Daniel Bertaux and Martin Kohli, "The Life Story Approach: A Continental View." *Annual Review of Sociology* 10:215–237, 1984.
5. In order to better understand the connections activists made between their sense of personal identity and the engagement in a social movement, I asked them to work with me in creating "life stories." People were already well

known to me. I interviewed them (using a tape recorder) for four to five hours, sometimes twice, at a location of their choice where we knew we would not be interrupted. Simply put, I asked people to tell me how they saw their lives in relation to their current activism on the abortion issue. I explained that my interests were to understand why women were so divided on the abortion issue, and to provide a more accurate portrayal of grassroots abortion activists since they tend to be overlooked or misrepresented in both popular and scholarly discussions of the issue. In general, the activists shared these concerns. I chose subjects who had taken during 1981–83, the period of my fieldwork, the most prominent roles in local activity and who reflected, in my estimation, the range of diversity encompassed in the active memberships of each group in terms of age, socioeconomic status, religious affiliation, household and marriage arrangements, style of activism, and the like. While most of these people continue to be active, each side continues to undergo rapid permutations both locally and nationally. Most of my interviews were with women since the membership of both groups is primarily female, as is the case throughout the country. The men I worked with were either husbands of activists or pro-life clergy. Altogether, I collected 21 life stories from right-to-life activists and 14 life stories from pro-choice activists. In the presentation of the data in the thesis I have changed names and obvious identifying features as I agreed to do at the time of the interview.

6. As Rayna Rapp notes in her essay "Family and Class in Contemporary America" (1982),

> If ever a concept carried a heavy weight of ideology, it is the concept of class in American social science. We have a huge and muddled literature that attempts to reconcile objective and subjective criteria, to sort people into lowers, uppers, and middles, to argue about the relation of consciousness to material reality. . . . "Social class" is a short-hand for a process, not a thing . . . by which different social relations to the means of production are inherited and reproduced under capitalism. . . . there are shifting frontiers which separate poverty, stable wage-earning, affluent salaries, and inherited wealth [170–171].

Recognizing this, as well as the complicated questions raised by the sticky question of the relationship of "class" to women's unpaid domestic labor, I use Rapp's definitions for middle-class families and households.

> Households among the middle class are obviously based on a stable resource base that allows for some amount of luxury and discretionary spending . . . Middle-class households probably are able to rely on commodity forms rather than kinship processes to ease both economic and geographic transitions.
>
> The families that organize such households are commonly thought to be characterized by egalitarian marriages [p. 181].

(For egalitarian marriages, see Schneider and Smith 1973.) This definition is consistent with those used in the studies I cite (see note 7) as evidence for the middle-class basis for the abortion movement as a whole. It offers a good general description of the households and families of activists I worked with in Fargo. I do not mean to dismiss class but rather want to underscore the point that the opposing positions on abortion are not isomorphic with distinctive groups of people situated differently in the social relations of production. I use the life histories in particular to show how much more complicated the process is, and the multiple settings from which identity is drawn.

7. See, for example, Daniel Granberg 1981; Harding 1981; and Tatalovich and Daynes 1981: 116–137. Granberg's random sample survey of members of the National Abortion Rights Action League (NARAL) and National Right to Life Committee (NRLC), which is the most thorough of all research to date, gives a breakdown of selected demographic and social status characteristics (see Granberg 1981, Table 1, p. 158).

8. In an article on new anthropological views of the family, authors Collier, Rosaldo, and Yanagisako write:

> One of the central notions in the modern American construct of The Family is that of nurturance . . . a relationship that entails affection and love, that is based on cooperation as opposed to competition, that is enduring rather than temporary, that is noncontingent rather than contingent upon performance, and that is governed by feeling and morality instead of law and contract. . . . a symbolic opposition to the market relations of capitalism [1982:34].

9. In assessing the way that abortion opponents view the world in relation to their ideology, authors Callahan and Callahan write:

> Both sides are prepared to argue that abortion is undesirable, a crude solution to problems that would better be solved by other means. The crucial difference, however is that those on the pro-choice side believe that the world must be acknowledged as it is and not just as it ought to be.
>
> By contrast, the pro-life group believes that a better future cannot be achieved . . . unless we are prepared to make present sacrifices toward future goals and unless aggression toward the fetus is denied, however high the individual cost of denying it. The dichotomies are experienced in our ordinary language when "idealists" are contrasted with "realists." [1984:221].

10. Several sessions at professional anthropology meetings in 1986 were indicative of this trend. A panel organized by the author and Linda Girdner entitled "Contested Domains of Reproduction, Sexuality, Family and Gender in America" was held at the American Ethnological Society meetings in April. At the December meetings of the American Anthropological Association, a session entitled "Speaking Women: Representations of Contemporary American Femininity" was organized by Joyce Canaan; at the same event, Susan Harding organized a panel on "Ethnographic America." Specific research presented at these sessions included Rayna Rapp's study of amniocentesis, Carole Vance's investigation of the pornography debates, Susan Harding's research on the Moral Majority, Shellee Colen's work on domestic childcare workers, Emily Martin's study of conflicting metaphors for birth and the female body, Joyce Canaan's work on adolescent sexuality in America, Linda Girdner's study of contested child custody disputes, and Judy Modell's research on adoption.

REFERENCES

Callahan, Daniel, and Sidney Callahan. 1984. "Abortion: Understanding Differences," *Family Planning Perspectives* 16(5):219–220.

Colen, Shellee. 1986. "Stratified Reproduction: The Case of Domestic Workers in America." Paper presented at the American Ethnological Society Meetings, Wrightsville Beach, NC.

Collier, Jane, Michelle Rosaldo, and Sylvia Yanagisako. 1982. "Is There A Family? New Anthropological Views." In *Rethinking the Family.* B. Thorne and M. Yalom, eds. New York: Longman.

Ginsburg, Faye. 1984. "The Body Politic: The Defense of Sexual Restriction by Anti-Abortion Activists." In *Pleasure and Danger: Exploring Female Sexuality.* C. Vance, ed. Boston: Routledge and Kegan Paul.

———. 1986. "Reconstructing Gender in America. Self-Definition and Social Action Among Abortion Activists." Ph.D. dissertation. City University of New York.

Gordon, Linda. 1982. "Why Nineteenth-Century Feminists Did Not Support "Birth Control" and Twentieth Century Feminists Do: Feminism, Reproduction and the Family." In *Rethinking the Family.* B. Thorne and M. Yalom, eds. New York: Longman.

Granberg, Daniel. 1981. "The Abortion Activists," *Family Planning Perspectives* 13(4).

Harding, Susan. 1981. "Family Reform Movements: Recent Feminism and Its Opposition," *Feminist Studies* 7(1).

Luker, Kristin. 1984. *Abortion and the Politics of Motherhood.* Berkeley: University of California Press.

Mannheim, Karl. 1952. "The Problem of Generations." In *Essays on the Sociology of Knowledge.* P. Kecskemeti, ed. New York: Oxford University Press.

Martin, Emily. 1986. "Mind, Body and Machine." Paper presented at the American Anthropological Association Meetings, Philadelphia, PA.

Rapp, Rayna. 1982. "Family and Class in Contemporary America." In *Rethinking the Family.* B. Thorne and M. Yalom, eds. New York: Longman.

———. 1986. "Constructing Amniocentesis: Medical and Maternal Voices." Paper presented at the American Anthropological Association Meetings, Philadelphia, PA.

Schneider, David M., and R. T. Smith. 1973. *Class Differences and Sex Roles in American Kinship and Family Structure.* Englewood Cliffs, NJ: Prentice-Hall.

Tatalovich, Raymond, and Byron W. Daynes. 1981. *The Politics of Abortion.* New York: Praeger.

Vance, Carole S. 1986. "Of Sex and Women, Meese and Men: The 1986 Attorney General's Commission on Pornography." Paper presented at the American Ethnological Society Meetings, Wrightsville Beach, NC.

Weiner, Annette. 1979. "Trobriand Kinship From Another View: The Reproductive Power of Women and Men," *Man* 14(2): 328–348.

THE MOVEMENT AGAINST CLITORIDECTOMY AND INFIBULATION IN SUDAN: PUBLIC HEALTH POLICY AND THE WOMEN'S MOVEMENT

Ellen Gruenbaum

Sudan is one of the countries where the most severe form of female circumcision persists and is practiced widely among both Muslims and Coptic Christians, in both urban and rural communities. Only the largely non-Muslim Southern Region is free of the practice, except among people of northern origin.

The most common form of the operation is referred to as pharaonic circumcision, consisting of the removal of all external genitalia—the clitoris, the clitoral prepuce, the labia minora and all or part of the labia majora—and infibulation (stitching together of the opening), so as to occlude the vaginal opening and urethra. Only a tiny opening is left for the passage of urine and menses. A modified version, Sunna circumcision, is less common, and consists of excision of the prepuce of the clitoris, generally also with partial or total excision of the clitoris itself (clitoridectomy), but without infibulation.

The operations customarily are performed by traditional or government-trained midwives on girls in the 5–7 year age range; the girls, however, may be older or younger, since it is common to circumcise two or three sisters at the same time. These occasions are ones of celebration, with new dresses, bracelets, and gifts for the girls. An animal may be slaughtered and a special meal prepared for the many guests and well-wishers who are expected to drop in. In wealthy families, musical entertainment is often arranged for an evening party. The girls themselves, though they may be fearful of the operation, look forward to the first occasion at which they will be treated as important people.

The origin of the practice is unknown, though its existence in the ancient civilizations of the Nile Valley in Egypt and Sudan has been documented. The practice survived the spread of Christianity to the ruling groups of the Nile Valley kingdoms in Sudan in the 6th century. Waves of Arab migration, intermarriage with the indigenous people, and the influence of Islamic teachers resulted in Islam's becoming the dominant religion of northern Sudan by about 1500. Pharaonic circumcision, along with other non-Islamic beliefs such as veneration of ancestors or saints and spirit possession cults, was successfully incorporated into the Sudanese Islamic belief system. The practice is deeply embedded in Sudanese cultures; and it should be recognized that the symbolic significance and cultural concomitants of female circumcision undoubtedly play important roles in individual repetition of the custom, as the work of Janice Boddy (1979) has shown.

Still, to say that it is a "custom" is not a sufficient explanation for the persistence of this damaging practice. Numerous physically harmful effects have been documented in the medical literature (Verzin 1975, Cook 1976, Shandall 1967). At the time of circumcision, girls may suffer from hemorrhage, infections, septicemia, retention of urine, or shock; deaths may result from these complications. The infibulated state may also result in retention of menses or difficulties in urination (due to scar tissue), and may be related to an apparently high prevalence of urinary tract and other chronic pelvic infections (Boddy

1979, Toubia 1981). At first intercourse, infibulation presents a barrier which is painfully torn unless cut open by husband, midwife, or doctor. Childbirth is complicated by the inelastic scar tissue of infibulation, which must be cut open by the birth attendant and restitched after delivery. Vasicovaginal fistulae, which can result from such obstructed labor, are by no means rare in Sudan. Such a fistula—a passage between the urinary bladder and the vagina created by damage to tissue between the two organs—results in a most embarrassing condition for the woman, who cannot retain her urine and therefore leaks constantly (Toubia 1981).

Why, then, in light of these physically harmful, even life-threatening, consequences, do women continue to perform these operations on their daughters? Much of the literature has gone no further than the observation that it is "customary," or as one Sudanese writer has put it, "the implicit and explicit message being that it is something we inherited from an untraceable past which has no rational meaning and lies within the realm of untouchable sensitivity of traditional people" (Toubia 1981:4).

Social scientists and feminists writing on the subject have pointed out that female circumcision forms part of a complex sociocultural arrangement of female subjugation in a strongly patrilineal, patriarchal society (*cf.*, Assaad 1980, Hayes 1975, El Saadawi 1980). The fact that it is women who carry out the practice, and who are its strongest defenders, must be analyzed in terms of their weaker social position.

Women in Sudan generally must derive their social status and economic security from their roles as wives and mothers. Among most cultural groups in northern Sudan, female virginity at marriage is considered so important that even rumors questioning a girl's morality may be enough to besmirch the family honor and to bar her from the possibility of marriage. In this context, clitoridectomy and infibulation serve as a guarantee of morality. Sudanese women hold that clitoridectomy helps to attenuate a girl's sexual desire so that she is less likely to seek premarital sex; infibulation presents a barrier to penetration. Any girl known to have been "properly" circumcised in the pharaonic manner can be assumed to be a virgin and therefore marriageable, while doubts can be raised about those who are not circumcised or have had only the modified Sunna circumcision.

Attempts to formulate policies against the practice have seldom recognized the significance of the linkage between the operations and the social goal of maintaining the reputations and marriageability of daughters in a strongly patriarchal society. In addition, the economic and social status of midwives, the group chiefly responsible for performing the operations, has seldom been seriously considered. Instead, government policies have tended to emphasize simple legal prohibitions; propaganda against the apparent ideological supports of the practice; spreading information on some of the physically harmful aspects of female circumcision; and tacit acceptance of a compromise policy of modification and "modernization" of the practice.

Some policies resulting from these emphases are undoubtedly useful. Certainly the recommendations of the 1979 Khartoum Conference (Seminar on Traditional Practices Affecting the Health of Women, sponsored by the Eastern Mediterranean Regional Office of the World Health Organization) are to be commended and supported. These recommendations included a call for clear national policies for the abolition of the practice in the countries where it persists; the passage of legislation in support of such policies; the intensification of general education on the dangers and undesirability of the practice; and intensification of educational programs for birth attendants and other practitioners to enlist their support. Because there is such strong social motivation for continuing the practice in Sudan, however, I would argue that the proposed public health education approach would have only a weak or slow effect. Policy on female circumcision requires rethinking.

In the following sections, I draw upon my experience in Sudan, where I carried out research on rural health services and lectured at the University of Khartoum. My goal here is twofold: to consider the reasons for failure of past anticircumcision policies, and to provide a critique of current policy efforts. In addition, I hope to provide insights into what is necessary for the development of viable policies.

ABOLITION EFFORTS IN SUDAN

The first efforts to eliminate the practice of clitoridectomy and infibulation in Sudan came during the British colonial period (1898–1956). When a British midwife was brought in to organize a midwifery training school in 1920, efforts were made to dissuade the traditional midwives enrolled in the training program from continuing the practice. But persuasion and example apparently had little effect.

In 1946, an edict was promulgated prohibiting pharaonic circumcision. This attempt to impose the colonialists' values on the culture of a subject people by force of law also failed completely, and was even met with violent resistance. Residents of the town of Rufa'a still talk about "our Revolution"—the day in 1946 when they tore the government prison to the ground to free a midwife who had been arrested for circumcising a girl. Government troops fired on the crowd, and injured some; yet even this failed to stem popular resistance to the British and to their attempts to outlaw the entrenched custom.

Resistance to the government ban did not require rebellion. Since the activity took place outside the purview of the foreign government, the practice simply continued as before. In fact, historically, the government seldom attempted the sort of enforcement that led to the Rufa'a "Revolution."

Another approach used by the British against the practice was propaganda. In 1945, the Sudan Medical Service issued and circulated a pamphlet, written in both English and Arabic, that condemned pharaonic circumcision and urged the Sudanese to abandon the practice. It was signed by the highest ranking British and Sudanese doctors, and was endorsed by Sudanese religious leaders. The Mufti of Sudan provided an authoritative Islamic legal opinion stating that female circumcision was not obligatory under Islam; and another endorsing religious leader advocated the substitution of Sunna circumcision (clitoridectomy). Thus, while the backing of the religious leaders was something less than total opposition to female circumcision, their opposition to the pharaonic form is important. (Few Sudanese queried in villages where I worked, however, were aware that the religious leaders had ever spoken against female circumcision.)

During this same period, the mid-1940s, several educated Sudanese women—teachers and midwives—undertook speaking tours in the provinces to publicize the bad effects of pharaonic circumcision. An Arabic poster used during the campaign declared that the Sunna circumcision came from the Prophet Mohammed, and should therefore replace the pharaonic form, ascribed to "Pharaoh the enemy of God" (Hall and Ismail 1981:93–95).

Today, after three decades of illegality, pharaonic circumcision of girls continues to be widely performed in both rural and urban areas. It is openly celebrated, with feasting and gift-giving. Midwives speak freely of their participation in the perpetuation of the practice. To my knowledge there have been no government efforts in recent years to enforce the legal prohibition.

There has, however, been some change in the methods used in performing the operations, although this has not been uniform. The dangerously unhygienic traditional methods, such as performing the operation over a hole in the ground, using knives for cutting, thorns and leg binding for infibulation, and plain water for cleansing, have been supplanted by the availability of better equipment and knowledge of more hygienic methods. The government-trained village midwife whose practice I observed did the operations on a wood and rope bed covered with a plastic sheet. She used xylocaine injections for local anesthesia, new razor blades, suture needles, dissolving sutures when available, and prophylactic antibiotic powder. Her equipment was sterilized with boiling water before use. After this initial use, however, she returned the instruments to the same bowl of previously boiled water, and did not resterilize them before using them in a second girl's operation. The midwife purchases most of the necessary supplies and medications out of her earnings; some of the basic equipment necessary for childbirth attendance is provided by the government, however, and some supplies are obtained informally through the local government health center.

CURRENT POLICY EFFORTS

In more recent years, opponents—ordinarily resorting to medical and psychological arguments against pharaonic circumcision—have recognized that complete eradication of the practice is an unrealistic short-term objective. While continuing to advocate eventual eradication, policymakers have tended to attempt to mitigate the effects by substituting the less drastic Sunna form of circumcision. This opinion, held unofficially by the government health service's leaders and many medical doctors with whom I spoke in the late 1970s, has meant that many doctors are willing to perform such operations themselves. They assume that, in terms of medical safety, it is better for them to perform clitoridectomies in their offices.[1]

As policy positions, both the eradication goal and the "modification" compromise are problematic. The view that the practice should or could be "eradicated," as if it were a disease, is a particularly medical view. While it is reasonable that arguments against circumcision stress physical risks, the problem nevertheless is one that is not necessarily amenable to medical solutions. The medical view implies not only that the practice is "pathological," but that its solution might lie in some sort of campaign-style attack on the problem. Social customs, however, are not "pathologies"; and such a view is a poor starting point for change, since it is not one necessarily shared by the people whose customs are under attack. While these people may be open to the view that a practice such as this may be harmful in some ways, to approach it as an evil or pathological situation is to insult those who believe strongly in it and consider it a means of promoting cleanliness and purity, and is unlikely to foster consideration of change. Furthermore, the decades of emphasis on medical reasons for discontinuing the practice have not in fact resulted in its abandonment. For example, in a study of medical records of 2526 women in Khartoum and Wad Medani, Mudawi (1977a) found only seven to be uncircumcised; 12 had been clitoridectomised only, and the remainder had been infibulated.[2] A questionnaire sample survey of about 10,000 women in Sudan found that 82% were infibulated (El Dareer 1979).

Another problem with the strategy of promoting a modified form of circumcision as a transitional program relates to the unfortunate ideological linkage of the modified type. Among Sudanese who practice pharaonic circumcision, it is widely believed that the practice is commanded by Islam. While this interpretation is disavowed by many Islamic scholars, the belief that both male and female circumcision were commanded by the Prophet Mohammed persists.[3] This widespread belief serves as strong ideological support for a practice known to predate Islam (Diaz and Mudawi 1977) and which is perpetuated largely because of its important social functions.

The use of the term "Sunna circumcision" for the less drastic operation, which many reformers are encouraging as the most feasible short-term alternative, has unfortunately reinforced the ideological linkage with Islam. To describe a practice as "Sunna" is to consider it religious law.[4] Since Sudanese Muslims are adherents of the Sunni branch of Islam (i.e., "those who follow the Sunna"), they do not want to say their practice is incongruent with Sunni tradition. The linguistic root of the words Sunni and Sunna is the same, and although "Sunna circumcision" does not literally imply linkage to Sunni Islam, they are commonly associated. Indeed, the ideological linkage between the term "Sunna circumcision" and the religion has been reinforced even by an eminent Sudanese gynecologist, Dr. Suliman Mudawi, who writes that, "The Sunna circumcision, or clitoridectomy, is the legal operation recommended by Islam, consisting of the excision of the glans clitoris and sometimes a small portion of the clitoris itself" (Mudawi 1977b).

Thus, now that the term "Sunna circumcision" is widely known, many people profess to practice it—since they wish to be regarded as faithful Sunnites—even when the operation is performed as before with infibulation after removal of clitoris and labia. Reform efforts advocating a modified operation, therefore, may have resulted in a change in nomenclature, rather than widespread change in the operations. Thus, reports that pharaonic circumcision with infibulation is gradually being abandoned in Sudan, which are based on questionnaire interviews or anecdotal material (e.g., Clark and Diaz 1977, Cook 1976), may be misleading, since some of those who say they have adopted the Sunna form simply may have begun calling pharaonic circumcision by another name.

In spite of the importance of ideological supports, it would not be sufficient to attack the presumed religious reasons. Change efforts must take into consideration the socioeconomic relations in which Sudanese women are enmeshed, and the social dilemmas to which families that try to change the practice would be exposed. After all, where a most significant aspect of marriage is control of female reproductive capacity, and where circumcision has come to be the mechanism for guaranteeing the perfect condition of that capacity, to dispense with circumcision is to violate a basic condition of an essential social relation. Thus, a religious scholar's testimony that female circumcision is not necessary for religious reasons would not be sufficient for a mother to risk her daughter's marriageability. Similarly, awareness of medical and psychological[5] hazards may be only weakly deterrent; a daughter's marriageability would scarcely be risked because of a psychological notion that she may suffer bad dreams or never experience orgasm. Marriage and children are more vital, closer to the meaning of life and to a woman's economic survival, than transitory emotional feelings.

While most women are economically active, either in subsistence production, wage employment, trade, or production of commodities, economic well-being—indeed, survival in many of the harsher rural areas—requires large family production units. A husband and children are necessary to a woman's economic security; not only do children contribute their labor at an early age to the family's economic production—especially in rural areas—but also they are security for old age. Commonly, women are to some degree dependent on their husbands for access to land or domestic animals, their labors, and/or their wages. A husband dissatisfied with his wife—either personally or because of reproductive inadequacy—is considered more likely to take a second wife. Although polygyny frequently enhances the prestige and wealth of the husband, it commonly weakens the individual woman's economic position and, if the other wife or wives bear children, lessens her own children's inheritance. Under Islamic law,[6] a divorced woman has no right to child custody after the age of seven for boys and the age of nine for girls, regardless of the reasons for divorce or on whose initiative the marriage was ended. Men have the right to unilateral divorce, but women do not. With these constraints it is not surprising that most women put considerable effort into pleasing their husbands and protecting their reputations, so as to safeguard their marriages.

Efforts to please husbands and safeguard virtue take many forms. Beautification methods, while pleasurable for a woman herself and usually done in pleasant camaraderie with other women, are primarily directed toward husbands, with the most sensuous techniques being reserved for married women. Even poor rural women spend considerable time and effort on the arts of decorative henna staining of hands and feet, removal of body hair, sauna-like incensing of the body, careful selection of clothing and ornaments, and decorative hair plaiting. They also prepare special scented substances for massaging their husbands.

Beyond these, the enhancement of a woman's ability to please her husband is considered to be most importantly achieved by clitoridectomy and infibulation. One midwife I spoke with claimed that clitoridectomy allowed for longer intercourse, pleasing to the man. This belief presupposes that a woman experiencing more sexual stimulation would be less patient, and can hardly be credited as a major factor in perpetuating clitoridectomy. On the other hand, the attenuation of *inappropriate* sexual desire, before marriage and extramaritally, should be considered one of the major goals of the practice.

It is infibulation, and especially reinfibulation, that is alleged to contribute most significantly to the sexual pleasure of men. Following childbirth, the midwife restitches the long incision made for the delivery of the baby. A tighter reinfibulation is expected to result in greater pleasure for the husband when intercourse is resumed following the customary 40-day postpartum recovery period. One reinfibulation I witnessed, performed by a government-trained midwife following a woman's thirteenth childbirth, left a completely smooth vulva, the urethral opening completely concealed, and only a pin-sized opening to the vagina. A number of women told me that such tight reinfibulation gives husbands greater sexual pleasure, the tightness lasting approximately three months after resumption of sexual intercourse. They claimed that husbands were more generous in their gifts (clothes, jewelry, perfumes) when the reinfibulation is very tight. It was clear, too, that such marital sexual satisfaction is considered important in avoiding the possibility of the husband exercising his legally guaranteed rights to unilateral divorce or polygynous marriage.

The attitudes of women toward the practice of clitoridectomy and infibulation are often contradictory. Occasionally, I encountered Sudanese women who were surprised to learn that American and European women are not circumcised. Others realized that Europeans did not circumcise women, but believed that all Muslims did. Although they found it hard to believe that Saudi Arabian women are not circumcised, such information did nothing to undermine their faith in the importance of the practice. To my comment that American women are left "natural," they replied, "But circumcision *is* natural for us."

There was, however, recurrent ambivalence expressed in many of the conversations I had on this topic. Without questioning the necessity of circumcision, a woman might sigh and say, "Isn't it difficult?" When discussing repeated reinfibulation with one small group of urban women (which included a new mother who had just been reinfibulated a few days before), I was urged, "Be sure and put all this in your report, about how difficult it is for us."

DEVELOPING VIABLE POLICY ALTERNATIVES

That women perpetuate practices painful and dangerous to themselves and their daughters and that inhibit their own sexual gratification must be understood in the context of their social and economic vulnerability in a strongly patriarchal society. Public health policymakers must allow for the fact that the circumcision of girls is a deeply rooted social custom. Even among urban-dwelling, educated families, there are those who would take their daughters back to the relatives in a rural village for circumcision, to ensure a traditional, thorough operation.

Although harmful sequelae have brought female circumcision to the attention of medical professionals, it is argued here that medical opinion can have little relevance in changing the situation. While more research into the psychological and medical hazards of circumcision could be useful for convincing influential educated people to back efforts toward change, the medical model and the efforts of the medical services system are limited in terms of policy development. Effective change can only come in the context of a women's movement oriented toward the basic social problems affecting women, particularly their economic dependency, educational disadvantages, and obstacles to employment (e.g., the dearth of child day-care facilities for urban workers). To improve women's social and economic security, marital customs must be challenged, and new civil laws are needed to offer additional protection to married and divorced women concerning child custody, rights in marital property, and financial support, going beyond the present provisions of Islamic and customary law. Further, general health conditions are very poor and must be improved. With an infant mortality rate conservatively estimated at 140 per 1000 (Sudan, Ministry of Health, 1975:6), and with a high prevalence of numerous disabling and life-threatening illnesses, especially dangerous to children, it is not surprising that Sudanese women—particularly in rural areas—seek to give birth to large numbers of children. The crude birth rate is approximately 49 per 1000 (Sudan, Ministry of Health 1975:5). Thus, basic health issues are important concerns of women.

The implications of reducing women's dependency through improvement of their economic opportunities are far-reaching. Any policy that would threaten the form or importance of the family and its functions would obviously excite widespread reaction. At the same time, Sudan's current laws and social values already offer some advantages to women in promising productive roles. Educated women are expected to hold full-time jobs and to have the right to the same pay and benefits as men in comparable jobs, although there are social barriers to women's participation in certain occupations. While many struggles remain to be fought on this front, the fact that wide networks of people benefit from each person employed in a stable job means that families generally back the educated woman who wants to work. Frequently, child care can be provided by relatives during working hours, and there is a general acceptance of the principle of equal pay for equal work. In addition, the government (the largest employer of the educated) gives eight weeks' paid maternity leave, often additional unpaid leave with position held, and makes special allowances for the needs of nursing mothers.

While these offer a good basis for developing women's position, many problems prevent women from taking full advantage of the opportunities that do exist. Working women complain (or, more often, do not complain, but simply carry on) that they must still perform all the usual housework after coming home, and are still expected to make time for all the traditional visiting and hospitality. Women college students find their neighbors and relatives consider them snobbish if they do not take the time for such visiting, regardless of the demands of their studies. This is especially hard on women medical students who must keep odd hours, and often spend the night at the hospital during their clinical training.

The family continues to be an extremely important factor, however, in the lives of even the most advantaged, educated, employed women. Since childbearing is expected to begin immediately after marriage, the employed woman most commonly depends on her mother or another female relative to provide child care. Family members become dependent on her income, and she may find herself locked into the necessity of working even when other social obligations make it difficult. Should her marriage falter and her husband divorce her, she may not only lose his support but custody of her children as well. Clearly, additional social services would help overcome these problems. For example, while government-sponsored child care centers presently exist in some towns, many women workers find them unavailable or too costly. Some form of social security benefits could reduce women's vulnerability to divorce and loss of support and child custody. But state subsidy of such services outside the family currently is neither a feasible nor a desired alternative in Sudan, where government policy favors investment in economic development over expansion of social service expenditures.

A full discussion of development strategies and their implications for women's position in the society would be outside the scope of this paper. It is important to realize, however, that while women share in the desire for economic development in their poor country, just as they desire increased incomes for their families and themselves, current development policies offer little to women. Sudan's development has been of the peripheral capitalist pattern of uneven development (O'Brien 1980). Investment has gravitated toward the center of the country in the most highly productive centers of primary products for export or import substitution. All too frequently, foreign investments have been self-serving, emphasizing high technology that the developed countries want to sell, or the production of products that the investors want to import. The high technology emphasis, which appeals to scheme managers and government officials seeking to "modernize," results in jobs for men rather than women, and sometimes even undercuts existing productive roles of women (see Sørbø 1977).

Sudanese and other Middle Eastern women have demonstrated their interest in changing their lot by the formation of women's organizations such as the Sudanese Women's Union. The Union has a history of militant action, as when Sudanese women took to the streets in the popular uprising that overthrew the military regime in 1964. While the issues such women's groups have chosen to address have long included modifying or abolishing circumcision, they have addressed themselves more urgently to other problems. In the 1950s and 1960s for example, the women's organization in Sudan was concerned with nationalist issues: the achievement of national independence, avoidance of control by U.S. imperialist interests, and the development of democratic government. In the early 1970s, the women's union was restructured under the ruling party (under Nimeiri's government, which came to power in a coup d'etat in 1969), and most of the communist and other politically radical women were purged or barred from leadership. Since then, the thrust of the organization has also changed somewhat. In the urban and "modern" sector rural areas (such as the Gezira Irrigation Scheme), the primary activities of the Union as they touch the lives of the ordinary women center on cultural and educational activities—embroidery classes, crafts shows, and the like and support for the ruling party; eradication of circumcision has not been a high priority.

The majority of women in the country, who live outside the towns and agricultural schemes or in the poor neighborhoods and rural villages in those areas, have not by and large been recruited into such organizations. Yet these women, too, have a number of very basic concerns: improved incomes, education for their children, clean water, and basic health services. Organizing these rural women, however, has proven difficult. In a prosperous village in the Gezira Irrigated Scheme, for example, the membership of the local branch of the Women's Union has not met in two years. One divorced woman, a Union member, tried to organize women in that village to take an active part in improving village sanitation. She was unable to mobilize support, however, even though a fully staffed health center (which should share responsibility for public health) is located in the village. Further, though this woman is part of the mandated one-third female membership of the village People's Council, she and the other women members are not ordinarily informed of meetings. Her participation as an individual in development is also blocked. Although she is literate, she is not highly enough educated to qualify for a white-collar job; and her brother has opposed her working in agriculture, a position that would threaten the prestige of the family.

This is not to say that women's organizations and programs are everywhere ineffective. In fact there is much enthusiasm in Gezira villages for the literacy campaigns and home economics courses offered by the Gezira Scheme's Social Development Department. But if the woman just mentioned must face such obstacles even in a relatively well off village that has resources to devote to local projects, the problems of the more remote and poorer villages, where literacy campaigns and women's organizations have not penetrated at all, are far greater.

Since, as history demonstrates, circumcisions can continue with or without governmental sanction, it is impossible to conceive of any efforts to change the custom having an effect unless they are supported by women themselves. These changes will come only as the result of many other societal changes, especially those that enable women to be less economically dependent on men and thus less oriented toward pleasing husbands.

POLICY CONTRIBUTIONS

To assert that changes in female circumcision must come from the women themselves and their social movement is not to say that policymakers have nothing to contribute. Indeed, there are several key areas where public policy and specifically health policy could contribute significantly.

First, further research is appropriate. Much of the writing thus far has been based on case studies, anecdotal material, or haphazard sampling (e.g., Assaad 1980, Hayes 1975). It would be useful to relate the place of circumcision and its celebration to the social position of women in societies where the practice is common. Studies should focus particularly on the significance of marriage, the importance of virginity and its relation to the maintenance of family "honor" (e.g., segregation of sexes, chaperoning, infibulation, manner of dress), and the economic participation of women and form of economic organization (especially whether the organization of production continues to emphasize family production units). Whether more clinical medical articles, describing the operations and their sequelae, would add anything to arguments against the practice is uncertain, although more information on the treatment of complications could be useful. Epidemiological studies of the apparently high rates of urinary and vaginal infections associated with circumcision also would be in order. Although I am aware of no data on a relationship between the operations and infertility or low fertility, such a relationship has nevertheless been suggested (*cf.*, Hosken 1980; Hayes 1975); Hayes (1975), in fact, considered lowered fertility a "latent function" of female circumcision. Certainly infertility might be expected in cases of obstructed intercourse (Sudan Medical Service 1945), and in association with the medical complications of circumcision. The existence of a demonstrable relationship between circumcision and infertility could provide a powerful argument against the operations in countries such as Sudan with strong pronatalist values.

Second, policies that promote the opportunities of women in education and employment could be beneficial in two ways. First, reducing women's dependence on marriage and motherhood as the only economically viable social roles could separate circumcision from basic economic survival and thus weaken support for it. Second, education and employment could be expected to enhance women's ability to act as a group by enabling them to become more involved in shaping their own destiny through access to political and economic power and greater opportunities for organizing themselves. Women then would be better able to influence and implement policies according to their own priorities. The realization of such opportunities may require not only that additional social security and other support services be provided but, in addition, that economic development policies be challenged. The high technology strategies which have so often resulted in skilled jobs for men while undermining women's traditional productive roles and ignoring the possibility of their involvement in new areas, may need to be revised.

The Role of Midwives

A particularly important locus of policy concerns should be the role of midwives, since they are the principal practitioners of circumcision. It is not enough to recommend that they be educated as to its harmful effects; it must also be recognized that fees, together with gifts such as soap, perfume, meat from the celebration slaughter and other foods, constitute important elements of a midwife's income. Government-trained midwives, if they are paid at all, receive only a very small monthly retainer fee from the local government. This is not paid in all areas and is too small to be considered even a meager salary. Untrained, traditional midwives receive no benefits from the government at all; even basic equipment for childbirth attendance is supplied only to the trained midwives, and both groups must purchase their own drugs and supplies, unless acquired informally through local health services facilities of the government. The fee-for-service payment system means that the midwife's income is directly dependent on the number of births attended and circumcision performed.

The current drive for the development of Primary Health Care for the achievement of WHO's goal of "Health for All by the Year 2000" could very usefully seek out midwives to be Community Health Workers. The additional training would benefit their midwifery practices, and whatever status individual midwives already have achieved as respected community members concerned with health could enhance their influence as health care providers. Further, since barriers to the effective health care of women by male health care providers now prevent women from receiving needed care, more female providers would fill a real need.[7]

Providing midwives with a wider role and some other income might help them heed educational efforts against circumcision by reducing the conflicts of interest with respect to income. Difficulties inherent in the training of midwives (involving a full year's study away from family, especially hard for married women and mothers) have been overcome. The same could be expected for Community Health Workers, whose training period is shorter. Such a strategy could help to achieve primary health care goals while improving midwifery at less cost than training and supporting two separate specialized individuals. Since midwives, as women, have access to women and children even in the most traditional communities, they could be expected to be very effective in promoting maternal and child health goals.

PERSPECTIVES ON INTERNATIONAL POLICYMAKING

Such recommendations should be considered in the context of the social dynamics of an underdeveloped country. The dependency relations between a country such as Sudan and the more powerful capitalist financial centers has surely played as much a part in molding priorities in social and health policy as have religion and cultural tradition.

Social scientists who seek to design rational, sensible, and culturally sensitive public health policies, must ask themselves several questions. What would be necessary to ensure the adoption of their proposals? What are the interests of the social classes with access to the most political power in a country? What image of their country do the relevant national ministries, organizations, and occupational groups wish to portray? What sort of research or program priorities might they want to block? Which would they prefer to support?

Similarly, international organizations and the aid missions of developed countries are limited by their own hidden agendas.[8] For example, USAID projects ordinarily must be demonstrated to have some beneficial effect on U.S. trade, U.S. geopolitical strategies, or other U.S. interests; beneficial effects on the people or the economies of the developing countries are desirable, but secondary. To suppose that an aid mission might withhold support from such programs as primary health care until serious work against female circumcision is undertaken is to pretend that aid missions are moral entities instead of international political and economic tools. For aid to be accepted by the host government, its terms ordinarily must be beneficial to the interests of ruling groups or to governmental stability. Aid must not, therefore, make the nation or the government appear backward, discriminatory, or as having anything less than the best interests of the entire populace at heart.

While international bodies such as the United Nations organizations are less likely to have such strongly political agendas, and can be assumed to be genuinely oriented to abstract goals such as peace and health, they, too, suffer from an inability to be critical of host governments. Programs must be invited and collaborative, although these organizations' apparently neutral political position gives them somewhat more leeway to provide guidance without seeming offensively imperialistic.

I believe it is a mistake to insist, as some outspoken critics do, that aid missions, international organizations, and even non-governmental and church groups take firm stands "to prevent the operations" (Hosken 1980). Such agencies and organizations would have no political interest in taking such a controversial stand except where host governments might ask them to do so as part of an indigenous movement against the practice. But even if the necessary forces could be mobilized in the developed countries to force the adoption of such a policy and such agencies and organizations *did* adopt this stance, a "backlash" phenomenon would all too likely follow. Heavy-handedness on the part of the developed countries is generally unwelcome in fiercely nationalistic underdeveloped countries such as Sudan. Thus, while its external relationships may be those of dependency and its economic system capitalist (including some state-capitalist structures and some use of "socialist" ideology), there is no loyalty to a particular power which extends beyond national interests or economic constraints. Even Saudi Arabia, with its stranglehold control of the supply of much of Sudan's energy and investment capital and its influential role in religious leadership of the Islamic countries, has thus far been able to impose only temporary or partial social programs—such as the crackdown on prostitution in Khartoum in 1976–77. The Nimeiri government, however, has stalled on such issues as the abolition of alcohol or imposition of an Islamic constitution, which might prove either widely unpopular or which might jeopardize the government's control over the largely non-Muslim south.

Policy research must be placed in this context. It is clear that the movement against clitoridectomy and infibulation must receive its primary momentum for national movements in which women themselves play a leading role. Thus, policy researchers should keep in mind that it is not appropriate merely to expose practices and make recommendations to outside organizations. Wherever possible, indigenous women and women's organizations should be involved in all stages of the research, from formulation of the problem to development of policy. Only in this way will such indigenous movements be sure to benefit from the research.

NOTES

1. In support of this point, one Sudanese doctor recently stated that before the Khartoum Conference in 1979, the medical profession's official policy "was not total abolition of female circumcision, but the promotion of clitoridectomy under more hygienic circumstances as a substitute for infibulation" (Toubia 1981).
2. It is ironic that this same author, a senior Sudanese gynecologist, has said, "Although the habit is still practised in some parts of the Sudan it is gratifying to note that it is gradually dying out." He is further quoted as saying. "The most effective line of attack was a medical one" (quoted in Toubia 1981:3).
3. The sayings attributed to the Prophet Mo-

hammed on this subject do not, however, endorse infibulation. "Reduce but do not destroy," is often quoted by reformers. Another saying, handed down by Um Attiya, is, "Circumcise but do not go deep, this is more illuminating to the face and more enjoyable to the husband" (Sudanese Medical Service 1945, in Foreword by the Mufti of the Sudan).

4. While "Sunna" may be translated as "rule" or "tradition," the Islamic ideology asserts that Islam is not simply a religion, but a "way of life." Hence, it is not uncommon for Sudanese Muslims to assume linkages between cultural traditions and religious beliefs, and to assume that their shared beliefs and practices are rooted in formal Islamic doctrine. In his statement against pharaonic circumcision in 1945, the Mufti of Sudan cited a religious authority who believed that "male circumcision was a Sunna and female circumcision was merely preferable" (Sudanese Medical Service 1945). This usage implies a greater obligation for that which is termed "Sunna." Therefore, to attach the term "Sunna" to female circumcision is to imply that *some* form of circumcision is expected by religious law.
5. The psychological effects of female circumcision have only recently received any systematic attention in Sudan (*see,* e.g., Baashar et al. 1979).
6. All matters concerning marriage, divorce, custody and inheritance in Sudan are governed by customary rather than civil law. A system of *shari'a* courts exists for the administration of Islamic law for cases where the individuals involved are Muslims.
7. It is interesting to note that in Sudan, where the great majority of primary health care workers at all levels are male, government statistics show males outnumbering females in 89 out of the 93 categories of treated illnesses that are not female-specific conditions (Sudan, Ministry of Health 1975a).
8. Dr. Nawal el Saadawi, an Egyptian physician and novelist who has written extensively on women in Arab societies, has criticized the "'them' helping 'us'" approach of some foreign groups: "That kind of help, which they think of as solidarity, is another type of colonialism in disguise. So we must deal with female circumcision ourselves. It is our culture, we understand it, when to fight against it and how, because this is the process of liberation" (El Saadawi 1980a).

REFERENCES

Assaad, Marie Bassili. 1980. "Female Circumcision in Egypt: Social Implications, Current Research, and Prospects for Change," *Studies in Family Planning* 11(1):3–16.

Baashar, T. A., et al. 1979. "Psycho-social Aspects of Female Circumcision. Seminar on Traditional Practices Affecting the Health of Women." World Health Organization, Regional Office for the Eastern Mediterranean.

Boddy, Janice. 1979. Personal Communication. [Based on her PhD research, University of British Columbia.]

Clark, Isobel and Christina Diaz. 1977. "Circumcision: A Slow Change in Attitudes," *Sudanow* (March 1977):43–45.

Cook, R. 1976. "Damage to Physical Health from Pharaonic Circumcision (Infibulation) of Females: A Review of the Medical Literature." World Health Organization, September 30, 1976.

Diaz, Christina and Suliman Mudawi. 1977. "Circumcision: The Social Background," *Sudanow* (March 1977):45.

El Dareer, Asma. 1979. "Female Circumcision and Its Consequences for Mother and Child." Contributions to the ILO African Symposium on the World of Work and the Protection of the Child. Yaoundé, Cameroun.

El Saadawi, Nawal. 1980a. "Creative Women in Changing Societies: A Personal Reflection," *Race and Class* 22(2):159–182.

———. 1980b. *The Hidden Face of Eve: Women in the Arab World.* London: Zed Press.

Hall, Marjorie and Bakhita Amin Ismail. 1981. *Sisters Under the Sun: The Story of Sudanese Women.* London: Longmans.

Hayes, Rose Oldfield. 1975. "Female Genital Mutilation, Fertility Control, Women's Roles and the Patrilineage in Modern Sudan," *American Ethnologist* 2(4):617–633.

Hosken, Fran P. 1980. *Female Sexual Mutilations: The Facts and Proposals for Action.* Lexington, MA: Women's International Network News.

Mudawi, Suliman. 1977a. "Circumcision: The Operation," *Sudanow* (March 1977):43–44.

———. 1977b. "The Impact of Social and Economic Changes on Female Circumcision." Sudan Medical Association Congress Series, No. 2.

O'Brien, John J. 1980. "Agricultural Labor and Development in Sudan." PhD dissertation, University of Connecticut.

Shandall, A. A. 1967. "Circumcision and Infibulation of Females," *Sudan Medical Journal* 5:178–212.

Sørbø, Gunnar M. 1977. *How to Survive Development: The Story of New Halfa.* Khartoum: Development Studies and Research Centre Monograph Series No. 6.

Sudan Medical Services. 1945. *Female Circumcision in the Anglo-Egyptian Sudan.* Khartoum: Sudan Medical Service, March 1, 1945.

Sudan Ministry of Health. 1975a. *Annual Statistical Report.* Khartoum: Ministry of Health.

———. 1975b. *National Health Programme 1977/78–1983/84.* Khartoum: Ministry of Health.

Toubia, Nahid F. 1981. "The Social and Political Implications of Female Circumcision: The Case of Sudan." MSc Proposal, University of College of Swansea, Wales.

Verzin, J. A. 1975. "Sequelae of Female Circumcision," *Tropical Doctor* (Oct., 1975).

FEMALE INFANTICIDE AND CHILD NEGLECT IN RURAL NORTH INDIA

Barbara D. Miller

INTRODUCTION

> Sitting in the hospital canteen for lunch every day, I can see families bringing their children into the hospital. So far, after watching for five days, I have seen only boys being carried in for treatment, no girls (author's field notes, Ludhiana Christian Medical College, November 1983).
>
> When the hospital was built, equal-sized wards for boys and girls were constructed. The boys' ward is always full but the girls' ward is underutilized (comment of a hospital administrator, Ludhiana Christian Medical College, November 1983).
>
> In one village, I went into the house to examine a young girl and I found that she had an advanced case of tuberculosis. I asked the mother why she hadn't done something sooner about the girl's condition because now, at this stage, the treatment would be very expensive. The mother replied, "then let her die, I have another daughter." At the time, the two daughters sat nearby listening, one with tears streaming down her face (report by a public health physician, Ludhiana Christian Medical College, November 1983).
>
> When a third, fourth, or fifth daughter is born to a family, no matter what its economic status, we increase our home visits because that child is at high risk (statement made by a public health physician, Ludhiana Christian Medical College, November 1983).

From Nancy Scheper-Hughes (ed.), *Child Survival,* pp. 95–112. Reprinted by permission of Kluwer Academic Publishers.

These quotations, taken from field notes made during a 1983 trip to Ludhiana, the Punjab, India are indicative of the nature and degree of sex-selectivity in health care of children there. Ethnographic evidence gleaned from the work of other anthropologists corroborates that intrahousehold discrimination against girls is a fact of life in much of the northern plains region of India (Miller 1981: 83–106). The strong preference for sons compared to daughters is marked from the moment of birth. Celebration at the birth of a son, particularly a first son, has been documented repeatedly in the ethnographic literature (Lewis 1965: 49; Freed and Freed 1976: 123, 206; Jacobson 1970: 307–309; Madan 1965: 63; and Aggarwal 1971: 114). But when a daughter is born, the event goes unheralded and anthropologists have documented the unconcealed disappointment in families which already have a daughter or two (Luschinsky 1962: 82; Madan 1965: 77–78; Minturn and Hitchcock 1966: 101–102). The extreme disappointment of a mother who greatly desires a son, but bears a daughter instead, could affect her ability to breastfeed successfully; "bonding" certainly would not be automatically assured between the mother and the child; and the mother's disappointed in-laws would be far less supportive than if the newborn were a son (Miller, 1986).

A thorough review of the ethnographic literature provides diverse but strongly suggestive evidence of preferential feeding of boys in North Indian villages (Miller 1981: 93–94), as well as preferential allocation of medical care to boys. Sex ratios of admissions to northern hospitals are often two or more boys to every one girl. This imbalance is not due to more frequent illness of boys, rather to sex-selective parental investment patterns.

The practice of sex-selective child care in northern India confronts us with a particularly disturbing dilemma that involves the incongruity between Western values that insist on equal life chances for all, even in the face of our universal failure to achieve that goal, versus North Indian culture which places strong value on the survival of sons rather than daughters. Public health programs in North India operate under the guidance of the national goal of "equal health care for all by the year 2000" which was declared by many developing nations at the Alma Ata conference in 1978. Yet the families with whom they are concerned operate with a different set of goals less concerned with the survival of any one individual than with the survival of the family. In rural North India the economic survival of the family, for sociocultural reasons, is dependent on the reproduction of strong sons and the control of the number of daughters who are financial burdens in many ways.

The chapter examines a variety of data and information sources on the dimensions and social context of female infanticide and daughter neglect in rural North India, an area where gender preferences regarding offspring are particularly strong. I review what is known about outright female infanticide in earlier centuries and discuss the situation in North India today, examining the empirical evidence and current theoretical approaches to the understanding of son preference and daughter disfavor. The next section considers the role of a public health program in the Punjab. In conclusion I address the issue of humanist values concerning equal life chances for all versus North Indian patriarchal values promoting better life chances for boys than girls, and the challenge to anthropological research of finding an appropriate theoretical approach to the study of children's health and survival.

INFANTICIDE: BACKGROUND

I consider infanticide to fall under the general category of child abuse and neglect which encompasses a range of behaviors. As I have written elsewhere:

> . . . it is helpful to distinguish forms of neglect from those of abuse . . . abuse is more "active" in the way it is inflicted; it is abuse when something is actually *done* to harm the child. In the case of neglect, harm comes to the child because something is *not done* which should have been. Thus, sexual molestation of a child is abusive, whereas depriving a child of adequate food and exercise is neglectful. One similarity between abuse and neglect is that both, if carried far enough, can be fatal (Miller 1981: 44–45).

Infanticide, most strictly defined, is the killing of a child under one year of age. Infanticide would be placed at one extreme of the continuum of effects of child abuse and neglect—it is fatal. At the opposite end of the continuum are forms of child abuse that result in delayed learning, slowed physical growth and development patterns, and disturbed social adjustment. Outright infanticide can be distinguished from indirect or "passive" infanticide (Harris 1977); in the former the means, such as a fatal beating, are direct and immediate, while in the latter, the means, such as sustained nutritional deprivation, are indirect.

Infanticide is further delineated with respect to the ages of the children involved. Most broadly defined, infanticide applies to the killing of children under the age of twelve months (deaths after that age would generally be classified as child *homicide,* although the definition and, hence, duration of childhood is culturally variable). *Neonaticide* usually pertains to the killing of a newborn up to twenty-four hours after birth and is sometimes given a separate analysis (Wilkey *et al.* 1982). The induced *abortion* of a fetus is sometimes categorized as a pre-natal form of infanticide that has been termed *"feticide"* in the literature.[1]

The discussion in this chapter encompasses both infanticide and child homicide, that is non-accidental deaths to minors from the time of birth up to the age of about fifteen or sixteen when they would become adults in the rural Indian context. For convenience, I will use the term infanticide to apply to the entire age range.

I have asserted (1981: 44) that where infanticide is systematically sex-selective, it will be selective against females rather than males. There are few cases of systematic male-selective infanticide in the literature that I reviewed. Some more recent work on the subject, however, has begun to reveal a variety of patterns. For example, a study conducted on several villages in a delta region of Japan using data from the Tokugawa era (1600–1868) reveals the existence of systematic infanticide which was sex-selective, but selective against males almost as frequently as females, depending on the particular household composition and dynamics (Skinner 1984).

Obviously all household strategies concerning the survival of offspring are not based solely on gender considerations, and it is doubtful that we can ever come close to a good estimation of just "how much" gender-based selective differential in the treatment of children exists, and how much of this is biased against females. Nevertheless, one part of the world where female-selective infanticide is particularly apparent is in North India, and across India's northwestern border through Pakistan . . . to the Near East, and perhaps in a diminished form also in North Africa. Looking toward the East from India, it seems that Southeast Asia is largely free of the son preference/daughter disfavor syndrome, as opposed to China where one result of the one-child policy . . . was the death of thousands of female infants.

FEMALE INFANTICIDE IN PRE-TWENTIETH CENTURY INDIA

The British discovery of infanticide in India occurred in 1789 among a clan of Rajputs in the eastern part of Uttar Pradesh, a northern state.[2] All of the infanticide reported by British district officers and other observers was direct female infanticide. A lengthy quotation from a mid-nineteenth century description by a British magistrate in the Northwest Provinces of India demonstrates how open was the knowledge of the practice of female infanticide at that time:

> There is at Mynpoorie an old fortress, which looks far over the valley of the Eesun river. This has been for centuries the stronghold of the Rajahs of Mynpoorie, Chohans whose ancient blood, descending from the great Pirthee Raj and the regal stem of Neem-rana, represents *la crème de la crème* of Rajpoot aristocracy. Here when a son, a nephew, a grandson, was born to the reigning chief, the event was announced to the neighboring city by the loud discharge of wall-pieces and matchlocks; but centuries had passed away, and no infant daughter had been known to smile within those walls.
>
> In 1845, however, thanks to the vigilance of Mr. Unwin [the district collector], a little grand-daughter was preserved by the Rajah of that day. The fact was duly notified to the Government, and a letter of congratulations and a dress of honour were at once dispatched from head-quarters to the Rajah.
>
> We have called this incident, the giving of a robe of honour to a man because he did not destroy his grand-daughter a *grotesque* one; but it is very far from being a ridiculous incident. When the people see that the highest authorities in the land take an interest in their social or domestic reforms, those reforms can give an impetus which no lesser influences can give them. The very next year after the investiture of the Rajah, the number of female infants preserved in the district was *trebled!* Fifty-seven had

> been saved in 1845; in 1846, one hundred and eighty were preserved; and the number has gone on steadily increasing ever since (Raikes 1852: 20–21).

A review of the secondary literature on female infanticide in British India reveals its practice mainly in the Northwest, and among upper castes and tribes. Not all groups practiced female infanticide, but there are grim reports that a few entire villages in the northwestern plains had never raised one daughter.[3] On the basis of juvenile (under ten years of age) sex ratios for districts in the Northwest Provinces, 1871, I have estimated crudely that for nineteenth-century Northwest India it would not be unreasonable to assume that one-fourth of the population preserved only half the daughters born to them, while the other three-fourths of the population had balanced sex ratios among their offspring (Miller 1981: 62). This assumption yields a juvenile sex ratio of 118 (males per 100 females) in the model population, which is comparable to current juvenile sex ratios in several districts of northwestern Indian and Pakistan (Miller 1981, 1984). It seems clear that female infanticide in British India was widespread in the Northwest rather than of limited occurrence.

The British investigated the extent and causes of female infanticide, and in 1870 passed a law against its practice. Other policy measures, based on their assessment of the causes of the practice, included subsidizing the dowries of daughters that were "preserved" by prominent families, and organizing conferences in order to enlighten local leaders and their followers about the need to prevent infanticide (Cave Browne 1857).

There are two areas of ignorance about the wider context of the historic practice of female infanticide in India. First, we know little about the apparent and gradual transition from direct to indirect infanticide. It appears that either deep-seated social change and/or British policy against the practice of female infanticide succeeded in bringing about the near-end of direct female infanticide by the beginning of this century. In the twentieth century we hear little about female infanticide in census reports, district gazetteers, or anthropological descriptions of rural life. What is needed is a careful tracing of the situation from roughly 1870 when the practice was outlawed to the present time in order to plot the dynamics of change from outright to indirect infanticide. Second, we need to know much more about the sociocultural determinants of female infanticide in British India. The British pointed to two causal factors—"pride and purse." The pride of upper castes and tribes is said to have pushed them to murder female infants rather than give them away as tribute to a more dominant group, or even as brides which is viewed as demeaning in rural North India today. By "purse" is meant dowry, and most groups that practiced infanticide did have the custom of giving large dowries with daughters.[4] But there is some contradictory evidence. In the undivided Punjab, it has been documented for the early twentieth century that dowry was not widely given among the rural Jats, a caste which nonetheless exhibited very high sex ratios (i.e., males over females) among its juvenile population. In fact, the Jats, a landed peasant caste, often secured brides through brideprice, which should have provided an economic incentive for parents to preserve daughters (Darling 1929; see also the discussion in Miller 1984). Further exploration of archival materials for the nineteenth century would help illuminate this matter.

FEMALE INFANTICIDE AND NEGLECT: THE CURRENT CONTEXT

It is beyond doubt that systematic indirect female infanticide exists today in North India. It is possible that outright infanticide of neonates is also practiced, though nearly impossible to document due to the extreme privacy of the birth event and the great ease with which a neonate's life may be terminated.[5] This section of the paper is concerned with indirect female infanticide, which is accomplished by nutritional and health-care deprivation of children, and which results in higher mortality rates of daughters than sons.[6]

There is a strong preference for sons in rural North India and there are several strong sociocultural reasons for this preference. Sons are economic assets: they are needed for farming, and for income through remittances if they leave the village. Sons play important roles in local power struggles over rights to land and water. Sons stay with the family after their marriage and thus maintain the parents in their old age; daughters marry out and cannot contribute to the maintenance of their natal households. Sons bring in dowries with their brides; daughters drain family wealth with their required dowries and the constant flow of gifts to their family of marriage after the wedding. Sons, among Hindus, are also needed to perform rituals which protect the family after the death of the father; daughters cannot perform such rituals.

Elsewhere I have argued that extreme son preference is more prevalent in North India than in the South and East, and that it is more prevalent among upper castes and classes than lower castes and classes (Miller 1981). By extension, daughter neglect would follow the same pattern. Some of the key research questions include: how extensive is daughter disfavor in different regions and among various social strata in India? How serious are its consequences in terms of mortality and in health status of the survivors (not to mention more difficult to diagnose conditions such as emotional and cognitive development)? Are these patterns changing through time? At this point, scattered studies help illuminate some aspects of these questions, but there is no study that addresses them all systematically either for one locale or for India as a whole.

First, let us consider the question of the extent of the practice in India. In a recent publication, Lipton (1983) suggests that fatal discrimination against daughters in India is a very localized, and thus minor, problem. But my all-India analysis (1981), using juvenile sex ratios as a surrogate measure of child mortality, shows that while the most afflicted area encompasses only two or three states of India, there are seriously unbalanced sex ratios among children in one-third of India's 326 rural districts, an area spanning the entire northwestern plains.[7] Simmons *et al.* (1982) provide results from survey data on 2064 couples in the Kanpur region of Uttar Pradesh (a state in northern India) which reveal that reported infant and child mortality rates for girls aged one month up to three years of age are much higher than the rates for boys. This finding is similar to, though less astonishing than, Cowan and Dhanoa's (1983) report that in a large sub-population carefully monitored in Ludhiana district, the Punjab, 85 percent of all deaths to children aged 7–36 months were female. Another dependable database that has been carefully analyzed by Behrman (1984) and Behrman and Deolalikar (1985) concerns an area of India where juvenile sex ratios are not notably unbalanced, south-central India in the area between Andhra Pradesh and Maharashtra. The authors have found that there is a noticeable nutrient bias in favor of boys in the intrahousehold allocation of food. This unequal distribution has a seasonal dimension: in the lean season boys are more favored over girls in the distribution of food in the family, while in the surplus season distribution appears quite equal.

Class/caste variations in juvenile sex ratios are also important. Simmons *et al.* (1982) unfortunately do not present findings on class or caste patterns. They mention that education of the parents is a positive influence on child survival in the first year of life, less so in the second and third. If parental education can be used as a crude indicator of class status, then it would seem that survival for both boys and girls would be more assured in better-off families. Demographic data from the Ludhiana area of Punjab state have been analyzed for class differences by Cowan and Dhanoa (1983). Among upper class, landed families (termed "privileged" by Cowan and Dhanoa), there is a large disparity between survival rates for male and female children and also in the nutritional status of those surviving (Table 1). These disparities are mirrored, though less severe, in the lower class, landless population. Cowan and Dhanoa found that birth order strongly affects the survival and status of daughters. Second-born and third-born daughters are classified by health care personnel as "high risk" infants, as are high birth order children of both sexes born to very large families, regardless of socioeconomic status. The extent of fatal daughter disfavor in this relatively affluent state of India is severe, and it contributes to Punjab's having infant (up to one year of age) mortality rates higher that those of poorer states where daughter discrimination is less severe (Miller 1985).

Caldwell's data on a cluster of villages in Karnataka (southern-central-India), with a total population of more than 5000, revealed "surprisingly small" differences in infant and child mortality by economic status, father's occupation and religion (1983:197). (This area of the country is characterized by balanced juvenile sex ratios at the district level.) The authors do not mention whether there are any sex differentials in child survival and health. Infant mortality rates are, however, much lower in households with an educated mother than those where the mother has little education. Girls tend to receive less food than boys, and family variables are mentioned as being involved in this matter.

Another report from a region with balanced juvenile sex ratios, a two-village study in West Bengal reported on by Sen and Sengupta (1983), produced some provocative findings. The authors did not look at mortality but rather at levels of undernourishment in children below five years of age according to caste and land ownership status of the household. Results were surprising: the village with a more vigorous land redistribution program had a greater nutritional sex bias, even among children in families who had benefited from the redistribution. In the second village, children in poor families had higher nutritional standards and a lower male-female differential than their counterparts in the first village.

Rosenzweig and Schultz (1982) used a subsample of rural households in India, presumably nationwide, and found that boys have significantly higher survival rates relative to girls in landless rather than in landed households. Horowitz and Keshwar report that survey data from a Punjab village (northern India) demonstrate more pronounced son preference among the propertied peasant castes, although the phenomenon is "nearly" as strong among agricultural laborers (1982: 12); they do not provide health or survival statistics, but use data on stated preferences of parents.

The above review indicates that, while we do not possess an ideal picture of the extent and nature of daughter disfavor, there is evi-

TABLE 1 Prevalence of 2nd/3rd Degree Malnutrition in 911 Children in Second and Third Year of Life, Ludhiana, the Punjab

	Number	*Sex Ratio*[a]	*With 2nd/3rd Degree Malnutrition*[b]	*Ratio of Male to Female Malnourished*
Privileged males	231	111.0	2	1:6.5
Privileged females	208		13	
Under-privileged males	244	102.5	11	1:2.6
Under-privileged females	228		29	
TOTAL	911	106.5	55	1:3.2

[a]Sex ratio refers to the number of males per hundred females.
[b]The numbers in this column were read from a graph and may be off by a small margin.
Source: Cowan and Dhanoa (1983: 352).

dence that its practice does exist widely in India and does tend to exhibit class/caste patterns—though the exact nature of these is in dispute. We know very little about the question of change through time since few good sources of longitudinal data exist, and those that do exist have not been examined for sex disparity information as yet.

SEX-SELECTIVE ABORTION

> Several years ago a Jain woman in her sixth month of pregnancy came to Ludhiana Christian Medical Hospital for an amniocentesis test. The results of the test showed that genetic defects such as Down's syndrome or spina bifida were not present in the fetus. The test indicated that the fetus was female. The woman requested an abortion and was refused. She went to a clinic in Amritsar, another major city in the Punjab, and had the abortion done (report by a physician, Ludhiana, November 1983).

This anecdote was told to me at Ludhiana Christian Medical College as an explanation why Ludhiana CMC no longer performs amniocentesis. There were so many requests for abortion of female fetuses following amniocentesis that the hospital made a policy decision not to provide such services.[8] Today a person with intent to abort a female fetus in Ludhiana must take the train about 90 miles to Amritsar where the service is available. An especially poignant aspect of the anecdote is the information that the woman was a Jain. Jainism supports nonviolence toward all life forms. Orthodox Jains sometimes wear cloths over their mouths so as not to swallow a fly, and Jains do not plow the earth for fear of inadvertently cutting in half a worm. But the Jain woman in the anecdote was willing to abort a female fetus in the sixth month of gestation, so strong was the cultural disfavor toward the birth of daughters.

At this time I do not have access to data on the number of female fetuses aborted each year in India, nor to data on the social characteristics of those people who seek to abort their female fetuses. Nonetheless, several considerations are important: how can we estimate the extent of the practice? What are the social and economic characteristics of those families seeking to abort female fetuses? What are the demographic characteristics of the families seeking sex-selective abortion? There are some clues.

In 1980 an article published in *Social Science and Medicine* provided some evidence of the extent of the phenomenon based on clinic records in a large city of western India (Ramanamma and Bambawale 1980). In one hospital, from June 1976 to June 1977, 700 individuals sought prenatal sex determination. Of these fetuses, 250 were determined to be male and 450 were female.[9] While all of the male fetuses were kept to term, fully 430 of the 450 female fetuses were terminated. This figure is even more disturbing in light of the fact that western India is characterized by a less extreme son preference than the Northwest.

There is an eager market in India for sex-selective abortion, although the cost of the service may make it prohibitive for the poorest villagers. A report in *Manushi* (1982) states that the service is available in Chandigarh, the Punjab, for only 500 rupees.[10] Another report mentions that the charge was 600 rupees at a clinic in Amritsar, the Punjab (*Washington Post* 1982). A recent visitor to Ahmedabad, Gujarat, reports a charge of only 50 rupees in a clinic there (Everett 1984). Whether the charge is 50 rupees or 500 rupees, the cost is minor compared to the benefits reaped from the possibility of having a son conceived at the next pregnancy, or compared to the money that would have been needed to provide a dowry for the girl were she to survive.

DETERMINANTS OF SON PREFERENCE AND DAUGHTER DISFAVOR

Why does son preference exist, and why does it often exist in tandem with the practices of sex-selective abortion, female infanticide, and female neglect? Anthropologists have proposed "explanations" for the practice of female infanticide in simple societies, but less work has been done for complex civilizations. Recent problems in China, provoked by the one-child policy, have attracted attention to the subject, but little scholarly thinking, with few exceptions. . . . A range of hypothesized causal factors has been suggested to account for female infanticide in the past few years. They can be divided into ecologic/economic determinants, social structural determinants and sociobiological determinants.

From the broadest population ecology perspective, Harris (1977) proposes that female infanticide, and by extension sex-selective abortion, will most likely occur when a society has reached a crisis level in its population/resources ratio, or right after that crisis when the society has moved into a necessarily expendable portion of the population in relation to resources. This theory has explanatory power for some cases, but we might bear in mind that infanticide is only one of many possible strategies for ameliorating a high population/resources ratio. Other options include migration, and the reduction of natural population growth through delayed marriage, abstinence, abortion, and other forms of birth control both traditional and modern.

My interpretation, based on the case of North India, gives more emphasis to economic demand factors. I have hypothesized that labor requirements for males versus females (themselves ecologically, agriculturally and culturally defined) are key in determining households' desires regarding number and sex of offspring (Miller 1981, 1984). Although I take the sexual division of labor as primary, I view it as creating a secondary and very powerful determinant in the domestic marriage economy. In the case of India, the contrast between dowry marriages and bridewealth marriages illustrates the "mirroring" of the sexual division of labor in marriage costs: generally where few females are employed in the agricultural sector, large dowries prevail, but where female labor is in high demand, smaller dowries or even bridewealth are the main form of marriage transfers.

Other more orthodox economic approaches stress rational decision-making on the part of the family based on perceived "market opportunities" of offspring (Rosenzweig and Schultz 1982) or intrafamily resource allocation systems (Simmons *et al.* 1982). Sen and Sengupta propose that land distribution patterns are an important determinant of sex differentials in children's nutritional status (1983).

The major exponents of a social structural theory are Dyson and Moore (1983). They identify the patriarchal nature of North Indian society as the basis for the neglect of daughters and other manifestations of low female status. They do not seek to explain why society in North India is strongly patriarchal—that is simply a given.

Dickemann, who studied female infanticide cross-culturally and particularly in stratified societies such as traditional northern India and China, provides a sociobiological interpretation for female infanticide (1979, 1984). Her early observation of the connection between hypergynous marriage systems and female infanticide was a particularly important contribution (1979). Dickemann views sex ratio manipulation among offspring as one reproductive strategy that will, under alternate resource conditions, result in maximum reproductive success for the family. She has recently stated that:

> Like other acts of reproductive management, infanticide-pedicide seems to be best understood at present, in all species, as one parameter of interindividual and interfamilial competition for the proportional increase in genes in the next generation . . . (1984: 436).

In terms of the explanatory power of evolutionary models with respect to the cause of violent mistreatment of human offspring, however, Hrdy and Hausfater (1984: xxxi) agree with Lenington (1981) that "only a portion of such cases" will be thus explained.

PUBLIC HEALTH AND PATRIARCHY

Ten years ago when I began my research on fatal neglect of daughters in rural India the problem was not widely accepted by scholars in the West or in India as a serious one.[11]

Today the practice of fatal daughter disfavor is more widely recognized by scholars as a serious social issue. Current concern in India about the growing recourse to sex-selective abortion, using information on sex of the fetus derived from amniocentesis, adds a new and important dimension to problems of female survival and the ethics of abortion (Ramanamma and Bambawale 1980; Kumar 1983).

Operating within such a patriarchal system, could any health care program seeking to provide equal health care for all have any success? There is controversy concerning the impact of health care programs in alleviating sex differences in child survival in patriarchal cultures, particularly North India. Some writers suggest that a simple increase in health care services will improve the situation for girls (Minturn 1984). Others have found evidence that increased services will be diverted to priority children, most often boys, and that only secondarily will low priority children, most often girls, benefit.[12] Finally, the introduction of new medical technologies—such as amniocentesis—can be manipulated to advance patriarchal priorities (Miller 1986).

Focus on the Punjab

The Punjab, India's wealthiest state, is located in the northwestern plains region adjacent to Pakistan. Its economy is agricultural with wheat the major food crop, but there is a well-developed industrial sector also. Within the Punjab, Ludhiana district is usually recognized as the most "developed" district. Ludhiana district also stands out because it houses one of the best medical colleges and community health programs in India, Ludhiana Christian Medical College. Ludhiana, and the Punjab district, are squarely in the area in northwestern India where juvenile sex ratios are the most masculine and excess female child mortality the greatest (Miller 1985).

Since the early 1970s, Ludhiana CMC has been monitoring the reproductive and health status of the surrounding population—first as a pilot project in three rural locations and one urban location, and later in the entire block of Sahnewal (an administrative subdivision of the district), with a population of about 85,000. The monitoring is part of a decentralized, comprehensive basic health care program that focuses on the welfare of mothers and children and includes both health care delivery at village centers and home-based educational programs. For each of the nearly 14,000 families in Sahnewal block, the CMC Ludhiana program maintains family folders containing information on all family members and their health status. Mortalities are carefully recorded in each folder and also in Master Registers kept in 49 village centers throughout the block. Some analysis of these data has been performed (Cowan and Dhanoa 1983) which provides startling figures on sex differentials of mortality for children aged 7–36 months in which female deaths constituted 85 percent of the total (1983: 341).

Cowan and Dhanoa note that one important result of their intensive home-based visiting approach in the rural Punjab is a reduction in the percentage of female child deaths (1983: 354). There is no doubt that their approach can be effective for saving the lives of high-risk children, though it requires great effort and entails much surveillance of private life. Two questions arise from this finding: a related result of increased survival for girls is an increase in the percentage of malnourished girls—girls' lives have been saved, but the quality of those lives may not be at all equal to that of males. Would even more intensive home visiting help alleviate this problem? Furthermore, some would argue that the death of unwanted children might be preferable to their extended mistreatment and suffering (Kumar 1983. . .).

We have not estimated the unit health care costs by sex and priority of the child, but the cost of saving the life of a low priority female child must far outweigh the cost of saving and improving the life of a high priority male. It is not unthinkable that the time will arrive when, with fiscal stringency the watchword of the day, the cost of intensive health care and survival monitoring for girls becomes a barrier to programs such as the one at Ludhiana CMC. Two arguments can be developed to counter policies which would limit special efforts to equalize life chances between boys and girls. First, one might look to the broader social costs of a society in which the sex ratio is seriously unbalanced. It cannot be proven that unbalanced sex ratios invariably lead to social disturbances, but there is much cross-cultural evidence to support this (Divale and Harris 1976). A balanced sex ratio does not guarantee social tranquility, but it could minimize some sources of social tension. Second, in a strongly son-preferential culture, women bear many children in the attempt to produce several sons. The pattern of selective care which promotes son survival to the detriment of daughter survival is built on "over-reproduction" and much child wastage. Mothers bear a physical burden in this system. The Ludhiana program seeks to keep children alive and wanted, and to promote family planning after a certain number and sex composition of children have been born in a household; this goal should reduce the physical burden on mothers created by extended childbearing.

HUMANISTIC VALUES, PATRIARCHAL VALUES, AND ANTHROPOLOGY

This chapter discusses an extreme form of sex-selective child care, one which is not universally found throughout the world though it is not limited to rural North India. Strong preference for sons which results in life-endangering deprivation of daughters is "culturally" acceptable in much of rural North India with its patriarchal foundation. It is not acceptable from a Western humanistic or altruistic perspective . . . nor from that of an emergent, international feminist "world view." But, how can anthropological research, with its commitment to nonethnocentric reporting of cultural behavior, contribute to an amelioration of the "worldview conflicts" that create inappropriate public health programs targeted at high-risk children, that sometimes only prolong the suffering of these disvalued ones?

. . . [P]erhaps positivistic anthropology and Western altruism can work together. First, let me hasten to soften the hard edges of the "conflict" in world views that Cassidy has constructed: there is no such thing as purely objective and nonethnocentric anthropological research and there is, increasingly, less and less culturally uninformed altruism being foisted on the Third World. All anthropologists, as Schneider so clearly states (1984), have their own unavoidable, culturally-influenced presuppositions and biases through which they choose subjects for research and through which they analyze their data. The best an anthropologist can do is state the nature of his/her presuppositions at the outset: mine, influenced by my white, middle class, American upbringing, are based on the precept that human life, its duration and quality, is something to which all persons should have equal access, although I am fully aware of the fact that scarcity (real or culturally defined) results in priorities about the quality of life that certain groups will receive. Thus I define female infanticide and skewed sex ratios as a social "problem." As an applied anthropologist I believe that socio-behavioral data can provide the key to successful public programs which seek to ameliorate the "problem."

My experience, though too brief, in working with Dr. Betty Cowan and Dr. Jasbir Dhanoa (two "altruists") in Ludhiana convinced me that there is hope for a realistic solution to the conflict between altruism and, in this case, extreme patriarchy, in the sensitive applications of social science knowledge and research. The public health program at Ludhiana is perhaps never going to dilute the force of Indian patriarchy, but knowledge about the patriarchal culture can help promote more effective health care. For instance, the Ludhiana hospital built equal-sized wards for boys and girls, on the Western model. But families bring their boys in for health care in much greater numbers than their girls; the girls' ward is relatively empty while the boys' ward is overflowing. Health care practitioners thus realized the need for very decentralized health care rather than only hospital-based services, including frequent home visiting, if health care was to reach girls.

Anthropologists can provide important information to health care intervenors which will allow those intervenors to be more effective in delivering their services. The most important issue in the Ludhiana area still to be resolved is the impact of class and caste stratification on female survival. Health care practitioners see daughter disfavor largely as a result of poverty. My own research would question poverty as the principal determinant in Ludhiana because there is a marked disparity in survival of boys and girls in the propertied class as well as in the unpropertied class. Although the larger picture is unclear because of lack of data across North India, it is obvious that policy implications differ greatly depending on class/caste dimensions of village life. If health care programs are to be targeted to "high-risk" groups, anthropologists can help by providing data on the nature of these groups and the potential implications of intervention in their lives.

NOTES

Much of my recent research on this subject has been supported by grants from the Wenner-Gren Foundation for Anthropological Research. I am grateful for the Foundation's support which enabled me to visit two hospitals in India during November 1983 in order to learn about their community health programs: Ludhiana Christian Medical College in the Punjab and Vellore Christian Medical College in Tamil Nadu. While in India, I received help from many people, but I especially want to thank Dr. Betty Cowan, Principal of Ludhiana CMC, and Dr. P.S. Sundar Rao, Chief of the Biostatics Department at Vellore CMC. An earlier version of this chapter was presented at a seminar sponsored by the Department of Anthropology and the Asian Studies Program at the University of Pittsburgh in March 1985, and I am grateful for the comments I received from those who attended. Finally, I must thank The Metropolitan Studies Program, The Maxwell School, Syracuse University, for support of my work.

1. A discussion of abortion and infanticide from a Western philosophical view is provided in Tooley (1983); compare his presentation with Potter's description of the Chinese view (this volume).
2. We know very little about the practice of female infanticide in India before the British era. The discussion that follows is extracted in large part from Miller (1981: 49–67).
3. Critics are quick to point out that without daughters, villages will not "survive." But in the case of North India, marriage is village exogamous, particularly for Hindus; that is, brides must come from a village other than the groom's. Villages without daughters would "survive" because they would bring in daughters-in-law. More anecdotally, the Community Health Program at Ludhiana CMC was started by a woman physician who was the third daughter of the Grewal lineage to be preserved; even without daughters, the Grewal lineage has "survived" for centuries.
4. Another effect, largely urban and upper-class, of the dowry system in North India is the murder of young wives by their in-laws in order to procure a second bride with her dowry (Sharma 1983).
5. Knowledgeable physicians who have worked with the community health care program in the rural areas surrounding Ludhiana, the Punjab, know that there is a preponderance of female neonatal deaths as compared to those of males. They are averse to labelling this as due to infanticide since an autopsy may well not reveal an intentional death as opposed to a stillbirth or an unintentional death. The physicians do know that neonatal deaths constitute a serious problem, and one that is the hardest for them to deal with due to the secrecy surrounding births in rural India.
6. A detailed discussion of the dynamics of son preference in India can be found in Miller (1981), and a comparison between Pakistan and Bangladesh in Miller (1984).
7. This pattern in Northwest India extends over the Indian border into Pakistan . . . .
8. The central government of India has banned prenatal sex determination tests in government hospitals throughout the country for the same reason.
9. The preponderance of females in the sample is probably due to sheer accident.
10. In 1984–85, one dollar equalled approximately twelve rupees.

11. There are some notable exceptions to this generalization (Bardhan 1974; Chandrasekhar 1972; Dandekar 1975; Visaria 1961), although none of these scholars emphasized the major role of sex-differential survival of children in creating the preponderance of males over females.
12. Srilatha (1983) reports that in a large study area in Tamil Nadu, South India, infant and child mortality rates have declined significantly in the last ten years, but the decline was dramatic for boys and only slight for girls. The implication is that improved health services may be differentially allocated to boys and girls in this area of India.

REFERENCES

Aggarwal, Partap C. 1971. *Caste, Religion and Power. An Indian Case Study.* New Delhi: Shri Ram Centre for Industrial Relations.

Bardhan, Pranab K. 1974. "On Life and Death Questions," *Economic and Political Weekly* 10 (32–34): 1293–1303.

Behrman, Jere R. 1984. "Intrahousehold Allocation of Nutrients in Rural India: Are Boys Favored? Do Parents Exhibit Inequality Aversion?" Unpublished manuscript, University of Pennsylvania, Department of Economics. (Revised 1985.)

Behrman, Jere R. and Anil B. Deolalikar. 1985. "How Do Food and Product Prices Affect Nutrient Intakes, Health and Labor Force Behavior for Different Family Numbers in Rural India?" Paper presented at the 1985 Meetings of the Population Association of America, Boston.

Caldwell, J.C., P.H. Reddy, and Pat Caldwell. 1983. "The Social Component of Mortality Decline: An Investigation in South India Employing Alternative Methodologies." *Population Studies* 37: 185–205.

Cave Browne, John. 1857. *Indian Infanticide: Its Origin, Progress, and Suppression.* London: W.H. Allen.

Chandrasekhar, S. 1972. *Infant Mortality, Population Growth and Family Planning in India.* Chapel Hill, NC: University of North Carolina Press.

Cowan, Betty and Jasbir Dhanoa. 1983. "The Prevention of Toddler Malnutrition by Home-based Nutrition Education." In *Nutrition in the Community: A Critical Look at Nutrition Policy, Planning, and Programmes.* D.S. McLaren (ed.), pp. 339–356. New York/London: John Wiley and Sons.

Dandekar, Kumudini. 1975. "Why Has the Proportion of Women in India's Population Been Declining?" *Economic and Political Weekly* 10(42): 1663–1667.

Darling, Malcolm Lyall. 1929. *Rusticus Loquitur or the Old Light and the New in the Punjab Village.* London: Oxford University Press.

Dickemann, Mildred. 1979. "Female Infanticide, Reproductive Strategies, and Social Stratification: A Preliminary Model." In *Evolutionary Biology and Human Social Behavior: An Anthropological Perspective.* N.A. Chagnon and W. Irons (eds.), pp. 321–367. North Scituate, MA: Duxbury Press.

———. 1984. "Concepts and Classification in the Study of Human Infanticide: Sectional Introduction and Some Cautionary Notes" In *Infanticide: Comparative and Evolutionary Perspectives.* Glenn Hausfater and Sarah Blâffer Hrdy (eds.), pp. 427–439. New York: Aldine Publishing Company.

Divale, William and Marvin Harris. 1976. "Population, Warfare, and the Male Supremacist Complex." *American Anthropologist* 78: 521–538.

Dyson, Tim and Mick Moore. 1983. "Gender Relations, Female Autonomy and Demographic Behavior: Regional Contrasts within India." *Population and Development Review* 9(1): 35–60.

Everett, Jana. 1984. Personal communication. (Dr. Everett is a political scientist at the University of Colorado, Denver.)

Freed, Stanley A. and Ruth S. Freed. 1976. "Shanti Nagar: The Effects of Urbanization in a Village in North India: 1. Social Organization," *Anthropological Papers of the American Museum of National History.* Vol. 53: Part 1. New York: The American Museum of Natural History.

Harris, Marvin. 1977. *Cannibals and Kings: The Origins of Cultures.* New York: Random House.

Horowitz, B. and Madhu Keshwar. 1982. "Family Life—The Unequal Deal." *Manushi* 11: 2–18.

Hrdy, Sarah Blaffer and Glenn Hausfater. 1984. "Comparative and Evolutionary Perspectives on Infanticide: Introduction and Overview." In *Infanticide: Comparative and Evolutionary Perspectives.* Glenn Hausfater and Sarah Blaffer Hrdy (eds.), pp. xii–xxxv. Aldine Publishing Company.

Jacobson, Doranne. 1970. "Hidden Faces: Hindu and Muslim Purdah in a Central Indian Village." Unpublished doctoral dissertation, Columbia University.

Kumar, Dharma. 1983. "Male Utopias or Nightmares?" *Economic and Political Weekly*, January 15: 61–64.

Lenington, S. 1981. "Child Abuse: The Limits of Sociobiology," *Ethnology and Sociobiology* 2: 17–29.

Lewis, Oscar. 1965. *Village Life in Northern India: Studies in a Delhi Village.* New York: Random House.

Lipton, Michael. 1983. "Demography and Poverty." World Bank Staff Working Papers, Number 623. Washington, DC: The World Bank.

Luschinsky, Mildred S. 1962. "The Life of Women in a Village of North India: A Study of Role and Status." Unpublished doctoral dissertation, Cornell University.

Madan, T.N. 1965. *Family and Kinship: A Study of the Pandits of Rural Kashmir.* New York: Asia Publishing House.

Manushi. 1982. "A New Form of Female Infanticide." 12: 21.

Miller, Barbara D. 1981. *The Endangered Sex: Neglect of Female Children in Rural North India.* Ithaca, NY: Cornell University Press.

———. 1984. "Daughter Neglect, Women's Work and Marriage: Pakistan and Bangladesh Compared." *Medical Anthropology* 8(2): 109–126.

———. 1985. "The Unwanted Girls: A Study of Infant Mortality Rates," *Manushi* 29: 18–20.

———. 1986. "Prenatal and Postnatal Sex-Selection in India: The Patriarchal Context, Ethical Questions and Public Policy." Working Paper No. 107 on Women in International Development (East Lansing, MI: Office of Women in International Development, Michigan State University).

Minturn, Leigh. 1984. "Changes in the Differential Treatment of Rajput Girls in Khalapur: 1955–1975," *Medical Anthropology* 8(2): 127–132.

Minturn, Leigh and John T. Hitchcock. 1966. *The Rajputs of Khalapur, India. Six Cultures Series,* Volume III. New York: John Wiley and Sons.

Raikes, Charles. 1852. *Notes on the North-Western Provinces of India.* London: Chapman and Hall.

Ramanamma, A. and Usha Bambawale. 1980. "The Mania for Sons: An Analysis of Social Values in South Asia," *Social Science and Medicine* 14B: 107–110.

Rosenzweig, Mark R. and T. Paul Schultz. 1982. "Market Opportunities, Genetic Endowments, and Intrafamily Resource Distribution: Child Survival in Rural India," *American Economic Review* 72(4): 803–815.

Schneider, David M. 1984. *A Critique of the Study of Kinship.* Ann Arbor, MI: The University of Michigan Press.

Sen, Amartya and Sunil Sengupta. 1983. "Malnutrition of Children and the Rural Sex Bias," *Economic and Political Weekly Annual Number,* May: 855–864.

Sharma, Ursula. 1983. "Dowry in North India: Its Consequences for Women," In *Women and Property, Women as Property.* Renee Hirschon (ed.), pp. 62–74. London: Croom Helm.

Simmons, George B., Celeste Smucker, Stan Bernstein, and Eric Jensen. 1982. "Post Neo-Natal Mortality in Rural India: Implications of an Economic Model," *Demography* 19(3): 371–389.

Skinner, G. William. 1984. "Infanticide as Family Planning in Tokugawa Japan." Paper prepared for the Stanford-Berkeley Colloquium in Historical Demography, San Francisco.

Srilatha, K.V. 1983. Personal communication. (Dr. Srilatha is an epidemiologist, Senior Training and Research Officer, Rural Unit for Health and Social Assistance, Vellore Christian Medical College, Tamil Nadu, India).

Tooley, Michael. 1983. *Abortion and Infanticide.* Oxford: Oxford University Press.

Visaria, Pravin M. 1961. *The Sex Ratio of the Population of India. Census of India 1961,* Vol. 1, Monograph No. 10. New Delhi: Office of the Registrar General.

Washington Post. August 25. 1982. "Birth Test Said to Help Indians Abort Females."

Wasserstrom, Jeffrey. 1984. "Resistance to the One-Child Family," *Modern China* 10(3): 345–374.

Wilkey, Ian, John Pearn, Gwynneth Petrie, and James Nixon. 1982. "Neonaticide, Infanticide and Child Homicide," *Medicine, Science and the Law* 22(1): 31–34.

XI

COLONIALISM, DEVELOPMENT, AND THE GLOBAL ECONOMY

We live today in a global world based on complex political and economic relationships. There are few places that remain untouched by international markets, the mass media, geopolitics, or economic aid. However, the global world, particularly the global economy, is not a new phenomenon. It has its roots in the sixteenth century, when the powerful countries of western Europe began to colonize populations in Asia, Africa, and the Americas. Part of this process involved the extraction of raw materials such as gold, sugar, rubber, and coffee, and the exploitation of the labor of indigenous populations for the profit of the colonizing nations.

Although most of the colonized world achieved independence by the 1960s, the economic domination of the capitalist world system that was initiated during the colonial period has not been significantly altered. In the late twentieth century an imbalanced relationship between the countries of the industrial, or "developed," world and the developing, or Third World, remains. How have the men and women of the developing world experienced the continuing impact of the penetration of capitalism and the integration of their societies into the global economy?

This question has been addressed in particular with regard to women, and two opposing views have been formulated. Chaney and Schmink (1980), in a review of studies on women and modernization, describe a minority position suggesting that women in the Third World are downtrodden and that capitalist development can help them improve their situation. Those who hold this opinion emphasize that women's economic and social status can be enhanced by an increase in female labor-force participation. Another perspective, stimulated by Ester Boserup's argument that in the course of economic development women experience a decline in their relative status within agriculture (1970: 53), suggests that colonialism and development have introduced "a structure and ideology of male domination" (Leacock 1979: 131). In many parts of the world, originally egalitarian gender relationships have been replaced by more hierarchical ones, and women have consequently been marginalized, removed from the positions of economic and political decision making that they held in the precolonial period.

Researchers have demonstrated the negative effects of colonialism and capitalist penetration in a number of different historical contexts. Silverblatt (1980: 160), for example, portrays the Spanish conquest of the Andes as a "history of the struggle between colonial forces which attempted to break down indigenous social relations and reorient them toward a market economy and the resistance of the indigenous people to these disintegrating forces." Her focus is on the impact of this struggle on the lives of Andean women.

In the pre-Inca and Inca periods Andean women had status and power that were manifested in their customary usufruct rights to land and in their ability to organize labor. After the conquest, Spanish law came up against Andean custom with regard to the property rights of women. In addition, "The Spanish system . . . ignored the deeply embedded Andean conception of the household embodying the necessary complementarity of male and female labor" (Silverblatt 1980: 168). The result of Spanish colonialism in the Andes was the strengthening of patrilineal and patrilocal ties at the expense of matrilineal and matrilocal ties. Women became both politically and religiously disenfranchised. Indeed, women who continued to practice traditional religion were persecuted. Despite this persecution, the religious practices survived and became a very important mechanism of cultural resistance and defense (Silverblatt 1980: 179).

The Spanish conquest of the Americas was a religious enterprise as much as a political and economic enterprise. In other parts of the world this religious dimension was also present. Grimshaw (in this book) presents a historical analysis of the efforts of Christian missionary wives to introduce native Hawaiian women to western notions of femininity, particularly the values of piety, purity, submissiveness, and domesticity that were given new meaning with the rise of the "cult of true womanhood" in nineteenth-century America. Missionary wives were horrified by the lack of education and relaxed sexuality of their Hawaiian female counterparts and set out to teach them a set of new ideas about marriage, child care, family, and religion. All these were founded in the gendered division of labor and society that predominated in their own cultural tradition. In the process, in Grimshaw's view, they attacked several aspects of traditional Hawaiian culture that gave women some measure of autonomy.

The work of these missionary wives was by no means easy because they faced a kinship system that emphasized relationships among a wide network of kin rather than the exclusive relationship between husband and wife. Though the education that was provided to Hawaiian women helped them adjust to the world into which they were progressively integrated, Grimshaw notes that many other aspects of Hawaiian society—especially the notions of masculinity and femininity—were ultimately resistant to change in an economic system that could not be easily transformed into a carbon copy of that on the American continent. As she argues, "The male breadwinner, the independent artisan, the small farmer, the wage earner, supporting a wife and family in modest but independent comfort, was a dream that faded before it could emerge."

Van Allen (in this book) also deals with the impact of Christianity on native populations, in her discussion of Igbo gender relations in Nigeria from the late nineteenth century to the 1970s. Here too an ideology of male domination was inculcated in mission schools. This ideology in turn sustained new economic and political structures that were introduced as part of the colonial system of government. In the traditional dual-sex political system of the Igbo, both men and women had access to political participation and public status, though the opportunities for wealth and power were always greater for men. For women, group solidarity and associations provided a basis for their power and activity in what were clearly public decision-making processes. When the British arrived they immediately attempted to alter a system that was characterized by "diffuse authority, fluid and informal leadership, shared rights of enforcement, and a more or less stable balance of male and female power." Operating with their own set of cultural assumptions about the appropriate roles for men and women, the British established a political structure in which women could not easily participate. The ultimate result, says Van Allen, was a social system that concentrated national political power in the hands of a small, educated, wealthy male elite. This eventually culminated in the "Aba Riots" (in British terms) or "Women's War" (in the Igbo language) of 1929. In this action Igbo women were using a traditional mechanism to express their frustrations, but the British interpreted their actions as instigated by men and failed to recognize that the roots of the women's demonstration lay in Igbo political structures that gave equal voice to men and women.

While the Igbo were ultimately not very successful in their protest efforts, Etienne and Leacock (1980) suggest that in other historical contexts women resisted colonization and acted to defend themselves. This was true, for example, of Seneca women in Pennsylvania and New York who withstood the attempts of Quakers to put agricultural production in the hands of men, to individualize land tenure, and to deny them political participation (Rothenberg 1980). A similar resistance to change has been documented for several other North American Indian groups (Grumet 1980). According to Weiner (1980: 43), the colonial period did not diminish the economic power of women in the Trobriand Islands in Melanesia "because no one ever knew that banana leaves had economic value." Women's wealth withstood a number of western incursions and, as a result, "served to integrate new kinds of Western wealth, as well as individual economic growth, into the traditional system."

The impact of culture contact and colonialism on the lives of women in the developing world has not been uniform. Indeed, Silverblatt (1980) stresses class distinctions—elite Inca women had different experiences from peasant women. However, it is evident that one aspect of colonialism was the imposition of European and American ideas about the appropriate roles of men and women. Programs designed to stimulate economic development in Third World societies continue to perpetuate culturally rooted assumptions about gender and the division of labor, particularly the definition of men as breadwinners and women as homemakers (Charlton 1984). Based on these assumptions, development planners, often with the support of local elites, direct their efforts at providing new skills and technology to men, even when women are the ones involved in subsistence production and trade (Chaney and Schmink 1980). As Schrijvers (1979: 111–112) has observed, "If women got any attention, it was as mothers and housekeepers in family-planning projects and in training programs for home economics. . . . Male-centered development programs often resulted in new divisions of labor between the sexes, by which the dependency of women on men greatly increased."

Lockwood (in this book) reviews the literature on the differential effects of the penetration of capitalism and development around the world, which sometimes work to the benefit of women and sometimes to their detriment. More specifically, she explores the relationship among gender ideology, women's control of material resources, family and kinship structures, and capitalist development. Based on a comparative analysis of two Tahitian cases where development programs were introduced in the 1960s, she argues that a gender ideology that empowers women is not sufficient to counter the increasing dependence on men that often results from developmental change. Rather, women must also control strategic resources in order to maintain status and power in both household and community in the face of capitalist penetration.

Like Lockwood, Wilson-Moore (in this book) shows that under certain conditions development programs can have a positive impact on women and their families. She explores the viability of homestead gardening as an economic strategy for women in Bangladesh where both men and women are involved in gardening, but use different methods and cultivate different crops. Women's gardens can be an effective foundation for the nutritional well-being of family members and do not necessarily have to compete with those of men. Development, in Wilson-Moore's view, is as much about feeding as it is about profit, and any program that is introduced should take into account the importance of subsistence as well as cash cropping in the context of the complementary gender roles in the local social system.

Agribusiness and multinational industrial production are other forms of international capitalism that bring mixed benefits for women in developing countries. Arizpe and Aranda (1981) argue that strawberry agribusiness, although a major employer for women in Zamora, Mexico, does not enhance women's status or create viable new opportunities for women. These researchers examine why women comprise such a high proportion of the employees in this business and cite cultural factors that constrain opportunities for women and continue to define women's work as temporary and supplementary. Employers take advantage of these constraints—they permit them to keep wages low and work schedules flexible. Arizpe and Aranda's conclusions support those of other researchers who point to a range of phenomena that make a female labor force attractive to multinational business and industry. "Women's socialization, training in needlework, embroidery and other domestic crafts, and supposedly 'natural' aptitude for detailed handiwork, gives them an advantage over men in tasks requiring high levels of manual dexterity and accuracy; women are also supposedly more passive—willing to accept authority and less likely to become involved in labour conflicts. Finally, women have the added advantage of 'natural disposability'—when they leave to get married or have children, a factory temporarily cutting back on production simply freezes their post" (Brydon and Chant 1988: 172).

As with agribusiness, the internationalization of capitalist production has led to the relocation in developing countries of many labor-intensive and export-oriented manufacturing and processing plants owned by multinational corporations. Many of these have provided new opportunities for employment, primarily for women. For example, in some electronics factories in Southeast Asia, women make up 80 percent to 90 percent of the labor force (Brydon and Chant 1988). However, just as with the assessment of the impact of development schemes on the lives of women in the developing world, there are two opposing views about the effect of multinationals. Some emphasize the benefits of jobs that provide women with greater financial stability (Lim 1983), while others see multinationals perpetuating or even creating new forms of inequality as they introduce young women to a new set of individualist and consumerist values. The sexually segregated work force remains in place within paternalistic industrial contexts that encourage turnover and offer no opportunities for advancement (Nash and Fernandez-Kelly 1983).

Fernandez-Kelly (in this book) analyzes workers' responses to the international political and economic system at the levels of household and factory along the Mexican side of the U.S.-Mexico border, where more than 100 assembly plants (*maquiladoras*) have been established. These industries primarily employ women. By working herself in the apparel industry, Fernandez-Kelly documents hiring practices and working conditions of factory women. Low wages, oppressive working conditions, lack of job mobility, and insecure job tenure make *maquiladoras* a precarious option, selected by women with few alternatives. Factory workers also suffer from the contradictions between idealized notions of women's roles and their actual involvement in wage labor, which causes conflict over mores and values.

Zimmer-Tamakashi (in this book) presents another situation where the introduction of wage labor and the shift from household to factory industry have problematic social implications, particularly for gender relations. She discusses the sexual politics of Papua New Guinea's educated elite, and the sexual competition among men of different tribal and national backgrounds. In a situation where men have access to cash and women have become more dependent on them, cases of domestic violence have increased. Women are experiencing a growing sense of gender oppression, and rape and violence against women have become "women's issues" largely ignored by male politicians. Those women who themselves enter the cash economy may experience more autonomy, but this too may generate domestic violence from men motivated by a fear of women's independence and their own economic uncertainty.

In the final analysis, much of the work on women in development tends to support Leacock's (1979) rather pessimistic assessment. Real development, from her perspective, "would mean bringing an end to the system whereby the multinational corporations continue to 'underdevelop' Third World nations by consuming huge proportions of their resources and grossly underpaying their workers" (1979: 131). This will require a truly international effort. The gendered approach to colonialism and development has demonstrated the close relationship between capitalist penetration, patriarchal gender ideologies, and the sexual division of labor. This relationship has been present since the early days of colonialism and has been perpetuated by a global economy that has created an international division of labor often oppressing both men and women, but especially women. As Chaney and Schmink (1980: 176) put it, development policies and programs frequently lead "not only to the degradation of the physical environment but also of the social environment, as various groups are systematically excluded from the tools of progress and their benefits."

REFERENCES

Arizpe, Lourdes and Josefina Aranda. 1981. "The 'Comparative Advantages' of Women's Disadvantages: Women Workers in the Strawberry Export Agribusiness in Mexico." *Signs* 7: 453–473.

Boserup, Esther. 1970. *Woman's Role in Economic Development.* New York: St. Martin's Press.

Brydon, Lynne and Sylvia Chant. 1988. *Women in the Third World: Gender Issues in Rural and Urban Areas.* New Brunswick, NJ: Rutgers University Press.

Chaney, Elsa M. and Marianne Schmink. 1980. "Women and Modernization: Access to Tools." In June Nash and Helen I. Safa (eds.). *Sex and Class in Latin America,* pp. 160–182. South Hadley, MA: J.F. Bergin Publishers.

Charlton, Sue-Ellen M. 1984. *Women in Third World Development.* Boulder: Westview Press.

Etienne, Mona and Eleanor Leacock. 1980. "Introduction." In Mona Etienne and Eleanor Leacock (eds.). *Women and Colonization: Anthropological Perspectives,* pp. 1–24. New York: Praeger.

Grumet, Robert Steven. 1980. "Sunksquaws, Shamans, and Tradeswomen: Middle Atlantic Coastal Algonkian Women During the 17th and 18th Centuries." In Mona Etienne and Eleanor Leacock (eds.). *Women and Colonization: Anthropological Perspectives,* pp. 43–62. New York: Praeger.

Leacock, Eleanor. 1979. "Women, Development, and Anthropological Facts and Fictions." In Gerrit Huizer and Bruce Mannheim (eds.). *The Politics of Anthropology: From Colonialism and Sexism Toward a View from Below,* pp. 131–142. The Hague: Mouton.

Lim, Linda Y. C. 1983. "Capitalism, Imperialism, and Patriarchy: The Dilemma of Third-World

Women Workers in Multinational Factories." In June Nash and Maria Patricia Fernandez-Kelly (eds.). *Women, Men and the International Division of Labor,* pp. 70–91. Albany: State University of New York.

Nash, June and Maria Patricia Fernandez-Kelly (eds.). 1983. *Women, Men and the International Division of Labor.* Albany: State University of New York.

Rothenberg, Diane. 1980. "The Mothers of the Nation: Seneca Resistance to Quaker Intervention." In Mona Etienne and Eleanor Leacock (eds.). *Women and Colonization: Anthropological Perspectives,* pp. 63–87. New York: Praeger.

Schrijvers, Joke. 1979. "Viricentrism and Anthropology." In Gerrit Huizer and Bruce Mannheim (eds.). *The Politics of Anthropology: From Colonialism and Sexism Toward a View from Below,* pp. 97–115. The Hague: Mouton.

Silverblatt, Irene. 1980. "Andean Women Under Spanish Rule." In Mona Etienne and Eleanor Leacock (eds.). *Women and Colonization: Anthropological Perspectives,* pp. 149–185. New York: Praeger.

Weiner, Annette. 1980. "Stability in Banana Leaves: Colonization and Women in Kiriwina, Trobriand Islands." In Mona Etienne and Eleanor Leacock (eds.). *Women and Colonization: Anthropological Perspectives,* pp. 270–293. New York: Praeger.

NEW ENGLAND MISSIONARY WIVES, HAWAIIAN WOMEN AND "THE CULT OF TRUE WOMANHOOD"

Patricia Grimshaw

One Sunday morning in early November 1825, Kaahumanu, awe-inspiring queen regent of the Hawaiian Islands, widow of the great warrior chief Kamehameha, was carried into the Christian mission chapel at Waimea for the morning service. The preacher was Samuel Whitney, his wife Mercy Partridge Whitney, New England Protestant missionaries supported by the American Board of Commissioners for Foreign Missions. The Whitneys had arrived with the first contingent of missionaries in 1820 and had laboured for four years, with their growing young family, on this unusual frontier. On this particular morning, Kaahumanu's bearers seated their chief's chair at the front of the chapel level with the preacher and, like him, facing the congregation (M. Whitney, Journal, 16 November 1825).

To the joy of the mission band, this powerful queen had already submitted to instruction in reading and writing and at a Honolulu school examination earlier in the year had written on her slate, 'This is my word and hand. I am making myself strong. I declare in the presence of God, I repent of my sin, and believe God to be our Father' *(Missionary Herald,* July 1825). This impressive matriarch, so enormous in size that Laura Judd, wife of the mission doctor, reported that 'she could hold any of us in her lap, as she would a little child, which she often takes the liberty of doing' (Carter 1899:26), had allotted tenancy rights for mission land and had expressed the encouraging belief that a ruler belonging to Christ's family should not only serve God personally but persuade her people to follow suit.

On this particular Sunday, however, Samuel and Mercy Whitney were not satisfied with Kaahumanu's behaviour. This proud chief had placed herself symbolically on the same

From Margaret Jolly and Martha Macintyre (eds.), *Family and Gender in the Pacific: Domestic Contradictions and the Colonial Impact* (Cambridge: Cambridge University Press, 1989), pp. 19–44. Reprinted with the permission of Cambridge University Press.

level as the preacher, God's representative. Moreover, it was essential that the minister face the entire congregation if play and disturbance were to be avoided. The missionary pair chided the queen who, her haughty and disdainful airs apparently a thing of the past, responded in a humble fashion. Kaahumanu admitted her ignorance, and 'begged them to tell her how to conduct herself at home, at church, in the house, eating and drinking, lying down or rising up' (M. Whitney, Journal, 16 November 1825).

Mercy Whitney, who recorded this incident in her daily journal, expressed special approbation for Kaahumanu's clear perception of the degree of changed behaviour now required of her. For acceptance into the full favour of the American missionaries Hawaiians could not simply attend church and mission school faithfully. To be recognised as good Christians they needed not only to regulate public and private behaviour according to the new moral laws of the fledgling state, but must also mediate every single aspect of their daily habits, trivial though these changes might seem, but all of which were evidence of the new heart, the reformed consciousness, that genuine conversion to Christ entailed.

The missionary general meeting in 1832 spelled out some of the mission's aims:

> Resolved, that while it is our main business to publish the word of God, we will discountenance the use and cultivation of tobacco; encourage improvements in agriculture and manufacture; habits of industry in the nation; neatness in the habits and dress of the inhabitants; punctuality in all engagements, especially in the payment of debts; justice and temperance in the rulers in the execution of the law, and loyalty, order and peace among their subjects, in all the relations and duties of life. (Sandwich Islands Mission 1832:133–4)

The women of the mission took as their special portion of this ambitious brief the 'transformation' of Hawaiian notions of femininity. Kaahumanu had at least realised the magnitude of the task they undertook and clearly saw adherence to mission ways to be ultimately in her own best political interests. The majority of Hawaiian women remained ignorant of or baffled by the essentially changed order that the American women sought to create. The story of three decades of intercultural contact in Hawaii—one of frustration for the mission women, and evasion by the Hawaiians—was fraught with considerable tension and unhappiness for both groups of women. Neither side could triumph: by the late 1840s, stalemate was reached. . . .

Mercy Whitney was one of the nearly eight women, predominantly from New England or the west of New York State, who left America for Hawaii (the 'Sandwich Islands') in the three decades from 1819 onwards. They were for the most part energetic, intelligent and well-educated women, daughters of farmers or small-business men, whose youthful ambition to serve on a mission field led them to marry departing missionaries. In the decades following the War of Independence, Protestant missionary outreach shifted from the native American Indians of their own west to encompass non-Christian peoples of the new lands opened to the imagination by explorers and travellers. Captain James Cook had visited and named the Sandwich Islands in 1778, on his third and last great Pacific expedition. Yankee traders had brought Hawaiian youths to New England port towns; some had displayed an interest in Christianity. The churches planned and prayed for the conversion of this 'interesting' people, and sent successive contingents of missionaries to accomplish this purpose (Andrew 1976).

It was no accident that young women were found to dedicate their lives to this missionary work. Women were centrally involved in the religious revivals which swept the northeast during the early decades of the century, the so-called 'second great awakening', which had provided metaphysical justification for a range of religious and charitable activity undertaken by women. Women were prominent in efforts to teach the young, reform slum dwellers, persuade men to temperance, rescue prostitutes and, increasingly, to free Southern slaves. To quit home and family in order to bring the strongly upheld benefits of Christian civilisation to non-believers on a distant, exotic frontier was an uncommon but nevertheless strongly valorised choice of reform endeavour (Grimshaw 1983). As Catherine Beecher wrote in her *Treatise on Domestic Economy* in 1842, 'To American women, more than to any others on earth, is committed the exalted privilege of extending over the world those blessed influences, which are to renovate degraded man, and "to clothe all climes with beauty"' (Hunter 1984:xiii).

Women's involvement in mission work was linked in an intricately complex fashion with the economic changes arising from early industrialisation in the northeast and a particular elaboration of notions of the family, and of femininity, that accompanied changes in material life. An appreciation of this social change makes more comprehensible the agenda which underwrote the mission women's activities in Hawaii. As the integrated household economy of small farms and independent artisanal industry began to break down with the introduction of mills and factories, a family structure involving the man as the sole breadwinner involved in paid, public employment, with the wife as the housekeeper removed from most productive labour, became dominant in growing urban areas. Married, middle-class women were portrayed in much prescriptive literature as the essential focus of an intimate, personal circle whose relationships contrasted radically with the alienated marketplace of male endeavour. Good family life would prove the catalyst for rejuvenation and reform in the fast-changing and potentially corrupt new social order. The articulation of proper femininity needed to fit women to their part in this haven of domesticity. Puritan traditions had sustained a significant role for women in the God-fearing family. The ante-bellum period saw an enhanced elaboration of 'the cult of true womenhood', in Barbara Welter's definition, involving piety, purity, submissiveness and domesticity (Cott 1977; Ryan 1981; Welter 1966; Sklar 1973; Smith-Rosenberg 1971).

The elevation of women's nature inherent in these fresh definitions of femininity contained within it the seeds of change in women's social and political roles. Women's supposed moral and spiritual value was used to stress a new competency for women in the public arena, initially within the orbit of social reform. Hence arose the decision of this particular group of American women to Christianise and raise the status of Hawaiian women to their own presumed level. Emerging from their own small worlds, sustained by both religious and national enthusiasm, they were innocent of notions of cultural relativism and prepared to designate every deviance from their own moral values as sinful, abroad no less than at home. When they reached their Polynesian destination it was inevitable that they would interpret what they saw within the set of cultural beliefs so deeply a part of their own identities.

The various contingents of American missionaries established themselves first in the port towns and eventually spread to the most dense centres of population in the five main islands. The Hawaiian society on the fringes of which they lived was in the process of change as a result of decades of intercultural contact with explorers, traders, beachcombers and, finally, the missionaries. Some months before the first missionaries arrived the religious system, the *kapu* laws, had been overthrown on the initiative of powerful chiefs, the islands' political leaders. Much of the social organisation of traditional Hawaiian culture persisted, however, changing shape radically in some aspects, minimally in others, from 1820 to 1850. For most of this time a chiefly elite, the landowners, dominated much of the daily life of the commoners, the *maka'ainana,* in a style reminiscent of feudal society. Commoners laboured as tenants on the chiefs' land, and surrendered much of the fruits of their labour to their superiors. The labour of commoners was not usually especially onerous since the land and sea provided plentiful nutritious food, but at times the acquisitiveness of chiefs, impressed by Western skills and goods, could drive the population to sustained and often excessive stints of labour. It appeared that pockets of impoverishment, physical deterioration and the neglect of the care of the young were the result, exacerbated by the acceptability of alcohol and nicotine to men, women and children. European diseases, too, took their toll, particularly the venereal diseases that were all too often the undesired result of Hawaiian women's sexual relationships with foreign visitors and which caused suffering and sterility.

The social status of Hawaiian women was closely intertwined with their class position and their place in the life cycle. Chiefly women wielded enormous power. As one missionary observed of the *konohiki,* or headmen of his district, 'some, by the way, are women, for Paul's injunctions are not observed on the Sandwich Islands. Women often usurp the reigns of government over large districts'. Before the ending of *kapu* such women had been subject to definitions of the female sex as profane or dangerous which were inherent in the Polynesian dichotomy of male and female qualities, and which had kept the sexes separate in both religious ritual and in such mundane areas as eating meals (Hanson 1982). . . . Chiefly women now were freed from such restrictions.

The lot of non-chiefly women was similarly relieved by the ending of *kapu,* but they still shared with their menfolk restrictions on their autonomy arising from their inferior social status as a group. Subject to some extent to male physical domination, their social position was not, however, noticeably inferior to that of non-chiefly men. Except when chiefs drove commoners to unaccustomed toil, women were if anything advantaged by the usual division of labour which persisted through the mission period. Men undertook the bulk of heavy labour in building, fishing and agriculture, and also cooked the meals. Women made mats and barkcloth, collected shellfish, and were more closely involved than men in the care of young children. Descent was traced through both the male and female lines, but although patrilocal residence was the norm, women's families of origin remained their significant point of reference. Sexual relations were little restrained in early youth, and marriages were easily terminated; chiefly men and women often had several spouses at the same time. Fertility was controlled by abortion and infanticide, and babies were often adopted among the extended kinship network which sustained significant material support systems (Goldman 1970; Sahlins 1958). Hawaiian women's share in productive labour, then, was not onerous; their sexuality was not heavily constrained; means of fertility control were normative; and the task of child socialisation was shared with kin.

It was not a figment of the American imagination, however, that the lives of Hawaiian women were not idyllic in precontact times, nor without tensions in the decades after 1820. Nothing in the Hawaiians' situation, however, appeared even remotely acceptable to the self-appointed evangelists who saw Hawaiian women as their life-long cause. The men of the mission automatically undertook the dominant roles as preachers and teachers of men, delegating to women a share in the teaching of children and a special obligation to female adults. Hiram Bingham, the foremost missionary in Honolulu, explained the strategy in this way. Separating Hawaiian women for instruction gave the mission women a full opportunity to read scripture, pray and 'conveniently to give sisterly and maternal counsel to multitudes of their own sex'. (Conventionally, mission women would have had to cede priority to men in a mixed gathering.) The separation similarly gave more scope for 'the awakened native talent and zeal' of Hawaiian women as well as men in church work. The separate instruction also produced 'a more perfect system of mutual watchfulness over the different members, and a more feasible mode of discipline' (Bingham 1981:365). The American missionary women's active participation in direct mission work was, in practice, heavily curtailed by their decision to segregate their own children from Hawaiian influence, and at various stages of their life cycle they participated only peripherally in formal teaching (Grimshaw 1983). The mission women's influence, however, emerged from all the various ways in which they transmitted their cultural prescriptions.

Arriving as they did at a critical period of Hawaiian cultural change, the American missionaries made rapid headway in persuading chiefs to a sympathetic interest in their religious system, and the adherence of Kaahumanu and other chiefs to church attendance and support of the mission effected a swift conversion of the population, remarkable when compared with the situation facing missionaries in the east. Granted that Western incursion was already setting in motion great change, the Christian chiefs undoubtedly believed that by welcoming the new religion and becoming leaders in the fledgling church their own political hegemony would be best preserved (Howe 1984; Daws 1974). Commoners began attending church because the chiefs commanded them to do so. As the Hilo missionaries told the home mission board in 1833, church attendance had not been voluntary, but in obedience to the commands of their chiefs. Hawaiians had 'put on the profession of true religion and engaged in the performance of its external duties', but all that had been secured was 'a prompt though thoughtless, servile and sycophantic audience' (Dibble *et al.* to ABCFM, 14 October 1833). Hawaiians were listless at meetings, according to Mary Parker, and could be moved neither to fear or anger. 'They submit wholly to what you say, ever having been accustomed to it.' If a chief told them to go to meeting, they immediately complied, but they simply did not know enough to become Christians (Parker, Journal (A), [?] June 1833). Meanwhile, despite new laws governing theft, murder and adultery, old ways of living, condemned over and over again by the missionaries, persisted.

The problem of how to bring about the genuine, deep-seated change in the hearts, minds and consciences of Hawaiians preoccupied mission thinking. In the last analysis, their strategy for reform came to rest on that institution so stressed in their own culture: the family. Family relationships on Hawaii appeared chaotic so that neither children, the citizens of tomorrow, nor adults could find reinforcement for decent behaviour in the one place where, as the missionaries saw it, altruistic and uplifting relationships were essential. 'It is impossible to conjecture who are husbands and wives, parents and children from their appearance assembled on the sabbath or at any other time', one missionary wrote. 'Nothing of that courtesy and attention is shown to each other by persons most intimately related as in the Christian population' (Dibble [*c.* 1831]). 'Where', asked Fidelia Coan, 'were the dutiful sons, virtuous daughters, chaste wives and faithful husbands of home?' (*Mother's Magazine,* 1837). Here, said a missionary at Waimea, was 'none of that mother's fondness of her darling child and that child's attachment to its affectionate mother which is seen in enlightened America' (Lyons to ABCFM, 6 September 1833).

Rather than in state, church or school, a reform endeavour should be shaped around the family life of Hawaiians and it was the mission women who spearheaded this effort. Above all, the women singled out the Hawaiian wife and mother as the agent for 'regeneration'. Hawaiian women were presented with the model of American femininity, the full force of the American's material wealth, skills, and the missionaries' undeniable altruism and forceful personal attributes. Hawaiian women should be rendered genuinely pious, sexually pure, dutifully submissive and domestically oriented as housewives and mothers. Then, as the centre of a better-ordered family, their influence would ripple outwards, redeeming not only wayward children and errant husbands, but the whole kingdom for godly living.

The foremost goal of the American mission women was to convert Hawaiian women to a genuine piety, the mainspring as they saw it of all worthy moral behaviour. The Americans led Hawaiian women in sex-segregated prayer meetings, held classes for women after the Sunday Services, or made time available in their own homes to hear Hawaiians 'tell their thoughts' on religious matters. Charlotte Baldwin, for example, during a period of increased religious interest, set apart a room in her house where, 'when not engaged in personal conversation, she could resort with pious females for prayer; and when she was not able to be with them, they prayed there by themselves' (Alexander 1952:91). One newly arrived single missionary, Maria Patton (later Chamberlain), found the American women's efforts impressive. At Lahaina in 1828 she witnessed Clarissa Richards 'sitting in the midst of 200 females addressing them on divine truths', women who sat with solemn expressions and 'big tears stealing down their cheeks' (Patton to sister, 19 May 1828). A determined effort was mounted for the souls of Hawaiian women. The souls of the heathen, they often told themselves, were of 'incalculable worth'.

For Hawaiian women to reach a direct and vital relationship with their Maker, however, wider instruction was needed than the bare elements of the Christian faith. Hawaiian women needed a formal Western education so that they could read the Bible and other spiritually uplifting literature and attain the spiritual refinement of sensibility and understanding gained through a liberal education. Most of the American women themselves had felt the benefits of an education in the new female seminaries of the northeast in their youth, and some had fought hard to attain this higher education. Hawaiian women, too, not just young children, would be offered the fruits of this learning.

And so, in daily or weekly sessions, the American mission women taught Hawaiians to read and write and count, and for the more forward scholars the curriculum included geography, geometry and philosophy. The Americans, devoid of customary teaching aids beyond the simple readers put out by the mission press, devised ingenious ways of matching the needs of the situation. Hawaiian women brought seeds to school for counting lessons, wrote on smooth sand with sticks and used home-made maps and globes which the mission women sat up at night to construct. Charlotte Baldwin at Waimea in the early 1830s daily held a school for female teachers (women who would in turn teach other Hawaiians), and on two days a week a school for three hundred women, as well as working with children (Baldwin, Report, 1832:2). Such onerous work loads were undertaken by brides until babies appeared, by the childless or by those whose children had been sent away to school.

Despite the distractions of infants in arms, Hawaiian women showed interest in acquiring basic literacy. Indeed they showed an aptitude which compared well with that of Americans in the opinion of Mercy Whitney, which was surprising considering 'their habits of sloth and indolence, being unaccustomed from infancy, to apply their minds to anything which required thought or the exercise of their mental faculties' (M. Whitney, Journal, 30 September 1834). The link between such pursuits and piety was frequently stressed. Sarah Joiner Lyman's attitudes in her educational work at Hilo was common. Many women in her school for females aged eight to sixty years might not be expected to make remarkable progress, but the school at least brought scholars more regularly under the means of grace (Lyman Journal, 24 January 1837).

When Maria Ogden first joined the mission station at Waimea in 1829, she wrote approvingly of the schoolroom for Hawaiian women. 'Their seats and writing tables are chiefly made of those boards, on which the natives used to spend much of their time, sporting in the surf' (Gulick to ABCFM, 27 April 1829). The use of surfboards in such an enterprise was both practical and symbolic. If women were to be pious they must be weaned away from pastimes that were far from moral and what better way to do so than by offering the substitute of education for their customary games and amusements? Hawaiians did not appear to the missionaries to have enough work to do, and some missionaries felt it valueless to urge them to greater labour while an autocratic government prevented the people from personal accumulation. Their free time was spent in swimming and surfing, in card-playing, boxing matches, games, cockfights, hulas and other traditional games of skill or chance. Not only were these games seen as a useless waste of time, but they were inextricably mingled with such sins as gambling and with sexuality of an overt kind which appeared subversive of Christian morals.

The women, whose labour appeared even less onerous than the men's, seemed particularly in need of those alternative pursuits which Christian education could offer: Bible-reading groups, church meetings, school examinations, Sunday school picnics and tea meetings, as well as formal classroom instruction. Choir work in particular attracted the American women's interest, since they so much missed the good music of their home congregations. Maria Patton described such a choir rehearsal at Lahaina where 'twenty-four genteely dressed Hawaiian ladies sat opposite the same number of gentlemen with an elegant table sporting three glass lamps placed between them' (Patton to sister, 20 August 1828).

With choirs, as in so many pursuits, American hopes were often thwarted. Mary Parker told a friend that she could hardly keep herself from laughing sometimes, the Hawaiians sang so laboriously. 'Nature seems not to have designed them for the best of singers' (M. Parker to Mrs Frisbie, April 1836). Her reaction to singing mirrored a deep-seated skepticism about the depth of genuine piety that the mission women's activity had really achieved. Newly arrived women could be impressed at the sight of a large group of Hawaiian women led in prayer by one of their number in a style not too far removed from expected forms. Those American women who had been years in the field however felt increasingly that the manifestation of piety was superficial. When a religious revival which swept the largest island and rapidly increased church membership (as opposed to mere attendance), many mission women were unmoved by the local missionaries' elation. 'We tremble, yet know not what to say, nor scarcely what to think', Sybil Bingham told a mission friend, musing on the 'fickleness' of the Hawaiian character (S. Bingham to N. Ruggles, 16 August 1838).

The essential thrust of the American women's strategy was to substitute piety for the sexuality which seemed to be the dominant drive in Hawaiian women's activities. The effort to induce notions of sexual purity extended far beyond prohibitions on 'promiscuous' bathing and sexually suggestive dances. While the American women saw monogamous marriage as the sole legitimate avenue for the expression of physical sex, their own notions of purity clearly accepted such sexuality in a relatively positive way. However to be confronted with a society in which matters concerning the body were explicitly, publicly and unselfconsciously presented was shocking. Nudity, urination, defecation and, above all, intimate sexual relations appeared scarcely subject to even minimal regulation, insensitive as they were to the cultural bases of Hawaiian sexual behaviour.

The Kailua missionaries complained in 1831 that 'the sin of uncleanness' clung to Hawaiians like leprosy, even to church members, despite the two-year probation period the ministers imposed. There was little concern or watchfulness over one another. Hawaiians congregated together in the same small house, and slept together on the one mat. Missionaries blamed 'the unceremonious manner of intercourse between the sexes, without any forms of reserve or any delicacy of thought and conversation—The idle habits of all, especially the women, and their fondness for visiting from home at night—and the force of long established habits' (*Missionary Herald,* July 1832). 'The degradation of the *females* in this spot deeply affects my heart', wrote Clarissa Richards. 'On this subject I could *write* much—but delicacy forbids' (C. Richards, Journal, 1822–3:40). The missionaries sought to establish and sustain monogamous marriage, acting wherever possible to stamp out premarital and extramarital sexuality and encouraging Hawaiians to cover nude bodies with decent clothing in Western style.

Instruction on the married state was spelled out clearly in a pamphlet *A Word Relating to Marriage,* prepared for mission purposes. Marriage meant one partner, in a relationship lasting for life. Prostitution, adultery and 'male and female impersonations' were sins of the flesh. Marriages forbidden by God, such as those between close blood relatives, were prohibited. Couples should not marry too young, but wait until their bodies grew stronger and their characters more developed. Partners should be close in age so that they shared many interests; they should know each other well, understand each other's commitments and love each other. They should have joint residence, and own all property together (Clark 1844). Divorce was sanctioned only in the case of adultery or wilful desertion where mediation had failed.

Missionaries did not require couples married Hawaiian style to submit to a Christian service lest every married person in the islands should feel perfectly free to consider their current relationships null and void, and to swap partners at will, but they insisted that all future liaisons be blessed by the church. Female and male chiefs, however, who had more than one spouse, were to choose one and relinquish the rest. One chiefly woman of Kailua claimed to have had no fewer than forty spouses, usually several at the same time (*Missionary Herald,* October 1829), and a male chief seven. Samuel Whitney asked him whether so many wives did not give rise to some anxiety. 'Yes, much', replied the chief. 'I can not sleep for fear some other man will get them!' (S. Whitney, Journal, 30 April 1826). Such irregularities were insupportable in the political leaders of the country. They were encouraged to introduce stringent punishments for bigamy and adultery; by the late 1820s in Lahaina, errant subjects were being forced to pay for their sins by making roads (men), or confinement in irons (women) (*Missionary Herald,* February 1829).

'Marriage is honorable in all, and the bed undefiled, but whoremongers and adulterers God will judge', thundered preachers from a favourite Hebrew text. It was easier to get Hawaiians to the altar, alas, than to restrain 'whoremongers and adulterers' thereafter. The most clearcut case of irregularity that the mission could bring under some degree of surveillance was the sexual trafficking between Hawaiian women and foreign sailors off visiting ships. Initially such exchange of sexual favours for material goods was welcomed by Hawaiian girls, who may even have hoped to absorb *mana* (sanctity or divine strength) from the god-like white men (Sahlins 1981b:40). As well as material goods, however, the exchange often entailed unwanted pregnancies, uncontrollable venereal disease, jealous male violence and, where a Hawaiian woman had been abandoned after several months of cohabitation, penury. Whatever the subtleties of sexual politics in this interchange, the mission women viewed it within the model of their own society as sheer exploitative prostitution. They wept when, a fresh ship in port, their young female scholars turned a deaf ear to instruction and went off in the boats with pleasurable excitement (Ogden to M. Chamberlain, n.d.). They were in the forefront of pressure on chiefs to try to prevent this trade, with an anger made more intense by their daily contact with girls whose bodies were covered with syphilitic sores and with women rendered sterile from venereal disease.

Hawaiian brides decked themselves out with clothes for weddings and prayer meetings. The rule that the body, particularly the breasts, ought to be clothed at all times, was one held without conviction, while the myriad rules governing appropriate dress to match various occasions was hardly won. One of Maria Chamberlain's first actions after acquiring some of the Hawaiian language was to exhort women at Waikiki, in faltering tongue, 'to be modest, to tell their neighbours it was a shame to go exposed and without kapa as we had recently seen some of them' (M. Chamberlain, Journal, 8 December 1829). Mary Parker's first sight of Hawaiians inspired a chill of disappointment:

'naked, rude and disgusting to every feeling' (M. Parker, Journal (A), 31 March 1833). The American women pressed clothes on to their parishioners, sewing early and late for chiefs and teaching the skill to as many women as would heed them. Their first success was to persuade women, at least in the sight of Westerners, to wear a cotton shift with a skirt of Hawaiian cloth wound around their waists, and eventually a style of dress patterned on their own nightgowns became common usage. Frequently clothes were removed for work or for bathing, and women would sit wet through in church services if they had been caught in rain, although they customarily removed wet clothing when they were outside.

At times success seemed imminent. At a school examination at Waimea in 1829, the women decked themselves out in silk gowns, black with white headdresses or green with yellow headdresses (Guilick to ABCFM, 27 April 1829). The high chief Kapiolani, defier of the goddess Pele, won acclaim, as was described by a mission daughter in this way:

> Her hair was becomingly arranged with side puffs, and a high tortoise shell comb, which was the admiration of our childish eyes. Her feet were always clad in stockings and shoes . . . on public occasions, or when visiting away from home, she wore a tight fitting dress, not even adopting the *'holuku'* (or 'Mother Hubbard') which afterwards became the national style. Silk and satin of the gayest colors were the chosen dress of the chiefs, but she preferred grave and quiet shades. (Taylor 1897:6)

Yet for the most part the women were pained at the sight of inappropriate dress, even among the chiefs: rich satin dresses with bare feet, expensive mantles over cotton shifts. Other Hawaiian women showed a tendency to see clothes as ornamentation rather than to cover nakedness. When straw hats were introduced to replace flower wreaths, women loaded them with bows of dyed kapa ribbon and extended the brims to enormous proportions. Leg of mutton sleeves, padded with cloth, ballooned out voluminously.

The proper balance in dress was a rare achievement indeed, as rare as the reordering of sexuality they had tried to impose. Marriage was no security against the sin of adultery, mourned Clarissa Armstrong in 1838. No less than nine quite young girls who attended meetings regularly and heard religious instruction every day had been guilty of adultery (Armstrong, Journal, 4 February 1838). Unless some honest way was laid out 'for the people to supply their new and clamorous wants', wrote Laura Judd from Honolulu in 1841, 'wives and daughters will continue to barter virtue for gain' just as the other sex resorted to extortion and theft (L. Judd to Mrs. R. Anderson, August 1841).

The American missionaries always looked askance at the marriage of Christian believers and non-believers, but particularly so when the non-believer was the wife. The problem involved in this case was the proper submission that a wife owed to husbandly authority: 'in the marriage contract', the mission asserted, 'the woman surrenders herself to the authority and control of the husband in a sense materially different from the surrender of the husband to the wife (though the husband's authority cannot contravene the authority of Christ which is always paramount)' (Sandwich Islands Mission 1837:13–14). It was this consideration that led them also to oppose older chiefly women's marriages to youths where there was a great disparity in rank, age or influence, 'for the wife would probably surrender her superiority reluctantly if at all; or the youth might exercise his authority in an unseemly manner'. If the older partner were a male chief, the tension would not be as severe. 'There is not the same danger of unwelcome usurpation, or competition for supremacy', as there was of discontent and unfaithfulness *(ibid.)*.

The concept of submissiveness as a feature of feminine behaviour and personality was not unproblematic for the mission women themselves, as the reminder that the Christian conscience was the ultimate arbiter of authority hinted. Most certainly the women did not equate 'submission' with any notion of passivity, weakness or ineffectualness. Courage, determination in a rightful cause, moderate assertiveness, were all qualities the American women often displayed and certainly valorised. Indeed such attributes were essential if women were to engage, as seemed essential, in charitable and religious concerns in the community. As daughters they had shown deference to their parents' opinions, and as wives they were undoubtedly prepared, should an irreconcilable difference arise, to yield to a husband's judgment, just as they assumed that a husband's interests preceded their own. Yet, partly because the gender division of labour was clearly spelt out in the marriage, and partly because much of their activism was conducted in a sex-segregated style, submissive behaviour in the conventional sense seemed rarely to be called for. The notion of women's moral leadership in the marriage offered in any case a countervailing source of power to that given the man by right.

The mission treatise on marriage instructed Hawaiians that the husband was head of the wife and should love, nurture and care for her. Wives, in turn, should reside in proper conduct under their husbands, and, through the fine example they set in living without sin and in the fear of the Lord, would influence their husbands to the good (Clark 1844:4). One reason that the mission women waged their campaign against Hawaiian women's customary amusements was the need to encourage those personal qualities of gentility that matched the submissive wife's role. 'The females, too, at the other end of the village are assembled for female fights, that is, *pulling hair, scratching* and *biting*', wrote two missionaries about the boxing craze among their community (Spaulding and Richards 1831). Women used alcohol and smoked to excess, in both cases inducing indelicate, hoydenish behaviour. Involving women in the organisational and educational work of the church—teaching, leading prayer groups, preparing parish functions—not only offered women alternative occupations but pointed them in the path of an effective community activism which could be reconciled with deference to the dominant sex.

Hawaiian women were begged to change their ways, and in particular wives were urged to combine their interests more closely with their husbands. 'The property of a husband and wife are perfectly separate', one missionary complained. '*Hoapili* [a chief] and his wife have two perfectly distinct establishments, they rarely eat together. No man ever uses his wife's book and vice versa and so of a slate and other property, each must have one of his own' (Andrews to ABCFM, 2 December 1835). When Hukona, one of Clarissa Richard's servants, was guilty of 'delinquency' while assisting Fanny Gulick, another mission wife, Clarissa insisted that the woman should remain with Fanny 'and that she live quietly with her husband and submit herself cheerfully to his authority and theirs'. She could return to visit the Armstrongs and her relations after Fanny's confinement, but Clarissa did not want Hukona to feel that her services were indispensable, 'if she does not love her husband, nobody wants her' (C. Richards to F. Gulick, April [1834]).

It was the kinship network, the 'relations', that many missionaries realised was the stumbling block to much submissive wifely behaviour. Their own culture upheld dutiful deference of young unmarried daughters to the authority of parents. Hawaiian women, however, sustained links with their family of origin which superseded their ties with their husbands throughout their lives. Their roles as sisters, daughters, nieces took precedence over the marriage bond and represented the reference point for status. American women expected a married woman to have status conferred by the husband. Hawaiian women were involved in strong bonds of reciprocity with their kin for material, emotional and physical support, and such demands frequently drew wives from the marital home. Increasingly, as European diseases ravaged the population, they were called upon to nurse sick relatives some distance from their homes. Maria Chamberlain articulated common exasperation with the strength of kinship ties. 'If we should give the natives in our family a whole hog or goat they would boil it up and share it with their friends and then perhaps go without any meat for 2 or 3 days' (M. Chamberlain to sister, 11 March 1830). The functional value of such behaviour escaped the missionaries.

However it was not merely the force of the kinship network which the Americans saw as undermining proper lines of authority. They abhorred the continuing power of the chiefs over the lives of individual members of the family except where this influence was exercised on behalf of the church. Mary Ives described such an incident that epitomised chiefly tyranny at Hana. A young girl had brought Mary two eggs to exchange for a needle. A chief, observing the transaction, seized the eggs and angrily told the girl she had no right to sell eggs without asking him. As the girl fled in shame, Mary recalled her, gave her a needle and remonstrated with the chief—who did not take her advice in good spirit (M. Ives to aunt, 21 January 1838). If a chief detained a Hawaiian in some place distant from his home and family, wrote Sarah Lyman, the man did not even express a wish to return, even if he was detained six months or a year. 'Such veneration they still have for chiefs' (Lyman, Journal, 4 January 1835). For women to be dutiful wives, continuity in cohabitation and regularity in material subsistence was essential, and the Americans looked forward to the time when the despotism of chiefs would be ended, while they expressed regret at individual chiefly acts in the meantime.

The teaching of submissiveness, then, was intimately related to the encouragement of women to lead a domestic-oriented existence based on a gender division of labour in the American mode. Mission teaching was explicit on this point. 'It is the husband's role to work out-doors—he farms and builds the home and prepares that which concerns the welfare of the body. The role of the wife is to maintain the house and all that is within. It is her responsibility to look after the husband's clothing and the food—the household chores—setting in place the sleeping quarters and all else that is within' (Clark 1844). The wife was advised against deficiency in this area. 'It is wrong to neglect work and to leave the husband to keep the household. It is right to remain within the house and to work without daydreaming, providing food, clothing and all that is essential for life together' *(ibid., 5)*. And by such domestic devotion, the wife would foster the husband's love for the children. The married couple should guide children, as Solomon said, on the correct path. If husband and wife loved each other, their love for their children would be great and the children would not abandon their parents in later life.

The reality of Hawaiian domestic life was far from the ideal projected by the Americans. When Abigail Smith arrived at Kaluaaha in 1833, she was driven to distraction by Hawaiian women coming to observe her performance of domestic chores. She begged them to go home to their household duties and the care of their children so she could get on with her own tasks undisturbed. They asserted cheerfully that they had no duties, and continued unabashed to occupy her yard and doorway (Frear 1934:71). On several occasions when Hawaiian women saw the Americans ironing they said, with heartfelt sympathy, 'I pity you'.

The simply constructed Hawaiian houses with their sparse furnishings, together with the plainness of diet and dress, militated against the mission plan. The Waimea missionaries tried to persuade the people 'to live like human beings', Lyons said, to put away dogs, give up tobacco, build better houses, make tables, seats, use separate dishes and eating utensils, make fences around their houses and cultivate the soil more extensively (Lyons, Report on Waimea Station, 1837:1). The chiefs built Western-style houses, and eventually a few of the better-off church families lived in Western style with thatched mud-walled cottages sporting separate sleeping places for children, a shelf of books, an engraved map on the wall, home-built furniture and wooden bowls and spoons *(Mother's Mag-*

azine, February 1839). But for the most part the Americans considered the Hawaiians' homes and diet totally unconducive to the performance of a day's domestic work by Hawaiian women. When the mission women went house-to-house visiting it was usually only the sick, the lame, the blind, the maimed or the old that they found at home—not a busy and welcoming Hawaiian housewife.

It seemed to the Americans that vast material improvement among commoners was dependent on breaking the hegemony of the chiefs. In the meantime, as they sought a cash crop which might give Hawaiian men employment and livelihood, they also looked for an avenue of household production for the women. One proposal was to induce Hawaiian women to spend more time sewing and knitting, since this not only afforded domestic occupation but provided the clothing so sorely needed by the whole population, and the clothes would generate occupation in mending, laundering, ironing and storing. The most concerted effort was the attempt to initiate clothmaking in the homes, that old skill of American women which was swiftly being overtaken by factory production back home. In 1834 a middle-aged spinster, Miss Lydia Brown, was sent to the islands to spearhead this enterprise. The mission board justified the appointment of Lydia, 'a woman of superior mind and character', in these terms. 'It is certainly of the utmost importance to make employment, and to create a necessity for it, for the people of the Islands. And it is very desirable to exert every influence on them that will be likely to produce among them industrious, orderly families.' The Hawaiians, therefore, should be trained in the domestic manufacture of cloth (Wisner to Missionaries, 23 June 1834). A number of Hawaiian women were intrigued by the process and keen to try it until they saw how coarse was the cloth of their own manufacture, and until more and more imported cottons made home spinning and weaving superfluous for the same reason as in America.

Persuading Hawaiian women to devote more time to childcare was similarly a frustrating task. 'In our opinion', stated the Lahaina mission report in 1833, 'all that ever has been written on the subject of a mother's influence, has come far short of giving it the high rank which it really holds. Could the influence of a pious mother be brought to bear upon the children of Hawaii, then these islands might be transformed . . . Otherwise it will be the work of ages to change the character of the nation's children' *(Missionary Herald,* September 1834). The children, all the missionaries agree, were growing up like wild goats in the field. The only way to get them to school was to seek them out and bribe them with books in exchange for attendance. To keep them in school, the teachers had to sustain the children's interest constantly, no small task considering that the knowledge which Hawaiian children attained appeared to bear no relevance for their future employment. If made the objects of anger or corporal punishment, the children deserted in decisive fashion. One missionary described their activities. 'From morning to night, ungoverned by their parents, almost naked, ranging the fields in companies of both sexes, sporting on the sand-beach, bathing promiscuously in the surf, or following the wake of some drunken sailors' (Dibble 1909:267). Something had to be done.

That something involved the formation of Maternal Associations on each station devoted to the task of explaining to Hawaiian women the serious business of rearing godly children. On occasions, with caution, a mission wife brought in one of her own offspring for brief display.

Instruction began with a sharp and anguished attack on abortion and infanticide. Abortions, 'base and inhuman practices' (Lyons to ABCFM, n.d. [*c.* 1836]), were suspected to be common but difficult to detect. Mercy Whitney, reporting that she had seen a child with an eye put out by his mother 'in endeavouring to kill him' before his birth, commented also on the common practice of former years, infanticide: 'They seemed to think but little more of killing a child, than they would an animal' (M. Whitney, Journal, 24 October 1828). Most mission women reported that the incidence of infanticide declined swiftly, however. This was very likely due to the high infant mortality rate from introduced diseases if for no other reason.

The mission publication *A Few Words of Advice for Parents* (Sandwich Islands Mission 1842) cautioned mothers against leaving their infants to cry in another's care while they went off wherever they wished. Infants should be fed only breast milk, not fish, or *poi,* or sugarcane juice. But beyond everything else, infants should not be given away to relatives, but reared by their biological parents in the one home. This common practice was seen not just as the chief cause of the high infant mortality, but the reason for the entire lack of discipline over older children. Sarah Lyman expressed the usual exasperation at this practice when, at a Maternal Association meeting at Hilo, she failed dismally to compile a neat list of mothers and children. Thirty women attended, but it proved impossible to discover exactly how many children they had as 'their *real* mother, grandmother, aunt, nurse and perhaps someone else' would all claim the one child (Lyman, Journal, 17 January 1837).

Consequently, as the children grew more independent, it proved impossible for parents to exert strong control over them. As one Hawaiian mother after another explained, if they were nasty to their children, the children simply rolled up their mats under their arms and moved on to be welcomed by a related household. One Hawaiian mother described how she had tried to hit her disobedient child with the rod—the child spat in her face, bit and scratched her, tore her clothes, and then ran away for several days *(Mother's Magazine,* October 1837). If Hawaiian mothers had been accustomed to govern their children instead of being governed by them, it might have been a simple matter to substitute alternative advice. But, said Fidelia Coan, 'The most simple directions we can give, presuppose, in many cases, more knowledge, more skill, more advancement in the art of governing a family than they have attained' *(ibid.).*

It was arguable, from observing non-Christian mothers, that good church members were a little less likely to give up their infants for adoption and attempted to control their children a little more firmly. Certainly where the wife was an unbeliever, and a Christian father exerted parental authority, his efforts were clearly undermined; the wife would intervene if he tried to whip a child and set up a fearful wailing. 'It is true here, as in civilized lands', wrote one missionary, 'that the female fills an important sphere and may be the means of doing *much* mischief or *much* good' (Forbes to ABCFM, 23 July 1836). For the most part, however, even Christian women resigned themselves to a continuation of usual practices. We hear your advice, but we forget it quickly, Hawaiians good-naturedly told the mission wives. Anyway, they were convinced that American children were born different: it was inconceivable that Hawaiian children could be so well-behaved.

On occasions Hawaiian women could express gratitude to American wives for their unswerving reform efforts. Maria Chamberlain had that experience one pleasant day in May, 1831. As an Hawaiian woman sat by Maria's baby's cradle brushing the flies off his face, she said to Maria that Hawaiians were fortunate that the missionaries had come with wives to the islands. Formerly, she said, Hawaiians had known nothing of taking care of children; gave newborn babies to others; knew nothing of domestic happiness. 'Husbands and wives quarrelled, committed adultery, drank, lied, stole . . . Now we wish to obey the word of God, to live together with love, to take care of our children and have them wear clothes as the children of the missionaries' (M. Chamberlain, Journal, 11 May 1831). Such praise was a rare treat and one which the mission women in any case came to regard with some skepticism. Penetrating the Hawaiian mind was a baffling task. 'It is exceedingly difficult to ascertain the true character of this people', wrote Nancy Ruggles after thirteen years in the islands. 'The expression of the lips merely, is no sure indication of the state of the heart' (N. Ruggles to Rev. and Mrs. S. Bartlett, 27 June 1833). Another missionary spelled out one of the major problems of communication. 'Unless every trifling particular is named they rarely have the judgement to carry out the principle themselves. They suppose they have complied when they observe the particular act forbidden' (Forbes to ABCFM, 10 October 1836). Scholars in the schools learned to pronounce the words, but that was all. They did not understand the essential *meaning*.

By the time the second decade of mission work was nearing its end without the reformation they craved becoming visible, many missionary women began to express the discouragement that had never, in any case, been far beneath the surface. They had God on their side; they had sacrificed a good deal to come to Hawaii; they felt exhausted in the cause; the population was ostensibly Christian and some change in women's behaviour had taken place. All Hawaiian women, however, fell far short of the desired model of true womanhood that they had tried so hard to impose. 'What in me hinders their salvation?' Lucia Smith plaintively asked her friend Juliette Cooke, as she watched women drift away from her instruction (L. Smith to J. Cooke, 5 May [1838]). Many another mission sister echoed her painful self-assessment.

Forceful and efficient fresh male missionaries who arrived in Hawaii in the 1830s were horrified by what they saw as the slow progress of the mission's work and began to question the decision of earlier missionaries to devote so much of the effort to the reformation of adults. Many felt a renewed onslaught should be made on the character formation of Hawaiian children. Lorrin Andrews, principal of the Lahainaluna Seminary which was founded on Maui in 1831 to offer advanced education to young Hawaiian men, was one who came to this opinion. '*We must begin with* children or the *most* of our labour must be lost as far as civilization and mental improvement are concerned', he told fellow missionaries with some vehemence (Andrews to ABCFM, 2 December 1835). He and his co-workers became disillusioned with their work with young men when they encountered sexual immorality both within the Seminary and among some graduate teachers in the community who used their new status to gain sexual favours from female pupils (Andrews *et al.* to ABCFM, 1836–37).

While others agreed about renewed emphasis on children, the teachers of day schools felt their task an impossible one. Children, said one missionary, lost the salutary effects of religious instruction by 'mingling with their vicious parents and others and observing all their heathenish and polluting habits and practices' (L. Lyons to ABCFM, Report, 1836). No sooner, reiterated another, did one alert children to their 'filthy and indecent appearance' and to the evils of quarrelling and lying than they returned to the 'beastly indifference' to the conventions of good behaviour, or even the sneers, of those with whom they associated back home. The solution seemed difficult, but obvious. The mission must educate children, but in sex-segregated boarding schools where they could be removed from their parents' influence (Hitchcock to ABCFM, April 1836). The missionaries on Hawaii knew that their fellow missionaries in Ceylon were finding this a constructive approach. The graduates of the girls' and boys' boarding schools in Ceylon were marrying and then re-entering their former communities as Christian leaders (Wisner to missionaries, 23 June 1834). A beginning on this policy was made. Lahainaluna was converted to a high school for young boys in 1837, and the Wailuku Girls' Seminary, for girls aged six to ten years, was opened at a discreet geographical distance.

At Wailuku, under the principal Miss Maria Ogden, Hawaiian girls received the training in true womanhood that the female missionaries had tried to offer adult women. Their daily schedule revealed much. Girls rose before dawn for prayers, set the tables, cleaned their rooms, washed, combed their hair and came down to breakfast at the sound of the bell. Some girls were rostered to wait at each meal. The girls sewed from 7:30 a.m. to 9:00 a.m., studied till midday, and again after lunch from 2:00 p.m. to 4:00 p.m. Another hour's sewing preceded supper at 5:00 p.m., followed by a scripture reading and prayer. On Saturdays the scholars scoured the dining room, schoolroom, tables, basins, aprons, plates, knives and forks; they washed and ironed their clothes, neat uniforms of sensible cottons. They learned at the school the basic elements of a formal education combined with an apprenticeship in female arts and crafts (Ogden to M. Chamberlain 27 June [?1837]). By 1839, however, Dr. Judd recommended some improvement not only in the quality of their diet but in the time allotted for physical exercise, when serious illness, resulting in deaths, occurred at the school. It seemed impossible, the missionaries concluded, 'to restrain them from rude and romping behaviour, and to confine them to those exercises deemed more proper for females without serious injury to health' (Dibble 1909:284; Judd 1960:95).

The 1840s saw a slow period of disengagement in active involvement in the mission by many missionary wives, which they lamented in an increasingly hopeless fashion. It was impracticable for most children to be confined for years in boarding schools—the one area where a small group of women remained involved. Their efforts with the Hawaiian women appeared to bear little fruit, and the Americans faced the gloomy experience of watching many of their most precious converts dying prematurely during the epidemics which swept the islands. 'Surely this people are melting away like dew . . . What we do for them must be done quickly', wrote Sarah Lyman (Lyman, Journal, 22 January 1838). Another missionary wrote, 'We bless the Lord and take courage but, oh, what a dying people this is. They drop down on all sides of us and it seems that the nation must speedily become extinct' (Gulick 1918:159). The mission women's nursing skills seemed more in demand than any other offering they could make. By the 1850s, there was often little to distinguish the mission women's daily round and preoccupations from many of their sisters' lives back home, the exotic character of their environment notwithstanding.

A young American, staying in the Hawaiian islands for his health in the 1830s, described his missionary aunt's activities, and the Hawaiian response, in an ironical yet sympathetic fashion:

> My aunt could work, scold, preach, wash, bake, pray, catechize, make dresses, plant, pluck, drive stray pigs out the garden. There was nothing useful in this wilderness which she could not do. She exercised an influence from her energy and practical virtue which bordered on absolute authority. As I walked with her through the village, her presence operated as a civilizing tonic. True, the effect in many cases was transient. But the natives knew what she expected. As she appeared, tobacco pipes disappeared, idle games or gambling were slyly put by. Bible and hymn books brought conspicuously forward and the young girls hastily donned their chastest dresses and looks. (Restarick 1924:50–1)

His characterisation of this intercultural relationship nicely captures both the single-minded effort of missionary women and the apparent conformity, but essentially evasive, response of Hawaiians. It also exemplifies the style of much outsiders' writing about mission women, the tendency to stress a comic element in the encounter. In truth, however, although the endeavour of the American missionary women could easily be described as comedy, it more nearly approaches tragedy.

The American women attempted what was, given the circumstances, a constructive role in the process of social change in Hawaii which it is easy to overlook. Hawaiian culture was being subjected to intense pressure to adapt to the rapid incursion of foreigners into their community. The missionaries were only one element in these first decades, and from an immediate economic perspective the least exploitative element in this capitalist and colonialist invasion. Granted that change in Hawaiian culture was inevitable, what in fact the American missionaries offered

Hawaiian girls and women was initiation into that range of skills and behaviour that would ensure some successful negotiation of the new order. Kaahumanu, the queen regent, was astute enough to recognise this fact.

The constructive nature of the American women's enterprise has been overlooked partly by the tendency of historians, themselves products of the same work-oriented society, to envy, and to enjoy vicariously, the lives of those Polynesian island dwellers who were innocent of puritanical drives. Yet there seems little basis in fact for describing Hawaiian women's lives as romantic or idyllic, either in their pre-contact world or in the period of change of the nineteenth century. This tendency to denigrate the missionary women's efforts is intensified by the trappings of Victorian gentility which necessarily surrounded their agenda, particularly with respect to sexuality. Yet the formal and informal education in Western forms which the mission women, alone of their sex, were prepared to offer would enable Hawaiian women to make out in a world increasingly dominated by this alien culture. Such Hawaiian women who were 'successful' in nineteenth-century Hawaii served an apprenticeship in the American mission programme.

Yet ultimately the American women's activities would prove of only marginal value to the vast majority of those Hawaiians who survived the ravages of imported diseases. Clearly a wide range of cultural beliefs and practices were bound to persist, and among these notions of masculinity, femininity and personal familial relationships would prove the most persistent. Moreover, the American prescriptions of femininity were based on an economic organisation which it proved impossible to replicate for indigenous Hawaiians. The male breadwinner, the independent artisan, the small farmer, the wage earner, supporting a wife and family in modest but independent comfort, was a dream that faded before it could emerge (Grimshaw 1986). Eventually large plantations and businesses headed by foreign capitalists dominated, employing non-Hawaiian labour for the most part. The bulk of Hawaiians remained excluded from the prosperity of this new Hawaii. The relative affluence of Hawaiian families and the Western gender division of labour desired by the Americans remained elusive goals. It was no wonder that their cultural constructs of gender characteristics proved unattainable.

The experience of American and Hawaiian cultural contact was an ironic one. The Americans sacrificed much personal comfort, suffered home-sickness, ill-health and heartache in their effort to transform Hawaiian lives. Yet they tended to attack, along with destructive elements in the processes of foreign incursion, many of the very aspects of Hawaiian culture which afforded Hawaiian women some measure of autonomy within their own social system. Meanwhile the Americans were powerless to reproduce for their protégés the framework which afforded American women informal power within American society.

REFERENCES

Alexander, M. C. 1952. *Baldwin of Lahaina*. Stanford, Stanford University Press.

Andrew, J. A. III. 1976. *Rebuilding the Christian Commonwealth: New England Congregationalists and Foreign Missions 1800–1830*. Lexington, University of Kentucky Press.

Andrews, L. Letter to ABCFM, 2 December 1835. ABCFM—Hawaii Papers, Missionary Letters.

Andrews, L., E. Clark and S. Dibble. Letter to ABCFM, 1836–1837. ABCFM—Hawaii Papers, Missionary Letters.

Armstrong, C. Journal, 1831–1838. Journal Collection, HMCS.

Baldwin, D. Report of Waimea Station, June 1832. Mission Station Reports. HMCS.

Bingham, H. 1981 [1848]. *A Residence of Twenty–one Years in the Sandwich Islands*. Rutland, Vermont, Charles E. Tuttle.

Bingham, S. Letter to N. Ruggles, 16 August 1936. Missionary Letters. HMCS.

Carter, H. A. P. 1899. *Kaahumanu*. Honolulu, R. Grieve.

Chamberlain, M. Journal, 1825–1849. Journal Collection, HMCS.

———. Letter to sister, 11 March 1830. Missionary Letters. HMCS.

Clark, E. 1844. *A Word Relating to Marriage,* translated by Carol Silva. Honolulu; Mission Press.

Cott, N. 1977. *The Bonds of Womanhood: 'Women's Sphere' in New England, 1780–1835.* New Haven: Yale University Press.

Daws, G. 1974 [1968]. *Shoal of Time: A History of the Hawaiian Islands.* Honolulu: University of Hawaii Press.

Dibble, S. 1909 [1834]. *A History of the Sandwich Islands.* Honolulu: Thomas G. Thrum.

———. Review of "A Visit to the South Seas" by Rev. C. S. Stewart [n.d.] [c. 1831]. ABCFM—Hawaii Papers, Missionary Letters.

Forbes, C. Letters to ABCFM, 23 July 1836 and 10 October 1836. ABCFM—Hawaii Papers, Missionary Letters.

Frear, M. D. 1934. *Lowell and Abigail: A Realistic Idyll.* New Haven: privately published.

Goldman, I. 1970. *Ancient Polynesian Society.* Chicago, University of Chicago Press.

Grimshaw, P. 1983. Christian Woman, Pious Wife, Faithful Mother, Devoted Missionary: Conflicts in Roles of American Missionary Women in Nineteenth–Century Hawaii. *Feminist Studies,* 9:489–522.

———. 1986. Paths of Duty: American Missionary Wives in Early Nineteenth–Century Hawaii. Unpublished Ph.D. thesis, University of Melbourne, Australia.

Gulick, O. and A. Gulick. 1918. *The Pilgrims of Hawaii.* New York, Fleming H. Revell Company.

Gulick, P. Letter to ABCFM, 27 April 1829. ABCFM—Hawaii Papers, Missionary Letters.

Hanson, F. A. 1982. Female Pollution in Polynesia. *JPS* 91:335–381.

Hanson, F. A. and L. Hanson. 1983. *Counterpoint in Maori Culture.* London: RKP.

Hitchcock, H. Letter to ABCFM: [?] April 1836. ABCFM—Hawaii Papers. Missionary Letters.

Howe, K. R. 1984. *Where the Waves Fall.* Sydney: Allen & Unwin.

Hunter, J. 1984. *The Gospel of Gentility: American Women Missionaries in Turn of the Century China.* New Haven: Yale University Press.

Ives, M. Letter to aunt, 21 January 1838. Missionary Letters. HMCS.

Judd, G. P. IV. 1960. *Dr. Judd: Hawaii's Friend.* Honolulu: University of Hawaii Press.

Judd, L. Letter to Mrs. R. Anderson, [?] August 1841. Missionary Letters. HMCS.

Lyman, S. Journal 1830–1863. Journal Collection. HMCS.

Lyons, L. Letter to ABCFM, 6 September 1833. ABCFM—Hawaii Papers, Missionary Letters.

———. Letter to ABCFM, n.d. [c.1836]. ABCFM—Hawaii Papers, Missionary Letters.

———. Report on Waimea Station. 1837 (typescript). Mission Station Reports. HMCS.

Missionary Harold. ABCFM Boston, 1821–1834.

Mother's Magazine. New York, 1836–1845.

Ogden, M. Letter to Maria Chamberlain, 27 June [?1837], Missionary Letters. HMCS.

Parker, M. Letter to Mrs. L. Frisbie, [?] April 1836. Missionary Letters. HMCS.

———. Journal (A): Voyages to Hawaii and Marquesas 1823–1833. Journal Collection. HMCS.

Patton (Chamberlain) M. Letters to sister, 19 May 1828 and 20 August 1828. Missionary Letters. HMCS.

Restarick, H. 1924. *Hawaii 1778–1920: From the Viewpoint of a Bishop.* Honolulu, Paradise of the Pacific.

Richards, C. Journal en Route to Hawaii 1822–1823. Journal Collection. HMCS.

———. Letter to Fanny Gulick, April [?1834]. Missionary Letters. HMCS.

Ruggles, N. Letter to Reverend and Mrs. S. Bartlett, 27 June 1833. Missionary Letters. HMCS.

Ryan, M. P. 1981. *Cradle of the Middle-Class: The Family in Oneida County, New York, 1790–1865.* Cambridge, Cambridge University Press.

Sahlins, M. 1958. *Social Stratification in Polynesia.* Seattle: University of Washington Press.

———. 1981. *Historical Metaphors and Mythical Realities: Structure in the Early History of the Sandwich Islands Kingdom.* Ann Arbor: University of Michigan Press.

Sandwich Islands Mission. 1832. *Extracts from the Minutes of a General Meeting of the Sandwich Islands Mission,* June 1832. Oahu: Mission Press.

———. 1837. *Extracts from the Records of the Hawaiian Association from 1832 to 1836.* Honolulu: Mission Press.

———. 1842. *A Few Words (of Advice) for Parents.* Lahainaluna: Lahainaluna High School Press.

Sklar, K. K. 1973. *Catherine Beecher: A Study in American Domesticity.* New Haven: Yale University Press.

Smith, L. Letter to Juliette Cooke, 5 May [1838]. Missionary Letters. HMCS.

Smith-Rosenberg, C. 1971. Beauty, the Beast, and the Militant Woman: A Case Study of Sex Roles and Social Stress in Jacksonian America. *American Quarterly,* 23:562–584.

Spaulding, E. and W. Richards. 1831. A Brief History of Temperance for Twelve Years at the

Sandwich Islands . . . , written 15 December 1831. ABCFM—Hawaii Papers, Missionary Letters.

Taylor, P. G. 1897. *Kapiolani.* Honolulu, Robert Grieve.

Welter, B. 1966. The Culture of True Womanhood, 1820–1860. *American Quarterly,* 18:151–174.

Whitney, S. Journal at Kauai 2 April–1 June 1826. ABCFM— Hawaii Papers, Missionary Letters.

Whitney, M. Journal, 1821–1860. Journal Collection. HMCS.

Wisner, B. Letter to Missionaries at the Sandwich Islands, 23 June 1834. ABDFM–HEA Papers: Letters to Missionaries.

"ABA RIOTS" OR IGBO "WOMEN'S WAR"? IDEOLOGY, STRATIFICATION, AND THE INVISIBILITY OF WOMEN

Judith Van Allen

The events that occurred in Calabar and Owerri provinces in southeastern Nigeria in November and December of 1929, and that have come to be known in Western social-science literature as the "Aba Riots," are a natural focus for an investigation of the impact of colonialism on Igbo women.[1] In the development and results of that crisis can be found all the elements of the system that has weakened women's position in Igboland—and in much of the rest of Africa as well.[2] The "Aba Riots" are also a nice symbol of the "invisibility" of women: "Aba Riots" is the name adopted by the British; the Igbo called it *Ogu Umunwanyi,* the "Women's War" (Uchendu 1965: 5; Okonjo 1974: 25, n. 40). This is more than a word game. In politics, the control of language means the control of history. The dominant group and the subordinate group almost always give different names to their conflicts, and where the dominant group alone writes history, its choice of terminology will be perpetuated. Examples of this manipulation of language abound in American history, as any examination of standard textbooks will reveal.

Reprinted from *Women in Africa: Studies in Social and Economic Change,* edited by Nancy J. Hafkin and Edna G. Bay with the permission of the publisher, Stanford University Press.

Calabar and Owerri provinces covered roughly the southeast and southwest quarters of Igboland, the traditional home of the Igbo peoples. In November of 1929, thousands of Igbo women from these provinces converged on the Native Administration centers—settlements that generally included the headquarters and residence of the British colonial officer for the district, a Native Court building and a jail, and a bank or white trader's store (if such existed in the district).[3] The women chanted, danced, sang songs of ridicule, and demanded the caps of office (the official insignia) of the Warrant Chiefs, the Igbo chosen from each village by the British to sit as members of the Native Court. At a few locations the women broke into prisons and released prisoners. Sixteen Native Courts were attacked, and most of these were broken up or burned. The "disturbed area" covered about 6,000 square miles and contained about two million people. It is not known how many women were involved, but the figure was in the tens of thousands. On two occasions, British District Officers called in police and troops, who fired on the women and left a total of more than 50 dead and 50 wounded. No one on the other side was seriously injured.[4]

The British "won," and they have imposed their terminology on history; only a very few scholars have recorded that the Igbo called this the "Women's War." And in most histories of Nigeria today one looks in vain for any mention that women were even involved. "Riots," the term used by the British, conveys a picture of uncontrolled, irrational action, involving violence to property or persons, or both. It serves to justify the "necessary action to restore order," and it accords with the British picture of the outpouring of Igbo from their villages as some sort of spontaneous frenzy, explained by the general "excitability" of these "least disciplined" of African peoples (Perham 1937:219). "Aba Riots," in addition, neatly removes women from the picture. What we are left with is "some riots at Aba"—not by women, not involving complex organization, and not ranging over most of southeastern Nigeria.

To the British Commissions of Enquiry established to investigate the events, the Igbo as a whole were felt to be dissatisfied with the general system of administration. The women simply were seen as expressing this underlying general dissatisfaction. The British explanation for the fact that women rather than men "rioted" was twofold: the women were aroused by a rumor that they would be taxed at a time of declining profits from the palm products trade; and they believed themselves to be immune from danger because they thought British soldiers would not fire on women (Perham 1937:213–217). The possibility that women might have acted because as women they were particularly distressed by the Native Administration system does not seem to have been taken any more seriously by the Commissions than women's demands in testimony that they be included in the Native Courts (Leith-Ross 1939:165).

The term "Women's War," in contrast to "Aba Riots," retains both the presence and the significance of the women, for the word "war" in this context derived from the pidgin English expression "making war," an institutionalized form of punishment employed by Igbo women and also known as "sitting on a man." To "sit on" or "make war on" a man involved gathering at his compound at a previously agreed-upon time, dancing, singing scurrilous songs detailing the women's grievances against him (and often insulting him along the way by calling his manhood into question), banging on his hut with the pestles used for pounding yams, and, in extreme cases, tearing up his hut (which usually meant pulling the roof off). This might be done to a man who particularly mistreated his wife, who violated the women's market rules, or who persistently let his cows eat the women's crops. The women would stay at his hut all night and day, if necessary, until he repented and promised to mend his ways (Leith-Ross 1939: 109; Harris 1940: 146–48).[5]

"Women's War" thus conveys an action by women that is also an extension of their traditional method for settling grievances with men who had acted badly toward them. Understood from the Igbo perspective, this term confirms the existence of Igbo women's traditional institutions, for "making war" was the ultimate sanction available to women for enforcing their judgments. The use of the word "war" in this specifically Igbo sense directs attention to the existence of those female political and economic institutions that were never taken into account by the British, and that still have not been sufficiently recognized by contemporary social scientists writing about the development of nationalist movements.

Conventionally, Western influence has been seen as "emancipating" African women through (1) the weakening of kinship bonds; (2) the provision of "free choice" in Christian monogamous marriage; (3) the suppression of "barbarous" practices (female circumcision, ostracism of mothers of twins, slavery); (4) the opening of schools; and (5) the introduction of modern medicine, hygiene, and (sometimes) female suffrage. What has not been seen by Westerners is that for some African women—and Igbo women are a striking example—actual or potential autonomy, economic independence, and political power did not grow out of Western influences but existed already in traditional "tribal" life. To the extent that Igbo women have participated in any political action—whether anticolonial or nationalist struggles, local community development, or the Biafran war—it has been not so much because of the influence of Western values as despite that influence.

TRADITIONAL IGBO POLITICAL INSTITUTIONS

In traditional Igbo society, women did not have a political role equal to that of men. But they did have a role—or more accurately, a series of roles—despite the patrilineal organization of Igbo society. Their possibilities of participating in traditional politics must be examined in terms of both structures and values. Also involved is a consideration of what it means to talk about "politics" and "political roles" in a society that has no differentiated, centralized governmental institutions.

Fallers (1963) suggests that for such societies, it is necessary to view "the polity or political system . . . not as a concretely distinct part of the social system, but rather as a functional aspect of the whole social system: that aspect concerned with making and carrying out decisions regarding public policy, by whatever institutional means." Fallers's definition is preferable to several other functionalist definitions because it attempts to give some content to the category "political." Examples will make this clear. Let us take a society that has no set of differentiated political institutions to which we can ascribe Weber's "monopoly of the legitimate use of physical force within a given territory," and yet that holds together in reasonable order; we ask the question, What are the mechanisms of social control? To this may be added a second question, based on the notion that a basic governmental function is "authoritative allocation": What are the mechanisms that authoritatively allocate goods and services? A third common notion of politics is concerned with power relationships, and so we also ask, Who has power (or influence) over whom?

The problem with all of these approaches is that they are at the same time too broad and too narrow. If everything in a society that promotes order, resolves conflicts, allocates goods, or involves the power of one person over another is "political," then we have hardly succeeded in distinguishing the "political" as a special kind of activity or area or relationship. Igbo women certainly played a role in promoting order and resolving conflicts (Green 1947: 178–216; Leith-Ross 1939: 97, 106–9), but that does not make them political actors. In response to each of those broad definitions, we can still ask, Is this mechanism of social control or allocation, or this power relationship, a *political* mechanism or relationship? In answering that question, Fallers provides some help. It is their relationship to public policy that makes mechanisms, relationships, or activities "political."

There are many different concepts of "public" in Western thought. We will consider only two, chosen because we can possibly apply them to Igbo politics without producing a distorted picture. There seem to be actions taken, and distinctions made, in Igbo politics and language that make it not quite so ethnocentric to try to use these Western concepts. One notion of "public" relates it to issues that are of concern to the whole community; ends served by "political functions" are beneficial to the community as a whole. Although different individuals or groups may seek different resolutions of problems or disputes, the "political" can nevertheless be seen as encompassing all those human concerns and problems that are common to all the members of the community, or at least to large numbers of them. "Political" problems are shared problems that are appropriately dealt with through group action— their resolutions are collective, not individual. This separates them from "purely personal" problems. The second notion of "public" is that which is distinguished from "secret," that is, open to everyone's view, accessible to all members of the community. The settling of questions that concern the welfare of the community in a "public" way necessitates the sharing of "political knowledge"— the knowledge needed for participation in political discussion and decision. A system in which public policy is made publicly and the relevant knowledge is shared widely contrasts sharply with those systems in which a privileged few possess the relevant knowledge—whether priestly mysteries or bureaucratic expertise—and therefore control policy decisions.

Traditional Igbo society was predominantly patrilineal and segmental. People lived in "villages" composed of the scattered compounds of relatively close patrilineal kinsmen; and related villages formed what are usually referred to as "village groups," the largest functional political unit. Forde and Jones (1950: 9, 39) found between 4,000 and 5,000 village groups, ranging in population from several hundred to several thousand persons. Political power was diffuse, and leadership was fluid and informal. Community decisions were made and disputes settled through a variety of gatherings (villagewide assemblies; women's meetings; age grades; secret and title societies; contribution clubs; lineage groups; and congregations at funerals, markets, or annual rituals) as well as through appeals to oracles and diviners (Afigbo 1972: 13–36).[6] Decisions were made by discussion until mutual agreement was reached. Any adult present who had something to say on the matter under discussion was entitled to speak, so long as he or she said something that the others considered worth listening to; as the Igbo say, "A case forbids no one." Leaders were those who had "mouth"; age was respected, but did not confer leadership unless accompanied by wisdom and the ability to speak well. In village assemblies, after much discussion, a small group of elders retired for "consultation" and then offered a decision for the approval of the assembly (Uchendu 1965: 41–44; Green 1947: chaps. 7–11; Harris 1940: 142–43).

In some areas, the assemblies are said to have been of all adult males; in other areas, women reportedly participated in the assemblies, but were less likely to speak unless involved in the dispute and less likely to take part in "consultation." Women may have been among the "arbitrators" that disputants invited to settle particular cases; however, if one party to the dispute appealed to the village as a whole, male elders would have been more likely to offer the final settlement (Green 1947: 107, 112–13, 116–29, 169, 199). Age grades existed in most Igbo communities, but their functions varied; the predominant pattern seems to have been for young men's age grades to carry out decisions of the village assembly with regard to such matters as clearing paths, building bridges, or collecting fines (Uchendu 1965: 43). There was thus no distinction among what we call executive, legislative, and judicial activities, and no political authority to issue commands. The settling of a dispute could merge into a discussion of a new "rule," and acceptance by the disputants and the group hearing the dispute was necessary for the settlement of anything. Only within a family compound could an individual demand obedience to orders; there the compound head offered guidance, aid, and protection to members of his family, and in return received respect, obedience, and material tokens of good will. Neither was there any distinction between the religious and the political: rituals and "political" discussions were interwoven in patterns of action to promote the good of the community; and rituals, too, were performed by various groups of women, men, and women and men together (Afigbo 1972; Meek 1957: 98–99, 105; Uchendu 1965: 39–40).

Matters dealt with in the village assembly were those of common concern to all. They could be general problems for which collective action was appropriate (for example, discussion might center on how to make the village market bigger than those of neighboring villages); or they could be conflicts that threatened the unity of the village (for example, a dispute between members of different families, or between the men and the women) (Harris 1940: 142–43; Uchendu 1965: 34, 42–43). It is clear, then, that the assembly dealt with public policy publicly. The mode of discourse made much use of proverbs, parables, and metaphors drawn from the body of Igbo tradition and familiar to all Igbo from childhood. Influential speech involved the creative and skillful use of this tradition to provide counsel and justification—to assure others that a certain course of action was both a wise thing to do and a right thing to do. The accessibility (the "public" nature) of this knowledge is itself indicated by an Igbo proverb: "If you tell a proverb to a fool, he will ask you its meaning." Fools were excluded from the political community, but women were not.[7]

Women as well as men thus had access to political participation; for women as well as for men, public status was to a great extent achieved, not ascribed. A woman's status was determined more by her own achievements than by those of her husband. The resources available to men were greater, however; thus, although a woman might rank higher among women than her husband did among men, very few women could afford the fees and feasts involved in taking the highest titles, a major source of prestige (Meek 1957: 203). Men "owned" the most profitable crops and received the bulk of the money from bridewealth. Moreover, if they were compound heads, they received presents from compound members. Through the patrilineage, they controlled the land. After providing farms for their wives, they could lease excess land for a good profit. Men also did more of the long-distance trading, which had a higher rate of profit than did local and regional trading, which was almost entirely in women's hands (Green 1947: 32–42).

Women were entitled to sell the surplus of their own crops. They also received the palm kernels as their share of the palm produce (they processed the palm oil for the men to sell). They might also sell prepared foods, or the products of women's special skills (processed salt, pots, baskets). All the profits were theirs to keep (Leith-Ross 1939: 90–92, 138–39, 143). But these increments of profit were relatively low. Since the higher titles commonly needed to ensure respect for village leaders required increasingly higher fees and expenses, women's low profits restricted their access to villagewide leadership. Almost all of those who took the higher titles were men, and most of the leaders in villagewide discussions and decisions were men (Green 1947: 169; Uchendu 1965: 41). Women, therefore, came out as second-class citizens. Though status and the political influence it could bring were "achieved," and though there were no formal limits to women's political power, men by their ascriptive status (membership in the patrilineage) acquired wealth that gave them a head start and a lifelong advantage over women. The Igbo say that "a child who washes his hands clean deserves to eat with his elders" (Uchendu 1965: 19). What they do not say is that at birth some children are given water and some are not.

WOMEN'S POLITICAL INSTITUTIONS

Though women's associations are best described for the south—the area of the Women's War—their existence is reported for most other areas of Igboland, and Forde and Jones made the general observation that "women's associations express their disapproval and secure their demands by collective public demonstrations, including ridicule, satirical singing and dancing, and group strikes" (1950: 21).

Two sorts of women's associations are relevant politically: those of the *inyemedi* (wives of a lineage) and of the *umuada* (daughters of a lineage). Since traditional Igbo society was predominantly patrilocal and exogamous, almost all adult women in a village would be wives (there would also probably be some divorced or widowed "daughters" who had returned home to live). Women of the same natal village or village group (and therefore of the same lineage) might marry far and wide, but they would come together periodically in meetings often called *ogbo* (an Igbo word for "gathering"). The *umuada's* most important ritual function was at funerals of lineage members, since no one could have a proper funeral without their voluntary ritual participation—a fact that gave women a significant measure of power. The *umuada* invoked this power in helping to settle intralineage disputes among their "brothers," as well as disputes between their natal and marital lineages. Since these gatherings were held in rotation among the villages into which members had married, they formed an important part of the communication network of Igbo women (Okonjo 1974: 25; Olisa 1971: 24–27; Green 1947: 217–29).

The companion grouping to the *umuada* was the *inyemedi,* the wives of the lineage, who came together in villagewide gatherings that during the colonial period came to be called *mikiri* or *mitiri* (the Igbo version of the English "meeting"). *Mikiri* were thus gatherings of women based on common residence rather than on common birth, as in the case of *ogbo.* The *mikiri* appears to have performed the major role in daily self-rule among women and to have articulated women's interests as opposed to those of men. *Mikiri* provided women with a forum in which to develop their political talents and with a means for protecting their interests as traders, farmers, wives, and mothers (Green 1947; Leith-Ross 1939; Harris 1940; Okonjo 1974). In *mikiri,* women made rules about markets' crops, and livestock that applied to men as well as women; and they exerted pressure to maintain moral norms among women. They heard complaints from wives about mistreatment by husbands, and discussed how to deal with problems they were having with "the men" as a whole. They also made decisions about the rituals addressed to the female aspect of the village's guardian spirit, and about rituals for the protection of the fruitfulness of women and of their farms. If fines for violations or if repeated requests to husbands and elders were ignored, women might "sit on" an offender or go on strike. The latter might involve refusing to cook, to take care of small children, or to have sexual relations with their husbands. Men regarded the *mikiri* as legitimate; and the use of the more extreme sanctions—though rare—was well remembered.

Though both *ogbo* and *mikiri* served to articulate and protect women's interests, it is probably more accurate to see these groups as sharing in diffused political authority than to see them as acting only as pressure groups for women's interests. Okonjo [1976] argues . . . that traditional Igbo society had a "dual-sex political system"; that is, there was a dual system of male and female political-religious institutions, each sex having both its own autonomous sphere of authority and an area of shared responsibilities. Thus, women settled disputes among women, but also made decisions and rules affecting men. They had the right to enforce their decisions and rules by using forms of group ostracism similar to those used by men. In a society of such diffuse political authority, it would be misleading to call only a village assembly of men a "public" gathering, as most Western observers unquestioningly do; among the Igbo, a gathering of adult women must also be accepted as a public gathering.

COLONIAL "PENETRATION"

Into this system of diffuse authority, fluid and informal leadership, shared rights of enforcement, and a more or less stable balance of male and female power, the British tried to introduce ideas of "native administration" derived from colonial experience with chiefs and emirs in northern Nigeria. Southern Nigeria was declared a protectorate in 1900, but ten years passed before the conquest was effective. As colonial power was established in what the British perceived as a situation of "ordered anarchy," Igboland was divided into Native Court Areas that violated the autonomy of villages by lumping together many unrelated villages. British District Officers were to preside over the courts, but they were not always present because there were more courts than officers. The Igbo membership was formed by choosing from each village a "representative" who was given a warrant of office. These Warrant Chiefs also constituted what was called the Native Authority. The Warrant Chiefs were required to see that the orders of the District Officers were executed in their own villages, and they were the only link between the colonial power and the people (Afigbo 1972: 13–36, 207–48).

In the first place, it was a violation of Igbo concepts to have one man represent the village; and it was even more of a violation that he should give orders to everyone else. The people obeyed the Warrant Chief when they had to, since British power backed him up. In some places Warrant Chiefs were lineage heads or wealthy men who were already leaders in the village. But in many places they were simply ambitious, opportunistic young men who put themselves forward as friends of the conquerors. Even where the Warrant Chief was not corrupt, he was still, more than anything else, an agent of the British. The people avoided using Native Courts when they could do so, but Warrant Chiefs could force cases into the Native Courts and fine people for infractions of rules. Because he had the ear of the British, the Warrant Chief himself could violate traditions and even British rules and get away with it (Anene 1967: 259; Meek 1957: 328–30).

Women suffered particularly under the arbitrary rule of Warrant Chiefs, who reportedly took women to marry without allowing them the customary right to refuse a particular suitor. They also helped themselves to the women's agricultural produce and domestic animals (Onwuteaka 1965: 274). Recommendations for reform of the system were made almost from its inception both by junior officers in the field and by senior officers sent out from headquarters to investigate. But no real improvements were made. An attempt by the British in 1918 to make the Native Courts more "native" by abolishing the District Officers' role as presiding court officials had little effect, and that mostly bad. Removing the District Officers from the courts simply left more power in the hands of corrupt Warrant Chiefs and the increasingly powerful Court Clerks. The latter, intended to be "servants of the court," were able in some cases to dominate the courts because of their monopoly of expertise—namely, literacy (Meek 1957: 329; Gailey 1970: 66–74).

THE WOMEN'S WAR

In 1925, the British decided to introduce direct taxation in order to create the Native Treasury, which was supposed to pay for improvements in the Native Administration, in accordance with the British imperial philosophy that the colonized should pay the costs of colonization. Prices in the palm trade were high, and the tax—on adult males—was set accordingly. Taxes were collected without widespread trouble, although there were "tax riots" in Warri Province (west of the Niger) in 1927.

In 1929, a zealous Assistant District Officer in Bende division of Owerri Province, apparently acting on his own initiative, decided to "tighten up" the census registers by recounting households and property. He told the Chiefs that there was no plan to increase taxes or to tax women. But the counting of women and their property raised fears that women were to be taxed, particularly because the Bende District Officer had lied earlier when the men were counted and had told the men that they were not going to be taxed. The women, therefore, naturally did not believe these reassurances. The taxation rumor spread quickly through the women's communication networks, and meetings of women took place in various market squares, which were the common places for women to have large meetings. In the Oloko Native Court Area—one of the areas of deception about the men's tax—the women leaders, Ikonnia, Nwannedie, and Nwugo, called a general meeting at Orie market. Here it was decided that as long as only men were approached in a compound and asked for information the women would do nothing. If any woman was approached, she was to raise the alarm; then the women would meet again to decide what to do. But they wanted clear evidence that women were to be taxed (Afigbo 1972; Gailey 1970: 107–8).

On November 23, an agent of the Oloko Warrant Chief, Okugo, entered a compound and told one of the married women, Nwanyeruwa, to count her goats and sheep.

She replied angrily, "Was your mother counted?" at which "they closed, seizing each other by the throat" (Perham 1937: 207). Nwanyeruwa's report to the Oloko women convinced them that they were to be taxed. Messengers were sent to neighboring areas, and women streamed into Oloko from all over Owerri Province. They "sat on" Okugo and demanded his cap of office. They massed in protest at the District Office and succeeded in getting written assurances that they were not to be taxed. After several days of mass protest meetings, they also succeeded in getting Okugo arrested, tried, and convicted of "spreading news likely to cause alarm" and of physical assault on the women. He was sentenced to two years' imprisonment (Gailey 1970: 108–13).

News of this victory spread rapidly through the market-*mikiri-ogbo* network, and women in many areas then attempted to get rid of their Warrant Chiefs and the Native Administration itself. Nwanyeruwa became something of a heroine as reports of her resistance spread. Money poured in from grateful women from villages scattered over a wide area but linked by kinship to Nwanyeruwa's marital village. Nwanyeruwa herself, however, was "content to allow" leadership in her area to be exercised by someone else. The money collected was used not for her but for delegates going to meetings of women throughout southern Igboland to coordinate the Women's War.

The British ended the rebellion only by using large numbers of police and soldiers—and, on one occasion, Boy Scouts. Although the shootings in mid-December and the growing numbers of police and soldiers in the area led the women to halt most of their activities, disturbances continued into 1930. The "disaffected areas"—all of Owerri and Calabar provinces—were occupied by government forces. Punitive expeditions burned or demolished compounds, took provisions from the villages to feed the troops, and confiscated property in payment of fines levied arbitrarily against villages in retribution for damages (Gailey 1970: 135–37).

During the investigations that followed the Women's War, the British discovered the communication network that had been used to spread the rumor of taxation. But that did not lead them to inquire further into how it came to pass that Igbo women had engaged in concerted action under grassroots leadership, had agreed on demands, and had materialized by the thousands at Native Administration centers dressed and adorned in the same unusual way—all wearing short loincloths, all carrying sticks wreathed with palm fronds, and all having their faces smeared with charcoal or ashes and their heads bound with young ferns. Unbeknownst to the British, this was the dress and adornment signifying "war," the sticks being used to invoke the power of the female ancestors (Harris 1940: 143–45, 147–48; Perham 1937: 207ff; Meek 1957: ix).

The report of the Commission of Enquiry exonerating the soldiers who fired on the women cited the "savage passions" of the "mobs"; and one military officer told the Commission that "he had never seen crowds in such a state of frenzy." Yet these "frenzied mobs" injured no one seriously, which the British found "surprising"; but then the British did not understand that the women were engaged in a traditional practice with traditional rules and limitations, only carried out in this instance on a much larger scale than in precolonial times.[8]

REFORMS—BUT NOT FOR WOMEN

The British failure to recognize the Women's War as a collective response to the abrogation of rights resulted in a failure to ask whether women might have had a role in the traditional political system that should be incorporated into the institutions of colonial government. Because the women—and the men—regarded the investigations as attempts to discover whom to punish, they volunteered no information about women's organizations. But would the British have understood those organizations if they had? The discovery of the market network had suggested no further lines of inquiry. The majority of District Officers thought that the men had organized the women's actions and were secretly directing them. The women's demands that the Native Courts no longer hear cases and that "all white men should go to their own country"—or at least that women should serve on the Native Courts and a woman be appointed a District Officer—were in line with the power of women in traditional Igbo society but were regarded by the British as irrational and ridiculous (Gailey 1970: 130ff; Leith-Ross 1939: 165; Perham 1937: 165ff).

The reforms instituted in 1933 therefore ignored the women's traditional political role, though they did make some adjustments to traditional Igbo male and male-dominated political forms. The number of Native Court Areas was greatly increased, and their boundaries were arranged to conform roughly to traditional divisions. Warrant Chiefs were replaced by "massed benches," which allowed large numbers of judges to sit at one time. In most cases it was left up to the villages to decide whom and how many to send. Though this benefited the women by eliminating the corruption of the Warrant Chiefs, and thus made their persons and property more secure, it provided no outlet for collective action, their real base of power (Perham 1937: 365ff).

In 1901 the British had declared all jural institutions except the Native Courts illegitimate, but it was only in the years following the 1933 reforms that Native Administration local government became effective enough to make that declaration at all meaningful. The British had also outlawed "self-help"—the use of force by anyone but the government to punish wrongdoers. And the increasingly effective enforcement of this ban eliminated the women's ultimate weapon: "sitting on a man." In attempting to create specialized political institutions on the Western model, with participation on the basis of individual achievement, the British created a system in which there was no place for group solidarity, no possibility of dispersed and shared political authority or power of enforcement, and thus very little place for women (Leith-Ross 1939: 109–10, 163, 214). As in the village assemblies, women could not compete with men for leadership in the reformed Native Administration because they lacked the requisite resources. This imbalance in resources was increased by other facets of British colonialism—economic "penetration" and missionary influence. All three—colonial government, foreign investment, and the church—contributed to the growth of a system of political and economic stratification that made community decision-making less "public" in both senses we have discussed and that led to the current concentration of national political power in the hands of a small, educated, wealthy, male elite. For though we are here focusing on the political results of colonialism, they must be seen as part of the whole system of imposed class and sex stratification.

MISSIONARY INFLUENCE

Christian missions were established in Igboland in the late nineteenth century. They had few converts at first, but by the 1930's their influence was significant, though generally limited to the young (Leith-Ross 1939: 109–18; Meek 1957: xv). A majority of Igbo eventually "became Christians," for they had to profess Christianity in order to attend mission schools. Regardless of how nominal their membership was, they had to obey the rules to remain in good standing, and one rule was to avoid "pagan" rituals. Women were discouraged from attending meetings where traditional rituals were performed or where money was collected for the rituals, which in effect meant all *mikiri, ogbo,* and many other types of gatherings (Ajayi 1965: 108–9).

Probably more significant, since *mikiri* were losing some of their political functions anyway, was mission education. The Igbo came to see English and Western education as increasingly necessary for political leadership—needed to deal with the British and their law—and women had less access to this new knowledge than men had. Boys were more often sent to school than girls, for a variety of reasons generally related to their favored position in the patrilineage, including the fact that they, not their sisters, would be expected to support their parents in their old age. But even when girls did go, they tended not to receive the same type of education. In mission schools, and increasingly in special "training homes" that dispensed with most academic courses, the girls were taught European domestic skills and the Bible, often in the vernacular. The missionaries' avowed purpose in educating girls was to train them for Christian marriage and motherhood, not for jobs or for citizenship. Missionaries were not necessarily against women's participation in politics; clergy in England, as in America, could be found supporting women's suffrage. But in Africa their concern was the church, and for the church they needed Christian families. Therefore, Christian wives and mothers, not female political leaders, were the missions' aim. As Mary Slessor, the influential Calabar missionary, said: "God-like motherhood is the finest sphere for women, and the way to the redemption of the world."[9] As the English language and other knowledge of "book" became necessary to political life, women were increasingly cut out and policy-making became less public.

ECONOMIC COLONIALISM

The traditional Igbo division of labor—in which women owned their surplus crops and their market profits, while men controlled the more valuable yams and palm products and did more long-distance trading—was based on a subsistence economy. Small surpluses could be accumulated, but these were generally not used for continued capital investment. Rather, in accord with traditional values, the surplus was used for social rather than economic gain: it was returned to the community through fees and feasts for rituals for title-taking, weddings, funerals, and other ceremonies, or through projects to help the community "get up." One became a "big man" or a "big woman" not by hoarding one's wealth but by spending it on others in prestige-winning ways (Uchendu 1965: 34; Meek 1957: 111).

Before the Pax Britannica, Igbo women had been active traders in all but a few areas (one such was Afikpo, where women farmed but did not trade).[10] The ties of exogamous marriage among patrilineages, the cross-cutting networks of women providing channels for communication and conciliation, and the ritual power of female members of patrilineages all enabled the traditional system to deal with conflicts with relatively little warfare (Anene 1967: 214ff; Green 1947: 91, 152, 177, 230–32). Conflict also took the nonviolent form of mutual insults in obscene and satirical songs (Nwoga 1971: 33–35, 40–42); and even warfare itself was conducted within limits, with weapons and actions increasing in seriousness in inverse proportion to the closeness of kinship ties. Women from mutually hostile village groups who had married into the same patrilineage could if necessary act as "protectors" for each other so that they could trade in "stranger" markets (Green 1947: 151). Women also protected themselves by carrying the stout sticks they used as pestles for pounding yams (the same ones carried in the Women's War). Even after European slave-trading led to an increase in danger from slave-hunters (as well as from headhunters), Igbo women went by themselves to their farms and with other women to market, with their pestles as weapons for physical protection (Esike 1965: 13).

The Pax increased the safety of short- and especially of long-distance trading for Igbo women as for women in other parts of Africa. But the Pax also made it possible for European firms to dominate the market economy. Onwuteaka argues that one cause of the Women's War was Igbo women's resentment of the monopoly British firms had on buying, a monopoly that allowed them to fix prices and adopt methods of buying that increased their own profits at the women's expense (1965: 278). Women's petty trading grew to include European products, but for many women the accumulated surplus remained small, often providing only subsistence and a few years' school fees for some of their children—the preference for sending boys to school further disadvantaging the next generation of women (Mintz 1971: 251–68; Boserup 1970: 92–95). A few women have become "big traders," dealing in £1000 lots of European goods, but women traders remain for the most part close to subsistence level. Little is open to West African women in towns except trading, brewing, or prostitution, unless they are among the tiny number who have special vocational or professional training (for example, as dressmakers, nurses, or teachers) (Boserup 1970: 85–101, 106–38). The "modern" economic sector, like the "modern" political sector, is dominated by men, women's access being limited "by their low level of literacy and by the general tendency to give priority to men in employment recruitment to the modern sector" (Boserup 1970: 99).

Women outside urban areas—the great majority of women—find themselves feeding their children by farming with their traditional digging sticks while men are moving into cash-cropping (with tools and training from "agricultural development programs"), migrant wage-labor, and trading with Europeans (Boserup 1970: 53–61, 87–99; Mintz 1971: 248–51). Thus, as Mintz suggests, "while the economic growth advanced by Westernization has doubtless increased opportunities for (at least some) female traders, it may also and simultaneously limit the range of their activities, as economic changes outside the internal market system continue to multiply" (p. 265). To the extent that economic opportunities for Africans in the "modern" sector continue to grow, women will become relatively more dependent economically on men and will be unlikely to "catch up" for a very long time, even if we accept education as the key. The relative stagnation of African economic "growth," however, suggests that the traditional markets will not disappear or even noticeably shrink, but will continue to be needed by the large numbers of urban migrants living economically marginal lives. Women can thus continue to subsist by petty trading, though they cannot achieve real economic independence from men or gain access to the resources needed for equal participation in community life.

It seems reasonable to see the traditional Igbo division of labor in production as interwoven with the traditional Igbo dispersal of political authority into a dual or "dual-sex" system. It seems equally reasonable to see the disruptions of colonialism as producing a new, similarly interwoven economic-political pattern—but one with stronger male domination of the cash economy and of political life.

To see this relationship, however, is not to explain it. Even if the exclusion of women from the colonial Native Administration and from nationalist politics could be shown to derive from their exclusion from the "modern" economic sector, we would still need to ask why it was men who were offered agricultural training and new tools for cash-cropping, and who are hired in factories and shops in preference to women with the same education. And we would still need to ask why it was chiefly boys who were sent to school, and why their education differed from that provided for girls.

VICTORIANISM AND WOMEN'S INVISIBILITY

At least part of the answer must lie in the values of the colonialists, values that led the British to assume that girls and boys, women and men, should be treated and should behave as people supposedly did in "civilized" Victorian England. Strong male domination was imposed on Igbo society both indirectly, by new economic structures, and directly, by the recruitment of only men into the Native Administration. In addition, the new economic and political structures were supported by the inculcation of sexist ideology in the mission schools.

Not all capitalist, colonialist societies are equally sexist (or racist); but the Victorian society from which the conquerors of Igboland came was one in which the ideology that a woman's place is in the home had hardened into the most rigid form it has taken in recent Western history. Although attacked by feminists, that ideology remained dominant throughout the colonial period and is far from dead today. The ideal of Victorian womanhood—attainable, of course, only by the middle and upper classes, but widely believed in throughout society—was of a sensitive, morally superior being who was the hearthside guardian of Christian virtues and sentiments absent in the outside world. Her mind was not strong enough for the appropriately "masculine" subjects: science, business, and politics.[11] A woman who showed talent in these areas did not challenge any ideas about typical women: the exceptional woman simply had "the brain of a man," as Sir George Goldie said of Mary Kingsley (Gwynn 1932: 252).[12] A thorough investigation of the diaries, journals, reports, and letters of colonial officers and missionaries would be needed to prove that most of them held these Victorian values. But a preliminary reading of biographies, autobiographies, journals, and "reminiscences," plus the evidence of statements about Igbo women at the time of the Women's War, strongly suggests that the colonialists were deflected from any attempt to discover or protect Igbo women's political and economic roles by their assumption that politics and business were not proper, normal places for women.[13]

When Igbo women forced the colonial administrators to recognize their presence during the Women's War, their brief "visibility" was insufficient to shake these assumptions. Their behavior was simply seen as aberrant and inexplicable. When they returned to "normal," they were once again invisible. This inability to "see" what is before one's eyes is strikingly illustrated by an account of a visit by the High Commissioner, Sir Ralph Moor, to Aro Chukwu after the British had destroyed (temporarily) the powerful oracle there: "To Sir Ralph's astonishment, the women of Aro Chukwu solicited his permission to reestablish the Long Juju, which the women intended to control themselves" (Anene 1967: 234). Would Sir Ralph have been "astonished" if, for example, the older men had controlled the oracle before its destruction and the younger men had wanted to take it over?

The feminist movement in England during the colonial era did not succeed in making the absence of women from public life noted as a problem that required a remedy. The movement did not succeed in creating a "feminist" consciousness in any but a few "deviants," and such a consciousness is far from widespread today; for to have a "feminist" consciousness means that one notices the "invisibility" of women. One wonders where the women are—in life and in print. That we have not wondered is an indication of our own ideological bondage to a system of sex and class stratification. What we can see, if we look, is that Igbo men have come to dominate women economically and politically: individual women have become economic auxiliaries to their husbands, and women's groups have become political auxiliaries to nationalist parties. Wives supplement their husbands' incomes but remain economically dependent; women's "branches" have provided votes, money, and participants in street demonstrations for political parties but remain dependent on male leaders for policymaking. Market women's associations were a vital base of support for the early National Council for Nigeria and the Cameroons (NCNC), the party that eventually was to become dominant in Igbo regions (although it began as a truly national party). And though a few market-women leaders were ultimately rewarded for their loyalty to the NCNC by appointment to party or legislative positions, market women's associations never attained a share in policymaking that approached their contribution to NCNC electoral success (Bretton 1966: 61; MacIntosh 1966: 299, 304–9; Sklar 1963: 41–83, 251, 402). The NCNC at first had urged female suffrage throughout the country, an idea opposed by the Northern People's Congress (NPC), dominated by Moslem emirs. Soon, however, the male NCNC leadership gave up pushing for female suffrage in the north (where women have never yet voted) in order to make peace with the NPC and the British and thus insure for themselves a share of power in the postindependence government. During the period between independence in 1960 and the 1966 military coups that ended party rule, some progress was made in education for girls. By 1966, consequently, female literacy in the East was more than 50 percent in some urban areas and at least 15 percent overall—high for Africa, where the overall average is about 10 percent and the rural average may be as low as 2 percent (MacIntosh 1966: 17–37; *West African Pilot,* April 29, 1959; Pool 1972: 238; UNESCO 1968).

Exhortations to greater female participation in "modern life" appeared frequently in the newspapers owned by the NCNC leader, Nnamdi Azikiwe, and a leadership training course for women was begun in 1959 at the Man O' War Bay Training Centre, to be "run on exactly the same lines as the courses for men, with slight modifications," as the *Pilot* put it. The motto of the first class of 22 women was, "What the men can do, the women can" (Van Allen 1974b: 17–20). But there was more rhetoric than reality in these programs for female emancipation. During the period of party politics, no women were elected to regional or national legislatures; those few who were appointed gained favor by supporting "party first," not "women first." Perhaps none of this should be surprising, given the corruption that had come to dominate national party politics (MacIntosh 1966: 299, 612–14; Sklar 1963: 402; Van Allen 1974b: 19–22).

BIAFRA AND BEYOND

On January 15, 1966, a military coup ended the Igbos' relationship with the NCNC: all political parties, and therefore their women's branches, were outlawed. A year and a half later—after the massacres of more than 30,000 Easterners in the North, the flight of more than a million refugees back to the East, a countercoup, and the division of the Igbo-dominated Eastern Region into three states—Biafra declared herself an independent state. In January 1970 she surrendered; the remaining Igbo are now landlocked, oilless, and under military occupation by a Northern-dominated military government.[14] Igbo women demonstrated in the streets to protest the massacres, to urge secession, and, later, to protest Soviet involvement in the war (Ojukwu 1969: 91, 143, 145–46, 245). During the war, the women's market network and other women's organizations maintained a distribution system for what food there was and provided channels for the passage of food and information to the army (Uzoma 1974: 8ff; Akpan 1971: 65–67, 89, 98–99, 128–30). Women joined local civilian-defense militia units and in May 1969 formed a "Women's Front" and called on the Biafran leadership to allow them to enlist in the infantry (Uzoma 1974: 5–8; Ojukwu 1969: 386).

During and after the war, local civilian government continued to exist more or less in the form that evolved under the "reformed" Native Administration. The decentralization produced by the war has by some reports strengthened these local councils, and the absence of many men has strengthened female participation (Peters 1971: 102–3; Adler 1969: 112; Uzoma 1974: 10–12). Thus, at tragic human cost, the war may have made possible a resurgence of female political activity. If this is so, women's participation again stems much more from Igbo tradition than from Western innovation.

It remains to be seen whether Igbo women, or any African women, can gain real political power without the creation of a "modern" version of the traditional "dual-sex" system (which is what Okonjo argues is needed) or without a drastic change in economic structures so that economic equality could support political equality for all women and men, just as economic stratification now supports male domination and female dependence. What seems clear from women's experiences—whether under capitalism, colonialism, or revolutionary socialism—is that formal political and economic equality are not enough. Unless the male members of a liberation movement, a ruling party, or a government themselves develop a feminist consciousness and a commitment to male-female equality, women will end up where they have always been: invisible, except when men, for their own purposes personal or political, look for female bodies.

NOTES

1. This paper is a revised version of papers presented at the 1971 African Studies Association meeting and at the 1974 UCLA African Studies Center Colloquium on "Women and Change in Africa: 1870–1970." I am grateful to Terrence O. Ranger, who organized the UCLA colloquium, and to the other participants (particularly Agnes Aidoo, Jim Brain, Cynthia Brantley, Temma Kaplan, and Margaret Strobel) for their encouragement, useful criticisms, and suggestions.
2. Today the Igbo, numbering about 8.7 million, live mainly in the East-Central State of Nigeria, with some half million in the neighboring Mid-Western State. The area in which they live corresponds approximately to Igboland at the time of the colonial conquest.
3. A number of Ibibio women from Calabar were also drawn into the rebellion, but the mass of the participants were Igbo.
4. Perham 1937: 202–12. Afigbo 1972 and Gailey 1970 give more detailed accounts of the Women's War than does Perham; all three, however, base their descriptions on the reports of the two Commissions of Enquiry, issued as Sessional Papers of the Nigerian Legislative Council (Nos. 12 and 28 of 1930), on the Minutes of Evidence issued with No. 28, and on intelligence reports made in the early 1930's by political officers. Afigbo, an Igbo scholar, provides the most extensive and authoritative account of the three, and he is particularly good on traditional Igbo society.
5. Similar tactics were also used against women for serious offenses (see Leith-Ross 1939: 97).
6. Though there is variation among the Igbo, the general patterns described here apply fairly well to the southern Igbo, those involved in the Women's War. The chief exceptions to the above description occur among the western and riverain Igbo, who have what Afigbo terms a "constitutional village monarchy" system, and among the Afikpo of the Cross River, who have a double-descent system and low female participation in economic and political life (P. Ottenberg 1959 and 1965). The former are more hierarchically organized than other Igbo but are not stratified by sex, having a women's hierarchy parallel to that of the men (Nzirimo 1972); the latter are strongly stratified by sex, with the senior men's age grade dominating community decision-making. Afikpo women's age grades are weak; there is no *mikiri* or, because of the double-descent system, *ogbo* (these terms are defined later in this paper . . . Afikpo women have not traditionally been active in trade; and female status among the Afikpo is generally very low. Afikpo Igbo, unlike almost all other Igbo, have a men's secret society that has "keeping women in their place" as a major purpose (P. Ottenberg 1959 and 1965).
7. I rely here chiefly on Uchendu 1965 and personal conversations with an Igbo born in Umu-Domi village of Onicha clan, Afikpo division. Some of the ideas about leadership were suggested by Schaar 1970. His discussion of what "humanly meaningful authority" would look like is very suggestive for studies of leadership in "developing" societies.
8. A few older men criticized the women for "flinging sand at their chiefs," but Igbo men generally supported the women though they nonetheless considered it "their fight" against the British. It is also reported that both women and men shared the mistaken belief that the women would not be fired upon because they had observed certain rituals and were carrying the palm-wrapped sticks that invoked the power of the female ancestors. The men had no illusions of immunity for themselves, having vivid memories of the slaughter of Igbo men during the conquest (Perham 1937: 212ff; Anene 1967: 207–24; Esike 1965: 11; Meek 1957: x).
9. For the missionaries' views and purposes, see Ajayi 1965, Basden 1927, Bulifant 1950, Maxwell 1926, and Livingstone n.d.
10. It is an unfortunate accident that the Afikpo Igbo, with their strong sexual stratification, have been used as examples of "the Igbo" or of "the effect of colonialism on women" in widely read articles. Simon Ottenberg's "Ibo Receptivity to Change" is particularly mislead-

ing, since it is about "all" Igbo. There is one specific mention of women: "The social and economic independence of women is much greater in some areas than in others." True, but the social and economic independence of women is much greater in virtually *all* other Igbo groups than it is in Afikpo, where the Ottenbergs did fieldwork. There are said to be "a variety of judicial techniques" used, but all the examples given are of men's activities. There is a list of non-kinship organizations, but no women's organizations are listed. Sanday's otherwise useful and thought-provoking article (1973) both takes the Afikpo as "the" Igbo and exaggerates the amount of change in female status that female trading brought about. Phoebe Ottenberg, Sanday's ultimate source on Afikpo women, described the change in female status as existing "chiefly on the domestic rather than the general level," with the "men's position of religious, moral, and legal authority . . . in no way threatened" (1959: 223). For examples of precolonial female trading in Igboland and elsewhere, see Little 1973 (particularly p. 46, n. 32); Uchendu 1965; Van Allen 1974b: 5–9; Dike 1956; and Jones 1963.

11. The fact that Englishwomen of the "lower classes" had to work in the fields, in the mills, in the mines, or on the street did not stop the colonialists from carrying their ideal to Africa, or from condemning urban prostitution there (just as they did at home) without acknowledging their contribution to its origin or continuation.
12. Mary Kingsley, along with other elite female "exceptions" who influenced African colonial policy (e.g., Flora Shaw Lugard and Margery Perham), held the same values that men did, at least in regard to women's roles. They did not expect ordinary women to have political power any more than men expected them to, and they showed no particular concern for African women.
13. For examples of this attitude among those who were not missionaries, see Anene 1967: 222–34; Crocker 1936; Meek 1957; Kingsley 1897; Perham 1960; and Wood 1960.
14. The attitude of the Northern emirs who now again dominate the Nigerian government is perhaps indicated by their order in June 1973 that single women get married or leave Northern Nigeria because Moslem religious authorities had decided that the North African drought was caused by prostitution and immorality. Landlords were ordered not to let rooms to single women, and many unmarried women were reported to have fled their home areas *(Agence France-Presse,* as reported in *The San Francisco Chronicle,* June 23, 1973). In late 1975 the military government appointed a 50-man body to draft a constitution for Nigeria's return to civilian rule. As of this writing women's protests have produced no changes in its membership.

REFERENCES

Adler, Renate. 1969. "Letter from Biafra," *The New Yorker,* Oct. 4.

Afigbo, A. E. 1972. *The Warrant Chiefs: Indirect Rule in South-Eastern Nigeria, 1891–1929.* London.

Ajayi, J. F. Ade. 1965. *Christian Missions in Nigeria, 1841–1891: The Making of a New Elite.* Evanston, Ill.

Akpan, Ntieyong U. 1971. *The Struggle for Secession, 1966–1970.* London.

Anene, J. C. 1967. *Southern Nigeria in Transition, 1885–1906.* New York.

Basden, G. T. 1927. *Edith Warner of the Niger.* London.

Boserup, Ester. 1970. *Woman's Role in Economic Development.* New York.

Bretton, Henry L. 1966. "Political Influence in Southern Nigeria," in Herbert J. Spiro, ed., *Africa: The Primacy of Politics.* New York.

Bulifant, Josephine C. 1950. *Forty Years in the African Bush.* Grand Rapids, Mich.

Crocker, W. R. 1936. *Nigeria: A Critique of British Colonial Administration.* London.

Dike, K. Onwuka. 1956. *Trade and Politics in the Niger Delta, 1830–1885.* London.

Esike, S. O. 1965. "The Aba Riots of 1929." *African Historian* (Ibadan), 1, no. 3.

Fallers, Lloyd Ashton. 1963. "Political Sociology and the Anthropological Study of African Politics," *Archives Européennes de Sociologie.*

Forde, Daryll, and G. I. Jones. 1950. *The Ibo- and Ibibio- Speaking Peoples of South-Eastern Nigeria.* London.

Gailey, Harry A. 1970. *The Road to Aba.* New York.

Green, M. M. 1947. *Igbo Village Affairs.* London.

Gwynn, Stephen. 1932. *The Life of Mary Kingsley.* London.

Harris, J. S. 1940. "The Position of Women in a Nigerian Society," *Transactions of the New York Academy of Sciences.* New York.

Jones, G. I. 1963. *The Trading States of the Oil Rivers.* London.

Kingsley, Mary H. 1897. *Travels in West Africa.* London.

Leith-Ross, Sylvia. 1939. *African Women: A Study of the Ibo of Nigeria.* London.

Little, Kenneth. 1973. *African Women in Towns.* London.

Livingstone, W. P. n.d. *Mary Slessor of Calabar.* New York.

MacIntosh, John P., ed. 1966. *Nigerian Government and Politics.* London.

Maxwell, J. Lowry. 1926. *Nigeria: The Land, the People and Christian Progress.* London.

Meek, C. K. 1957. *Law and Authority in a Nigerian Tribe.* London.

Mintz, Sidney W. 1971. "Men, Women, and Trade," *Comparative Studies in Society and History,* 13.

Nwoga, D. I. 1971. "The Concept and Practice of Satire among the Igbo," *Conch,* 3, no. 2.

Nzirimo, Ikenna. 1972. *Studies in Ibo Political Systems: Chieftaincy and Politics in Four Niger States.* Berkeley, Calif.

Ojukwu, C. Odumegwu. 1969. *Biafra.* New York.

Okonjo, Kamene, 1974. "Political Systems with Bisexual Functional Roles—The Case of Women's Participation in Politics in Nigeria." Paper presented at the Annual Meeting of the American Political Science Association, Chicago.

———. 1976. "The Dual-Sex Political System in Operation: Igbo Women and Community Politics in Midwestern Nigeria," In Nancy J. Hafkin, and Edna Bay, eds., *Women in Africa: Studies in Social and Economic Change.* Stanford.

Olisa, Michael S. O. 1971. "Political Culture and Political Stability in Traditional Igbo Society," *Conch, 3, no. 2.*

Onwuteaka, J. C. 1965. "The Aba Riot of 1929 and Its Relation to the System of 'Indirect Rule,'" *The Nigerian Journal of Economic and Social Studies,* November.

Ottenberg, Phoebe V. 1959. "The Changing Economic Position of Women Among the Afikpo Ibo," in W. R. Bascom and M. J. Herskovits, eds., *Continuity and Change in African Cultures.* Chicago.

———. 1965. "The Afikpo Ibo of Eastern Nigeria," in James L. Gibbs, Jr., ed., *Peoples of Africa.* New York.

Ottenberg, Simon. 1959. "Ibo Receptivity to Change," in W. R. Bascom and M. J. Herskovits, eds., *Continuity and Change in African Cultures.* Chicago.

Perham, Margery. 1937. *Native Administration in Nigeria.* London.

———. 1960. *Lugard: The Years of Authority, 1898–1945.* London.

Peters, Helen. 1971. "Reflections on the Preservation of Igbo Folk Literature," *Conch, 3, no. 2.*

Pool, Janet E. 1972. "A Cross-Comparative Study of Aspects of Conjugal Behavior Among Women of Three West African Countries," *Canadian Journal of African Studies, 6, no. 2.*

Sanday, Peggy R. 1973. "Toward a Theory of the Status of Women," *American Anthropologist, 75, no. 5.*

Schaar, John H. 1970. "Legitimacy in the Modern State," in Philip Green and Sanford Levinson, eds., *Power and Community.* New York.

Sklar, Richard. 1963. *Nigerian Political Parties.* Princeton, N.J.

Uchendu, Victor C. 1965. *The Igbo of Southeast Nigeria.* New York.

United Nations Economic and Social Council (UNESCO). 1968. "Problems of Plan Implementation: Development Planning and Economic Integration in Africa."

Uzoma, Chinwe. 1974. "The Role of Women in the Nigerian/Biafran Civil War as Seen Through My Experiences Then." Unpublished personal communication to Judith Van Allen.

Van Allen, Judith. 1972. "'Sitting on a Man': Colonialism and the Lost Political Institutions of Igbo Women," *Canadian Journal of African Studies,* 6, no. 2.

———. 1974a. "African Women—Modernizing into Dependence?" Paper presented at the conference on "Social and Political Change: The Role of Women," sponsored by the University of California, Santa Barbara, and the Center for the Study of Democratic Institutions.

———. 1974b. "From Aba to Biafra: Women's Associations and Political Power in Eastern Nigeria." Paper presented at the UCLA African Studies Center Colloquium on Women and Change in Africa, 1870–1970.

———. 1974c. *"Memsahib, Militante, Femme Libre: Political and Apolitical Styles of African Women,"* in Jane Jaquette, ed., *Women in Politics.* New York.

Wood, A. H. St. John. 1960. "Nigeria: Fifty Years of Political Development among the Ibos," in Raymond Apthorpe, ed., *From Tribal Rule to Modern Government.* Lusaka, Northern Rhodesia.

THE IMPACT OF DEVELOPMENT ON WOMEN: THE INTERPLAY OF MATERIAL CONDITIONS AND GENDER IDEOLOGY

Victoria S. Lockwood

During the colonial era, European nations expanded their cultural, economic, and political hegemony over much of the non-western world (see Wolf 1982). To gain access to the material wealth of their colonies, the Europeans established conditions under which native populations had little choice but to produce crops or other commodities for markets, or to work for wages on European plantations or in mines. As these processes escalated and other western interventions intensified, capitalist relations of production began to subsume indigenous economies in most parts of the world.

Since that time, capitalism has proven a versatile, dynamic, and ever-expanding political economic system. Today, even the most remote and isolated village has been touched and transformed by it. The general terms often applied to that transformation—"development" and "modernization"—describe not only the processes of market integration (and shifts to capitalist production relations), but also the dynamic restructuring of social institutions, social relations, and worldview that accompanies it.

Although there is great diversity in how this structural and ideological transformation has taken place around the world, research focused on gender issues in development has identified several important themes. First, men and women rarely participate in development the same way; in other words, they do not have access to the same kinds of development-generated opportunities and choices. Second, men and women rarely share equally in the various "costs" and "benefits" of development. Indeed, a growing number of studies suggest that women's social, economic, and political position relative to that of men actually deteriorates with capitalist development, or that, at best, its effects on women are highly mixed (Boserup 1970; Etienne and Leacock 1980; Nash 1977; Fernandez-Kelly 1981; Charleton 1984; Bossen 1975, 1984; Caulfield 1981; Afonja 1981).

At the same time, a number of cases in which women's position and status have improved show that there are important exceptions to this general trend. In other words, it is clear that, "The changes brought about by colonialism, or, later, capitalist productive relations, are not *automatically* detrimental to women" (Rapp 1979: 505, cited in Di Leonardo 1991: 15; my emphasis). Thus, ". . . we must be wary of simplistically portraying men as the winners and women as the losers" (Moore 1988: 79). As the rapidly growing body of literature on women and development points out, the situation is much more complex than that.

The highly variable impact of development on non-western women raises a number of important questions. How, specifically, does development (capitalist integration) differentially affect men and women, and why does women's position frequently deteriorate? And, in those cases where women's position has improved, is it possible to identify particular material/structural or ideological factors that have contributed in the development process to maintaining women's position or to promoting gender equity?

My goal in this article is twofold: first, to discuss these questions in the context of recent research; and second, to present a comparative case study of two rapidly modernizing, neighboring Tahitian islands[1] that sheds light on these issues.

Original material prepared for this text.

VARIABILITY IN DEVELOPMENT'S IMPACT ON WOMEN

Most scholars agree that it is difficult to generalize about the impact of development on non-western women. As Moore (1988: 74) notes, "Women are not a homogeneous category, and the circumstances and conditions of their lives in the varying regions of the world are very different." Nevertheless, it is possible to identify the factors that play a major role in shaping how women in any particular society are affected by integration into capitalist markets and production systems. These factors interact in highly complex ways to shape the choices and options—the "opportunity structures"—open to women.

But first, in order to understand how men and women—even husbands and wives in the same family—can differentially experience development, it is important to remember that families are internally stratified units and that family members do not necessarily share the same priorities or goals (see Wilk 1989). Gender and age differences structure patterns of unequal access to authority, decision-making prerogatives, and control over family activities and resources. Those that do have access—most often senior males or male heads of households—may be in a favored position to participate in new and prestigious economic activities (e.g., commercial agriculture). In contrast, other family members, such as wives, may find that "modernization" simply means working longer hours at devalued household tasks that bring in little or no money, and having less say over the affairs of their families.

Forms of Capitalist Integration

One of the key factors affecting women's position is the *manner* in which different communities participate in capitalist markets and are integrated into global capitalism (see Mukhopadhyay and Higgins 1988). In rural areas, previously subsistence-based families may begin producing cash crops for local or export markets, become involved in other kinds of commodity production (i.e., crafts), or seek jobs in nearby towns. If jobs are available, families may abandon agriculture wholly or in part. As they become more dependent on money and imported foods and the cost of living increases, some rural villagers leave the countryside, migrating to nearby cities in search of wage work. Sometimes the search for work ultimately takes rural migrants to foreign industrialized nations where they are absorbed into the low-skilled, lowly-paid urban work force.

Each of these forms of capitalist integration has different implications for men and women depending on how the sexual division of labor is renegotiated to reflect new economic conditions; that renegotiation will be shaped by ideological notions of the types of work "appropriate" for men and women. Cash-crop agriculture may be defined as the domain of men, while women continue to produce food crops. Women may specialize in the production and sale of crafts if craft production was a female activity before market integration. If men migrate to find wage jobs, women may be left at home to feed and support families. If families migrate, men may find work in the city, but women who cannot find jobs may resort to street peddling or other marginal activities in the urban informal sector.

Degree of Structural Transformation

The *degree* to which a particular society has been incorporated into capitalist relations of production also plays a role in shaping how women are affected by development. Some communities have resisted or avoided full incorporation and maintained pre-capitalist institutions and values (see, for example, Rodman 1993; Petersen 1993); this is true in many rural "peasant" communities in the Third World where families produce for markets or hold wage jobs, yet simultaneously maintain kin-based relations of production and property ownership. In other communities, pre-capitalist institutions have largely been replaced by capitalist relations of production; this is true in areas of the most extensive commercial and missionary intervention.

These structural changes include shifts from kin- or family-based systems of property ownership to individual ownership. Land and labor become commodified and production becomes oriented to market sales and making money; wealth accumulation becomes a major goal. Those who are able to accumulate capital become an elite who are in a position to concentrate control over land and the other means of production. These processes result in the formation of class structures and the promotion of individualistic, competitive, and profit-oriented value systems characteristic of capitalist societies.

The impact of development on women will, in part, be shaped by how far this structural transformation has advanced. If, for example, increasing pressure on land has caused a system of land tenure to shift from matriclan ownership to individual ownership, women may find that they have lost control over land while men who participate in cash-cropping or other market-oriented activities are increasingly gaining individual control. On the other hand, where communities have resisted this shift to individual ownership, women may find that their property rights have not diminished.

Existing Systems of Gender, Family, and Social Relations

Another critical factor shaping the impact of development on women is the local system of gender and family relations, including patterns of gender stratification and ideology. There is great diversity in these systems around the world ranging from the relatively egalitarian, horticultural societies of island New Guinea (Lepowsky 1993), to the highly gender stratified and segregated Islamic societies of the Middle East (see Abu-Lughod 1986). Variability in gender structures is accompanied by fundamental differences in how different societies conceive of femaleness and maleness, and in what they perceive to be the basic mental and physical capabilities of men and women. Gender ideology, as well as family and kinship structures, will play a major role in determining the kinds of behaviors and socioeconomic roles that are considered appropriate (and consistent with family responsibilities) for women.

THE WESTERN GENDER BIAS IN DEVELOPMENT

Appreciating the complexity of forces that shape the options open to men and women as their communities develop explains little, however, about the frequently negative impact of development on women. If development were in fact a gender-neutral phenomenon, one would expect that the *relative* social, economic, and political position of men and women would remain the same—both men's and women's situations would either improve or deteriorate in more or less the same ways. But this rarely happens. Numerous studies now point to several important processes of gender discrimination embedded in western-style, capitalist development, processes that have contributed to women's deteriorating position in many developing regions. In some cases, development has introduced forms of gender bias that did not previously exist in non-western communities; in others, introduced gender biases have intensified existing gender asymmetries.

Women and "Modernization"

Prior to the 1970s and the surge of scholarly interest in women's issues, it was widely (and ethnocentrically) assumed that modernization ("westernization") promoted more egalitarian gender relations, and greater rights and freedoms for women. In an influential article, Laurel Bossen (1975) noted, "The Western industrialized nations [were] thought to be closest to an ideal of modern egalitarian treatment for women . . . Hence modern changes that [brought] societies closer to the Western pattern and standard [were] presented as advantageous to women" (1975: 587). Evidence of women's increasing equality included legal freedoms; the right to vote, run for office, and own property; as well as greater participation in the wage labor force. The latter was thought to promote female economic independence from "traditional family structures." In contrast, women in rural developing areas were thought to be "servile, dependent, and decidedly inferior to . . . men" (1975: 587).

Bossen effectively argues that neither the egalitarian view of western gender relations nor the servile, inferior view of Third World women reflects reality. While western women may possess certain legal rights, they do not enjoy full equality with men, nor are they as socially valued or esteemed as men. At the same time, research in less technologically sophisticated, non-western cultures has shown that, in some cases, women may be highly valued and possess many of the same socioeconomic and political prerogatives as men (see Lepowsky 1993 on the Vanatinai of New Guinea; Geertz 1961 on the Javanese; Kluckhohn and Leighton 1946 on the Navajo; and Etienne and Leacock 1980). Thus, as Bossen (1975: 589) notes "... it does not follow that the greater wealth and superior technology controlled by modern societies corresponds to greater equality among its members, female or otherwise."

"Modernized Patriarchy"

The gender biases that characterize western capitalist societies—and which were more severe in the Victorian era—were first introduced in many non-western regions during the colonial era. They have continued to reappear, however, as one "subtext" of many western-designed or oriented development programs.

One of these gender biases is a structural feature of western, capitalist relations of production in which the formal economic ("productive") and domestic/reproductive spheres are artificially distinguished, and the latter is devalued. In capitalist societies, "The concept of labor [is] reserved for activity that produces surplus value" (i.e., cash-earning activities) (Mies 1982a: 2; see also Sacks 1974). Thus, "work" becomes commodity or cash-crop production, or wage employment, activities that were typically dominated by men after their introduction; men, then, become associated with a formal, "productive" sphere that is often physically (spatially) separated from the activities of the household/domestic sphere.

Many of the typical activities of women—giving birth to and caring for children, maintaining the household and its affairs, production for family use/consumption—are not defined as "productive" in capitalist systems because they generate nothing of monetary value, and thus women do not "work." Thus much of the work that women do perform in the domestic domain becomes "invisible." An important example of this is that agricultural development efforts in Africa and elsewhere have frequently focused on men, even though "invisible" women farmers actually produce 50 percent of the world's food for direct consumption (Escobar 1995: 172–173).

Capitalist enterprises benefit from the structural separation of the productive and domestic domains because, since women do no work, they do not have to be compensated for their labor; they also benefit in that women (and sometimes children) serve as a relatively inexpensive, available, and easily dismissed pool of labor. If the demand for labor increases in the capitalist system or families cannot support themselves on one income, women may move into wage labor, but they are typically paid less than men. The rationale of capitalist employers is that women are "temporary" (and less skilled) workers who really belong at home with the children.

This capitalist economic rationale for the devaluation and domestication of women was reinforced during the colonial era (and since) by patriarchal, Victorian-era notions of appropriate male/female activities and relations, and by notions of female inferiority (physically and intellectually). In the Society Islands, for example, English missionaries believed that cultivation (previously practiced by both Tahitian men and women) was "unsuitable to [the female] sex" and that pre-contact women's other economic activities were "derogatory to the female and inimical to an improvement in morals"; they decided that "men should dig, plant, and prepare the food, and the women make cloth, bonnets, and attend to the householdwork" (Ellis 1981, III: 392–393, cited in Thomas 1987). Being relegated to making bonnets at home was quite a step down, particularly for high-ranking Tahitian women, who had figured prominently in the affairs and sociopolitical machinations of their chiefdoms—and sometimes even led warriors into battle—before the arrival of the Europeans (Oliver 1974; Lockwood 1988).

The model of Christian family life advanced by missionaries and colonial officials provided a supporting ideological framework for the structural separation of the male-dominated productive domain and the devalued, female domestic domain. The Bible describes the moral and correct family as consisting of a male head of family who is father and provider, and a female wife and mother who is his helpmate and subordinate. Women's financial dependence on the male "breadwinner" is a cornerstone of their secondary status.

Western gender biases not only domesticated non-western women, they frequently also introduced a "value structure that defines women's primary task in society as biological and social reproduction"; when this occurs in conjunction with a system—capitalism—that "allocates higher rewards to production roles in the public domain . . . men [achieve] an edge over women" (Afonja 1986: 134). That edge frequently supported patriarchal gender and family systems.

Relegation to a devalued, "nonproductive" domestic sphere was frequently accompanied in many cases by women's loss of control over productive resources and property; these were vested in the male "breadwinner" and head of the family. And that loss of control had a critical, negative impact on women's social position, authority, and status. In capitalist systems, control over the means of production (resources, capital, technology) is the material basis of differential authority and power; this is true not only in the community at large, but also in the internally stratified family. Following Schlegel (1977), "power" can be defined as the ability to control one's own and others' persons and activities, as well as the ability to make the decisions and shape the affairs/policies of the family or social group. Where women do not participate in productive activities or control resources or income, they are not only financially dependent on men, they are also relatively powerless and politically subordinate to men (see Freidl 1975, 1991).

By introducing structures and ideologies that privilege men and "domesticate" women, western-style development has frequently limited the options available to women and contributed to a decline in their status in the family and community.[2] In these cases, development becomes more than simply a means for promoting market integration or raising the standard of living, it becomes a vehicle for institutionalizing "modernized" patriarchy (Escobar 1995: 177).

Contemporary Negative Trends for Women

Several of the major trends in Third World development today reflect these gender biases. In rural areas, the devaluation and domestication of women has contributed to the *feminization of subsistence agriculture.* When new cash crops and technologies were introduced (during the colonial era and more recently), it was typically assumed that men were the farmers, and new opportunities, credits, and modern technology were made available to them. In many areas of Africa and Latin America where women had in fact been the major farmers, women were pushed into subsistence cultivation for family consumption. Defined as part of the "domestic" domain, subsistence production became both devalued and "invisible." As women assumed "the burden for providing for 'family' consumption" . . . they were "often prevented from engaging in cash-crop production themselves, and the frequent bias of government schemes and incentives in favour of male farmers (and the cash crops they produce) lead to further discrimination and disadvantage for women" (Moore 1988: 75). The cost to women of the feminization of subsistence agriculture was often exacerbated by changes in land tenure and other systems of property rights that effectively negated women's rights and institutionalized systems of individual (often male) ownership and inheritance.

Women are frequently pushed into subsistence production not only by male domination of cash-crop production (and of resources and technology), but also by male domination of most wage jobs and by male out-migration. In rural areas, where jobs are available on plantations or on commercial farms, women are typically hired as lowly-paid domestics, while men have access to the higher-paying and more prestigious jobs. When men migrate from rural areas to towns in search of wage work, rural women are frequently left at home with the double burden of caring for the house and children, and fulfilling familial subsistence needs.

Not only does subsistence production become devalued and invisible in the domestic domain, but women's other productive—and even cash-earning—activities frequently do as well. In many developing regions, women have found ways to earn small amounts of cash income by producing marketable crafts or other commodities (i.e., prepared foods) in their homes ("cottage industries").

In the Yucatan, for example, Mayan women weave hammocks (Littlefield 1978), and in India women make lace (Mies 1982b). But these women's situation is much like that of other poor, female commodity producers who work out of their homes. They are dependent on outside suppliers who bring them the raw materials for their craft, and they are exploited by commercial middlemen and exporters who pay them little yet reap large profits for themselves. Because women have few income-earning options outside the domestic domain and are largely bound to this domain by gender and family structures, they are unable to alter the conditions of that exploitation. Because this work is frequently defined as "domestic activity women do in their spare time," instead of as productive labor (Moore 1988: 84 citing Mies 1982b), these contributions to family livelihood are devalued and become invisible.

It is important to note that in both the cases where rural women seek wage jobs or produce commodities at home, the prevailing perception that women are domestics who make no productive contributions to the family has little to do with reality. Indeed, the entire artificial conceptualization of a female "domestic" domain in opposition to a formal, male "productive" domain is largely a myth in most developing regions (see Lamphere in this volume). Nevertheless, the "myth" remains strong and western gender ideology supports it. The dual beneficiaries are men, whose dominant position as "provider" and head of the family remains intact and unthreatened, and capitalist enterprises, which hire female "domestics" cheaply.

Another major trend in Third World development has been the *feminization of the industrial labor force* (see Fernandez-Kelly in this volume). It has been estimated that 80 percent of the workers in world market factories (typically owned by western multinational corporations) are young women (13–25 years old) (Moore 1988: 100; see also Nash and Fernandez-Kelly 1983). Young women are hired because of their ". . . apparently innate capacities for the work—'nimble fingers'—their docility, their disinclination to unionize, and the fact that women are cheap because, while men need an income to support a family, women do not" (Moore 1988: 101). Women are also paid less (as noted above), and hired at the lowest levels (skilled and management positions go to men), because they are seen as temporary workers. It appears that wage earning and financial contributions to families frequently do enhance young women's personal autonomy (see Ong 1987; Kung 1994). But often there are also significant social costs, and rarely does women's position improve in the male-dominated family.

These cases suggest that even though women's income earning is a *potential* material foundation for enhanced authority and status in the household, that potential may not be realized. Young female Taiwanese factory workers, for example, turn over their wages to their fathers, the heads of patriarchal Chinese families (Kung 1994). And in other cases, women's income may be so meager (due to low wages) or devalued that it is seen only as a "domestic supplement." Thus gender ideologies and family structures may redefine or "mystify" women's actual productive and income contributions—effecitvely negating them.

MAINTAINING WOMEN'S POSITION: THE INTERPLAY OF MATERIAL CONDITIONS AND GENDER IDEOLOGY

The relatively smaller number of cases in which women's position has not deteriorated illustrates how key material factors, supported by prevailing gender ideology and family systems, have worked to enhance women's autonomy, authority, and power in the family and community. In rural Java, for example, shifts to an export agricultural economy during the Dutch colonial period (and since) were not associated with major changes in the sexual division of labor, or in women's relatively high status and economic independence (Stoler 1977). Both men and women played important roles in labor-intensive, wet rice cultivation, and women were also significantly involved in trading activities. Through agricultural wage labor and trading, women became significant income earners in the household: "... women clearly control family finances and dominate the decision-making process" in the domestic domain, but Stoler notes that the domestic and public domains actually merge and overlap (1977: 85). In poorer households, women's income gives them both independence and authority in the family; in wealthier households, women's earnings could become the "material basis for social power" (84); where they are able to buy land or expand lucrative trading operations, women achieved both economic and political power.

Similarly, women in male-dominated Yoruba society (Nigeria) have achieved economic independence by participating in commercial enterprises and trade, and by owning houses (Barnes 1990). In this society where marriages are brittle and women do not inherit property from husbands, owning a house is an important form of social security for women. Income from commercial enterprises is used to purchase a house; the house then generates capital from rents. By owning the house, Yoruba women achieve the status of senior authority figure in the household. This is possible because even though Yoruba gender and family structures strongly favor men, women and men "are [seen as] equally capable of performing society's valued and essential tasks" (Barnes 1990: 255). Thus, when a woman owns a house, she is able to undermine the conditions that promote her structural subordination and achieve some social power. Female "home owners" also achieve political clout in their urban neighborhoods and sometimes become community leaders.

All the cases that have been cited in which development-related socioeconomic change did not promote women's increasing subordination have two significant characteristics in common. First, women were able to exert control over strategic productive resources (usually through ownership), and/or they were able to earn *and* control cash income (capital). And second, prevailing gender ideologies *supported* (did not redefine or negate) female participation in production and income earning, as well as female control over the products of their labor, including income. Whether women's productive efforts take place in the "formal" public domain or in the domestic domain (or in that large amorphous area where the two domains are actually one in many cases), they are socially defined as "producers," and they *control* key resources and income.

The cases of rural Tahitian women on the islands of Tubuai and Rurutu (Austral Islands, French Polynesia) show how different forms of market integration may have strikingly different consequences for women (even in the same society). They also show how women's control of resources and income plays a critical role in shaping their differential authority, decision making, and "power" in the household and community.

DIFFERENT OUTCOMES FOR WOMEN ON NEIGHBORING TAHITIAN ISLANDS

Rurutu and Tubuai are neighboring islands in rural French Polynesia. They are culturally similar, sharing the relatively homogeneous, Neo-Tahitian sociocultural patterns that coalesced in the region following centuries of French colonial and Christian missionary intervention. They have also both experienced the intense French government efforts to "modernize" and develop its overseas Pacific territory over the last three decades. In addition, the islands are similar in their geographic and population sizes (about 2,000 people; 300 households).

The push for regional development began in the early 1960s. In the rural outer islands, development programs were aimed at modernizing agriculture by transforming Tahitian taro farmers and fishermen into export producers for the rapidly growing Papeete market. Various heavily subsidized projects were implemented on different islands; they included copra and coffee production, European vegetable cultivation, and other kinds of commodity production (e.g., crafts).

Rural modernization also included the building of schools and clinics, rural electrification and telephone services (late 1980s), and integration of rural populations into the French family welfare and legal systems. Each rural island was designated a "municipality" and provided with a budget to employ a significant number of islanders on the government payroll (as road or maintenance workers, clerks, teachers, or secretaries). In the absence of commercial and tourist development on these remote islands, there are few other kinds of jobs. Today, about 45 percent of all families on Rurutu and Tubuai include an employed member, usually the male household head; about 25 percent of all jobs are held by women. Despite income earning from jobs or commodity production, most families continue to rely on agriculture/fishing to fulfill their subsistence needs.

Through their various cash-earning activities, as well as government social programs, many rural Tahitian families have achieved relatively high incomes and a level of material affluence unknown in many parts of the "developing" world (see below). At the same time, however, the cost of living in this import-dependent society is extremely high, and consumption standards are constantly rising. Consequently, and despite their high incomes, cash is ever-scarce and highly coveted. Most families today pursue any and all economic activities possible to generate cash income.

Pre-Modernization Gender Relations and Stratification

Before the introduction of development programs in the 1960s, rural families on both Tubuai and Rurutu mainly cultivated gardens (taro and other root crops, coconuts, bananas) and fished to fulfill subsistence needs. Small amounts of cash were earned through copra production or vanilla cultivation, or from sporadic sales of manioc starch, fresh foods, or pandanus craft items to passing schooners. Land was owned jointly by cognatic groups of kin; both men and women inherited rights in the land owned by their parents and grandparents.

Patterns of Tahitian domestic organization and gender relations reflected French colonial and Christian missionary efforts to transform Tahitians in their own images. As noted earlier, missionaries specifically sought to bring Tahitian society more into line with Victorian-era mores and practices (Thomas 1987). In accord with those patterns, as well as with Christian precepts, men were defined as the "breadwinners," "providers," and heads of their families. Men performed most agricultural labor and fished. Women's appropriate (and moral) domain was the household, where they spent their time caring for children, doing the housework, and weaving pandanus mats (and making bonnets) (Ellis 1831, III: 392–393, cited in Thomas 1987). Islanders today sometimes describe women's domain as "interior" (household) and men's domain as "exterior," the fields and ocean.

Men dominated cash-earning opportunities where they were available. Men processed copra and planted vanilla gardens, and controlled the cash earnings (see Lockwood 1988; Oliver 1981). Although women's efforts were concentrated in the household itself, they also worked in their husbands' gardens, fished from the reef, and performed many other kinds of "productive" labor. Nevertheless, a general pattern of male authority and preeminence (and female subordination) in the household was promoted by Christian teachings and the Bible, and by male control of increasingly coveted cash income. Although wives were usually in charge of daily expenditures for food and other necessities, husbands dispersed these monies to their wives as they saw fit.

Despite these structural changes, Tahitians somehow failed to become indoctrinated in Victorian-era attitudes about women's relative inferiority. Although Tahitians were (and are) devout believers in the familial/domestic prescriptions of the Bible, their own understandings of the nature of men and women differed substantially from those of the French and the missionaries. Most importantly, they did not have a belief in individuals' superiority or inferiority based on gender criteria.[3] This was reflected in a psychological study of Tahitian men and women conducted in the early 1960s (Levy 1973). Levy (1973: 236) concluded that in Tahitian worldview, women and men are seen to be much alike in their capabilities and talents, and to have no major personality, behavioral, or intellectual differences. He note that Tahitians acknowledged that men's and women's *lives* were different—because of women's role in reproduction and because they perform different tasks—but that's all.

Indeed, one of the major themes of Tahitian gender ideology is male/female interdependence, and not hierarchy (superiority/inferiority) as in many western societies. Thus, although Tahitian women were economically and politically subordinate in the post-contact, male-dominated household, they were not (and are not today), treated as inferiors. In contemporary communities, women receive a great deal of respect and admiration from both men and other women for their roles as managers of the family and domestic domain, and for their devoted care of their children (see Langevin 1990). Despite their "domesticity," they are out-spoken at community meetings and exhibit little deference to men.

Rural Development: Differing Paths for Tubuai and Rurutu

The economic profiles of Tubuai and Rurutu began to diverge in the early 1960s when government development planners charted different courses for each island. Tubuai was chosen as a major target for agricultural development, specifically European green vegetable and potato cultivation. It also became the administrative center for the five Austral Islands, and the site for the one high school in the group. A small airstrip was built to facilitate transport and contact with Tahiti.

Today, Tubuai Islanders are heavily involved in commercial agriculture, as well as other kinds of commodity production and export; these activities are largely the domain of men, although women are needed to perform substantial amounts of secondary labor in agricultural fields. Tubuai is today the regional potato producer, exporting over 1,200 tons (metric) to Papeete each year; it also exports about 550 tons of vegetables annually. The commodification of land and labor, shifts to individual land ownership (from the previous kin-based system), and the spread of new ethics of wealth accumulation and consumerism are increasingly observable. Of all of the Austral Islands, Tubuai is the most developed and affluent; in 1994, average familial income was about $2,000/month (Lockwood 1993). It is also the most westernized as measured in the number of islanders who have attended the French-staffed high school and who aspire to a western material lifestyle.

In the mid-1980s and despite the fact that they were not "farmers," Tubuai women began to sign up with the Agricultural Service in large numbers to plant potatoes. Women's access to land was assured by their own familial lands, and they also had access to the same financial subsidies and credits as male farmers. By the early 1990s, 43 percent of all potato farmers were women (Lockwood 1993).

Tubuai women had always earned small amounts of money from selling crafts or a few vegetables to other families, and a few held jobs as teachers, secretaries, or maintenance workers. But, for most women, potato cultivation was the first opportunity to earn significant amounts of income of their own; most women—who typically cultivate on a smaller scale than men—earn between $1,000 and $1,500 during the three-month potato season. Because Tahitians believe that income earned by an individual belongs to that individual, wives are able to make their own independent decisions about how their money will be expended. Indeed, many female potato farmers explain that they decided to plant potatoes to have their own money to do as they like; women's money is, however, almost always used to buy food, clothes, and other items for their families.

Thus by the early 1990s, Tubuai women were adopting new "modern" socioeconomic roles and breaking down barriers in the traditional sexual division of labor that defined women as "domestics." They had also achieved a level of financial autonomy.

The Island of Rurutu

The island of Rurutu's development trajectory has been significantly different. Because of its rugged interior terrain, agricultural development projects were not promoted, although in recent years limited efforts have been made to expand the potato project and green vegetable cultivation there. (In 1990, islanders exported about 35 tons of onions and 60 tons of taro, tarua, and bananas.) A small airstrip was built on the island, and government services and jobs were created much as on Tubuai.

Most families on Rurutu earn money from the craft production of their female members and craft items are Rurutu's major export. Crafts include pandanus mats, satchels, and hats, Tahitian quilts (*tifaifai*), and shell and flower necklaces—items once made exclusively for household use. Rurutu women produce crafts as part of their domestic work in their own households, or while participating in a *pupu*, a cooperative work group of 10–20 women who usually belong to the same church. Their reputation for fine craft production extends throughout the territory.

Rurutu women have organized cooperatives to help sell their crafts, and these are supported and subsidized by various government programs. (Craft cooperatives are present on most outer islands, but they are most highly developed on Rurutu.) Women are active agents in making arrangements to sell their items in Papeete though relatives, or if necessary, through a retailer at the central urban market. The minimal use of non-kin middlemen means that female producers retain almost all of the market price of their products. In the early 1990s, Rurutu's annual craft exports were valued at about $400,000 (one-third the value of Tubuai's potato crop).

How Rurutu women came to specialize in craft production to an extent that far exceeds that of other rural islands, however, is not clear (and informants could not explain it). As noted earlier, most rural Tahitian women weave mats and make quilts for household use. This specialization probably began to emerge in the pre-development decades; at that time, the populations of neighboring islands earned small amounts of cash selling copra, coffee, or manioc starch. Rurutu families had little of these items to sell; they could, however, sell mats and hats to the local Chinese family-owned general stores for export to Papeete. Thus, in the absence of other significant options, it is likely that women launched themselves into commercial craft production and in so doing, they became central agents in the generation of their families' incomes.

Although Rurutu is integrated into regional markets through craft and other kinds of small-scale production, it is today less "westernized" than Tubuai. As commercial agriculture is little developed, the traditional, family-based system of land ownership is not threatened by the kinds of changes taking place on Tubuai. Ethics of familial sharing and participation in cooperative work groups (*pupus*) are widespread on Rurutu, but have generally disappeared on Tubuai. Because families do not participate in potentially lucrative vegetable exports, most make significantly less money than Tubuai families (the average monthly income is $1,500). Consequently, there is less western-style consumerism. And because until recently, Rurutu children were required to board at the Tubuai high school in order to attend it, fewer Rurutu Islanders have received as many years of formal French education as Tubuai Islanders.

And clearly, on Rurutu, there has been little change in the traditional division of labor. The division between the female's "interior" world and the male's "exterior" world is strictly maintained. Interestingly, it is women who chastise other women who violate these "proper" roles by "doing men's work" in the gardens; women are highly protective of their domain. Compare to more "modern" Tubuai women, then, Rurutu women appear to be both "traditional" and domestic.

THE GENDER CONSEQUENCES OF DIFFERENT DEVELOPMENT PATHS[4]

Although Rurutu women may not be doing anything "new," they have achieved an important role in income generation (and control) that is unparalleled on the more modernized Tubuai. Careful examination of household budgets and income on both islands revealed that women on Rurutu are indeed significant "providers." On Rurutu, women bring in more than 50 percent of all income in almost half of all families (45.5 percent). In other words, it is almost equally likely in Rurutu families that the wife/mother is the breadwinner as it is that the husband/father is the breadwinner. On Tubuai, women are the breadwinners in only 26 percent of all families.[5]

And in this society where women *retain control* of the income they generate, Rurutu women are given credit for their productivity. This was summed up by one Rurutu man who said that women today differed from those of his grandmother's generation because they helped to "provide" for the family (the male role). I had not heard Tubuai women described this way, although they are certainly involved in many productive activities. It became clear that a general ethic of women as "providers" existed on Rurutu that was not articulated on Tubuai.

Rurutu women's status as "providers" was reflected in a subtle shift away from the typical pattern of husbands as heads of families to "joint husband/wife" family heads. In 49 percent of all Rurutu families the husband was declared head of the family, while in 41 percent, husbands and wives were joint household heads. In comparison, Tubuai had a much higher proportion of male household heads (68 percent) and husbands and wives were "joint" heads in only 25 percent of all families.[6] Rurutu women also played a greater role than Tubuai women in decision making about household budgets and expenditures.[7]

There were also significant differences between the two islands in how women and men were perceived and valued. Informants were asked to compare men and women in terms of various characteristics including intelligence, who worked harder, and several other personality traits. They were also asked who was "superior": men, women, or both (equal). Tubuai and Rurutu islanders generally agreed on most of the characteristics of men and women, with the exception of intelligence and superiority. On Rurutu, the majority of informants (58 percent) thought that women were more intelligent, while on Tubuai, the majority (64 percent) thought that men and women were equally intelligent.[8] (Only 29 percent of Tubuai Islanders thought that women were more intelligent.) And, on both Rurutu and Tubuai, the majority thought that men and women were "equal" (56 percent and 82 percent respectively); but on Rurutu, 23 percent of all informants thought that women were superior, whereas this was true of only 2 percent of all Tubuai informants. (It is also interesting to note that no one thought men worked hardest; both sets of islanders thought either women worked hardest, or that men and women worked equally hard.)

The higher valuation of Rurutu women can also be seen in women's greater political participation on the island. In 1994, three women served on the 16-member, island municipal council; one woman had been elected as a district mayor (the island has three districts). On Tubuai, islanders could remember no woman ever serving on the municipal council, and no woman has ever been elected mayor or district mayor.

There was also a tendency for both male and female Rurutu Islanders to extoll the virtues of women to a greater extent than on Tubuai, although women were clearly held in high regard on both islands. When asked to compare the thoughts and mentality of men and women, Rurutu informants (male and female) described women as more expressive and outgoing (men were reserved), as better organizers, and generally as "seeing farther" than men. Women were described as more active in church and community groups than men, and they tended to take on the organizational roles in those activities. Both men and women described men's thoughts as centered on their taro gardens and fishing; once these tasks were successfully accomplished, men relaxed or got together with other men to drink; they were described as having "few concerns" other than farming and fishing. Women, however, were described as constantly thinking about how to make ends meet, how to generate the money that was needed for a household purchase, or how to organize the next church event. They "saw further" in that they were constantly contemplating the future needs of their families.

It should be noted that although Rurutu women's economic roles and income generation have promoted greater gender equity in familial authority and decision making and in community leadership than on Tubuai, they are not associated with other differences in family organization, fertility, or gender-based land-use patterns. On both islands, most families are nuclear in structure (about two-thirds of all families), have an average household size of five to six people, and produce approximately five children. Between 20 and 30 percent of all families reside on and cultivate the wife's land (most familial); the rest utilize the husband's land.

CONCLUSION

As the discussion has shown, many of the western gender biases described above were introduced into Tahitian society, promoting the structural domestication of women, including their economic dependence on male "providers" and heads of families. But at the ideological level, Tahitians never accepted notions of male superiority and female inferiority, continuing to see men and women in a largely egalitarian, interdependent way that afforded mutual respect for both. Consequently, and despite other kinds of changes in their society, women never lost their rights to own and control land and other resources, they were never divested of the right to control the income they earned, and they were given credit for the productive contributions they made regardless of their "domesticity."

On Rurutu, development introduced conditions under which women would oftentimes become the breadwinners in their families. That critical role has been translated into enhanced authority and decision-making prerogatives for women, and a higher social valuation. In contrast, although Tubuai women are economically active and "development-oriented," their financial contributions to the household remain minimal compared to those of men (in most cases). Thus, in the "quest for money," Tubuai women are not seen as "provisioners"; they also remain financially dependent on husbands in the majority of cases. Consequently, men are still defined as the heads of households in most families. And although women's social esteem and status is generally high on Tubuai, it is not as high as on Rurutu.

The cases of Tubuai and Rurutu highlight the interplay of both material conditions and gender ideology in shaping how capitalist development affects women. They suggest that a gender ideology that "empowers" women (i.e., Tahitian women's generally high status) is *not* sufficient—in and of itself—to ensure that women will not be subordinate to, and dependent on, men in developing regions of the world. The Rurutu data reinforce the conclusion drawn from other cases where women's position has not deteriorated: Women's control of strategic material resources and capital—the material basis of "power" in all capitalist systems—is a *necessary* condition for achieving a position of relative authority and power in both the household and community. It is important to note, however, that the extent to which women are able to control resources and capital will in part be determined by prevailing gender ideologies and family structures. Thus one can conclude that where women in developing regions are able to produce a strong material base, and where gender ideology empowers them to control it for their own ends, they will be in a position to achieve greater gender equity with men.

NOTES

1. In 1994–1995, a comparative study of the differential impact of capitalist development on women was undertaken on the neighboring Tahitian islands of Tubuai, Rurutu, and Raivavae. Two other anthropologists, Jeanette Dickerson-Putman and Anna Laura Jones, contributed to the project. The study was funded by a gratefully acknowledged grant from the National Science Foundation (SBR-9311414).
2. Women's relative lack of opportunity compared to men can also be seen in their strikingly lower rates of literacy and educational attainment (particularly in Latin America, the Middle East, and Africa) (see Moore 1988), as well as in higher rates of female morbidity and mortality (Charleton 1984).
3. Pre-contact Tahitians (both male and female) were ranked relative to one another in terms of the amount of *mana*, or supernatural power, they possessed (see Oliver 1974). *Mana*, and thus social rank, was determined by birth and genealogical distance from high-ranking chiefs; males and females were ranked in this highly stratified society by these criteria and not by gender. High-ranking women clearly dominated lower-ranking men.
4. In this comparative study, 164 Tubuai households and 181 Rurutu households were included (approximately 55–60 percent of all island households). These households were chosen to be representative of the populations at large in terms of two criteria: 1) major household economic activity/socioeconomic status (income), and 2) stage in the developmental cycle of the family (young, middle, elderly families). Informants included male and female household heads, as well as couples.
5. Tubuai households (N = 139): In 103 (74 percent) women earn less than half of all income; in 36 (26 percent) women earn more than half of all income. Rurutu households (N = 134): In 73 (54.5 percent) women earn less than half of all income; in 61 (45.5 percent) women earn more than half of all income. This is a statistically significant difference: Chi-square = 11.47; $p < .00071$; df = 1. (Families of single male or female heads were not included.)
6. For Tubuai (N = 134 households), husbands were declared head of the family in 91 households (68 percent), husbands and wives were joint heads in 34 households (25 percent), and wives were declared the head in 9 households (7 percent). For Rurutu (134 households), husbands were declared head in 66 households (49 percent), husbands and wives were joint heads in 55 households (41 percent), and wives were declared the head in 13 households (10 percent). The difference between the two islands is statistically significant (Chi-square = 9.66; $p < .0079$; df = 2). (Households of single household heads were not included in the analysis.)
7. Although on both islands the predominant pattern is for either wives, or husbands and wives together, to oversee day-to-day household expenditures, this is more often true on Rurutu (82 percent of all families) than on Tubuai (74 percent). Similarly, wives contribute to decision-making about large consumer purchases in 87 percent of all Rurutu families, but in 75 percent of Tubuai families.
8. Tubuai informants (N = 58): Most intelligent—women (17 or 29 percent; men (4 or 2 percent), both (37 or 64 percent). Rurutu informants (N = 33): Most intelligent—women (19 or 58 percent), men (2 or 6 percent), both (12 or 36 percent). The difference between the two islands is statistically significant (Chi-square = 7.20, $p < .0272$; df = 2).

REFERENCES

Abu-Lughod, Lila. 1986. *Veiled Sentiments: Honor and Poetry in a Bedouin Society*. Berkeley: University of California Press.

Afonja, Simi. 1986. "Changing Modes of Production and the Sexual Division of Labor Among the Yoruba." In E. Leacock and H. Safa (eds). *Women's Work: Development and the Division of Labor by Gender*. S. Hadley: Bergin & Garvey.

Barnes, Sandra. 1990. "Women, Property and Power." In P. Sanday and R. Goodenough (eds.). *Beyond the Second Sex*, pp. 253–280. Philadelphia: University of Pennsylvania Press.

Boserup, Ester. 1970. *Women's Role in Economic Development.* London: George Allen and Unwin.

Bossen, Laurel. 1975. "Women in Modernizing Societies." *American Ethnologist* 2 (4): 587–601.

———. 1984. *The Redivision of Labor: Women and Economic Choice in Four Guatemalan Communities.* Albany: State University of New York Press.

Caulfield, Mina. 1981. "Equality, Sex, and the Mode of Production." In G. Berreman (ed.). *Social Inequality: Comparative and Developmental Approaches*, pp. 201–219. New York: Academic Press.

Charleton, Sue Ellen. 1984. *Women in Third World Development.* Boulder: Westview.

Deere, Carmen D. 1977. "Changing Social Relations of Production and Peruvian Peasant Women's Work." *Latin American Perspectives* 4 (1 & 2): 38–47.

Di Leonardo, Michaela, ed. 1991. *Gender at the Crossroads of Knowledge: Feminist Anthropology in the Postmodern Era.* Berkeley: University of California Press.

Escobar, Arturo. 1995. *Encountering Development: The Making and Unmaking of the Third World.* Princeton, NJ: Princeton University Press.

Etienne, M. and E. Leacock, eds. 1980. *Women and Colonization: Anthropological Perspectives.* Cambridge: J.F. Bergin.

Fernandez-Kelly, Maria P. 1981. "The Sexual Division of Labor, Development, and Women's Status." *Current Anthropology* 22 (4): 414–419.

Friedl, Ernestine. 1975. *Women and Men: An Anthropologist's View.* Prospect Heights, IL: Waveland Press.

———. 1991. "Society and Sex Roles." In E. Angeloni (ed.). *Annual Editions, Anthropology 91/92*, pp. 112–116. Guilford, CT: Dushkin Publishing.

Geertz, Hildred. 1961. *The Javanese Family.* New York: Free Press.

Kershaw, Greet. 1976. "The Changing Roles of Men and Women in the Kikuyu Family by Socioeconomic Strata." *Rural Africana* 29: 173–194.

Kluckhohn, C. and D. Leighton. 1946. *The Navaho.* Cambridge, MA: Harvard University Press.

Kung, Lydia. 1976. "Factory Work and Women in Taiwan: Changes in Self-Image and Status." *Signs* 2: 35–58.

———. 1994. *Factory Women in Taiwan.* New York: Columbia University Press.

Langevin, Christine. 1990. *Tahitiennes de la Tradition a l'Integration Culturelle.* Paris: Editions L'Harmattan.

Lepowsky, Maria. 1993. *Fruit of the Motherland: Gender in an Egalitarian Society.* New York: Columbia University Press.

Levy, Robert. 1973. *Tahitians: Mind and Experience in the Society Islands.* Chicago: University of Chicago Press.

Linnekin, Jocelyn. 1990. *Sacred Queens and Women of Consequence: Rank, Gender and Colonialism in the Hawaiian Islands.* Ann Arbor: University of Michigan Press.

Littlefield, Alice. 1978. "Exploitation and the Expansion of Capitalism: The Case of the Hammock Industry of Yucatan." *American Ethnologist* 5 (3): 495–508.

Lockwood, Victoria. 1988. "Capitalist Development and the Socioeconomic Position of Tahitian Peasant Women." *Journal of Anthropological Research* 44 (3): 263–285.

———. 1989. "Tubuai Women Potato Planters and the Political Economy of Intra-Household Gender Relations." In R. Wilk (ed.). *The Household Economy: Reconsidering the Domestic Mode of Production*, pp. 197–220. Boulder, CO: Westview.

———. 1993. *Tahitian Transformation: Gender and Capitalist Development in a Rural Society.* Boulder, CO: Lynne Rienner.

Mies, Maria. 1982a. "The Dynamics of the Sexual Division of Labor and the Integration of Rural Women into the World Market." In L. Beneria (ed.). *Women and Development: The Sexual Division of Labor in Rural Societies*, pp. 1–28. New York: Praeger.

———. 1982b. *The Lace Makers of Narsapur.* London: Zed Press.

Moore, Henrietta. 1988. *Feminism and Anthropology.* Minneapolis: University of Minneapolis Press.

Mukhopadhyay, C. and P. Higgins. 1988. "Anthropological Studies of Womens' Status Revisited: 1977–1987." *Annual Review of Anthropology* 17: 461–495.

Nash, June. 1977. "Women and Development: Dependency and Exploitation." *Development and Change* 8: 161–182.

Nash, June and Maria Fernandez-Kelly, eds. 1983. *Women and Men and the International Division of Labor.* Albany: State University of New York Press.

Oliver, Douglas. 1974. *Ancient Tahitian Society.* (3 vols.) Honolulu: University of Hawaii Press.

Oliver, Douglas. 1981. *Two Tahitian Villages: A Study in Comparison.* Honolulu: The Institute for Polynesian Studies.

Ong, Aihwa. 1987. *Spirits of Resistance and Capitalist*

Discipline: Factory Women in Malaysia. Albany: State University of New York Press.

Ong, Aihwa. 1988. "The Production of Possession: Spirits and the Multinational Corporation in Malaysia." *American Ethnologist* 15 (1): 28–42.

Petersen, Glenn. 1993. "Some Pohnpei Strategies for Economic Survival." In *Contemporary Pacific Societies: Studies in Development and Change,* V. Lockwood, et al., eds., pp. 185–196. Englewood Cliffs, N.J.: Prentice-Hall.

Rapp, Rayna. 1979. "Anthropology: Review Essay." *Signs* 4 (3): 497–513.

Rodman, Margaret. 1993. "Keeping Options Open: Copra and Fish in Rurual Vanuatu." In *Contemporary Pacific Societies: Studies in Development and Change,* V. Lockwood, et al., eds., pp. 171–184. Englewood Cliffs, N.J.: Prentice-Hall.

Sacks, Karen. 1974. "Engels Revisited: Women, the Organization of Production and Private Property." In *Woman, Culture and Society,* M. Rosaldo and L. Lamphere, eds., pp. 207–222. Stanford: Stanford University Press.

Sanday, Peggy. 1974. "Female Status in the Public Domain." In M. Rosaldo and L. Lamphere (eds.). *Woman, Culture and Society,* pp. 189–206. Stanford: Stanford University Press.

Schlegel, Alice. 1977. *Sexual Stratification: A Cross-Cultural View.* New York: Columbia University Press.

Stoler, Ann. 1977. "Class Structure and Female Autonomy in Rural Java." *Signs* 3: 74–89.

Strathern, Marilyn. 1984. "Domesticity and the Denigration of Women." In O'Brien, D. and S. Tiffany (eds.). *Rethinking Women's Roles: Perspectives from the Pacific.* Berkeley: University of California Press.

Thomas, Nicholas. 1987. "Complementarity and History: Misrecognizing Gender in the Pacific." *Ocenia* 57 (4): 261–270.

Wilk, Richard, ed. 1989. *The Household Economy: Reconsidering the Domestic Mode of Production.* Boulder: Westview Press.

Wolf, Eric. 1982. *Europe and the People Without History.* Berkeley: University of California Press.

DOING THEIR HOMEWORK: THE DILEMMA OF PLANNING WOMEN'S GARDEN PROGRAMS IN BANGLADESH

Margot Wilson-Moore

Recently a number of development agencies in Bangladesh (for example, CARE, CIDA, Helen Keller International, the Mennonite Central Committee, Save the Children, UNICEF, USAID) have planned and implemented independent projects or program components directed specifically toward homestead gardening as an alternative to field crop production. For the growing cadre of marginal and landless farmers with little or no cultivable land outside of the household, homestead gardening constitutes a subsistence strategy with considerable potential for improving family nutrition and cash generation.

Original material prepared for this text.

Traditionally a complement to field crop production, homestead gardens provide a much-needed supply of nutritious, interesting, and vitamin-rich foods for home consumption. Additionally, the sale of homestead garden produce makes substantial amounts of cash available for rural farm families. The discussion that follows considers homestead gardening within the broad context of international development in Bangladesh and more particularly in relation to the burgeoning literature on the role of women in development. This discussion focuses specifically on homestead gardening as a viable development strategy for rural women.

International development aid constitutes a major influence for change today. In

Bangladesh millions of foreign aid dollars comprise a large proportion of the national budget. Since 1974 to 1975, Bangladesh has received not less than $700 million from the United States each year in international aid, and these donations represent two to three and one-half times the total revenue budget generated in-country. However, the results in terms of quantifiable improvements are relatively few, and despite these substantial foreign aid contributions Bangladesh continues to demonstrate a negative balance of payments (greater than $5 million in 1984 to 1985) and a negative balance of trade ($135 million US in 1984 to 1985).

Environmental stress, population pressure, illiteracy, and historical explanations such as exploitation and isolation have been espoused as general causes for the persistent poverty in Bangladesh. Similarly, behavioral causes, such as a closely structured hierarchy and system of patronage, rugged individualism, and failure of Bangladeshis to "trust" one another and work cooperatively, have been offered as causes of the destitution and privation that characterize daily life in Bangladesh (Maloney 1986).

Whatever the causes, pervasive poverty and widespread destitution are commonplace, and in terms of standard "development" criteria, such as per capita income, literacy rate, mortality and fertility rates, economic diversification, and physical and social infrastructure, Bangladesh can only be termed a development failure. Historically, vast transfers of resources out of the area have significantly depleted the resource base while more recent problems of overpopulation, land fragmentation, and environmental disasters have drawn the attention of the international aid community.

Women's issues have received considerable attention from the international donor community in recent years, but to understand the "state of the art" of women and development research[1] in Bangladesh, it is necessary to trace its roots in broader issues of development theory and feminism. Early development theory tended to overlook the special needs of women, anticipating perhaps a "trickle-down" of benefits from men toward whom most programs are directed. Feminist critiques of development theory revolve primarily around this issue—the failure of development theory to address the problems of women directly. Women are either categorized with men or ignored altogether. Women are routinely subsumed within the rubric of more general development processes that are expected to address the issues of both men and women.

A variety of critiques of development theory exist (for an in-depth discussion see Jaquette 1982; Barnes-McConnell and Lodwick 1983; Wilson-Moore 1990), and the ongoing dialogue among these critiques has generated a vast and critical literature addressing the issue of women and development in the Third World. The feminist critique of development theory is firmly grounded in feminist thought, and the theoretical perspectives that have emerged in feminist development theory clearly reflect theoretical underpinnings in feminist theory. Feminist theoretical models predict relationships between various spheres of women's lives[2] and generate research questions and information useful, indeed imperative, for appropriate development planning for women.

Too often, however, women and development researchers fail to incorporate feminist theory into their research designs or neglect to articulate the underlying feminist assumptions that influence their work. Theorizing is, in large part, left to feminist academicians who usually rely on ethnographic (rather than development) literature for constructing and testing their models. As a result feminist theory, women, and development research have progressed, in recent years, along separate and divergent paths. Despite the actuating influence of feminist theory on women and development research and their common concerns with the situation of women, discourse between these two bodies of literature is remarkably scant.

Women and development research tends to be of a highly practical nature, concentrating on the immediate and pragmatic problems faced by women in developing nations. Resources and institutional support are then directed toward these identified needs. A women's component may be incorporated into existing development programs, or alternatively projects may be designed specifically and solely for women. Often, however, development programs do not meet the needs of the women for whom they are designed. Many focus on "individual solutions," such as education to improve women's opportunities for urban wage employment, increase their access to innovative technology, or improve their subsistence production skills. Too often the systemic constraints on Third World people in general and on women in particular, such as high rates of unemployment and lack of child-care facilities, are overlooked.

The role of women in socioeconomic development has been the subject of much interest in Bangladesh (cf. Hossain, Sharif, and Huq 1977; Islam 1986) and has focused the attention of the aid community on those development issues particular to women, especially those at the lowest economic levels who are often the poorest of the poor. Khan et al. (1981) have shown that in 1981 326 government and nongovernment programs for women were registered with the Ministry of Women's Affairs. The majority provide training in knitting, sewing, embroidery, handicrafts, and garment-making. Unfortunately, however, although directed toward poor and destitute women, the income-generating potential of these skills is minimal (Khan et al. 1981:24) and the emphasis on low payment and domestic-like work only serves to perpetuate women's subordinate status and economic circumstance.

In 1986 Schaffer found that the focus of more than 100 development projects directed specifically toward women had expanded to include self-help and income generation, family planning and health, education and literacy, agriculture development projects, rural employment and industry, and female leadership training. The majority of these projects focus on integrating women into existing programs, although a few "women only" projects exist. Most donor agencies philosophically support development activities for women (Schaffer 1986:4); however, a number of cultural attitudes toward women constrain them. The view of women's work as minimal and unimportant is compounded by the women's own perception of their work as noneconomic and therefore without value.

Beyond this, religious proscriptions that predicate family honor on women's virtue and legislate women's appropriate place as inside the household necessitate development on an outreach basis (providing inputs and training to women in their own homes), while effectively preventing agencies from recruiting female staff to provide that outreach service.

Initially, little specific information was available about women in Bangladesh, and the resulting imperative for more and better data regarding women's roles, statuses, and activities generated a predominantly descriptive focus in the early research. This is especially true in the rural areas where early village studies (cf. Raper 1970; Zaidi 1970) provided only brief references to women's activities. Other village studies followed (cf. Arens and Van Beurden 1980; BRAC 1983; Chowdhury 1978; Hartmann and Boyce 1983; Mukherjee 1971), but still little direct reference was made to women.

More recently a number of authors have commented on the "invisibility" of women's economic contribution in Bangladesh (cf. Chen 1986; Huq 1979; Islam 1986; Smock 1977; Wallace et al. 1987). Women's labor routinely includes postharvest processing of field crops, such as rice, jute, mustard seed, lentils and millet; care of animals; homestead gardening; and minor household maintenance, to name only a few. Because the labor of rural women takes place primarily inside the household, it often goes unnoticed. Nevertheless, their economic contribution is substantial (Chen 1986; Wallace et al. 1987). The importance of these kinds of studies is in shifting the focus away from the view of women as dependent and helpless. Instead, they are recognized as actors, engaged in economic pursuits in both rural and urban areas. As such they cease to be "welfare cases" and become instead an appropriate target for "mainstream" development processes.

In addition to their traditional domestic roles increasing numbers of women from landless and marginal families are being forced by economic circumstance to leave their homes to seek wage labor. At the same time technology, especially mechanized rice processing, is displacing rural women from their traditional roles in postharvest processing of field crops (Begum 1989). Cooperative programs are encouraging and supporting female entrepreneurs, but the success of these schemes often accrues from their constituting an extension of existing female roles that do not "encroach upon the traditional domain of men . . . [and are] not conceived as a threat to men's interests" (Begum 1989: 527).

Homestead gardening as a development strategy for women fits easily within these dictates because it neither encroaches on nor threatens men's traditional subsistence activities. Homestead gardening is an integral part of women's work in Bangladesh (cf. Chen 1983; Hannan 1986; Hassan 1978; Huq 1979; Hussain and Banu 1986; Scott and Carr 1985) and provides an opportunity for women to make sizable contributions to the rural farm family in terms of nutritious food for consumption as well as income generated from the sale of excess produce.

Homestead gardening is *not* the exclusive purview of women, although much of the research to date suggests that it is (Chen 1986; Huq 1979). This misconception is likely a result of research bias toward women. In Bangladesh women's issues have become a primary concern of development planners, and as a result women's roles are often considered without reference to other members of the community and to men in particular. The result is a misrepresentation of women as the principle, even exclusive, actors in certain sectors of the subsistence economy; in this case as the cultivators of homestead gardens. By contrast data from my own research (Wilson-Moore 1989, 1990) show that both men and women are involved in vegetable cultivation, although some clear differences exist between what men and women do in the garden.

Men and women grow different crop varieties at different times of the year—men in winter, women in summer. The fact that the crops grown by women tend to be more indigenous in nature and those cultivated by men more likely to be imported varieties may be an artifact of men's more active participation in the public sphere. Because men are active in the marketplace, they may simply be exposed to new varieties of vegetables most often and are therefore more predisposed to experimentation. In a similar vein it may be argued that women are in some sense a reservoir of traditional information and cultivation patterns, reflective of a time before imported varieties and development inputs were available.

A clear distinction also exists between male and female patterns of vegetable cultivation in which men's patterns are reminiscent of field crop production patterns characterized by monocropping and the rows and beds of European gardens. Women's gardens, by contrast, have a jumbled appearance and may represent the indigenous patterns commonly in practice prior to outside influence (for a discussion of cross-cultural gardening traditions see Brownrigg 1985).

Women's gardens are found inside or immediately adjacent to the household. Requirements for housing, cooking, stabling of animals, and postharvest processing and storage of field crops necessitate that individual plants or small clusters of plants be scattered throughout the homestead, dotted around the central courtyard and household structures. Small plots may be located around the periphery of larger homesteads, usually immediately outside of the circle of infacing buildings.

Gourds are encouraged to grow over trellises, along the walls, and across the roofs of buildings. Other climbing plants may be trained to grow up the trunks of nearby trees. Shade-loving plants are grown under the cover of fruit and fuelwood trees, and those more tolerant of direct sun are planted in the clear places.

Plant species are highly diverse. Because there are no beds or rows, tall and medium height trees, smaller bushy shrubs, upright plants, creepers, and root crops form the horizontal layers characteristic of this type of garden. Weeding is infrequent, and it is often difficult to differentiate the homestead garden from the surrounding undergrowth. In fact an untrained observer might not recognize this type of homestead garden at all.

Husbands often fail to recognize the gardening efforts of their wives, even when the proof was crawling across the roofs and walls of the homestead and into the cooking pot at meal times. That men fail to acknowledge women's productive labor in gardens may lie partially in more general societal attitudes toward women as producers (they are not seen as such) but also in the scattered appearance of their homestead gardens, which prevents their immediate recognition by uninterested, or uninitiated, observers, be they husband, anthropologist, or development worker.

Women cultivate vegetable varieties that spring up readily, can be produced from seed preserved from the previous year, and are well-adapted to the seasonal vagaries of the climate, flourishing inside and around the homestead with a minimum of care or input. Women often stagger the planting times so that everything does not mature at once. In fact related women in separate households may coordinate their planting times, as well as the varieties planted, to maximize their production through sharing.

Vegetable gardens cultivated by women tend to have a high diversity of plant species but a small number of plants of any particular type. Accordingly, the quantities are smaller yet more varied, and they are intended for family consumption. High diversity and low volume production is the predominant characteristic of women's gardening patterns in Bangladesh and throughout Asia, a strategy well-suited to fulfilling family consumption needs.

It is no coincidence that the vegetables grown most commonly in homestead gardens are the ones villagers prefer to eat. These vegetables can be eaten on a daily basis without becoming unappetizing. Alternatively the diversity of vegetables produced in the homestead garden also helps to offset the boredom of eating the same food every day. In fact villagers prefer to have a variety of foods, even if that means eating something that they dislike from time to time.

In this way the garden acts as a living larder, providing fresh produce on a daily basis. As individual plants become ripe the women harvest them and prepare them for consumption. If more vegetables become ripe than can be consumed within the household at one time, they may be given away, traded with neighbors, or sent to the market for sale.

Homestead gardening as a development strategy for women is predicated on a view of women's production as valuable and essential to the nutritional and economic welfare of the rural farm family. Furthermore, the minimal overlap between men's and women's gardening patterns ensures that as a development strategy homestead gardening also does not compete with men's traditional activities in field crop cultivation or vegetable production. Thus, homestead gardening conforms to two primary stipulations (Begum 1989; Schaffer 1986) for success and would seem an ideal development strategy for women.

Unfortunately, these stipulations do not necessarily guarantee a positive result, and outcomes of garden programming may prove surprising if the planners have not "done their homework" prior to implementation. In this regard Brownrigg has (1985) emphasized the necessity of in-depth locally based research and observes that when such research is omitted or conducted in a cursory manner programs often fail to meet the needs of the target population. Barnett (1953) has argued that acceptance of innovation is based on the ability of recipient populations to analyze new ideas and technologies and to identify some similarity with existing culture traits. Accordingly, the more identifiable an innovation is, the more easily it can be matched with a trait already existing in the cultural lexicon, and the more readily it will be adopted.

Social science, and anthropology in particular, has much to contribute. Participant observation is a field methodology well-suited to producing detailed information about existing indigenous practices; information often not available through any other means; and information appropriate, perhaps imperative, for planners who wish to build on and enhance those existing practices. By focusing on extant patterns planners can effectively determine which goals are attainable and which populations are most appropriately targeted.

In the context of Bangladesh, for example, homestead garden programs intended to improve family nutrition and increase consumption of vitamin-rich vegetables are most appropriately directed toward women because their production is intended, in the first instance, for home consumption. If, on the other hand, program goals include increasing family income through sale of garden produce, men may constitute a more appropriate target group because their vegetable production is traditionally intended for the market. Finally, a program goal of increased access to cash for women requires careful consideration because women's limited access to the market and ramifications of cash generation on family nutrition are two important, potentially negative, dimensions of income-generating schemes for women.

Women routinely remain secluded within the household in Bangladesh. As a result, marketing of women's garden produce constitutes something of a dilemma. Produce must be transported and sold by a male family member or neighbor. Women are able to retain control over the cash generated in this way by providing a shopping list (for household essentials such as oil or kerosene) when they turn over the produce for sale. Accordingly, the money is recycled back into the family budget on a daily basis and does not accumulate. It fails to be assigned a "value" by men or women and as a result goes unrecognized. That this particular economic contribution fails to affect women's status in any appreciable way has been discussed elsewhere (Wilson-Moore 1989).

Beyond the lack of recognition that greets women's economic enterprise in the garden, Boserup (1970) has shown that when women's economic activities become profitable (especially in terms of cash generation), men tend to take them over (see also Chaney and Schmink 1976). Male takeovers of the income-generating component of women's homestead gardening and the displacement of women from their traditional roles in vegetable production necessitates only a small shift in production activities. However, the ramifications in terms of family nutritional well-being may be far reaching. Rural farm families depend on women's homestead production for a ready supply of varied and vitamin-rich vegetable foods, a complement nutritionally and aesthetically to the masebhate (rice and fish) mainstays of the Bangladeshi diet.

Redirecting women's vegetable production toward the market would necessitate a change in production technique, disrupting the traditional patterns of women's homestead garden production and interfering with that ready supply of vegetable foods. The traditional pattern that produces small quantities of diverse vegetable foods intended for consumption within the homestead would have to be replaced by high-output, low-diversity cropping. Furthermore, there is little evidence to suggest that rural families would use the cash earned in this way to "buy back" or replace vegetable foods in the diet. Rather, high-status processed foods such as tea, white sugar, white flour, and bread are more apt to make an appearance when cash becomes available for their purchase.

Maintaining a balance between growing vegetable crops in large volume for sale and in sufficient variety for home consumption represents a problem in terms of the space and time constraints of homestead production. However, the existing, complementary yet rarely overlapping patterns of men's and women's traditional vegetable production seems well-suited to the respective cash generation and consumption needs of the family. Accordingly, planners concerned with pervasive poverty and widespread nutritional deficiency diseases in Bangladesh may wish to consider the benefits of developing each of these gardening strategies as they mutually, yet independently, support the rural farm family.

NOTES

1. Throughout this paper the terminology women and development has been used as a generic term for women's development in an effort to avoid more specific references such as women in development (WID) or development for women. These advocate, in the first case, the incorporation of a women's component into existing programs and, in the second, separate programming by women for women (see Jaquette 1982; Barnes-McConnell and Lockwick 1983; Wilson-Moore 1990 for a more comprehensive discussion of these terms).
2. For example, see Boserup (1970), Friedl (1975), and Sanday (1973, 1974) for models that predicate women's status on women's participation in the work force and their economic contribution to the family.

REFERENCES

Arens, Jenneke and Jos Van Beurden. 1980. *Jhagrapur: Poor Peasants and Women in a Village in Bangladesh.* Calcutta: Orient Longman.

Barnes-McConnell, Pat and Dora G. Lodwick. 1983. *Working with International Development Projects: A Guide for Women–in–Development.* East Lansing: Michigan State University, Office of Women in International Development.

Barnett, Homer. 1953. *Innovation: The Basis of Culture Change.* New York: McGraw-Hill.

Begum, Kohinoor. 1989. "Participation of Rural Women in Income-Earning Activities: A Case Study of a Bangladesh Village," *Women's Studies International Forum* 12(5):519–528.

Boserup, Ester. 1970. *Women's Role in Economic Development.* New York: St. Martin's Press.

BRAC (Bangladesh Rural Advancement Committee). 1983. *Who Gets What and Why: Resource Allocation in a Bangladesh Village.* Dhaka: BRAC Publication.

Brownrigg, Leslie. 1985. *Home Gardening in International Development: What the Literature Shows.* Washington, DC: League for International Food Education.

Chaney, Elsa and Marianne Schmink. 1976. "Women and Modernization: Access to Tools." In June Nash and Helen Safa (eds.). *Sex and Class in Latin America.* New York: Praeger.

Chen, Martha Alter. 1986. *A Quiet Revolution: Women in Transition in Rural Bangladesh.* Cambridge: Schenkman Publishing.

Chowdhury, Anwarullah. 1978. *A Bangladesh Village: A Study of Social Stratification.* Dhaka: Centre for Social Studies.

Friedl, Ernestine. 1975. *Women and Men: An Anthropologist's View.* New York: Holt, Rinehart and Winston.

Hannan, Ferdouse H. 1986. *Past, Present and Future Activities of Women's Desk.* Comilla: Bangladesh Academy for Rural Development.

Hartmann, Betsy and James K. Boyce. 1983. *A Quiet Violence: Views from a Bangladesh Village.* London: Oxford University Press.

Hassan, Nazmul. 1978. *Spare Time of Rural Women: A Case Study.* Dhaka: University of Dacca, Institute of Nutrition and Food Science.

Hossain, Monowar, Raihan Sharif, and Jahanara Huq (eds.). 1977. *Role of Women in Socio-Economic Development in Bangladesh.* Dhaka: ABCO Press.

Huq, Jahanara. 1979. "Economic Activities of Women in Bangladesh: The Rural Situation." In Women for Women (eds.). *The Situation of Women in Bangladesh,* pp. 139–182. Dhaka: BRAC Printers.

Hussain, S. and S. Banu. 1986. *BARD Experiences in Organization of Women in their Involvement in Agricultural Related Activities.* Comilla: Bangladesh Academy for Rural Development.

Islam, Shamima. 1986. "Work of Rural Women in Bangladesh: An Overview of Research." Paper presented at workshop on women in agriculture. Comilla: Bangladesh Academy for Rural Development.

Jaquette, Jane S. 1982. "Women and Modernization Theory: A Decade of Feminist Criticism," *World Politics* 34(2):267–284.

Khan, Salma, Jowshan Rahman, Shamima Islam, and Meherunnessa Islam. 1981. *Inventory for*

Women's Organizations in Bangladesh. Dhaka: UNICEF.

Maloney, Clarence. 1986. *Behavior and Poverty in Bangladesh.* Dhaka: University Press Limited.

Mukherjee, Ramkrishna. 1971. *Six Villages of Bengal.* Bambay: Popular Prakashan.

Raper, Arthur. 1970. *Rural Development in Action: The Comprehensive Experiment at Comilla, East Pakistan.* Ithaca: Cornell University Press.

Sanday, Peggy. 1973. "Toward a Theory of the Status of Women," *American Anthropologist* 75(5): 1682–1700.

———. 1974. "Female Status in the Public Domain." In Michelle Z. Rosaldo and Louise Lamphere (eds.). *Woman, Culture, and Society,* pp. 189–206. Stanford, CA: Stanford University Press.

Sattar, Ellen. 1979. "Demographic Features of Bangladesh with Reference to Women and Children." In Women for Women (eds.), *The Situation of Women in Bangladesh,* pp. 1–22. Dhaka: BRAC Printers.

Schaffer, Teresita C. 1986. *Survey of Development Project and Activities for Women in Bangladesh.* Dhaka: Provatee Printers.

Scott, Gloria L. and Marilyn Carr. 1985. *The Impact of Technology Choice on Rural Women in Bangladesh: Problems and Opportunities.* Washington, DC: World Bank Working Paper No 731.

Smock, Audrey Chapman. 1977. "Bangladesh: A Struggle with Tradition and Poverty." In Janet Z. Giele and Audrey C. Smock (eds.). *Women: Roles and Status in Eight Countries,* pp. 83–126. New York: John Wiley and Sons.

Wallace, Ben J., Rosie M. Ahsan, Shahnazz H. Hussain, and Ekramul Ahsan. 1987. *The Invisible Resource: Women and Work in Rural Bangladesh.* Boulder: Westview Press.

Wilson-Moore, Margot. 1989. "Women's Work in Homestead Gardens: Subsistence, Patriarchy, and Status in Northwest Bangladesh," *Urban Anthropology* 18(203):281–297.

———. 1990. "Subsistence, Patriarchy, and Status: Women's Work in Homestead Gardens in Northwest Bangladesh." Ph.D. dissertation, Southern Methodist University, Dallas, Texas.

Zaidi, S. M. Hafeez. 1970. *The Village Culture in Transition: A Study of East Pakistan Rural Society.* Honolulu: East-West Press.

MAQUILADORAS: THE VIEW FROM THE INSIDE

María Patricia Fernández Kelly

Since the end of World War II, and particularly during the last two decades, there has been an increasing trend for the large monopolies of the highly industrialized nations to transfer more parts of their manufacturing operations to underdeveloped areas of the world (Palloix, 1975: 57–63). The industrial countries have thus become administrative and financial headquarters for the international management of refined manufacturing activities (Fröbel, Heinrichs, and Kreye, 1976). Large numbers of working people throughout the underdeveloped world are experiencing directly the impact of multinational investment.

There is a somewhat mechanical tendency to interpret social events in underdeveloped areas as an automatic effect of the requirements of capital accumulation at a global level, without regard for local diversity or independent activity, particularly among working classes and class fractions (O'Brien, 1975). Participant observation contributes to understanding the effects of, and workers' responses to, the international political and economic system at the level of the factory and the household. It shows workers as more than the cheap labor they appear to be when viewed from a global demands-of-capital view-

From *My Troubles Are Going to Have Trouble with Me,* Karen Brodkin Sacks and Dorothy Remy, eds. Copyright 1984 by Rutgers, The State University. Reprinted by permission of Rutgers University Press.

point. Yet insights derived from political economic theory can inform ethnographic data collection and illuminate the details often missed in broader analytical efforts.

Along the Mexican side of the United States—Mexico border, there has been a huge expansion of manufacturing activities by multinational corporations. This has incorporated large numbers of women into direct production in the last fifteen years. As a result of implementation of the Border Industrialization Program since 1965, more than one hundred assembly plants, or *maquiladoras,* have sprung up in Ciudad Juarez, across the border from El Paso, Texas. This set of programs has made it possible for multinational firms to collaborate with Mexican state and private enterprise to foster the emergence of a booming export industry along the border. More than half of the plants are electric or electronic firms. Most of the rest are apparel assembly plants (see Newton and Balli, 1979).

The importance of the program in recent years may be appreciated by noting that *maquiladoras* account for about half of U.S. imports from underdeveloped countries under assembly industry tariff provisions, as compared with only 10 percent in 1970. In 1978 they provided the Mexican economy with more than ninety-five thousand jobs and $713 million in value added in this class of production in all of Latin America (Newton and Balli, 1979: 8). They rank third, behind tourism and petroleum sales, as a contributor to Mexican foreign exchange. The objective circumstances that have determined the growth of the *maquiladoras* industry are the availability of what appears to be an inexhaustible supply of unskilled and semiskilled labor, and extremely high levels of productivity.

The plants themselves are small, and most subcontract from corporations with their headquarters in the United States. Although nationally recognized brands are represented in Ciudad Juarez, the vast majority of these industries are associated with corporations that have regional rather than national visibility. The low level of capital investment in the physical plant often results in inadequate equipment and unpleasant working conditions.

While all *maquiladoras* employ an overwhelming majority (85 percent) of women, the apparel industry hires women whose position in the city makes them especially vulnerable to exploitative labor practices. They tend to be in their midtwenties, poorly educated, and recent migrants to Ciudad Juarez. About one-third of the women head households and are the sole supports of their children.

LOOKING FOR A JOB: A PERSONAL ACCOUNT

What is it like to be female, single, and eager to find work at a *maquiladora?* Shortly after arriving in Ciudad Juarez, and after finding stable lodging, I began looking through the pages of newspapers, hoping to find a want ad. My intent was to merge with the clearly visible mass of women who roam the streets and industrial parks of the city searching for jobs. They are, beyond doubt, a distinctive feature of the city, an effervescent expression of the conditions that prevail in the local labor market.

My objectives were straightforward. I wanted to spend four to six weeks applying for jobs and obtaining direct experience about the employment policies, recruitment strategies, and screening mechanisms used by companies to hire assembly workers. I was especially interested in how much time and money an individual worker spent trying to get a job. I also wanted to spend an equal amount of time working at a plant, preferably one that manufactured apparel. This way, I expected to learn more about working conditions, production quotas, and wages at a particular factory. I felt this would help me develop questions from a workers' perspective.

In retrospect, it seems odd that it never entered my head that I might not find a job. Finding a job at a *maquiladora* is easier said than done, especially for a woman over twenty-five. This is due primarily to the large number of women competing for jobs. At every step of their constant peregrination, women are confronted by a familiar sign at the plants—"no applications available"—or by the negative responses of a guard or a secretary at the entrance to the factories. But such is the arrogance of the uninformed researcher. I went about the business of looking for a job as if the social milieu had to conform to my research needs.

By using newspapers as a source of information for jobs, I was departing from the common strategy of potential workers in that environment. Most women are part of informal networks which include relatives, friends, and an occasional acquaintance in the personnel management sector. They hear of jobs by word of mouth.

Most job seekers believe that a personal recommendation from someone already employed at a *maquiladora* can ease the difficult path. This belief is well founded. At many plants, managers prefer to hire applicants by direct recommendation of employees who have proven to be dependable and hard working. For example, the Mexican subsidiary of a major U.S. corporation, one of the most stable *maquiladoras* in Juarez, has an established policy not to hire "outsiders." Only those who are introduced personally to the manager are considered for openings. By resorting to the personal link, managers decrease the dangers of having their factories infiltrated by unreliable workers, independent organizers, and "troublemakers."

While appearing to take a personal interest in the individual worker at the moment of hiring, management can establish a paternalistic claim on the worker. Workers complain that superintendents and managers are prone to demand "special services," like overtime, in exchange for granting personal "favors" such as a loan or time off from work to care for children. Yet workers acknowledge a personal debt to the person who hired them. A woman's commitment to the firm is fused with commitment to the particular personnel manager or superintendent who granted her the "personal favor" of hiring her. Anita expressed the typical sentiment, "If the group leader demands more production [without additional pay], I will generally resist because I owe her nothing. But if the *ingeniero* asks me to increase my quota on occasion, I comply. He gave me the job in the first place! Besides, it makes me feel good to know that I can return the favor, at least in part."

Only those who are not part of the tightly woven informal networks rely on impersonal ways to find a job. Recently arrived migrants and older women with children looking for paid employment for the first time find it especially difficult. As a "migrant" to Ciudad Juarez, I too lacked the contacts needed for relatively stable and well-paid jobs in the electronics industry. Instead, I too entered the apparel industry.

This was not a random occurrence. Ciudad Juarez electronics *maquiladoras* tend to employ very young, single women, a preferred category of potential workers from management's point of view. Workers also prefer electronics because it has large, stable plants, regular wages, and certain additional benefits. In contrast, the apparel-manufacturing sector is characterized by smaller, less stable shops where working conditions are particularly strenuous. Many hire workers on a more or less temporary basis, lack any commitment to their employees, and in the face of a fluctuating international market, observe crude and often ruthless personnel recruitment policies.

One such firm advertised for direct production workers in the two main Juarez newspapers throughout the year, an indication of its high rate of turnover. Despite a grand-sounding name, this small plant is located in the central area of the city rather than in one of the modern industrial parks, hires only about one-hundred workers, and is surrounded by unpaved streets and difficult to reach by public transportation. The shoddy, one-story plant, with its old-fashioned sewing machines and crowded work stations, reflects the low level of capital investment made in it.

I went into its tiny office in the middle of summer to apply for a job. As I entered, I wondered whether my appearance or accent would make the personnel manager suspicious. He looked me over sternly and told me to fill out a form now and to return the following morning at seven o'clock to take a dexterity test. Most of the items were straightforward: name, age, marital status, place of birth, length of residence in Ciudad Juarez, property assets, previous jobs and income, number of pregnancies, and general state of health. One, however, was unexpected: what is your major aspiration in life? All my doubts surfaced—would years of penmanship practice at a private school in Mexico City and flawless spelling give me away?

I assumed the on-the-job test would consider of a short evaluation of my skills as a seamstress. I was wrong. The next morning I knocked at the door of the personnel office where I filled out the application, but no one was there. In some confusion, I peeked into the entrance of the factory. The supervisor, Margarita, a dark-haired woman wearing false eyelashes, ordered me in and led me to my place at an industrial sewing machine. That it was old was plain to see; how it worked was difficult to judge. I listened intently to Margarita's instructions. I was expected to sew patch pockets on what were to become blue jeans from the assortment of diversely cut denim parts on my left. Obediently I started to sew.

The particulars of "unskilled" labor unfolded before my eyes. The procedure demanded perfect coordination of hands, eyes, and legs. I was to use my left hand to select the larger part of material from the batch next to me and my right to grab the pocket. There were no markers to show me where to place the pocket. Experienced workers did it on a purely visual basis. Once the patch pocket was in place, I was to guide the two parts under a double needle while applying pressure on the machine's pedal with my right foot.

Because the pockets were sewed on with thread of a contrasting color, the edge of the pocket had to be perfectly aligned with the needles to produce a regular seam and an attractive design. Because the pocket was diamond shaped, I also had to rotate the materials slightly three times while adjusting pressure on the pedal. Too much pressure inevitably broke the thread or produced seams longer than the edge of the pocket. The slightest deviation produced lopsided designs, which then had to be unsewed and gone over as many times as it took to do an acceptable pocket. The supervisor told me that, once trained, I would be expected to sew a pocket every nine to ten seconds. That meant 360 to 396 pockets every hour, or 2,880 to 3,168 every day!

As at the vast majority of apparel-manufacturing *maquiladoras,* I would be paid through a combination of the minimum wage and piecework. In 1978 this was 125 pesos a day, or U.S. $5.00. I would, however, get a slight bonus if I sustained a calculated production quota through the week. Workers are not allowed to produce less than 80 percent of their assigned quota without being admonished, and a worker seriously endangers her job when unable to improve her level of output. Margarita showed me a small blackboard showing the weekly bonus received by those able to produce certain percentages of the quota. They fluctuated between 50 pesos (U.S. $2.20) for those who completed 80 percent of the quota, to 100 pesos for those who completed 100 percent. Managers call this combination of steep production quotas, minimum wages, and modest bonuses an "incentive program."

I started my test at 7:30 A.M. with a sense of embarrassment about my limited skills and disbelief at the speed with which the women in the factory worked. As I continued sewing, the bundle of material on my left was renewed and slowly grew in size. I had to repeat the operation many times before the product was considered acceptable. I soon realized I was being treated as a new worker while presumably being tested. I had not been issued a contract and therefore was not yet incorporated into the Instituto Mexicano del Seguro

Social (the national social security system). Nor had I been told about working hours, benefits, or system of payment.

I explained to the supervisor that I had recently arrived in the city, alone, and with very little money. Would I be hired? When would I be given a contract? Margarita listened patiently while helping me unsew one of many defective pockets and then said, "You are too curious. Don't worry about it. Do your job and things will be all right." I continued to sew, aware of the fact that every pocket attached during the "test" was becoming part of the plant's total production.

At 12:30, during the thirty-minute lunch break, I had a better chance to see the factory. Its improvised quality was underscored by the metal folding chairs at the sewing machines. I had been sitting on one of them during the whole morning, but until then I had not noticed that most of them had the Coca Cola label painted on their backs. I had seen this kind of chair many times in casual parties both in Mexico and in the United States. Had they been bought, or were they being rented? In any event, they were not designed to meet the strenuous requirements of sewing all day. Women brought their own colorful pillows to ease the stress on their buttocks and spines. Later on, I was to discover that chronic lumbago is a frequent condition among factory seamstresses (Fernández, 1978).

My questions were still unanswered at 5 P.M., when a bell rang to signal the end of the shift. I went to the personnel office intending to get more information. Despite my overly shy approach to the personnel manager, his reaction was hostile. Even before he was able to turn the disapproving expression on his face into words, Margarita intervened. She was angry. To the manager she said, "This woman has too many questions: Will she be hired? Is she going to be insured?" And then to me, "I told you already, we do piecework here; if you do your job, you get a wage; otherwise you don't. That's clear isn't it? What else do you want? You should be grateful! This plant is giving you a chance to work! What else do you want? Come back tomorrow and be punctual."

This was my initiation into applying for a job. Most women do not job-hunt alone. Rather, they go with friends or relatives and are commonly seen in groups of two or three around most factories. Walking about the industrial parks while following other job seekers was especially informative. Very young women, between sixteen and seventeen, often go with their mothers. One mother told me she sold burritos at the stadium every weekend and that her husband worked as a janitor but that their combined income was inadequate for the six children. Her daughter Elsa was sixteen. "I can't let her go alone into the parks," the mother explained. "She's only a girl and it wouldn't be right. Sometimes girls working in the plants are molested. It's a pity they have to work, but I want to be sure she'll be working in a good place."

At shift changes, thousands of women arrive at and leave the industrial parks in buses, taxis, and *ruteras* (jitney cabs). During working hours only those seeking jobs wander about. Many, though not the majority of these, are "older women." They face special difficulties because of their age and because they often support their children alone. Most of them enter the labor force after many years dedicated to domestic chores and child care. Frequently, desertion by their male companions forces their entry into the paid labor force. A thirty-one year old mother of six children explained. "I have been looking for work since my husband left me two months ago. But I haven't had any luck. It must be my age and the fact that I have so many children. Maybe I should lie and say I've only one. But then the rest wouldn't be entitled to medical care once I got the job." Women need jobs to support their children, but they are often turned down because they are mothers.

I finally got a job at a new *maquiladora* that was adding an evening shift. I saw its advertisement in the daily newspapers and went early the following morning to apply at the factory, which is located in the modern Parque Industrial Bermudez. Thirty-seven women preceded me. Some had arrived as early as 6 A.M. At 10, the door that separated the front lawn from the entrance to the factory had not yet been opened, although a guard appeared once in a while to peek at the growing contingent of applicants. At 10:30 he finally opened the door to tell us that only those having personal recommendation letters would be permitted inside. This was the first in a series of formal and informal screening procedures used to reduce the number of potential workers. Thirteen women left immediately. Others tried to convince the guard that, although they had no personal recommendation, they knew someone already employed at the factory.

Xochitl had neither a written nor a verbal recommendation, but she insisted that her diploma from a sewing academy gave her claim to a particular skill. "It is better to have proof that you are qualified to do the job than to have a letter of recommendation, right?" I wondered whether the personnel manager would agree. The numerous academies in Ciudad Juarez offer technical and vocational courses for a relatively small sum of money. The training does not guarantee a job because many *maquiladora* managers prefer to hire women with direct experience on the job, or as one manager put it to me, "We prefer to hire women who are unspoiled, that is, those who come to us without preconceptions about what industrial work is. Women such as these are easier to shape to our own requirements."

Xochitl's diploma was a glossy document dominated by an imposing eagle clutching a terrestrial globe. An undulating ribbon with the words "labor, omnia, vincit" complemented the design. Beneath it was certification of Xochitl's skills. A preoccupied expression clouded Xochitl's face while she looked at her certificate again. The picture on its left margin, of a young girl with shiny eyes, barely resembled the prematurely aged woman in line with me. At thirty-two, Xochitl was the mother of four children. She took up sewing at home to supplement the money her husband made peddling homemade refreshments. When there was work available (which was not always), she sewed from 6 A.M. until 3 P.M. She could complete three beach dresses, for which is she received 22 pesos (U.S. $0.80) a day. The dresses were then sold in the market for approximately 150 pesos. She resented her contractor's high profit but felt she had no other choice. Most of her income was spent on food, clothing, and in attempts to furnish her two-room adobe house. She had already been standing outside the factory for over 3½ hours. All this time she could have been sewing at home and minding the children. Her husband might not approve of her looking for work in the factory, either. He felt it was one thing to sew at home, another to work in a factory.

The young, uniformed guard seemed unperturbed by the fluctuating number of women standing by the door. To many of us, he was the main obstacle lying between unemployment and getting a job from someone inside. To the women, he appeared arrogant and insensitive. "Why must these miserable guards always act this way?" nineteen-year-old Teresa asked. "It would seem that they've never had to look for a job. Maybe this one thinks he's more important than the owner of the factory. What a bastard!"

Teresa turned to me to ask if I had any sewing experience. "Not much," I told her, "but I used to sew for a lady in my hometown."

"Well then, you're very lucky," she said, "because they aren't hiring anyone without experience." She told me that she and her sister worked with about seventy other women for three years in a small shop in downtown Juarez. They sewed pants for the minimum wage but had no insurance. When the boss could not get precut fabric from the United States for them to sew, he laid them off without pay. For the last three months they had been living on the little their father earned from construction work, painting houses, selling toys at the stadium, or doing other odd jobs. "We are two of nine brothers and sisters (there were twelve of us in total but three died when they were young)."

"I am single, thanks be to God, and I do not want to get married," she informed me. "There are enough problems in my life as it is!" But her sister Beatriz, who was standing in line with us, had married an engineer when she was only fifteen. Now she is divorced and has three children to support. "They live with us too. Beatriz and I are the oldest in the family, you see; that's why we really have to find a job."

"I also used to work as a maid in El Paso. I don't have a passport, so I had to cross illegally as a wetback, a little wetback who cleaned houses. The money wasn't bad. I used to earn up to thirty-five dollars a week, but I hated being locked up all day. So I came back and here I am."

I asked Beatriz if her husband helped support her children.

"No," she said emphatically, "and I don't want him to give me anything, not a cent, because I don't want him to have any claim or rights over my babies. As long as I can support them, he won't have to interfere."

I asked if there were better jobs outside of *maquiladoras*. "I understand you can make more money working at a *cantina;* is that true?"

Both of them looked at me suspiciously. *Cantinas* are an ever-present reminder of overt or concealed prostitution. Teresa acknowledged that she could earn more there but asked:

> What would our parents think? You can't stop people from gossiping, and many of those *"cantinas"* are whorehouses. Of course, when you have great need you can't be choosey, right? For some time I worked there as a waitress, but that didn't last. The supervisor was always chasing me. First he wanted to see me after work. I told him I had a boyfriend, but he insisted. He said I was too young to have a steady boyfriend. Then, when he learned I had some typing skills, he wanted me to be his secretary. I'm not stupid! I knew what he really wanted; he was always staring at my legs. So I had to leave that job too. I told him I had been rehired at the shop, although it wasn't true. He wasn't bad looking, but he was married and had children. . . . Why must men fool around?

The guard's summons to experienced workers to fill out applications interrupted our conversation. Twenty women went into the narrow lobby of Camisas de Juarez, while the rest left in small, quiet groups. For those of us who stayed, a second waiting period began. One by one we were shown into the office of the personnel manager, where we were to take a manual dexterity test, fitting fifty variously colored pegs into fifty similarly colored perforations on a wooden board in the shortest possible time. Clock in hand, the personnel manager told each woman when to begin and when to stop. Some were asked to adjust the pegs by hand; others were given small pliers to do so. Most were unable to complete the test in the allotted time. One by one they came out of the office looking weary and expressing their conviction that they would not be hired.

Later on, we were given the familiar application form. Again, I had to ponder what my greatest aspiration in life was. But this time I was curious to know what Xochitl had answered.

"Well," she said, "I don't know if my answer is right. Maybe it is wrong. But I tried to be truthful. My greatest aspiration in life is to improve myself and to progress."

Demonstrating sewing skills on an industrial machine followed. Many women expressed their doubts and concern when they rejoined the waiting women in the lobby. Over the hours, the sense had increased that all of us were united by the common experience of job seeking and by the gnawing anxiety that potential failure entails. Women compared notes and exchanged opinions about the nature and difficulty of their respective tests. They did not offer each other overt reassurance or support, but they made sympathetic comments and hoped that there would be work for all.

At 3:30 P.M., seven hours after we arrived at the plant, we were dismissed with no indication that any of us would be hired. They told us a telegram would be sent to each address as soon as a decision was made. Most women left disappointed and certain that they would not be hired. Two weeks later, when I had almost given up all hope, the telegram arrived. I was to come to the plant as soon as possible to receive further instructions.

Upon my arrival I was given the address of a small clinic in downtown Ciudad Juarez. I was to bring two pictures to the clinic and take a medical examination. Its explicit purpose was to evaluate the physical fitness of potential workers. In reality, it was a pregnancy test. *Maquiladoras* do not hire pregnant women in spite of their greater need for employment. During the first years of its existence, many pregnant women sought employment in the *maquiladora* program knowing they would be entitled to an eighty-two day pregnancy leave with full pay. Some women circumvented the restrictions on employing pregnant women by bringing urine specimens of friends or relatives to the clinic. Plant managers now insist on more careful examinations, but undetected pregnant women sometimes get hired. The larger and more stable plants generally comply with the law and give maternity leave, but in small subcontracted firms, women are often fired as soon as the manager discovers they are pregnant.

After my exam at the clinic, I returned to the factory with a sealed envelope containing certification of my physical capacity to work. I was then told to return the following Monday at 3:30 P.M. to start work. After what seemed like an unduly long and complicated procedure, I was finally hired as an assembly worker. For the next six weeks I shared the experience of approximately eighty women who had also been recruited to work the evening shift. Xochitl, Beatriz, and Teresa had been hired too.

WORKING AT THE *MAQUILADORA*

The weekday evening shift began at 3:45 and ended at 11:30 P.M. A bell rang at 7:30 to signal the beginning of a half-hour dinner break. Some women brought sandwiches from home, but most bought a dish of *flautas* or *tostadas* and a carbonated drink at the factory. On Saturdays the shift started at 11:30 A.M. and ended at 9:30 P.M., with a half hour break. We worked, in total, forty-eight hours every week for the minimum wage, an hourly rate of about U.S. $0.60.

Although wages are low in comparison to those of the United States for similar jobs, migrants flock to zone 09, which includes Ciudad Juarez, because it has nearly the highest minimum wage in the country (only zone 01, where Baja California is located, has a higher rate). Legally, *maquiladoras* are also required to enroll their workers in the social security system and in the national housing program (Instituto Nacional a la Vivienda). As a result, investment per work hour reached U.S. $1.22 in 1978. For women who have children, the medical insurance is often as important as the wage.

Newcomers receive the minimum wage but are expected to fulfill production quotas. My new job was to sew a narrow bias around the cuff openings of men's shirts. My quota of 162 pairs of sleeves every hour meant one every 2.7 seconds. After six weeks as a direct production operator, I still fell short of this goal by almost 50 percent.

Sandra, who sat next to me during this period, assured me that it could be done. She had worked at various *maquiladoras* for at last seven years. Every time she got too tired, she left the job, rested for a while, then sought another. She was a speedy seamstress who acted with the self-assurance of one who is well-acquainted with factory work. It was difficult not to admire her skill and aloofness, especially when I was being continuously vexed by my own incompetence.

One evening Sandra told me she thought my complaints and manner of speech were funny and, at the end of what turned out to be a lively conversation, admitted to liking me. I was flattered. Then she stared at my old jeans and ripped blouse with an appraising look and said, "Listen Patricia, as soon as we get our wage, I want to take you to buy some decent clothes. You look awful! And you need a haircut." So much for the arrogance of the researcher who wondered whether her class background would be detected. Sandra became my most important link with the experience of *maquiladora* work.

Sandra lived with her parents in "las lomas" in the outskirts of the city. The area was rugged and distant, but the house itself indicated modest prosperity. There were four ample rooms, one of which was carpeted. The living room walls were covered with family photographs. There were an American television and comfortable chairs in the room. There were two sinks in the kitchen as well as a refrigerator, blender, beater, and new American-made washing machine (waiting until the area got its hoped-for running water). Sandra's father was a butcher who had held his job at a popular market for many years. Although in the past, when his three daughters were small, it had been difficult to stay out of debt, better times were at hand. He had only two regrets: his failing health and Sandra's divorce. He felt both matters were beyond his control. He considered Sandra a good daughter because she never failed to contribute to household expenses and because she was also saving so she could support her two children, who were currently living with her former husband. Sandra had left him after he beat her for taking a job outside the home.

Even with Sandra's help, I found the demands of the factory overwhelming. Young supervisors walked about the aisles calling for higher productivity and greater speed. Periodically, their voices could be heard throughout the workplace: "Faster! Faster! Come on girls, let's hear the sound of those machines!"

My supervisor, Esther, quit her job as a nurse for the higher wages as a factory worker because she had to support an ill and aging father after her mother's death three years earlier. Although her home was nice and fully owned, she was solely responsible for the remaining family debts. She earned almost one thousand pesos a week in the factory, roughly twice her income as a nurse.

The supervisor's role is a difficult one. Esther, like the other supervisors, often stayed at the plant after the workers left, sometimes until one in the morning. She would verify quotas and inspect all garments for defects, some of which she restitched. She would also prepare shipments and select materials for the following day's production. Management held supervisors directly responsible for productivity levels as well as for workers' punctuality and attendance, putting the supervisors between the devil and the deep blue sea. Workers frequently believed that supervisors were the ones responsible for their plight at the workplace and regarded abuse, unfair treatment, and excessive demands from them as whims. But while workers saw supervisors as close allies of the firm, management directed its dissatisfaction with workers at the supervisors. Many line supervisors agreed that the complications they faced on their jobs were hardly worth the extra pay.

One young woman at another factory told me, "Since I was promoted to a supervisory capacity I feel that my workmates hate me. We used to get along fine. I would even go so far as to say that we shared in a genuine sense of comaraderie. Now, they resent having to take orders from me, a former assembly worker like themselves. They talk behind my back and ask each other why it was I and not one of them who was promoted" (Fernández, 1978).

For some months this woman labored under considerable stress. Her problems were compounded when she had to decide who among her subordinates would have to be laid off as a result of plant adjustments. Caught between the exigencies of management and the resentful attempts of workers to manipulate her, she came close to a nervous breakdown. A short time afterward she asked to be transferred to her old job. From her point of view it was not worth being "a sandwich person."

Although my supervisor, Esther, was considerate and encouraging, she still asked me to repair my defective work. I began to skip dinner breaks to continue sewing in a feeble attempt to improve my productivity level. I was not alone. Some workers, fearful of permanent dismissal, also stayed at their sewing machines during the break while the rest went outside to eat and relax.

I could understand their behavior; their jobs were at stake. But presumably my situation was different. I had nothing to lose by inefficiency, and yet I felt compelled to do my best. I started pondering upon the subtle mechanisms that dominate will at the workplace, and about the shame that overwhelms those who fall short of the goals assigned to them. As the days passed, it became increasingly difficult for me to think of factory work as a stage in a research project. My identity became that of a worker; my immediate objectives, those determined by the organization of labor at the plant. I became one link in a rigidly structured chain. My failure to produce speedily had consequences for others operating in the same line. For example, Lucha, my nineteen-year-old companion, cut remnant thread and separated the sleeves that five other seamstresses and I sewed. Since she could only meet her quota if we met ours, Lucha was extremely interested in seeing improvements in my level of productivity and in the quality of my work. Sometimes her attitude and exhortations verged on the hostile. As far as I was concerned, the accusatory expression on her face was the best work incentive yet devised by the factory. I was not surprised to find out during the weeks I spent there that the germ of enmity had bloomed between some seamstresses and their respective thread cutters over matters of work.

Although the relationship between seamstresses and thread cutters was especially delicate, all workers were affected by each other's level of efficiency. Cuffless sleeves could not be attached to shirts, nor could sleeves be sewed to shirts without collars or pockets. Holes and buttons had to be fixed at the end. Unfinished garments could not be cleaned of lint or labeled. In sum, each minute step required a series of preceding operations effectively completed. Delay of one stage inevitably slowed up the whole process.

From the perspective of the workers, the work appeared as interconnected individual activities rather than as an imposed structure. Managers were nearly invisible, but the flaws of fellow workers were always present. Bonuses became personal rewards made inaccessible by a neighbor's laziness or incompetence. One consequence of these perceptions was that workers frequently directed complaints against other workers and supervisors. In short, the organization of labor at any particular plant does not automatically lead to feelings of solidarity.

On the other hand, the tensions did not inhibit talk, and the women's shared experiences, especially about longings for relief from the tediousness of industrial work, gave rise to an ongoing humorous dialogue. Sandra often reflected in a witty and self-deprecatory manner on the possibility of marriage to a rich man. She thought that if she could only find a nice man who would be willing to support her, everything in her life would be all right. She did not mind if he was not young or good looking, as long as he had plenty of money. Were there men like that left in the world? Of course, with the children it was difficult, not to say impossible, to find such a godsend. Then again, no one kept you from trying. But not at the *maquiladora.* Everyone was female. One could die of boredom there.

Sandra knew many women who had been seduced and then deserted by engineers and technicians. Other women felt they had to comply with the sexual demands of fellow workers because they believed otherwise they would lose their jobs. Some were just plain stupid. Things were especially difficult for very young women at large electronics plants. They needed guidance and information to stay out of trouble, but there was no one to advise them. During the first years of the *maquiladora* program, sexual harassment was especially blatant. There were *ingenieros* who insisted on having only the prettiest workers under their command. They developed a sort of factory "harem." Sandra knew of a man—"Would you believe this?"—who wanted as much female diversity as possible. All of the women on his crew, at his request, had eyes and hair of a different color. Another man boasted that every woman on his line had borne him a child. She told me about the scandals, widely covered by the city tabloids, about the spread of venereal disease in certain *maquiladoras*. Although Sandra felt she knew how to take care of herself, she still thought it better to have only female fellow workers. The factory was not a good place to meet men.

Fortunately, there were the bars and the discotheques. Did I like to go out dancing? She did not think I looked like the type who would. But it was great fun. Eventually Sandra and I went to a popular disco, the Cosmos, which even attracted people from "the other side" (the United States), who came to Juarez just to visit this disco. It had an outer-space decor, full of color and movement, and played the best American disco music. If you were lucky, you could meet a U.S. citizen. Maybe he would even want to get married, and you could go and live in El Paso. Things like that happen at discotheques. Once a Jordanian soldier in service at Fort Bliss had asked Sandra to marry him the first time they met at Cosmos. But he wanted to return to his country, and she had said no. Cosmos was definitely the best discotheque in Juarez, and Sandra could be found dancing there amidst the deafening sound of music every Saturday evening.

The inexhaustible level of energy of women working at the *maquiladoras* never ceased to impress me. How could anyone be in the mood for all-night dancing on Saturdays after forty-eight weekly hours of industrial work? I had seen many of these women stretching their muscles late at night trying to soothe the pain they felt at the waist. After the incessant noise of the sewing machines, how could anyone long for even higher levels of sound? But as Sandra explained to me, life is too short. If you don't go out and have fun, you will come to the end of your days having done nothing but sleep, eat, and work. And she didn't call that living. Besides, where else would you be able to meet a man?

Ah men! They were often unreliable, mean, or just plain lazy ("wasn't that obvious from the enormous number of women who had to do factory work in Ciudad Juarez?"), but no one wanted to live alone. There must be someone out there worth living for—at least someone who did not try to put you down or slap you. Sandra could not understand why life had become so difficult. Her mother and father had stayed married for thirty years and they still liked each other. There had been some difficult times in the past, but they had always had each other. She knew a lot of older folks who were in the same situation. But it was different for modern couples.

At 11:15, Sandra's talks about men stopped, and we prepared to go home. We cleaned up our work area and made sure we took the two spools and a pair of scissors we were responsible for home with us to prevent their being stolen by workers the following morning. As soon as the bell rang at 11:30, we began a disorderly race to be the first to check out our time cards. Then we had to stand in line with our purses wide open so the guard could check our belongings. Women vehemently resented management's suspicion that workers would steal material or the finished products. The nightly search was an unnecessary humiliation of being treated as thieves until proven innocent by the guard.

Once outside the factory, we walked in a group across the park to catch our bus. There was a lot of laughing and screaming, as well as teasing and exchanging of vulgarities. Most of the time we could board an almost-empty bus as soon as we reached the main avenue. Sometimes, when we had to wait, we became impatient. In jest, a woman would push another worker toward the street, suggesting provocative poses for her to use to attract a passerby to offer a ride. When a car did stop, however, they quickly moved away. To joke was one thing, but to accept a ride from a man, especially late at night, was to look for trouble.

Individually, the factory women appeared vulnerable, even shy, but as a group, they could be a formidable sight. One night a man boarded the bus when we were already in it.

His presence gave focus to the high spirits. Women immediately subjected him to verbal attacks similar to those they often received from men. Feeling protected by anonymity and by their numerical strength, they chided and teased him; they offered kisses and asked for a smile. The exchanged laughing comments about his physical attributes and suggested a raffle to see who would keep him. The man remained silent through it all. He adopted the outraged and embarrassed expression that women often wear when they feel victimized by men. The stares of whistling women followed him as he left the bus.

Although I only saw one such incident, I was told that it was not uncommon. "It is pitiful," a male acquaintance told me; "those girls have no idea of what proper feminine behavior is." He told me he had seen women even paw or pinch men while traveling in buses and *ruteras*. According to him, factory work was to blame: "Since women started working at the *maquiladoras* they have lost all sense of decorum." The women see it as a harmless game fostered by the temporary sense of membership in a group. As Sandra liked to remind me, "Factory work is harder than most people know. As long as you don't harm anybody, what's wrong with having a little fun?"

CONCLUSIONS

In telling of my experience, I have tried to acquaint the reader with a new form of industrial employment from a personal viewpoint. Textile and garment manufacturing are, of course, as old as factories themselves, but *maquiladoras* epitomize the most distinctive traits of the modern system of production. They are part of a centralized global arrangement in which central economies such as the United States have become the locus of technological expertise and major financial outflows, while Third World countries increase their participation in the international market via the manufacture of exportable goods.

This global system of production has had unprecedented political and economic consequences. For example, the fragmentation of labor processes has reduced the level of skill required to perform the majority of assembly operations required to manufacture even the most complex and sophisticated electronics products. In turn, the geographical dispersion of production has curtailed the bargaining ability of workers of many nationalities vis-à-vis large corporations. At times, workers in Asia, Latin America, and the Caribbean seem to be thrust into competition against one another for access to low-paying, monotonous jobs. Labor unions and strikes have limited potential in a world where factories can be transferred at ease to still another country where incentives are more favorable and wages cheaper.

More than two million workers are presently employed in export-processing zones located in less developed countries. Perhaps most significant is the fact that between 85 percent and 90 percent of them are women. Under the Border Industrialization and *Maquiladora* Programs, Mexico is participating in this global arrangement by offering attractive stimuli and customs leeway to multinational corporations mainly involved in electronics and garment manufacturing. More than 156,000 women are employed in *maquiladoras*. In spite, or perhaps because, of Mexico's increasing economic difficulties, the number of such plants will increase in the next years. Several devaluations of the Mexican currency have placed the country in a competitive position with respect to Taiwan and Hong Kong as a source of cheap labor.

From the point of view of business, *maquiladoras* are a great success. But as the preceding narration suggests, the experiences of working women employed at the plants give reason for concern. Low wages, strenuous work paces, the absence of promotions, the temporary nature of employment, and unsatisfactory working conditions combine to make *maquiladoras* a precarious alternative. Such factories thrive only in labor markets characterized by very few occupational choices.

It is evident from the testimony of workers that women seek *maquiladora* jobs compelled by their need to support families whether they be formed by parents and siblings or by their own children. Male unemployment and underemployment play an important part in this. Multinationals tend to relocate assembly operations to areas of the world where jobless people automatically provide an abundant supply of cheap labor. Sandra's longing for male economic support and regrets over the irresponsibility of men represent a personal counterpoint to a structural reality where men are unable to find remunerative jobs while women are forced, out of need, to join the ranks of the industrial labor force.

The same testimony demonstrates that *maquila* women would prefer to withdraw from the exhausting jobs available to them and give full attention to home and children. Husbands and fathers frequently press women to leave their jobs to adjust to a conventional understanding of what gender roles should be. Nevertheless, when women retire from wage labor to become housewives and mothers, they often face dire alternatives. Later, they may have to seek new forms of employment because of the inability of their men to provide adequately for their families. Older and with children to provide for, they then face special constraints in a labor market that favors very young, single, childless women. The life profile of *maquiladora* women is, then, a saga of downward mobility, a fate contrary to the optimistic expectations of industrial promoters.

The segregation of the labor market on the basis of sex tends to weaken the bargaining position of both men and women as wage earners. But perhaps more important is the observation that the same segregation produces a clash between ideological notions about the role of women and their actual transformation into primary wage earners. This has given rise to tensions perceived both at the household and community levels. *Maquiladora* workers have become notorious in that they challenge conventional mores and values regarding femininity. Concerns about young women's morality, virtue, and sexual purity are, in part, reflections of widespread anxiety and fear that, as a result of wage earning, women may end up subverting the established order. *Maquiladora* workers may see their riotous behavior toward a man in a bus as an innocuous diversion. Others, however, see it as a clear sign that women are losing respect for patriarchy.

Maquiladoras are hardly a mechanism for upward mobility, hardly the bold entrance to middle-class respectability, hardly the key to individual economic autonomy. All these are issues that should be of concern to government officials and social planners. Yet, while *maquiladoras* have taken advantage of women's vulnerability in the job market, they have also provided a forum where new forms of consciousness and new challenges are present. For younger *maquila* workers who are living with parents and siblings and have few or no children of their own, wage labor offers the cherished possibility of retaining at least part of their income for discretionary purposes.

REFERENCES

Fernández, M. P. 1978. "Notes from the Field." Ciudad Juarez, Mexico. Mimeo.

Fröbel, J. R., J. H. Heinrichs, and O. Kreye. 1976. "Tendency Towards A New International Division of Labor Force for World Markets Oriented Manufacturing." *Economic and Political Weekly* 11: 71–83.

Newton, J. R., and F. Balli. 1979. "Mexican In-Bond Industry." Paper presented to the seminar on North-South Complementary Intra-Industry Trade. UNCTAD United Nations Conference, Mexico, D.F.

O'Brien, Philip. 1975. "A Critique of Latin American Theories of Dependency." In I. Oxaal, T. Barnett, and D. Booth, eds., *Beyond the Sociology of Development*. London: Routledge and Kegan Paul.

Palloix, C. 1975. "The Internationalization of Capital and the Circuit of Social Capital." In H. Radice, ed., *The International Firms and Modern Imperialism*. New York: Penguin.

"WILD PIGS AND DOG MEN": RAPE AND DOMESTIC VIOLENCE AS "WOMEN'S ISSUES" IN PAPUA NEW GUINEA

Laura Zimmer-Tamakoshi

INTRODUCTION

Male violence against women is a concern of feminists in both developed and developing countries (Counts, Brown & Campbell 1992; Davies 1994). Leaders in many developing countries, however, have been slow in recognizing the extent and nature of the problem. This is in part because of insufficient research and cultural norms allowing for a "certain amount of wife-beating" and forced sex within marriage (United Nations 1989). It is also the result of women's weaker political presence in developing countries and male resentment over a few women's gains in economic and social independence. Nevertheless, prompted by alarm over increased violence against women, concern over the deleterious effects of violence on women's participation in development, and negative images of Papua New Guinea in the world press, in 1982 the Papua New Guinean government directed its Law Reform Commission to begin research into domestic violence. The resulting, and for a developing country, unprecedented publications revealed that a majority of Papua New Guinean wives have been hit by their husbands, most more than once a year, with urban wives suffering a higher level of violence than their rural counterparts (Toft, ed. 1985, 1986a, and 1986b; Toft and Bonnell 1985). Less systematically researched, rape is also a concern as Papua New Guinea tops the United States with a reported rate of 45 rapes per 100,000 persons versus 35 per 100,000 in the United States and well above the lower incidences of reported rapes in Japan and other industrial and non-industrial nations (Herman 1989: 23). In 1990 there were, 1,896 rapes reported in Papua New Guinea, a country with less than 4 million in population (Dinnen 1993). Such statistics do not capture the severity of the problem, however, as most of these rapes were committed by three or more rapists (with upwards of 15, 20 or 40 males participating in any particular gang rape), and, as in the United States and elsewhere, many rapes are unreported, especially those committed by the victims' husbands, lovers, dates, or close relatives (Dinnen 1996; Finkelhor and Yllo 1985; Russell 1984; Toft 1985; Toft 1986a; Zimmer 1990).

This chapter examines violence against women in Papua New Guinea, reviewing past and present patterns of rape and domestic violence and adding to a multidimensional theory concerning the prevalence and increase of such violence. While traditional attitudes toward violence contribute to its acceptance, recent research has targeted the psychological and economic pressures of development and inequality as fueling violence against women, particularly as they affect differently the circumstances and attitudes of males and females. Josephides (n.d.), for example, argues that in Papua New Guinea, "Much of men's violence towards women is motivated by a fear that women are gaining a new kind of independence," and that men's violence is an attempt to terrify and control the women. Both Josephides and Bradley (1994), who worked at the Papua New Guinea Law Reform Commission from 1986 to 1990, see the violence as stemming not only from men's insecurities about their wives' potential independence but also their own uncertain situations and the effects of urban lifestyles

Original material prepared for this text.

(including alcohol abuse and reduced social support networks) on male-female relations. Other factors are increased eroticism and sexual conflicts as old taboos disappear and men (and sometimes women) place greater demands on their spouses and sexual partners (Jenkins 1994; Rosi and Zimmer-Tamakoshi 1993).

Supporting these arguments with cases and other material, I also develop a needed political dimension to better understand violence against women in Papua New Guinea (and elsewhere, as I discuss in the concluding section of this chapter). While individuals commit violence and it is individuals who experience the traumas and dislocations of change and development, the intersection of sex and class politics also informs and fuels sexual and domestic violence. With a small number of Papua New Guineans enjoying an elite lifestyle and under pressure from the "grassroots" to bring about an economic miracle on their behalf, elite women have become targets of disaffection not only from men and women in the lower classes but also from men in their own class. Feeling harassed on all sides, by unsympathetic constituents and, from their perspective, "demanding" or *bikhet* (uncontrollable, conceited) wives and girlfriends, many elite males have taken the path of least resistance and higher political capital, scapegoating elite women and using violence to assert control over them (Rosi and Zimmer-Tamakoshi 1993; Zimmer-Tamakoshi 1993b and 1995). Thus, I not only contend, along with others, that 1) women's opportunities for self-expression and economic independence threaten the self-esteem and security of men who do not have such opportunities and 2) that such men use violence against women to assert or regain a sense of dominance, I also argue that 3) violence against women is rife among Papua New Guinea's elite (a fact demonstrated by the Law Reform Commission reports) even when one excludes what Josephides has referred to in person as anti-feminist *rascals* (or criminals) some of who are members of elite society (as has been reported by Dinnen 1993; Harris 1988; and Zimmer-Tamakoshi n.d.) and 4) that the violence is partly motivated by class and sexual tensions that paint elite females as symbols of all that is wrong with contemporary Papua New Guinean society. Finally, violence against women does not occur in isolation from other forms of violence. Political tensions in Papua New Guinea are grounded in a weak state that is unable to assure even basic services to its population or to control public disturbances such as tribal conflicts over land. As has been argued for Papua New Guinea (A. Strathern 1993) and other parts of the world (Riches 1986), expressions of conflict such as the resumption of tribal warfare in the New Guinean highlands have strategic value in the context of a weak state. In a weak state violence may be a rational means of social advantage when there are no higher-level powers strong enough or interested enough in interfering with lower-level clashes. In the case of violence against women, men who want to can assert their dominance over women with little fear of resistance as long as there is widespread envy or fear of those women, and state officials charged with protecting them are unable or unwilling to do so.

WILD PIGS AND DOG MEN

Rape and domestic violence are not common in every New Guinean society (see Goodale 1980 and Mitchell 1992), but, fearing violence, most Papua New Guinean women walk in groups when going to and from their gardens or to office, school or marketplace. Because husbands and boyfriends are likely perpetrators of violence against them, women also seek the protective company of family and friends when they are at home. Women's fear of violence, especially sexual violence, is fanned with vivid stories of past attacks on women and fresh accounts in the daily press. Around village hearths in the night, women and girls listen to the hushed and often admonitory tones of older persons telling them tales (captured in early anthropological monographs) of gang rape and mutilation of women's genitals as ways men "used to" punish errant wives and daughters (Meggitt 1964: 204, 207; Newman 1964: 266; Read 1952: 14); how wife-swapping or preying on other men's wives were tolerated as long as neither was too blatant an attack on a man's self-esteem (Berndt 1962: 160, Brown 1969: 94; Langness 1969: 45 and 1974: 204; Read 1954: 866); and how rape did and does occur in the varied contexts of women being found alone on a garden path or at work in their gardens, in war, and when a man tires of his lover, wishes to end an adulterous affair or lessen his culpability in either case by instigating a gang rape of the woman (Berndt 1962: 168). Outside the highlands, Tolai women shudder when they hear how Tolai men's cults once celebrated masculinity with the sexual abuse of widows and other women without male protection (Bradley 1982, 1985; Parkinson 1907: 473). And in West New Britain, Lakalai women do not mourn changes in the men's ceremonial season, which once included the casual rape of women in their own villages (Chowning 1985: 85).

Although many men's cults and their predations on women have died out as Christianity has taken over (Bradley 1985 and Chowning 1985), violence against women continues. Today, the contexts in which violence occurs are more but there are parallels in the circumstances of some of the victims and the motivations of their attackers. Finding a woman alone on a garden path is now varied in cases like one in 1983 in which a former rugby league star and two other assailants beat and raped a three-months-pregnant woman when they found her alone on the Daulo Pass where she was stranded after the vehicle in which she was a passenger broke down (PNG *Post Courier* 1984a). Tiring of his lover, a young man may arrange to have her gang-raped as did a young man in the city of Lae when he forced his girlfriend to have sex with his friends after he had sex with her (PNG *Post Courier* 1984c). Another traditional form of violence—humiliating the enemy by raping their women—was echoed in the same month when a man was held by two assailants and forced to watch while a third man raped his wife in Rabaul village (PNG *Post Courier* 1984g). In the same month, a gang of about 15 youths, all under the age of 20, raped a nine-year-old girl, her mother, and another woman while the women's husbands were beaten and held at knife-point. The gang then broke into a nearby house and stole $6,000 worth of cash and goods (PNG *Post Courier* 1984b, d, e, f, g). The gangs' actions replicated attacks against the enemies' women in warfare, but in this instance there was the added twist that some of the younger rapists were trying to prove their right to membership in the gang by raping white women (see Harris 1988 on *rascal* gang entry requirements). Echoes of using rape and beatings to punish errant wives or daughters abound in the case of "Bill and Maria" (Case 2 below) in which "Bill" (all names are pseudonyms for obvious reasons) rapes his wife in a public carpark as a means of asserting his dominance and punishing her independence.

In many traditional Papua New Guinean societies, particularly in the Highlands, violence against women was part of a socio-political context in which political eminence was achieved through the control and distribution of wealth, and older men and women controlled access to land and marriage, two main ingredients in the acquisition of wealth. Marriage was important for both males and females for it was through marriage that one acquired a helpmate, produced children, and paid off one's debts to society. For men of ambition, marrying several women was virtually the only means of becoming a 'Big Man,' as women's gardening and pig-raising activities and daughters' brideprices brought men the necessary "wealth" (pigs, yams, shells) to fund networks of supporters and to outgive competitors within and outside their clans. To marry at all required the support of older men and women, who gathered together the brideprice. The process of attracting brideprice supporters began during a man's childhood and youth, when he and his peers participated in lengthy initiations designed to test and strengthen their obedience and relationships to their supporters. During initiation, young men were told many falsehoods about women as a way of keeping them away from women until their elders were ready to support their marriages. Such fabrications included depictions of women, particularly young women, as dangerous and untrustworthy creatures who were to be feared and avoided if possible (Counts 1985; Dickerson-Putman n.d.; Faithorn 1976; Gelber 1986; Zimmer-Tamakoshi 1996a). Boys learned that "over-indulgence in sexual relations with women depletes a man's vital energies leaving his body permanently exhausted and withered" (Meggitt 1964: 210) and that contact of any kind with women causes a man "to accumulate debilitating dirt in his body" (Newman 1964: 265). Young women's powers of seduction were portrayed as so great that young men were warned not to look at a young woman because "if you look at her, and she looks at you, then you will copulate" (Berndt 1962: 103; Read 1954: 867; Langness 1967: 165).

Part of the ideology initiates learned included notions of male superiority and dominance over women. Men's superiority was said to reside in their greater capacity for self-control. Initiates were taught that mature men do not act "like wild pigs" having sex indiscriminately or like "women" acting on whim and self-interest rather than promoting the social good (Gelber 1986, Chapter Two; Lindenbaum 1976: 56). Young men who were disrespectful of or doubted their elders' injunctions risked permanent bachelorhood as they depended on older men and women for brideprice help (Bowers 1965; Glasse 1969: 26; Waddell 1972: 46), and few prospective in-laws would allow their daughters to marry "dog men," men with inordinant desires for sex who spent their lives "sniffing" after other men's wives and destroying the village peace.

Promoting male solidarity, notions of male superiority allowed for effective regulation of access to and control over women. In most Papua New Guinean societies, the importance of female labor to men was such—and still is—that men have variously portrayed women as men's "hands" (Lindenbaum 1976: 59), "tradestores" (M. Strathern 1972: 99), "tractors" (Langness 1967: 172), and "capital assets" (Cook 1969: 102). Recent ethnographies suggest it was more young women's sexuality and labor than older women's that was at issue, as older women had rewards and reasons of their own to support their husbands' activities and to promote the well-being of their children's clans as well as their own (Counts 1985; Dickerson-Putman n.d.; M. Strathern 1980; Zimmer-Tamakoshi 1996a). Just as parents warned sons against the dangers of women, so too did they warn daughters against unregulated association with young men. They also taught their daughters that safety lay in cooperating with their elders to achieve fruitful marriages and honorable lives. Women—young or old—who rebelled against such beliefs or interfered with men's activities and plans, risked beatings and punitive rapes (Berndt 1962; Josephides 1985; Meggitt 1964; Read 1954; and M. Strathern 1972). Believing women to be weak-willed, husbands justified beating their wives fairly regularly as a way of getting them to fulfill their obligations to them. Also believing women to be by nature deceitful and seductive, men readily blamed rape victims for bringing the rapes on themselves. Women were thus wise to build large networks of supporters in their own and their husbands' groups who might rise to their defense in the case of rape or an overzealous wife-beater.

Today, introduced notions of women's inferiority and men's right to dominate them, men's greater access to cash incomes and women's increasing dependence on men, the weakening of parents' economic control over sons and daughters (especially those living and working in urban areas), and opportunities (primarily through education) for a few women to achieve both economic and social independence all contribute to an increasing incidence of violence against women in Papua New Guinea. Grafted onto old beliefs, the views of some Christian missions—that women be subservient to and mindful at all times of their husbands' and, much less so, their parents' wishes—and foreign media portrayals of women as erotic sex objects, docile housewives, or man-eaters, further alienate young Papua New Guineans from one another as women are shrouded in further mystifications. During my first year of fieldwork with a group of Highlanders known as the Gende, an urban gang member bragged to me about his sexual exploits which included kidnapping and raping young girls and even a married woman. In response to my shocked expression, he assured me that "They liked it! It was like it is in a James Bond movie—sexy! The woman fights with James Bond and tries to kill him and then he forces her to have sex with him and she is his woman from then on. Sometimes he kills her if she is a really bad woman." When I asked if he had killed anyone, he said he had killed the one woman because he feared she would tell her husband that he had raped her (which he denied, insisting that it wasn't rape and that "She liked it! I'm sexy!").

In the material realm, men's control of economic resources has tightened in both village and town as the proceeds from most cash crops are controlled by men, men dominate the job market, and men's educational opportunities are greater than women's. Women's dependence on men is greatest among urban women. One result of this dependence is that urban husbands—especially prosperous ones—are more likely to fight with their wives, to cheat on them, and to abuse them both physically and sexually (Ranck and Toft 1986; Rosi and Zimmer-Tamakoshi 1993; Zimmer-Tamakoshi 1993a). Several Gende women I know left husbands who beat them, drank too much, and wasted their salaries on other women, saying they'd rather marry a village husband who worked with them in the gardens and not against them in town. In the case of low-income husbands who are less attractive to other women, a wife's threat to return to the village to find another husband is taken very seriously, and such a husband is less likely even than a villager to beat his wife (Ranck and Toft 1986; Zimmer-Tamakoshi 1996b).

The weakening of parental control over the beliefs and actions of the younger generation and its relationship to violence against women can be illustrated in the experience of another Gende woman. This young woman's husband, also Gende, grew up in Port Moresby and is more western in his outlook on life than she is. Jealous of his womanizing and pressured by her relatives to get him to pay off the remaining brideprice he owes them, she has stayed in town, playing cards most of the time her husband is working and being the butt of his anger or lust whenever he is home. While she usually suffers his abuse quietly, on one occasion he forced her to have sex during her period, a heinous act in the eyes of more traditional Gende. Hysterical and threatening suicide, the young woman cut off one of her fingers with an axe, thereby demonstrating her shame. A parallel experience occurred a generation before to the girl's aunt. Married to a migrant but living in the village, the aunt was forced by her young husband—on a rare visit home—to have sex during her period. Ashamed and angry, the aunt moped around the village for a day and then left for her garden house—several miles distance from the village—where she hung herself. Unsuspecting, her family did not find her until it was too late. When the women cleaned her body for burial, they discovered menstrual blood mixed with semen smeared over her lower body and skirt as well as bruises on her arms and chest where her husband had apparently held her down forcefully. While such actions would have resulted in the young man's death in the past, the aunt's husband stayed in town, away from the girl's parents and male relatives, hiding behind the power of Australian colonial law and her parents' belief that the young man would be more useful to them if he continued working and paid them a large compensation payment for their daughter's death.

How far outside the normal realm of parental control (and protection) young persons can get is illustrated in "Violet's" case. In this case, parental pressures and absence are only part of the story. Other factors responsible for "Violet's" fate are her naive hopes for love and romance, and a sociocultural environment in which many young men no longer fear women so much as see them as sexual prey.

Case 1—"Violet"

I have written elsewhere on the motives and circumstances of young village women moving to town in the hope of attracting suitors who can pay the large brideprices expected by the women's families and fulfill women's dreams of a prosperous lifestyle (Zimmer-Tamakoshi 1993a). Living with younger kinsmen, married sisters, or even non-relatives, these girls are poorly chaperoned and often end up victims of sexual assault and bondage. One such victim was Violet. When she first came to Port Moresby, Violet stayed with an older sister and brother-in-law in a house provided by the company her brother-in-law worked for. Violet spent her days looking after her sister's children while her sister worked as a checker in a local supermarket. Evenings, Violet attended the local movie theater with girlfriends or stayed home to watch T.V. with her sister's family. As soon as she moved in with her sister, Violet became the target of her brother-in-law's unwanted sexual advances. On numerous occasions feigning illness in order to spend the day at home and threatening to kill her if she revealed what he was doing, Violet's brother-in-law had sex with Violet. When Violet became pregnant, her sister wanted to send her back to the village, but Violet feared the censure and disappointment of her parents. Violet obtained an illegal abortion and moved in with a girlfriend.

Supporting herself by prostitution and frequenting the notorious "Pink Pussycat" and other cocktail lounges, Violet continues to hope that she will one day meet and marry a "nice man" who will take her out of her misery. The types of men Violet is most likely to meet, however, are married men looking for an evening's distraction or university students preying on naive husband-hunters. The violent and sexually-charged atmosphere of both the University and the city are well-known to anyone who has spent time in either location. In a paper on the situations of women students at the University of Papua New Guinea, Joan Oliver reported that "women students had a pervasive fear of attack, harassment, threats, bashings, rape and breaking into rooms by male students or strangers" (1987: 159; see also Still and Shea's report of 1976). She further reported that because of their fears many women either drop out of school or become engaged to male protectors who not infrequently soon have the women pregnant (1987: 170).

With the proportion of female students at UPNG hovering at 10 percent, male students are in keen competition with one another for the friendship of female classmates. The competition works itself out along divisions of language and region as, for example, Chimbu *wantoks* (persons who speak Chimbu) jealously attempt to guard all Chimbu girls for themselves and Papuans (from southern Papua New Guinea) fight off any non-Papuans who might try to have a relationship with a Papuan girl. Since having sex with a female student risks reprisal from her campus *wantoks*—but not the police!—many University men satisfy their sexual desires by visiting Port Moresby's night spots and bringing back girls like Violet to the University playing fields and dorms where they have sex with them—often forced. These escapades may also bring reprisals, of course, as happened when a gang of University students raped a young girl from a nearby squatter settlement on the University football field while her younger brother was made to watch. Class antagonism as well as ethnic outrage was evident as men and boys from the settlement stalked the campus paths and housing areas for weeks after threatening to rape female students and teachers at UPNG for what the "spoiled, *bikhet* school boys" had done.

MERI WANTOK AND *MERI UNIVERSITI*

As suggested in the previous paragraph, a broad set of factors that seems conducive to high levels of violence against women in Papua New Guinea is the extra-local politics of sexuality. This set of factors includes the intersections of elite and urban sexual politics with nationalist and class interests and rhetoric. In a paper on nationalism and sexuality in Papua New Guinea, I argued that the practice of holding educated women, or *meri universiti,* responsible for all that is wrong with contemporary Papua New Guinean society is both a political maneuver to ease class and inter-ethnic tensions and jealousies in Papua New Guinea's culturally diverse society (Zimmer-Tamakoshi 1993b) and a satisfying fiction for the majority of Papua New Guineans who feel left out of "progress" and "development." Symbolizing privilege and, in some instances, sexual freedom (or anarchy), *meri universiti* and *skull meri* (school girls) are both envied for their perceived opportunities and hated as selfish betrayers of their cultural roots, while "grassroots" women and more circumspect elite women who show (or appear to show) greater concern for their kin and language groups are accorded respect as *meri wantok* and *meri bilong ples.*

There is as much diversity within the elite as without, particularly between educated men and women. Unlike their male counterparts, who come from all parts of the nation, Papua New Guinea's small class of educated elite women come almost entirely from coastal and off-shore island areas that have been long involved with the outside world. As a result, they are more likely than their male peers to come from educated and economically privileged backgrounds, and as a group they are more western in demeanor and appearance than most Papua New Guinean women. Another difference between educated men and women (and between educated women and the majority of Papua New Guinea's population) is that many educated elite women come from matrilineal societies in which women's status tends to be higher relative to many patrilineal societies and women are freer in their relations with men. On one occasion, when I was having dinner at the Bird of Paradise hotel in Goroka, I was surprised to learn that the couple at the table beside me were married (but not to each other!), were travelling together throughout the Highlands on government business, and that their spouses on Bougainville Island were satisfied with the phone calls the pair made at each stop on their tour of duty. It was difficult to imagine such easy professionalism in a partnership involving a Highlands man and woman. Rumors and jealous spouses would prevent this as Highlanders (and many other Papua New Guineans) believe it is impossible for men and women to be together for long without engaging in sex. Unusual, such behavior becomes a focus of the anger and jealousies that exist between the sexes and between class, ethnic, and racial groupings in Papua New Guinea.

Increasing the distance between elite men and themselves some elite women have opted for marriage with non-Papua New Guineans or to forgo marriage entirely. Several examples are two of the three women to ever sit as members of National Parliament and a former president of the National Council of Women, all married to or in long-term relationships with white, expatriate males. Such high-profile interracial relationships on the part of women embarrass the male leadership as the majority of Papua New Guineans see them as signs of elite immorality and weakness (e.g. elite men's inability to control their women) and collaboration of the elite with outsiders and former colonials. There have been attempts to control elite women's freedoms at all levels of Papua New Guinean society from the government down, including public censure, violence, and the refusal of full citizenship rights to foreign spouses and recurrent threats to disenfranchize the children of mixed marriages.

An example of the public scapegoating of elite or educated women is the "mini-skirt debate." The "mini-skirt debate" began back in the early seventies—prior to Papua New

Guinea's independence in 1975—with Tolai religious and political leaders in East New Britain calling for a campaign against immodest dress and claiming that school girls and young women were provoking an increasing incidence of rape and STD's in East New Britain by wearing provocative western-style clothing and makeup. The debate entered the pages of Papual New Guinea's *Post Courier* where it has continued off and on for years. The response of young women to men's condemnation of their dress is summed up in one early letter to the editor signed "Four Tolai Girls" (PNG *Post Courier* 1973a). As quoted in Hogan (1985: 56–57):

> [The young women] had no doubts that the banning of mini-skirts would have wider implications. For its writers, wearing mini-skirts signified that they wanted greater control over their lives. They accused the initiators of the circular of having political motivations—of using the issue of public morality for their own political purposes . . . and [of knowing] that with education women would be able to judge the decisions of men.

Three male Tolai students at the University of Papua New Guinea added their opinions to the debate by writing that the four Tolai girls were blindly following the dictates of western culture and wanting "to keep on 'pleasing' and 'praising' the colonial administration without stopping and asking themselves a single question" (PNG *Post Courier* 1973b).

The political advantages of focusing on the behaviors of a few elite women and suggesting that they are the root cause of problems both for women and the country as a whole are the obvious appeal to the masses, the small cost of blaming persons who do not constitute a large constituency, and the ease of following a time-honored tradition of blaming women for problems that men create or holding them up as suspicious characters bent on interfering in men's relations with one another. The anti-colonial sentiment and racial undercurrents in elite men's condemnation of elite women is also a popular cause in a nation that is trying to unite a diversity of regions and language groups into one strong nation (see Lindstrom 1992).

Two cases that illustrate the sexual politics of Papua New Guinea's educated elite and the sexual competition among men of different tribal and national backgrounds are the cases of "Bill and Maria" and "Lita." Although their cases are well-known to me, I can only sketch in the barest of details here in this brief chapter. Readers who wish to read more detailed cases are referred to Susan's Toft's harrowing account of marital violence of two couples living in Port Moresby (1985) and Andrew Strathern's grisly report on sadistic rape in Hagen (1985).

Case 2—"Bill and Maria"

I have written about Bill and Maria in a paper on love and marriage among the educated elite in Port Moresby (Rosi and Zimmer-Tamakoshi 1993). I described how this young couple—both highlanders, both finishing their education at UPNG and the parents of two young children—were suffering severe pressures and tensions in their marriage, with the result that they fought often and violently. Much of the tension was caused by inlaws: Maria's father demanding a large brideprice for his educated daughter, and Bill's village-based family critical of Maria's lack of traditional skills and anxious that the couple pay most of the brideprice and childwealth payments themselves. Raised on a government station and exposed in her religious and educational experience to western ideas about appropriate and desirable marital relations, Maria was hurt and angered by Bill's drinking, numerous infidelities, and by his toying with the idea of marrying a second wife back in the highlands to raise pigs for exchange purposes.

What I did not discuss in that paper was the fact that Bill ended most arguments with his wife by raping her, sometimes in public places. On one occasion, after coming home drunk and disheveled in the early morning hours, Bill dragged Maria out of bed and raped her—spread-eagled over a car hood in a University parking lot—while loudly accusing her of being the cause of all his troubles, of having affairs with other men, and of dressing and behaving too provocatively to be a good wife. While there was little truth to his accusations, his use of these particular criticisms to justify his brutality reveals important contradictions in the lives of educated men, contradictions arising from the complex politics of sexuality in contemporary Papua New Guinea. On many occasions, Bill expressed pride in Maria's education and her poise in social situations involving both Papua New Guineans and expatriates. At one large garden party, for example, at which scores of University professors and students had gathered, Bill and Maria joined easily into the festivities, eating, drinking, dancing, and talking with the other guests—together and singly. As the evening progressed, however, Bill began following Maria around, demanding that she join the group of women who were sitting on woven mats on the perimeter of the night's action. These women—the wives of older and more conservative faculty and staff—were dressed modestly in *meri wantok* fashion in form-hiding *meri blouses* and ankle-length *laplaps,* and spent the evening quietly talking with one another and tending small children they had brought with them to the party. Also on the fringes, but drinking heavily, were some of Bill's male relatives—several students and several older men who did maintenance work at the university. These men ogled skimpily dressed expatriate women and the more daring *meri universiti* at the same time they criticized Bill for allowing Maria to wear a short, tight skirt and form-revealing blouse.

At the University club and at parties, I many times heard men slander particular women, their clothing choices, and their alleged sexual habits. If the women were not related to the men, they would also discuss ways of going about seducing or raping the woman. Add to this the disapproving and often envious statements of men's lesser-educated kin—telling their more advantaged brothers to avoid marrying women who waste money on makeup and fancy clothes like spoiled white women at the same time as they express their desire to have sex with such women—and a situation arises in which it seems impossible for men like Bill to have it both ways—a wife who is attractive in new and sophisticated ways but one who does not attract the desire or censure of men who are her husband's associates, friends, relatives, or enemies.

Case 3—"Lita"

Further illuminating the sexual side of interethnic and interracical politics in urban Papua New Guinea, Lita's case is interesting because she is one of a small number of Papua New Guinean women who have discarded traditional relationships in order to express themselves in new and unusual ways. Pretty, bright, and poised in the presence of men of all ages and nationalities, Lita was engaged to a middle-aged expatriate when I first met her in one of the classes I was teaching at UPNG. Spurning her age-mates and vocal about her preference for white men—whom she claimed were gentler and more supportive of women's interests (for similar sentiments see the case of "Barbara" in Rosi and Zimmer-Tamakoshi 1993)—Lita accepted the gifts and attentions of her lover while at the same time playing the field at local discos and bars frequented by expatriate and Papua New Guinean businessmen and leaders.

Halfway through the semester, Lita began a secret love affair with one of her teachers at UPNG—an expatriate who was much younger than her fiance. When the affair became public knowledge and both expatriate lovers were spying on the other and attempting to engage the sympathies and help of Lita's friends, Lita's *wantoks* abducted her from apartment, severely beat and raped her, warning her to cease having affairs with either man and to choose someone from her own ethnic and racial background to marry. When I learned about the attack from some of Lita's classmates, I was dismayed by their lack of sympathy for her. Saying that she should not have embarrassed her *wantoks* and other Papua New Guineans by choosing white lovers over black, the majority felt she had only gotten what she deserved and that she was lucky her *wantoks* had not killed her.

Lita's social background is similar to Maria's in that both women were raised in urban or peri-urban settings by parents who are employed in the government sector and who—in their commitment to a more western, or "modern" ethic—have raised their daughters to expect more egalitarian and open relations with men than is the norm in most parts of Papua New Guinea. Unfortunately for both young women, most of their *wantoks* do not agree and feel that the young women's "immodest" and "loose" behavior is injurious to ethnic and racial pride. Furthermore, both young women's *wantoks* are for the most part far less prosperous than either young woman's family, and there are economic and class tensions to contend with. When Lita informed her parents she was engaged to a foreigner, they at first protested it would never work. Promised a large brideprice, however, they and many of their village *wantoks* allowed that the marriage might be a good idea. Lita's *wantoks* at UPNG, however, took her engagement as an insult to them as more suitable partners, and when she compounded the insult by having affairs with two expatriates at the same time, it was too much to bear. In Maria's case, while her father and brothers have threatened to have her husband arrested for his repeated brutality, her *wantoks* side with Bill, contending that Maria is at least partly to blame for his behavior and that her husband and father should see to it that she conform to the clothing and behavioral norms of most highlanders rather than some small segment of PNG and expatriate society.

RAPE AND DOMESTIC VIOLENCE AS "WOMEN'S ISSUES"

As the foregoing suggests, violence against women has long been accepted in many Papua New Guinean societies as a legitimate means of controlling women and expressing or affecting men's relations with other men. From studies done in the 1980s by the Law Reform Commission (Toft, ed. 1985, 1986b) and other ethnographic sources we know that in the past both women and men agreed to men's right to chastise women with beatings and sometimes rape. Today, when some women's increased opportunities for self-expression and economic independence are perceived as threatening men's relations and the general good, many men and even many women consider violence to be an acceptable "comeuppance" for young women like Maria and Lita, and a means of preserving ethnic and national unity and pride. Nevertheless, there has been a sea change in women's attitudes toward violence against them and not only amongst elite women. Since the Second World War and the expansion of Papua New Guinea's towns and cities, urban dwellers have voiced their concerns over high rates of urban crime and domestic violence. Urban women have been especially concerned with the ever-present threat of pack rape and domestic violence associated with urban men's greater alcohol consumption, male sexual jealousy, and money problems (Toft 1986a: 12–14). In 1981, the National Council of Women passed a resolution stating that crimes against women seemed to be increasing and that there were inadequate controls to protect women. The Council then requested the government to investigate the problem, and on August 18, 1982, the Papua New Guinea Minister for Justice passed to the Law Reform Commission a Reference on Domestic Violence (Toft, ed. 1986a). The ensuing studies revealed many things about the nature, extent, and causes of domestic violence in Papua New Guinea as well as changing attitudes toward violence against women. Positive correlations were shown to exist, for example, between a decreasing acceptance of domestic violence and a person's sex, degree of urbanization, and levels of education and income (Toft 1986a: 23–26). Significantly, both urban low-income women and elite women are far less prepared than rural women to admit fault in failing to meet obligations to their husbands or to believe they "deserve" occasional beatings. Although the majority of urban men—especially educated men—also say it is unacceptable to hit wives, their apparent change in attitude is not reflected in their behavior.

Statistics are a weak measure of reality, however, and it is in case studies that we learn the depth of experience and motivations behind women's change of attitudes. In a study of two cases of marital violence in Port Moresby, Toft (1985) shows how men's violence against women interferes with the women's abilities, needs, and desires to function well in urban environments. One informant, "Rose," was regularly hit by her husband, who also phoned her at work in jealous piques and sometimes beat her so badly she could not work or take care of their young children. In a paper on Gende women in town, I make the point that while many urban women are technically unemployed, they fulfill many obligations to their village kin and in-laws and must be free to move about the urban environment without fear (Zimmer-Tamakoshi 1996b). Women in low-income households, for example, are almost always in town to protect their husbands' incomes from dissipation (e.g., alcohol, cards, prostitutes) and to see that their children get a better education than is always possible in the village. To achieve these ends, women meet husbands at their place of work on pay day for the handing over of the pay packet, they search the urban markets and stores for bargains to make their husbands' small incomes pay for both household and extra-household exchange demands, and they do without their school-age children's help in the daily round of collecting firewood and water for use in substandard squatter settlements at the edge of town. Such women have little patience with violent husbands whose utility to them is marginal at best. Women with more education have potentially greater opportunities to live life differently than their mothers' generation. Often, however, their desires and potential are not realized as violence, and fear of violence keeps them out of work. Female graduates of Papua New Guinea's teachers' colleges, for example, rarely teach for more than a year or so after graduating, even though they express, during their training, a strong desire and ability to be career teachers. A major constraint against their fulfilling their self-expectations is the threat of male violence against them, causing many to flee into early marriages and the comparative safety of compliance with men's wishes (Wormald and Crossley 1988).

Women's growing sense of gender oppression and their anger over their wasted potential reveals itself in diverse and often unusual ways. Young women like "Violet," impregnated by her brother-in-law and more or less abandoned by her family, may turn to prostitution to earn a living and make men pay for what they would otherwise take anyway. In urban contexts where women and girls have few options, "selling their bodies" to husbands or customers makes economic sense however much self-violence its represents (see also Borrey 1994). Cases like "Donna's" (see below), in which women are packraped because they represent a threat to men's interests or, as in this case, a threat to Papua New Guinean pride, are more and more seen as deliberate assaults against women as a whole and not individual women.

Case 4—"Donna"

Donna was a successful Filipina business woman married to one of the expatriate lecturers at UPNG and living on campus in one of the homes provided for UPNG faculty and their families. Resentment against expatriate women is high in Papua New Guinea, because most expatriate women live enviable lifestyles and many fill full- or part-time positions in the work force that Papua New Guineans feel should be given to Papua New Guinean workers, especially male workers. Openly critical of what she felt were lax working habits on the part of her Papua New Guinean employees, Donna earned even more enmity than usual.

Sometime in the late '80s, Donna and her husband were eating dinner when a gang of rascals broke through their dining room windows, beat the husband, and abducted Donna. Taking Donna by car to a remote location, the gang raped her and then left her, naked and badly injured. After crawling and stumbling back to the University, Donna left the country to be joined soon after by her husband. Newspapers and gossip revealed that Donna had been the victim of a pay-back rape for her racial slurs and her successful competition against Papua New Guinean businessmen. While her rape shocked the University community, particularly the expatriates, many persons—expatriate and Papua New Guinean, male and female—blamed Donna for being too outspoken and too obviously successful for a female expatriate business woman.

As time went on, however, public outcry began to divide itself along sexual rather than racial lines, and all women were more fearful as they went about their daily activities. In another much-reported case in the city of Lae, several Papua New Guinean men raped and then murdered a respected and well-liked white helicopter pilot when the man she was trying to sell her car to drove her to a secluded place where he was joined by the other men. During the trial, there were demonstrations throughout Papua New Guinea in favor of a strong penalty—"Death," *"Katim bol bilong ol"* ("cut their balls off!")—and when the defendants were let off with light sentences there was a spontaneous demonstration of several thousand women in Port Moresby protesting "men's disregard for women."

While in the mid-1980s Papua New Guinea's male-dominated government supported the Law Reform Commission studies and a subsequent public awareness campaign on violence against women, rape and domestic violence are now "women's issues" in Papua New Guinea and no longer even a small part of male politicians' rhetoric. This shift became brutally apparent in 1987 when an all-male Parliament booed Rose Kekedo and other women from the floor when they tried to present the Law Reform Commission's interim report on domestic violence (*The Times of Papua New Guinea* 1992). In 1987 and since there have been no women in Papua New Guinea's Parliament. Papua New Guinea has never had more than a few women in higher government positions, and at most there have been only three Papua New Guinean women in Parliament at the same time (1977–1982). Significantly, none of these women ever felt the need to run a feminist campaign, until recently that is. Since 1987, as the numbers of female candidates and winners continues to shrink (Wormald 1992), female leaders such as former Parliamentarians Josephine Abaijah and Nahau Rooney have taken public positions on women's issues, focusing most on the concerns of "grassroots" women as crucial to Papua New Guinea's future and, of course, their own re-election. Rape and domestic violence top the list of concerns, however, as they affect all women (Waram 1992a and 1992b). Women's organizations have joined the campaign against violence with women leaders in Port Moresby choosing the theme "Violence Against Women" for their May 1993 International Women's Day Celebration (*The Times of Papua New Guinea* 1993b) and provincial women's leaders in East New Britain embarking on a campaign against violence and making plans to open a women's crisis center by 1994 (*The Times of Papua New Guinea* 1993a).

Similar situations exist in other Pacific countries where violence against women is less prevalent but nonetheless serious and feared by women who see it destroying their families and any hopes they have for establishing new opportunities and relationships for themselves (Dominy 1990; Lateef 1990; Ralston 1993; Trask 1989; Zimmer-Tamakoshi 1993b and 1995). Women in Vanuatu and the Solomon Islands have been especially vocal, decrying the effects of colonialism and modernity on their societies (most notably alcohol abuse, consumerism, gambling, and class and sex inequalities), but, above all, the impact of male dominance on women's hopes and aspirations (see Billy, Lulei, and Sipolo 1983;

Griffen 1976; Molisa 1983, 1987, 1989). Asserting what it is that women want, Vanuatu poet and feminist Grace Mera Molisa both unites and speaks for women throughout the Pacific in her poem "Colonised People" (1987: 9–13), part of which is reprinted here:

> Women too
> have a right
> to be Free.
>
> Free to think
> Free to express
> Free to choose
> Free to love
> and be loved
> as Woman Vanuatu.

She does not, however, any more than my argument has, lay the blame for women's plight simply on the shoulders of men. While she blasts male leaders for scapegoating female politicians who threaten their grasp of power in "Hilda Lini" (1987: 26–27), she also condemns women for envying other women's successes and going along with men's definitions of things in "Delightful Acquiescence" (1989: 24):

> Half of Vanuatu
> is still colonised
> by her self.
>
> Any woman
> showing promise
> is clouted
> into acquiescence.

REFERENCES

Berndt, Ronald M. 1962. *Excess and Restraint: Social Control Among a New Guinea Mountain People.* Chicago: University of Chicago Press.

Billy, A., H. Lulei, and J. Sipolo, eds. 1983. *"Mi Mere": Poetry and Prose by Solomon Islands Women Writers.* Honiara.

Borrey, Anou. 1994. "Youth, Unemployment, and Crime." Paper presented at the National Employment Summit, 11–12 May, Port Moresby.

Bowers, Nancy. 1965. "Permanent Bachelorhood in the Upper Kaugel Valley of Highland New Guinea." *Oceania* 36: 27–37.

Bradley, Christine. 1982. "Tolai Women and Development." University College of London. Unpublished Ph.D. Thesis.

———. 1985. "Attitudes and Practices Relating to Marital Violence Among the Tolai of East New Britain." In Susan Toft (ed). *Domestic Violence in Papua New Guinea,* pp. 32–71. Port Moresby: Papua New Guinea Law Reform Commission Monograph No. 3.

———. 1994. "Why Male Violence Against Women is a Development Issue: Reflections from Papua New Guinea." In Miranda Davies (ed). *Women and Violence,* pp. 10–26. London: Zed Books, Ltd.

Brown, Paula. 1969. "Marriage in Chimbu." In R.M. Glasse and M.J. Meggitt (eds.). *Pigs, Pearlshells, and Women: Marriage in the New Guinea Highlands,* pp. 77–95. New Jersey: Prentice Hall, Inc.

Chowning, Ann. 1985. "Kove Women and Violence: The Context of Wife-Beating in a West New Britain Society." In Susan Toft (ed.). *Domestic Violence in Papua New Guinea,* pp. 72–91. Port Moresby: Papua New Guinea Law Reform Commission Monograph No. 3.

Cook, E. A. 1969. "Marriage Among the Manga." In R.M. Glasse and M.J. Meggitt (eds.). *Pigs, Pearlshells, and Women: Marriage in the New Guinea Highlands,* pp. 96–116. New Jersey: Prentice Hall, Inc.

Counts, Dorothy Ayres. 1985. "*Tamparonga:* 'The Big Women' of Kaliai." In J.K. Brown, Virginia Kerns, and Contributors. *In Her Prime: A New View of Middle-Aged Women,* pp. 49–64. South Hadley, MA: Bergin and Garvey Publishers, Inc.

Counts, Dorothy Ayers, Judith K. Brown, and Jacquelyn C. Campbell, eds. 1992. *Sanctions and Sanctuary: Cultural Perspectives on the Beating of Wives.* Boulder: Westview Press.

Davies, Miranda, ed. 1994. *Women and Violence: Realities and Responses Worldwide.* London: Zed Books Ltd.

Dickerson-Putman, Jeanette. n.d. "From Pollution to Empowerment: Women, Age, and Power Among the Bena Bena of the Eastern Highlands." In J. Dickerson-Putman (ed). *Women, Age, and Influence,* under review by *Pacific Studies.*

Dinnen, Sinclair. 1993. "Big Men, Small Men and Invisible Women." *Australian and New Zealand Journal of Criminology* (March 1993) 26: 19–34.

———. 1996. "Law, Order, and State." In Laura Zimmer-Tamakoshi (ed.). *Modern PNG Society.* Bathurst, Australia: Crawford House Press.

Dominy, Michelle. 1990. "Maori Sovereignty: A Feminist Invention of Tradition." In J. Linnekin and L. Poyer (eds.). *Cultural Identity and Ethnicity in the Pacific,* pp. 237–257. Honolulu: University of Hawaii Press.

Faithorn, Elizabeth. 1976. "Women as Persons: Aspects of Female Life and Male-Female Relations Among the Kafe." In P. Brown and G. Buchbinder (eds.). *Man and Woman in the New Guinea Highlands,* pp. 86–95. Washington, DC: American Anthropological Association.

Finkelhor, David and Kersti Yllo. 1985. *License to Rape: Sexual Abuse of Wives.* New York: Holt, Rinehart, and Winston.

Gelber, Marilyn G. 1986. *Gender and Society in the New Guinea Highlands: An Anthropological Perspective on Antagonism Toward Women.* Boulder, CO: Westview Press, Inc.

Glasse, R. M. 1969. "Marriage in South Fore." In R.M. Glasse and M.J. Meggitt (eds.). *Pigs, Pearlshells, and Women: Marriage in the New Guinea Highlands,* pp. 16–37. Englewood Cliffs, NJ: Prentice Hall, Inc.

Goodale, Jane C. 1980. "Gender, Sexuality, and Marriage: A Kaulong Model of Nature and Culture." In C. MacCormack and M. Strathern (eds.). *Nature, Culture and Gender,* pp. 119–142. Cambridge: Cambridge University Press.

Griffen, V., ed. 1976. *Women Speak Out! A Report of the Pacific Women's Conference, October 27–November 2.* Suva.

Harris, Bruce. 1988. *The Rise of Rascalism—Action and Reaction in the Evolution of Rascal Gangs.* Port Moresby: Papua New Guinea Institute of Applied Social and Economic Research.

Herman, Dianne F. 1989. "The Rape Culture." In Jo Freeman (ed.). *Women: A Feminist Perspective,* pp. 20–44. Mountain View, California: Mayfield Publishing Company.

Hogan, Evelyn. 1985. "Controlling the Bodies of Women: Reading Gender Ideologies in Papua New Guinea." In Maev O'Collins et al. *Women in Politics in Papua New Guinea,* pp. 54–71. Working Paper No. 6. Canberra Department of Political and Social Change, Australian National University.

Jenkins, Carol (and The National Sex and Reproduction Research Team). 1994. *National Study of Sexual and Reproductive Knowledge and Behaviour in Papua New Guinea.* Papua New Guinea Institute of Medical Research Monograph 10.

Josephides, Lisette. 1985. *The Production of Inequality: Gender and Exchange Among the Kewa.* London: Tavistock.

———. n.d. "Gendered Discourses of Tradition and Change." Unpublished paper.

Langness, L. 1967. "Sexual Antagonism in the New Guinea Highlands: A Bena Bena Example." *Oceania* 37: 61–177.

———. 1969. "Marriage in Bena Bena." In R.M. Glasse and M.J. Meggitt (eds.). *Pigs, Pearlshells, and Women: Marriage in the New Guinea Highlands,* pp. 38–55. Englewood Cliffs, NJ: Prentice Hall, Inc.

———. 1974. "Ritual, Power, and Male Dominance." *Ethos* 2: 189–212.

Lateef, S. 1990. "Current and Future Implications of the Coups for Women in Fiji." *The Contemporary Pacific* 2 (1): 113–130.

Lindenbaum, Shirley. 1976. "A Wife is the Hand of Man." In P. Brown and G. Buchbinder (eds.). *Man and Woman in the New Guinea Highlands,* pp. 54–62. Washington, DC: American Anthropological Association.

Lindstrom, Lamont. 1992. *Pasin Tumbuna: Cultural Traditions and National Identity in Papua New Guinea.* Culture and Communications Working Paper. Honolulu: Institute of Culture and Communications, East-West Center.

Meggitt, Mervyn J. 1964. "Male-Female Relationships in the Highlands of Australian New Guinea." *American Anthropologist* 66: 204–224.

Mitchell, William E. 1992. "Why Wape Men Don't Beat Their Wives: Constraints Toward Domestic Tranquility in a New Guinea Society." In Counts, Brown, and Campbell (eds.). *Sanctions and Sanctuary: Cultural Perspectives on the Beating of Wives,* pp. 89–98. Boulder: Westview Press.

Molisa, Grace Mera. 1983. *Black Stone.* Suva.

———. 1987. *Colonised People.* Port Vila, Vanuatu.

———. 1989. *Black Stone II.* Port Vila, Vanuatu.

Newman, Philip L. 1964. "Religious Belief and Ritual in a New Guinea Society." *American Anthropologist* 66: 257–272.

Oliver, Joan. 1987. "Women Students at the University of Papua New Guinea in 1985." In S. Stratigos and P.J. Hughes (eds). *The Ethics of Development: Women as Unequal Partners in Development,* pp. 156–172. Port Moresby: University of Papua New Guinea Press.

Parkinson, R. 1907. *Thirty Years in the South Seas* (trans. by N.C. Barry from *Dreissig Jahre in der Sudsee*). Stuttgart: Strecker and Schroder. Typescript in the Papua New Guinea Collection, University of Papua New Guinea.

PNG Post Courier. 1973a. "Four Tolai Girls." June 13.

———. 1973b. "Three Mataungan Students." June 28.

———. 1984a. "Gang Rapist Jailed for Seven Years." April 13, p. 9.

———. 1984b. "Pack Rape! Horror Attack on Two Families." October 4, p. 1.

———. 1984c. "Two More Attacks." October 23, p. 2.

———. 1984d. "Another Youth is Charged." October 25, p. 2.

———. 1984e. "Badili Horror: Sixth Youth Charged." October 26, p. 2.

———. 1984f. "Badili Attack Man Charged." October 30, p. 2.

———. 1984g. "Young Girl Raped." October 31, p. 2.

Ralston, Caroline. 1993. "Maori Women and the Politics of Tradition: What Roles and Power Did, Do, and Should Maori Women Exercise?" *The Contemporary Pacific* 5 (1): 23–44.

Ranck, Stephen and Susan Toft. 1986. "Domestic Violence in an Urban Context with Rural Comparisons." In S. Toft (ed.). *Domestic Violence in Urban Papua New Guinea,* pp. 3–51. Law Reform Commission of Papua New Guinea, Occasional Paper No. 19.

Read, Kenneth E. 1952. "Nama Cult of the Central Highlands, New Guinea." *Oceania* 23: 1–25.

———. 1954. "Marriage Among the Gahuka-Gama of the Eastern Central Highlands, New Guinea." *South Pacific* 7: 864–871.

Riches, David, ed. 1986. *The Anthropology of Violence.* Oxford: Basil Blackwell.

Rosi, Pamela and Laura Zimmer-Tamakoshi. 1993. "Love and Marriage Among the Educated Elite in Port Moresby." In R. Marksbury (ed.). *The Business of Marriage: Transformations in Oceanic Matrimony,* pp. 175–204. The University of Pittsburgh Press.

Russell, Diana E. H. 1984. *Sexual Exploitation.* Beverly Hills, CA: Sage Publications.

Still, K. and J. Shea. 1976. *Something's Got to be Done So We Can Survive in This Place: The Problem of Women Students at UPNG.* Education Research Unit Research Report 20. Port Moresby: University of Papua New Guinea.

Strathern, A. 1985. "Rape in Hagen." In S. Toft (ed.). *Domestic Violence in Papua New Guinea,* pp. 134–140. Law Reform Commission of Papua New Guinea Monograph No. 3.

———. 1993. "Violence and Political Change in Papua New Guinea." *Pacific Studies* 16 (4): 41–60.

Strathern, M. 1972. *Women in Between: Female Roles in a Male World, Mt. Hagen, New Guinea.* London: Seminar Press.

———. 1980. "No Nature, No Culture: The Hagen Case." In C. MacCormack and M. Strathern (eds.). *Nature, Culture and Gender,* pp. 174–222. Cambridge: Cambridge University Press.

The Times of Papua New Guinea. 1992. "The Status of Women in Papua New Guinea." 9 January, p. 19.

———. 1993a. "East New Britain Women Embark on Campaign Against Violence." 4 March, p. 5.

———. 1993b. "Women Celebrate Their Day on Monday." 4 March, p. 2.

Toft, Susan. 1985. "Marital Violence in Port Moresby: Two Urban Case Studies." In S. Toft (ed.). *Domestic Violence in Papua New Guinea,* pp. 14–31. Papua New Guinea Law Reform Commission Monograph No. 3.

Toft, Susan, ed. 1985. *Domestic Violence in Papua New Guinea.* Papua New Guinea Law Reform Commission Monograph No. 3.

———. 1986a. *Domestic Violence in Urban Papua New Guinea.* Papua New Guinea Law Reform Commission Occasional Paper No. 19.

———. 1986b. *Marriage in Papua New Guinea.* Papua New Guinea Law Reform Commission Monograph No. 4.

Toft, Susan and S. Bonnell, eds. 1985. *Marriage and Domestic Violence in Rural Papua New Guinea.* Papua New Guinea Law Reform Commission Occasional Paper No. 18.

Trask, Haunani-Kay. 1989. "Fighting the Battle of Double Colonization: The View of an Hawaiian Feminist." *Ethnies* 8–9–10 (1): 61–67.

United Nations. 1989. *Violence Against Women in the Family.* Vienna: Centre for Social Development and Humanitarian Affairs.

Waddell, Eric. 1972. *The Mound Builders: Agricultural Practices, Environment and Society in the Central Highlands of New Guinea.* Seattle: University of Washington Press.

Waram, Ruth. 1992a. "Violence: A Crime Against Women." *Papua New Guinea Post Courier* 13 February, 24–25.

———. 1992b. "Women's Day Snubbed, While Many Centres Go Without Celebrations." *Papua New Guinea Post Courier* 26 March, 25 and 28.

Wormald, Eileen. 1992. "1992 National Election—Women Candidates in the Election." *The Times of Papua New Guinea* 28 May, 23–26.

Wormald, Eileen and Anne Crossley, eds. 1988. *Women and Education in Papua New Guinea and the South Pacific.* Port Moresby: University of Papua New Guinea Press.

Zimmer, Laura J. 1990. "Sexual Exploitation and Male Dominance in Papua New Guinea." In a special issue on *Human Sexuality. Point* 14: 250–267.

Zimmer-Tamakoshi, Laura. 1993a. "Bachelors, Spinsters, and 'Pamuk Meris.'" In R. Marksbury (ed.). *The Business of Marriage: Transformations in Oceanic Matrimony,* pp. 83–104. University of Pittsburgh Press.

———. 1993b. "Nationalism and Sexuality in Papua New Guinea." *Pacific Studies* 16 (4): 61–97.

———. 1995. "Passion, Poetry, and Cultural Politics in the South Pacific." In R. Feinberg and L. Zimmer-Tamakoshi (eds.). *Politics of Culture in the Pacific Islands,* special issue *Ethnology* 34 (2 & 3): 113–128.

———. 1996a. "Empowered Women." In W. Donner and J. Flanagan (eds.). *Social Organization and Cultural Aesthetics: Essays in Honor of William H. Davenport,* pp. 84–101. University of Pennsylvania Press.

———. 1996b. "Papua New Guinean Women in Town: Housewives, Homemakers, and Household Managers." In L. Zimmer-Tamakoshi (ed.). *Modern PNG Society.* Bathurst, Australia: Crawford House Press.

———. n.d. "Patterns of Culture in the Tower of Babel: Letters from Port Moresby, Papua New Guinea." Accepted for publication in *Journal de la Societe des Oceanistes.*

FILM LIST

BIOLOGY, GENDER, AND HUMAN EVOLUTION

Jane Goodall Studies of the Chimpanzee. "Tool Using." National Geographic Society. 1978. 24 minutes.
Describes how young chimpanzees play with objects and how this play prepares them for making and using tools as adults.

Among the Wild Chimpanzees. National Geographic Society. 1984. 59 minutes.
Features Jane Goodall as researcher and examines infant chimpanzee development and behavior, male-female dominance, and hunting.

Ax Fight. Penn State. 1971. 30 minutes.
Portrays conflict between hosts and visitors among the Yanomamo.

The Two Brains. PBS Brain Series. 1984. 60 minutes.
Examines the unique functions of each hemisphere of the human brain and the possible effects of culture on the brain. Describes differences between male and female brains that seem to result from sex hormones and shows how some brain abnormalities may chemically affect the brain.

Sex and Money. Filmakers Library. 1989. 50 minutes.
Focuses on transsexual individuals in the United States and the Netherlands. Dr. John Money addresses differences between gender identity and gender roles. Contains explicit sexual material.

Argument About a Marriage. DER. 1966. 18 minutes.
Views a conflict that arises between two !Kung bands concerning the legitimacy of a marriage, discusses a charge of infidelity, and illustrates use of verbal aggression among the !Kung.

Sex and Gender with Evelyn Fox Keller. PBS Video. 1990. 30 minutes.
Evelyn Fox Keller, a theoretical physicist and feminist historian of science, describes how gender plays a significant role in Western scientific theory and method.

DOMESTIC WORLDS AND PUBLIC WORLDS

Kypseli: Women and Men Apart—A Divided Reality. University of California, Berkeley. 1976. 40 minutes.
Examines gender roles in a Greek peasant village.

Afghan Women. University of California, Berkeley. 1975. 17 Minutes.
Examines the role of women in a rural community in northern Afghanistan.

Some Women of Marrakech. Granada Disappearing World Series. Thomas Howe Associates. 1976. 55 minutes. Re-edited for Odyssey, 1981.
Discusses the importance of marriage and family for women in Morocco and shows the impact of religion and class on women's lives.

Women, Work and Babies. NBC production. 1985. 60 minutes.
Discusses gender ideology in the United States and problems of working mothers.

The Double Day. IWFP. Cinema Guild. 1975. 51 minutes.
Discusses burdens of working women in Latin America.

Clotheslines. Filmakers Library. 1981. 32 minutes.
Shows the love-hate relationship that women have with cleaning the family clothes.

Not Baking. University of California. 1995. 9 minutes.
A woman explores her inability to bake. Archival footage demonstrates the tremendous force of America's baking tradition.

THE CULTURAL CONSTRUCTION OF GENDER AND PERSONHOOD

A Man, When He is a Man. Women Make Movies. 1982. 66 minutes.
Set in Costa Rica, this film illuminates the so-

cial climate and cultural traditions that nurture machismo and allow the domination of women to flourish in Latin America.

Sexism in Language: Thief of Honor, Shaper of Lies. University of California. 1995. 29 minutes.

Analyzes the gender bias that permeates everyday language.

Small Happiness. Women of a Chinese Village. New Day Films. VHS Video cassette. 1984. 58 minutes.

Provides historical perspective on marriage, birth control, work, and daily life.

The Women's Olamal: The Organization of a Maasai Fertility Ceremony. Documentary Educational Resources. 1984. 115 minutes.

Presents a picture of women's lives in the male-dominated society of the Maasai in Kenya.

Maasai Manhood. ISHI. 1983. 53 minutes.

Describes a male initiation ritual among pastoral Maasai of Kenya.

Rivers of Sand. University of California, Berkeley. 1975. 83 minutes.

Portrays male supremacy among the Hamar of Ethiopia, including male initiation.

Killing Us Softly. Cambridge Documentary Films. 1979. 30 minutes.

Details psychological and sexual themes in American advertising.

Slim Hopes. Media Education Foundation. 1995. 30 minutes.

Offers a new way to think about eating disorders such as anorexia and bulimia and provides a critical perspective on the social impact of advertising. New film by Jean Kilbourne.

Men's Lives. New Day Films. 1974. 43 minutes.

Discusses American concepts of masculinity and links gender ideology, power, and capitalism.

Beyond Macho. Films for the Humanities and Sciences. 1985. 26 minutes.

Explores roles for men that have evolved in response to feminism and economic changes in the United States through an examination of the lives of two men, one a nurse and the other a "house-husband."

Men and Masculinity. OASIS. 1990. 30 minutes.

Covers the thirteenth National Conference on Men and Masculinity and discusses a broad range of men's movement issues in the United States, including antipornography activism, challenges to homophobia, and domestic violence.

Stale Roles and Tight Buns. OASIS. 1988. 29 minutes.

Uses advertising images to show how men are stereotyped in the media and how myths develop that limit men's and women's roles.

Becoming a Woman in Okrika. Filmakers Library. 1990. 27 minutes.

A coming-of-age ritual in a village in the Niger Delta.

Surname Viet Given Name Nam. Women Make Movies. 1989. 108 minutes.

Explores the multiplicity of identities of Vietnamese women in Vietnam and in California.

Faces of Change: Andean Women. University of California, Berkeley. 1975. 19 minutes.

Describes cultural ideals of female subservience among Aymara.

Dear Lisa: A Letter to My Sister. New Day Films. 1990. 45 minutes.

Based on interviews with 13 women and girls from various backgrounds, the film explores women's roles in the United States in relation to childhood, play, work, parenting, and family culture. It also touches on questions of body image, the "second shift," self-esteem, and sexual assault.

Period Piece. Jay Rosenblatt Film Library. 30 minutes.

Focuses on girls' first menstrual periods. Women aged 8–84 who are from diverse cultural backgrounds describe their experiences with first menstruation. Their stories expose culturally-constructed ideas about womanhood, family dynamics, and attitudes toward menstruation.

The Smell of Burning Ants. Film Arts Foundation. 1995. 21 minutes.

The film depicts the often painful aspects of male socialization in the west.

Monday's Girls. Women Make Movies. 1993. 50 minutes.

Documents the rite of passage to adulthood of two Nigerian girls.

Juggling Gender. Women Make Movies. 1992. 27 minutes.

Through a focus on a bearded lesbian performer, the film explores the fluidity of gender and the construction of gender identity.

CULTURE AND SEXUALITY

Women Like Us. Women Make Movies. 1990. 49 minutes.

Portrays older lesbian women in Great Britain, their feelings and lifestyles, and discusses the implications of sexual orientation for family and work relations.

On Being Gay. TRB Productions. 1986. 80 minutes.
Through a monologue by Brian McNaught, this film addresses myths about homosexuality and such topics as growing up gay in a straight world, Bible-based bigotry, stereotypes, transvestitism, transsexualism, and AIDS.

Metamorphosis: Man into Woman. Filmakers Library. 1990. 58 minutes.
Features a transsexual confronting gender stereotypes in society.

Man Oh Man—Growing Up Male in America. New Day Films, Inc. 1987. 19 minutes.
Focuses on being a man in contemporary American society, with an emphasis on the difficulties of living up to cultural ideals of manhood.

Choosing Children. Cambridge Documentary.
Explores three situations in which lesbians have had children.

Masai Manhood. Films Incorporated Video. 1983. 52 minutes.
Focuses on the lives of Masai men and the Eunoto ceremony that marks their transition from warrior to elder.

De Mujer a Mujer. Women Make Movies. 1995. 46 minutes.
Latina women discuss their experiences and feelings about sexuality and maturation.

Friends and Lovers. World Cultures on Film and Video, University of California. 1994. 28 minutes.
Gay men discuss their feelings about intimacy in an age of AIDS and challenge our assumptions about relationships and sexuality.

EQUALITY AND INEQUALITY: THE SEXUAL DIVISION OF LABOR AND GENDER STRATIFICATION

Hunters and Gatherers

N!ai: The Story of a !Kung Woman. Penn State University. 1980. 59 minutes.
Features the biography of a !Kung woman from early childhood to middle age and the impact of colonial penetration on her life.

The Warao. University of California, Berkeley. 1978. 57 minutes.
Ethnographic account of division of labor among the Warao of the Orinoco River Delta in Venezuela.

Before We Knew Nothing. World Cultures on Film and Video, U. of California. 1989. 62 minutes.
An exploration of the roles and activities of Ashaninka women in the Amazon rain forest.

Horticulturalists

Seasons of the Navajo. PBS Video. Peace River Films. 1984. 60 minutes.
Presents one family's kinship with the earth through seasons, touching briefly on Navajo matriliny and women's work and craft responsibilities.

Summer of Loucheux: A Portrait of a Northern Indian Family. New Day Films. 1983. 28 minutes.
Portrays a young woman who joins her family at their summer fishing camp.

The Trobriand Islanders of Papua New Guinea. Films Incorporated Video. 1990. 52 minutes.
Focuses on the distribution of women's wealth after a death and the month of celebration following the yam harvest.

Agriculturalists

Luisa Torres. Chip Taylor Communications. 1980. 28 minutes.
The recollections of a Hispanic woman in northern New Mexico; discusses division of labor, marriage, use of medicinal plants, and other aspects of daily life.

Kheturni Bayo: North Indian Farm Women. Penn State. 1980. 19 minutes.
Examines the roles and the duties of the women in a typical extended family of landowning peasants in Gujarat, India.

Pastoralists

Masai Women. Thomas Howe Associates. 1983. 52 minutes.
Examines the role of women among pastoralists in Kenya.

Women of the Toubou. University of California, Berkeley. 1974. 25 minutes.
Examines gender roles among nomads of the Sahara.

Boran Women. University of California, Berkeley. 1975. 18 minutes.
Shows women's daily work in Kenyan society, including caring for cattle, milk storage, and child care.

Deep Hearts. University of California, Berkeley. 1980. 53 minutes.
Documentary on the Bororo Fulani in Niger, Africa. Focuses on ritual dances in which men compete in a beauty contest.

Miscellaneous

Asante Market Women. Penn State. 1983. 52 minutes.
Power of Ghanaian market women from a matrilineal and polygynous society.

From the Shore. Indiana University. 1989.
Explores the formation of a fishing cooperative among women in the coastal village of Shimoni, Kenya, in defiance of the traditional roles of women.

With These Hands. Filmakers Library. 1987. 33 minutes.
Shows how African women are overworked, how cash crops interfere with their food production, and how their political empowerment might overcome constraints to agricultural production.

Shunka's Story. University of California, Berkeley. 1977. 20 minutes.
Portrait of a Tzotzil Maya woman in Mexico, conveying her thoughts about her life, culture, and children.

Maids and Madams. Filmakers Library. 1985. 52 minutes.
Describes the plight of Black female domestic servants in South Africa and analyzes the relationship between gender, class, and apartheid.

A Kiss on the Mouth. Women Make Movies. 1987. 30 minutes.
Examines female prostitution in urban Brazil.

My Husband Doesn't Mind if I Disco. World Cultures on Film and Video, University of California. 1995. 28 minutes.
The negotiation of role and gender ideology in Tibet.

GENDER, PROPERTY, AND THE STATE

Who Will Cast the First Stone? Cinema Guild, Inc. 1988. 52 minutes.
Examines the impact of Islamization on women in Pakistan, in particular the Hudood Ordinances under which adultery, rape, or extramarital sex are considered a crime against the state, punishable by stoning to death.

No Longer Silent. International Film Bureau. 1986. 57 minutes.
Analyzes dowry deaths in India, as well as the cultural preference for boys and female infanticide.

Modern Brides. South Asian Area Center, University of Wisconsin. 1985. 30 minutes.
Features two young women, one with an arranged marriage and one with a "love match," and discusses the bride's capacity to work as a substitute for dowry.

Las Madres: The Mothers of Plaza de Mayo. Direct Cinema Ltd. 1986. 64 minutes.
Focuses on Argentinean mothers who, beginning in 1977, defy laws against civil demonstrations to protest the disappearance of their children under the military dictatorship.

Donna: Women in Revolt. Women Make Movies. 1980. 65 minutes.
An examination of the history and development of Italian feminism through the personal stories of women involved in the women's rights movement at the turn of the century, the resistance during World War II, and of present day feminists.

Weaving the Future: Women of Guatemala. Women Make Movies. 1988. 28 minutes.
A perspective on women in Guatemala's liberation struggle, exploring the pivotal role of women in building a just society amid political strife and poverty.

Gabriella. Women Make Movies. 1988. 67 minutes.
Examines the work of a mass organization of diverse women's groups in the Philippines.

GENDER, HOUSEHOLD, AND KINSHIP

Dadi's Family. Odyssey. 1981. 58 minutes.
Describes family tensions in a patrilineal joint household in northern India.

A Wife Among Wives. University of California, Berkeley. 1981. 70 minutes.
Turkana women discuss polygyny.

The Vanishing Family: Crisis in Black America. University of California, Berkeley. 1986. 64 minutes.
CBS News production with Bill Moyers that examines the disintegration of the black family in America, emphasizing individual responsibility rather than the structural conditions affecting employment rates and use of welfare.

Tobelo Marriage. University of California, Berkeley. 1990. 106 minutes.
Chronicles a marriage ritual in Eastern Indonesia, including exchange of valuables, negotiations, and preparatory activities.

Asian Heart. Filmakers Library. 1987. 38 minutes.
Deals with marriage brokering between clients from Denmark and Filipino "mail order brides."

A Village in Baltimore. Doreen Moses. 1730 21st St. N.W. Washington, DC 20009. 1981. 63 minutes.
Conveys the problems and conflicts of chang-

ing identities and traditions among Greek immigrants in the United States, focusing on dowry, marriage, and other social events.

A Family to Me. New Day. 1986. 28 minutes.

Portrays four nonstereotypical American families, their philosophies of childrearing, and family organization.

All Dressed in White. University of California. 1994. 18 minutes.

Explores the complex relationships among religion, ethnicity, and gender by investigating one key symbol: the wedding dress. Based on stories of four women in a Catholic Indian family from Goa who have migrated from Goa to Singapore and then to California.

GENDER, RITUAL, AND RELIGION

Out of Order. Icarus Films. 1983. 88 minutes.

Presents personal narratives of six women in various stages of convent life.

Behind the Veil: Nuns. Wombat Productions. 1984. 115 minutes.

Examines the history of women in the Christian Church.

The Living Goddess. University of California, Berkeley. 1979. 30 minutes.

Studies the Newar of Nepal, focusing on a ritual cult in which young virgin girls are thought to embody the spirits of goddesses.

The Shakers. University of California, Berkeley. 1974. 29 minutes.

Traces the growth and decline of the Shaker community.

A Sense of Honor. Films Incorporated. 1984. 55 minutes.

Made by an Egyptian anthropologist, the film describes the impact of Islamic fundamentalism on the lives of women in Egypt.

Rastafari: Conversations Concerning Women. Eye in I Filmworks. 1984. 60 minutes.

Examines the roles and relations of men and women in the Jamaican Rastafarian movement.

A Veiled Revolution. Icarus. 1982. 27 minutes.

Attempts to discern the reasons behind the movement in Egypt by young educated women to resume wearing traditional Islamic garb.

Saints and Spirits. Disappearing World Series. 1978. 25 minutes.

Explores the religious life of Muslim women in Marrakech, Morocco, including domestic rituals and pilgrimage to a mountain shrine.

An Initiation Kut For A Korean Shaman. Laurel Kendall and Diana Lee and the Center for Visual Anthropology. University of Hawaii Press. 1991. 36 minutes.

Portrays the initiation of Chini, a young Korean woman demonstrating her ability to perform as a shaman and shouting out the spirits' oracles.

Mammy Water: In Search of Water Spirits in Nigeria. University of California. 1991. 59 minutes.

Focuses on the worship of a local water goddess by the Ibibio-, I jaw-, and Igbo-speaking people of southeastern Nigeria.

Hidden Faces. Women Make Films. 1990. 52 minutes.

The conflict between feminist ideals and Islamic values and traditions of the veil and clitoridectomy.

GENDER, POLITICS, AND REPRODUCTION

No Longer Silent. International Film Bureau. 1986. 57 minutes.

Discusses dowry deaths in India, as well as the cultural preference for boys and female infanticide.

Blood of the Condor. Penn State. 1969. 70 minutes.

Describes U.S.-imposed sterilization of Quechua Indian women.

Rites. Filmakers Library. 1990. 52 minutes.

Considers three major contexts in which female "genital mutilation" occurs: cosmetic, punitive, and rite of passage. Particularly emphasizes the health risks and psychological consequences of female circumcision.

China's One-Child Policy. Nova Special. 1985. 60 minutes.

A documentary on China's population policy, its implementation, unpopularity, and its relation to gender ideology.

Nyamakuta—The One Who Receives: An African Midwife. Filmakers Library. 1989. 32 minutes.

Portrays a traditional African midwife who incorporates pharmaceuticals with local practices to improve health standards in her village.

Kutambura, Struggling People. Films, Inc. 1987. 30 minutes.

Focuses on women's efforts to ensure economic opportunity for their families in Zimbabwe. Family planning is emphasized as the key to raising womens' self-esteem and standard of living.

Birth and Belief in the Andes of Ecuador. University of California. 1995. 28 minutes.

A portrait of women in four Andean communities, documenting their beliefs and practices surrounding childbirth and infant care. Cultural construction of the female body, ideas about conception, motives for post-partum seclusion, and gender differences in the "natures" and needs of infants are all shown to be part of this ethnomedical system.

On the Eighth Day. Women Make Movies. 1992. Two Parts, 51 minutes each.

A two-part film series which explores the social, economic, and political influences and impacts of new reproductive and genetic technologies.

Something Like War. Women Make Movies. 1991. 52 minutes.

The film explores the intersection of the reality of women's lives and the family planning project enforced by the government.

COLONIALISM, DEVELOPMENT, AND THE GLOBAL ECONOMY

The Four Seasons in Lenape Indian Life. 1983. Spoken Arts Inc. 4 film strips with sound cassettes.

Treatment of experiences of women and men under colonialism through stories of Old Elm Bark Woman.

Women in a Changing World. University of California, Berkeley. 1975. 48 minutes.

Impact of modernization on women in Bolivia, Kenya, Afghanistan, and Hong Kong.

Women in the Third World. PBS Video. 30 minutes.

Examines living conditions of women in the developing world, emphasizing their central economic roles.

Women at Risk. Filmakers Library. 1991. 56 minutes.

Presents portraits of women refugees in Asia, Africa, and Latin America.

The Global Assembly Line. New Day Films. 1986. 58 minutes.

A portrayal of the lives of working women and men in the "free trade zones" of developing countries and North America. Focuses on Mexico and the Philippines.

Bringing It All Back Home. Women Make Movies. 1987. 48 minutes.

Analyzes how the patterns of international capital investment and the exploitation of Third World women workers in free-trade zones are being brought home to the First World, as Britain's declining industrial regions have been designated "enterprise zones" to attract the multinationals.

The Price of Change. Icarus. 1982. 27 minutes.

A picture of changing attitudes of and toward women in Egyptian society, focusing particularly on work outside the home.

Sweet Sugar Rage. Third World Newsreel. 45 minutes.

Illustrates the harsh conditions under which women live and work and the efforts of the Sistren theatre collective to change these conditions in a creative way.

Women Under Siege. Icarus. 1982. 26 minutes.

Illustrates women's lives and political goals in a Palestinian refugee camp near the Israeli border.

A State of Danger. Women Make Movies. 1989. 28 minutes.

Offers a perspective on the Intifada, presenting women's testimonies on their experiences with the Israeli military.

Hell to Pay. Women Make Movies. 1988. 52 minutes.

Presents an analysis of the international debt situation through the eyes of the women of Bolivia.

Holding Our Ground. International Film Bureau, Inc. 1988. 51 minutes.

Features women and children in the Philippines who pressure the government for land reform, establish their own money lending system, and build shelters for street children.

South Africa Belongs to Us. University of California, Berkeley. 1980. 35 minutes.

Describes economic and emotional burdens borne by black women in South Africa.

Maria's Story. Filmakers Library. 1990. 53 minutes.

Portrays an FMLN guerilla, Maria Serrano, who has been living in the countryside for 11 years. Discusses her role in the revolution as well as the impact of the revolution on her family.

Reassemblage. Women Make Movies. 1982. 40 minutes.

A study of the women of rural Senegal that addresses issues of the ethnographic representation of cultures.

Time of Women. Women Make Movies. 1988. 20 minutes.

A portrait of the life of women in an Ecuadorian village where men are absent as migrants. The film looks at the impact of national economic policies on these rural women.

Fair Trade. Indiana University. 1989.

Profiles Tanzanian women and their struggle to become small entrepreneurs, and looks at the impact of development organizations and the aid that they extend to women through capital loans.

Where Credit Is Due. Indiana University. 1989.
Features the problem that Kenyan women have with the banking system, which generally refuses loans to women, and describes the Kenya Women's Finance Trust as an example of a credit cooperative for women borrowed from rural traditions of women's support groups.

My Husband Doesn't Mind if I Disco. University of California. 1995. 28 minutes.
Explores the impact of change on the lives of women in a community in eastern Tibet. The video examines the effects on the women of their exposure to feminism under the Maoists.

Once This Land Was Ours. Women Make Movies. 1991. 19 minutes.
The feminization of poverty in rural agricultural India.

Troubled Harvest. Women Make Movies. 1990. 30 minutes.
This documentary traces the female workers' experience with the fruit industry in Mexico and Latin America.